Sheep, Goat, and Cervid Medicine

Sheep, Goat, and Cervid Medicine

THIRD EDITION

Editors

David G. Pugh, BSA, DVM, MS, MAG, DACT, DACVN, DACVM

Owner
Large Animal Medicine
Southern Traxx Veterinary Services
Waverly, Alabama, United States

A. N. Baird, DVM, MS, DACVS

Professor of Surgery, Large Animal Chief-of-Staff
Department of Veterinary Clinical Sciences
Purdue University
West Lafayette, Indiana, United States

Misty A. Edmondson, DVM, MS, DACT

Associate State Veterinarian
Alabama Department of Agriculture and Industries
Montgomery, Alabama, United States

Thomas Passler, DVM, PhD, DACVIM

Associate Professor
Department of Clinical Sciences
Auburn University, College of Veterinary Medicine
Auburn, Alabama, United States

With 249 illustrations

ELSEVIER

Edinburgh London New York Oxford
Philadelphia St Louis Sydney 2021

First edition 2002
Second edition 2012

SHEEP, GOAT, AND CERVID MEDICINE, THIRD EDITION ISBN: 978-0-323-62463-3

Cover photos of goats and sheep courtesy of Kim Benson

ISBN: 978-0-323-62463-3

Content Strategist: Jennifer Catando
Content Development Specialist: Kim Benson
Project Manager: Manchu Mohan
Design: Brian Salisbury
Marketing Manager: Bergen Farthing

Printed in India

Last digit is the print number: 9 8 7 6 5 4 3

For my parents, Terry and the late Jack Pugh, who taught Helen, Joel, and me to love the Lord, work hard, and try our best.
For my wife, partner, and best friend, Ms. Jayne Moore Pugh, who taught our three children the same ideas for life.
For our three wonderful children, Rebekah, Natalie, and Dylan, their spouses, Brent, Aaron, and Chasity, and our four grandchildren, Ella, Eli, Layne, and Leah, all of whom we are so very proud.
For the Lord, who has given me a multitude of blessings.
Keep the faith.

David G. Pugh

To the memory of my parents Aubrey and Arline, who taught me to always give my best and that with opportunity comes responsibility. I hope they would be proud.
To Debra, my love and my life, who graciously agreed to sacrifice time while I tackled another book.
To our children, Taylor (Purdue DVM 2021), Tanner (Casper College 2017, Fightin' Texas Aggie 2019), and Kaycee (TBD 2024), who have given us many great memories and the hope of many more to come.
Thank you to my great friend of over 30 years, David Pugh, for inviting me to participate in this project and his never-ending work to make this book the best it could be.
And thanks to God, through which all this is possible.

A. N. Baird

To my parents, Barbara Fechner and the late Hans Passler, for their love and emotional, moral, and financial support. They instilled in me the work ethic, perseverance, and desire to succeed in all tasks large or small.
To my wife Nicole and son William. It is their love and smiles that I look forward to when I come home every day. I would be lost without you and appreciate your support of the extracurricular activities in my career!
And to my host family, Roger, Peggy, Nathan, Nick, and Nora Borgmeyer and their respective spouses and children, who have always treated me like their own and have fostered my desire to become a veterinarian. They successfully turned a city slicker into a country boy!

Thomas Passler

To my parents, John and Priscilla Abrams, who taught me, John, and Kristy the importance of family, the value of hard work, and to always do our best in everything.
To my husband, Jason, for always pushing me to follow my dreams and for giving me mine.
To our two amazing children, Wyatt and Laken, who make everything worthwhile. We are so proud of you both and thank God for you every day.
To my teacher, mentor and friend, David Pugh, for all of the wonderful veterinary and life lessons and for all of the fun along the way. Thank you for all that you have done to help me. I will be forever grateful and will always Keep the Faith.

Misty A. Edmondson

List of Contributors

The editors would like to acknowledge and offer grateful thanks for the input of all previous edition contributors, without whom this new edition would not have been possible.

A. N. Baird, DVM, MS, DACVS
Professor of Surgery, Large Animal Chief-of-Staff
Department of Veterinary Clinical Sciences
Purdue University, West Lafayette
Indiana
United States

Jenna E. Bayne, DVM, PhD, DACVIM (LA)
Clinical Assistant Professor
Veterinary Diagnostic and Production Animal Medicine
Iowa State University College of Veterinary Medicine, Ames
Iowa
United States

Kenneth R. Brown, JD, DVM
Program Director
Veterinary Services
Rural Veterinary Outreach, Bell
Florida
United States

Chris Cebra, VMD, MA, MS, DACVIM
Department Chair, Clinical Sciences
Carlson College of Veterinary Medicine, Oregon State University, Corvallis
Oregon
United States

Margaret Cebra, VMD, DACVIM
Corvallis
Oregon
United States

Manuel F. Chamorro, DVM, MS, PhD, DACVIM
Assistant Professor
Department of Clinical Sciences
Auburn University, College of Veterinary Medicine, Auburn
Alabama
United States

Lionel J. Dawson, BVSc, MS, DACT
Professor
Department of Veterinary Clinical Sciences
Oklahoma State University, Stillwater
Oklahoma
United States
Professor
American Institute for Goat Research
Langston University, Langston
Oklahoma
United States

Misty A. Edmondson, DVM, MS, DACT
Associate State Veterinarian
Alabama Department of Agriculture and Industries, Montgomery
Alabama
United States

Virginia R. Fajt, DVM, PhD
Clinical Professor
Veterinary Physiology and Pharmacology
Texas A&M University College of Veterinary Medicine and Biomedical Sciences, College Station
Texas
United States

Eric J. Fish, DVM, PhD, DACVP
Clinical Pathologist
IDEXX Laboratories
Westbrook
Maine
United States

Nar Kaji Gurung, PhD, PAS, DACAN
Associate Professor
Agricultural and Environmental Sciences
Tuskegee University, Tuskegee
Alabama
United States
Affiliate Professor
Department of Animal Sciences
Auburn University, Auburn
Alabama
United States

Meredyth Jones, DVM, MS, DACVIM
Associate Professor, Food Animal Medicine and Surgery
Large Animal Clinical Sciences
Oklahoma State University, Stillwater
Oklahoma
United States

President
Large Animal Consulting & Education, Perkins
Oklahoma
United States

Richard J. McMullen Jr., DVM, DACVO, DECVO
Associate Professor
Department of Clinical Sciences
Auburn University, College of Veterinary Medicine, Auburn
Alabama
United States

Matt Miesner, DVM, MS, DACVIM (LAIM)
Associate Clinical Professor
Veterinary Clinical Sciences
Kansas State University College of Veterinary Medicine, Manhattan
Kansas
United States

Roger Merkel, BS, MS, PhD
American Institute for Goat Research
Langston University, Langston
Oklahoma
United States

Benjamin W. Newcomer, DVM, PhD, DACVPM (Epidemiology), DACVIM, DABT
Associate Professor
Department of Clinical Sciences
Auburn University, College of Veterinary Medicine, Auburn
Alabama
United States

Daniel K. Newhard[†], DVM
Cardiology Resident
Department of Clinical Sciences
Auburn University, College of Veterinary Medicine, Auburn
Alabama
United States

Thomas Passler, DVM, PhD, DACVIM
Associate Professor
Department of Clinical Sciences
Auburn University, College of Veterinary Medicine, Auburn
Alabama
United States

Paul J. Plummer, DVM, PhD, DACVIM, DECSRHM
Executive Director
National Institute for Antimicrobial Resistance Research and Education, Ames
Iowa
United States

Jenny Pope, DVM, DACVP
Veterinary Pathologist
Thompson-Bishop-Sparks State Diagnostic Laboratory
Alabama Department of Agriculture and Industries, Auburn
Alabama
United States

David G. Pugh, BSA, DVM, MS, MAG, DACT, DACVN, DACVM
Owner
Large Animal Medicine
Southern Traxx Veterinary Services, Waverly
Alabama
United States

Emily Reppert, DVM, MS, DACVIM
Assistant Professor
Veterinary Clinical Sciences
Kansas State University College of Veterinary Medicine, Manhattan
Kansas
United States

Jessica Rush, DVM, MS, DACT
Assistant Professor
Department of Clinical Sciences
Food & Fiber Animal Services, J.T. Vaughan Large Animal Teaching Hospital, College of Veterinary Medicine
Auburn University, Auburn
Alabama
United States

Clifford F. Shipley, DVM, DACT
Associate Clinical Professor Emeritus
Veterinary Clinical Medicine
University of Illinois, Urbana
Illinois
United States

Lindsay A. Starkey, DVM, PhD, DACVM (Parasit)
Assistant Professor
Pathobiology
Auburn University, Auburn
Alabama
United States

Kelly M. Still Brooks, DVM, MPH, DACVPM, DABVP-Food Animal
Assistant Professor
Dairy and Livestock Production Medicine
Colorado State University, Fort Collins
Colorado
United States

Jenna Workman Stockler, BS, DVM
Graduate Teaching Assistant
Clinical Sciences
Auburn University, Auburn
Alabama
United States

Ricardo M. Stockler, DVM, MS, DABVP Dairy Practice
Assistant Clinical Professor of Farm Animal Ambulatory
Clinical Sciences
Auburn University College of Veterinary Medicine, Auburn
Alabama
United States

[†]Deceased

Sandra D. Taylor, DVM, PhD, DACVIM
Associate Professor
Department of Veterinary Clinical Sciences
Purdue University, West Lafayette
Indiana
United States

Heather Walz, DVM, PhD, DACVP
Veterinary Pathologist
Thompson-Bishop-Sparks State Diagnostic Laboratory
Alabama Department of Agriculture and Industries, Auburn
Alabama
United States

Paul H. Walz, DVM, MS, PhD, DACVIM
Professor
Department of Pathobiology
Auburn University, College of Veterinary Medicine, Auburn
Alabama
United States

Ann B. Weil, MS, DVM, DACVAA
Clinical Professor of Veterinary Anesthesiology
Department of Veterinary Clinical Sciences
Purdue University, West Lafayette
Indiana
United States

Preface

The first edition of *Sheep and Goat Medicine* was published in 2002, with me as the only editor and primary author. The second edition, published in 2012, was improved over the first edition by asking Dr. Baird to also be an editor. His work helped the content tremendously. In this, the third edition of the book *Sheep and Goat Medicine*, we have added Cervid and changed the name to *Sheep, Goat, and Cervid Medicine.* This new rendition, with the addition of cervids (deer, elk, etc.), came about by way of a phone conversation in 2015 with Dr. Baird, when I asked him, "If Elsevier asks us to re-edit/write 'The Book' again, how would you change it?" He said, "Add deer and other cervids, as farm raising those critters is becoming a big industry here in the Midwest (USA)." Great recommendation! I had an interest in cervids, as part of my MS degree dealt with mercury toxicity in WTD (White Tailed Deer), but I remained very limited in my cervid knowledge base. I also had a difficult time finding readily accessible information that could help me with cervid medicine for our university practice. In late 2016, Ms. Jennifer Flynn-Briggs, of Elsevier, contacted me about editing/writing a new edition of the book. We discussed the addition of cervids and settled on the term "Cervid Medicine," as the book *Nutrient Requirements of Small Ruminants: Sheep, Goats, Cervids, and New World Camelids (2007), NAS/NRC* had set the precedence to use that term to encompass many of the "cervidae" family that may be encountered by practicing veterinarians. Once they agreed to that change, I told the folks at Elsevier I would only take on the task if Dr. Baird would reprise his role from the second edition, and if we could add two other exceptional large-animal veterinarians as editors, Drs. Misty Edmondson (Professor of Large Animal Medicine, Auburn University) and Thomas Passler (Associate Professor and Food Animal Medicine Section Chief). Like Dr. Baird, both Drs. Edmondson and Passler had superbly written chapters in the second edition of this book. Both these clinicians, like Dr. Baird, had a wealth of small ruminant knowledge and experience. Dr. Passler's PhD was in virology of white-tailed deer, and Dr. Edmondson had been a food animal clinician at Auburn University's CVM (College of Veterinary Medicine) from 2004 to 2018 and she had assumed the role as the predominant small ruminant veterinarian much of that time. Thankfully, the folks from Elsevier agreed. We formatted the editing process, where each editor would plan, pick new authors where needed, oversee the writing, and edit the final version of certain chapters. Dr. Baird oversaw Chapters 3, 4, 10, 11, and 18 (Fluid Therapy and Parenteral Nutrition, Oral-Esophageal Diseases, Diseases of the Integumentary System, Diseases of the Musculoskeletal System, and Anesthetic and Pain Management, respectively) and contributed to the surgery sections for each chapter; Dr. Edmondson oversaw Chapters 5, 8, 12, 15, and 16 (Diseases of the Gastrointestinal System, Theriogenology of Sheep, Goats, and Cervids, Diseases of the Urinary System, Diseases of the Mammary Gland, Diseases of the Hematologic, Immunologic, and Lymphatic Systems [Multisystem Diseases], respectively); Dr. Passler oversaw Chapters 7, 9, 13, 14, and 17 (Diseases of the Respiratory System, Diseases of the Endocrine System, Diseases of the Neurologic System, Diseases of the Eye, and Diseases of the Cardiovascular System, respectively); and I oversaw Chapters 1, 2, 6, 19, 20, Appendix 1 and Appendix 2 (Physical Examination, Handling, and Restraint of Sheet, Goats, and Cervids, Goats, and Cervids, Feeding and Nutrition, Internal Parasites of Sheep, Goats, and Cervids, Herd and Flock Health, Field Necropsy and Diagnostic Tests, Commonly Used Drugs and Vetrinary Feed Directive in Sheep, Goats, and Cervids, and Reference Intervals and Conversions). The authors were charged with re-writing where needed, updating all information, and adding cervids to each chapter and the appendices. In addition to the editors, we asked Dr. Cliff Shipley (2017 ACT (American College of Theriogenologists) Theriogenologist of the Year, Professor of the University of Illinois, and noted small ruminant veterinarian) to help us add some of the deer and other cervid information to Chapters 1, 4, 8, 10, 11, and 19, and he did a great job. Dr. Kelley Steury, a diagnostic specialist at the Al State Diagnostic Laboratory, found many of the figures used in multiple chapters, mainly of white-tailed deer. We have added new authors and/or co-authors to all chapters except Chapters 3 and 13. Chapter 20 (Necropsy) was added to the second edition, written by Dr. John Roberts (Auburn University), and was an excellent tool for use on necropsy in sheep and goats. In this third edition, Drs. Heather Walz and Jenny Pope covered necropsy on sheep and goats very well and aimed much of the new material and many of the figures toward cervid and field necropsy. In a very far-sighted and novel move, Drs. Walz and Pope wrote their chapter with the potential use of all the editions. We added many very knowledgeable and experienced clinicians. I have always had a (bad?) habit of wanting to learn from new folks, and the authors.

I am very blessed to have been able to work with three awesome and very talented editors. The book would not have happened if it were not for Drs. Baird, Edmondson, and Passler. They all are such a credit to the veterinary profession, and it was a joy to be able to watch, read, and learn from them. I was able to read the entire book after all authors, then editors, had finished each chapter. I learned so much, and hope all the readers/users of this book do, as well.

Finally, I would be remiss if I didn't mention several clinicians who, either directly or indirectly, contributed to this undertaking. Dr. Christine Navarre (chapter author in the first two editions); the late Drs. Bob Carson, Alan Heath, and Tom Powe; and Drs. Dwight Wolfe, Darrel Rankins, Jim Wenzel, Gatz Riddel, Debra Taylor, Julie Gard, and Hui-Chu Lin all had a great and positive influence on the all three editions of this book.

Keep the Faith

David G. Pugh, BSA, DVM, MS, MAG, DACT, DACVN, DACVM
Southern Traxx Veterinary Services
Waverly, AL 36879

Contents

1

Physical Examination, Handling, and Restraint of Sheep, Goats, and Cervids

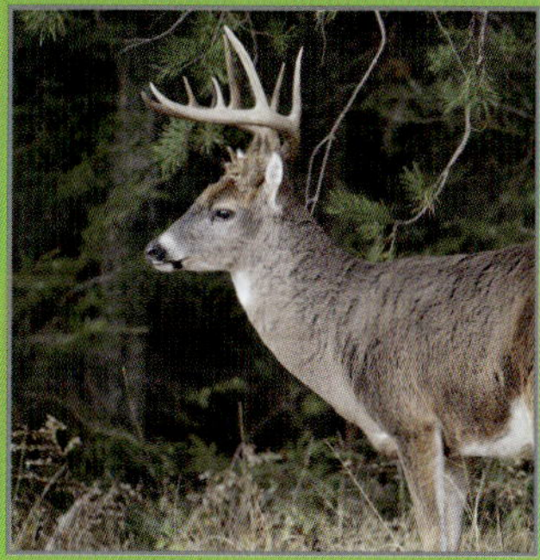

RICARDO M. STOCKLER, JENNA WORKMAN STOCKLER, CLIFFORD F. SHIPLEY, AND DAVID G. PUGH

Introduction

In general, there are three parts to any physical examination: history, distance examination, and the actual "hands-on" systematic examination. This three-part approach is true for individual patients and for a herd or flock evaluation.

A systematic method allows the practitioner to assess all body systems in an organized and comprehensive manner. The development of a problem list and their localization to a body system in conjunction with a thorough history and understanding of the patient`s husbandry and the farm management practices will undoubtedly offer enough evidence for the practitioner to create a list of acceptable differential diagnoses. All of the aforementioned (history, physical examination, and farm management practices) will lead to a diagnosis, the institution of a treatment plan, and improvement of the herd or flock management practices.

History

Questioning the owner or farmhand for basic information such as breed, age, sex, production level, and purpose (pet, wool, leather, meat, milk, antler size, etc.) is imperative. Medical history including when the perceived problem started, initial signs and symptoms, duration of the current disease, core vaccination history, as well as reproduction and production status are critical questions to ascertain the answers to. On-farm treatment details regarding antimicrobials administered, amount and route of administration, and response to therapy are important moving forward with the treatment of the disease. The authors realize owner experience and ability to provide specific details vary significantly from farm to farm, however, any information gathered is known to be relevant and should be taken into consideration. Questions regarding housing and detailed dietary routine are also important aspects to consider in any individual clinical case. When assessing a herd or flock problem, full understanding of overall husbandry (housing, feeding, animal movement, population density, etc.), as well as herd health information (see Chapter 19) are imperative and will further guide the veterinarian towards a solid diagnosis.

Visual Examination

Initial evaluation of the group or individual is critical; at this time the practitioner has the ability to appreciate individual animal or group behavior and interaction in their natural environment. Small ruminants (sheep, goats, and cervidae) are prey animals by nature and want to remain with the group even if they are sick. The veterinarian should be suspect of those animals that segregate themselves, do not interact as usual (pets), or are physically unable to ambulate. It should not be assumed that all animals within the herd or flock are well just because the individual patient appears to be keeping up with the rest of the group.

Visual examination allows the veterinarian to observe any of the following: abnormal respiratory pattern, the presence of ocular or nasal discharge, lethargy, active diarrhea or a stained perineal area, rumen tympany, rumination activity via cud chewing, lameness, swollen joints, and submandibular edema ("bottle jaw"). Further assessments can be made related to body condition score, conformation, and mental status. Mentation and neurological assessment/clinical signs not limited to depression, head pressing, opisthotonos, strabismus, and circling (see Chapter 13) are syndromes commonly noted in small ruminants with many disease processes.

Body condition scoring of both the herd or flock and the individual animal is a great tool to prompt more attention to on-farm problems, such as inappropriate dietary management and internal parasitism. Both distance examination and hands-on palpation are necessary for complete body condition scoring (BCS) of the herd or flock (Table 1.1; see Chapter 19). Cervids are often scored similar to sheep and goats but, to the authors' knowledge, no official BCS system has been proposed or accepted for white-tailed deer or mule deer. A score from 1 to 5 is also used, taking into consideration overall appearance, fat deposits over the ribs, hook and pin bones and over-the-chest area (Table 1.1). Using a scoring system similar to sheep would be acceptable assuming that the parameters are clearly defined. A cervid's hair coat will usually not hide body condition to a great extent, so a practiced eye should be able to determine with some accuracy a BCS for the individual

TABLE 1.1 Body Condition Scoring of Sheep, Goats, and Cervids.

Body Condition Score	Spinous Processes	Transverse Processes	Loin Eye Muscle	Fat Cover Over Loin Eye Muscle
Score 1	Sharp and prominent	Sharp	Shallow	None
Score 2	Sharp and prominent	Smooth, slightly rounded	Medium depth	Little
Score 3	Smooth and rounded	Smooth, well covered	Full	Medium
Score 4	Palpable as firm line with pressure	Not palpable	Full	Thick
Score 5	Not palpable	Not palpable	Very full	Very thick

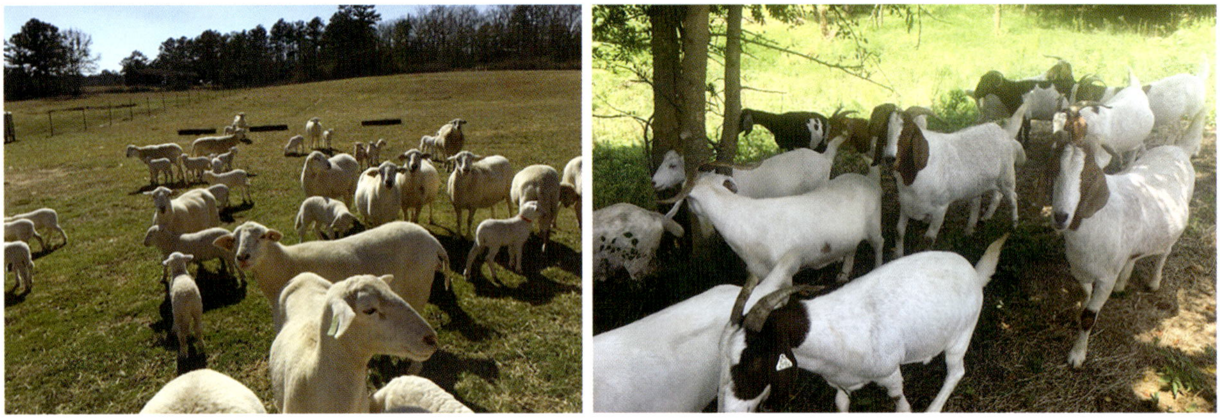

• **Fig. 1.1** Distance observation as an assessment of overall health of the flock/herd. Body condition scoring and disposition of the individuals are evaluated during this time.

animal as well as for the herd. An attentive observer may identify additional sick animals that may have initially been overlooked by the owner/producer (Figure 1.1).

Farmed cervids may also have rough hair coats from "barbering." This is a condition that may occur when one or more animals eat/chew/pick at others' hair. It may manifest itself as one or all animals in a group. Careful observation of the pattern and frequency of the hair loss will lead to a proper diagnosis. Hair is broken or pulled out and there is no itch involved. The cervids also cannot pull hair where they can't reach (head if self-inflicted) or where they resist such activity from others.

Once the thorough history is gathered and a focused observation performed, the clinician than proceeds to the medical systematic "hands-on" physical examination.

Systematic Physical Examination

Several approaches may be taken to accomplish this step. Consistency in execution of the examination makes it extremely doubtful the practitioner will overlook any system. Having knowledge of the normal physiological parameters is imperative. Table 1.2 shows a comprehensive summary of values the practitioners is expected to remember.

For biosecurity purposes, the veterinarian and assistant(s) must always wear gloves and protective clothing when handling animals. Human protection against zoonotic pathogens and the transmission of communicable diseases between cohorts of animals and between farms must be conveyed to assistants and instituted by the attending veterinarian.

Head and Neck Examination

Objectives:

1. Symmetry
2. Skin condition
3. Oral and ocular examination

Evaluation of symmetry of the head, neck, ears, eyes, and muzzle is important as potential abnormalities due to congenital defects, trauma, or neurological disease may be diagnosed. Swelling under the chin is frequently consistent with submandibular edema, often associated with hypoproteinemia associated with protein-losing enteropathy due to heavy parasitism. Masses that lead to abscessation and are adjacent to a peripheral lymph node, submandibular or pre-scapular may be linked to *Corynebacterium pseudotuberculosis* infection. Swelling at the level of the larynx may be an indication of goiter caused by an enlarged thyroid gland (see Chapter 9). Horns and wattles should also be evaluated as they are normal structures in many breeds. A central whorl of hair is usually found in polled goat breeds, whereas horned breeds may have palpable horn buds with overlying whorls of hair. Wattles can be present in both males and females.

Overall skin and hair or wool condition must be evaluated. Alopecia, the presence of ectoparasites (lice, mites, and ticks), dermatitis (see Chapter 10), and location of the lesions assist the veterinarian in making a diagnosis and guiding further diagnostic testing. Presence of crusting or vesicular lesions at the mucocutaneous junctions of the face are often a sign of contagious ecthyma, a zoonotic disease.

Oral examination is conducted with the help of a flashlight and speculum; in some cases sedation may be warranted. Evaluating for

TABLE 1.2 **Normal Physiological Parameters of Sheep and Goats.**

Parameter	Sheep	Lambs	Goats	Kids	Cervids[a]
Rectal temperature (°F)	102–103.5	102.5–104	100.5–103.5	102–104	99–106
Rectal temperature (°C)	39–39.7	39.5–40	38–39.7	39.5–40	37.5–41.6
Pulse (beats per minute)	70–80	80–130	70–90	90–150	85–225
Respiration (breaths per minute)	12–20	20–40	15–30	20–40	16–20
Rumen contraction rate (per minute)	1–2	–	1–2	–	1–3
Puberty (months)	5–12	–	4–12	–	6–16
Estrus (hours)	36	–	12–24	–	24
Estrus cycle (days)	16–17	–	18–23	–	17–22

[a]In cervids, the physiological parameters vary greatly depending on environmental factors and the circumstances of those parameters, e.g., during sedation or anesthesia.

structural abnormalities (e.g., presence of cleft palate), teeth condition, presence of prognathism and brachygnathism, and mucosal lesions such as vesicles or ulcerations is easily achieved during the examination. The presence of a foul oral odor could be an indication of disease associated with the oral cavity, gastrointestinal system (specifically the rumen), or respiratory tract. Teeth eruption and wear patterns can be easily used to estimate the age of sheep and goats (Table 1.3, Figure 1.2). Conversely, cervidae are mostly aged via eruption and wear of the premolars and molars. Typically, eruption of premolars starts at 1.5 years wear and full eruption and wear of molars occurs by 3.5 years. Wear is then evaluated until all premolars and molars reach the gum line at approximately 10 years of age and various wear patterns of the cusp and dentine help to determine the age of the animal (Table 1.3).

Detailed aging information is available from most wildlife and hunting agencies. The most accurate way to determine age is to submit to a laboratory for examination of annular rings.

The use of this method to age the animal becomes less accurate once all of the permanent incisors have erupted and are in wear. Abnormal wear patterns or poor dentition (loose teeth, absence of teeth, and tooth root abscess) may be contributors to a chronic weight loss complaint, especially in situations of competition for food (see Chapter 4).

The assessment of hydration status and FAMACHA scoring is accomplished during the ocular examination. Eyeball recession and eyelid skin tenting are the two reliable methods to subjectively determine the hydration status of the animal. FAMACHA scoring (see Chapter 6, Box 6.2 & Figure 6.2 and Chapter 19) is recommended to be part of the routine care of any herd or flock as an important aspect of parasite management and control. The conjunctival membrane color is used to estimate systemic perfusion. (Figure 1.3). Oral mucous membranes should not be used for this assessment as many breeds have a pigmented oral cavity and the rough nature of the mouth may portray an erroneous estimation. As a general rule, pale membranes may indicate anemia, most likely due to intestinal parasitism (*Haemonchus contortus* infection) or coccidiosis. Jaundice or icteric mucous membranes may indicate a hemolytic crisis or liver disease, such as copper toxicity, and congested (red in color) membranes may be indicative of fever, septicemia, or toxemia.

TABLE 1.3 **Estimating Age of Sheep, Goats, and Cervids by Teeth Eruption.**

Estimating Age of Sheep and Goats Using the Incisors (I)		Estimating Age of Cervids Using the Premolar and Molar Eruptions[a]
Deciduous	Eruption Age	**Fawn–6 months old**
I1	Birth–1 week	Five or fewer teeth present and the third premolar (tooth 3) has three cusps
I2	1–2 weeks	1½ years of age
I3	2–3 weeks	Tooth 3 (third premolar) has three cusps. Tooth 6 has erupted and is slightly visible just above the gum line
I4	3–4 weeks	2½ years of age
Permanent		Lingual crest on all molars are sharp and pointed. Tooth 3 now has two cusps. Back cusp of tooth 6 is sharp and pointed
I1	1–1.5 years	4½ years of age
I2	1.5–2 years	Lingual crest on tooth 4 rounded off, and in tooth 5 blunt. The dentine in tooth 4 is twice as wide as the enamel. The dentine in tooth 5 is wider than the enamel.
I3	2.5–3 years	6½ years of age
I4	3.5–4 years	Tooth 4 is worn completely smooth; no enamel ridge should be visible in the center of tooth 4. Small enamel ridge will be present in center of tooth 5 and tooth 6. Lingual crest on tooth 5 is almost worn away and rounded in tooth 6

[a]Cain and Wallace: A Guide to Age Determination of White-Tailed Deer Austin, TX: Texas Parl and Wildlife, 2003.

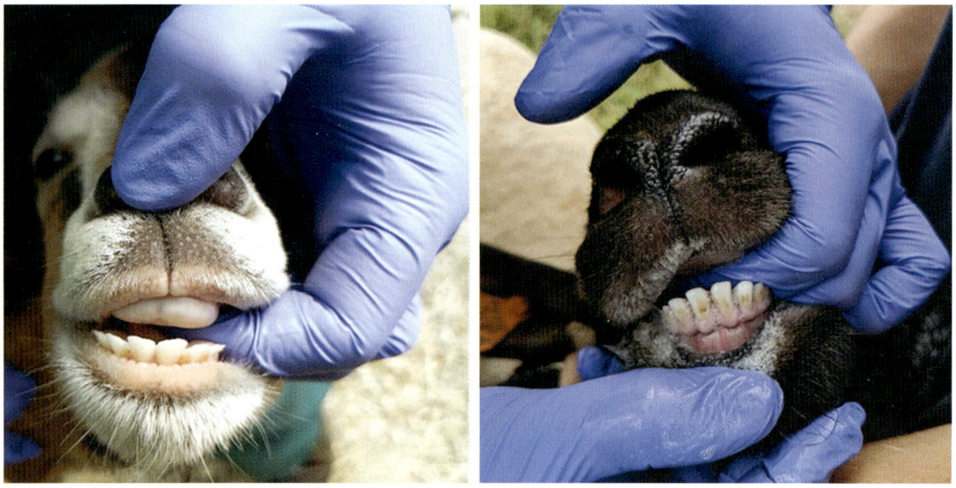

• **Fig. 1.2** The practitioner may insert the index finger inside of the sheep/goat mouth, laterally, and with the other hand lower the bottom lip allowing exposure of the incisors. The approximate age may be determined according to Table 1.3.

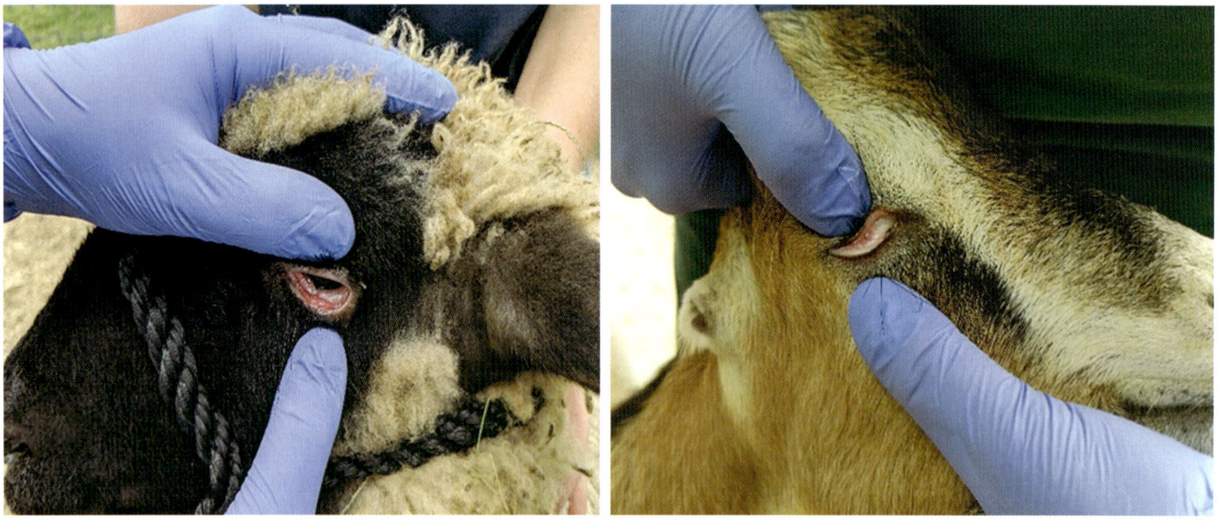

• **Fig. 1.3** To FAMACHA score sheep and goats, the practitioner gently pushes the upper eyelid medially and rolls the lower eyelid ventrally to access conjunctival membrane color.

Cardiovascular Examination

Objectives:

1. Auscultate both left and right side skin conditions
2. Presence of jugular vein distention
3. Peripheral perfusion
4. Peripheral edema

Auscultation of both the left and right side of the thorax is imperative. Assessment of rate, rhythm, character, and intensity of the heart sounds should be performed. Auscultation of the heart is accomplished by moving the stethoscope over the location of the valves and determining the point of maximal intensity. The pulmonic valve (low third intercostal space, below the elbow), the aortic valve (high fourth intercostal space, above the elbow), and the left (mitral) atrioventricular (AV) valve (at the low fifth intercostal space, at the level of the elbow) are found on the left chest. The right AV valve or tricuspid valve (high fourth intercostal space, above the elbow) should be auscultated on the right side.

As a general rule, normal heart rate should vary between 70 and 90 beats per minute in adults and between 80 and 130 beats per minute in neonates. There is physiological variation according to environmental conditions (i.e., ambient temperature) and situations that cause hyperexcitability (i.e., aggressive handling or movement). Anemia, murmurs, pain, heart failure, and infectious and inflammatory processes are certain conditions known to effect the heart rate.

Observing for jugular pulses and palpation of distal appendages, such as tip of the ears and limbs are indicators of appropriate peripheral perfusion when warm. Distention of the jugular veins and the presence of pulsations may indicate heart failure. Peripheral edema is known to be consistent with either hypoproteinemia or congestive heart failure and warrants further investigation (see Chapter 17).

Respiratory Evaluation

Objectives:
1. Observe and record rate at a distance first
2. Auscultate both left and right side

The clinician must be aware that the respiratory system should be examined in conjunction with the cardiovascular system and drawing major conclusions without examining both may impair the ability to accurately determine a diagnosis.

On average, the normal respiratory rate should vary between 10 and 30 breaths per minute in adults and between 20 and 40 breaths per minute in neonates. The rate can be obtained by observing the movement of the coastal arch and nostrils from a distance. In cervids, similar rates to sheep and goats can be expected, however, cervids are highly sensitive to excitement and may be hard to evaluate except at a distance. Neonates may "hold" their breath (mule deer fawns especially) when hiding as a reflex to avoid predators.

As noted for the cardiovascular system, environmental conditions and systemic illness are known to influence respiratory rate and must be taken into consideration when appropriate. Animals in apparent respiratory distress, either dyspneic or tachypneic, with open mouth breathing, flaring the nostrils, abducted elbow stance, and with excessive abdominal effort must be evaluated critically and efficiently. Air flow should be symmetric from both nostrils. Mild, clear, serous nasal discharge is a common finding, especially in sheep; however, excessive clear to mucoid to purulent exudate must be explored.

Bilateral auscultation of the lung fields should be performed in a systematic approach. The margins of the lung fields are as follows: the cranial border is deep to the triceps, the dorsal border extends from the point of the shoulder to the last rib, and the caudoventral border arches from the point of the elbow to the last rib. Bronchial sounds usually are loudest over the craniodorsal lung fields at the level of the tracheal bifurcation. Generally, tracheal sounds should be absent. When tracheal disease is present, wheezes can be auscultated, indicating tracheal collapse; obstructive lesions and crackling sounds are characteristic of tracheitis. Elicitation of a cough can be achieved with minimal compression of the trachea and pharyngeal region. The normal animal will cough one to two times, while the diseased patient coughs repeatedly and often with forced effort.

Crackles are auscultated when air moves through inflammatory fluid in the alveoli, whereas wheezes are reverberations of air moving through inflamed, narrowed airways. One must remember that significant lung pathology may be present and not necessarily appreciated on auscultation. Coughing, nasal discharge, dyspnea with a fever, and severe open mouth breathing may be the only indication of lung pathology.

Upper airway diseases, such as rhinitis, tracheitis, foreign body, and compressive lesions, are usually characterized by a loud, harsh, dry, nonproductive cough of acute onset. Lower airway diseases, such as pneumonia, pulmonary edema, lung abscessation, and lungworm infection, are characterized by a chronic, soft, productive cough. Animals with lower airway disease typically cough infrequently and will swallow after coughing, which is different from animals with upper airway diseases who typically do not swallow after coughing.

Cervids can be difficult to assess due to restraint in drop chutes (poor access) or because they are highly excited. Many that have respiratory disease may have advanced disease that has consolidated portions of the lung, leading to "dead" spots that show no air movement/sounds. They are poor anesthetic as well, so evaluation is difficult at best. Ultrasound, transtracheal wash, radiographs, and other diagnostic tools can be used as well, but risk/benefit ratio and economics must be taken into consideration (see Chapter 7).

Gastrointestinal Examination

Objectives:
1. Examination extends from mouth to rectum
2. Auscultation, palpation, and observation

The gastrointestinal system is one of the largest and most important in the body. Evaluation should be performed in a systematic and stepwise fashion from the mouth to rectum. The mouth should be examined for the presence of vesicles, ulcerations, swellings, and ptyalism. Inspection of the teeth for wear and soundness is important, and the upper dental pad should also be evaluated for evidence of abnormal wear. Although not easy to examine, and sedation or anesthesia may be necessary for a complete examination, the molars should be sound and present as their role in mastication of forages before swallowing and in proper cud chewing is critical. The use of a mouth gag and a bright light source is helpful. It is important to take into consideration that wear patterns may present in different ways and are dependent on the environmental conditions and primary diet of the herd or flock. The practitioner can then make a judgment of whether the wear pattern is abnormal or normal for the living conditions of the animal. Often, culling of lambs or kids is needed due to poor dentition.

The neck area is examined via thorough palpation. Masses, enlarged lymph nodes, or swelling may be causing esophageal compression and subsequent obstruction/choke. Rumen tympany, ptyalism, bruxism, and pain are common clinical signs that may be associated with esophageal disease.

It is wise if the clinician examines one side of the animal first, as this will help to avoid missing any aspect of the examination. On the left side of the animal, the rumen constitutes the major forestomach. Due to its size, the rumen may give an asymmetrical appearance to the abdominal contour favoring a larger "bulge" to the left side, which is considered normal and is expected. Healthy rumen striation consists of a gas cap dorsally, fiber mat in the middle, and fluid (digested ingesta) ventrally. Using the stethoscope, the practitioner should auscultate and perform succussion (i.e., shaking) of the abdomen. Within the left paralumbar fossa, rumen contractions can be auscultated in the healthy animal (sheep, goats, and cervids) at a rate of one to two primary contractions (active rolling of the ingesta) and one secondary rumination (eructation) per minute. A solid understanding of the individual or herd/flock dietary management and medical history, along with a physical examination, helps the practitioner determine the primary cause of rumen fill. Ballottement of the paralumbar fossa while listening with the stethoscope is imperative to support abnormal findings related to the striation of the rumen, displaced abomasum, and ascites. Auscultation of the right paralumbar fossa will allow the practitioner to evaluate the cecum, spiral colon, and small intestines. Illness associated with of any of these structures will lead to fluid and gas accumulation and distension of the viscus in the upper right quadrant. Dilation lower on the right side of the animal may be related to abomasal impaction, late gestation, or a severe rumen impaction.

If bilateral abdominal distention is seen, one may suspect vagal indigestion syndrome (chronic indigestion, failure of the omasal transport, or pyloric stenosis), ileus, or free fluid accumulation. This fluid accumulation could be caused by diffuse peritonitis, ascites due to protein losing enteropathy, liver failure, or severe congestive heart failure.

Body temperature should be taken rectally observing common biosecurity practices. Normal temperature typically varies from 100.5° F to 103.5° F. In general, sheep tend to have a higher body temperature than goats, and cervids typically fall in the same range (101.5° F–102.5° F) with variations due to age, activity level, and environmental temperature. The practitioner must distinguish between true hyperthermia and a febrile response. A febrile response is more likely to be associated with an inflammatory or infectious process, whereas hyperthermia is going to be associated with the location of the patient (e.g., barn, paddock, pasture, etc.), behavior (e.g., hyperexcitability does increase body temperature), and environmental conditions (e.g., high temperature and humidity).

The authors would like to stress that obtaining body temperature should be the first procedure to be performed when examining sheep and goats and the results interpreted in conjunction with other clinical signs.

Fecal consistency and staining of the perineum, tail, and back of legs is a good way to assess the history of diarrhea. A thorough history of dietary management and fecal examination (fecal float or fecal egg count) is the only way the practitioner will reliably make a diagnosis and then recommend a targeted treatment.

In young stock, the authors recommend full examination of the umbilical structures both externally and internally. The use of ultrasound imaging if pain or swelling is found is highly valuable. Any signs or history of diarrhea in lambs, kids, or fawns must be addressed quickly as it can be life threatening. Lastly, atresia ani and atresia coli have been reported in kids and lambs, so the practitioner needs to be sure there is a patent anus and fecal passage present (see Chapter 5).

Urogenital Examination

Objectives:

1. Examination from a distance
2. History
3. Ultrasound imaging

The examination commences at the external genitalia of both males and females. In males, the prepuce should be free of adhesions, swelling, or any signs of trauma. The preputial opening should be evaluated for the presence of crystals, blood, excessive dryness, scabs, or ulcerations since any of these may be indicative of urethral calculi, obstructive urolithiasis, or ulcerative posthitis.

Urine samples in both sheep and goats can often be obtained by briefly occluding the nostrils. Young cervids can be encouraged to urinate with gentle stimulation. Older cervids that are bottle raised may be able approached for a "free catch" urine sample.

The penis is difficult to examine without the use of sedation or anesthesia (cervids). The authors strongly recommend the use of acepromazine or a benzodiazepine (see Chapters 8, 12, and 18) for sedation and relaxation. Rams and bucks can be placed in lateral recumbency or sitting up on their rump (preferred method) by an assistant, then the practitioner pushes the prepuce caudally while pushing the sigmoid flexure cranially. Once exteriorized, the practitioner can hold the penis using gauze. The surface of the penis should be examined for color, scabs, and any traumatic lesions. Palpation of the penis may reveal the presence of uroliths, swelling, or a focal area of pain. The urethral process in sheep and goats should be examined closely for the presence of a urolith or sandy grit, which may be indicative of urolithiasis or urethral blockage. Cervids do not have a urethral process.

Frequently, the presentation of a sheep or goat with suspected urogenital disease involves standing in a stretched out position, intermittent straining, vocalization, and wagging of the tail when attempting to urinate. This stance is often confused by owners and their perception is that the animal is constipated when in all actuality the animal has a urinary obstruction. History of inability to urinate followed by relaxation and acute abdominal distention may indicate rupture of the urinary bladder, whereas caudal ventral edema (often reported by the owner as "broken penis") may indicate distal urethral rupture.

It is important to take into consideration, contrary to what is commonly done in small animal practice, catheterization of the urethra is difficult in does and ewes owing to the presence of the urethral diverticulum at the floor of the pelvis and close to impossible in bucks and rams. Multiple anatomic locations in male anatomy (urethral process, sigmoid flexure, urethral diverticulum) are difficult to traverse with a catheter. Attempts to pass a urinary catheter can actually cause more harm due to severe trauma caused by the procedure.

The testicles are gently palpated to ensure they are not adhered to the scrotum, and there are no signs of epididymitis, orchitis, and poor testicular tone, which are often associated with suboptimal sperm production. In breeding males, the phrase "big is beautiful, mobility meaningful, resilience respectable, softness suspicious" is helpful to remember when evaluating males for breeding soundness. In addition, the scrotum should be free of traumatic lesions with intact skin. Signs of dermatitis due to ectoparasites, frostbite, or asymmetry are undesirable findings (see Chapter 8).

In females, the labia of the vulva is examined for their color, size, and presence of discharge. Pale mucous membranes may be an indication of anemia, whereas hyperemia and swelling may indicate the onset of estrus or an impending parturition. If calculi or sandy grit is found attached to the hairs below the urethral orifice, urolithiasis is suspected and the practitioner must evaluate further. Reproductive history is important when it comes to evaluating a potential vaginal or uterine discharge. Color, consistency, and volume are a good start as they may characterize a late estrus discharge, a postpartum normal lochia, or an infection. Lochia is considered a normal finding between days 0 and 21 post parturition. The finding of large protruding vulvar labia or clitoris, or a short anogenital distance is suggestive of an intersex condition (see Chapter 8).

In both males and females with suspected obstructive urolithiasis, an enlarged bladder may be palpable extending from the pelvis to the abdomen; in this case, the authors recommend further examination using ultrasound imaging. Caution should be used when applying manual pressure to the abdomen because there is a risk of rupturing the bladder and causing more pain to the patient (see Chapter 12).

Musculoskeletal Examination

Objectives:

1. Examination from a distance
2. History
3. Knowledge of foot conditions
4. Imaging examination

First, posture and locomotion are evaluated at a distance for both sheep and goats, as well as cervids. The animals are then observed as they walk away from and towards the practitioner. It is important to note that lameness issues often present in a variety of ways and because of the prey mentality of small ruminants, the lameness may be very subtle. The patient may prefer to not bear weight on the limb at rest and use it sparingly while in motion, or may bear weight at rest and hop on three legs while in motion.

All claws should be observed for appropriate wear, hoof-wall separation due to white line disease, and defects in the sole. The interdigital space should be checked for pain, exudate, or a foul odor. The coronary bands should be observed for pain, swelling, ulceration, or separation from the foot. Separation of the hoof wall from the hoof in cervids is a common sequelae to hemorrhagic disease survivors. All joints should be palpated and checked for appropriate range of motion. Older and/or heavier small ruminants may have "clicking" within their joints indicating chronic osteoarthritis or overuse of the joint(s). This may or may not be an abnormal finding but should be recorded in the medical record.

In young stock, septic joints are typically diagnosed before swelling is ever a problem. It is an extremely painful condition affecting one or more joints and likely a sequelae from failure of passive transfer. Many of these patients present with non–weight-bearing lameness rather than swelling being noticed at one or more of the joints.

In goats, hygromas and synovitis secondary to caprine arthritis encephalitis infection can be differentiated on clinical examination. Hygromas are nonpainful, whereas synovitis typically is a painful condition.

Fractures must be evaluated immediately. The age of the animal, location of the fracture, and intended purpose (pet or production animal) will allow for an appropriate treatment plan and prognosis. Prognosis is also easily determined by radiographic examination (see Chapter 11).

Nervous System Examination

Objectives:
1. History
2. Examination—localizing the lesion

It is imperative for the practitioner to always wear gloves when interacting with an animal showing neurological disease. In general, the neurological examination should start by obtaining a thorough history of the patient. The examiner should have a full understanding of the animal's diet and behavior within the past 24 to 48 h, housing and environment, new additions to the herd, travel, and interaction with wildlife.

From a distance, gait, posture, and overall behavior when interacting with herd or flock mates and with humans must be noted. Known traumatic events must be taken into consideration.

Clinical signs will help the practitioner to localize the lesion to the peripheral or central nervous system.

In sheep, goats, and cervids, infectious peripheral nerve disorders are less common than traumatic events leading to peripheral nerve damage. The peripheral nerves and their most likely clinical presentation when traumatized are summarized in Table 1.4. Often, one or more lesions is appreciated on clinical examination and this is attributable to multiple nerve roots or pathways being affected (e.g., complicated dystocia followed by traumatic obstetric maneuvers).

Sciatic and obturator nerve paresis and paralysis are the most common peripheral pelvic limb disorders. Radial nerve paralysis is the most common nerve palsy affecting the thoracic limb in sheep, goats, and cervids.

TABLE 1.4 Typical Clinical Signs Associated With Peripheral Nerve Disease.

Peripheral Nerves	Clinical Signs
Femoral nerve	Inability to bear weight and advance the limb, absent patellar reflex
Sciatic nerve	Knuckled fetlock with dropped hock and intact patellar reflex
Peroneal nerve	Hyperflexed fetlock, overextending the hock, and inability to extend digit
Obturator nerve	Inability to adduct limbs
Tibial nerve	Knuckling of fetlock but no dropped hock
Radial nerve	Inability to advance the limb

TABLE 1.5 Typical Clinical Signs Associated With Central Nerve Disease.

Area Affected	Clinical Signs
Cortical and cerebral	Changes in mentation with normal gait, posture, and spinal reflexes
Cortical	Head pressing, propulsive walking, convulsions, and blindness
Cerebellar and spinal cord	Altered gait and posture with normal mentation
Cerebellar	Ataxia with normal strength and proprioception, truncal sway, hypermetria and head tremor
Spinal cord	Increased extensor tone and exaggerated spinal reflexes or paresis to paralysis with decreased spinal reflexes
Brain stem	Change in mentation, gait, posture, and spinal reflexes may or may not be present. Cranial nerve deficits which may manifest as head tilt, flaccid tongue, facial paralysis, circling, or ptosis

The central nervous system is divided into four major anatomic sites to which clinical signs may be localized: cortical, cerebral, cerebellar, and spinal cord. Diseases at any of these locations may be characterized by alterations in mentation, gait, posture, and spinal reflexes. The common clinical signs associated with the location in the nervous system are summarized in Table 1.5.

Chapter 13 discusses in detail differential diagnoses for each location, treatment, and prognosis associated with nervous system diseases.

Mammary Gland Examination

Objectives:
1. Production history
2. Reproduction history
3. Examination

If in lactation, both halves of the mammary gland, teats, and teat sphincter are observed and palpated for symmetry, size, conformation, temperature, and consistency. Infectious and noninfectious mastitis is detrimental to the production life of the female, and can be a life-threatening disease if not treated promptly and correctly.

It is recommended to first and foremost gather a complete history and observe the young stock. Problems associated with the udder can be appreciated first in the lambs or kids that are weak, show poor body condition, or are failing to gain weight. Malnourished neonates can be an indication of poor milk production or a painful udder in the dam that has resulted in the dam not allowing the neonate to nurse.

The presence of edema that extends symmetrically and cranial ventral to the udder is a common finding shortly after parturition, especially in first-time ewes or does. A diffusely hard or firm udder noted in the first few days after lambing may indicate ovine progressive pneumonia (OPP) infection in sheep or caprine arthritis encephalitis (CAE) in goats. Low milk production and no signs of clinical mastitis are a common occurrence in most cases of OPP and CAE (see Chapter 16).

Aside from palpation of the mammary gland, if the doe is in lactation, the practitioner must remove a few streams of milk from both sides to assess patency of the sphincter. Color, consistency, and presence of abnormal clots or flakes in the secretion should prompt the practitioner to investigate further. The California Mastitis Test (CMT) can be used to determine if a subclinical mastitis is present and if further culture of the secretion is necessary.

Prepartum mastitis, although uncommon in small ruminants, can be caused by a herd/flock mate suckling or by a pathogen. This condition must be evaluated and treated promptly as it can severely affect colostrogenesis and ability to lactate after the birth of the offspring (see Chapters 15 and 19).

Lymphatic Examination

Objectives:

1. History of *Corynebacterium pseudotuberculosis* (CL) in the herd
2. Examination

It is part of the physical examination to palpate all the peripheral lymph nodes. Submandibular, retropharyngeal, parotid, prescapular, prefemoral, and supramammary (in females) are the most common palpable lymph nodes. It is important to note that often the practitioner will be unable to physically feel them, either because they are too small, or in wool breeds of sheep, the thick wool will impair access to them.

The authors recommend that attention be paid to lymph nodes that are enlarged and draining purulent exudate. CL infection is known to be the most common disease associated with draining lymph nodes in small ruminants and is extremely contagious in nature and is considered a zoonotic pathogen. Cervids commonly have lymph node involvement with Fusobacterium infections (see Chapter 16).

Integumentary Examination

Objectives:

1. Examination
2. Environment

Lesions like abrasions, lacerations, papules, pustules, scabs, and hair or wool loss are clinical signs associated with and indicative of dermatological issues. Always take into consideration the season and type of environment where the animals are being housed. Haired breeds of sheep e.g., Barbados, Katahdin, St. Croix, etc.) and goats will shed winter coats in the spring. Wooly sheep (e.g., Dorset, Suffolk, Merino, Corriedale, etc.) need to be sheared at least once a year, during the summer months. Wool blindness is a term often used by producers in reference to sheep with excessive wool above their eyes leading to their sight being physically impaired. In these cases, shearing of the periorbital area must be performed to avoid further damage, such as severe dermatitis and eye damage.

In cases where the practitioner encounters a flock with more than one case of poor wool quality, nutrition issues should always to be discussed. Hairiness or abnormal wool pigmentation, such as presence of brown fibers over the nape of the neck in wool sheep, may indicate border disease infection. Table 1.6 summarizes the most common clinical signs associated with skin or coat diseases in sheep and goats (see Chapter 10).

TABLE 1.6 Typical Clinical Signs and Their Associated Differential Diagnosis.

Clinical Signs	Potential Common Etiologies
Pruritus	Mange, allergy, and scrapie
Hair loss	Ringworm, mange, and nutrition
Skin nodules	Abscesses, pustules, and demodectic mange
Dandruff	Dry environment and often poor or improper nutrition
Crustiness	Chorioptic mange (under the dew claws), fungal or bacterial dermatitis
Sunburn	Hairless parts of the body in white animals (often seen on the top line, tip of nose, ears). Must differentiate from photosensitization
Barbering	Chewing, biting, pulling of hair or wool by self or others

Restraining and Handling

Handling Sheep, Goats, and Cervids

Biosecurity. The practitioner should always be aware of potential zoonotic diseases during routine handling of small ruminants. Protective clothing and gloves should be worn at all times when visiting a herd or flock, and while interacting with animals. Clothes must be changed and footwear thoroughly washed between farms as it can easily serve as a fomite for infectious and contagious pathogens. As mentioned earlier, part of the physical examination is to learn about the herd health status through the use of historical information. This information will help the practitioner to identify the potential risk for the presence of zoonotic disease within a flock or herd. Segregation of sick animals and dedicated areas for lambing or kidding are strongly recommended to avoid and prevent pathogen transmission.

To prevent the introduction of new diseases to an established herd or flock, a prepurchase examination performed by a veterinarian is strongly recommended. Although prepurchase examinations do not guarantee the future health of that individual at the future farm, it serves as an assurance that at that point in time there is a healthy female or breeding male. Aside from obtaining historical data from the herd/flock as a whole, the veterinarian must also ask directed questions concerning vaccination history, dietary protocols, and if any previous health events have occurred. It is also imperative that the practitioner question whether any treatments have been performed and by whom. Also, the veterinarian may decide to perform diagnostic tests including serology (for caprine arthritis encephalitis, caseous lymphadenitis, paratuberculosis, etc.), serum biochemistry, complete blood count, and a fecal examination. A reproductive or breeding soundness examination in both males and females may be indicated. It is strongly recommended that the new owner quarantine new animal additions a minimum of 4 weeks with no physical or visual contact with existing animals. Thirty days is known to be sufficient for most of the diseases that are worrisome and for those animals to show clinical signs. The authors understand that quarantine may be logistically difficult for some herds/flocks. Quarantine allows new animals the chance to acclimate to the environment, diet, and behavior patterns, allowing a stress free and productive atmosphere (see Chapter 19).

Behavior and Facilities. The use of behavior patterns and handling principles like "flight zone" and "point of balance", as well as providing appropriate facilities are the hallmark to successfully and safely working with sheep, goats, and cervids.

Once one enters the animal's flight zone, to the point where they feel threatened, the animal will walk/run away and face the person to assess the situation. The way the farmer or the veterinarian handles this situation is exactly the way the animal will handle it. That is, if the practitioner enters the flight zone calmly, the animal will behave calmly; if the person aggressively and loudly runs or walks towards the animal, the normal behavior is to also run. It is imperative to remember sheep, goats, and cervids are typically small and fast, yet extremely strong. They can injure themselves and/or injure the people that are attempting to work with them. In tightly enclosed spaces, some cervids will choose to fight and have been known to cause injury or death, especially males with antlers.

The level of the shoulder is known to be the point of balance. When working a herd or flock, the location where the people managing the animals are standing or moving about makes a significant difference in how effectively and timely the job can be executed. Standing in front of the chute or alleyway intended for the animals to walk through is counterproductive. If the desire is to encourage the animals to walk forward, the practitioner must stay behind the point of balance (behind the level of the shoulder). If the goal is to encourage the animal to back up, then the individual may walk past the level of the shoulder; this will invariably make the animals walk backwards. Having knowledge of behavior patterns in sheep and goats is a fundamental part of successful handling (Table 1.7).

TABLE 1.7 Typical Behavior Characteristics of Sheep and Goats.

	TYPICAL BEHAVIOR CHARACTERISTICS		
Activity	**Sheep**	**Goats**	**Cervids**
Food preference	Grass and succulent herbage	Browse (weeds, leaves, twigs)	Browse broadleaf herbaceous weeds, leaves and tender twigs, and grass
Food variety	Accept monotonous diet	Require variety	Require variety
Habitat selection	Lowlands or hilly grasslands	Climb rocks and elevations	Hardwoods, croplands, brush lands, and pastures
Antagonistic behavior	Butt head on	Sideways hooking motion	
Fighting	Butt	Rear on hind legs	Bite and push
Sexual behavior	Less herding	Herding of females	Fallow deer tend to maintain sexual segregation and make lion-like vocalizations
Newborn young behavior	Remain by dam ("lying in")	Freezing some distance from the dams ("lying out")	First days, they hide in tall grass becoming more active the second week of life
Alarm signal	Snort and stamp forefoot	Frequent high pitched "sneeze"	Snort or whistle, groan, or bleat when predators are around
Alarm	Form compact bunch	Form thin line	Run
Hornless condition	Fertile	Sterile (usually) in males	N/A
Tail	Hangs down	Stands up	Down when calm/up with alarm
Beard	Absent	Present in buck and some females	Absent
Wattles	Absent	May be present	Absent
Hear a low flying plane	Frightened and likely to run	Often stand and watch	Alarm/run
Stress	Results from isolation or subjugation to unfamiliar environment	More of a problem in young kids and doelings	Segregation or confinement

Another crucial aspect of managing small ruminants is that the farmer must be able to gather, restrain, and handle animals with minimal stress. Injury prevention for both animals and personnel is crucial. Small ruminants will readily follow one another and will move away from things that frighten them. They move better around slight corners or curves and will not move toward an area that appears to be a dead end. Sheep and goats will move away from buildings and prefer to move uphill. Lit areas are preferred as the animals will resist movement into dark barns, alleys, and chutes. Handling areas should be well lit and free of objects that may project shadows into the visual path. Solid sides in alleyways will help maintain forward momentum and minimize attempts at escape.

Well-planned working facilities to deal with a flock of sheep for example, are known to provide the desirable details mentioned above. Commercially available chute systems (Figure 1.4A) placed in an appropriate, well-lit location that is free of random loose objects, allows the flock to ease their way into the holding area. This is considered one of the best-known ways to work a flock (Figure 1.4B).

If a chute system is not available, the farmer should consider moving the flock into a small paddock or stall as a group (Figure 1.5). It is wise to always try to work the flock together, even though you may not need all animals present in that group. Sheep have an extremely strong flocking instinct, therefore, if one animals is seen segregated and away from the flock, the practitioner and famer must investigate further. Once the group is in a small area, the practitioner carefully and calmly enters the area to attempt to catch an individual animal. Always remember they can be flighty animals and if necessary, they will give their full potential to escape by head butting or jumping.

To catch a sheep, the handler can cup a hand under the animal's jaw, grasping the bony part of the jaw—not the throat.

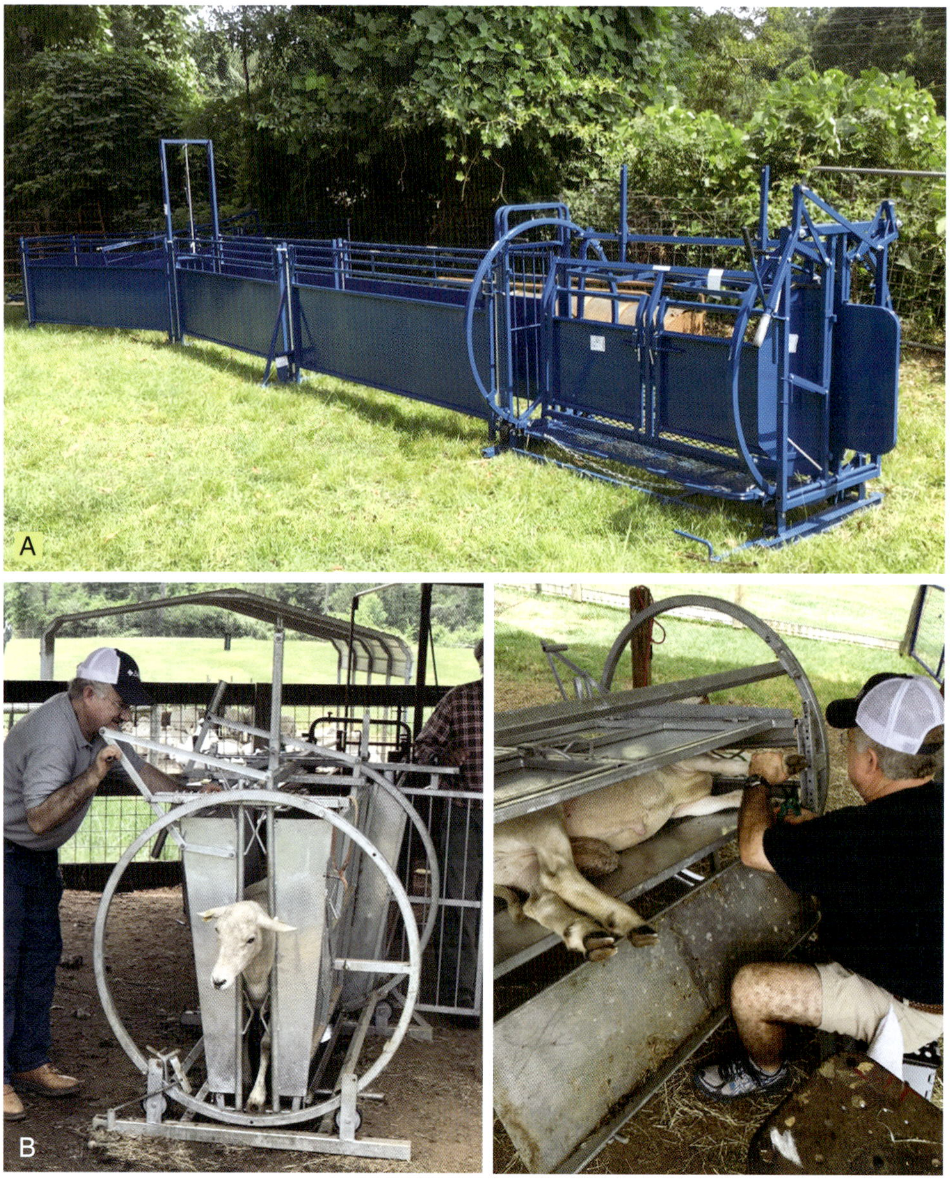

• **Fig. 1.4** **A.** Commercially available chute restraint system to facilitate herd work. (Photo courtesy Sims Pond Farm.) **B.** Operating the chute system to safely restrain the animals allowing routine livestock procedures to be performed. (Photo courtesy Hunt Road Katahdin Sheep Farm.)

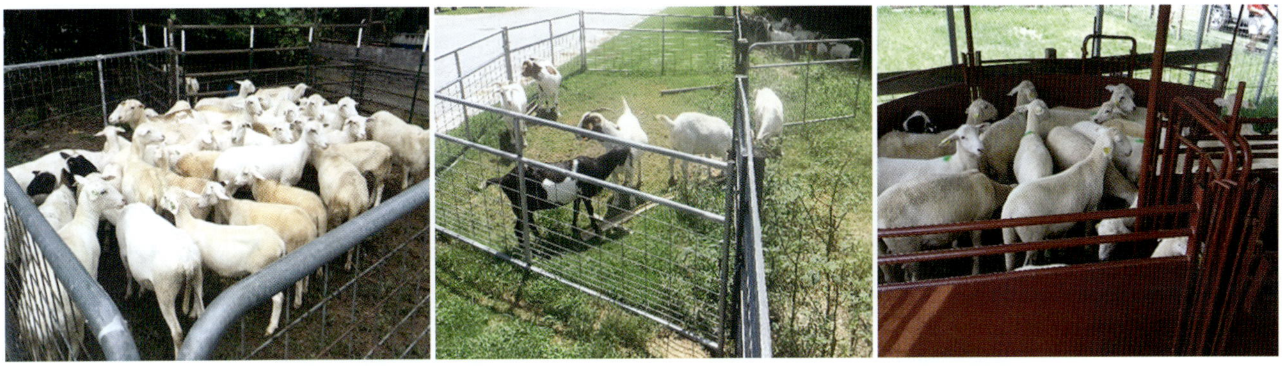

• **Fig. 1.5** Depicted in this image is an example of a corral area. If a chute system is not available, small groups are moved into these smaller areas allowing herd work to be performed.

Once it has been caught, a second hand should be placed behind the head below the animal's ears. It is important to note that for better control, the animal's nose should be pointed upward to stop its forward motion, as sheep have a lot more power when the head is down. The handler should never grab the sheep by the wool or hair. A crook or lariat also is an acceptable catching device. A sheep can be handled using various handling points—for example, under the mandible, tail, and flank (Figure 1.6). After it has been caught, a sheep can be "tipped" on its rump for examination, shearing, foot trimming, and other routine procedures (Figure 1.7).

Goats are different in many respects when it comes to handling and to the facilities needed to work them. Goats are not as concerned about herding, but rather they develop close relationships with certain herd mates and can be seen playing and socializing. Goats typically spread out while browsing and ruminating. To catch a goat, the use of the horns as "handles" is an acceptable way to get a hold on them (Figure 1.8A, B); restraint by their ears is painful and considered abusive. Goats housed with a collar or halter can be caught using this, with the handler looping an arm around the animal's neck. It is strongly recommended not to hold a goat by its hindlimbs as it may possibly dislocate a hip joint in an attempt to escape.

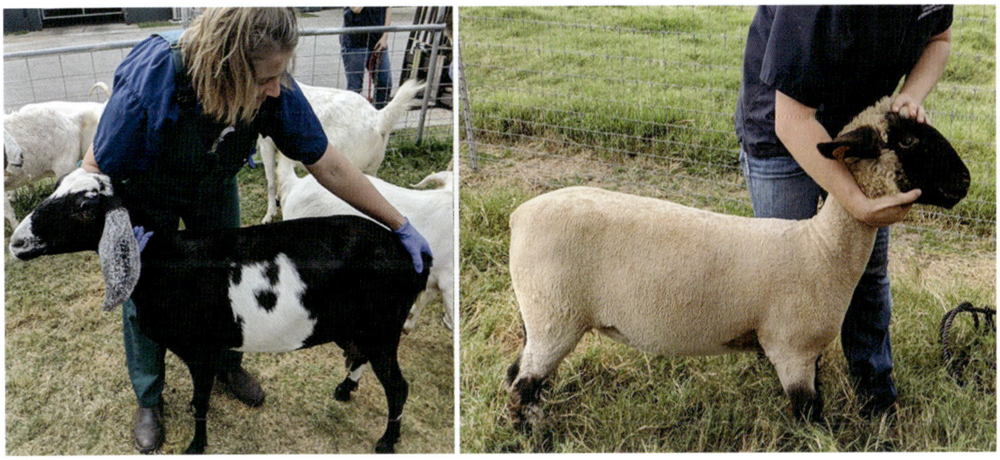

• **Fig. 1.6** Proper method of individual animal restraint.

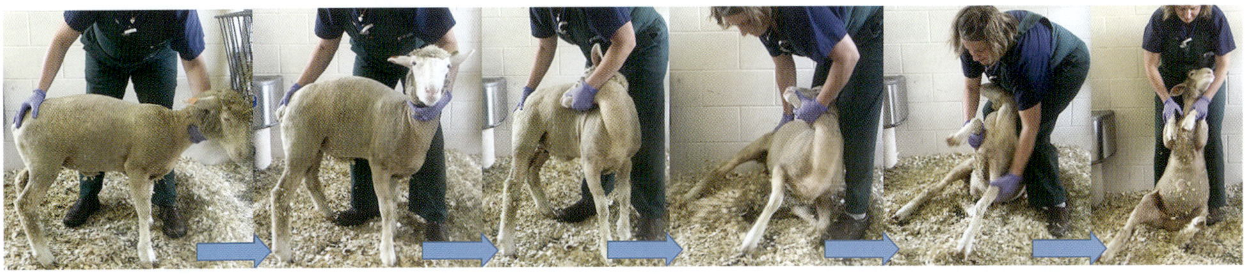

• **Fig. 1.7** Series of images on how to tip a sheep and place it on its rump. This is a common method used to restrain adult sheep, allowing a multitude of livestock procedures to be performed (e.g., foot trimming, shearing).

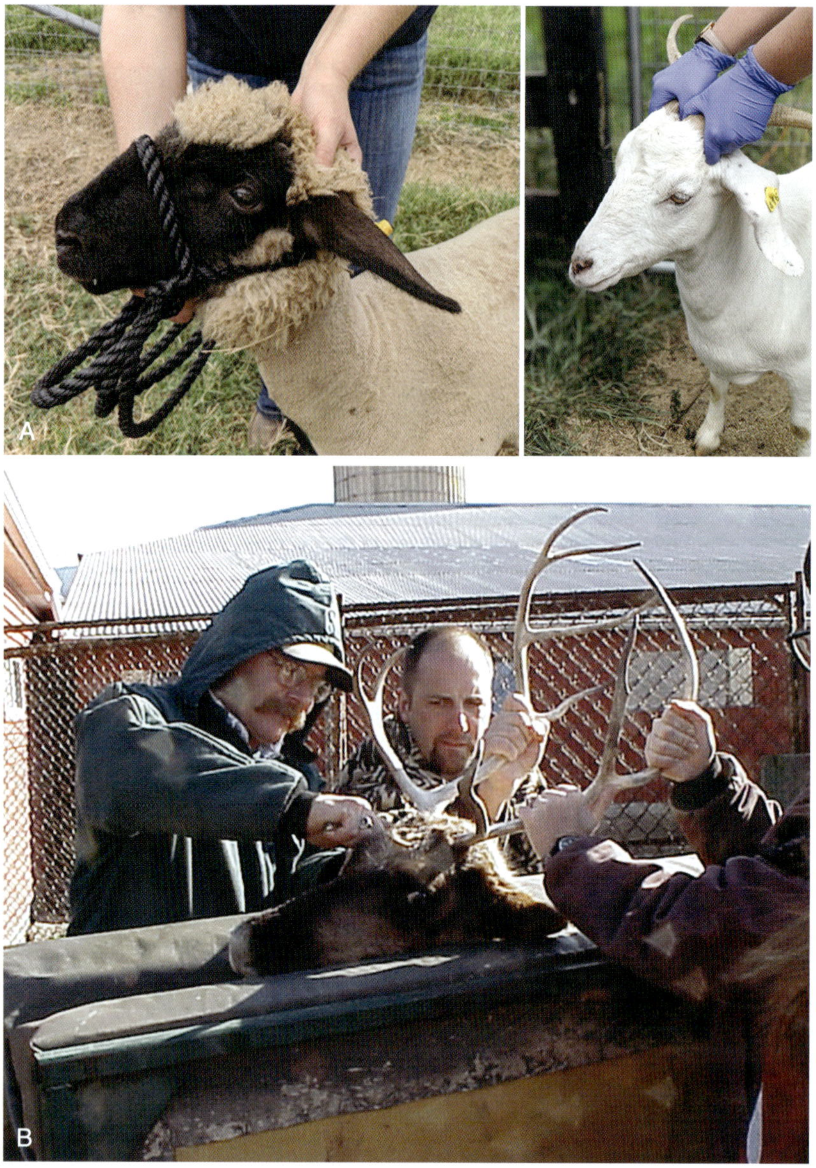

• **Fig. 1.8** **A.** This image shows how to properly restrain a sheep and a goat by the head. In horned breeds, it is important to note that the horns must be held at the base. **B.** This image shows a restraint table with solid cushioned sides for cervids and manual restraint of the horns.

Special handling facilities for cervids will include a drop chute (Figure 1.9) and a box system leading to the chute, or box stalls with remote door opening to minimize animal-human contact (Figure 1.10). Animals may actually be calmer in the dark and work better through the facility. Training the animals to use the facility is very important and will result in less stress to the animals and handlers. Small fawns may be restrained manually, but larger fawns and adults may injure themselves or the handlers if not sedated or restrained in a chute. Cervids can strike with their front feet, or males in hard antler may charge and attempt to gore a handler. Shields may be used, but properly designed facilities usually do not require handlers to enter small confined areas. Extremely tame cervids may lie down and refuse to move in some cases and may have to be manually pushed or prodded into a chute or pen.

Fencing for cervids may be dictated by state statute. Most cervid fencing comes in 8- or 10-foot heights and is high-tensile

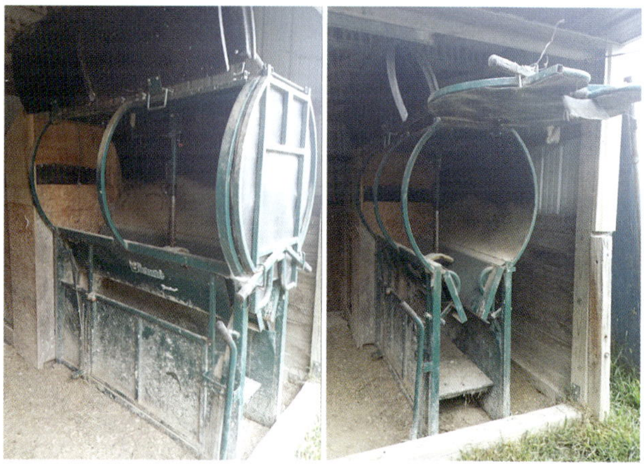

• **Fig. 1.9** Commercially available chute restraint system to facilitate herd work of cervids.

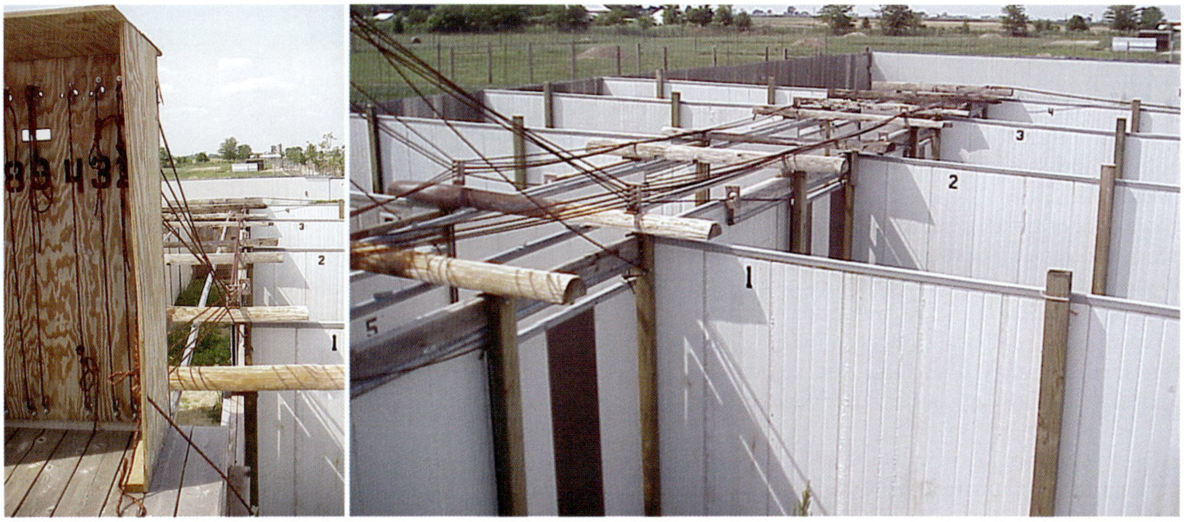

• **Fig. 1.10** Deer-holding working facilities with individual stalls with solid walls and automatic doors.

net wire. White-tailed deer rarely use shelters. Fawns will hide under or behind objects placed in the pasture for shade and adults will seek out shade in hot weather, but most will not use buildings or shelters as do sheep, goats, or cattle. Mule deer do tend to use buildings more, primarily in the summer to escape flies and excessive heat.

Bottle-raised fawns will need approximately 6 to 8 square feet of area minimum per head while in a pen. As they grow, the deer are typically turned out into larger areas. Stocking densities are usually given in animals per acre with ranges from 4 to 10 adults per acre. The authors believe that stocking density for cervids should be based on animal units used in sheep and cattle production which takes into account local climate and soil conditions. Overstocking should be discouraged and leads to destruction of trees, shrubs, grasses, and forbs. If all the forage has been destroyed, the pen is overstocked, and a reduction in animal numbers should be carried out.

Restraining for Examination and Procedures

General Considerations. There is no single best way the practitioner should use to restrain small ruminants for an examination or to perform a common livestock procedure. Using the information above, and typically if the animals are well socialized and behaved, often the job can be done without extra personnel or elaborate restraining devices. If a large herd or flock is being worked and there has previously been minimal animal handling, planning ahead on how to best use a facility and restraining devices is highly recommended for human and animal safety, as well as efficiency.

Once the animal is caught, the practitioner can place a sheep or goat into lateral recumbency if needed. With goats, the practitioner leans over the goat (in this case, from the left) and grasps the goat's left pelvic limb with the right hand and the goat's left thoracic limb with the left hand. The goat is then lifted and leaned into the practitioner and placed on the ground. The practitioner's knee can be paced on the animal's neck (Figure 1.11).

When the head is examined, one should always pay attention to horned animals, as they can suddenly use the horns as a safety mechanism, putting humans at risk of serious injuries. The ability to control the head of a horned goat or cervid depends on the temperament of the animal, as well as on the skill and strength of the handler (Figure 1.8A, B). After the head is stabilized, the animal's ears, eyes, nose, and mouth can be inspected, blood can be drawn from the jugular vein, or a subcutaneous or intramuscular injection can safely be given. For an oral examination, the use of

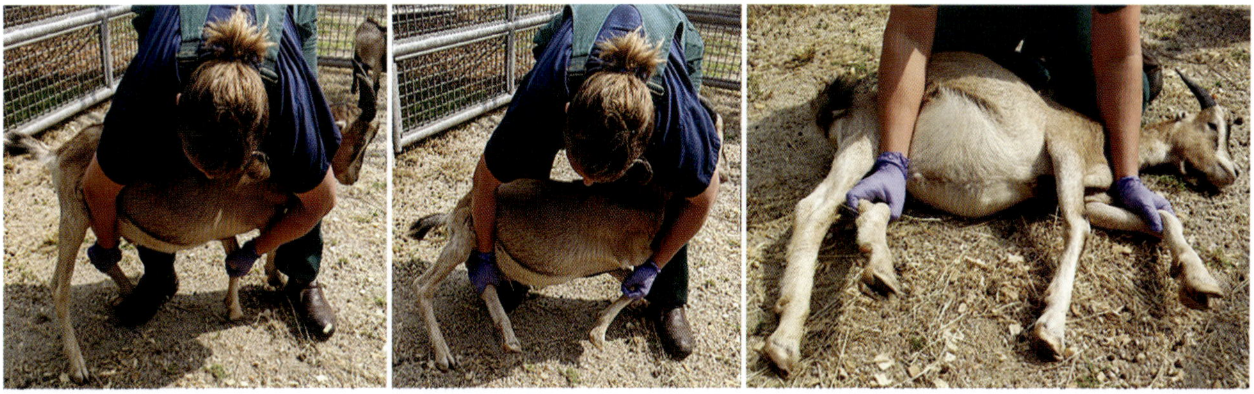

• **Fig. 1.11** This series of images shows how to place a goat in lateral recumbency. The practitioner may carefully apply pressure on the neck using his/her knee. Attention to the horns is imperative to avoid trauma.

a speculum and light source is strongly recommended to ensure a clear view of the oral cavity and prevent the animal from biting instruments or the practitioner's fingers.

Once again, small fawns may be manually restrained as described previously. Larger fawns and adults cannot usually be safely handled in any way other than a drop chute/box or under sedation/anesthesia.

The choice of appropriate restraint technique is dependent on the preference and experience of the clinician. Restraint will also depend on the clinical condition and disposition of the patient, as well as the procedure needing to be performed. For welfare reasons, the practitioner should always be mindful that restraint methods are used for safety of humans and animals and often chemical restraint is necessary rather than the use of excessive force.

Once the practitioner has concluded the examination and prior to the institution of any treatments, it is imperative to consider the animal's intended use (e.g., leather, meat, breeding, exhibition, or pet). Injection reactions can be detrimental to the quality of the carcass of animals intended for human consumption and can be aesthetically unappealing in animals intended for shows and exhibitions. Meat producers prefer that injections be placed in the neck, which yields a meat cut of low value. Breeders prefer the axilla, in which a nodular mass of scar tissue will not be visible and cannot be readily mistaken for caseous lymphadenitis. Subcutaneous injections should always be used in preference to intramuscular, obviously taking into consideration that the label of the medication in question calls for a subcutaneous route of administration. Less pain and mild to no muscle damage are known to be the major reasons for the preferred subcutaneous route.

Oral medications are often used. With the head properly stabilized as described above, a drenching gun, oral or dose syringe (with a metal tip), orogastric intubation, and balling guns are typically the instruments used to deliver oral medications to sheep, goats, and cervids. The dose syringe, drench gun, and balling guns are to be inserted well into the cheek pouch via the commissure of the lips, and the medication delivered slowly but consistently, always allowing the animal to swallow. The practitioner should avoid tilting the head upward to prevent aspiration pneumonia and choking.

Almost all cervidae except bottle-raised animals (and even most of them) resent restraint and will struggle, fight, and risk injury to themselves and those attempting restraint. Small fawns may be restrained by lifting them off the ground with an arm behind rear legs, an arm in front of the shoulders and under neck, and squeezing tightly against the body. Covering of the eyes with a mask will help reduce struggling and stress and is recommended in all sizes of cervids even when anesthetized (Figure 1.12). Capturing and handling cervids for more than a few minutes will put them at risk of capture myopathy and as such, their temperature should be monitored and a plan in place to avert or treat. Ice packs, cold water, alcohol, enemas, intravenous (IV) fluids, etc. have all been used to treat hyperthermia. Strict attention to the weather and working the animals at the appropriate time of day is essential. Cervidae can be successfully examined in a drop chute designed for restraint, but this must be carried out quickly to avoid injury and capture myopathy. If a detailed physical examination is warranted and the animal is deemed healthy enough to undergo general anesthesia or profound sedation, it is probably more appropriate to anesthetize/sedate than to use physical restraint. Appropriate selection of tranquilizers and anesthetics that can be reversed or are known to cause the least number of side effects should be used. Supplemental oxygen may be helpful but is not always available or appropriate in field situations where almost all cervid work occurs.

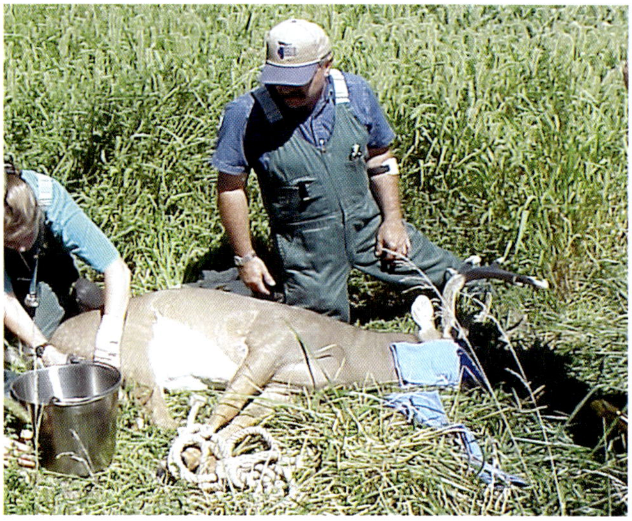

• **Fig. 1.12** Field anesthesia of cervids. The practitioner should use a towel to cover and protect the eyes, along with leg ropes to tie the legs as an adjunct restraint method. Care should be taken to avoid injury. The clinician should consider applying a sterile ophthalmic ointment to the eyes in order to avoid corneal drying during prolonged procedures.

Recommended Reading

1. Nagy DW, Pugh DG: Handling and examining sheep and goats. In Pugh DG, editor: *Sheep and goat medicine,* ed 2, Philadelphia, 2012, Saunders, pp 117.
2. Reynolds JP, Terra RL: *Ruminant History, Physical Examination, Welfare Assessment, and Records.* In Smith BP, editor: *Large animal internal medicine,* ed 5, Amsterdam, 2015, Elsevier, 2-12.
3. Washburn KE: Food animal neurology, *Vet Clin North Am Food Anim Pract* 33:409–426, 2017.
4. Washburn, KE: Localization of neurologic lesions in ruminants, *Vet Clin: Food Animal Practice* 33(1):19–25, 2017.
5. Fthenakis G, Menzies P: Therapeutics and control of sheep and goat disease, *Vet Clin: Food Animal Practice* 27:1–246, 2011.
6. Sherman DM, Robinson RA: Clinical examination of sheep and goats, *Vet Clin North Am Large Anim Pract* 5:409–426, 1983.
7. Grandin T: Design of loading facilities and holding pens, *Appl Anim Behav Sci* 28:187–201, 1990.
8. Heffelfinger JR: *Deer of the southwest,* ed 1, College Station, Texas, 2006, A&M University Press.
9. Hutson GD: Behavioural principles of sheep handling. In Grandin T, editor: *Livestock handling and transport,* Wallingford, UK, 1993, CAB International, 127–146.
10. Cain A, Wallace M: *A guide to age determination of white-tailed deer,* Austin, TX, 2003, Texas Parks and Wildlife. https://tpwd.texas.gov/publications/pwdpubs/media/pwd_bk_w7000_0755.pdf.
11. Body condition score for deer. https://www.purinamills.com/deer-feed/education/detail/body-condition-score-for-deer.
12. Body condition scoring for white tail deer and mule deer. http://www.albertadeer.com/pdfs/AWMDA-Body-Condition-Scoring.pdf.

2

Feeding and Nutrition

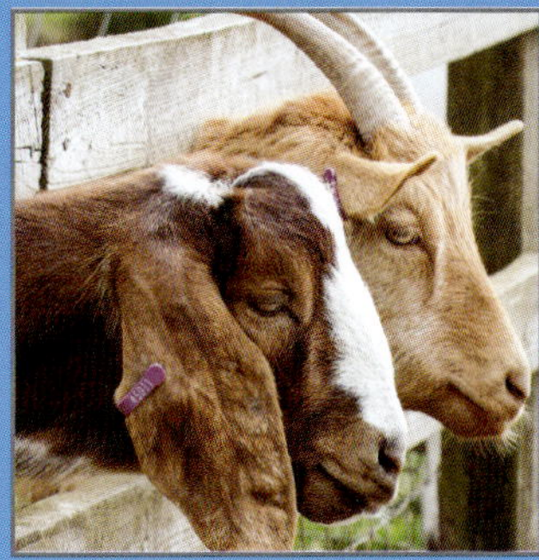

NAR KAJI GURUNG, JESSICA RUSH, AND DAVID G. PUGH

A well-designed program is paramount to the successful implementation of all other aspects of flock health, production, and profitability. This third edition, now entitled *Sheep, Goat, and Cervid Medicine*, has been expanded to include cervid species. In the context of this chapter, sheep, goats, and cervids will be collectively referred to as "small ruminants". The goal in feeding sheep, goats, and cervids is optimal health as reflected in productivity, reproduction, and performance. The information presented here is based on peer-reviewed research data, but many interpolations and approximations are suggested for users.

Small ruminants can convert browse, forages, and other feedstuffs barely usable for more commonly encountered livestock species, into usable animal products (e.g., meat, milk, fiber, antlers, etc.), or to reach peak performance (e.g., pet, show, breeding). These small ruminant species exhibit a high degree of mobility of the lips and tongue, which allows selective consumption of plants and other foodstuffs available in the environment. Like other ruminants, small ruminant species can be characterized by their grazing preferences.[1] Sheep are grass or roughage grazers and tend to graze higher-quality portions of the plant. Goats, as active foragers, tend to select highly digestible portions of grasses and can use browse that is woody or stemmy and will readily consume flowers, fruits, and leaves. In general, goats select grass over legumes and browse over grass with preference to graze along fence lines and in rough or rocky pasture areas. Goats typically perform poorly compared with sheep or cattle on flat, improved, monoculture pastures but usually flourish in areas featuring browse or numerous plant species to graze. Goats tend to be particular about their diet, and may refuse to consume feedstuffs that have been soiled. If given a choice, many meat goats (e.g., Kiko, Spanish, Boer, Tennessee Wooden Leg) prefer a diet of 15 to 20% grasses and 80 to 85% browse[1] and are effectively utilized for brush management in many regions of the world. Goats maintained for brush control should be closely monitored for changes in bodyweight (BW), body condition score (BCS—Figure 2.1; see Chapter 1, Table 1.1; Chapter 19, Table 19.3, and https://www.purinamills.com/deer-feed/education/detail/body-condition-score-for-deer), hair coat, and signs of toxicosis.

The cervids are obligate herbivores with diets including grass, small shrubs, and leaves. They forage selectively on easily digestible vegetation rather than consuming all available food.[2] Deer in the "wild" have diets that are comprised of mainly forbs and browse (80% or more), about 5% grasses, and 15% fruits and acorns.[3] Among cervids, the white-tailed deer is a concentrate selector, whereas wapiti and caribou/reindeer are classified as having intermediate type diets.[4,5]In captivity, white-tailed deer are usually raised as grazers or allowed to selectively browse.

Table 2.1 shows probable dietary preference differences between some free grazing/browsing small ruminants as a percent of their diet.[5a,6] Whenever browse, with its deeper root systems, is the predominant forage consumed, mineral uptake may be greater than that expected with consumption of grasses grown on the same land. Sheep, goats, and cervids also are excellent converters of browse and brush to meat, fiber, and milk, but they are raised mostly as grazing animals. The digestibility of browse is variable, but in many instances may be as high as 70%, which could support many classes of goat or cervid production.

Water

Water is an essential nutrient and the major constituent of an animal's body. If an animal were deprived of all nutrients, it would succumb to water deprivation first. Although small ruminants may survive despite loss of most of their body fat and up to 40 to 50% of their total body protein, a water loss of only 10% can prove fatal.

Small ruminants may be very particular about sources and quality of their water. A fresh, clean, nonstagnant source of water should be available at all times. Water sources should be easily accessible, safe, should be monitored so they are not a source of toxins and/or pathogenic organisms, and kept clean. A paved surface, or clean, dry rocks of 8 to 10 feet diameter around the water tanks/troughs helps prevent unsanitary conditions and may decrease the incidence and spread of disease (e.g., foot rot) in sheep, goat, and farm-raised cervid operations. Anecdotally, in paddocks, dominant buck deer may limit water access to subordinate bucks, thus water consumption must be more closely monitored under some management conditions.

Daily water intake can be affected by several factors, including age, growth rate and stage of production, diet, etc. Pregnancy and lactation increase water requirements and consumption. In addition, water intake is greater for females carrying twins than for those carrying only a single fetus.[7] Likewise, lactating ewes or does consume twice as much water as that typical for nonlactating females: 7 to 15 L/day versus 3.5 to 7 L/day, respectively (e.g., a lactating doe will require about 1 L/~quart of water for every 1/2 L/pint of milk produced). When high-protein diets are being fed or when mineral consumption increases, water consumption also increases. Sheep may increase their water intake 12-fold during summer over that during the winter months.[7] Animals grazing

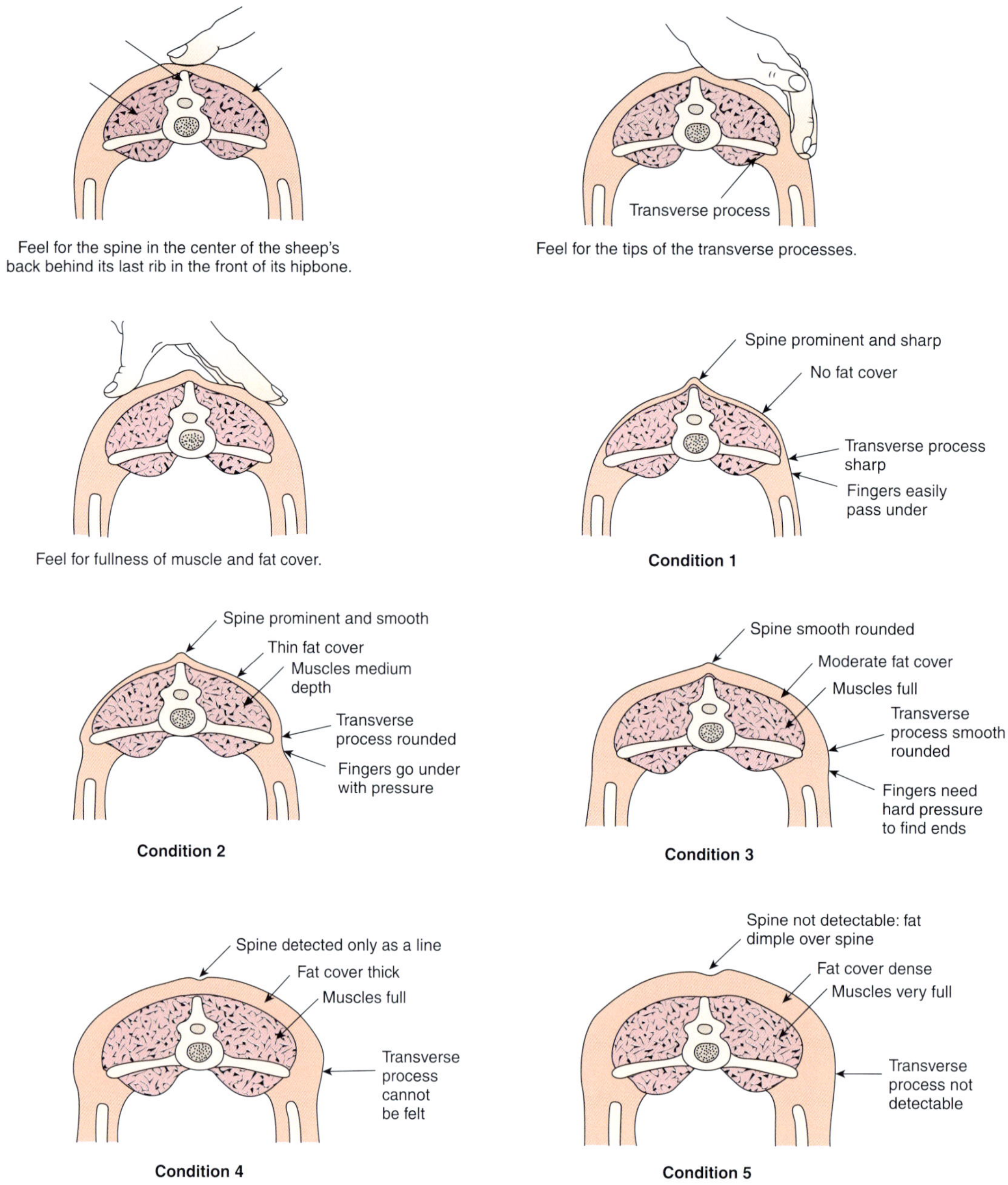

• **Fig. 2.1** Body condition scores (BCSs) for sheep. These drawings show a cross-section through the lumbar region and depict the fat covering (or lack thereof). **(A)** BCS of 1. The spinal and transverse processes are sharp and no fat is detectable on the loin area. Plan: Complete physical examination, parasite evaluation, clinical chemistries, and possible other tests (specialized testing: CL, Johne's, OPP/CAE, etc.), slow introduction of good quality hay, parasite control; additional therapy should be used with care as hepatic function may be compromised. **(B)** BCS of 2. Animals are still thin, with prominent spinal ridge and slightly rounded transverse processes. The examiner's fingers can be passed under the edge of the transverse processes. Plan: Proceed as with BCS 1, however, some grain can be slowly introduced into the diet. Increasing grain intake before breeding (flushing) will be of some benefit. **(C)** BCS of 3. Animals have a smooth, slightly rounded spinal ridge and transverse processes. Slight pressure is required to palpate the transverse process. Plan: Similar to BCS 2; however, many animals should be maintained in this "preferred" level of fat covering. Increasing grain intake before breeding (flushing) will be of some benefit. **(D)** BCS of 4. These animals are fat. The spinal processes are barely palpable. Plan: Consider decreasing feed intake and body fat covering in all but pregnant animals. Be cautious of pregnancy toxemia in late gestation. Increasing grain intake before breeding (flushing) will be of little or no benefit. **(E)** BCS of 5. These animals are obese, with a midline concavity running over the spinal process. Plan: Decreasing feed intake in all but pregnant animals. Be cautious of pregnancy toxemia in late gestation. Increasing grain intake before breeding (flushing) will be of no benefit. NOTE: Because these scores are broad, many owners or managers round up to half-scores (e.g., 2.5) if the animal has more fat covering then one score but not quite as much as the next whole number score. (Personal communication, Jayne Pugh, RD, LD, MEd, SouthernTraxx Farm.)[1] (Reprinted with permission from the Oregon State University Extension Service: Thompson J, Meyer H: *Body Condition Scoring of Sheep* Oregon State University. OSU Extension Catalog: https://catalog.extension.oregonstate.edu. EC 1433, 1994.)

TABLE 2.1 Diet Preference Differences Between Different Ruminants.[4–7]

	TYPE OF DIET (%)		
Animal Species	Grasses	Broadleaf Weeds and Legumes	Browse (Shrubs or Trees)
Sheep	45–55	30–40	10–20
Goats	20–30	10–30	40–60
White-tailed deer	10–30	30–50	30–50
Elk, red, and fallow deer	30–60	40–50	10–30

lush spring pastures, for which the forage water content may exceed 80%, consume markedly less water than those restricted to dry hay, which may only contain 12 to 15% water. Water quality also can affect daily water consumption. For maintenance, individual goats and sheep usually consume 3.5 to 15 L of water/day.[8]

Water varies in quality according to the amount and type of contaminant. The most common dissolved substances in water are calcium, magnesium, sodium chloride, sulfate, and bicarbonate.[8] If the salts of these minerals are present in high enough concentrations, depressed performance, illness, and occasionally death can result. In addition to causing various specific problems in animals, dissolved salts have additive effects on suppression of production and health. As salt concentrations increase, water consumption usually is depressed, with young animals generally being more affected than adults. Over time, animals tend to adapt to water with high concentrations of dissolved salts. However, rapid or abrupt changes from water with relatively low dissolved salt concentrations to water with high concentrations of dissolved substances are poorly tolerated.[8–11] High sulfate concentrations in the range of 3500 to 5000 parts per million (ppm) may result in suppressed copper absorption from the intestine. Nitrates and, less commonly, nitrites occasionally are encountered in toxic concentrations from ground water. Most safe, drinkable water has a pH of 7 to 8. As the alkalinity of water increases, its suitability for consumption decreases.

Although water contaminated with coliform bacteria has been associated with disease in humans, only rarely is coliform contamination of drinking water implicated as an agent of disease in sheep and goats. In general, only very young animals are affected. Goats tend to adapt to high ambient temperatures better than do other domestic ruminants and require less water evaporation to control body temperature.[12] In addition, goats possess the ability to reduce urine and fecal water losses during times of water deprivation. Water requirement data for cervids are not available but Nagy and Peterson[12] showed that some deer species (mule deer and reindeer) have water "economy" which may be superior to sheep.

Farmed small ruminants should have access to a continuous supply of fresh, clean, palatable water, which is free from excessive concentrations of sulfur, iron, toxins and other pollutants to ensure that productivity is not compromised.

Energy

Energy generally is the first limiting nutrient under most practical conditions where sheep and goats are maintained throughout the world. Energy requirements vary greatly depending on level and stage of production, level of activity, and intended animal use. Except in situations in which rapid growth rates are desired or milk production is to be maximized, the energy requirement usually can be met with medium-to high-quality forage. Under maximal production pressures however, some sort of supplementation may be required. Energy-deficient diets can result in poor growth rates, lower BCSs, decreased fiber production, reduced fiber diameter, decreased immune function, subfertility, and increased susceptibility to parasitic diseases and other pathologic conditions. Angora goats and many wool breeds of sheep are prone to various fiber production changes, whereas cashmere goats may be less susceptible. The onset of puberty in small ruminants appears to be associated with lean/fat ratio, and reproduction partially is determined by energy balance in sheep, goats, and cervids. Small ruminants with less body fat and muscle are usually older at first estrus cycles, have lower pregnancy rates, and have lower twinning rates.

The greater portion of the energy that is utilized by sheep and goats comes from the breakdown of structural carbohydrates from roughage. Therefore, roughage should constitute the bulk of their diet. Energy can be expressed in terms of the net energy system (calories) or in terms of total digestible nutrients (TDN) as a percentage of the feed. The two expressions are interchangeable with use of various prediction equations; in this chapter, TDN is used as the measure. Currently, most feed and forage testing laboratories estimate TDN using the Van Soest fiber analysis. A more comprehensive formula was developed by Weiss[13] and is used by most commercial labs for estimating TDN for forages and total mixed rations. A representative sample is analyzed for neutral and acid detergent fiber contents, and then TDN is predicted based on one or both of these values. This system works effectively for most forages but is less reliable for feeds that are high in starch (e.g., corn). In general, warm-season, perennial grass hays are approximately 50 to 54% TDN, whereas many of the cereal grains usually are 80 to 90% TDN. Most forages in the green, vegetative state are approximately 62 to 70% TDN on a dry matter basis. Steamy, dry, poor-quality hay is less than 50% TDN. By comparing these typical values with the requirements of various classes of sheep and goats, keepers can ascertain when supplemental energy sources are needed for forage-based rations. For example, a 150-lb ewe requires a diet containing 52.5% TDN for maintenance and 66% for the first few weeks of lactation, with a steady increase from 53 to 66% TDN during gestation. Therefore, the dry (nonlactating), nonpregnant ewe could use low-quality forage, but the pregnant or lactating ewe needs a diet of lush, vegetative forage. If a good-to-excellent forage is unavailable, some type of energy supplement is required for the ewe in late pregnancy or while lactating. Similar supplementation may be indicated for goats: a 110-lb doe requires a diet containing 53% TDN for maintenance but higher amounts during pregnancy and lactation.[6]

A variety of options are available for energy supplementation. Cereal grains are commonly used, corn being the most common as it is dense in energy, and most of that energy is in the form of starch. When appreciable levels of starch are supplemented to ruminants consuming forage-based diets, the general response is a decrease in forage intake and digestibility. However, the energy status in the sheep or goats receiving corn supplementation will be improved because of the energy from the corn. Goats are less adaptive to high concentrate diets compared to cattle and sheep. Several other cereal grains are available for use as energy supplements for ruminants consuming forage-based diets (e.g., grain sorghum, oats, barley, rye). Other nontraditional energy supplements are soybean hulls, corn gluten feed, and wheat middlings. Soybean hulls, the outermost layer of the soybean, are composed of abundant quantities of digestible fiber. Unlike corn, soybean hulls do not suppress fiber digestion but may increase hay digestibility. Even though soybean hulls have TDN values ranging from 65 to 70% less than corn, they produce similar results when used as an energy supplement for ruminants consuming forages. Wheat middlings, a byproduct of wheat milling, elicit similar responses. Beet pulp, citrus pulp, and brewer's grains all are byproduct feedstuffs that can be effectively used in both sheep and goat feeding. These byproduct-type feeds often are much more economical than corn. All byproduct feeds should be analyzed for composition and used accordingly in diet formulation.[1]

Another source of energy supplementation is fat. In general, total fat content should not exceed 8% of the diet, or 4 to 5% as supplemental fat. High levels of fat supplementation depress fiber digestion by bypass fats and may be used in dairy goat diets, but are not generally used for meat goats. In the southern United States, where cotton production is prevalent, whole cottonseed, which contains approximately 24% fat, is used as an energy supplement for both sheep and goats. In animals of both species, the diet should be supplemented with no more than 20% of the daily intake as whole cottonseed, assuming that the remainder of the diet contains no fat.[1] Energy requirements of free-ranging cervids are difficult to determine, but are discussed in the 2007 *Nutrient Requirements of Small Ruminants; Sheep, Goats, Cervids and New World Camelids*.[6] However, energy requirements and adequacy of farmed cervids may be extrapolated from the National Research Council (NRC)[6] and by using BCS (see Chapter 1, and https://www.purinamills.com/deer-feed/education/detail/body-condition-score-for-deer).

Protein

As a general rule, a minimum of 7% dietary crude protein is needed for normal rumen bacterial growth and function for sheep, goats, and deer. Crude protein (CP) for fawns should be up to 20% for body mass development as well as for achieving optimal first-year antler growth. The CP level for bucks should be on an average 16%. If dietary protein drops below 7%, forage intake and digestibility are depressed. Protein deficiency is associated with decreased fiber production, slowed growth, decreased immune function, anemia, depressed feed use, edema, and death. All of the protein reaching the small intestine is found in bacteria or protozoa or dietary protein that escaped ruminal digestion. The quality (amino acid content) of the bacterial protein is surprisingly quite good. Therefore, the quantity of dietary protein provided to adult ruminants is much more important than the quality. The opposite is true of the pre-ruminant lamb or kid. If lambs or kids are fed a milk replacer, it should be composed of milk byproducts to provide an adequate amino acid composition for maximal growth.[1]

Crude protein content varies widely among the various feedstuffs. Warm-season, perennial grass hay samples can range from less than 6% to more than 12% crude protein, whereas legumes in the vegetative state may occasionally be more than 28% crude protein. The protein content of plants declines with maturity. As with energy needs, crude protein requirements vary with the animal's stage of production. For maintenance, ewes and does of most weight classes require a diet containing 7 to 8% protein. During lactation, both ewe and doe require 13 to 15% crude protein in the diet, depending on the number of offspring suckling. Supplementation of protein may be necessary for heavy-producing animals. Whenever grass hay is fed, protein deficiency should be a concern, particularly for growing or lactating animals. The most consistent sign of protein deficiency in lactating animals is poor weight gain or slow growth in their lambs or kids, particularly with twins or triplets.[6] Many plants browsed by small ruminants are legumes and will average 17 to 20% crude protein.

Typical protein supplements include the oilseed meals (cottonseed meal, soybean meal), commercially blended supplements containing both natural protein and nonprotein nitrogen (NPN) (e.g., range cubes, pellets, or molasses-based products), and various byproducts (e.g., whole cottonseed, corn gluten feed, dried distiller's grains). Protein should be fed to meet, but not greatly exceed, requirements. Excess protein usually results in increased feed costs and higher rates of disease (e.g., heat stress, pizzle rot). The excess protein cannot be stored in the body.[1]

Providing NPN is an inexpensive way to increase the protein concentration of rations for sheep or goats. NPN includes any source of nitrogen in the nonprotein form, but the most commonly used type is urea. Whenever NPN is used, the diet should have sufficient amounts of highly fermentable energy components. Feeding grain with NPN can result in a decrease in rumen pH. In this altered environment, the ability of the ruminal urease enzyme to ferment urea is depressed, resulting in a slower release of or breakdown to ammonia and carbon dioxide (CO_2). Slowing this metabolic pathway allows for more efficient protein synthesis by the rumen microbes. By contrast, diets of poor-quality roughage result in a higher rumen pH and enhanced urease activity. These conditions result in a quicker release of ammonia, a poorer "marriage" of chains of carbon atoms and nitrogen for microbial protein synthesis, and a potential increase in the incidence of urea or ammonia toxicity. Whenever NPN is added to the diet, feeds containing a urease enzyme should be limited or avoided. Such urease-containing feeds include raw soybeans and wild mustard. Signs of urea or ammonia toxicity, which may be fatal, include dull or depressed demeanor, muscle tremors, frequent urination and defecation, excessive salivation, increased respiration, ataxia, and tetanic spasms. Treatment includes the infusion of a 5% acetic acid solution (vinegar and water) into the rumen through a stomach tube. In severe cases, rumenotomy and fluid therapy may be required.

The following guidelines are useful when feeding urea as a protein source:

1. Never use urea for more than one-third of the protein in the diet or more than 3% of the grain portion of the diet.
2. Ensure that a highly fermentable source of carbohydrates (e.g., corn, milo) is fed along with NPN.
3. Avoid the sudden introduction of urea into the diet. Introduce over a minimum of 8 to 10 weeks.
4. NPN and silage should not be fed to sheep and goats until the rumen is fully developed.
5. Ensure proper mixing of feedstuffs whenever urea is used.
6. Urea is not fed as frequently to goats compared with cattle. However, it is acceptable to feed urea with corn if it is more of an economical option compared to another protein source (cottonseed or soybean meal).
   For example, if 1 lb of urea plus 6 lb of ground corn is cheaper than 7 lb of cottonseed meal or soybean meal, then the former diet may be efficiently fed. However, if 7 lb of either the cottonseed or the soybean meal is less expensive, the urea should be avoided.
7. If the crude protein of the diet is greater than 14% of the dietary TDN, NPN is of little value. For example, if TDN is

45%, which is typical of many dry hays during winter, NPN is of limited or no value if the crude protein of the diet is greater than 6.3% (45 × 0.14 = 6.3).

Because of variable dietary intake and its relationship to body condition scoring, NPN is best used in sheep or goats with BCSs greater than 2.5 out of 5; they should be avoided in animals with a BCS of less than 2. If NPN is offered to animals, it should be fed daily because less is used for protein synthesis if the supplement is fed less frequently. In one report, the inclusion of NPN in poorly digestible forage diets for lambs resulted in increased weight gain and wool production, and decreased signs of parasitic nematode infestation.[14,15] The fiber production is also impacted by season, breed type, species, frequency of shedding, scurf, and fiber CP. The antler growth in cervids is also impacted by protein level in the diet.[16,17] There is lack of data for protein needs for wool- and fiber-producing ruminants.

Protein requirements of cervids, as with other small ruminants, change throughout the year according to season, physiological needs, age, and activity. The metabolizable protein needs of cervids are published by NRC.[6] Doe deer need higher amounts of protein intake when pregnant and lactating, while adult bucks require more protein for antler growth.[18] The hardened antlers of a white-tailed deer contain about 45% protein.[18] If dietary protein intake is deficient during the spring and summer (in North America), bucks will produce smaller antlers. Regardless of age, bucks need on average 16% protein in their diets from spring through summer for optimal antler growth.[19] However, buck fawns require higher concentrations of protein (up to 20% of the ration) than older bucks to achieve optimal first-year antler growth.[19]

TABLE 2.2 Macromineral and Micromineral Requirements of Goats.[1,7]

Mineral	Minimum	Maximum
Macrominerals, % of Diet		
Calcium (Ca)	0.30	0.80
Phosphorus (P)	0.25	0.40
Sodium (Na)	0.20	—
Potassium (K)	0.80	2.0
Chloride (Cl)	0.20	—
Sulfur (S)	0.20	0.32
Magnesium (Mg)	0.18	0.40
Microminerals, ppm in Diet		
Iron (Fe)	50	1000
Copper (Cu)	10	80
Cobalt (Co)	0.10	10
Zinc (Zn)	40	500
Manganese (Mn)	40	1000
Selenium (Se)	0.10	0.30
Molybdenum (Mo)	0.10	3
Iodine (I)	0.50	50

Minerals

Clinicians generally consider seven macrominerals and eight microminerals when assessing mineral nutrition for sheep and goats. The designations *macro* and *micro* do not reflect the relative importance of the mineral but rather characterize the amount of each that is required as a proportion of the diet. Macromineral needs usually are expressed as percentage of the diet, whereas micromineral needs generally are expressed as ppm or mg/kg (example: 100 ppm is equal to 1.6 ounces per 1/2 ton[15]). The seven commonly assessed macrominerals are calcium, phosphorus, sodium, chlorine, magnesium, potassium, and sulfur. The eight microminerals are copper, molybdenum, cobalt, iron, iodine, zinc, manganese, and selenium. Trace mineral deficiency is less common than energy, protein, or macromineral deficiency. Such deficiencies evolve slowly over time and rarely lead to the dramatic effects on productivity and body condition seen in protein deficiency.[6] In some cases of mineral deficiency, liver biopsy is the diagnostic tool of choice. The technique for liver biopsy is covered in Chapter 5. Hair analysis is of limited diagnostic value.[15] Serum may be useful for zinc concentrations if special trace mineral tubes are used for blood collection. Whole blood may be useful for diagnosing dietary selenium status. Mineral nutrition should be assessed from a local standpoint as some soils are inherently deficient in certain minerals or are acidic, thus, the plants grown in these areas are likely to be mineral deficient. As many plants mature, most minerals have lower bioavailability to animals grazing on them, while many browse or forbs have higher mineral bioavailability than grasses.[15] Various other factors can also affect soil mineral levels, including soil salinity. Table 2.2 shows minimum and maximum requirements for macro- and microminerals for goats.[19] The mineral requirements for cervids have not been completely determined,[6,18,20] but other ruminant guidelines may be applicable.

Calcium and Phosphorus

Calcium (Ca) and phosphorus (P) are interrelated in body functions and are therefore discussed together. Nearly all of the calcium in the body, and most of the phosphorus, is found in the skeletal tissues. Diets deficient in calcium and phosphorus may delay growth and development in young lambs and kids and predispose them to metabolic bone disease (e.g., rickets, osteochondrosis) (see Chapter 11).[21] Likewise, calcium and phosphorus deficiencies in lactating ewes and does can dramatically reduce milk production. Calcium and phosphorus are very important minerals for antler growth in cervids, as hardened antlers are composed of about 22% calcium and 11% phosphorus.[18,20–22]

Between these two minerals, phosphorus is usually the most expensive macromineral. When supplying mineral to a 150-lb (68.2 kg) goat, it is estimated that 46% of the annual cost is phosphorus alone.[15]

Serum phosphorus concentrations are not highly regulated but are still maintained between 4 and 7 mg/dL for sheep and between 4 and 9.5 mg/dL for goats. Phosphorus deficiency is the most commonly encountered mineral deficiency in range- or winter-pastured animals, as most forage tends to be high in calcium and relatively low in phosphorus, and is true especially for legumes. Beet pulp and legumes, such as clover and alfalfa, are good to excellent sources of calcium. For lactating dairy goats and sheep, supplemental calcium and phosphorus are necessary to meet high demands for milk production. Range goats may need less supplemental phosphorus than sheep because of their preference to browse the parts of plants that tend to accumulate phosphorus. Phosphorus serum concentrations of less than 4 mg/dL may indicate phosphorus deficiency.[6] Phosphorus deficiency results in slow growth, listlessness, an "unkempt" appearance, depressed fertility, and depraved appetite or pica.[6]

Small ruminants fed high-grain or high-concentrate diets typically need supplemental calcium and little to no additional phosphorus. Grains are relatively low in calcium but contain moderate to high concentrations of phosphorus. Although serum calcium is tightly held in a narrow range, serum concentrations consistently below 9 mg/dL are suggestive of chronic calcium deficiency.[6] Chronic parasitism can lead to a decrease in body stores of both calcium and phosphorus.[6] Common calcium supplements include oyster shells and limestone. Defluorinated rock phosphate is an excellent source of phosphorus. Dicalcium phosphate and steamed bone meal (when available) are good sources for both. The calcium-to-phosphorus ratio should be maintained between 1:1 and 2:1.[6]

Phosphorus is the most limiting mineral for growth and reproduction for wild herbivores.[22,23] While the research data is limited, the phosphorus requirement for body growth of 6.5 g P/kg BW gain for goats is recommended for cervids,[6] however, the phosphorus requirement for bucks is related to antler weight and antler growth rate with the maximum demand in the final 20% of the growth period (approximately 49 days). Diets with 0.64% calcium and 0.56% phosphorus appear to be optimal for body and antler growth in some studies.[24]

Sodium and Chlorine

Sodium and chlorine are integral components of many bodily functions. Salt (sodium chloride [NaCl]) is the carrier for most ad libitum mineral supplements. If salt is not offered ad libitum, it should be incorporated into a complete ration at a level of 0.5% of the diet. Sodium, predominantly an extracellular ion, is important for normal water metabolism, intracellular and extracellular function, and acid-base balance. Sodium is seldom a problem except when animals are fed grain-based diets. Conversely, chloride is an intracellular ion, functioning in normal osmotic balance, and is a component of gastric secretions. Sheep or goats that are deficient in salt intake routinely chew wood, lick the soil, or consume other unlikely plants or debris. The NaCl content of feeds may be increased to 5%, particularly for feeding males, to help increase water intake and reduce the incidence of urolithiasis (see Chapter 12).[1]

Sheep and goats, and probably cervids, have a natural drive for NaCl in the diet. An important consideration is the decision to use a salt-containing mineral mixture to ensure that mineral intake is consistent, since individual consumption may vary drastically. Furthermore, improperly prepared salt mixtures or blocks, feed supplements, liquid feeds, or certain types of food or water contamination may be associated with drastically altered mineral consumption.

Salt may be used as an intake limiter for energy-protein supplements for sheep and goats. A 10 to 15% NaCl mixture of two parts ground corn and one part soybean meal contains approximately 20% crude protein. The addition of salt usually limits intake of this mixture to 0.45 kg/day in the adult goat or sheep. Whenever using salt-limited feeding, the keeper should take care to introduce the feedstuffs slowly over 2 to 3 weeks and provide access to adequate quantities of fresh clean water. Only white salt should be used as an intake limiter. If trace mineral salt or ionized salt is used, mineral (e.g., copper, iodine) toxicity is likely, particularly in sheep. The sodium requirement for cervids is recommended as 9.0 mg/kg BW for maintenance[25] and 3.2 mg/kg BW for reindeer/caribou. Sodium deficiency is common worldwide while chlorine deficiency has not been shown.[26] Chlorine requirements are not available for cervids, but the sheep and goat values are recommended.

Magnesium

Magnesium is important for normal functioning of the nervous system and required for many enzymatic reactions. Skeletal magnesium can be used by the animal during times of deficiency, but the skeletal magnesium reserve is much smaller than the calcium reserve. Many fast-growing heavily fertilized cereal grains or grass pastures are deficient in magnesium. Magnesium absorption is depressed by high concentrations of plant potassium or rumen ammonia. Legume and legume-grass mixed pastures are good sources of magnesium. A magnesium deficiency can lead to a clinical manifestation known as *grass tetany* in either sheep or goats.[6] Magnesium toxicity is very rare. The magnesium data are not available for cervids. The value for goats is recommended.

Potassium

Potassium functions as an intracellular ion and is required for normal acid-base balance and is an integral component of many enzymatic pathways. The requirement is between 0.5 and 0.8% of the diet, depending on the stage of production. Most grains contain less than 0.4% potassium, whereas fresh green forages generally contain more than 1%. Dormant forages, however, may have much lower potassium concentrations.[1]

Potassium deficiency or toxicity is rare in sheep and goats. However, deficiency may occur in highly stressed animals being fed diets composed mostly of grain. Therefore, in stressful situations (such as weaning), supplemental potassium may be indicated for animals fed predominantly on grain.[6]

Sulfur

Sulfur, a component of many bodily proteins, is found in high concentrations in wool and mohair, in keeping with the large amounts of sulfur-containing amino acids (cystine, cysteine, and methionine) in keratin. Sulfur deficiency can reduce mohair production in Angora goats.[28,29] The general recommendation is to maintain a 10:1 nitrogen-to-sulfur ratio in sheep and goat diets.[6] Ideal ratios are 10.4:1 for maximal gains and 9.5:1 for maximal intake in growing goats.[28] However, a ratio as low as 7.2:1 has been suggested for optimal mohair production.[29,30] If the forage has a low sulfur content, or if large quantities of urea are used in the diet, weight gain and fiber production can be increased by providing supplemental sulfur.

In both sheep and goats, sulfur deficiency may result in anorexia, reduced weight gain, decreased milk production, decreased wool growth, excessive tearing, excessive salivation, and, eventually, death. Browsing animals, such as goats, may ingest enough tannins to decrease sulfur availability. Sulfur deficiency also depresses digestion, decreases microbial protein synthesis, decreases use of NPN, and lowers the rumen microbial population. Whenever NPN is fed to fiber-producing animals, sulfur supplementation is indicated. With the possible exception of oats and barley, the sulfur content of most cereal grains usually is low to deficient, although corn-soybean diets usually meet requirements for the ruminal synthesis of sulfur-containing amino acids.[1]

Sulfur toxicity is occasionally seen in settings where calcium sulfate is used as a feed intake limiter. It also occurs when ammonium sulfate is fed as a source of NPN or as a urinary acidifier. If sulfur is supplemented in the form of sulfate, toxicity may occur, particularly if the sulfur content is greater than 0.4% of the diet.[6] Sulfate can be reduced to sulfide in the rumen or lower bowel. Sulfide in large enough concentrations can result in polioencephalomalacia that is only partially responsive to thiamine (see Chapter 13).

In the southeastern United States, the use of ammonium sulfate as fertilizer has markedly increased due to the rising cost of commercial nitrogen. If signs of marginal trace mineral deficiencies begin to appear in any group of sheep or goats, forage sulfur concentrations should be measured. An excess of dietary sulfur can lead to deficiency of any of several trace minerals (e.g., copper, zinc) without causing any overt toxicity problems. Some feed byproducts such as distillers' dried grains with solubles contain higher levels of sulfur, so caution must be taken to adjust the right amount of inclusion in the diet.[1]

Copper

Copper deficiencies can be primary, as a result of low intake, or secondary, caused by high concentrations of molybdenum, sulfur and/or iron, or other substances in feedstuffs. In the rumen, copper, molybdenum, and sulfur form thiomolybdates, which reduce copper availability. Specifically, the ability of copper to function as part of the enzyme systems needed for specific biochemical reactions is depressed. This impairment in metabolism results in clinical signs of deficiency. Other factors that alter copper absorption include high concentrations of dietary cadmium, iron, selenium, zinc, and vitamin C as well as alkaline soils. Zinc supplementation in the diet to a concentration higher than 100 ppm will reduce availability and liver stores of copper. Roughage grown on "improved" (fertilized, limed) pastures is more likely to be deficient as liming reduces copper uptake by plants. Many fertilizers contain molybdenum which can further complicate copper availability. Good-quality lush grass forages have less available copper than most hays. Legumes have more available copper than most grasses. Liver copper reserves last up to 6 months in sheep.[6,31]

Copper Deficiency. Signs of copper deficiency include microcytic anemia, depressed milk production, lighter or faded-looking hair color, poor-quality fleeces, heart failure, infertility, increased susceptibility to disease, slowed growth, enlarged joints, lameness, gastric ulcers, and diarrhea. Copper deficiency also depresses the immune response of the animal. These signs appear to be more severe with primary copper deficiencies than with a lowered copper-molybdenum (Cu:Mo) ratio. The Cu:Mo ratios of at least 4:1 are considered ideal.[31] Liming can increase molybdenum in forage and disturb the Cu:Mo ratio. Sheep with copper deficiency have inferior wool that lacks both tensile strength and crimp and is characterized as "stringy" or "steely". Growing lambs and kids are most susceptible to copper deficiency, followed by lactating females.[1]

Several breed differences have been observed with regard to copper metabolism. For example, some Finnish-Landrace sheep may have lower serum copper concentrations than in Merinos, which in turn have lower serum copper levels than in British breeds at similar levels of intake.[32] Milk usually is deficient in copper, whereas molybdenum is concentrated in milk.

Anecdotal reports indicate that goats offered only sheep mineral that contains molybdenum, but little to no added copper, may succumb to copper deficiency. The risk of this deficiency may be magnified in pygmy goats and young, growing animals. Merino sheep and dwarf goat breeds require 1 to 2 ppm more copper than other breeds. Copper is absorbed more efficiently by young animals than by adults.[6]

Very young lambs or kids born from copper-deficient ewes and does can present with *enzootic ataxia* or *swayback*. The swayback condition of lambs or kids usually is seen at birth but may be diagnosed in animals up to 3 months of age. Neonates may experience a progressive ascending paralysis due to impairment of the central nervous system development. Manifestations of this ataxia include muscular incoordination, especially in the hind legs, and failure to nurse. Most neonates die within 3 to 4 days of onset of the first clinical signs and symptoms. The prognosis of older animals depends on the severity of the condition. Rear limb ataxia, muscle atrophy, and weakness are noted in lambs or kids from 2 weeks to 3 months of age.[1]

A definitive diagnosis is made with necropsy. Histopathologic examination of the spinal cord reveals myelin degeneration and cavitations of cerebral white matter. Liver copper concentrations are invariably depressed, typically less than 8 ppm. Prevention and treatment consist of copper supplementation (using oral supplements, copper needles, a trace mineral mixture, or injectable copper) and maintaining an appropriate dietary copper-to-molybdenum ratio.

If copper deficiency is suspected, the copper, molybdenum, sulfur, and iron concentrations of the diet should be determined. To confirm copper deficiency, the nutritionist or clinician should measure body tissue concentration. Serum copper commonly is used to determine body copper status, however much of the copper is bound in the clot, making plasma a more reliable indicator of body copper status. Unfortunately, from a body assessment standpoint, blood copper concentrations may be falsely increased by stress or disease. If serum copper is overtly low and animals were not stressed during sampling, copper deficiency is likely. If serum copper concentrations are used for assessment, and copper concentrations fall within normal ranges, additional copper supplementation is of little or no value. An exception is in those cases in which serum copper is normal but dietary molybdenum is high, or the Cu:Mo ratio is less than 4:1. In such cases, the assayed copper may not be available for use in body metabolism. The dietary Cu:Mo ratio should be maintained between 5:1 and 10:1. Liver is the best tissue to use in determining body copper status, but it is a poor indicator of short-term copper balance. If liver copper is marginal, but plasma or serum copper is in the normal range, the animal may have a favorable response to copper supplementation. In such instances, dietary copper probably is deficient, and the liver stores of copper are being depleted. If a herd problem seems likely, the clinician should sample not only a cross-section of ages and production status, but also as many symptomatic animals as possible.

Forage samples should be taken for copper and trace mineral analysis. Core samples of hay should be properly collected. Feed samples should be placed in plastic bags, not brown paper boxes or bags. Dietary copper should range between 4 and 15 ppm. In areas where copper deficiency is a problem in goats, a mineral mixture with 0.5% copper sulfate should be offered on a free-choice basis, however, this level of copper may be toxic for sheep.[6] In extremely deficient areas, copper needles can be administered orally, or copper can be injected parenterally (see Chapters 8, 11, and 13).

Copper Toxicity. Copper toxicity is a much larger problem in both wool and hair sheep than in goats or cervids. Angora goats appear to be more susceptible than either meat or dairy goats.[15]

In sheep, the magnitude of difference between copper deficiency and copper toxicity is quite small. Copper toxicity can occur in sheep as a result of simple mixing errors during the formulation of mineral premixes, or from feeding mineral mixes formulated for species other than sheep. It can also be exacerbated by the ingestion of toxic plants (e.g., lupines, alkaloid-containing species) and stress. Sources of toxic copper concentrations include premixes, trace mineral supplements made for species other than sheep, copper sulfate–containing foot baths, feedstuffs containing high levels of copper (horse, hog, or chicken feeds), and some nontraditional feedstuffs (broiler litter). Signs of copper toxicity include increased respiration, depression, weakness, hemoglobinuria, and icterus, with sudden death in some instances. Gross histopathologic findings in affected animals include signs of a massive hemolytic crisis and dark, hemoglobin-filled kidneys. Treatment includes administration of D-penicillamine (26 mg/kg once a day for 6 days) and ammonium tetrathiomolybdate (1.7 mg/kg intravenously [IV] every other day for three treatments). The control of methemoglobinemia should be specifically addressed (see Chapter 12). As reported earlier, goats, like cattle, are more resistant to copper toxicity than sheep, with diets of 100 to 150 ppm fed to Nubian goats showing improved growth and performance without any adverse signs of toxicity.[33] The 2007 NRC[6] recommends the same copper requirements for cervids as for sheep and goats.

Cobalt

Cobalt (Co) is used by rumen bacteria in the formation of vitamin B_{12}. Co is the only known animal requirement as a constituent of vitamin B_{12} which has 4% cobalt in its chemical structure.[30] It is deficient in some highly organic or poorly drained soils. Cobalt deficiency in sheep or goats is characterized as a classic B_{12} deficiency, with signs and symptoms including lack of appetite, emaciation, anemia, and "wasting disease". Cobalt deficiency is associated with white liver disease, although phosphorus and copper deficiencies and chronic parasitism also play roles in pathogenesis. Animals with this condition have excessive ophthalmic discharge, and their skin becomes extremely pale. Necropsy reveals a fatty liver (see Chapter 5).

To determine whether a cobalt deficiency exists, the clinician must evaluate the complete diet. In cobalt deficiency, serum or urinary methylmalonic acid is increased, while serum vitamin B_{12} and liver cobalt concentrations are depressed. Diagnosis may be difficult, however, because of the normally low tissue concentration of cobalt. A diet with a cobalt concentration of 0.1 ppm is adequate in most instances, but dietary levels below 0.06 ppm should be considered deficient. The 2007 NRC Committee[6] recommends 0.11 mg Co/kg Dry Matter (DM, which is 0% water) for maintenance for goats and 0.10 to 0.20 mg Co/kg DM for sheep. If a frank deficiency exists, a cobalt-supplemented trace mineral mixture should be fed ad libitum. Cobalt toxicity is of minimal concern with most sheep and goat operations under typical conditions in North America.[6]

Iron

Iron deficiency in sheep and goats is quite rare under grazing conditions. However, lambs or kids raised in total confinement, deprived of access to pasture, and housed in earth-floored stalls or paddocks may become deficient. Iron deficiency is exacerbated when young animals are fed a milk replacer deficient in iron as newborn kids and lambs are born with minimal iron stores. Iron is an important component of hemoglobin, and a deficiency can result in microcytic-hypochromic anemia. Iron deficiency is a rare problem in adults, except in cases of excessive parasitism.

In kids and lambs with diagnosed iron deficiency, iron dextran (150 mg given intramuscularly) at 2- to 3-week intervals may prove a valuable therapy.[27] Parenteral iron dextran may be toxic, and caution is indicated with its use.[27] If selenium deficiency also exists, the use of iron dextran can result in painful muscle reactions. The dietary iron requirement generally is 30 to 40 ppm. The maximum tolerable level of dietary iron is 500 mg/kg DM for sheep and goats,[33] but limited data is available for cervids.[34] Anecdotally, iron concentrations in water high enough to "stain white linen" may provide aid to the depressed absorption and possible deficiency of zinc, copper, manganese, and selenium.

Iodine

Iodine (I) deficiency is more common in certain geographic regions of North America, particularly the "Northern Tier" of the United States. Iodine availability is depressed by methylthiouracil, nitrates, perchlorates, soybean meal, and thiocyanates. Minerals that interfere with iodine absorption include rubidium, arsenic, fluorine, calcium, and potassium. Iodine appears to be most available for use by the body during winter months and during lactation. The form or "state" in which iodine exists in the feed alters availability—iodates are absorbed more readily than iodides. Signs of iodine deficiency are goiter, poor growth, depressed milk yield, pregnancy toxemia, and reproductive abnormalities including abortion, stillbirth, retained placentas, irregular estrus, infertility, depressed libido, and birth of small, weak, and either hairless or short- and fuzzy-haired newborns. Lambs or kids born to iodine-deficient dams may have enlarged thyroid glands. Affected kids can be treated with 3 to 6 drops of iodine (Lugol's solution) daily for 7 days. An iodine deficiency has been reported as goiter in neonates.[1]

An enlarged thyroid in the kid commonly is a congenital problem unassociated with dietary iodine. After a thorough examination of the diet, if iodine deficiency is still suspected, the clinician can measure the serum or plasma thyroxine levels, which are lowered in deficient states, to assess the body status. Iodine is readily absorbed, so most sources will work well in salt-mineral mixtures or feed supplements. Iodine levels of 0.8 ppm for lactating animals and 0.2 ppm for nonlactating ewes or does usually are sufficient for normal function. Applying iodine (1 to 2 mL of tincture of iodine or Lugol's solution) to the skin of a pregnant female once each week is a labor-intensive but rewarding method of preventing iodine deficiency-induced hypothyroidism. Hyperiodinism occasionally is associated with the feeding of kelp or related plants in mineral mixtures. This clinical problem may be encountered in the occasional pet or dairy goat. Simply removing the iodine source may be all that is required for treatment of toxicity.[6] A 0.26 mg I/kg DM is recommended for growth for white-tailed deer in the United States.[6] The recommendations for iodine for cervids for other physiologic states are the same as for sheep and goats[6] (see Chapters 8 and 9).

Zinc

Zinc deficiency-related disease or dysfunction has been reported in sheep and goats. Zinc availability is improved with the presence of vitamin C, lactose, and citrate in the diet. Oxalates, phytates, and large dietary concentrations of calcium, cadmium, iron, molybdenum, and orthophosphate all depress zinc availability. Zinc concentrations usually are higher in legumes than in grasses, but legumes invariably contain large concentrations of calcium, which can depress zinc availability. The bran and germ of cereals usually contain high levels of zinc but tend to be less available. Signs of zinc deficiency include dermatitis and parakeratosis, depressed milk production, impaired appetite, poor feed utilization, slowed growth, increased susceptibility to foot rot, diminished hair growth on legs and head, swollen joints, poor growth, decreased reproductive performance, reduced testicular development, impaired vitamin A metabolism, and increased vitamin E requirements. Male goats appear to be more sensitive to the potential for adverse effects of marginal zinc intake.

When zinc deficiency is suspected, the clinician should carefully sample all constituents of the diet. Serum or plasma should be properly collected into tubes specifically designed for trace mineral analysis in royal blue top or trace mineral tubes. Hemolysis alters the accuracy of serum and plasma samples because red blood cells have high zinc concentrations. Liver samples yield the most reproducible measurements of the zinc status of the animal. Both polystyrene containers and brown paper bags may be contaminated with zinc and should not be used for sample collection. Diets containing 20 to 50 ppm of zinc usually are sufficient, except for animals that consume a high percentage of legumes in their diets. In these instances, a chelated form of zinc is indicated. Providing trace mineral–salt mixes with 0.5 to 2% zinc usually prevents deficiency.[1] The difference between required and toxic amounts is quite large, so zinc toxicity is rare under most conditions.[6] The sheep and goat values are recommended for cervids[6] (see Chapters 10 and 11).

Selenium

The absorption of selenium from the small intestine is enhanced by adequate dietary levels of vitamins E and A, and histidine. Large dietary quantities of arsenic, calcium, vitamin C, copper, nitrates, sulfates, and unsaturated fats inhibit selenium absorption. Legumes usually are a better source of selenium than are grasses, which in turn are superior to cereal grains.

The signs of selenium deficiency include retained placentas and nutritional muscular dystrophy, particularly of the skeletal and cardiac muscles of fast-growing young lambs or kids. Other signs associated with insufficient selenium include poor growth, weakness or premature birth of lambs or kids, depressed immune function, mastitis, and metritis. Most often, selenium deficiency is observed in lambs between birth and 8 weeks of age.

Serum selenium concentrations are difficult to interpret because they may reflect dietary intake over the past 2 to 4 weeks. Whole blood selenium is reflective of dietary selenium intake over the past 100+ days.[1,35]

Liver biopsy is the most accurate method for diagnosing selenium deficiency[35] (see Chapter 5). From a practical standpoint, the authors preference is to use whole blood selenium to determine selenium adequacy. Diets containing 0.1 to 0.3 ppm of selenium usually are adequate. The upper limit (0.3 ppm) should be fed during the final trimester of pregnancy. Mineral-salt mixes should contain between 24 and 90 ppm selenium in deficient regions. Of course, dietary limits may be restricted to different levels in different countries and regions of the United States. In cases of frank deficiency, injectable vitamin E and selenium preparations may be given. However, selenium supplementation through feed is more effective than by injection. Selenium toxicity may occur, but deficiency is the more prevalent problem. Toxicity is characterized by wool break, anorexia, depression, incoordination, and death.[6] There are limited studies on selenium requirements of cervids so NRC[6] recommends sheep and goat values for cervids. However, most North American plants contain high levels of selenium due to the type of soils and the accumulation of capacity of the plants, so the serum and liver selenium levels are adequate in northern cervids (see Chapter 8 and 11).

Vitamins

Because a healthy rumen and intestinal tract normally synthesize B vitamins, the only vitamins needed in the diets of nonstressed animals are the fat-soluble vitamins: A, D, E, and K. Supplemental water-soluble vitamins may be required in animals with altered rumen function, parasitized, on low-fiber/high-concentrate diets, high dietary sulfate intake, or being given long-term antibiotic therapy.[15]

Vitamin A

Vitamin A is involved in numerous bodily functions. It is essential for growth, proper skeletal development, normal reproduction, vision, and epithelial tissue integrity. Signs of vitamin A deficiency include weight loss, depressed immune function, night blindness, decreased fertility, and hair loss. Vitamin A can be stored in the liver for 4 to 6 months or longer. Green, vegetative forage meets the daily vitamin A requirement for sheep and goats, which is 105 international units (IU)/kg BW/day for nonlactating animals.[6] During late gestation, the requirement increases to 150 IU/kg/day, and for lactation, 175 IU/kg/day. For conversion purposes, one retinol equivalent (RE) is equal to 3.33 IU. Plants are not a source of preformed vitamin A but instead contain carotenoid precursors for vitamin A.[6] Formulated feeds should contain near 5000 IU/lb of vitamin A for small ruminants.[15]

Hay that is brown and dry, or has been stored for long periods probably is deficient in vitamin A. Vitamin-mineral supplements that also contain oxidizing agents (e.g., copper, iron) are subject to oxidative destruction during storage. Although the label may indicate that vitamin A is present, its activity may be minimal. There is no controlled data on vitamin requirements for cervids, but based on extrapolations of requirements for sheep, the vitamin A requirement would be from 21.1 to 35.2 RE/kg BW.[36] Cervids may be provided with additional RE to enhance the growth and development of antler.[23,37]

Vitamin D

Vitamin D requirements generally are met when the animals are exposed to sunlight. In confinement feeding operations or during sustained overcast or cloudy conditions, vitamin D should be supplemented. Vitamin D deficiency can occur in heavily woolled lambs raised with limited access to sunlight or sun-cured forages. Winter months tend to be the most common time for marginal blood vitamin D concentrations.

Vitamin D along with calcium and phosphorus, is important for normal bone integrity. Deficiencies can result in rickets (see Chapter 11). Plants, both fresh and in the form of hay, particularly sun-cured hay, contain abundant quantities of ergocalciferol (vitamins D_2 and D_3). The vitamin D requirement for sheep is 5 to 6 IU/kg BW/day, except for early-weaned lambs, which have a requirement of 6 to 7 IU/kg/day.[6] For conversions, 1 IU of vitamin D equals 0.025 μg of crystalline D_3.[6] Vitamin D requirements for cervids may be extrapolated from sheep data, as limited information is available. Vitamin D would be critical for antler growth and development. Short day length and cloudy days may pose a problem with adequacy unless vitamin D is added to diets of farmed-raised cervids. Properly managed habitats involving brush management can also help provide adequate amounts of this nutrient. Formulated feeds should contain near 2000 IU/lb of vitamin D activity for small ruminants.[15]

Vitamin E

Vitamin E is a biologic antioxidant that plays a major role in maintaining cell membrane integrity. It is closely associated with selenium in its mode of action, and a deficiency of either can lead to white muscle disease, depressed immune function, and subfertility in sheep and goats. Lambs from vitamin E–deficient ewes may exhibit stiffness, paralysis, and pneumonia. If a higher-than-expected incidence of infection and disease is noted in the herd or flock, the keeper or clinician should investigate adequacy of vitamin E intake. In selenium-deficient areas, young lambs generally should be given extra vitamin E and selenium by injection. Vitamin E is poorly stored in the body, making daily intake crucial. Most good-quality forages contain vitamin E, however females consuming poor-quality hay, particularly in selenium-deficient areas, will require supplementation. Feeds rich in vitamin E include alfalfa meal, cottonseed meal, and brewer's grains. Some feedstuffs (e.g., corn, feeds containing high levels of sulfur, onions) decrease vitamin E availability.[1] The 2007 NRC[7] recommendation for vitamin E requirements of small ruminants is 5.3 IU/kg BW/day. This recommendation is for all classes of sheep and goats.[6] Although vitamin E requirements of cervids are not fully understood, those of cervids raised in captivity maybe five- to tenfold greater than other livestock species. Formulated feeds should contain near 80 IU/lb of vitamin E for small ruminants[17] (see Chapters 8 and 11). Although vitamin E requirements of cervids are not fully understood, those of cervids raised in captivity may be five- to tenfold greater than other livestock species.[38]

Vitamin K

If a ruminant animal is healthy, the keeper does not need to supplement vitamin K. Vitamin K is important for normal blood clotting and vision. In healthy animals it is produced in sufficient quantities in the rumen and lower gut. The vitamin requirements for sheep and goats is shown in Table 2.3.[6]

TABLE 2.3 Vitamin Needs of Sheep and Goats.[7]

Vitamins	Suggested Feeding Rates
A	5000 IU/lb of feed
D	2000 IU/lb of feed
E	80 IU/lb of feed
K	Properly functional rumen can produce adequate amounts of vitamin K so not generally recommended

IU, International Unit.

Mineral Feeding

A salt block or loose salt is just that—a block or loose mixture of NaCl. Trace mineral salt in block or loose form is composed of usually 98 to 99% NaCl with added trace microminerals. The adequacy or content of certain minerals in the block or loose salt mixture generally is not specified. The nutritionist or clinician should carefully evaluate the type of salt-mineral supplement that is being offered to sheep or goats.[1]

Most adult ewes consume around 0.3 to 0.8 kg of a mineral mix per month, or approximately 10 to 28 g daily. Sheep and goats maintained in dry lots usually consume more than this, whereas those that graze or browse on range consume less. Although commonly used, salt blocks are inappropriate for both sheep and goats, and their use can lead to inadequate mineral intake and the occasional broken tooth.[1]

Complete mineral mixtures should be used for animals grazing poor-quality forages, and for breeding, pregnant, and lactating animals. A useful mixture of 40% dicalcium phosphate and 60% trace mineral salt offered ad libitum generally provides an effective yet inexpensive salt-mineral supplement. If vitamin E supplementation is required, 1 kg (21/4 lb) of a vitamin E supplement containing 44,100 IU/kg can be combined with 22.7 kg (50 lb) of trace mineral salt. If animals consume 10 to 17 g of the mixture daily, requirements for vitamin E should be met. In situations in which the amount consumed may not be adequate to meet these requirements, the keeper can monitor intake by weighing the mineral being offered weekly. If animals are not consuming enough of the supplement, the addition of corn, molasses, or soybean meal may enhance intake. If too much of the mixture is being consumed, the addition of white salt will curtail intake. Mineral feeders should be located where they can remain dry to avoid "caking". Mineral supplementation should be based in individual farm practices, forage analysis, stage of production, and breed. As a general guide, mineral supplementation should be year-round.[1]

Feed Additives

To date, very few feed additives have been approved by the U.S. Food and Drug Administration (FDA) for use in sheep and goats. For a list of approved antibiotics, see Appendix l. An explanation of the Veterinary Feed Directives is discussed in Appendix l.

Two ionophores, lasalocid and monensin, are approved by the FDA as feed additives for control of coccidiosis in sheep and goats, respectively. Both are approved for confinement feeding only, and neither is approved for use in animals whose milk is to be used for human consumption in the United States. Feeding these ionophores to ewes or does 30 days before they give birth can reduce the shedding of infective oocysts and may decrease pasture contamination and resultant coccidiosis infection in young lambs or kids. Both agents have value in improving weight gain and feed efficiency in adults and young growing animals. Ionophores also enhance propionic acid fermentation in the rumen, thereby increasing the pool of glucose precursors and aiding in the prevention of pregnancy toxemia in late-term ewes and does. These drugs have the added benefit of decreasing the incidence of free-gas bloat in animals on high grain–low forage diets (e.g., show lambs, feedlot lambs).[1]

Decoquinate is another anticoccidial feed additive that is licensed for use in sheep and goats in the United States. However, it is not approved for use in animals producing milk for human consumption. Decoquinate acts early in the life cycle of coccidia, before they can cause gastrointestinal damage, thereby preventing some of the more serious consequences of infection. Decoquinate is very safe and can be added to feed, mineral mixtures, and milk or milk replacers. Lambs or kids at risk for the development of coccidiosis secondary to stress or environmental contamination and ewes or does in late gestation are likely candidates for the use of this feed additive. To maximize their effectiveness, decoquinate-containing feeds should be provided continually for a minimum of 28 days (see Chapter 6 and Appendix 1).

The dewormer, morantel tartrate, is approved as a feed additive for goats to control gastrointestinal nematodes. Anthelmintic feed additives are valuable for use in animals that are difficult to handle individually because of temperament or lack of facilities. However, if anthelmintics are fed continuously and consistent therapeutic intake is not met, anthelmintic resistance will occur.

The anionic salts ammonium chloride and ammonium sulfate are urinary acidifying agents that help prevent certain types of urolithiasis when added to the diets of rams, bucks, and wethers. Urolithiasis may occur in males consuming high-grain diets due to a smaller urethral diameter as compared with females. This is particularly true in pet goats, breeding bucks or rams, and feedlot lambs. These anionic salts tend to be unpalatable and in effective doses of 200 mg/kg/day, their use may result in depressed feed intake.

The term *yeast culture* refers to yeast and the medium on which it is grown. This product can be dried, preserved, and used as a feed additive. Although the mode of action has not yet been determined, the feeding of some yeast cultures may stimulate dry matter intake and fiber digestion, especially in mildly stressed animals. These yeast cultures may stimulate the growth of ruminal bacteria, which utilize lactic acid. The quality of these preparations should be examined closely before their use. Yeast culture may be useful in easing animals into grain-rich diets and minimizing rumen upset during the diet transition phase.

Buffers are salts that resist pH changes, whereas neutralizing agents neutralize acid and therefore increase pH. Some feed-grade buffers include sodium bicarbonate, sodium sesquicarbonate, sodium bentonite, and calcium carbonate. Magnesium oxide, sodium carbonate, and sodium hydroxide are neutralizing agents. Buffers and neutralizing agents can be added to high-grain diets (e.g., diets fed to feedlot lambs, show lambs, and dairy animals) to help limit the rapid changes in ruminal pH associated with the ingestion of excessive concentrates. Sodium bicarbonate probably is the most widely used of these agents. The response to feeding buffers appears to be variable, except when they are used in dairy animals receiving high-grain diets. Buffers are of less value when forage-based diets are fed. In dairy goats and sheep, buffering agents improve milk production, minimize milk fat depression, decrease the incidence of lactic acidosis–rumenitis complex, and improve overall health. These buffers may be fed ad libitum to dairy goats, included in a total mixed diet at around 1%, or top-dressed onto the feed.[1]

Fiber

Fiber is an important component of the diet of a ruminant animal. Without adequate fiber in the diet, normal rumination does not occur. In sheep, feeding a concentrate-based diet with limited amounts of fiber results in "wool pulling" as the animals seek a roughage source. To promote a healthy rumen, the dietary fiber content generally should be greater than 50%.

Fiber also is required in the diet to maintain acceptable levels of milk fat. The particle size of the fiber is important. It is generally accepted that a minimum particle size of 1 to 2.5 cm is appropriate to stimulate normal rumination, although the effect of smaller particles is not well documented in sheep and goats. Pelleted roughage does not meet the requirement for fiber size. Animals being fed pelleted forage or lush pasture should be offered hay.[1,15,39]

Pelleted Feeds

The process of pelleting compacts feeds by forcing them through a die. Pelleting of feeds decreases waste, enhances feed utilization, allows for easier storage and mechanization, and decreases labor. However, it usually increases the total feeding cost. Compacting the feed ingredients reduces or eliminates 'fines' and dust particles, thereby increasing palatability. The pelleting process reduces separation and feed sorting by the animal, preventing the intake of only certain parts of the total feed. Because pelleting usually entails grinding, particle size usually is reduced, somewhat improving digestibility. However, feeding pellets can result in decreased milk fat in dairy animals, an increased incidence of ulcers and choke, and urolithiasis in males. Pelleted rations may increase the incidence of phosphatic calculi, owing to decreases in saliva production, thus lowering phosphate excretion by the gastrointestinal tract (GIT). Pelleted rations can therefore increase urinary excretion of phosphorus. Pelleted rations also are associated with increased mucoprotein excretion in the urine. Pelleting also may reduce the content of vitamins A, E, and K, or destroy these nutrients outright, in the feed. In formulating pelleted feeds, manufacturers should fortify these nutrients in the pellet. The animal keeper or producer should weigh the costs versus benefits of pelleted feedstuffs.[1]

Feed Analysis

Both sheep and goats can derive nutritional value from numerous feeds. A listing of a wide array of feeds and their nutritional content can be found in the 2007 NRC[6] recommendations for small ruminants. For simplicity, energy values are reported as TDN. Most commercial labs are using a comprehensive TDN formula developed by Weiss[13] for forages and total mixed rations. Many feeds have limitations on their use because of such factors as fat content, palatability, moisture content, antinutritional factors, and other attributes beyond the scope of this discussion.

To analyze the nutrient content of a given feedstuff, the clinician must obtain a representative sample. For hay analysis, random sampling of approximately 10% of the bales is adequate. With large round bales, a core sample into the round surface of the bale to a depth of approximately 78 cm is ideal. Most sampling devices provide an approximate 2.5-cm-diameter core from the bale. All the core samples should be combined into one container and thoroughly mixed. From this combined mix, the clinician should properly package a subsample of approximately

0.22 kg and send it to a laboratory for analysis. Samples of silage and other high-moisture feeds should be frozen before shipment to the testing laboratory. To analyze bulk feeds that are stored in bins or other storage facilities, the clinician should take several random grab samples as the feed is being augered or unloaded.

Forage can be evaluated by appearance, albeit with much less accuracy than with some sort of laboratory analysis. Green, leafy forage that is free of mold or weeds usually is more nutritious. Goats tend to select leaves when fed hay; thus, hay analysis may not always apply to nutritional intake.

After a representative sample arrives at the laboratory, it is analyzed for a variety of nutritive components. First, the sample is assayed for moisture content. Most feeds contain approximately 10 to 15% moisture, or possibly less in arid environments. The dry matter of a feed is therefore important, and for comparison, the nutrient content of the feed is reported as percent dry matter. If the moisture content exceeds 15%, mold contamination is typically a problem. In addition, total ash content also may be determined and amounts of individual minerals measured. Total ash content may be of value for analysis of various byproduct feeds in which dust or soil contamination may be a problem.[1]

Fiber refers to the diet's cellulose, hemicellulose, lignin, and poorly to slowly digestible portions of feedstuffs. Most laboratories use the Van Soest procedure, which is based on the use of detergents. The first step is to boil the sample in a neutral detergent solution and separate the cell contents from the fiber. The undissolved fraction is referred to as the *neutral detergent fiber* (NDF). This NDF fraction is then boiled in an acid detergent solution to dissolve the hemicellulose, which leaves behind the *acid detergent fiber* (ADF). This fraction is dissolved in 72% sulfuric acid, which solubilizes the cellulose. The remaining lignin and silica are separated by ashing the sample. The NDF is an estimate of the amount of hemicellulose, cellulose, and lignin the sample contains, whereas the ADF estimates the amount of only cellulose and lignin. As the NDF content of a feedstuff rises, the bulkiness of the feed also increases—that is, NDF is negatively correlated with dry matter intake.[15] As the ADF content of a feed rises, its digestibility is decreased. Pelleting or grinding usually results in a greater dry matter intake, even for feedstuffs with relatively high NDF content. Based on the determined levels of the various fiber fractions, prediction equations are used to compute TDN content and various other values for energy content (e.g., metabolizable energy, net energy).

The last major nutrient that is measured is crude protein. The sample is analyzed for nitrogen content, and then crude protein is calculated as percent nitrogen multiplied by 6.25. The crude protein value cannot indicate if any or how much of the protein has been damaged by heat. Heat damage often results in decreased digestibility. This method of protein analysis does not differentiate between NPN and natural protein. Protein content reported as digestible protein is formulated from crude protein content. Unfortunately, digestible protein is of limited practical value in developing rations. Additionally, samples may sometimes be analyzed for fat. Table 2.4 illustrates sample hay analyses.

Different testing laboratories use different equations to predict energy values. One such equation in common use is as follows:

$$\text{TDN }(\%) = 88.9 - [0.793 \times \text{ADF }(\%)]$$

The equation balances using either the ADF (39%) or the TDN (58.09%) values from the analysis provided in Table 2.4. In contrast with this simple equation, the various net energy prediction equations use cubic and quadratic terms, which are much more complex. One of the most commonly used prediction equation for TDN was developed by Weiss[13] for plant origin feed ingredients, forages, and total mixed rations given below.

TABLE 2.4 A Sample Analysis for Fescue Hay.

Constituent	Content Determined on Dry-Matter Basis
Moisture	12.75%
Dry matter	87.25%
Crude protein	12.31%
Fiber	
NDF	62.00%
ADF	39.00%
Total digestible nutrients[a]	58.09%
Net energy: lactation*	1.31 mcal/kg
Net energy: maintenance*	1.25 mcal/kg
Net energy: grain*	0.58 mcal/kg

NDF, Neutral detergent fiber; *ADF*, acid detergent fiber.
[a]Calculated from prediction equations.

$$\text{TDN} = 0.98 \times (100 - \text{NDFn} - \text{CP} - \text{ash} - \text{EE}) + \text{e-}0.012 \times \text{ADIN} \times \text{CP} + 2.25 \times (\text{EE-1}) + 0.75 \times (\text{NDFn-Lig}) \times [1\text{-}(\text{lig/NDF}).667] - 7$$

where

Neutral detergent fiber nitrogen-free (NDFn) = NDF-NDICP (% of DM)

Neutral detergent insoluble crude protein (NDICP) = Neutral detergent insoluble nitrogen (NDIN) × 6.25

ADIN is expressed as a percent of total nitrogen (ADIN/N × 100). All other values are as a percent of DM.

The NDF fraction can be used to estimate the animal's voluntary dry matter intake:

Dry matter intake (% of BW) = 120 divided by NDF (%)

Again, using the information from Table 2.4, the equation is solved as follows:

Dry Matter intake = 120 divided by 62 = 1.94 of body weight

Thus, animals provided with the hay in Table 2.4 would consume approximately 1.9% of their BW in dry matter.

Another nutritional measure that may be reported on a forage analysis is *relative feed value* (RFV), which is calculated as follows:

RFV = digestible dry matter (%) × dry matter intake (%) divided by 1.29

Where digestible dry matter (%) = 88.9 – (0.779 × ADF [%]). For this example, therefore, the equation is completed as follows:

$$\text{RFV} = (58.52 \times 1.94) \text{ divided by } 1.29 = 88$$

RFVs can exceed 100 and often do so for good-quality alfalfa. However, this measure does not take into account the crude protein content of the forage, which must be evaluated separately. The poorer the quality of a forage, the longer it requires for digestion. Poor-quality forage remains in the rumen for a longer period, thereby indirectly limiting feed intake. Keepers purchasing feeds would do well to make decisions based on RFV. During diet formulation, however, TDN and protein concentrations most often are used as guidelines.

Balancing a Ration

Substitution Method

The substitution method for balancing a ration works best when only two or three feedstuffs are used in the animal nutritional plan. In this chapter, pounds, rather than kilograms, are used in demonstrating this method of ration calculation. In the following example, a diet composition is determined for a group of ewes with an average BW of 150 lb. These animals also are in late gestation, with a high expectation for twinning. Some grass hay is available and has been analyzed to contain 51% TDN and 8.8% crude protein. Both corn and soybean meal can be purchased as needed. Daily requirements can be determined from the NRC recommendations.[7] Dry matter intake is predicted to be 4.0 lb/day, and the ewes require 2.7 lb of TDN and 0.42 lb of protein. If x = lb of hay, then $4.0 - x$ = lb of corn. TDN can then be determined as follows:

$$\text{RFV} = (0.51)\ (x) + 0.881\ (4.0 - x) = 2.7$$

Where 0.51 and 0.881 are, respectively, the proportion of TDN in the hay and in the corn and 2.7 is the daily TDN requirement in pounds. Solving for x indicates that feeding 2.2 lb of hay and 1.8 lb of corn per day (dry matter basis) will provide the ewe's energy needs.

The next step is to determine the protein adequacy. The provided hay contributes 0.19 lb of protein (2.2 × 0.088); the corn contributes 0.18 lb of protein (1.8 × 0.1). Total daily intake of protein is therefore 0.37 lb (0.19 + 0.18). However, because the protein requirement was determined to be 0.42 lb, the diet is still deficient by 0.05 lb (0.42 − 0.37), a protein source such as soybean meal can be used to supplement the grain (corn). The net gain in protein for this substitution is 0.34 lb for every pound of soybean meal substituted for corn (0.44 − 0.1). Dividing the deficiency (0.05 lb) by the net gain in protein gained by substituting soybean meal for corn (0.34 lb) indicates that the ration can be balanced by adding 0.15 lb of soybean meal and subtracting 0.15 lb of corn. The final daily ration is therefore 1.65 lb of corn, 0.15 lb of soybean meal, and 2.2 lb of hay.

For conversion of this ration composition on an as-fed basis, and for simplicity's sake in this example, all feeds are assumed to be 90% dry matter. Therefore, the amount of each feedstuff should be divided by 0.9, resulting in 1.8 lb of corn, 0.17 lb of soybean meal, and 2.4 lb of hay.

From a practical standpoint, we recommend offering the ewe free-choice hay, supplemented with 2 lb of a corn–soybean meal mixture that contains 90% corn and 10% soybean meal. This ration is fed until lambing commences, at which time the diet is reformulated to meet the demands of lactation.

Fixed Ingredients Method

Presented next is a method of balancing a ration using a fixed set of ingredients. In this example, three different grain sources are used: corn, oats, and wheat. The diet is balanced for 30-lb kids growing at a rate of 0.20 lb/day. In addition, cottonseed hulls are available as a roughage source and cottonseed meal is a source of protein. The wheat was purchased at a bargain price but feeding wheat in large amounts is associated with potential problems. Therefore, wheat is limited to 15% of the diet. In this example, the owners have requested that equal quantities of corn and oats be used in the diet formulation. The daily requirements for these goats are as follows: dry matter intake of 0.9 lb, protein intake of 0.119 lb, and TDN intake of 0.59 lb. First, the nutrients being provided by the fixed level of wheat should be taken into account:

$$\text{Daily intake} = 0.09 \text{ lb} \times 15\% = 0.135 \text{ lb of wheat/day}$$
$$\text{TDN from wheat} = 0.135 \text{ lb} \times 0.8735 = 0.12 \text{ lb of TDN}$$
$$\text{Protein} = 0.135 \times 0.151 = 0.020 \text{ lb of protein}$$

Subtracting these amounts from the requirement yields the following results:

$$\text{Dry matter} = 0.90 - 0.135 = 0.765$$
$$\text{TDN} = 0.59 - 0.12 = 0.47 \text{ lb}$$
$$\text{Crude protein} = 0.119 - 0.020 = 0.02 \text{ lb}$$

An equation similar to that in the previous example, in which x = pounds of cottonseed hulls and $0.765 - x$ = 1:1 mixture of corn and oats, is now used to solve for TDN:

$$0.45\ (x) + 0.8275\ (0.765 - x) = 0.47$$

where 0.451 is the TDN content of the cottonseed hulls and 0.8275 is the TDN content of a mixture of equal parts of corn (0.881) and oats (0.774), [0.881 + 0.774] ÷ 2 = 0.8275. Solving for x reveals that balancing the ration requires 0.52 lb of cottonseed hulls and 0.24 lb of the corn+ oats mix, which equates to 0.12 lb (0.24 lb ÷ 2) of each.

So far, the ration consists of 0.52 lb of cottonseed hulls, 0.135 lb of wheat, 0.12 lb of corn, and 0.12 lb of oats. The hulls provide 0.022 lb of protein (0.52 lb × 0.042), the corn provides 0.012 lb of protein (0.12 lb × 0.10), and the oats provide 0.016 lb of protein (0.12 × 0.132). Total protein in the ration thus far is 0.05 lb (0.022 + 0.012 + 0.016). The requirement is 0.099 lb, leaving a deficit of 0.049 lb.

Cottonseed meal can be substituted for some of the grain. An equal mix contains 11.6%, so the net gain of the substitution is 32.7% (44.3 to 11.6%). Therefore, to balance the ration, the keeper should add 0.15 lb (0.47 lb ÷ 0.327) of cottonseed meal and take out 0.075 lb of corn and 0.075 lb of oats from the diet. The final daily ration is shown in Table 2.5.

Pearson Square

The Pearson square is a simple tool that is quite useful for blending two ingredients on the basis of one nutrient.[1,15] In the following

TABLE 2.5 Final Daily Ration Determined Using a Fixed Set of Ingredients.

Component	lb Dry Matter	lb as Fed[a]	% as Fed
Cottonseed hulls	0.52	0.58	58.0
Wheat	0.135	0.15	15.0
Corn	0.045	0.05	5.0
Oats	0.045	0.05	5.0
Cottonseed meal	0.15	0.15	17.0

[a]To calculate "lb as fed" values, the keeper should determine the percentage of dry matter and divide it into the amount of dry matter being fed (e.g., cottonseed hulls, 0.52 lb at 90% dry matter, or 0.52 ÷ 0.9 = 0.58 lb of feed). In this example, all feeds are 90% dry matter

example, corn and soybean meal are blended to attain a concentrate mixture of 16% crude protein. The square is formed by placing the percentage of the nutrient that is desired in the center and then placing the percentages of the nutrient present in the two feeds at the left corners:

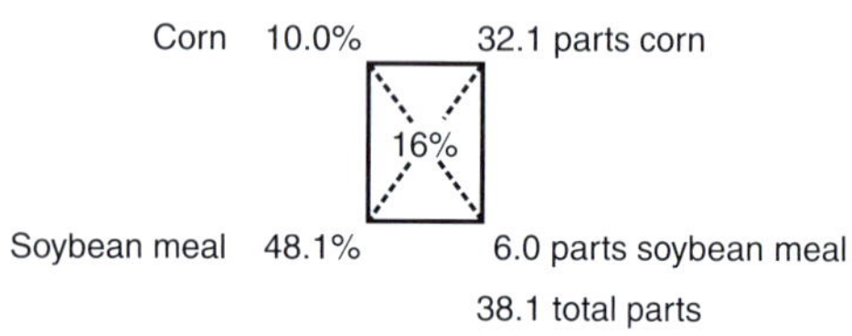

The square is solved by subtracting diagonally across the square without regard to the sign of the differences (in other words, *no* negative numbers) and recording the difference at the right corners. Using the individual and total parts, the percentage of each ingredient can be calculated:

$$32.1/38.1 = 84.25 \text{ corn}$$
$$6/38.1 = 15.75 \text{ soybean meal}$$

Therefore, a mixture composed of 84.25% corn and 15.75% soybean meal mixture yields a feed with a crude protein content of 16%. This quick method can be used to determine content for any class of nutrient.

Calculating Requirements for Phosphorus and Calcium Supplementation

The next example illustrates a method for calculating requirements for phosphorus and calcium supplementation, using the 84.25% corn–15.75% soybean meal mixture from the previous example. Values for the calcium and phosphorus content of these two feedstuffs are from the 2007 NRC recommendations for small ruminants.[6]

	Calcium Content	Phosphorus Content
Corn grain, grade 2	0.02%	0.33%
Soybean meal, mechanically extracted	0.26%	0.62%

All values are provided on a dry matter basis. Calcium supplementation is with limestone, and phosphorus supplementation is with dicalcium phosphate. The corn–soybean meal mixture composes 97% of the diet. This allows for the addition of a calcium and phosphorus source (dicalcium phosphate); a calcium source (limestone) can be added for needed trace minerals, as well as a urine acidifier (if needed). Corn therefore makes up 81.7% of the diet (84.25% × 0.97), whereas soybean meal composes 15.3% of the diet (15.75% × 0.97). Based on an assumed requirement of 0.5% for phosphorus and the percentage of phosphorus in dicalcium phosphate (18.5%), the amount of phosphorus supplementation (as dicalcium phosphate) can be calculated by multiplying each feed ingredient by the percent phosphorus in that feed and adding the results

$$0.5 = (81.75 \times 0.0033) + (15.3 \times 0.0062) + (X \times 0.185)$$

where 0.5% is the daily phosphorus requirement, 81.75% is the percentage of corn in the diet, 0.0033 is the percentage of phosphorus found in corn, 15.3% is the percentage of soybean meal in the diet, 0.0062 is the percentage of phosphorus found in soybean meal, X is the amount of dicalcium phosphate required for supplementation, and 0.185% is the percentage of phosphorus in dicalcium phosphate. The equation is solved as follows:

$$0.5 = 0.27 = 0.095 + (X \times 0.185\%)$$
$$0.5 = 0.365 = (X \times 0.1850)$$
$$(0.5 - 0.365) \text{ divided by } 0.185 = X$$
$$X = 0.75$$

Therefore, dicalcium phosphate must make up 0.73% of the diet to satisfy the phosphorus requirement.

It is now possible to solve for the required calcium supplementation in the form of limestone, based on a daily requirement of 0.6% and the percentages of dicalcium phosphate in the diet (0.73%) and of calcium in limestone (38%):

$$0.6 = (81.75 \times 0.0002 + (15.3 \times 0.0026)$$
$$+ (0.73 \times 0.22) + (X \times 0.38\%)$$

Where 0.6% is the daily calcium requirement, 81.75% is the percentage of corn in the diet, 0.0002 is the percentage of calcium found in corn, 15.3% is the percentage of soybean meal in the diet, 0.0026 is the percentage of calcium found in soybean meal, 0.73% is the percentage of dicalcium phosphate in the diet, 0.22% is the percentage of calcium in dicalcium phosphate, X is the amount of limestone required for supplementation, and 0.38% is the percentage of calcium in limestone. The equation is solved as follows:

$$0.6 = 0.016 + 0.04 + 0.16 + (X \times 0.38)$$
$$0.6 = 0.216 + (X \times 0.38)$$
$$(0.6 - 0.216) \text{ divided by } 0.38 = X$$
$$X = 1$$

Therefore, limestone must make up 1% of the diet to satisfy the calcium requirement.

The ration calculated in the previous examples would therefore be composed of the following:

- Corn 81.7%
- Soybean meal 15.3%

- Dicalcium phosphate 0.73%
- Limestone 1%
- Total ration 98.73%

Values for this ration are on an as-fed basis. With the standard addition of 0.5 lb (equivalent to 0.5%) of sodium chloride and 0.05 lb (equivalent to 0.05%) of trace minerals, the resultant mixture is 99.28% complete on a dry matter basis.

Langston University in Langston, Oklahoma, sponsors a website that allows owners, producers, caregivers, nutritionists, and veterinarians to balance total rations, calculate calcium and phosphorus requirements, estimate supplemental concentrate, and other diet and nutritional calculations for goats (http://www.luresext.edu/?q=content/nutrient-requirement-calculator-and-ration-balancer).[15]

The Pearson Square and simultaneous algebraic equations are common methods of ration balancing, but the use of computers has made the ration-balancing job much easier. There are many programs available for balancing rations for sheep and goats in the United States,[40] including Iowa State University Brands software, FeedForm from Cornell University, CAPRICORN 2010 developed by the University of California at Davis, the University of Maryland software for sheep and goats, Montana State University's Sheep Ration Program, and Langston University's nutrient requirement calculator and ration balancer for goats. There is a Canadian web-based program called SheepBytes Ration Balancer. Some of the software is available free of charge while others are fee-based.

Body Condition Scoring

Theoretically, animals in livestock enterprises should be provided with the exact amount of nutrients required for each stage of production; however, this usually is not practicable under field conditions. The animals will therefore be subject to seasonal periods of undernutrition and overnutrition. A useful tool in assessing the overall nutritional status of the flock or herd is body condition scoring. Cervids are difficult to check for BCS due to handling difficulty. The scoring system most commonly used for sheep and goats has a range of 1 to 5, with a BCS of 1 assigned to extremely thin animals and a BCS of 5 to those that are extremely obese. One BCS change is equal to 11% BW change in sheep.[41–43] BCS is accomplished by palpating a relaxed sheep or goat for the degree of fat covering on the spinous processes and transverse processes in the lumbar region[1] (Figure 2.1; see Chapter 1). Because more than 85 to 90% of all healthy ewes receive a score of 2, 3, or 4, half-scores often are assigned for greater accuracy.[42–44] For example, if the general score is higher than a 3 but not quite a 4, the animal should be assigned a BCS of 3.5. Ideally, a majority of the flock should have a BCS of 2.5 to 3 at breeding and parturition.

If the flock animals were scored 45 days before parturition, and the average was less than 2.5 to 3, the keeper should increase the flock's energy intake so that an average BCS of 2.5 to 3 is attained by the time of parturition. Animals in thin body condition at parturition give birth to weaker babies and generally produce less milk during early lactation. An ideal BCS is especially important in accelerated breeding systems, in which the females are rebred within 60 to 90 days of parturition. Likewise, if the average BCS at 30 days before breeding is less than 3, the keeper should consider "flushing" the females (recommended flushing regimens are discussed later in the chapter). Moreover, condition scoring all of the females allows the keeper to move the thin females, those with a BCS less than 2, into one feeding group while leaving the others, those with a BCS higher than 3, in another feeding group. This allow the thin females to receive additional supplementation without the risk of over conditioning in the remainder of the ewes.

The BCS of goats can be used on two scales: a scale of 1 to 5 is used for meat, dairy, and fiber goats, but when goats are used for vegetation management or for a browsing project, a scale of 1 to 9 is used.[43] Goats should at a BCS 3 to 3.5 at the browsing initiation (6 out of a possible BCS 9) and not below a BCS 2.5 (4 out of possible BCS 9) at any time.[44,45] Most healthy goats should have a BCS of 2.5 to 4.0 while a BCS of 1.0, 1.5, or 2.0 indicates a management or health problem. BCS must be determined by touching and feeling an animal. BCS in goats is described in Chapter 1, and in Chapter 19.

A body condition scoring system of 1 to 5 is used in reindeer and caribou, 1 indicating emaciated and 5 as obese. BCS is measured for degree of fatness and performed by palpating the rump, ribs and withers.[44,45] The BCS system is popular in field conditions for assessing the relative body conformation of red deer hinds in New Zealand, but it lacks sufficient precision to truly reflect the magnitude of live weight changes for individual hinds during late pregnancy (150 to 220 days).[46] See also Chapter 1, Table 1.1, https://www.purinamills.com/deer-feed/education/detail/body- condition-score-for-deer, and for both white-tail deer and mule deer, http://www.albertadeer.com/pdfs/AWMDA-Body-Condition-Scoring.pdf. Feeding and management of cervids using BCS is similar to other small ruminants.[23]

Feeding Programs

In North America, most farm flocks of sheep and goats are maintained on pasture- or range-based systems. Worldwide, approximately 80% of all nutrients for sheep and goats are derived from forage.[1] Both species are adept at converting forage into high-quality products for human consumption and use. Whenever sheep, and possibly goats, graze large pastures or range, their maintenance energy requirements may be more than 60% higher than those of animals raised in dry lots.[6] The more walking required or the larger the range, the more work the animal must perform to consume enough forage to support maintenance, growth, lactation, and fiber production.

Pastures

Producing and providing good-quality forage ultimately will reduce feeding costs and increase overall health, and usually results in a more profitable farming operation. In a typical fall breeding–spring lambing operation, supplemental grain feeding can be kept to a minimum if a good forage management program is followed.[15,47]

A variety of perennial grasses (e.g., fescue, orchard) can be used by sheep and goats. Strategic incorporation of legumes (e.g., clover) and some annual grasses (e.g., ryegrass or small grains) can provide excellent nutrition for the flock. The addition of 30% legumes to a grass pasture improves the nitrogen content of the soil and increases pasture productivity. A pasture with 30% legumes is expected to increase animal productivity by 20% compared with a similar quality pasture with no legumes. Clover can be part of temporary pasture programs, or overseeded onto winter pastures. Legumes improve the nutritional value of a pasture but may predispose animals grazing the pasture to formation of calcite calculi or bloat. Pastures that are approximately 40 to 50% clover should be avoided within 1 month of breeding through parturition, owing to the potential for intake of excessive phytoestrogens. Still, the benefits far outweigh the problems when legumes are used judiciously.[1]

When possible, a pasture grazing system should include warm-season perennial grasses for use by the ewes after weaning. During early gestation, these same grasses can be used as mature forage. Approximately 60 days before parturition and through the first 90 days of lactation, the females can graze on cool-season annual grasses. In some environments, the warm-season grasses then begin their seasonal production. With this system, very little supplemental feeding is required. So long as quantity of the various forages is not limited, grain supplementation usually is not required. In practice, however, weather typically limits forage quantity for 60 days or more each year. A good-quality, pasture-based forage feeding system often requires minimal energy and protein supplements for nonlactating, nongrowing animals. Stockpiled forages can be an economical source of nonharvested feedstuffs and are most efficiently utilized when "strip grazed". With use of winter annual pastures for grazing, allowing the forage to reach a height of 8 inches before access by animals, strip grazing, and limiting grazing all enhance efficiency of utilization.

For proper forage management, adequate acreage in grazeable land and several pastures are needed for a rotational grazing program. Forage requires some periods of rest from grazing to maintain optimal productivity. Therefore, pasture rotation is essential.

The pasture layout does not need to be elaborate or to comprise many small paddocks. However, pastures do need to be divided for proper maximization of forage production. Approximately six to ten separate paddocks or pastures are desirable, and further subdivisions can be added as needed. The divisions should be based on the productivity of the soil and natural breaks in the topography. They will not necessarily be of equal size. The forage should be grazed in a way that optimal leaf material is produced. Depending on the time of year and amount of moisture, the length of time grazing an area and rest between each rotation will vary. For example, the keeper may decide to have the flock graze each of ten paddocks for an average of 3 days at a time. At the end of the rotation, the first paddock has had 30 days of rest and should have good forage regrowth. This type of grazing management may not necessarily increase animal gains, but it may increase the land's carrying capacity as well as the overall quality of the pastures. Pasture rotation systems that increase grass production do not necessarily aid in parasite control. Between four and six ewes (and their lambs) and five to eight does (and their kids) can be maintained on the same amount of land that will support one cow and her calf. In woodland or brushy areas, the same land that will nutritionally support one cow and her calf will provide enough forage for approximately ten does and their kids.

A complete mineral supplement should be offered at all times. An adequate mineral supplement for animals grazing grass pasture contains 15 to 30% salt, 6 to 12% calcium, 6 to 12% phosphorus, and 1 to 4% magnesium (except in early spring when magnesium should be 8 to 14% of the minerals). Trace minerals suitable for the area and soil type also should be offered.

Range

Many of the world's sheep and goats graze on range lands. The common goal for all range land enterprises is to use as much standing forage as possible, with minimal use of harvested forage or other supplements. When grazing sheep and goats, the grazing height should be 4 inches above the ground to reduce internal parasite infection and pasture maintenance.[48] Supplemental feeding should be practiced only when nutrient demands far exceed the nutrient supply of the forage. Some deficiencies are acceptable because of the female's ability to regain body condition during the period from weaning until breeding.

The amount and type of supplementation needed are variable across range conditions. The two most important factors in supplementation decisions are stage of animal production (e.g., growth, gestation, lactation) and weather conditions (e.g., moisture or snow cover). A good range mineral mixture includes equal parts of dicalcium phosphate and trace mineral salt. The trace mineral–salt component should be designed for the local forage and soil types. When supplements are fed in troughs, they should be moved at least once a week to avoid trampling of grazing areas and manure accumulation, and to reduce parasite infections. In general, phosphorus should be supplemented under most range land conditions. Regardless of its composition, the salt-mineral supplement should be made available on a free-choice basis as the only source of salt.

Additional supplements containing protein or energy may be used as needed. Body condition scoring can help in making the decision to supplement energy.[48] If the level of desirable performance can be attained by using a supplemental grain in amounts equal to 0.5% of BW or greater, feeding grain can be economical. If greater quantities of grain are needed, negative effects on forage use (e.g., depressed digestibility of forage) are possible. Several grain byproducts are acceptable supplements for ruminants consuming a forage-based diet. For example, soybean hulls and wheat middlings can provide economical supplies of energy without negative effects on forage use. Protein supplements in the form of soybean meal or cottonseed meal are often used and may actually enhance the digestibility of moderate- or poor-quality forage.[48,49]

Whenever hand feeding is difficult, *salt-limited* rations may be useful for range-fed sheep or goats used for brush control. Depending on requirements, supplemental energy (e.g., corn, oats) or protein (e.g., cottonseed meal, soybean meal) should be ground and mixed with salt in a 3:1 to a 6:1 salt-to-grain ratio, depending on intake. If intake is too great, more salt should be added. If intake is too low, salt should be reduced. In all cases, only white salt (NaCl) should be used. The use of salt-limited feeds decreases trace mineral intake. If trace mineral deficiencies exist while using salt-limited feeds, the keeper should add a suitable trace mineral salt to the feed in quantity such that trace mineral consumption does not exceed 0.02% of the animal's weight. Salt-limited supplemental feeding should be introduced slowly over 2 to 3 weeks. Animal performance should be monitored daily, particularly in times of stress (predator attacks, weather changes).

Confinement Feeding

Confinement feeding of sheep or goats in various small vegetation-free enclosures or dry lots is used in certain locales for all or part of the year. In climates with colder winters and areas that lack winter grazing, some producers move sheep, and occasionally goats, to a sheltered dry lot or barn for protection. Such situations usually require more start-up money for construction of a barn to house animals, feeding floor or lot, and water system than that would be needed for range or pasture operations. Confinement management also may increase the incidence of some contagious diseases, external parasites (particularly during winter), feeding costs, bedding costs, and the need to handle and dispose of manure. Nevertheless, the advantages can more than outweigh the disadvantages in operations where a cheap source of feed and labor is available.

When properly performed, confinement or dry lot feeding can all but eliminate two of the most serious problems with sheep and goat production: internal parasites and predators. However, during confinement feeding, some access to outdoor dry lots is needed to improve hoof and udder health and to decrease the need for supplemental vitamin D. Because no grazing is allowed and feedstuffs (hay, silage, grains) are fed in bunks or other types of feeders, production losses resulting from parasites can be curtailed. Also, less energy is required for maintenance, as walking to a feed bunk uses less energy than is required for grazing. Animals require 2 to 4 h to consume the same amount of dry matter from hay that is consumed in 16 to 22 h of grazing pasture. Heavy-woolled breeds of sheep in full fleece require 1.5 times more space in a confined area than those that have been shorn. Adult sheep and goats require 0.6 and 0.3 m, respectively, of linear bunk space per animal.

With confinement systems, ewes and does are more easily separated by age (ewe lambs, adult ewes) and production (lactating, dry or early lactation, late lactation). The ability to feed groups separately can improve the use and efficiency of available feedstuffs while helping to decrease the incidence of some production diseases (e.g., pregnancy toxemia, hypocalcemia). A dry lot program can be used not only during winter, but also when pasture becomes scarce, or for feeding young lambs or kids for rapid gains.

In dry lot feeding, sheep or goats may be fed hay, silage, "haylage" (hay silage), or green chop. For hay feeding, "square" bales are associated with less waste, but they tend to be more expensive than larger, round bales. Nutrient loss from round bales can be as high as 50%. Storing hay in a shelter above the ground, and feeding hay above the ground in a rack or feeder will reduce waste.

The dietary habits of sheep and goats vary and affect intake. However, dietary preference appears to be a more important limiting factor in the use of certain feedstuffs in goats. The smell, taste, and variety of feeds also affect intake. Silage can be fed to sheep and goats, but animals of both species may take time to adapt to its smell and consistency. Silages should not be fed to sheep and goats until their rumen is fully developed. Sheep and goats appear to be more susceptible to infection from *Listeria monocytogenes*; silage that has been poorly packed, exposed to air, or has not attained a low enough pH (less than 4.5) may be contaminated with *Listeria* or mold. Such silage should be avoided, as should bundle-fed, uneaten, frozen, moldy, or spoiled silage. Hay silages (haylage) and corn silage should have pH values of 3.8 to 4.5 and 4.0 to 4.2, respectively. Corn silage will invariably be deficient in both protein and calcium. (Note: Adding 20 lb of urea, 2 lb of limestone, and 4 lb of dicalcium phosphate per ton of silage will improve nutritional content.)

Feed bunk design should minimize animal contamination. Adults and kids (lambs) should be prevented from crawling into feed containers and soiling the feed.

Dry lot feeding is of value in implementing a parasite control program. If oral anthelmintics of the benzimidazole class are to be used in a deworming program, forcing the animals to fast or feeding dry hay for 12 to 24 h before deworming and then providing dry lot feeding for as long as 72 h will improve the results. This technique also allows for parasite egg-laden feces to be "cleaned" or passed from the bowel before the animals are placed on a safe pasture. Animals may then be moved to pasture after deworming in a relatively parasite-free state, reducing pasture contamination.

Farmed cervid diets should be predominantly composed of leafy natural browse, legumes (e.g., clover or alfalfa), and good quality grass hays. As with other small ruminants, cervids should be grouped by production status. Grain or grain-based pellet feed is also commonly fed in cervid confinement systems. Many pelleted feeds are commercially available as supplements for browse-, grass-, and legume-fed confined cervids (Clifford Shipley, University of Illinois, Personal communication via e-mail). Integrating sound, herd health, and dietary principles implemented, along with the use of BCS to adjust intake, is critical in feeding all small ruminants. Examples of confinement or dry lot rations are shown in Table 2.6.

Feeding the Adult Male

Males should enter the breeding season in good body condition without excessive fat. Rams and bucks should be maintained at a prebreeding body condition score of 3 to 4, because they may lose more than 10 to 12% of their BW in 1 1/2 months of a breeding season. Body condition scores should be assessed as part of a breeding soundness evaluation approximately 2 months prior to breeding.

TABLE 2.6 Example Rations for Dry Lot Feeding for Nondairy Animals (lb/day).

	150-POUND EWE						70-POUND DOE					
	MAINTENANCE		GESTATION		LACTATION		MAINTENANCE		GESTATION		LACTATION	
Ingredient	A†	B†	A	B	A	B	A	B	A	B	A	B
Alfalfa hay	2.9		4.25		5.5		2.0		2.8		2.6	
Grass hay		2.9		3.6		4.8		1.67		2.3		2.2
Corn			0.25	0.75	1.0	1.0		0.33		0.5	0.4	0.4
Soybean meal				0.15		0.75						0.4

†*A* and *B* are different sample diets for each stage of production.

It usually is beneficial to feed a concentrated energy-protein supplement to the males beginning approximately 4 to 6 weeks before the breeding season. Depending on the body condition and size of the males and quality of forage, a daily ration of 6 to 8 lb of forage and 1 to 2 lb of 12 to 14% crude protein concentrate usually suffices. A good-quality supplement for grass-based forage is 80% corn and 20% soybean meal. After the breeding season, some concentrate may need to be fed to help the animals regain an adequate body condition. Breeding males should be fed supplements as early as 6 to 7 weeks or at least 3 weeks before breeding in order to produce fertile semen which begins 40 to 60 days before it is deposited in the female reproductive tract. Cervid bucks tend to lose large amounts of weight pre- and post-breeding season, thus, greater nutrient requirements during the recovery period must be addressed in order to prepare them for the following season's antler growth and breeding season (Communication via e-mail, Clifford Shipley, University of Illinois).

For the remainder of the year, adult males can be maintained on good-quality hay. If grass forage is fed, animals should have free access to a mixture of 50% dicalcium phosphate and 50% trace mineral salt. If legumes constitute a significant portion of the diet, a mixture of 50% trace mineral salt, 25% dicalcium phosphate, and 25% defluorinated rock phosphate can be offered. In both instances, these mineral-salt mixtures should be the only source of salt offered to encourage adequate intake. The trace mineral component should be designed for the local soil types. For sheep, low-copper mineral mixtures are optimal, but goats can safely consume trace mineral mixtures made for cattle. Because of the possibility of urolithiasis in males, the keeper should take steps to prevent stone formation by adding ammonium chloride or other urine acidifiers to the mineral mixture.

Feeding the Female

Breeding females have different nutrient requirements as the stage of production changes. Although requirements are much lower for maintenance than for lactation, meeting these requirements is important for efficient production. Body condition scoring all females every 2 to 3 weeks is an important and cost-effective management tool. Mineral feeding as described for the adult male is applicable for the female.

Maintenance

During maintenance, the objective is to maintain the female's weight and health and replenish any losses experienced during lactation. Most pasture or range settings provide adequate levels of nutrient intake to maintain dry, nonpregnant sheep and goats for this entire period. If extremes in environmental conditions occur (e.g., drought, snowfall), some supplemental feeding is required.

Breeding

At the time of breeding, the practice of *flushing* females has been used with some success. The basic premise is that increased nutrition, specifically energy, just before and during the early breeding season increases the ovulation rate and thus the lambing or kidding rate. The female's age and body condition, and the time of year all affect the response to flushing. Mature females in marginal body condition usually respond best to flushing. Moreover, the practice appears to be more beneficial in attempts to breed the group early or late, as opposed to during the peak of breeding season. Over-conditioned females either do not respond or appear to respond only marginally to flushing. Flushing can be accomplished by the provision of lush pastures or by supplementation with approximately 0.14 kg (0.33 lb) to 0.45 kg (1 lb) of a 10 to 12% crude protein grain per head per day. It is best to begin the hypernutrition approximately 2 weeks before the males are introduced and continue for an additional 2 to 3 weeks into the breeding season.

The benefits of flushing include increased body condition, increased ovulation rate, and increased number of lambs born. Adequate body condition is necessary for acceptable conception rates. Outside certain biologic limits, a flushing effect is not observed. For example, an extremely thin (BCS 1) female probably will not achieve an increased ovulation rate because she is too thin to have normal reproductive cycles. However, within normal ranges (BCS 2.5 to 3) the ovulation rate appears to respond to a short-duration increase in energy and, to a lesser extent, to increased protein intake (Figure 2.1; see Chapter 19). Flushing does not always increase lambing or kidding rates. However, it does increase the number of females cycling early in the breeding season, resulting in birth of a greater proportion of the offspring early in the lambing or kidding season. In females, a BCS at or just under 2.5 to 3 is optimal for most breeding flocks.

Early to Middle Gestation

After the female has conceived, early gestation is the time of partial fetal and placental development. Nutrition is important for adequate development, but requirements are not greatly increased over those of maintenance. If the diet is lacking in energy, protein, and certain minerals, placental development may be poor, resulting in poor fetal growth. A reduction in lamb survival rates at birth can result from inadequate feeding during early gestation. Likewise, adequate nutrition is required for proper attachment of the embryo to the uterus. Midterm stress abortions can occur in Angora goats as a result of energy deficiency. This stress effect is more common in range conditions, particularly after a weather change, predator attack, or decreased feed intake. The incidence can be minimized by not breeding the female until she has attained 60 to 70% of her projected mature weight, and by maintaining a steady nutritional state during pregnancy.[27]

During early gestation, ewes and does can be maintained on winter range, pasture, or moderate-quality hay, but grass-quality grass hay, grass-legume, or small-grain pasture would be best. If corn silage is fed, ewes and does at this stage may need 1/4 to 1/3 lb of a protein supplement daily. Some supplemental grain may be needed with seasonal decreases in feed availability or with weather-associated increases in feed requirements. Females should be fed to maintain a BCS of 2.5 to 3 during early gestation. The scores should be assessed every 2 to 3 weeks, and any flock condition score change acted on immediately.[1]

Late Gestation

The nutrition of the female during the last 6 weeks of gestation is extremely important. Approximately 70% of fetal growth occurs during this period. Inadequate nutrition can result in poor colostrum production, low birth weight in both lambs and kids, lower energy reserves in the newborn animals, and increased death losses, especially during cold and inclement weather. Birth weight is an important factor affecting newborn survival. It can be influenced by breed, number born, age of dam, and the dam's preparturient diet. Extremely low birth weights, less than 4–5 lbs, in lambs can result in increased mortality during the first 24 h of life. Conversely, overfeeding of energy can result in obesity and contribute to dystocia. Proper nutrition is crucial. In general, more problems result from underfeeding than from overfeeding during late gestation.

The process of converting dietary energy into fetal growth is quite inefficient. Because 70 to 80% of fetal growth occurs during the final 6 weeks of gestation, the dam's energy requirements increase substantially. In many instances, the only way to provide the extra nutrition is to increase the amount of concentrate being offered. This sharp increase in energy requirements is compounded if the pregnancy involves multiple fetuses. A large uterus filled with several fetuses physically limits rumen capacity. In such cases, the mature female may not be able to consume enough forage to meet her needs. The keeper may then wish to feed a supplement of between 1/3 to 1 lb and between 3/4 to 2 lb of grain per day for goats and sheep, respectively. A ration of free-choice grass hay, 1 to 2 lb of a 20% protein range cube (depending on female size), usually will suffice.

During late gestation, feeding regimens should be designed to minimize use of energy supplied by body fat reserves. This consideration is especially crucial for ewes during late gestation. Excessive catabolism of body fat can result in pregnancy toxemia. The dam is at greater risk for this condition with concurrent stress from an environmental factor or disease. Pregnancy toxemia is characterized by a buildup of ketones in the blood secondary to accelerated fat catabolism. Affected ewes appear listless and have a distinct acetone smell to the breath.

Maintaining the flock at BCSs of 2.5 to 3 and promoting adequate energy intake during late gestation will help prevent pregnancy toxemia. During late gestation, ewes with a single fetus may consume as much as 3.5 to 4% of their BW in dry matter in grain or excellent-quality forages. Intake may reach 5% in some does. If poor-quality forage is fed, these pregnant females may be able to consume only 2 to 3% of their BW in dry matter. Treatment can be successful, but as is the case with all nutritional problems, prevention is the best strategy. Ewes should be fed approximately 1 kg (2.2 lb) of a cereal grain (e.g., corn, oats) during the final month of gestation to prevent pregnancy toxemia.

Goats also can develop pregnancy toxemia but appear to be more resistant (see Chapter 5 and 8). Dairy goats that are grazing or being fed good-quality grass hay can be fed 0.5 to 1 kg (1 to 2 lb) of a 16% crude protein grain per 100 lb of BW daily during the final 11/2 months of gestation. The amount of grain may need to be adjusted depending on body condition.

In addition to promoting the birth of healthy lambs and/or kids, and preventing pregnancy toxemia, adequate nutrition during this time frame promotes significant mammary development during the last 30 days of gestation. Stillbirths, pregnancy toxemia, and poor milk production all are indicators of feeding an energy-deficient diet in late gestation. Adequate nutrition should be provided to support milk and colostrum production.

Feed or mineral supplements that contain added ionophore, antibiotics, or decoquinate may help control or prevent coccidiosis, abortion, and pregnancy toxemia (see earlier under "Feed Additives," as well as Chapters 5 and 6 and Appendix 1). The addition of antibiotics in feeds requires a veterinary feed directive as of 2017 (see Appendix l).

Lactation

In both sheep and goats, milk production peaks within 2 to 3 weeks after parturition and then declines rather rapidly to a low by 8 to 10 weeks after parturition. In dairy-breed animals, this drop in milk production is less profound. A dam nursing a single kid or lamb produces less milk than a female nursing twins or triplets. This is because one lamb or kid is unable to consume the full amount being produced, allowing a reduction in total mammary output. A dam nursing twins produces approximately 30% more milk than one nursing a single. Likewise, a lactating dairy goat being milked two to three times per day for maximal production also produces greater amounts. A dairy goat usually weighs 10% of a dairy cow's weight but may require 12 to 14% of the nutrients. Lactating does may be capable of consuming 4 to 5% or more (up to 10 to 11% in some females) of their BW in dry matter, making feed intake the most important limiting factor affecting milk production.

Milk production during the first 4 weeks of lactation is important for good lamb and kid growth. If milk production is lacking, the lamb or kid can compensate by increasing solid feed consumption. Because feed is less digestible than milk, suckling animals cannot consume enough feed to make up for a milk deficiency and may therefore exhibit suppressed growth rates during early lactation.

Underfeeding energy during late gestation or early lactation results in greater-than-expected death losses in lambs, particularly twin lambs. Depressed milk production results in lambs that are "scruffy," poorly kept, thin, and weak. Necropsy findings in affected lambs are nondescript — the GIT is filled with straw and the animal has little or no abdominal fat. Lambs older than 1 month are less likely to starve as they begin to eat on their own (see Chapter 20).

During peak lactation it is nearly impossible for a doe or ewe to consume enough feed to meet her nutrient demands. During this time, good- to excellent-performing dairy animals use body fat to make up for this deficit and therefore experience a downward shift (often by more than 1 point) in BCS. This degree of loss is the reason why an adequate body condition before parturition is paramount. To make efficient use of her body fat, a doe or ewe must have adequate levels of protein in the diet. Whenever diets containing large quantities of cereal grain are fed, some form of a rumen buffer should be included in the diet or offered on a free-choice basis.

Because feed intake can limit production in heavy-producing dairy animals, increasing the diet's energy density in early lactation may be required. The addition of fat to the diet is an excellent way to increase the energy density of the diet. As a general rule, supplemental fats should not exceed 4 to 5% of the diet. Oil seed (whole cottonseed), when locally available, is an excellent source of additional energy in the diet. Approximately 2 to 3% of the added fat can effectively come from oil seeds. If more fat is needed, 2 to 3% more fat can be added in the form of specialty-feed fats, including calcium or magnesium salts or fatty acids. These specialty fats are expensive but, for the most part, bypass the rumen. The fatty acids and calcium or magnesium salts are broken apart for digestion in the small intestine.

Obviously, the concentrate portion of the grain can be adjusted on the basis of BCSs. These recommendations show the importance of adequate protein concentrations for maximal milk production. Whole cottonseed can be included in the diet of lactating animals as an excellent source of both energy (greater than 90% TDN) and protein (21 to 23% crude protein). Whole cottonseed should account for no more than 20% of the diet. The requirements of most lactating ewes can be met by feeding 3.2 to 3.6 kg (7 to 8 lb) of a 12 to 14% crude protein, 55 to 60% TDN diet. If hay is fed, a grass-legume or legume-only hay helps supply protein demands. If silage (approximately 2 to 3 lb) is fed, then a protein supplement (1/4 to 1/2 lb), grain supplement (1 to 1.5 lb), and ground limestone (0.02 to 0.04 lb) should be offered. If grass hay is offered (approximately 2 to 4 lb), then a protein supplement (1/3 lb) and grain (1 to 2 lb) should be provided. With the exception of dairy goats or ewes, milk production decreases quickly. By 8 to 10 weeks postpartum, it has become an insignificant nutrition source for the suckling lambs or kids. Up to this point, the dam's requirements can be met by grazing moderate- to good-quality pasture or range. If animals are grouped and fed by production, first-lactation dams with one kid or lamb should be fed with mature females with twins. Also, if these first-lactation dams have twins, they should be fed with mature dams with triplets.

Some dairy goats are susceptible to production of "off-flavor" milk. Cabbage, onions, wild garlic, and some species of weeds or browse all can negatively affect milk flavor. If certain feed sources cannot be avoided, feeding these off-flavor producers just after milking may limit some of their ill effects. Still, avoiding the offending feedstuffs is the best method of prevention. Other non-feed influences on milk flavor are disease (metritis, mastitis), filthy living conditions, and gastrointestinal upset.

Feeding the Lamb or Kid

Bottle Feeding

Rearing orphaned lambs or kids on milk replacer is quite expensive and labor-intensive. If at all possible, keepers should attempt to graft the orphans onto another dam, feeding them on milk replacer only if this cannot be accomplished. Ideally, orphans need to consume small quantities of milk many times per day, which generally is not possible for most sheep and goat producers. Many cervid farms prefer to "bottle feed" doe fawns to adapt them to human handling. Bottle feeding buck fawns should be discouraged, as they may be unpredictably aggressive if kept as pets. Most producers feed "bottle babies" only one to three times each day (see Chapter 19). Many dairy kids or lambs are removed from their dams somewhere between birth and 72 h of age and fed as orphans. The most economical way to raise orphans is to get them onto a dry concentrate feed as soon as possible.

The newborn needs to receive 10 to 20% of its BW in colostrum, preferably within 3 to 12 h after birth. If it is not available from the dam, frozen colostrum supplies can be thawed and used. Colostrum absorption decreases rapidly from birth through 36 h of age. Hemolytic crisis has been observed in some lambs fed cow colostrum. Still, cross-species colostrum is better than no colostrum. Dairy cow colostrum usually is available but is relatively dilute in its immunoglobulin content. Any colostrum fed to an orphan should be free of caprine arthritis encephalitis (CAE) and Johne's disease. If lambs or kids are unable to nurse, they need to be tubed. To pass a tube for feeding, lay a 14–18 French, rubber feeding urethral catheter along the lamb or kid from the tip of the nose, along the neck so the tip lies at the last rib. Mark the tube at the level of the nose. Gently open the neonate's mouth and pass the tube over the tongue, into the esophagus, and until the mark is just in front of the mouth. The tube can usually be palpated just to the left of the larynx as it passes into and down the esophagus.

After the initial amount of colostrum is fed, additional feeding should be withheld for as long as 5 h in newborn animals that are to be bottle-raised. This strategy encourages sucking, easing the transition and aiding in training to a bottle, nipple pail, or bucket. If the owner wishes to feed by hand, a lamb nipple attached to a soda bottle is an effective system. The nipple should be placed in the mouth by the handler while the newborn's jaw moves in a chewing motion. This usually stimulates the nursing reflex in all but very weak newborn animals. Lambs or kids left with their dams for more than 2 days require longer training to become accustomed to a bottle or pail.

When a doe or ewe has too little milk to support more than one newborn, it is imperative that sufficient colostrum be given to all. The keeper should then leave the strongest, most vigorous newborn with the dam and raise the weakest artificially. Although immunoglobulins may not be absorbed after 12 to 36 h, colostrum is a rich source of vitamin A, energy, protein, and local gut-acting antibodies. It also acts as a laxative. If possible, colostrum should be fed for 2 to 3 days.

If lambs or kids are to be hand-fed, feeding 10 to 20% of their BW in the form of good-quality milk replacer divided into four equal daily feedings usually is adequate. Milk replacers for goats should be around 20% protein and 20% fat, with most of the protein supplied by an animal source (whey proteins). If the milk replacer appears brown, the protein sources may have been overheated, resulting in decreased digestibility. Antibiotics are commonly added to help reduce the incidence of bacterial respiratory and enteric diseases. Milk replacers should be fortified with vitamin A (20,000 to 30,000 IU/kg of dry matter), vitamin E (30 to 40 mg/kg of dry matter), and vitamin D (2500 to 3500 IU/kg of dry matter). If lamb milk replacers are used for goats, they should be diluted, because they contain more fat than naturally occurs in goat milk. Good-quality milk replacers designed for calves may be fed to goats and lambs in small quantities in several feedings (10 to 20% of BW divided into four to six equal feedings). When mixing milk replacers, the keeper should take care to ensure that the powder and water are properly mixed into a suspension. Frequent feeding of small quantities will help reduce the incidence of bloat. By the third week of life, some kids or lambs can be switched to a twice-daily feeding regimen. Because milk replacers are expensive, animals should be weaned as soon as possible. If lambs or kids are underfed or fed a poorly digestible replacer, they may become emaciated, weak, or comatose, and death is possible. Inadequately fed lambs or kids have lower-than-normal blood glucose and at necropsy will be found to be devoid of fat stores. The abomasum in starved neonates often becomes impacted with hair or poorly digestible items.[1]

The most efficient and least labor-intensive system is to place the orphans on a self-feeder using refrigerated milk or milk replacer (see Chapter 19). This strategy helps limit milk consumption so that the orphans nurse more frequently throughout a 24-h period. A self-feeder regimen in effect imitates the normal dam-newborn nursing regimen. Keeping the milk cold also may help prevent spoilage and lessen the extent to which the milk replacer separates out of suspension. In addition, kids or lambs using a self-feeder should have access to an extremely palatable dry feed. In orphaned lambs or kids, solid feed should be introduced as soon as possible. Offering 1/4 lb per day of a mixture of corn, oats, alfalfa pellets, molasses, and soybean meal that provides 14 to 16% crude protein works well. Top-dressing the feed with a dry milk replacer also may stimulate early intake of the dry feed. Other ingredients known to be extremely palatable to young ruminants are soybean hulls and various sources of bran, including wheat bran (see Chapter 19).

Creep Feeding

The term *creep feeding* refers to the use of supplemental feed for the nursing lamb or kid. The goals of a creep-feeding program are to promote an adequate intake with a palatable feed and to provide all necessary nutrients in the most economical regimen possible. Winter-born lambs or kids are more often creep fed. Similarly, show animals are creep fed to grow them bigger and faster. Both lambs and kids use feedstuffs more efficiently before weaning.

Lambs and kids will only nibble at the creep feed until they are 3 to 4 weeks old. Nevertheless, the creep feed should be made available as soon as possible to help orphans get used to eating from one location and to help establish rumen function. The feeder should be placed in a dry, well-lighted area where lambs or kids can easily gain access but still retain visual contact with their dams, and kept clean, with a minimum of 2 feet of bunk space per lamb or kid. A variety of methods can be employed to maximize the acceptance of the creep area. Strategies include hanging a light over the creep feeder, retaining one or two dams and their offspring in the area for a few days (with limited feed, of course), and putting all of the animals in a small, confined space adjacent to the creep area.[15]

Creep feeds do not have be complex, but must be palatable because of competition with milk. Pelleting or coarse grinding feeds usually increases intake. Fine grinding usually results in decreased intake as animals' age, particularly lambs. Pellets should be small enough for consumption. In goats, pellet size larger than 5 to 7 mm may decrease intake. After the lambs or kids have begun to consume the creep feed, cheaper ingredients can be used for a more cost-effective regimen. Until the animals reach 3 to 4 weeks of age, however, palatability is the key to successful creep feeding. If increased performance is to be attained from creep feeding lambs, they must consume more than 0.23 kg (0.5 lb) daily from 3 weeks of age to weaning. Low-fiber creep feeds, usually about 10%, containing 16 to 20% protein usually work best. Enhanced performance may be attained if salt (0.5% of the creep feed), ammonium chloride (0.2 kg/440 kg of feed, or 10 lb/ton) and vitamin E are added to most creep feeds. Some examples of creep feeds are shown in Table 2.7.

In general, creep feeding should provide an additional 0.5 kg of gain for each 1.8 to 3.2 kg (4 to 7 lb) of feed consumed. The level of efficiency will vary from one set of conditions to another, but generally, when feed costs are low and sale prices are high, creep feeding usually is profitable. The creep feeding is generally more cost-effective with lambs than kids. In the final analysis, the feasibility of creep feeding is determined simply as a matter of feed costs versus animal sale prices.

TABLE 2.7 Sample Creep Diets for Lambs and Kids.[a]

Element	Sample 1 (%)	Sample 2 (%)	Sample 3 (%)	Sample 4 (%)
Ground corn	33	60	63	40
Oats	—	—	—	11
Soybean hulls	—	—	10	—
Soybean meal	6	8.5	10	6.5
Alfalfa hay	55	25	—	35
Bran	—	—	10%	—
Molasses	5	5	5	6
Trace mineral salt	0.5	0.5	0.5	0.5
Ammonium chloride	0.5	0.5	0.5	0.5
Limestone	—	0.5	1	0.5

[a]Diets 1, 2, and 3 should be fed with an excellent quality hay offered on a free-choice basis Diet 4 is a complete, pelleted feed

Weaning

Lambs and kids can be weaned as early as 3 or 4 weeks, but better results may be obtained if weaning is delayed until 8 to 12 weeks. Because of labor constraints, many keepers attempt to wean milk replacer–fed young as early as possible. Milk replacers typically contain 30 to 32% fat, 22 to 24% CP, and 22 to 25% lactose. Kids of most meat and dairy breeds should weigh at least 9.1 to 11.4 kg (20 to 25 lb) and consume 0.23 kg (0.5 lb) per day of a 16 to 18% crude protein grain at weaning.[1]

Because weaning is such a stressful event, the immediate goal should be to get the lamb or kid accustomed to eating out of feed bunks and drinking from a water trough. The decision to wean lambs or kids depends on age, season of birth, whether they have been consuming creep feed, existing parasite or predator problems on the farm, market price, and available labor. Feed bunk location is important in encouraging newly weaned animals to consume adequate amounts of dry matter. If excellent-quality forage is available, it can be used as the sole source of feed. A good strategy is to place the feed bunks perpendicular to the fence line so that the weanlings are forced to see and possibly investigate the feed as they walk, usually continually, the fence line. For the first 2 days of the weaning period, good-quality hay should be offered on a free-choice basis. The weanlings should then be introduced to a concentrate feed offered at a level of approximately 1% of BW per day. A lamb weighing 31.8 kg (70 lb) consumes approximately 0.32 kg (0.75 lb) per day. After the lambs or kids have been introduced to the grain, the keeper can gradually increase the amount.

Some managers prefer to remove all grain supplements and place the dam on a poor-quality forage 1 week before weaning. This reduces milk production and decreases the incidence of mastitis. By 7 months, most dairy breed kids should weigh between 27.3 and 36.4 kg (60 to 80 lb). A good-quality mineral mixture should be offered on a free-choice basis. Potential replacement animals should be identified and fed a regimen to minimize excessive fat deposition and maximize postweaning growth rates. The same guidelines described for mineral feeding in the male (50% dicalcium phosphate and 50% trace mineral salt) are applicable for weanlings.

Finishing

Finishing of lambs for slaughter can be accomplished in a variety of ways. No one perfect diet for finishing has been defined. Instead, each feeding facility accomplishes the goal by using feedstuffs that are available and economical to the geographic area. Feedlots designed specifically for goats are not as common as those designed for lambs. Most goats are slaughtered off forage-based diets with little use of concentrate feeding.

At slaughter, the lamb should have approximately 0.23 to 0.46 cm of backfat. However, the amount of backfat often depends on specific market preferences. Slaughter weights have a wide range because of the variation in frame size among North American sheep, although they generally fall between slightly below 45.4 kg (100 lb) and 68 kg (150 lb). Ideally, the lambs should be marketed at the proper degree of finish, regardless of their weight. Feeding beyond the lamb's ideal finish results in higher cost of gain because of decreased feed efficiency. Adding lean muscle is much more energy efficient than adding body fat. Blackface sheep and meat goat breeds generally finish at greater BWs.

If high-quality forage is available, lambs can be finished on it. This regimen generally works best for smaller, younger lambs. Older, heavier lambs require some concentrate feeding. For example, a small-framed lamb born in January in the southeastern United States could be ready for slaughter in June having been grazed on only cool-season annual grasses (ryegrass) or grass-legume pastures. By contrast, a large-framed, spring-born lamb in the western United States may come off range in the fall at 6 months weighing 31.8 to 41 kg (70 to 90 lb) and need a concentrate-based diet to be finished by 1 year.

Many lambs in North America are finished in a feedlot or dry lot. These lots vary in size and may be open areas, confinement barns, or a combination of both. An excellent feeding regimen is stepwise feeding, whereby lambs, and occasionally kids, are given more grain as they get larger. By the end of the finishing period, many animals typically are consuming approximately 80% concentrate and 20% roughage. However, when given free access to both roughage and concentrate, lambs consume approximately 60 to 70% concentrate and 30 to 40% roughage. A variety of cereal grains, including corn, oats, barley, milo, and to some extent wheat, can be used by lambs. Amounts used are based on local economics. A protein supplement may be included depending on the amount of protein being provided by the roughage source. Alfalfa commonly is used as a roughage source because of its wide availability, and animals feeding on it may not need additional protein. Mineral and vitamin premixes also are added to some diets. Because the finishing period usually involves instituting diets that emphasize grains, the nutritionist or clinician must be aware that excessive grain intake can predispose animals to urolithiasis, enterotoxemia, and bloat.

Processing of grains, with the possible exception of sorghum, does not appreciably increase lamb performance. Cracking, rolling, or flaking milo to break the hard seed coat increases its usability in lambs. Feeding other grains whole tends to decrease the incidence of acidosis and other digestive disturbances. Pelleting bulky rations may be of some benefit because of the increased level of consumption. Pelleted feeds help ensure a more uniform intake and they are less dusty and easier to handle. The most important factor to consider with regard to pelleting or other processing is the potential for the lamb or kid to "sort" the feed and consume only a portion of the diet. Sorting feed is more of a problem with self-feeding and group feeding. Thus, pelleted feeds are best used in free-choice, self-feeding systems. For example, if the protein, mineral, and vitamin premix is a loose meal, cracking the grain may be beneficial in minimizing sorting, despite its lack of effect on usability. Such feed formulations, however, are more expensive, and their use may be associated with an increased incidence of some diseases.

As stated earlier, goats generally are not finished in commercial settings. In North America, most meat goats are slaughtered by the consumer, in small, local processing facilities, or within niche marketing systems. With some exceptions, goats tend to be sold in small groups over the course of the year. Because of this method of marketing, goats generally are kept on a forage-based diet rather than maintained with year-round feeding of grain. Still, some feedlots, or "grain on grass" operations, do exist. If a group of kids is placed on a concentrate-based diet for finishing, the same basic principles discussed previously for lambs apply. Table 2.8 provides examples of growing and finishing diets for lambs and kids. Growing diets, which contain 14.5% protein and 68% TDN, are used for younger, lighter lambs and kids.

TABLE 2.8 Sample Grower and Finisher Diets for Lambs and Kids.

Element	Grower 1 (%)	Grower 2 (%)	Grower 3 (%)	Finisher 1[a] (%)	Finisher 2[a] (%)	Finisher 3[a] (%)
Corn	33.5	28.5	32.1	73.2	76.0	74.6
Alfalfa	55	—	—	20	—	—
Grass hay	—	50	—	—	17	—
Cottonseed hulls	—	—	40	—	—	14
Soybean meal	5.5	15	21	—	—	4
Molasses	5	5	5	5	5	5
Trace mineral salt	0.5	0.5	0.5	0.5	0.5	0.5
Limestone	—	0.5	0.9	0.8	1.0	1.4
NH_4Cl	0.5	0.5	0.5%	0.5	0.5	0.5

[a]Finisher diets should contain enough limestone (or other calcium source) to provide a 2:1 calcium-to-phosphorus ratio.

Finishing diets, which contain 10% protein and 80% TDN, are more effectively fed to older, heavier animals.

Regardless of the species being fed, the introduction of energy-dense diets in a feedlot setting is stressful and associated with many metabolic diseases. The nutritionist or clinician should ensure that animals being fed in the finishing stages be slowly introduced to these diets and vaccinated for *Clostridium perfringens* serotypes C and D infection and possibly other diseases (e.g., contagious ecthyma, pasteurellosis) that are locally problematic. On arrival at the finishing facility, animals should be offered free access to a good-quality legume-grass hay, fresh clean water, and a mineral mixture. Animals should be introduced to the finishing diet slowly over a 2- to 4-week period. For males, ammonium chloride or other urine acidifiers should be fed to prevent urolithiasis (see Chapter 12). Rumen buffers, antibiotics, ionophores (see earlier under "Feed Additives"), and free-choice hay all are effective in minimizing some production diseases.

Feeding Yearlings

Females

Each sheep and goat enterprise is unique in terms of overall goals. Some operations place importance on breeding ewes and does so that they have their first offspring by 1 year of age. Other farms or ranches may find it much more practical and economical to breed their animals to have their first offspring as 2-year-olds. A ewe's lifetime production can be as much as 20% greater if she is bred as a ewe lamb rather than as a yearling.[50]

If the goal is to have the females lamb or kid as yearlings, nutrition is crucial from weaning to breeding. Yearlings should be maintained on a steady growth plane.

Depending on their weaning weights, most females need to gain between 0.11 and 0.23 kg (0.25 to 0.5 lb) per day from weaning until breeding. Replacement yearlings should be kept on the best available pasture. In most instances, this management approach will require some supplemental energy or concentrate feeding. Concentrate feeding of 1/2 to 2 lb (depending on breed, species, size, and so on) of a 12 to 14% crude protein should be offered in settings of poor-quality forage. Overfeeding young females, however, can result in excessive fat deposition in the mammary glands and decreased lifetime milk production.

If females are to be bred as yearlings, a moderate growth rate is most desirable. The female should obtain 65% of her projected mature weight by the time of breeding. In reality, a range of weights probably exists within which small-framed sheep and goats may have acceptable conception rates at 55 to 60% of their projected mature weights, whereas some large-framed animals may need to be closer to 70% of their mature weights. So long as a good, well-planned forage system is available, females can achieve desired weight gains with little or no grain supplementation. Sheep or goats that can successfully breed out of season should be bred at 13 months so they can lamb or kid at 18 months. This approach requires less nutritional input than breeding 7-month-old females, but still provides an acceptable generation interval for increased female productivity. After the females have been bred, moderate and steady weight gain is desirable until parturition, with a weight goal of 85 to 90% of the projected mature weight by 1 year of age.

Good-quality grass pasture will need to be supplemented with additional energy and protein sources. Animals maintained on grass-legume mixtures will require less supplementation.

Regardless of the breeding system, animals should be weighed and body condition scored regularly whenever possible. If the BCSs of the group begin to drop below 2.5, the keeper should offer a source of supplemental energy. Conversely, if the scores rise above 3.5, less energy supplementation is needed. A good-quality mineral mixture as described for adult males is appropriate for use in yearlings.

Males

Feeding developing males is quite straightforward. They should be developed using as much forage as possible, with just enough supplemental feeding to produce desirable gains (0.34 kg or 0.75 lb/day). This goal is easily accomplished with good genetics. Growing males should be offered a good-quality mineral mixture as described previously, with the keeper taking steps to prevent urolithiasis and other production-related diseases.

Feeding Show Animals

All show animals should be offered a good-quality mineral mixture and given free access to fresh, clean water.

Lambs

Feeding show lambs should be as simple as possible while providing the desired rate of gain and appropriate "bloom". Ideally, the lamb should be fed 30 to 40% of its total daily intake as good-quality hay or forage; the remaining 60 to 70% of the diet should be in the form of a concentrate or grain mixture (Table 2.9). A lamb can eat as much as 3 to 4% of its BW daily. At least 0.45 kg (1 lb) of hay per day should be fed with the concentrate. Lambs should be gradually exposed to increasing concentrate portions of the feed, taking 10 to 14 days to make the transition from little grain to the full amount. Feeds should never be switched abruptly, and fresh, clean water should always be offered on a free-choice basis.

Mature Sheep

Mature show ewes and rams should consume approximately 1.36 to 2.27 kg (3 to 5 lb) of concentrate per day, depending on their size. They also should be offered good-quality hay on a free-choice basis. The requirements for mature sheep are found in the 2007

TABLE 2.9 Concentrate Mixes for Show Lambs.[a]

Element	Sample 1 (%)	Sample 2 (%)
Corn	50	45
Oats	35	—
Soybean hulls	10	40
Soybean meal	10	10
Molasses	4	4
Mineral mix	1	1

[a]Animals should be introduced to high-grain diets slowly over 2 to 3 weeks.

NRC recommendations for small ruminants.[6] Adult show animals should be maintained in good condition but should not be obese. A good exercise regimen is necessary to prevent overconditioning. When possible, forcing animals to graze or walk some distance from grain to hay to water may prove valuable.

Show Goats

The feeding of young meat goats for show is similar to the feeding of show lambs, as discussed previously. The recommended approach is to use a simple diet that provides the desired level of gain and degree of bloom.

Feeding for Fiber Production

Sheep

Wool production is highly heritable; however, nutrition can affect wool growth and character. Within certain biologic limits, energy intake is directly proportional to wool production,[49–52] although separating protein effects from energy effects is difficult. So long as the minimal protein requirement is met, additional dietary protein does not appear to increase wool growth. Wool does contain an abundance of the sulfur-containing amino acid, cystine. Accordingly, feedstuffs rich in sulfur-containing amino acids are important for optimizing wool growth.

In general, the effects of nutrition on wool production are associated with quantity rather than quality. Increased nutrient intake can increase wool production, within limits. However, quality can be affected during periods of severe nutrient deprivation. Under these conditions, fiber diameter is decreased. Extreme underfeeding can result in weak fiber with limited value.[1,6]

The nutritional status of the ewe during gestation can influence the wool production of subsequent offspring. Kelly and colleagues[51] bisected embryos to produce clones that were then placed in ewes fed at maintenance or submaintenance energy and protein levels from days 50 to 140 of gestation. The lambs that were born to ewes fed a submaintenance diet produced 0.136 kg (0.3 lb) less wool from 0.4 to 1.4 years of age. The wool from these lambs was coarser than that produced by lambs born to ewes fed at a maintenance level. These effects have been attributed to decreased hair follicle development in fetuses whose dams were fed deficient diets, and they continue for the rest of the offspring's life.[52]

Goats

Angora goats produce large quantities of fiber per unit of BW. The 2 to 3.6 kg (4.5 to 8 lb) of mohair obtained with each cutting can greatly increase nutritional demands. As with wool, mohair production can be improved with increased energy intake. However, protein appears to elicit more of an effect on mohair growth than that on wool growth. Whereas cashmere wool appears to be only minimally affected by dietary manipulation, increasing dietary protein above requirements increases mohair volume and fiber diameter.[1] In Angora does fed isocaloric diets containing either 12% or 19% protein, an increase in grease fleece weight (of approximately 0.57 kg [1.25 lb]) and fiber diameter were noted with the higher protein intake.[49] Mohair also contains abundant amounts of sulfur, so sulfur-containing amino acids are important in Angora goat nutrition. Qi and co-workers[28,29] indicated that the NRC-recommended[6] 10:1 nitrogen-to-sulfur ratio for maximal mohair production may be on the low side and suggested that a ratio of 7.2:1 may be more useful. Therefore, if NPN is used as a protein source, sulfur supplementation is necessary.

Ranged Angora goats should receive nutritional supplementation during late gestation and early lactation. Salt-limited feeds can be used to control both energy and protein consumption under range conditions. Cottonseed or soybean meal (or other protein sources), corn, and salt (noniodized, nonmineralized) can be added at a 1:3:1 ratio. The keeper should introduce the supplement slowly, adding more white salt if the animals are overconsuming and decreasing salt if they are under-consuming. This salt-limited feeding system can be an effective way to increase energy and protein intake for range-fed goats (and possibly sheep). Careful intake monitoring is important.

Adequate shelter should be provided to fiber-producing animals, particularly young animals and Angora goats, that have just been sheared. In early spring or late fall, animals may be susceptible to cold stress for as long as 4 weeks after shearing. The provision of shelters or wind breaks and an additional 0.23 to 4.5 kg (0.5 to 1 lb) per day of an energy supplement (cracked corn) above the normal feeding regimen can help minimize freezing and stress loss.

Feeding Pet and Geriatric Sheep and Goats

Pet sheep and goats can live much longer than animals in production units. The principles of nutrition presented throughout this chapter apply to the proper feeding of pet animals as well. The only dietary formulation, manipulation, or plan that appears to be associated with increased longevity is lowered intake. Thus, keepers should strive to maintain a proper body condition and weight in pet animals to help them achieve a long healthy life.

Obesity is a constant and major problem in the pet population and includes both sheep and goats. Pet goats tend to be more commonly affected by overfeeding-related diseases than are sheep or goats in production units. With the exception of feedlot animals and those being prepared for shows, pet sheep and goats are overrepresented in cases of obesity, bloat, acidosis or ruminitis, and urinary calculi. The increased prevalence of these disorders is related to a lack of knowledge about feeding in many owners, inactivity of the animals, and pet status with its lack of performance or production goals. A barn or paddock layout that necessitates walking, client education, and proper diet design all are essential to combat obesity and will increase the pet animal's long-term health. Forcing animals to walk (e.g., for grazing or access to water, salt, or minerals) will enhance the chances of the weight loss program's success. Weight loss programs should never be instituted in pregnant animals and should be avoided until after midlactation.

A weight loss program should begin with a complete physical examination, an accurate weight measurement, determination of BCS, and a complete blood count and serum chemistry analysis when possible. If the animal has no overt disease, the weight loss program should set goals for weight and BCS and a plan to attain these goals in approximately 4 to 8 months. A generic weight loss diet modification might be as follows: (1) first 4 to 6 weeks: feed moderate-quality grass hay at 2% of BW (accurate weight of animal and hay); (2) second 4 to 6 weeks: feed moderate-quality grass hay at 2% of target weight. (Note: The hay should be 8 to

10% crude protein; free-choice water and a mineral mixture designed for the farm should be provided; and accommodation for some form of exercise should be made.)

BW and condition loss are common problems among geriatric animals. A complete physical examination, complete blood count, and serum chemistry analysis may be indicated to identify ongoing disease processes. Older animals may require special feeding to address dental disease, parasite damage to the bowel, and other general health problems. Good-quality hay, moistened pellets, lush forage, and palatable concentrates often are required for animals with dental disease (see Chapter 4).

Allowing older animals ready access to feed, particularly if their social status has changed, along with longer periods of noncompetitive time to consume it, will help maintain good body condition. Because many geriatric animals have arthritic conditions, minimizing excess BW, properly trimming feet, and placement of water and feed such that animals are not forced to walk great distances all are valuable in case management. Diets designed for the geriatric horse can be used for some geriatric small ruminants but should be avoided for any sheep or to goats with a history of hepatic disease, as the copper concentration is greater than 10 ppm. If the animal has renal disease, the protein content of the diet should be maintained at 7 to 8%, and the calcium-to-phosphorus ratio should be kept at 1:1. A good-quality granular mineral mixture of equal parts dicalcium phosphate and trace mineral salt should be offered on a free-choice basis.

If older animals are losing weight, the keeper can slowly increase caloric intake by 7 to 10% in the form of fat. However, protein, fats, and copper should be restricted in animals with hepatic disease. Animals with hepatic or renal disease may benefit from the addition of B vitamins, given orally or parenterally. If renal disease is present, the protein requirement should be met but not exceeded. If anorexia is a problem, varying the diet, offering lush grazing, and adding energy-dense feeds are useful strategies. Obviously, all husbandry practices that aid in overall health (e.g., proper shelter, deworming) will enhance long-term survival.

Nutritional Disorders

The most common nutrition-related diseases seen in late gestation in goats and sheep are pregnancy toxemia (discussed in Chapter 8), hypocalcemia, and hypomagnesemia.

Hypocalcemia

Hypocalcemia can be a problem in dairy goats and, to some extent, in ewes, meat and fiber goats, and pet animals. This condition usually becomes apparent shortly before or after parturition and is a result of low concentrations of serum calcium. Some cases also are complicated by hypophosphatemia and hypermagnesemia or hypomagnesemia. Ewes appear to be most susceptible in late gestation and early lactation, particularly when experiencing some sort of stress (e.g., hauling, predator attack, lack of feed). Sheep may succumb to hypocalcemia from 6 weeks before to 10 weeks after parturition. The greatest demand for calcium for the nondairy animal occurs 3 to 4 weeks before parturition in females with more than one fetus, as a result of the calcification of fetal bones. Goats may have hypocalcemia before parturition. In high-producing dairy goats, the disease generally occurs after the dam gives birth. With any abrupt demand for calcium, the body requires 1 or more days to accrue the necessary enzymes capable of mobilizing bone stores of calcium. High intake of calcium, phosphorus, or some cations (potassium, sodium) decreases the production of parathyroid hormones. During decreased parathyroid function, less 1,25-dihydroxycholecalciferol is produced. Lack of this hormone results in lowered absorption and mobilization of calcium from the intestines and bones. Low dietary calcium or increased amounts of dietary anions enhances the production and release of parathyroid hormones.

Clinical Signs. Early in the course of the disease, affected animals exhibit a stiff gait, tremors, and tetany. They also experience decreased rumen motility and may be ataxic or constipated. As the disease progresses, increased heart and respiratory rates increase, regurgitation of rumen content, bloat, and depression to the point of opisthotonos may be noted. Corneal and pupillary light reflexes are normal at first but become depressed before disappearing entirely. The rectal temperature usually remains in the normal range but may be slightly low.

Diagnosis. Diagnosis usually is based on a history and signalment conducive to development of hypocalcemia, as well as on response to therapy. Serum calcium concentrations less than 4 to 5 mL/dL in sheep and goats are fairly diagnostic of this condition.

Treatment. In clinical cases, immediate treatment is needed, usually in the form of IV administration of calcium borogluconate (50 to 100 mL of a 23% solution). Subcutaneous delivery of these calcium solutions or the oral administration of a calcium gel designed for cattle, but based on sheep or goat BW, will help prevent relapse. If the subcutaneous route is chosen to develop a "reservoir" of calcium for affected animals, solutions containing dextrose or numerous electrolytes should be avoided, as the use of some of these preparations has been associated with abscess formation. During treatment, cardiac monitoring is indicated, and therapy should be slowed or stopped if arrhythmias develop. If the treatment is successful, the animal will stand and urinate within 20 minutes. If left untreated, affected animals usually die.

Prevention. To prevent or minimize the risk of hypocalcemia, particularly in dairy goats, the diet should be low in calcium, with a low cation-to-anion ratio. The dietary modifications used for the prevention of milk fever in cattle may be of value in dairy sheep and goats. Therefore, reducing or eliminating diets rich in cations (alfalfa) or in calcium and phosphorus in the late dry period may aid in prevention. Many legumes are rich sources of potassium and calcium and can therefore contribute to hypocalcemia. Immediately after parturition, the levels of calcium in the diet should be increased. This strategy improves calcium reabsorption for bones and absorption from the intestine. Hauling or other forms of stress should be minimized in sheep and goats during the final 3 weeks of gestation. Even with this strategy, some incidence of hypocalcemia may occur.[1,6]

Hypomagnesemia

Hypomagnesemia, manifesting as grass tetany, can be a problem in sheep and, to a lesser extent, goats grazing on lush, rapidly growing forage. This is rarely seen with browsing goats. It usually occurs during the early spring on pastures that are well fertilized with nitrogen and potassium. A combination of elevated nitrogen and potassium levels in the forage leads to a reduced absorption of magnesium from the GIT.

The primary problem in hypomagnesemia is reduced absorption by the animal, rather than low plant concentrations. Sheep, and goats that graze lush cereal grains (e.g., wheat, rye), particularly in early lactation or late gestation, are predisposed to this condition. Any type of stress (e.g., weather changes, transportation, and predator attack) can increase blood concentrations of free fatty acids, and excess blood from fatty acid concentrations depresses blood magnesium. Other forms of hypomagnesemia occur during winter when animals are fed poor-quality grass hay (with low magnesium content) and in lambs or kids fed only low-magnesium milk replacers. Kids or lambs with access to grain or legume-grass hay are more resistant to hypomagnesemia. Ewes with poor dentition and those that lose excessive weight during winter are prone to develop the condition.

Clinical Signs. Hypomagnesemia generally occurs in ewes 2 to 4 weeks after lambing. It is more common in females that had twins. Affected animals are excitable and may exhibit paddling convulsions, clonic-tonic muscle spasms, and an increased respiratory rate. They also may simply be found dead in the pasture. Rectal temperature commonly is normal. Convulsions may be triggered by any number of stimuli, from being chased by predators to acute changes in weather patterns. Lambs or kids with the milk replacer–associated form of hypomagnesemia usually are anorexic and hyperexcitable and may salivate profusely.

Diagnosis. Diagnosis often is based on signalment and history, as well as response to treatment. Serum magnesium levels less than 1.5 mg/dL may be indicative of this disease and levels less than 1 mg/dL should be considered diagnostic. Postmortem serum samples are of limited value. Magnesium concentrations in cerebrospinal fluid (for 12 h after death), urine (for 24 h after death), or anterior eye chamber fluid (for 48 h after death) are useful postmortem tests.[1]

Treatment. Treatment consists of the intravenous administration of a solution which contains 20 to 25% calcium borogluconate and 4 to 5% magnesium (50 mL). Oral calcium magnesium gel and subcutaneous injection of calcium-magnesium salts both are beneficial to prevent relapse.

Prevention. Because grass tetany results from a reduction in available magnesium, a number of methods can be used to increase consumption. Properly balanced fertilizers and magnesium compounds can be applied to the soil to increase plant concentrations of magnesium. The addition of such compounds is helpful but not very economical, because as noted, the primary problem with the occurrence of hypomagnesemia is reduced absorption by the animal, rather than low plant concentrations. Therefore, prevention is best accomplished by offering high-magnesium mineral supplements before the growth of lush spring forage and several weeks prior to lambing or kidding. Most mineral supplements with high levels of magnesium are unpalatable, so feeders should be checked frequently to ensure proper consumption. To enhance intake, the keeper can mix magnesium oxide with molasses, corn, salt, or other feedstuffs. Daily consumption is important, because magnesium in a readily usable form is poorly stored in the body. An average adult lactating ewe needs 7 to 9 g of magnesium oxide daily. An economical supplement is a 1:1 mix of trace mineral salt and magnesium oxide, but this combination appears to be unpalatable. A more acceptable substitute may be equal parts of ground corn, trace mineral salt, and magnesium oxide. Other palatable grains can be used in place of the corn. Legumes (e.g., alfalfa, clover, bird's foot, kudzu) are much better sources of both calcium and magnesium, and their inclusion in a pasture helps reduce the incidence of hypomagnesemia.[6] Maintaining a high soil pH (greater than 5.5) enhances magnesium availability and intake by plants. The inclusion of vitamin D (5 to 10 IU/kg/day) in a milk replacer helps prevent hypomagnesemia in lambs or kids fed indoors.

Urolithiasis

Urolithiasis is a common and frustrating problem for owners of male sheep and goats, particularly pet goats, and for clinicians involved in their management. This condition is encountered in intact or castrated male goats and sheep.[1] In Chapter 12, the pathophysiology and clinical signs of urolithiasis and therapeutic modalities of relevance are covered in greater detail than that provided here.

Formation of phosphatic calculi is seen with management practices that allow feeding of high-concentrate, low-roughage, low calcium-to-phosphorus ratio, high-magnesium diets, and alkaline urine. High-grain diets result in the excretion of large amounts of phosphorus in the urine. Oxalate calculus formation is associated with the consumption of oxalate-containing plants (Table 2.10). Urinary stones are composed of salts and minerals arrayed in a crystal lattice surrounding an organic nidus. The nidus forms when urine mucoproteins or mucopolysaccharides and saturated urine precipitate to form crystals. Urinary mucoprotein-mucopolysaccharide production is increased with ingestion of estrogenic compounds, inadequate levels of vitamin A, consumption of certain feedstuffs (e.g., cottonseed meal, milo), use of pelleted diets, and rapid growth of the animal.[1,6,27,53]

Dietary risk factors for urolithiasis include high-grain–low-roughage diets, decreased formation of saliva, an increased amount of phosphorus excreted in the urine, and increased levels of dietary magnesium. Calcium-to-phosphorus ratio should be maintained between 2:1 and 2.5:1. Cereal grains have an abnormal calcium-to-phosphorus ratio of 1:4 to 1:6.[15,27] Low-forage, high-concentrate diets traditionally are deficient in vitamin A or its precursors. Vitamin A deficiency can result in desquamation of

TABLE 2.10 Plants With a High Oxalate Content.

Common Name	Species Designation
Halogeton	*Halogeton glomeratus*
Lamb's quarters or fat hen	*Chenopodium album*
Pokeweed	*Phytolacca Americana*
Russian thistle	*Salsola kali*
Purslane	*Portulaca oleracea*
Bassia	*Bassia hyssopifolia*
Pigweed	*Amaranthus retroflexus*
Soursob	*Oxalis cernua* and *Oxalis pes-caprae*
Greasewood	*Sarcobatus vermiculatus*
Dock and orchard sorrel	*Rumex acetosella* and *Rumex acetosa*
Cultivated rhubarb	*Rheum rhaponticum*
Sugar beet leaves	*Beta vulgaris*
Fungi	*Aspergillus niger* and *Aspergillus niger*

cells lining the urinary bladder, which may serve as a nidus for stone formation. Clinical signs may include dysuria, stranguria, hematuria, urine dribbling, vocalization, prolonged urination, tail flagging, colic, and bruxism. A complete examination should be performed, an appropriate diagnosis made, and immediate medical or surgical therapy instituted[1] (see Chapter 12).

Access to fresh, clean water is crucial to the prevention of this condition. Water should be abundant, fresh, clean, palatable, and readily accessible. In many geographic regions, maintaining water supplies requires more attention during winter months. The addition of sodium chloride to the diet (3 to 5% of the dietary dry matter intake) will increase water consumption, and the excess chloride ions may reduce production of calculus-forming salts.[27] Diets and feedstuffs rich in cations (e.g., alfalfa, molasses-sweet feed) should be avoided. An anionic diet increases the urinary excretion of hydrogen ions, decreases urinary pH, increases urinary excretion of calcium, and decreases the precipitation of struvite.[27] The diet should be balanced for macrominerals (i.e., calcium, phosphorus, magnesium, and sulfur). The addition of calcium carbonate or calcium chloride to the diet to attain a 2 to 2.5:1 calcium-to-phosphorus ratio, with the dietary magnesium content kept to $< 0.6\%$, may be required. Pelleted rations probably should be avoided or used at a minimum in animals with a history of urolithiasis or in those prone to it, because such feed is associated with both an increase in mucoprotein matrix formation and urinary excretion of phosphorus. All cereal grains (e.g., corn, oats, milo) are high in phosphorus and relatively low in calcium, so their consumption should be minimized. If cereal grains are fed, calcium should be added to the diet to maintain the proper calcium-to-phosphorus ratio (2:1). The addition of chlortetracycline or tetracycline and beta-carotene or vitamin A to complete diets, mineral mixtures, or feed supplements also can be helpful. Diets containing 30% green forage probably are sufficient in beta-carotene content.[27,53] In cases of calcium oxalate or calcium carbonate calculi, feeding legumes (e.g., alfalfa, clover, kudzu) should be limited. All of the plants listed in Table 2.10 are associated with formation of oxalate calculi, so their ingestion should be avoided or minimized. Management practices used to minimize oxalate stone formation include slow introduction to new grazing or browse and control of plants that accumulate oxalates (e.g., by application of 2,4-Dichlorophenoxyacetic acid to pastures).[1]

Dietary protein should be fed to meet, but not greatly exceed, requirements for maintenance or growth, because excessive protein intake (e.g., pet goats, feedlot lambs) can result in an increased urinary output of the mucoprotein. Dietary estrogenic compounds, including phytoestrogens, should be minimized or avoided because they may be associated with an increase in secondary sex gland size, and in the output of urinary mucoprotein. Many legumes (e.g., white clover) contain estrogenic compounds or have inappropriate calcium-to-phosphorus ratios and a larger-than-necessary protein content, contributing to formation of some types of stones. Although legumes in hay and forage may improve growth and productivity, they should be used and fed to calculi-prone males with caution. Urine pH should be maintained at or slightly less than 6.8. The addition of cationic salts to the diet may aid in reducing urinary pH and aid in reducing the incidence of urolithiasis. Many anionic salts appear poorly palatable, but can be added to the feed or mixed with honey and sprayed onto forage to ensure adequate intake. Calcium chloride or ammonium chloride can be fed at 1 to 2% and 0.5 to 2% of the total diet, respectively. When individual medication is cost-prohibitive, providing a loose mineral mixture with an anionic salt can provide some protection (e.g., 2.5 lb of ammonium chloride well mixed with 50 lb of trace mineral salt, provided as the only source of available salt). Vitamin C (3 to 4 mg/kg/day) also can help maintain pH balance, but administering the vitamin often enough for it to be of practical value may be difficult and may predispose animals to urinary oxalate crystal formation. All urinary stones should be submitted for laboratory analysis to aid in the development of a preventive plan for the rest of the flock.[1]

Gastrointestinal Parasites

Dietary manipulation and or supplementation of specific nutrients has gained attention in aiding the control of internal parasites.[54–56] Feeding practices that increase stocking rates and pasture parasite contamination with nematode parasite eggs magnify internal parasitism in grazing animals. Sheep, goats, and cervids share most of the same species of internal cestodes, nematodes, and trematodes (see Chapter 6). GIT parasitism has a negative effect on both energy and amino acid metabolism and also increases requirements of these nutrients in sheep and goats. This effect is due to an increase in GIT protein turnover, a nutritional cost for increased immune stimulation by the parasites, direct GIT blood loss, and possibly a reduced feed intake.[6,52,57–59] GIT parasites appear to have a greater effect on protein requirements than on energy. Increasing dietary metabolizable protein intake in the face of subclinical parasitism may help meet production goals in some instances.[57–60] Compared with most other amino acids, the sulfur-containing amino acids are influenced to a greater extent by parasitism, which can have a negative effect on wool and fiber production.

The strategy of feeding supplemental metabolizable protein improves resilience and resistance to parasites in sheep, particularly if the protein source is not degraded in the rumen.[61–63] The quality of the diet appears to be more significant than the quantity.[64] Feeding the bypass protein fish meal (8%) to parasitized sheep in late gestation has been shown to reduce *Trichostrongylus colubriformis* and *Trichostrongylus circumcincta* burdens by a factor of three to four and to improve body condition and BW.[58] Rumen-protected methionine also has a positive effect on wool production and weight gain in *T. colubriformis*–infected lambs.[65] Supplementation with soybean meal and energy also will be beneficial to maximize resilience.[1,6] Dietary supplementation appears to affect parasitism most profoundly if targeted. That is, when specific nutrients are deficient in the diet and the animal's stage of development, or when health status dictates requirements for those nutrients are greatest, then those nutrients (e.g., protein, carbohydrates, copper, and phosphorus) are supplemented. An example of targeted supplementation is the addition of protein to the diet during early pregnancy, which may promote immunity to parasitism at parturition in sheep.[56,63,66,67] In animals with access to forage containing plants with condensed tannins, expected benefits include reduced gastrointestinal parasite burden, altered parasite life cycle, reduced parasite larval numbers, and stimulation of the host's immune system.[68–70] Many plants containing condensed tannins also are legumes, which also will improve protein intake (e.g., sulla, lucerne, peanut skins, *Sericea lespedeza*).[70] However, tannin feeding is not without drawbacks. Some associated problems include depression of food intake, and binding of dietary proteins and digestive enzymes resulting in a decrease in protein supply and digestion, and injury to parts of the GIT.[71] With feeding of condensed tannins, a balance must be drawn to maximize the positive effects on gastrointestinal parasite control while minimizing some of their deleterious effects. Much of the browse and forbs currently used in small ruminant production systems will have 17 to 20% crude protein and significant amounts of condensed tannins. An added benefit is that animals browsing above ground level may have reduced exposure and ingestion of infective nematode parasite larvae. Mineral nutrition also appears to be critical in enhancing internal parasite control.[72–74] The administration of copper oxide boluses to sheep and goats appears to aid in nematode parasite control; however, dietary supplementation of copper sulfate has failed to achieve the same goal.[72,73]

Ensuring adequate nutrient intake (energy, protein, macrominerals, and trace minerals), supplementation with rumen bypass protein, targeted nutritional supplementation, allowing access to browse containing condensed tannins, good grazing strategies (e.g., reduced stocking rates, pasture rotations), logical anthelmintic usage (e.g., targeted parasite control, use of only effective anthelmintics), and selecting and breeding animals with superior parasite resistance are needed in implementing a parasite control program[67,71] (see Chapter 6).

References

1. Rankins DL Jr, Pugh DG: Feeding and nutrition. In Pugh DG, Baird AN, editors: *Sheep and goat medicine*, ed 2, Maryland Heights, MO., 2012, Elsevier, pp 8–49.
2. Van Soest PJ: *Nutritional ecology of the ruminant*, ed 2, Ithaca, NY, 1994, Cornell University Press.
3. Tomeček JM, Redmon LA: *Supplemental feeding of white-tailed deer*, College Station, Texas, 2016, A&M Agrilife Extension, EWF-032.
4. Hofmann RR: Evolutionary steps of ecophysiological adaptation and diversification of ruminants: a comparative view of their digestive system, *Oecologia* 78:443–457, 1989.
5. Hiller I: *The white-tailed deer*, College Station Texas, 1996, A & M University Press.
5a. Peischel A: *Tennessee' goat and sheep, pasture/browsing planner*, Nashville, 2014, Tennessee State University.
6. National Research Council: *Nutrient requirements of small ruminants sheep*, goats, cervids, and new world camelids, Washington, DC, 2007, National Academies Press.
7. *Water Requirements for Livestock*, Alberta, 2000, Agriculture Food and Rural Development Extension Bulletin.
8. Bauder J: When is Water Good Enough for Livestock? Montana State Extension Bulletin, 2000.
9. Guyer PQ: Livestock water quality, University of Nebraska Extension Service Bulletin G79-46A, 1979.
10. Meyer KB: *Water Quality in Animals*, Purdue University Extension Bulletin WQ9, 1999.
11. Maloiy GMO, Taylor CR: Water requirements of African goats and haired sheep, J Agric Sci 77:203, 1971.
12. Nagy KA, Peterson CC: Scaling of water flux rate in animals, University of California Publication, *Zoology* 12:1–172, 1988.
13. Weiss WP: Predicting energy values of feeds, *J. Dairy Sci* 76:1802–1811, 1993.
14. Knox MR, Steel JW: The effects of urea supplementation on production and parasitological responses of sheep infected with *Haemonchus contortus* and *Trichostrongylus colubriformis*, *Vet Parasitol* 3:123–135, 1999.
15. Hart SP: *Goat Nutrition*, in Proceedings of the 33rd Annual Goat and Haired Sheep Field Day, Langston, OK, 2018, Agricultural Extension, Langston University, pp 73–99.
16. Bubenik GA, Schams D White RJ Rowell J, Blake J, Bartos L: Seasonal levels of reproductive hormones and their relationship to the antler cycle of male and female reindeer (*Rangifer tarandus*), *Biochem, Physiol* 116(B2):269–277, 1997.
17. Pierce RA, Jr., Vandeloecht B, Flinn E: *Nutritional requirements of white-tailed deer in Missouri*, University of Missouri Extension Bulletin, 2012. https://extension2.missouri.edu/g9487.
18. Harmel DE, Williams JD Armstrong WE: *Effects of genetics and nutrition on antler development and body size of white-tailed deer*, Austin, TX, 1979. Texas Parks and Wildlife Department.
19. National Research Council: *Mineral tolerance of domestic animals*, Washington, DC, 1980, National Academy Press.
20. Bubenik GA, White RG, Bartos L: Antler growth in male and female reindeer and its relationship to seasonal blood level of alkaline phosphatase, *Folia Zool* 49:161–166, 2000.
21. Hart SP, Kott R: Targeted grazing for vegetation management. In Merkel RC, Gipson TA, Sahlu T, editors: *Meat goat production handbook*, Langston, OK, 2015, Langston University, pp 233–242.
22. Grasman BT, Hellgren EC: Phosphorus nutrition in white-tailed deer: nutrient balance, physiological responses, and antler growth, *Ecology* 74:2279–2296, 1993.
23. Verme, LJ, Ullrey DL: Physiology and nutrition. In Halls LK, McCabe RE, Jahn LR, editors: *White-tailed deer: ecology and management*, Harrisburg, PA, 1984, Stackpole Books, pp 91–118.
24. Perkins JR: *Supplemental feeding*, Texas parks and wildlife department fisheries and wildlife division, PWD BK W7000-033, 1991.
25. Robbins, CT: *Wildlife feeding and nutrition*, New York, 1993, Academic Press.
26. McDowell, LR: *Minerals for grazing ruminants in tropical regions*, ed 3, Bulletin. Gainesville, 1997, University of Florida.
27. Bratzlaff K, Henlein G, Huston J: Common nutritional problems feeding the sick goat. In Naylor JM, Ralston SL, editors: *Large animal clinical nutrition*, St. Louis, 1991, Mosby.
28. Qi K, Lu CD, Owens FN: Sulfate supplementation of growing goats: effects on performance, acid-base balance, and nutrient digestibilities, *J Anim Sci* 71:1579, 1993.
29. Qi K, Lu CD, Owens FN, Lupton CJ: Sulfate supplementation of Angora goats: metabolic and mohair responses, *J Anim Sci* 70:2828–2837, 1992.
30. Miller JK, Ramsey, N, Madsen FC: The trace elements. In Church DC, editor: *The ruminant nutrition: digestive physiology and nutrition*, Englewood Cliffs, NJ, 1988, Prentice Hall.
31. Hayter S, Wiener G: Variation in the concentration of copper in the blood plasma of Finnish-Landrace and Merino sheep and their crosses with reference to reproductive performance and age, *Anim Prod* 16:261, 1973.
32. Solaiman SG, Maloney MA, Qureshi MA, Davis G, Andrea GD: Effects of high copper supplements on performance, health, plasma copper and enzymes in goats, *Small Rumin Res* 41:127–139, 2001.
33. NRC (National Research Council): *Mineral tolerance of animals*, ed 2 rev, National Research Council of the National Academies, Washington, DC, 2005, The National Academies Press.
34. Grace ND, Wilson PR: Trace element metabolism, dietary requirements, diagnosis and prevention of deficiencies in deer, *NZ Vet J* 50:252–259, 2002.
35. Humann-Ziehank E, Renok K, Mueller AS, Roehrig P, Wolfsen J, Ganter M: Comparing functional metabolic effects of marginal and sufficient selenium supply in sheep, *J Trace Elem Med Biol* 27(4):380–390, 2013.
36. Van Saun RJ: Nutrient requirements of South American camelids, *Small Rumin Res* 61(2/3):153–164, 2006.
37. Price L, Allen S: Exploring the mechanisms regulating regeneration of deer antlers, *Phil Trans R Soc London B* 359:809–822, 2004.
38. Dierenfeld ES: Vitamin E in exotics: effects, evaluation and ecology, *J Nutr* 124:2579S–2581S, 1994.
39. Holland C, Kezar W: *Pioneer forage manual*. A nutritional guide, Des Moines, IA, 1995, Pioneer Hi-Bred International.
40. Schoenian S. *Maryland Small Ruminant Page*, 2018. https://www.sheepandgoat.com/rationsoftwarehort.

41. Morrical DG: *Feeding ewes better for increased production and profit*, Animal Science White Papers, 2, Ames, 2003, Iowa State University.
42. Thompson J, Meyer H: *Body condition scoring of sheep*, Oregon State University. OSU Extension Catalog, 1994. https://catalog.extension.oregonstate.edu. EC 1433.
43. Peischel, A. Environmental enhancement. In Solaiman SG, editor: *Goat science and production*, Oxford, 2010, Blackwell Publishing.
44. Gerhart KL, White RG, Cameron RD, Russell DE: Body composition and nutrient reserves of Arctic caribou, *Can J Zool* 74:136–146, 1996a.
45. Gerhart KL, White RG, Cameron RD, Russell DE: Estimating fat content of caribou from body condition scores, *J Wildl Manage* 60:713–718, 1996b.
46. Asher GW, Mulley RC, O'Neill KTP, Scott IC, Jopson NB Littlejohn RP: Influence of level of nutrition during late pregnancy on reproductive productivity of red deer. I. Adult and primiparous hinds gestating red deer calves, *Anim Reprod Sci* 86:261–283, 2005.
47. Hart S: Grazing systems and management for goat production. In Tuskegee, AL, editor: *3rd national goat conference proceedings*, Tuskegee University, 2018.
48. Ensminger ME, Oldfield JE, Heinemann WW: *Feeds and nutrition*, ed 2, Clovis, CA: Ensminger Publishing, 1990.
49. Sahlu T, Fernandez JM, Lu CD, Manning R: Dietary protein level and ruminal degradability for mohair production in Angora goats, *J Anim Sci* 70:1526–1533, 1992.
50. Allden WG: Undernutrition of the Merino sheep and its sequelae: II. The influence of finite periods of arrested growth on the subsequent wool growth, fleece development, and utilization of feed for wool production of lambs, *Austr J Agric Res* 19:639, 1968.
51. Kelly RW, Macleod I, Hynd PI, Greeff JC: Nutrition during fetal life alters annual wool production and quality in young Merino sheep, *Austr J Exp Agric* 36:259, 1996.
52. Adams NR, Liu SM: Principles of nutrient partitioning for wool, growth, and reproduction: implications for nematode parasitism, *Austr J Ag* 43:1399–1407, 2003.
53. Belknap EB, Pugh DG: Diseases of the urinary system. In Pugh DG, editor: *Sheep and goat medicine*, Philadelphia, 2002, WB Saunders, pp 255 276.
54. Knox MR, Torres-Acosta JFJ, Aguilar-Caballero AJ: Exploiting the effect of dietary supplementation of small ruminants on resilience and resistance against gastrointestinal nematodes, *Vet Parasitol* 139:385–393, 2006.
55. Houdjik JGM: Influence of periparturient nutritional demand on resistance to parasites in livestock, *Parasite Immunol* 30:113–121, 2008.
56. Houdjik JGM, Kyriazakis I, Kidane A, Athanasiadoua S: Manipulating small ruminant parasite epidemiology through the combination of nutritional strategies, *Vet Parasitol* 186:38–50, 2012.
57. Sykes AR, Greer AW: Effects of parasitism on the nutrient economy in sheep: an overview, *Austal J Exp Agric* 43:1393–1398, 2003.
58. Sykes AR: Parasitism and production in farm animals, *Anim Prod* 59:155–172, 1994.
59. Coop RL, Kyriazakis I: Nutrition-parasite interaction, *Vet Parasitol* 84:187–204, 1999.
60. Sylvester HJ, Griffith EH Jacob ME, Foster DM: Factors associated with strongyle infection in goats at the individual and farm level, *JAVMA* 253:907–917, 2018.
61. Donaldson JD, van Field MFJ, Sykes AR: The effect of nutrition on the periparturient status of mature sheep, *Anim Sci* 67:523–533, 1998.
62. Kidane A, Houdijk JG, Tolkamp BJ, Athanasiadou S, Kyriazakis I: Consequences of infection pressure and protein nutrition on periparturient resistance to *Teldorsagia circumcincta* and performance in ewes, *Vet Parasitol* 165:78–87, 2009.
63. McClure SJ: Dietary impacts on the resistance of Merino lambs to *Trichostrongylus colubriformis, NZ Vet J* 57:102–108, 2009.
64. Coop RL, Kyriazakis I, Huntley JF, et al: *The influence of protein and amino acid on the resilience of sheep to intestinal parasitism, Proceedings of the 4th International Congress for Sheep Vets*, Armidale, New South Wales, Australia, 1997, pp 196–198.
65. Valderrabano J, Gomez-Rincon C, Uriarte J: Effect of nutritional status and fat reserves on the periparturient immune response to *Haemonchus contortus* infection in sheep, *Vet Parasitol* 141:122–131, 2006.
66. Kahn LP, Knox MR, Gray GD, Lea JM, Walkden-Brown SW: Enhancing immunity to nematode parasites in single-bearing Merino ewes through nutrition and genetic selection, *Vet Parasitol* 112:211–225, 2003.
67. Min BR, Hart SP: Tannins for suppression of internal parasites, *J Anim Sci* 81(Suppl 2):E102–E109, 2003.
68. Athanasiadou S, Kyriazakis I, Jackson F, Coop RL: Direct anthelmintic effects of condensed tannins towards different gastrointestinal nematodes of sheep: in vitro and in vivo studies, *Vet Parasitol* 99:205–219, 2001.
69. Zafar I, Mufti KA, Khan MN, et al: Review. Anthelmintic effects of condensed tannins, *Int J Agric Biol* 4:438–440, 2002.
70. Athanasiadou S, Kyriazakis I: Plant antimetabolites: antiparasitic effects and their role in ruminant production systems, *Proc Nutr Soc* 63:631–639, 2004.
71. Kahn LP, Knox MR, Walkden-Brown SW, Lea JM: Regulation of the resistance to nematode parasites of single- and twin-bearing Merino ewes through nutrition and genetic selection, *Vet Parasitol* 114:15–31, 2003.
72. Burke JM, Orlik S, Miller JE, Terrill TH, Mosjidis JA: Using copper oxide wire particles or sericea lespedeza to prevent peri-parturient gastrointestinal nematode infection in sheep and goats, *Livestock Sci* 132:13–18, 2010.
73. Burke, JM, Miller JE: Dietary copper sulfate for control of gastrointestinal nematodes in goats *Vet Parasitol* 154:289–293, 2008.
74. Hooper KJ, Bobe G, Voracheck WR, et al: Effect of selenium yeast supplementation on naturally acquired parasitic infection in ewes, *Biol Trace Elem Res* 161:308–317, 2014.

3

Fluid Therapy and Parenteral Nutrition

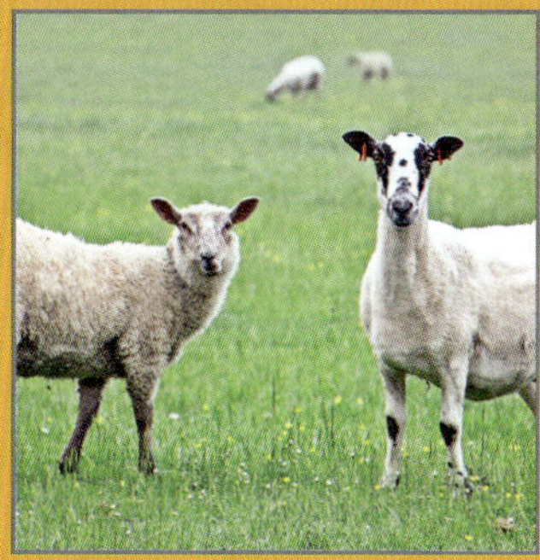

SANDRA D. TAYLOR AND A. N. BAIRD

Introduction

Fluid therapy is an important component of management for many diseases that affect sheep, goats, and cervids. Dehydration and hypovolemia can occur secondary to decreased fluid intake or excessive fluid loss from diarrhea, hemorrhage, excessive salivation, third space loss, and polyuria. Serum electrolyte disturbances and acid-base imbalance can occur in conjunction with fluid depletion and must be considered when making a fluid therapy plan. Hypoglycemia is of particular concern in neonates given their lack of glycogen storage capacity. Other indications for fluid therapy include diuresis in cases of toxin exposure and acute kidney injury (AKI), failure of passive transfer (FPT), hypothermia, malnutrition, and trauma. A variety of fluid compositions are available for intravenous (IV) administration and are dependent on the underlying disease process, the fluid deficit, rate of loss, serum electrolyte and glucose concentrations, and acid-base status. Parenteral nutrition (PN) is not commonly used in sheep, goats, and cervids due to budgetary constraints, but should be considered in animals with prolonged anorexia, dysphagia, severe gastrointestinal disease, or pregnancy toxemia.

Body Fluid Physiology

Total body water is the sum of fluids contained in the intracellular and extracellular fluid compartments and makes up approximately 60% of body weight in adult small ruminants.[1]

The extracellular fluid compartment is subdivided into interstitial and intravascular compartments, with interstitial fluid including transcellular fluid, cerebrospinal fluid, joint fluid, and fluid within the gastrointestinal tract. Approximately two-thirds of total body water is intracellular fluid (40% of body weight), and one-third is extracellular fluid (20% of body weight). Of the extracellular fluid components, 75% is interstitial fluid while 25% is intravascular fluid. Total body water can vary with age and fat content. Neonatal sheep, goats, and cervids have more extracellular fluid than adults, with total body water approaching 80% of body weight. Fat has a relatively low water content, so overconditioned animals contain lower total body water compared to lean animals.[2]

Dehydration is loss of total body water, and occurs when water losses exceed water gains. When dehydration is mild, normal physiologic mechanisms may be adequate to restore water balance by activating thirst. Fluid replacement is necessary during moderate to severe dehydration. In dehydration, the immediate source of water lost from the body is the extracellular fluid compartment, with the majority of water lost from the interstitial pool. This will be followed by a fluid shift from intracellular to extracellular compartments in order to preserve the effective circulating blood volume, protecting against development of hypovolemic shock. With continuing dehydration, electrolytes are depleted and tissue hypoxia can occur.

Clinical Assessment

When performing a physical examination, it is important to determine hydration status. Clinical signs of dehydration include enophthalmos (eyeball recession), tacky mucous membranes, and prolonged cervical skin tenting. The general demeanor of the animal is also correlated with the degree of dehydration. Estimating the severity of dehydration is important in order to calculate the fluid deficit and formulate a fluid therapy plan. Extrapolation from an experimental study in calves can be used to assess hydration status in small ruminants and cervids (Table 3.1).[3] Less than 4% dehydration cannot be determined from a physical examination, but may be used to calculate a fluid deficit when there is a history of fluid loss. Increases in packed cell volume (PCV) and total plasma protein concentration may be observed in dehydrated animals, but these findings are non-specific. Furthermore, animals with anemia and hypoproteinemia (e.g., gastrointestinal parasitism), as well as concurrent dehydration might present with a normal PCV and total plasma protein concentration; thus, alterations in these laboratory values must be interpreted with caution. It is also important to assess tissue perfusion during a physical examination. Clinical signs of hypovolemia (decreased intravascular fluid volume) include tachycardia, tachypnea, cool extremities, poor peripheral pulse pressure, and decreased urine output. Blood lactate concentration is often elevated in hypovolemic patients since decreased tissue perfusion leads to anaerobic metabolism, of which lactate is a byproduct.

Routine laboratory testing, including serum biochemistry and venous blood gas analyses, can be helpful in guiding fluid and electrolyte therapy. Serum concentrations of electrolytes (sodium, potassium, chloride, calcium, magnesium, and phosphorous), glucose, urea nitrogen, creatinine, and bicarbonate can be altered due to an underlying disease process or from dehydration. Prerenal azotemia is a common finding in dehydrated animals, and might lead to AKI if left untreated. Hypoglycemia is a common

TABLE 3.1 Physical Examination Parameters Associated With Percentage of Dehydration, Extrapolated from Experimental Induction of Dehydration and Diarrhea in Calves.

	4–6% (mild)	7–9% (moderate)	≥ 10% (severe)
Globe recession	2–3 mm	3–4 mm	6–8 mm
Oral mucosa	Moist	Tacky	Dry
Cervical skin tent	4–5 s	5–7 s	≥ 8 s
Demeanor	Standing, bright	Sternal, quiet	Lateral, depressed

Constable PD, Walker PG, Morin DE, et al: Clinical and laboratory assessment of hydration status of neonatal calves with diarrhea, *J Am Vet Med Assoc* 212:991, 1998.

finding in sick neonates and requires immediate dextrose administration. With respect to acid-base status, acute diarrhea, obstructive urolithiasis, and grain overload often result in metabolic acidosis, while intestinal obstructions typically cause hypochloremic metabolic alkalosis (see Appendix II).

Fluid Plan

Route of Administration

The two primary routes of fluid and electrolyte administration in small ruminants and cervids are oral and IV. In cases of mild to moderate (< 8%) dehydration in animals with a healthy gastrointestinal tract, oral fluids are preferred given their low cost and utilization of normal physiology. Oral fluids are most commonly administered through an orogastric tube, but small amounts can be given through a syringe. Pre-ruminant animals can be fed through a feeding tube that does not extend beyond the mid-esophageal region; this allows stimulation of the esophageal groove and subsequent diversion of milk into the abomasum for digestion and absorption. Finally, fluid can be administered through a rumenostomy in rare cases (see Chapter 5). Two other routes of fluid administration less frequently used are intra-peritoneal and intra-osseous. Intra-peritoneal fluid administration may be performed with a catheter via the flank or caudal ventral paramedian area of the animal. Care should be taken to avoid the intestinal tract when placing the intra-peritoneal catheter. This is most useful in neonates needing small volumes of fluid that can be physically restrained while the fluids are given. This technique can also be useful in neonates that are difficult to maintain with an IV catheter because of activity or housing with the dam and other neonates. Intra-osseous fluids can be administered when collapse of the vascular system prevents IV access. Intra-osseous fluid administration usually involves placing a cannulated screw through cortical bone to access the medullary cavity. This creates a high pressure-low volume system and should be limited to animals either in life threatening shock with no vascular access or those suffering from thrombophlebitis.

In cases of moderate to severe (≥ 8%) dehydration or in dehydrated animals with a diseased gastrointestinal tract (e.g., enterocolitis, ileus, obstruction, etc.), IV fluid administration is necessary. Catheterization of the jugular vein is a relatively simple procedure, with 16-gauge, 3.25-inch (8.3-cm) catheters

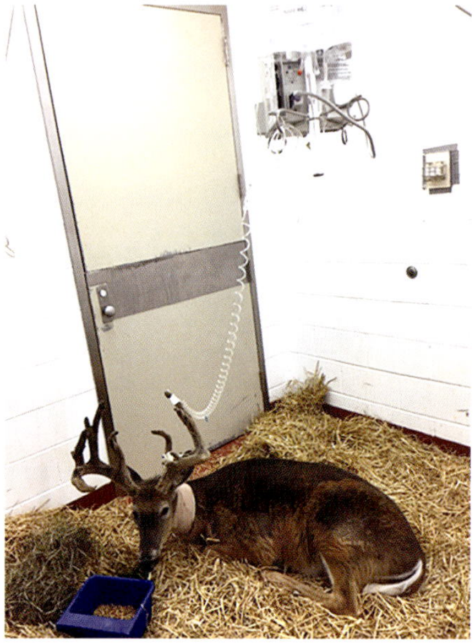

• **Fig. 3.1** Fluid line secured to the antlers of a 4-year-old male white-tailed deer.

appropriate for most adults and 18-gauge, 2-inch (5.1-cm) catheters appropriate for most neonates.[4] A detailed description of proper jugular catheterization technique is described elsewhere.[5] Fluid lines can be taped to horns or antlers when possible to decrease the likelihood of damage occurring to the fluid line (Figure 3.1); however, goats are especially keen to chew through fluid lines and should be monitored closely.

Volume and Rate

When formulating a fluid plan, the fluid deficit, maintenance requirement, and estimate of ongoing fluid losses (if present) must all be considered (Table 3.2). It is also important to determine if the animal requires a "shock dose" (resuscitation dose) of IV fluids, which is indicated in cases of severe dehydration or hypovolemia.

Deficit. The fluid deficit is calculating by multiplying the animal's weight in kg by the estimated percentage of dehydration (Table 3.2):

$$\left(\text{Body Weight in kg}\right) \times \left(\text{Estimated Percentage of Dehydration}\right) = \text{Fluid Deficit in L}$$

TABLE 3.2 Fluid Plan Components Including Deficit, Maintenance, Ongoing Losses, and "Shock Dose," with Associated Formula or Fluid Rate.

Fluid Plan Components	Formula/Rate
Deficit	(BW* in kg) × (% dehydration) = Deficit (L)
Maintenance	Adults: 50 mL/kg/day Neonates: 80 mL/kg/day
Ongoing losses	Estimated amount per day
"Shock dose"	50–80 mL/kg

*BW = body weight.

As a general rule, approximately half of the fluid deficit is given immediately, with the remainder of the deficit replaced within 6 to 8 h. If hypoproteinemia is present, the fluids should be given at a slower rate to minimize the potential for edema formation.

Maintenance. Maintenance fluid requirements are based on fluids lost through normal physiologic processes, including urination, defecation, respiration, sweat, salivation, and lacrimation. Maintenance fluid requirements are somewhat variable depending on physiologic demands (e.g., pregnancy, lactation, age), but the following rates are typically adequate when formulating a fluid plan and are based on water requirements in goats (Table 3.2)[6]:

Adults: 50 mL/kg/day (2 mL/kg/h)
Neonates: 80 mL/kg/day (3.5 mL/kg/h)

Ongoing Losses. The most common cause of ongoing fluid loss in small ruminants is diarrhea, which is often caused by gastrointestinal parasitism (e.g., trichostrongylosis, coccidiosis).[7,8] Acute or chronic hemorrhage can occur secondary to *Haemonchus contortus* infection, with severity of disease associated with the number of larvae present.[9] If anemia develops quickly, hypovolemia might be seen on initial presentation. In cases of chronic haemonchosis, anemia develops more slowly and is not often associated with dehydration; however, in both situations, a whole blood transfusion might be indicated. A precise measure of ongoing losses is difficult, so estimations based on observation are typically used. Less common causes of ongoing fluid loss in small ruminants include excessive salivation (e.g., oral lesions from foot-and-mouth disease), saliva loss (e.g., esophageal obstruction), third-space loss (e.g., neoplasia, chronic parasitic pneumonia), and polyuria (e.g., chronic renal disease).

In severely dehydrated and/or hypovolemic animals, a "shock dose" may be administered IV to expand the intravascular volume and facilitate tissue perfusion. The "shock dose" for sheep, goats, and cervids is 50 to 80 mL/kg, half of which may be given as a bolus. The remainder of the "shock dose" may be given over the course of 2 to 3 h and should be included in the fluid deficit replacement calculation.

Continuous rate infusion (CRI) is ideal in most cases in which IV fluids are required; however, this might be impossible in certain settings or circumstances. For example, even when syringe cases are stacked together as a barrier to protect the fluid line, it is not uncommon for goats to chew through the line. In addition, the benefits of housing a sick neonate with its dam might outweigh the benefit of CRI fluid administration. In these cases, intermittent fluid boluses may be administered every 2 to 3 h after dividing to calculate the total volume needed for this period. Fluid boluses are contraindicated when administering PN or fluids containing > 2% dextrose, as severe hyperglycemia might result.

Fluid Type

The two main fluid types used in veterinary medicine are crystalloids and colloids. Crystalloids are solutions that contain electrolytes and solutes that can enter all body fluid compartments. Crystalloid fluids can be classified as isotonic, hypotonic, or hypertonic

Isotonic Crystalloids. Isotonic crystalloids contain an osmolarity (mOsm/L) that is similar to extracellular fluid (e.g., plasma), which allows for initial intravascular volume expansion followed by absorption of fluid, electrolytes, and non-electrolyte solutes over 20 to 30 minutes. In general, 25% of the administered volume remains in the intravascular space, while 75% is absorbed and distributes into the interstitium. Replacement solutions include lactated Ringer's solution, Hartmann's solution, Normosol-R (Hospira, Inc., Lake Forest, IL), Plasma-Lyte A (Baxter, Deerfield, IL), Plasma-Lyte 148, and Vetivex pHyLyte (Dechra Veterinary Products, Overland Park, KS) (lactated Ringers and Hartmann's are generic) Injection pH 7.4 (Table 3.3). Although 0.9% sodium chloride is isotonic, it is "unbalanced" in electrolyte composition compared to plasma, and its acidic pH precludes its use for many conditions, especially those resulting in metabolic acidosis. Indications for 0.9% sodium chloride administration include metabolic alkalosis (e.g., gastrointestinal obstruction or stasis), obstructive urolithiasis, ruptured urinary bladder, and some cases of hyperosmolar syndrome. Isotonic bicarbonate (1.3% $NaHCO_3$; 150 mEq HCO_3^-/L) is an alkalinizing solution that can be used to correct metabolic acidosis (e.g., D-lactic acidosis in lambs and kids, rumen acidosis secondary to grain overload, and pregnancy toxemia).[10,11] To determine the HCO_3^- deficit in such cases, the following formulas can be used:

$$\text{Adults: mEq } HCO_3^- \text{ deficit} = \text{base deficit} \times \text{body weight (kg)} \times 0.3$$

$$\text{Neonates: mEq } HCO_3^- \text{ deficit} = \text{base deficit} \times \text{body weight (kg)} \times 0.6$$

The base deficit is obtained from a venous blood gas analysis or can be estimated by subtracting the serum TCO_2 (plasma bicarbonate) from 24 mEq/L. Approximately half of the HCO_3^- deficit should be replaced within 2 to 4 h. Patient reassessment may indicate that the remainder of the HCO_3^- deficit should be replaced over the following 8 to 12 h, but in many cases, fluid therapy and concurrent treatments have corrected the

TABLE 3.3 Isotonic Crystalloid Replacement Fluid Sodium, Potassium, and Chloride Concentrations (mEq/L) and Osmolarity (mOsm/L) and pH.

	Sodium	Potassium	Chloride	Osmolarity	pH
LRS*/Hartmann's	130	4	109	272	6.5
Normosol-R	140	5	98	294	6.6
Plasma-Lyte A	140	5	98	294	7.4
Plasma-Lyte 148	140	5	98	294	5.5
Vetivex pHyLyte	140	5	98	294	7.4
0.9% NaCl	154	0	154	308	5.5

*LRS: lactated Ringer's solution

acidosis. Isotonic bicarbonate can be made by adding 154 mL of 8.4% $NaHCO_3$ to 1 L of sterile water.

Hypotonic Crystalloids. Hypotonic crystalloids contain a lower osmolarity than extracellular fluid, rapid administration of which can result in intracellular fluid shifts and subsequent cerebral edema. For this reason, hypotonic crystalloids are never used to correct dehydration or hypovolemia. Hypotonic maintenance solutions include Normosol-M, Plasma-Lyte 56, 0.45% sodium chloride/2.5% dextrose, Vetivex 18 (0.18% sodium chloride, 4% glucose monohydrate), and 5% dextrose in water (D5W). Normosol-M, Plasma-Lyte 56, 0.45% sodium chloride/2.5% dextrose, and Vetivex 18 contain less sodium compared to isotonic replacement fluids, with Normosol-M and Plasma-Lyte 56 also containing more potassium. Maintenance fluids are appropriate for animals on long-term (i.e., > 3 days) maintenance fluid therapy, because their relatively lower sodium and higher potassium concentrations compared to isotonic replacement fluids more closely mimic normal plasma concentrations. It is important to remember that although D5W has an osmolarity of 252 mOsm/L, the glucose is immediately oxidized to CO_2 and water, resulting in administration of free water *in vivo*; therefore, D5W is rarely used.

Hypertonic Crystalloids. Hypertonic crystalloids have a higher osmolarity relative to extracellular fluid, and are considered a supplement to isotonic crystalloids. The most common hypertonic solution available in veterinary medicine is hypertonic saline (7 to 7.5%) and is given at a dose of 4 mL/kg.[12,13] Administration of hypertonic saline results in a rapid increase in plasma osmolarity, followed by a fluid shift from the interstitial fluid compartment into the intravascular space. Thus, hypertonic saline might be indicated in hypovolemic shock, but must be followed with isotonic replacement fluids. Hypertonic crystalloids should be avoided in cases of acute hemorrhage, as increases in blood pressure can inhibit clot formation.

Crystalloid Additives. In many cases, crystalloids should be supplemented with electrolytes or dextrose. Calcium borogluconate (23% solution) can be added at 25 mL/L in anorexic patients or those with hypocalcemia. Bicarbonate-containing solutions should not be mixed with calcium as this will result in precipitate formation. Anorexic animals should also receive potassium chloride (KCl) at 20 to 40 mEq/L since hypokalemia is a common sequelae of decreased feed intake. Hypophosphatemia may be associated with starvation or pregnancy toxemia, and is most safely treated orally (see later). However, for severe hypophosphatemia, 0.6 mL/kg of 10% sodium monophosphate can be given IV slowly.[14] Dextrose supplementation is necessary in cases of hypoglycemia caused by anorexia in neonates, and in adults with pregnancy toxemia. Neonatal lambs and kids do not have sufficient glycogen stores to tolerate anorexia and can become hypoglycemic within hours of decreased milk intake. A commercially available 50% dextrose solution can be added to isotonic fluids to make a 1 to 10% dextrose solution, depending on the degree of hypoglycemia. Generally, the rate of administration should be 2 to 4 mg/kg/min, but might need to be given more quickly during a hypoglycemic crisis. Animals with pregnancy toxemia might also present with severe hypoglycemia and require aggressive dextrose administration. Undiluted 50% dextrose can be administered IV, or can be added to isotonic crystalloids to make a 10% dextrose solution (200 mL of 50% dextrose/L). The rate of administration should be 2 to 4 mg/kg/min, which can break the cycle of negative energy balance. In cattle, rapid administration of 50% dextrose undiluted as an IV bolus contributes to hypophosphatemia through insulin-regulated activation of phosphorus uptake by skeletal muscle cells.[15] It is unknown if this occurs in small ruminants or cervids, but serum phosphorus concentrations should be monitored if this therapy is chosen. Once an animal with pregnancy toxemia is stabilized, dextrose can be administered IV as a 1 to 2.5% isotonic solution to provide a source of energy. Although CRI fluids are preferred, boluses of 200 to 280 mL of 2.5% dextrose solution (5 to 7 g glucose) administered every 4 h have been recommended as a treatment option.[16] Calcium borogluconate and KCl may also be added to CRI fluids, especially when anorexia persists. Some patients with pregnancy toxemia require PN to provide sufficient energy during late gestation. It is important to monitor blood glucose concentrations every 2 to 4 h in animals receiving IV dextrose. If hyperglycemia develops, insulin (long-acting protamine zinc) can be given at 0.4 mg/kg subcutaneously (SC), with subsequent monitoring of blood glucose concentrations.

Colloids. Colloids are fluids that contain high molecular weight compounds that remain in the intravascular space following IV administration. These compounds act similarly to albumin by maintaining osmotic pressure within the vascular space, and are often used to maintain intravascular fluid volume in animals with hypoproteinemia. Plasma and whole blood are considered natural colloids, while hetastarch, tetrastarch, and dextrans are synthetic colloids. Commercial plasma and synthetic colloids are often cost-prohibitive in small ruminants and cervids, but should be considered in select cases. Plasma is recommended for neonates with FPT at a dose of 20 to 40 mL/kg.[17]

Whole blood transfusions are indicated in patients with anemia and clinical signs of hypoperfusion, including weakness, pale mucous membranes, tachycardia, and tachypnea. In general, whole blood transfusions in small ruminants and cervids are recommended when the PCV is ≤ 12% in cases of chronic anemia, or ≤ 15% in acute cases.[18] In cases of acute hemorrhagic shock, at least half of the estimated blood loss should be replaced if possible. Otherwise, the following formula should be used to determine the amount of blood to transfuse, assuming blood volume is 8% of body weight in kg:

$$\text{Blood volume to be replaced }(\text{L}) = \text{body weight }(\text{kg})\ x\ 0.08\ x \frac{\text{Desired PCV} - \text{Recipient PCV}}{\text{Donor PCV}}$$

Whole blood should be administered at 1 to 5 mL/kg/h IV for the first 30 minutes, followed by 10 to 20 mL/kg/h until the desired volume is replaced. Vital signs should be monitored every 5 minutes throughout the transfusion; signs of anaphylaxis (Type I hypersensitivity) include pyrexia, tachycardia, respiratory distress, urticaria, facial edema, muscle fasciculations, hiccupping, salivation, and lacrimation. Treatment for anaphylaxis includes discontinuation of the transfusion and administration of 0.03 mg/kg epinephrine IV. If urticaria or facial edema develops, diphenhydramine at 2 mg/kg can be given IV slowly. Blood donors should be healthy, non-pregnant adults and confirmed negative for caprine arthritis encephalitis virus (CAEV), brucellosis, tuberculosis, Q fever *(Coxiella burnetii)*, *Anaplasma ovis*, *Mycoplasma ovis*, and *Corynebacterium pseudotuberculosis*.[18] As a general rule of thumb, the donor can safely donate 15 mL/kg of blood at one time.

A whole blood transfusion might also be indicated for hypoproteinemia when the cost of commercial plasma is prohibitive. Caution should be used in hemoconcentrated animals, given the risk of iron toxicity.

Oral Fluids

Oral fluids are practical and cost-effective, and can be used to rehydrate small ruminants and cervids with mild to moderate dehydration. However, a healthy gastrointestinal tract is necessary to achieve proper absorption of fluids and electrolytes, and to prevent further morbidity in cases of gastrointestinal disease. The healthy rumen is capable of absorbing large volumes of water and electrolytes, with optimum absorption occurring when the plasma osmolality (mOsm/kg) is slightly higher than rumen osmolality.[19] Therefore, administration of oral fluids that are hypo-osmotic is ideal. Commercially available oral rehydration solutions for calves can be used in small ruminants and cervids. These solutions contain variable concentrations of electrolytes with or without dextrose and alkalizing agents (e.g., bicarbonate, acetate, propionate). Alternatively, oral electrolyte solutions can be made by adding the following per liter of water:

- 7 g NaCl
- 1.5 g KCl
- 0.5 g $CaCl_2$

Correction of electrolyte and acid-base disturbances can also be achieved through oral fluid therapy. In sheep and goats with diarrhea and subsequent metabolic acidosis, a combination of IV and oral alkalizing fluids can be beneficial.[10,20] Small ruminants and cervids with hypokalemia may be supplemented orally with 10 g KCl per 100 kg body weight, every 12 h. Animals with starvation or prolonged anorexia might have hypophosphatemia, which can be treated with 1 to 2 sodium phosphate enemas (4.5 oz/13 mL each) in oral fluids.[4] Given the high osmolarity of the enema solution, each 13 mL bottle should be diluted in at least 50 mL of water. Finally, does and ewes with early signs of pregnancy toxemia may benefit from oral propylene glycol as a glucose precursor (15–30 mL every 12 h). Rumen transfaunation and oral vitamin B complex supplementation are also recommended.

Although a fluid plan should be calculated as described above to determine the amount of fluids that should be administered, oral fluids (in L) can be safely administered at a dose of 3.5% of body weight in kg. For example, a 20 kg goat can safely receive 0.7 L (700 mL) of oral fluids at one time.

Parenteral Nutrition

Parenteral nutrition is an effective means to provide nutrients to animals with prolonged anorexia, dysphagia, or an unhealthy gastrointestinal tract that cannot tolerate enteral feeding. Intravenous dextrose supplementation only provides up to 25% of the patient's maintenance energy requirement, so animals with anorexia for > 3 days should be considered candidates for PN. Total PN (TPN) contains dextrose, amino acids, and lipids and is designed to meet the total energy requirement of the patient. Partial PN (PPN) refers to solutions with only partial components (e.g., no lipids) or to solutions given at a rate that only partially meets the patient's total energy requirement. The cost of TPN often precludes its use in sheep, goats, and cervids, so PPN is used more commonly.

It is important to use aseptic technique when mixing PN solutions, with amino acids added first, followed by lipid (if applicable), and then dextrose.[4] If possible, a dedicated port in a double-lumen polyurethane catheter should be used for PN, with IV fluids and/or medications delivered through a separate port. Animals on PN are at high risk for development of thrombophlebitis and septicemia, so it is critical to maintain an aseptic fluid line and injection site adapter. The PN solution and associated fluid lines should be changed daily. While on PN, the patient should be monitored closely for fluctuations in serum glucose concentrations, electrolyte abnormalities, or acid-base disturbances. If TPN is used, increases in serum lipids might occur. A fluid pump should be used to deliver PN accurately. It is important to remember to adjust the rate of IV fluid administration based on the rate of PN administration if both are given concurrently. If insulin is being administered to control hyperglycemia associated with PN administration, insulin therapy should be discontinued 24 h prior to discontinuation of PN. The rate of PN should be gradually decreased over 24 to 48 h before it is discontinued.

The recommended formulation for PPN in sheep, goats, and cervids is:[4]

- 5 L balanced isotonic crystalloid fluids
- 500 mL 50% dextrose (1.7 kcal/mL = 850 kcal)
- 1 L 8.5% amino acids (0.34 kcal/mL = 340 kcal)
- 20 mL B-complex vitamins
- ± KCl (20 to 40 mEq/L)
- ± Calcium borogluconate 23% (25 mL/L)

The rate of PN is based on the daily caloric requirements during illness, and utilizes the following equation: 140 kcal/kg$^{0.75}$ body weight in kg. To calculate, enter the animal's body weight in kg into a scientific calculator, and then press the "xy" or "^" key; enter 0.75, followed by enter (=). Multiply this number by 140 to obtain the kcal/day required for maintenance energy. The PPN solution above contains 0.24 kcal/mL. It is recommended to start PPN at 25% of the patient's daily requirement and increase by 25% every 12 to 24 h. For example, a sick 20 kg goat has a daily caloric requirement of 1324 kcal/day ($20^{0.75} \times 140$). Twenty-five percent of this requirement = 331 kcal/day. Given that the PPN solution above contains 0.24 kcal/mL, the PPN rate should be set to 57 mL/h initially ([331 kcal/24 h] / 0.24 kcal/mL), and then increased by 25% every 12 to 24 h. An easier estimate using this PPN formulation is to start at a rate of 6% of body weight in kg, divided by 24 to set a rate in mL/h. For example, 6% of 20 kg = 1.2 L, divided by 24 h = 50 mL/h.

If TPN is indicated and affordable, the following formula is recommended:[5]

(Remove 400 mL from balanced isotonic crystalloid fluids before adding the following:)

- 100 mL 50% dextrose (1.7 kcal/mL = 170 kcal)
- 200 mL 8.5% amino acids (0.34 kcal/mL = 68 kcal)
- 100 mL 20% lipids (2 kcal/mL = 200 kcal)
- 4 mL B-complex vitamins
- ± KCl (20 to 40 mEq/L)
- ± Calcium borogluconate 23% (25 mL/L)

This TPN solution provides 0.44 kcal/mL. As above, initiating treatment at 25% of the daily caloric requirement is recommended. Therefore, a sick 20-kg goat has a daily requirement of 1324 kcal/day ($20^{0.75} \times 140$). Twenty-five percent of this requirement = 331 kcal/day. Given that this TPN solution contains 0.44 kcal/mL, the TPN rate should be set to 31 mL/h initially ([331 kcal/24 h] / 0.44 kcal/mL). Using this TPN formulation, an estimation that uses a starting rate based on 4% of body weight in kg can be used; for example, 4% of 20 kg = 0.8 L, divided by 24 h = 33 mL/h.

Take Home Points

1. The most common cause of dehydration and hypovolemia in small ruminants is diarrhea from gastrointestinal parasitism.

2. Small ruminants and cervids with > 8% dehydration should be treated with IV fluid therapy.
3. When formulating a fluid plan, the fluid deficit, maintenance fluid rate, and ongoing losses (if applicable) must be considered.
4. Hypotonic fluids should never be used to correct dehydration or hypovolemia.
5. Dextrose supplementation at 2 to 4 mg/kg/min IV is indicated in hypoglycemic neonates and in adult females with pregnancy toxemia.
6. Oral fluid therapy is a practical and cost-effective method for treating mild to moderate dehydration in animals with a healthy gastrointestinal tract, given the rumen's vast capacity for fluid and electrolyte absorption.
7. Parenteral nutrition, either total or partial, should be considered in animals with prolonged anorexia or pregnancy toxemia.

References

1. Macfarlane WV, Morris RJ, Howard B: Water economy of tropical merino sheep, *Nature* 178:304, 1956.
2. Reece WO: Body water: properties and functions. In: Reece WO, editors: *Dukes' physiology of domestic animals*, ed 13, Ames, IA, 2015, John Wiley & Sons, Inc., p 103.
3. Constable PD, Walker PG, Morin DE, Foreman JH: Clinical and laboratory assessment of hydration status of neonatal calves with diarrhea, *J Am Vet Med Assoc* 212:991, 1998.
4. Jones M, Navarre C: Fluid therapy in small ruminants and camelids, *Vet Clin North Am Food Anim Pract* 30:441, 2014.
5. Walz PH, Taylor, D: Fluid therapy and nutritional support. In Pugh DG, Baird AN, editors: *Sheep and goat medicine*, ed 2, Maryland Heights, MO, 2012, Elsevier Saunders, p 50.
6. National Research Council: *Nutrient requirements of small ruminants: sheep, goats, cervids, and New World camelids*, Washington, DC, 2007, The National Academies Press.
7. Larsen JW, Anderson N, Vizard AL, Anderson GA, Hoste H: Diarrhoea in merino ewes during winter: association with trichostrongylid larvae, *Aust Vet J* 71:365, 1994.
8. Keeton STN, Navarre CB: Coccidiosis in Large and Small Ruminants, *Vet Clin North Am Food Anim Pract* 34:201, 2018.
9. Le Jambre LF: Relationship of blood loss to worm numbers, biomass and egg production in Haemonchus infected sheep, *Int J Parasitol* 25:269, 1995.
10. Bleul U, Schwantag S, Stocker H, et al: Floppy kid syndrome caused by D-lactic acidosis in goat kids, *J Vet Intern Med* 20:1003, 2006.
11. Braun U, Rihs T, Schefer U: Ruminal lactic acidosis in sheep and goats, *Vet Rec* 130:343, 1992.
12. Silverstein DC, Aldrich J, Haskins SC, et al: Assessment of changes in blood volume in response to resuscitative fluid administration in dogs, *J Vet Emerg Crit Care (San Antonio)* 15:185, 2005.
13. Smith GJ, Kramer GC, Perron P, Nakayama S, Gunther RA, Holcroft JW: A comparison of several hypertonic solutions for resuscitation of bled sheep, *J Surg Res* 39:517,1985.
14. Constable P: Fluid and electrolyte therapy in ruminants, *Vet Clin North Am Food Anim Pract* 19:557, 2003.
15. Grunberg W, Morin DE, Drackley JK, Barger AM, Constable PD: Effect of continuous intravenous administration of a 50% dextrose solution on phosphorus homeostasis in dairy cows, *J Am Vet Med Assoc* 229:413, 2006.
16. Rook JS: Pregnancy toxemia of ewes, does, and beef cows, *Vet Clin North Am Food Anim Pract* 16:293, 2000.
17. Divers TJ: Blood component transfusions, *Vet Clin North Am Food Anim Pract* 21:615, 2005.
18. Balcomb C, Foster D: Update on the use of blood and blood products in ruminants, *Vet Clin North Am Food Anim Pract* 30:455, 2014.
19. Dobson A, Sellers AF, Gatewood VH: Dependence of Cr-EDTA absorption from the rumen on luminal osmotic pressure, *Am J Physiol* 231:1595, 1976.
20. Angell JW, Jones GL, Voigt K, Grove-White DH: Successful correction of D-lactic acid neurotoxicity (drunken lamb syndrome) by bolus administration of oral sodium bicarbonate, *Vet Rec* 173:193, 2013.

4 Oral-Esophageal Diseases

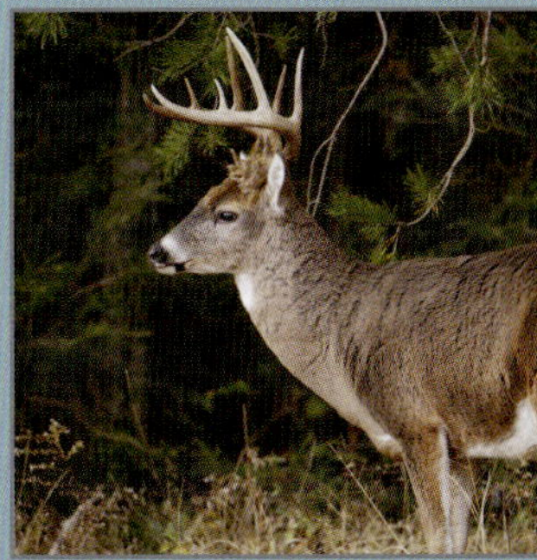

A.N. BAIRD AND CLIFFORD F. SHIPLEY

Although oral-esophageal conditions make up a very small part of small ruminant practice, when present they can cause a significant productive and economic loss to the flock or herd in question. When a practitioner is called upon to investigate oral-esophageal conditions it is very important to gather a thorough history of illness, management procedures, and treatments; to observe the animals as they move and eat (looking for normal eructation and rumination); and to evaluate the body condition of several animals. A cursory examination of the oral cavity can be done with the aid of physical restraint, a mouth gag, and a good light. The gingiva is normally pale pink in color. Some cases of gingivitis are seen and frequently are associated with more serious tooth problems and even tooth loss in the year or two to come. While mild gingivitis is very common, it is uncommon to see any significant oral disease related to mild cases. More severe redness and edema diffusely throughout the mouth may affect deeper tissues causing periodontal disease which will lead to tooth loss and the inherent conditioning problems. If this becomes a significant problem in a given group, one should perform regular oral exams to identify changes in the teeth and determine if any management or diet changes can be made that might help the herd performance.[1]

A thorough oral examination of small ruminants can be a challenge. The small ruminant has a relatively narrow intermandibular space and the mouth does not open as widely as some other species. Sedation or a short-acting anesthetic should be considered when one needs to perform a very thorough oral examination on an individual animal (see Chapter 18 and Appendix l). With appropriate restraint, the lips can be reflected to expose the buccal surface of the incisors and gingiva. Further retraction of the lips may lead the animal to open the mouth so you can see the lingual surface of the incisors and part of the tongue. The incisors should be checked for normal tooth eruption, along with wear and loss of teeth. One should also note any abnormal inclination of the incisors that lead to incorrect occlusion with the dental pad. The animal will usually be moving the mouth in a chewing motion so a prolonged study of the oral cavity is not practical. Palpation of the cheeks can give some insight as to the health of the cheek teeth. Direct visualization of the cheek teeth requires a mouth gag and light source. Even then, a thorough examination is difficult because the animal will continue to chew against the mouth gag. The cheek teeth should be checked for abnormal wear, such as wave mouth and loss of teeth, which lead to long growth of opposing teeth or food impaction in empty spaces. Molars will often be black because of grass staining, which has no deleterious effect.[2] The mandible should also be carefully palpated to determine any bony swelling which may coincide with tooth root disease.[1]

Dental care such as floating or clipping abnormally growing teeth may be considered on a case-by-case basis. One probably does not want to start a management program that includes a lot of such dental care. It can be time consuming and may serve to propagate more bad teeth in the herd. It also runs the risk of making tooth problems worse if the sensitive pulp cavity is exposed in the shortened tooth. In the case of shortening a cheek tooth that is overgrown because of a missing apposing tooth, this floating is only a short-term help since the missing tooth is really the reason for the problem. Each owner must make management decisions in animals with sufficiently abnormal teeth where grazing and maintaining body condition is a problem. That decision centers on supplemental feeding to maintain the animal in production versus culling. The owner must make that decision based on costs of supplemental feeding, as well as replacement costs and confinement facilities to allow supplemental feeding.[1]

Loss of incisors is very important to the productive life of an animal in most management systems which require a lot of grazing. The normal mouth should consist of short, closely arranged incisors. Incisors may become short and peg-like in some young animals because of rough grazing. This may become a problem in the long run due to decreased grazing efficiency in these animals. Long teeth with spaces between may be a predictor of teeth that will be lost in the future and cause significant nutritional problems.

Small ruminants will frequently have chronic conditions before being brought to the attention of a veterinarian, largely because they are grouping animals and individual changes in food intake, body condition, and production are not noticed as quickly in the group as they are in animals that are raised more as individuals. Sheep with poor teeth may have lost a lot of weight before being noticed by owners, since they stay with the flock and are seen to eat (although not very efficiently) and move normally.[3]

Cervids may have increased numbers of teeth and jaw problems due to their proclivity to run into fences and other solid objects when frightened, resulting in injuries. They almost always need tranquilization or anesthesia, and proper handling equipment for proper examination and treatment (see Chapter 1). Traumatic injuries commonly encountered in cervid production range from broken mandibles and maxillas to broken teeth and serious degloving injuries of the lip and face. Wiring, pinning, and other repair have good overall success if carried out in a timely manner (see Chapter 11). Soft tissue injury to the muzzle can be treated with surgical debridement and wound closure with absorbable sutures (Figure 4.1 and 4.2). Daily care is very difficult due to their nature, so repair and turn out are generally best with observation done remotely without exciting the animal. Tame

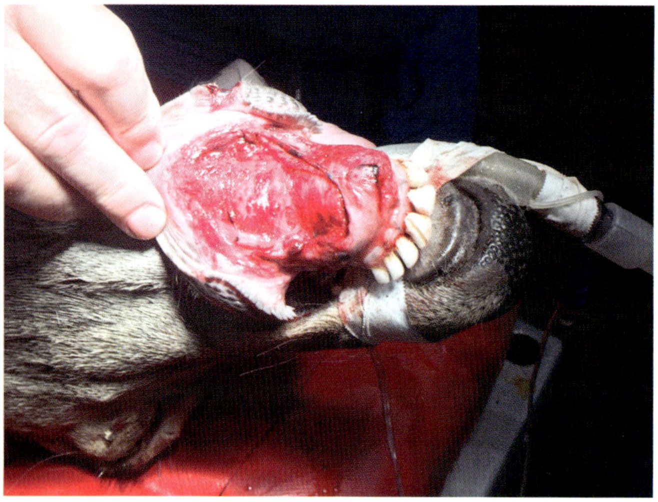

• **Fig. 4.1** A 4-year-old red deer with a lip avulsion.

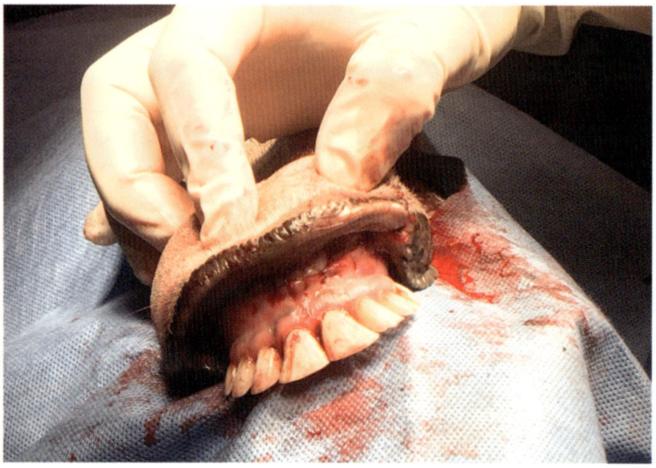

• **Fig. 4.2** The same red deer as in Figure 4.1, postoperatively. The doe was pregnant at the time of injury and maintained the pregnancy to deliver healthy twin fawns, in spite of injury, anesthesia, and surgery.

animals generally do well with care as in other domestic species although they may develop resentment to regular treatment and will be better if left alone or treated with a remote delivery system. Animals that cannot chew may be offered "gruel" (e.g., 1 lb alfalfa pellets with ½ to 1 gallon of water, depending on desired consistency) or other feeds that they can consume.

Diagnostic Procedures

Ultrasonography has become increasingly popular in all aspects of veterinary medicine including small ruminant and cervid practice.[4–7] While ultrasound examinations have been used for some time in reproductive examination, there are more and more reasons to use it in any soft tissue abnormality. Conditions discussed in this chapter on head, oral cavity, and esophagus are no exception. Ultrasonography can delineate abscess cavities, follow draining tracts, look for foreign bodies, and also help in evaluation of esophageal obstruction. Color Doppler and three-dimensional ultrasonography technologies are making this modality even more useful.[8] It is also a helpful imaging tool when obtaining biopsies of soft tissue masses or lymph nodes. The wool in the area will inhibit good contact with the probe, so clipping will be more important in sheep than goats, although depending on the location and length of hair, the goat will often need to be clipped to allow a meaningful study of the area. Thoroughly soaking the area to be examined with alcohol followed by ultrasound gel is helpful to obtain a good quality image since it removes small air pockets and provides uniform coupling of the gel with the skin. Superficial lesions such as lymph nodes or palpable masses are best visualized with a high frequency probe 8.0 to 7.5 MHz range. Deeper structures such as muscle abscesses and retropharyngeal lymph nodes often require imaging with lower frequency, such as with a 5.0-MHz probe to get better penetration of the ultrasound beam into the deeper tissues. The trade-off is a loss in resolution, but visualization of the deeper tissues is gained. The sonographic appearance of abscesses can vary. Depending on maturity and contents, an abscess can look anechoic (black) to hypoechoic (gray) with ultrasound imaging. If the abscess contains thick caseous material, the abscess can appear hypoechoic and similar in echotexture to a lymph node. Gas within an abscess will often appear as small, hyperechoic foci that have a "comet-tail" associated with them. Abscesses with a very fluid-like center often appear black, or anechoic.

Ultrasound imaging to search for a foreign body is often very rewarding. Foreign material such as wood can be missed on plain film radiographs but easily seen with ultrasonography. Foreign material such as wood, bone, or metal will produce a linear, hyperechoic focus with "shadowing." The foreign material strongly reflects the ultrasound beam so that a black shadow, or "tail," is formed below the foreign body. Draining tracts often have fluid or gas within them that can be followed with ultrasound imaging. The foreign body itself is often surrounded by a hypoechoic rim of fluid. Ultrasound-guided biopsy of a soft tissue mass is extremely useful in obtaining a sample for histopathologic evaluation and diagnosis. The biopsy instrument can be visualized using ultrasound imaging to guide the needle to the correct location and avoid vasculature within the mass to be biopsied. Ultrasound-guided biopsies are commonplace in veterinary medicine but underutilized in ruminants and other large animals.

Radiography adds information to conditions of the head, particularly the teeth. Tangential views, typically lateral (Figure 4.3) and dorso-ventral (Figure 4.4) projections are often needed to make an accurate diagnosis and to localize an abnormality. Oblique views are especially helpful when looking at tooth conditions. In oblique views, tooth roots can be evaluated without superimposition of the contralateral arcade. The angle of obliquity is approximately 30 degrees (from lateral) with the x-ray beam directed ventral to dorsal. The affected side should be placed against the cassette. In the 30-degree left ventral–right dorsal view, the right mandible and left maxilla will be profiled on the image. Oftentimes it is helpful to also take the opposite oblique view so that the tooth roots of both arcades can be compared without superimposition of other teeth. Occasionally a 45-degree oblique can be useful to evaluate the crowns of the teeth without superimposition. Tooth root abscesses, broken teeth, skull fractures, and nasal or sinus masses are a few conditions about which skull radiography provides important diagnostic information.

Contrast radiography can be quite useful when looking at conditions of the esophagus.[9] Barium is the contrast media of choice unless a perforation is suspected, in which case an iodine-based contrast agent should be used. A contrast study of the

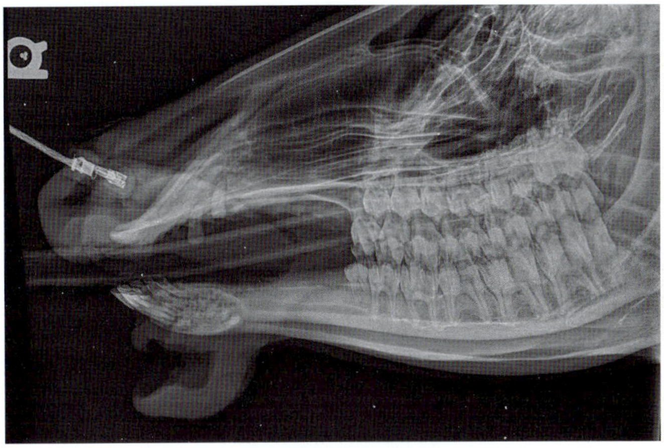

• **Fig. 4.3** Lateral radiograph of a 4-year-old red deer showing normal dentition as well as the sparse covering of incisors and lip avulsion. The animal is under general anesthesia so the endotracheal tube is in place and the pulse oximeter is seen attached to the tongue.

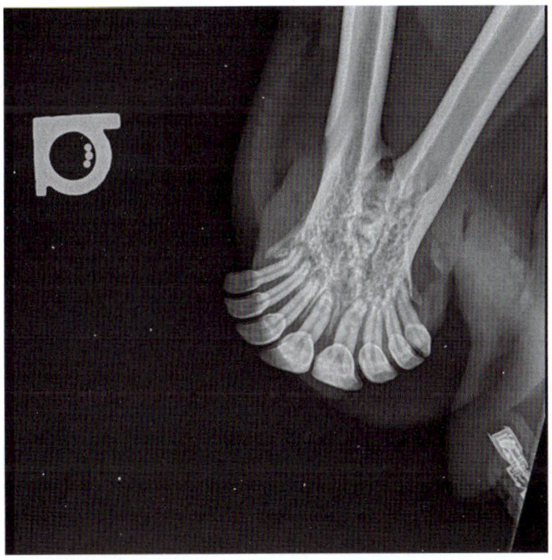

• **Fig. 4.4** An intra-oral ventro-dorsal radiograph of the deer in Figure 4.3 showing normal incisors and mandibular symphysis.

esophagus (esophagram) will determine types of diverticulae, locations, and some information on obstructions of the esophagus. While it is not likely to become a common procedure in small ruminants, computed tomography and three-dimensional reconstruction have been used in veterinary medicine to discover and describe esophageal diverticula.[10]

Fistulogram is another valuable contrast study that can be used in evaluating draining tracts. This procedure can determine the extent of a draining tract, outline radiolucent foreign bodies, and identify a piece of infected bone or other structure that needs to be removed surgically. A fistulogram is performed by injecting an iodinated contrast agent into the hole of the draining tract. Typically, a small catheter such as a polyethylene urinary catheter is used so that it can be inserted a short way into the tract. Enough contrast should be injected to completely fill the draining tract. If the opening of the draining tract is ventral to the bulk of the tract, a Foley catheter can be used with the balloon inflated to keep the contrast within the tract. Another method to overcome gravity's effect on the contrast is to perform the study under general anesthesia with the animal positioned so that the opening is dorsal. Towel clamps can also be used to help close the opening around the catheter. In all cases, an initial film/image should be made before contrast is injected. The clinician may need multiple films to make sure the draining tract is completely filled. In some instances, the radiograph is exposed toward the end of the injection so that it is under pressure.

Endoscopic examinations may be useful for the diagnosis of pharyngeal and esophageal conditions.[11] The small relative size of the sheep, goat, and cervid nasal passage prohibits nasal endoscopy with most of the endoscopes of 10 mm or greater diameter that are used in large animal practice. Smaller diameter "pediatric" endoscopes may be used but again adequate restraint for a thorough examination that is safe for the animal and the equipment is difficult to accomplish in the nonsedated small ruminant. The oral pharyngeal region and esophagus may be examined endoscopically through the mouth using a tube speculum to protect the endoscope from the damage by the teeth, but we still advise heavy sedation or anesthesia for the best results and safety.

Oral Cavity

The muzzle and oral cavity of sheep, goats, and cervids are characterized by very mobile lips which are thin relative to larger ruminants such as cattle. There is an obvious philtrum in the upper lip. The tongue and palate are smoother than that of cattle. The mouth is relatively narrow in sheep, goats and cervids, when compared with cattle, which makes examination of the teeth and oral cavity more difficult. Consistent with all ruminants, the dental pad is located rostral to the palate where upper incisors are found in other species.[12] Small ruminants have three pairs of lower incisors and one pair of lower canine teeth which look and function just like the incisors. (Therefore, for the purpose of this discussion, we may take the liberty to refer to those canine teeth as incisors when discussing the front teeth as a group.) The dental formula for sheep, goats, and most cervids is: 2(Di0/3, Dc0/0, Dp3/3) for deciduous teeth and 2(I0/3, C0/1, P3/3, M3/3) for permanent teeth. Some elk and reindeer may retain upper canines. Deciduous teeth are in place by 4 weeks of age in sheep and goats. Aging based on tooth eruption is performed by looking at the incisors and canine which make up the four pairs of rostral mandibular teeth in sheep and goats. Aging of deer over 1 year relies on cheek teeth eruption and wear, or more accurately, microscopic evaluation of cementum annuli of the first incisor. The eruption time in these teeth may vary by 6 months or more, depending mostly on nutrition (Table 4.1). The canine is the most unpredictable of these teeth in time of eruption and may even be absent in some mature sheep. One study determined that up to 15.4% of 266 sheep studied lacked either one or both canine teeth which can interfere with aging by tooth eruption.[13]

The periodontal ligament holding incisors is relatively large compared to other animals of similar size. This wider ligament allows the movement in the incisors normally seen in ruminants. The normal incisors in sheep and goats are loose enough to be moved a couple of millimeters with gentle digital pressure. The movement minimizes trauma to the cartilaginous dental pad with occlusion and actually aids in cutting plant stuffs when grazing. However, this also predisposes the small ruminants to loss of the incisors over time with grazing. The loss of the incisors can be problematic to the individual animal that loses the teeth, as well as it being a serious herd management problem with certain rough

TABLE 4.1. Ages of Permanent Tooth Eruption in Sheep, Goats, and White-tailed Deer.

	AGE OF ERUPTION	
Permanent Tooth	**Sheep & Goats**	**White-tailed Deer**
Incisor 1	1 to 1.5 years	5 to 6 months
Incisor 2	1.5 to 2 years	10 to 11 months
Incisor 3	2.5 to 3 years	10 to 11 months
Incisor 4	3.5 to 4 years	10 to 11 months
Premolars	1.5 to 2 years	6 months to 2.5 years
Molar 1	3 months	6 months
Molar 2	9 to 12 months	6 months
Molar 3	1.5 to 2 years	1.5 to 2 years

All cervids have similar eruption dates but vary between and even among different species. Most aging of cervids after 11 months based on teeth is done after harvest by examination of wear and eruption of cheek teeth, or alternatively by microscopic evaluation of the first incisors.

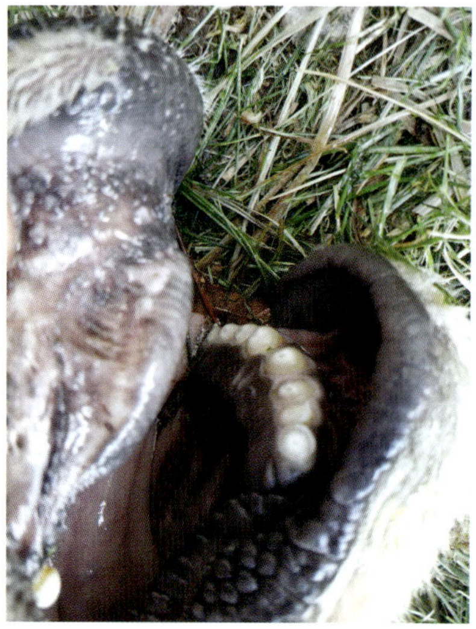

• **Fig. 4.5** Worn incisors in a 19-year-old white-tailed deer.

grazing pastures, if a large percentage of the flock suffers incisor loss, especially at a relatively young age. The loss of incisors can lead to poor performance by the individual animal or herd due to poor nutrition.[1] Loss of incisors is not as dramatic an issue for goats, which are primarily browsers, as opposed to sheep that graze closely. Goats will normally lose incisors at an older age than sheep but maintain body condition better than sheep after incisor loss.[14]

Incisor loss may be due to sandy soils and wear on teeth from picking up soil when grazing. The teeth also wear on sides as well as the crown, prompting one to think other reasons exist for the excessive wear of the incisors. Acid soils may contribute to this tooth loss as tooth dentine is demineralized when exposed to calcium and phosphate ions at a pH consistent with some forage and soils.[15]

One study of sheep from one herd culled due to disease or slaughter for meat found 34% of the animals had abnormalities of the incisors but only one-third of that group showed clinical disease and all those sheep also had significant conditions of the molars. Other sheep presented for necropsy had significant disease of the molars at a rate of 84%. One-third of those animals also had advanced incisor disease. Primary dental abnormalities are seldom treated but can be responsible for weight loss, culling, and disease.[16] Farm-raised deer may develop wear of incisors as they age, since they do not face many of the natural challenges of deer in the wild (Figure 4.5). This incisor wear and loss must not be overlooked in older farm-raised does that start to lose condition. The same deer in the wild would not likely survive.

Dental health and the resultant ability (or inability) of sheep to graze is a very important factor in cull rates of sheep. This is especially true in some countries where grazing may be a more important nutritional factor than those in which a lot of supplemental feeding is done. In some management systems it is financially feasible to move older ewes with a poor dentition to supplemental feeding to get another year or two of production from that ewe rather than to cull and have to replace the ewe in the flock. This true cost of incisor loss includes increased costs of supplemental feed, lost productive years of ewes, replacement costs for culled ewes, lost production of wool and offspring in ewes with poor dentition, and decreased prices of ewes sold with unsound mouths. "Broken mouthed" is a term used to describes sheep with one or more missing incisor while "gummy" describes a sheep with all the incisors missing.[2]

Contrary to the looseness of the incisors, the cheek teeth are very stable with ligamentous support and bone so as to serve the purpose of grinding food stuff and cud. Improper wear of cheek teeth may occur as a herd problem when ewes develop higher than normal rates of pregnancy toxemia related to inability to take in enough nutrition to normally maintain the pregnancy and body condition. Abnormal wear or lost cheek teeth may lead to cheek and gingival abrasions from the remaining teeth growing in the absence of apposing teeth, and thus causing trauma to the oral cavity. The inefficient chewing and painful oral cavity will eventually lead to poor body condition.[1]

As mentioned earlier, sheep are more adversely affected by lost incisors than goats; however, goats still have dental issues that can affect body condition. They may have cheek teeth that wear unevenly causing sharp points that can damage soft tissues of the mouth and make chewing painful. Some may have tooth root abscesses that make the teeth cold-sensitive, thus decreasing water intake. The cheek teeth normally have sharp edges on the lateral aspect of the maxillary teeth and medial aspect of the mandibular teeth. If these areas are associated with soft tissue injury, abnormal chewing and loss of condition, the abnormal points may need to be reduced by filing or cutting, either with dental floats of appropriate size to file the hooks, or cutting with pliers or gigli wire. Goats that are having trouble with cheek teeth may chew only on one side of the mouth or else drop food. Some will act hungry but will not eat because of mouth pain. Oral tumors such as sarcoma, adenosarcoma, osteoma, fibrosarcoma, and fibroma may cause loose teeth, lost teeth, and mouth pain in some older goats. Cheek tooth root abscesses may show some firm swelling of the area of the affected root. Some respond at least temporarily to broad-spectrum antibiotics for several weeks. Most will not be healed by antibiotics alone and it is often difficult to financially justify surgical extraction or peri-apical curettage on any but the most valuable goats.[14] Cheek teeth abnormalities are more difficult to determine because examination and visualization of the cheek teeth can be a challenge. While gingivitis may lead to abnormal wear and even loss of cheek teeth, the first clinical sign of cheek tooth loss may be loss of body condition. Upon closer observation, one may see cheek swelling from impacted food stuffs or palpate lost teeth. With loss of teeth, the opposing teeth then grow longer without normal wear. Food may impact where the tooth was lost or sharp points form on the remaining tooth that may damage soft tissue structures of the cheek, gum, and tongue.[17]

Sheep with poor dentition that has caused lacerations in the oral cavity will lose body condition because the oral pain prevents proper food intake. Some may have saliva wetting the jaw from drooling. Halitosis may also be noted. Cheek teeth abnormalities frequently cause swellings in the cheek from either oral lesions or impacted food stuffs. Occasionally, the swelling may be retained cud which can be mistaken for some soft tissue swelling by visual observation alone. Oral examination has already been described. Molar teeth abnormalities may lead to short jerky jaw movement sometimes with the mouth slightly open. With excessive quidding, fibrous feed may be seen at the commissure of the mouth. Radiographs can be helpful to evaluate cheek teeth with the appropriate oblique view to avoid superimposition of tooth roots. The best information can be gained if the animal is under general anesthesia for the radiographic study. Palpation of the mandible may detect missing teeth or sharp points on cheek teeth. Cheek tooth abscesses with draining tracts are not frequently seen in sheep.[3]

The mandible may develop osseous swellings that can be readily discovered on physical examination by palpation of the mandible. Some of these swellings are due to periostitis around tooth roots. Many are of little significance and resolve without treatment. Indeed, some may go unnoticed by the owners. Ones that become too large to ignore, or cause grazing issues, are probably due to abscessation of tooth roots. These are seldom herd problems and while surgical intervention may improve the condition, it is often more involved than is reasonable for all but the most valuable of small ruminants. Conflicting results have been achieved by antibiotic therapy but that is usually worth an attempt to improve the animal's condition, especially in cases such as pregnant females, in order to get healthy offspring.[1]

Fluorosis

The skeletal lesions of fluorosis are not usually apparent until after dental fluorosis is appreciated in the animal. The dental abnormalities are noted because the toxic level of fluoride disrupts the normal deposition of mineral in developing teeth. The dental abnormalities are therefore dependent on the length of time of exposure and the age of the animal. The clinical signs are not apparent until long after the exposure to the fluoride. The clinical signs seen of abnormal dental development include a faster wearing of the teeth that have discolored, and chalky and pitted enamel. The dental abnormality observed may be as simple as a groove around a pair of teeth when the animal is exposed to toxic levels of fluoride for a short time period.[17] Goats with chronic fluorosis have reduced serum levels of copper, iron, manganese, and nickel compared with normal goats.[18] Sheep with chronic fluorosis show altered tissue levels of copper, magnesium, manganese, calcium, and zinc.[19]

Malocclusion

Malocclusion of the incisors with the dental pad can have a negative effect on grazing efficiency and therefore, body condition and production. Brachygnathia (parrot mouth) occasionally occurs as a congenital defect in which the incisors meet caudal on the dental pad, or in severe cases, behind the dental pad on the palate.[1] Some reports suggest brachygnathia inferior is heritable (far from simple) with an oligogenic pattern including dominant and recessive loci with further modifying loci likely. Craniofacial abnormalities seen with brachygnathia inferior may be related to viral infections, plant alkaloids, or teratogenic drugs.[20,21] Surgical treatment for this condition has been described in horses[22] but the cost of treatment and low chance of perfect results would make this feasible in very few small ruminants. The equine upper incisors allow an anchor point to secure retardation wires to treat these cases. However, the lack of upper incisors in ruminants make growth retardation of the maxilla more difficult. The possible heritable nature of the condition leads one to question the ethics of treatment. If an owner chooses to have this condition treated, the clinician should treat early and refer to equine references for more details. The best course of action for these animals is probably to simply cull the animal and decrease losses. More often, the incisors are anterior to the dental pad which does interfere with grazing. This can be from the angle or length of the incisors, or the relative lengths of the mandible and maxilla. The length and angle of the incisors change with age. The angulation of the incisors leading to abnormal occlusion is thought to be more a product of periodontal disease than any heritable predisposition by some authors.[1] However, others believe incisor malocclusion of both undershot mandible (brachygnathia) and overshot mandible (prognathia) are hereditary.[2] Abnormal dentition has been reported in cervids suspected to be secondary to trauma, or possibly genetic as a result of in-breeding.[23]

Chlamydia pecorum has been shown to cause fetoplacental lesions and abortion in goats. The aborted kids had brachygnathia as well as other skeletal abnormalities including anasarca, intramuscular edema, and palatoschisis.[24] Brachygnathia may be seen with other more significant, even life-threatening congenital anomalies. Severely affected animals may be stillborn.[25] Temporomandibular joint luxation has been reported in a goat. The animal presented for weight loss and inappetence. The mandible was displaced to the side, teeth were malaligned, and the animal was resistant to open the mouth. A radiographic examination of this goat confirmed the temporomandibular luxation and the goat was culled rather than treated.[26]

Pharyngeal Lesions

Growing lambs can have a necrotic stomatitis caused by *Fusobacterium necrophorum*. This has also been reported in goats.[27] This may be related to poor hygiene when lambs are being raised on milk replacer or following trauma from oral dosing with medication or oral fluids. Breaks in the oral mucosa become infected. The lamb will be a poor grower because of oral pain leading to decreased feed intake. They also often have wet matted hair around the mouth from excessive salivation. Respiratory signs may be seen as the infectious agent migrates to the lungs where abscesses form. Pleuritis occurs with the abscesses and this is not often responsive to treatment. The breath is malodorous. Penicillin (50,000 International Units [IU]/kg) for at least a week is the treatment of choice. Prevention is superior to treatment and simply involves good hygiene in bottle-raising lambs and taking proper care when using a dosing instrument to give any oral medications.

Pharyngeal lesions are common after balling gun use or drenching young lambs. Unfortunately, this injury may not be appreciated until the wound has abscessed and either compressed the larynx to cause abnormal breathing or even migrated to the cervical vertebral canal causing neurologic signs. Thorough examination and visualization (or endoscopy) require at least very heavy sedation and is best done under general anesthesia.[3] Pharyngeal abscesses from any organism can develop secondary to trauma of the pharynx while administering oral medication, whether liquid or capsule formulations. Trauma to the pharyngeal wall by the tip of the instrument cannot only allow secondary infection of the wound, but often introduces medication directly into the tissue planes where it acts as a foreign substance causing irritation and an inflammatory reaction. The infection may migrate to the cervical spinal cord where swelling places compression on the cord leading to paresis.[3,28] It may otherwise cause compromised breathing or painful swallowing. The pharyngeal discomfort will lead to decreased food intake so that weight loss may be one of the first signs noticed by owners. The history of recent drenching (less than 2 weeks earlier) will assist with the diagnosis. By the time clinical signs are seen, the prognosis for response to treatment with antibiotics is poor. One should likely consider euthanasia. Certainly, proper techniques and prevention will be much better than attempted treatment.[3]

Herd outbreaks of pharyngeal abscesses can be sometimes seen following administration of medications via a drenching gun. Some reports describe a morbidity of up to 15%. Some animals show acute signs that lead to death (malignant edema) while others may linger several months with weight loss before dying or being euthanatized. Some have an abscess that forms in the mouth or pharynx which then fistulates to drain through the skin of the face.[28]

Actinobacillosis will occasionally be associated with facial subcutaneous abscesses which can drain through the skin, or rarely, into the pharyngeal region. When this occurs, it is usually due to sheep grazing pastures with thorns or some potential traumatic plant that causes oral lesions which become infected. As long as no clinical signs of decreased food intake or difficult breathing occur, no treatment is required. If breathing noise occurs due to pharyngeal compression, treat with steroids and antibiotics, although the prognosis is poor if this occurs.

A common presentation in white-tailed deer is feed impaction of the cheek (Figure 4.6). This condition can be a one-time event or may turn into a chronic impaction that may lead to pressure necrosis of the cheek with subsequent stoma, loss of teeth, infection, and even death. Several theories exist and it may be due to one or more of these factors: meningeal worm *(Parelaphostrongylus tenuis)* migration affecting cranial nerve function, malalignment of teeth, injury, infection (usually from *Fusobacteria* spp.), or arterial worm *(Elaeophora schneideri)*.[29] A thorough examination may reveal the problem but not always. Treatment with antiinflammatories, antibiotics (usually long acting that will be effective against *Fusobacteria* spp.), and deworming to kill migrating larvae may be effective in some cases. It should be noted that meningeal worm infection in cervid species other than white-tailed deer is almost always fatal.

The molars and premolars of most cervidae erupt and wear in a regular fashion and will be worn out by 10 or so years of age. Aging tools exist to help the practitioner to properly age most cervids, or it may be appropriate in some cases to send complete central incisors, including all of the root to the laboratory for aging by microscopic evaluation of cementum annuli. Some cervidae will live to 20 years or longer in captivity if proper nutrition is available. Incisor eruption, wear, and angle are generally considered to not be an accurate way to age cervids. Most are concentrate selectors and as such, may not establish wear patterns that we see in grazing species. Likewise, their mouths and lips are developed for the selection of highly nutritious small parts of growing plants and shrubs.

Malocclusion does occur in cervids but is infrequent. The most common defect that has been observed is "undershot jaws" or brachygnathia. Most of these animals do well in a pen-reared situation but should probably not be retained in a breeding program as inheritance may be possible (Figure 4.7).

Necrotic stomatitis due to *Fusobacterium necrophorum* or *Fusobacterium varium* may be the number one killer of white-tailed fawns in certain areas of the country. Infection is thought to be due to eruption of teeth causing openings for the bacteria to enter or from fawns mouthing objects as they start to explore and eat solid feed. Severe infections that get into bone are usually fatal. If caught early, aggressive treatment with high doses of penicillin or another antibiotic that is effective against the bacteria may be successful. Supportive care and supplemental feeding or tubing may

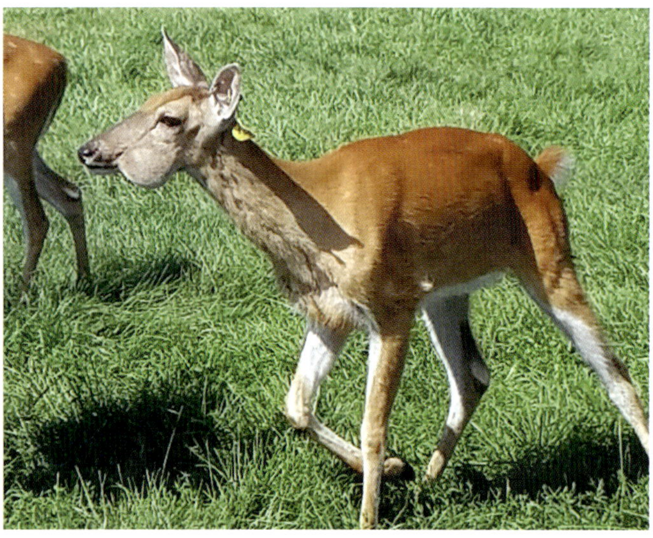

• **Fig. 4.6** Feed impaction in the cheek of a white-tailed deer.

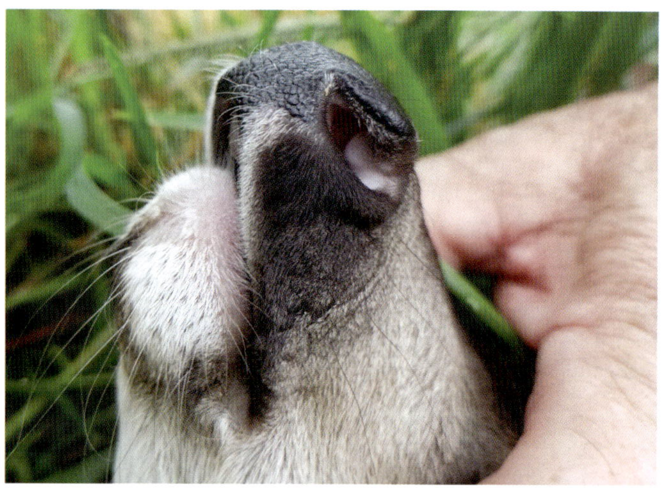

• **Fig. 4.7** Brachygnathia in a white-tailed deer.

increase the odds of survival. Septicemia and pneumonia are also common sequelae to infection, and abscesses, both internally and externally, are also seen frequently.[30]

Conditions of the Head and Neck

There are reports of 2- to 4-year-old sheep developing a firm swelling of the rostral mandible, known as dentigerous or odontogenic cysts. The incidence may be high enough to have a significant effect on the flock as a whole. The swellings are osseous and result in the displacement or absence of one or more teeth. Radiographically, the swelling demonstrates a classic "cystic" appearance with teeth in or near the cystic area. Microscopically, one appreciates a cavity of thin alveolar bone lined with stratified epithelium and filled with sterile fluid. The cause of this cystic lesion is not known. The swelling is seen occasionally in flocks with abnormal wear of temporary teeth. Some investigators have suggested this disease to be a type of dental malpositioning and maleruption. One yet unproven theory is that the cysts are due to an abscess of the periodontal tissues during the development of the permanent incisors.[31] The affected animals are usually culled when the tooth loss prevents normal grazing to maintain body condition. A rostral mandibulectomy is a treatment option for this condition only if the owner wishes to alleviate the animal's pain and is willing to supplement feeding, since the animal would be rendered unable to graze. Odontogenic cysts have been reported in sheep[31] and it is reasonable that they may be seen in goats and deer. However, they are seen much more frequently in dogs[32] and less so in horses,[33] calves,[34] and people.[35]

A differential list for soft tissue swellings of the head and neck region includes thymic hyperplasia, thymoma, wattle cysts, salivary mucocele, caseous lymphadenitis (CLA), as well as some esophageal lesions which will be covered elsewhere in this chapter.[17,36] Thymic hyperplasia is seen as soft swelling on the ventral aspect of the neck in very young goats. This is a normal enlargement that may be seen as early as 2 weeks of age and will usually resolve by 6 months. This does not require any treatment. The clinician needs only to recognize the cause of this swelling should the owner inquire.

A thymoma is a tumor that affects older goats. The swelling associated with this tumor may be observed at the thoracic inlet or some of the tumors will be in the thoracic cavity. Thymomas often have no clinical significance and are an incidental finding at necropsy. They can become large enough at the thoracic inlet to impinge on the esophagus and cause signs of esophageal obstruction such as bloat due to difficulty in swallowing or eructation.

Wattle cysts are swellings at the base of a wattle. The wattle itself serves no real purpose and some producers may request wattle removal for cosmetic reasons if they are not symmetrical. The presence of wattle cysts may also cause a producer to want the cyst removed in a show animal. While the location of the swelling is diagnostic for the wattle cysts, the size may range from barely noticeable to several centimeters in diameter at the base of the wattle. The cysts are inherited and therefore will be seen more often in some family lines. Aspiration of these cysts is not curative. Histopathology of the removed cysts reveals stratified squamous epithelium with mature hair follicles.

Another differential for facial swellings are salivary cysts also known as salivary mucoceles. These cause fluid-filled swellings that do not cause pain to the animal. They are either on the side of the head or the intermandibular area depending on whether they are associated with the parotid or submandibular salivary glands. The cysts can be surgically removed and the salivary duct ligated.[36] Occasionally, the duct may be lacerated and result in a chronic draining tract which discharges saliva excessively when the animal eats. These should also be treated by ligation of the duct and subsequent shrinkage of the associated gland.

CLA will cause enlargement and abscessation of lymph nodes of the head and neck. The causative agent of CLA is *Corynebacterium pseudotuberculosis*. The disease is on all continents and can affect all breeds of goats. The spread may have been enhanced by the popularity and importation of Boer goats over the last 20 years. The organism can survive for several months in the environment after drainage of an abscess. Then, other animals are infected by contamination of an open wound. The wound does not have to be more than a skin break from head butting or even browsing forage. The organism can be spread by contaminated equipment such as shears or tattoo pliers or affected animals. The incubation period is 2 to 6 months. Sheep more often than goats will have internal lymph node abscesses and abscesses of internal organs with hematogenous spread of CLA. Animals with external lymph node abscesses may not show other clinical signs but those with internal abscesses may exhibit progressive weight loss or even respiratory signs if the thoracic nodes are involved.[17] Further discussion of diagnosis and treatment (control) will be found elsewhere.

Head and neck soft tissue swellings are very common in white-tailed deer. Bucks engage in hard antler fight almost continuously during rut, and infections around the antlers and regional lymph nodes are common.[29] These infections can be from almost any bacteria, but most frequent isolates that the authors have seen are *Fusobacteria* spp., and *Trueperella pyogenes*. If an abscess is diagnosed, drainage should be done with lavage of the cavity with appropriate agent. Sometimes systemic antibiotics are warranted as these infections may be spread through the lymphatic system or migrate to the brain through the calvarium. Use of a long-acting antibiotic at time of treatment is best and then long-term follow-up treatment using remote delivery is usually done.

Soft tissue swelling in fawns and does is also common and is typically due to the same bacteria as with the bucks. Treatment is essentially the same. Prevention is difficult but people have used autogenous vaccines in high-risk endemic herds. Clean, dry pens and not overstocking is very important in the control of these abscesses.

Viral Diseases

Foot-and-Mouth disease

Foot-and-mouth disease (FMD) is a highly contagious viral disease of tremendous economic and biosecurity importance to the cloven-hoof livestock industry as a whole. The etiologic agent is a picornavirus. Small ruminants may have mild clinical signs but more importantly may serve as a source of infection for other animals.[37,38] Therefore, small ruminants must be included in vaccination programs in areas battling disease outbreaks in other species.[39] However, work in the Sudan suggested small ruminants were not nearly as important to the spread of FMD as cattle.[40]

Sheep may put other species at risk through movement and contact because of mild clinical signs usually exhibited or carrier animals that have recovered from the clinical disease.[41] Young sheep and goats that are infected will show more severe signs and suffer a higher death rate. The oral lesions of FMD include vesicles that progress to mucosal erosions.[37,38] When sheep show oral lesions, the differential lists must also include contagious ecthyma (orf) as well as traumatic oral lesions that have no infectious component.[38]

The ulcers are also seen at the coronary band as per the name FMD.[42] The first clinical signs seen may be acute severe lameness in sheep.[43,44] Erosions are commonly seen on dental pads.[43] However, up to 27% of sheep known to be infected with FMD did not show clinical signs of erosions or lameness.[45] Sheep are susceptible to infection by respiratory contact and contamination of skin breaks with the virus.[46]

Laboratory testing is required to determine the specific vesicular disease since clinical signs are similar. In the United States (and many other countries), government authorities should be enlisted to help with diagnosis and disposition when FMD is suspected. FMD is the most important disease constraint to international trade of livestock and animal products. The virus is sensitive to pH ranges below 6 and above 9 but is resistant to alcohol, ether, chloroform, and detergents.[46]

Deer are susceptible to FMD and display the characteristic signs that are seen in other cloven-hooved animals (see earlier description). The main concern is with wild deer carrying and spreading the disease to cattle, sheep, goats, and swine. Contained farmed herds would be treated as any other susceptible domestic species. In a 1924 FMD outbreak in California, 22,000 black-tailed deer were killed to stop the spread of the disease. In some deer and traditional domestic livestock-dense areas of the country, it may be necessary to kill a substantial number of wild deer to control the spread of the disease.[29]

Contagious Ecthyma (ORF)

Contagious ecthyma (also known as orf and sore mouth) is a quite common disease of sheep and goats caused by a poxvirus. The classic clinical signs are crusty scabs affecting the mucocutaneous junction of the nose and mouth. There may also be proliferative lesions affecting the oral mucosa.[47] The oral lesions are usually seen in young animals born into endemic herds. Immunologically naïve older animals may develop clinical signs when exposed to clinically normal carrier animals.[48] Orf lesions are differentiated from oral lesions of FMD and Bluetongue by the clinical signs of crusty scabs as opposed to erosions and ulcerative lesions. The clinical signs of contagious ecthyma are usually self-limiting in 3 to 6 weeks. Severely affected animals may require supportive care and assisted feeding if the mouth is sore enough to prevent nursing or if ewes have udder lesions significant enough to prevent the young from nursing. Humans can be infected by the virus as well as act as vectors transmitting the virus from one animal to another so extreme care should be taken to use protective gloves when handling affected animals.[49,50]

Animals usually show immunity for 2 to 3 years after a clinical case of orf although some may show clinical signs 1 year after disease. Lesions are usually milder and respond more quickly during subsequent infections.[36] Eighteen outbreaks of orf over 4 years in India (6 sheep, 12 goat) had morbidity rates of 18.93% for goats and 21.50% in sheep while mortality rates were 2.53 and 1.10% in those species, respectively. Kids were more likely to have lesions on the gums and tongue than older animals.[51] Contagious ecthyma is endemic in northeastern Brazil.[52] One lamb flock affected by an orf outbreak in addition to the signs of crusty nostrils, lips, and muzzle had significant facial swelling with pitting edema. The disease ran its course but the healed animals showed some hair loss at the sites of the facial edema.[53] While most cases of orf have healing of the clinical lesions in weeks there is a report of sheep showing clinical signs for as long as 6 months. The scabs of the chronic form were well adhered to the skin and caused bleeding when removed.[54]

One survey of 48 goat flocks in Argentina found that 81.2% identified contagious ecthyma as an infectious disease problem on the premises.[55] There has been a report of orf in five sheep from three flocks in the United States that exhibited proliferative skin lesions on the limbs that were painful to touch and caused the sheep to be reluctant to move. The lesions did not spontaneously resolve as is the case with most cases of orf. The disease also appeared to be less contagious than classic orf in sheep. All these animals were euthanized after lack of response to imperative treatment with antibiotics and topical medications, or spontaneous resolution of signs. This stresses that while this disease is usually diagnosed on clinical signs and course of disease, not all cases are classic.[56]

Contagious ecthyma has been reported in several species of cervidae and there are case reports of human disease (orf) that have been contracted from exposure to cervidae.[29] Pox virus has also been reported from white-tailed deer in Florida.[29] Diagnosis is rare and treatment is limited to benign neglect unless secondary bacterial infection is suspected, in which case systemic antibiotics may be helpful. Prevention through vaccination may be helpful in affected herds, but proof of disease and the subsequent use of either sheep vaccine or an autogenous vaccine should be carefully considered before implementing.

Bluetongue

Bluetongue is an arthropod-transmitted orbivirus that affects all ruminants. Clinical signs are seen more often in sheep than other ruminants. Animals infected by Bluetongue can show reproductive disorders but the disease is discussed here because vasculitis causes clinical signs associated with the head and oral cavity, as well as other organs. Rarely, the tongue may indeed be cyanotic (or blue), but more commonly, there will be edema present in the muzzle. Oral lesions may include erosions progressing to ulcers of the dental pad and commissures of the lips. While this is not a thorough description of Bluetongue, it is included here because the disease belongs on the differential list of viral diseases causing oral lesions. Treatment is basically supportive care, especially feeding, in cases where the mouth becomes very sore due to the oral ulcers.[57]

Bluetongue causes economic losses from mortality, reduced production, poor wool growth, and reduced reproductive performance including ram infertility.[44] In domestic ruminants, sheep may be more frequently affected with clinical signs than other animals. The clinical signs of bluetongue are associated with injury to small blood vessels. Fetal infection can be due to transplacental transmission.[58,59]

Bluetongue vaccines are being developed and show some promise, but at time of writing, there are no commercially available vaccines.[60,61] Successful vaccines may be useful in Bluetongue endemic areas to limit the economic impact of this condition.

Bluetongue (BT) virus and epizootic hemorrhagic disease virus (EHD) cause similar disease in white-tailed and mule deer and are difficult to distinguish from each other. Hemorrhagic disease is the most appropriate terminology but regionally, it is usually referred to as BT or EHD. This arthropod-borne orbivirus causes severe losses in both wild and farmed cervidae and has several serotypes that affect the animal systemically. Morbidity and mortality rates may vary depending on region and serotype, but morbidity of 90% or more is commonly reported, with matching mortality rates. Control of the midge through management of breeding sites, flight paths, and feeding areas may be effective. Application of insecticides directly to the animals or to site barriers where the midges land may also be effective. Fogging, misting, or spraying of premises with insecticides is done by many producers in endemic areas. Worries of resistance and killing of nontarget species are the two main concerns with this approach. Vaccination is currently either through autogenous vaccines or experimental vaccines. Serotype cross protection is not effective, so vaccines either have to contain the proper antigens or have core antigen capability. New vaccines are expected in the very near future that will hopefully prevent this disease (Lee Constaedt, Personal Communication, March 23, 2018).

Diseases of the Esophagus

The esophagus is dorsal to the trachea in the anterior one-third of the neck, then is found just to the left of the trachea until moving dorsal again near the thoracic inlet. The thoracic esophagus passes in the mediastinum, dorsal to the base of the heart and tracheal bifurcation. Then it continues straight back through the mediastinum ventral to the aorta and through the esophageal hiatus of the diaphragm. The outer layer of the esophagus in the cervical region is adventitia, while serosa covers the thoracic and peritoneal parts of the esophagus. The muscular tunic of the esophagus is made of striated muscles in outer and inner layers of spiral fibers. The muscular layer readily separates from the submucosa and mucosa when incised. The submucosa is very loose while the mucosa is normally in longitudinal folds in the normal relaxed esophagus. The folds obviously flatten as the esophagus dilates for passage of food material. The vascular supply to the esophagus is segmental with little collateral circulation which makes it very important to preserve vasculature when performing surgical intervention with the esophagus.[12,62]

Esophageal Obstruction

The lumen of the esophagus narrows at the thoracic inlet and again at the esophageal hiatus of the diaphragm.[62] These two areas are the common areas where choke will occur. Obstruction of the esophagus is less common in small ruminants than in cattle. A review of esophageal obstruction in cattle suggested manual retrieval of obstructing material from the anterior esophagus rather than pushing the obstruction into the rumen when the distal esophagus was occluded.[63,64] Esophageal obstruction is more common in sheep than goats. Fortunately, choke in sheep is usually due to feed pellets being consumed too quickly for saliva to moisten it. As such, most of the obstruction caused by feed will resolve relatively quickly as the feed becomes moist in the esophagus. Affected animals may look anxious and be salivating because of the inability to swallow. Because of the normal ruminant physiology and need to eructate, the ruminant with a complete esophageal obstruction will develop ruminal bloat.[65] The practitioner should first attempt to pass a stomach tube to resolve the obstruction. A mouth gag should be used to hold the mouth open and the well-lubricated stomach tube should be carefully passed to avoid causing more trauma to the esophagus. If this is not successful and the animal is bloating, one should quickly perform a rumenostomy to relieve the bloat or at least decompress the rumen via a large gauge needle (or intravenous catheter) placed into the rumen through the left flank. While the catheter may be quicker, it may also allow contamination of the abdominal cavity with rumen contents.

The emergency rumenostomy can be performed with a small volume of lidocaine for local anesthesia in the left flank. A 2-inch skin and body wall incision is adequate to grasp the distended rumen and exteriorize it enough to secure the serosal layer to the muscular body wall with four sections of continuous absorbable suture. The rumen may then be incised and the mucosal layer sutured to the skin. This rumenostomy can be reversed once the esophageal obstruction and secondary bloat have been resolved (see Chapter 5).

If the obstruction does not resolve on its own in a reasonable period of time (hours), further intervention is warranted. One may again carefully attempt to pass a stomach tube to break down the obstruction. Another method is to anesthetize the animal and intubate with the cuff inflated to prevent aspiration as one passes a stomach tube to the obstruction to lavage the esophagus in an effort to hydrate and break down the obstruction. One may also attempt to massage the obstruction toward the mouth during this lavage. Obstructions of prolonged duration may lead to mucosal damage of the esophagus and subsequent scarring with stricture formation.[66] A stricture may lead to future obstructions and mean a poor prognosis for the animal.

Esophagotomy

If the esophageal obstruction does not resolve with conservative management, surgery may be indicated.[67] An esophagotomy is not a commonly done procedure, and as such, the practitioner may wish to refer any animal valuable enough to pursue this treatment rather than attempt it under less than ideal situations. This is especially true since an esophagotomy is not an emergency procedure in the ruminant; a more commonly done and less difficult rumenostomy can prevent life-threatening aspects of esophageal obstruction allowing release of ruminal gases and allowing a path to meet caloric and hydration needs of the animal with a complete esophageal obstruction.[68] With that said, the esophagotomy is best done with the animal under general anesthesia for ease of exposure and closure (see Chapter 18). The surgery is done with the animal in dorsal recumbency. An orogastric tube is passed to the level of the obstruction to help identify the proper location. Alternatively, an endoscope may be placed into the esophagus to the level of the obstruction. This allows visualization of the obstruction as well as transillumination of light to direct the incision and dissection. It is preferable to make the esophageal incision immediately distal to the obstruction in healthy esophageal tissue. An obstruction near the thoracic inlet may dictate that the esophageal incision be made proximal to the obstruction. This allows for primary closure of the healthy tissue or gives the option of leaving the esophageal incision open as an esophagostomy to facilitate feeding while allowing the inflamed part of the esophagus to return to normal before the temporary esophagostomy heals by second intention. This point is actually less critical in ruminants since the rumenostomy can provide the same feeding access.

Primary closure of an esophagotomy incision can be more difficult to manage in ruminants than other species because of the eructation done by ruminants. Non-ruminant species would be held off food and water while providing parental fluids for several days to allow healing of the incision. Upon incision, the mucosa easily separates from the muscular layer of the esophagus. The mucosa is the holding layer of the esophageal closure. It is recommended that the mucosa be closed with small suture in a simple continuous pattern with knots in the lumen. The muscular layer can then be closed. Care should be taken to preserve the blood supply of the esophagus. The skin and muscles should be closed in a routine manner. A drain should be placed next to the esophagus to remove (and detect) any leakage from the esophageal closure.[69]

Megaesophagus

Megaesophagus was reported in a 2-year-old goat that presented with intermittent regurgitation and swelling of the distal neck. The diagnosis was made by endoscopic examination and positive contrast radiographs. The animal was not treated.[70] The diagnosis is suspected based on clinical signs but contrast radiography is useful in making the definitive diagnosis.[71]

Megaesophagus has been reported in two sheep and two goats,[72] a ram,[73] and is uncommonly seen in other ruminants.[65] The most common clinical sign associated with megaesophagus is regurgitation soon after eating.[73]

Miscellaneous Esophageal Conditions

The esophagus can have diverticulum formation following trauma from intraluminal obstruction or extraluminal injury. The diverticulum can cause obstruction by allowing food stuffs to pack into the lesion. The diverticula are described as traction or pulsion depending on shape. Clinical signs may be distention of the esophagus noted in the neck area or recurrent, usually mild, esophageal obstruction. The practitioner may see the diverticulum with endoscopy, but contrast radiographs are the best way to identify the type and full extent of the diverticulum.

There is a report of a kid presenting shortly after birth with a subcutaneous swelling that when aspirated contained milk. Aspiration would decrease the size of the swelling but it enlarged again after nursing. Further examination determined the kid to have a congenital fistula of the proximal esophagus that communicated with the subcutaneous space.[74] This particular lesion is certainly rare but goats tend to be prone to a number of congenital conditions.

The authors acknowledge the work of Dr. Debra K Baird on the previous edition of book in this chapter.

References

1. Spence J, Aitchison G: Clinical aspects of dental disease in sheep. In Boden E, editor: *Sheep and goat practice*, London, 1991, Bailliere Tindall.
2. Bruere AN, West DM: Dental abnormalities. In *The sheep: health, disease & production*, Palmerston North, New Zealand, 1993, Foundation for Continuing Education of the NZ Veterinary Association.
3. Scott PR: Digestive system. In *Sheep Medicine*, London, 2007, Manson Publishing.
4. Patel KK, Howe L, Heuer C, Asher GW, Wilson PR: Pregnancy and mid-term abortion rates in farmed red deer in New Zealand, *Anim Reprod Sci* 193:140–152, 2018.
5. Tan YK, Khairuddin NH, Hiew MWH: Urinary bladder rupture secondary to obstructive urolithiasis in a Jamnapari goat, *J Vet Malays* 29(2):20–24, 2017.
6. Haro M, Zongo M Bazie A, et al: Ultrasonographic imagery of mammary gland of the goat in lactation, *Int J Biol Chem Sci* 11(3):1307–1314, 2017.
7. Scott PR: Thoracic ultrasonography as an adjunct to clinical examination in sheep, *Small Rumin Res* 152:107–118, 2017.
8. Fasulkov I, Karadaev M, Vasilev N, Nikolov M: Application of colour Doppler and three-dimensional (3D) ultrasonography for visualization of mammary gland structures in goats, *Small Rumin Res* 162:43–47, 2018.
9. Jhirwal SK, Satyaveer S, Munna L: Surgical management of oesophageal diverticulum in a heifer buffalo, *Intas Polivet* 17(2): 619–620, 2016.
10. Park HyunAh, Kim JuWon, Park HeeMyung: Characteristics of esophageal diverticula using computed tomography and three-dimensional reconstruction in a Maltese dog, *J Vet Med Sci* 74(9):1233–1236, 2012.
11. Tejas S, Parikh PV, Patil DB, et al: Endoscopic diagnosis of oesophageal affections in 12 dogs, *Indian J Vet Surg* 37(2):130–132, 2016.
12. Habel RE: Ruminant digestive system. In Getty R, editor: *Sisson and grossman's the anatomy of the domestic animals*, ed 5, Philadelphia, 1975, W. B. Saunders.
13. Cocquyt G, Broeck W, van den Driessen B, Simoens P: Variations of the canine teeth in sheep, *Vlaam Diergeneeskundig Tijdschr* 72(5):332–339, 2003.
14. Matthews J: The geriatric goat. In *Diseases of the Goat*, ed 3, Oxford, 2009, Wiley-Blackwell.
15. Bloxham GP, Purton DG: Demineralisation and incisor wear: an *in vitro* study, *NZ J Agric Res* 34:277–279, 1991.
16. Erjavec V, Crossley D: Initial observations of cheek tooth abnormalities in sheep in Slovenia, *Vet Rec* 167(4):134–137, 2010.
17. West DM, Spence JA: Disease of the oral cavity. In Martin WB, Aitken ID, editor: *Disease of sheep*, ed 3, Oxford, 2000, Blackwell Science Ltd.
18. Altug N, Arslan S, Yuksek N, et al: The levels of trace elements and selected vitamins in goats with chronic fluorosis. *Turk J Vet Anim Sci* 37(5):529–534, 2013.
19. Aydin N, Dede S, Tanritanir P: The distribution of minerals in some tissues of sheep with fluorosis, *Fluoride* 47(1):43–48, 2014.
20. Kerkmann A, Kuiper H, Ganter M, Distl O: Review of literature and results from test matings of East Friesian milk sheep affected with brachygnathia inferior, *Berl Munch Tierarztl Wochenschr* 121(7/8):292–305, 2008.
21. Lievaart-Peterson K, Luttikholt SJM, van den Brom R, Vellema P: Schmallenberg virus infection in small ruminants — first review of the situation and prospects in Northern Europe, *Small Rumin Res* 106(2/3):71–76, 2012.
22. DeBowes RM: Brachynathia. In White NA, Moore JN, editors: *Current practice of equine surgery*, Grand Rapids, 1990, JB Lippincott.
23. Flis M: Double anomaly in the male roe deer dentition (*Capreolus Capreohts* L) — a case study, *Zycie Weter* 89(2)151–152, 2014.
24. Giannitti F, Anderson M, Miller M, et al: Chlamydia pecorum fetal and placental lesions in sporadic caprine abortion, *J Vet Diagn Invest* 28(2):184–189, 2016.
25. Kaçar C, Ozcan K, Takci I, Gürbulak K, Ozen H, Karaman M: Diprosopus, craniorachischisis, arthrogryposis, and other associated anomalies in a stillborn lamb, *J Vet Sci* 9(4):429–431, 2008.
26. Faez Firdaus JA, Chung LimTeik, Abba Y, et al: Left temporomandibular joint luxation in a Boer goat — a case report, *Int J Livest Res* 5(5):98–102, 2015.
27. Yeruham I, Elad D: Necrotizing stomatitis associated with *Fusobacterium necrophorum* in two goats, *J Vet Med B Infect Dis Vet Public Health* 51(1):46–47, 2004.
28. Sant'Ana FJF de, Garcia EC, Rabelo RE, Costa YL da, Schild AL, Riet-Correa F: Oropharyngeal and neurologic lesions in sheep associated with the use of drenching guns, *Pesquisa Veterinaria Brasileira* 27:7, 282-286, 2007.
29. Davidson WR, Nettles VF: Field manual of wildlife diseases in the southeastern united states, ed 2, Athens, GA, 1997, Southeastern Cooperative Wildlife Disease Study, College of Veterinary Medicine, University of Georgia.
30. Brooks JW, Kumar A, Narayanan S, et al: Characterization of Fusobacterium isolates from the respiratory tract of white-tailed deer (*Odocoileus virginianus*), *J Vet Diagn Invest* 26(2):213–220, 2014.

31. Gardner DG, Orr MB: Dentigerous cysts (ovine odontogenic cysts) in sheep, *N Z Vet J* 38:148–150, 1990.
32. Verstraete FJM, Zin BP, Kass PH, Cox DP, Jordan RC: Clinical signs and histologic findings in dogs with odontogenic cysts: 41 cases (1995-2010), *J Am Vet Med Assoc* 239(11):1470–1476, 2011.
33. Delaunois-Vanderperren H: Congenital odontogenic keratocyst in a filly, *Equine Vet Educ* 25(4):179–183, 2013.
34. Alcigir ME, Vural SA: A case of odontogenic inflammatory dentigerous cyst in a calf: macroscopic and histopathological findings, *Bulg J Vet Med* 15(2):137–141, 2012.
35. Hetal P, Abhineet L: Unilateral maxillary swelling: a retrospective study, *Indian J Otolaryngol Head Neck Surg* 62(4):403–407, 2010.
36. Matthews J: External swellings. In *Disease of the goat*, ed 3, Oxford, 2009, Wiley-Blackwell.
37. Smith BP: Foot-and-mouth disease. In Smith BP, editor: *Large animal internal* medicine, ed 3, St. Louis, 2002, Mosby.
38. Watson P: Differential diagnosis of oral lesions and FMD in sheep, *In Pract* 26(4):182–191, 2004.
39. Mansoor MK, Al-Rawahi AH, El-Tahir HA, et al: Concurrent vaccination of goats with foot and mouth disease (FMD) and peste des petits ruminants (PPR) booster vaccines, *Trop Anim Health Prod* 50(1):1–3, 2018.
40. Raouf YA, Yousif H, Almutlab AA, et al: Role of small ruminants in the epidemiology of foot-and-mouth disease in Sudan. *Bull Anim Health Prod Afr* 5(1):145–156, 2017.
41. Donaldson AI, Sellers RF: Foot-and-mouth disease. In Martin WB, Aitken ID, editors: *Disease of sheep*, ed 3, Oxford, England, 2000, Oxford, Blackwell Science Ltd.
42. Cottral GE, Callis JJ: Foot-and-mouth disease. In Commission on Foreign Animal Disease, editor: *Foreign animal diseases, their diagnosis and control*, Richmond, VA, 1975, US Animal Health Association.
43. Geering WA: Foot-and-mouth disease in sheep, *Aust Vet J* 43: 485–489, 1967.
44. Scott PR: Miscellaneous diseases. In *Sheep medicine*, London, 2007, Manson Publishing.
45. Gibson CF, Donaldson AI, Ferris NP: Response of sheep vaccinated with large doses of vaccine to challenge by airborne foot-and-mouth disease virus, *Vaccine* 2:157–161, 1984.
46. Donaldson AI: Foot-and-mouth disease: the principal features, *Ir Vet J* 41:325–327, 1987.
47. Michelsen PGE: Contagious ecthyma. In Smith BP, editor: *Large animal internal medicine*, ed 3, St. Louis, 2002, Mosby.
48. Nettleton PF, Gilray JA, Yirrell DL, Scott GR, Reid HW: Natural transmission of orf virus from clinically normal ewes to orf-naïve sheep, *Vet Rec* 139:364–366, 1996.
49. Kromer C, Bierschenk C, Czerny CP, Schön MP, Buhl T: Orf (ecthyma contagiosum) in a sheep and a shepherd, *Lancet Infect Dis* 18(1):122, 2018.
50. Bergqvist C, Kurban M, Abbas O: Orf virus infection, *Rev Med Virol* 27(4):e1932, 2017.
51. Ramesh A, Babu SS, Saravanabave K, Vadivoo VS, Premalatha N: Confirmatory diagnosis of contagious ecthyma by PCR and electron microscopy, *Indian Vet J* 86(8):770–772, 2009.
52. Nobrega JE Jr, Macedo JT, Araujo JA, et al: Contagious ecthyma in sheep and goats in the semiarid of Paraiba, Brazil, *Pesqui Vet Bras* 28(3):135–139, 2008.
53. Casey MJ, Robinson JHM, Sammin DJ: Severe facial oedema associated with orf in an Irish sheep flock, *Vet Rec* 161(17):600, 2007.
54. Housawi FMT: Chronic and acute natural sheep orf infection: comparative clinic-pathological observations, *Vet Med J Giza* 56(1):89–96, 2008.
55. Bedotti DO, Sanchez Rodriguez M: Observations on animal health problems of goats in the west of the province of La Pampa (Argentina), *Vet Argent* 19(182):100–112, 2002.
56. Smith GW, Scherba G, Constable PD, Hsiao V, Behr MJ, Morin DE: Atypical parapoxvirus infection in sheep. *J Vet Intern Med* 16(3):287–292, 2002.
57. Michelsen PGE: Bluetongue. In Smith BP, editor: *Large animal internal medicine*, ed 3, St. Louis, 2002, Mosby.
58. Maclachlan NJ, Drew CP, Darpel KE, Worwa G: The pathology and pathogenesis of bluetongue, *J Comp Pathol* 141(1):1–16, 2009.
59. Worwa G, Hilbe M, Ehrensperger F, et al: Experimental transplacental infection of sheep with bluetongue virus serotype 8, *Vet Rec* 164(16):499–500, 2009.
60. Niedbalski W, Fitzner A: New generation vaccines against bluetongue virus, *Med Weter* 74(6):377–382, 2018.
61. Pandey AB, Nandi S, Audarya SD, et al: Monovalent inactivated bluetongue virus type 1 vaccine induced neutralising antibody response in sheep, *Ind J Small Rumin* 24(1):89–94, 2018.
62. König HE, Liebich HG: Digestive system. In König HE, Liebach HG, editors: *Veterinary anatomy of domestic mammals*, ed 3, Stuttgart, 2007, Schattauer.
63. Patil AS, Venkanna B, Vaagheesh C, et al: Retrospective studies on occurrence and surgical management of esophageal obstruction in bovines, *Intas Polivet* 18(2):286–292, 2017.
64. Mahesh V, Pramodh JK, Ranganath L, et al: Clinical management of esophageal choke — a clinical study of 25 cattle, *Intas Polivet* 17(2):607–610, 2016.
65. Guard C: Choke and esophageal disorders In BP, editor: *Large animal internal medicine*, ed 3, Smith., St. Louis, 2002, Mosby.
66. Husnik R, Kralova-Kovarikova S, Schanilec P, et al: Stricture as a complication of esophageal obstruction by a foreign body, *Veterinarstvi* 61(12):691–697, 2011.
67. Raut SU, Aher VD: Surgical management of oesophageal obstruction in a goat, *Intas Polivet* 18(2):307–308, 2017.
68. Sankar P, Kumar RVS, Lakshmi ND, et al: Surgical management of cervical esophageal obstruction in a goat (*Capra hircus*) — a case report, *Ind J Anim Res* 44(2):153–154, 2010.
69. Stick JA: Esophageal obstruction. In White NA, Moore JN, editors: *Current practice of equine surgery*, Grand Rapids, 1990, JB Lippincott.
70. Mozaffari AA, Vosough D: Idiopathic megaesophagus in a goat: clinical and radiologic features, *Iran J Vet Surg* 2(4):94–97, 2007.
71. Silva Junior LC, Arruda LCP, Silva DGB, et al: Clinical and radiographic analyses of a goat with megaesophagus, *Arquivo Brasileiro de Medicina Veterinaria e Zootecnia* 63(3):761–764, 2011.
72. Nascimento EM, Campos EM, Maia LA, et al: Megaesophagus in sheep and goats, *Ciencia Rural* 46(3):1450–1455, 2016.
73. Braun U, Steiger R, Flückiger M, Bearth G, Guscetti F: Regurgitation due to megaesophagus in a ram, *Can Vet J* 31:391–392, 1990.
74. Prasad A, Dharmaceelan AS, George RS, William BJ: Congenital esophageal diverticulum in a kid, *Tamilnadu J Vet Anim Sci* 4(1):29, 2008.

5 Diseases of the Gastrointestinal System

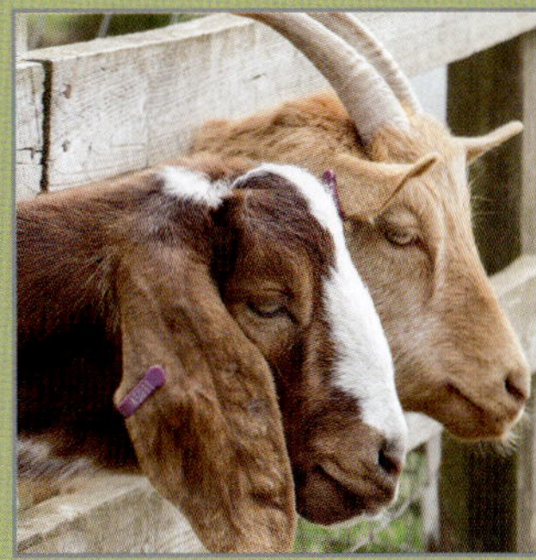

JENNA E. BAYNE AND MISTY A. EDMONDSON

Infectious and noninfectious diseases of the gastrointestinal tract (GIT) are very common in small ruminants. A complete history and thorough physical examination are of utmost importance in the characterization of gastrointestinal disease in small ruminants, with attention made during the physical examination to body condition score (BCS), abdominal contour, manure characteristics, and motility of the reticulorumen. Combined use of auscultation, percussion, and ballottement over the entire abdomen should be carried out, especially given preclusion of rectal palpation in sheep, goats, and most cervids. Even with a complete physical examination, localizing the exact nature of GIT disease can be difficult. The physical examination can be augmented using ancillary tests, including the assessment of clinicopathological parameters including rumen fluid evaluation, as well as the use of imaging modalities. If indicated, an exploratory laparotomy can serve both as a diagnostic and therapeutic tool.

Diagnostic Procedures

Basic Laboratory Studies

Basic clinicopathological analyses include a complete blood cell count (CBC), serum biochemistry, and urinalysis. These tests, along with diagnostic imaging, help define the differential list generated from the physical examination. Furthermore, they can be helpful in determining the severity of disease, prognosis, and response to therapy with serial evaluation. Rarely, a specific disease is identified based on clinicopathological tests. Usefulness of the CBC includes the evaluation of the erythrogram and leukogram to characterize the severity of anemia, dehydration, and inflammatory response. Interpretation of the packed cell volume (PCV) should be done in conjunction with total protein concentration as well as the estimation of dehydration on physical examination. An anemic or dehydrated hypoproteinemic animal may have a normal PCV and total protein. Both the CBC and serum biochemistry can be helpful in determining the presence and severity of an inflammatory disease process. Changes in the total and differential white blood cell counts indicate acute or chronic inflammation, ranging from neutropenia and a degenerative left shift to a mature neutrophilia. Increases in globulins or fibrinogen suggest a chronic inflammatory disease. Low protein levels, especially albumin, need to be further evaluated for the potential of chronic blood loss due to gastrointestinal parasitism, infiltrative bowel disease, liver dysfunction, third-space compartmentalization, or protein loss through the kidneys. Liver disease should be suspected if liver enzymes or bilirubin levels are increased. However, liver enzyme concentrations can be normal in the presence of chronic liver disease. Also, albumin levels rarely drop in ruminants with liver disease as they do in other species. Liver function tests may be performed, including measurement of bile acids and blood ammonia concentrations. Point-of-care (POC) meters for the stall-side measurement of blood glucose, L-lactate, and ketone concentrations have been evaluated in cattle and small ruminants.[1–4] Urine strips for the detection of ketone bodies are also useful in monitoring ewes and does at risk for pregnancy toxemia. Changes in electrolytes are common with gastrointestinal diseases, especially in anorexic animals or those with profound diarrhea. Electrolyte measurements are also useful in the formulation of treatment plans. Although abomasal disease is rare in small ruminants, a metabolic alkalosis with hypochloremia and hypokalemia may be observed. Gastrointestinal stasis can result in hypokalemia, hypochloremia, and a mild hypocalcemia. In the case of surgical intestinal obstructions, small ruminants can develop severe metabolic acidosis due to ischemic necrosis of tissues and shock. The major biochemical changes commonly associated with diarrhea are metabolic acidosis, with the loss of sodium and bicarbonate in diarrheic feces, and the presence of azotemia and hypoproteinemia. Renal disease should be ruled out in these cases.

Normal ranges for clinicopathologic laboratory values are available in Appendix II, Tables 1 to 5 and are published elsewhere. However, familiarity should be made with normal values of both a CBC and serum biochemistry as established by the laboratory commonly used for analyses in their practice.

Rumen Fluid Analysis

Rumen fluid analysis is useful in characterizing the health of the forestomach and aids in differentiation of diseases, including types of vagal indigestion, ruminal acidosis, and potential intoxications. Collection of rumen fluid can be via orogastric or nasogastric intubation or percutaneous rumenocentesis. Regardless of method chosen, proper restraint of the animal and suitable equipment (Figure 5.1) should be used to avoid trauma to the esophagus or abdominal viscera and damage of equipment (e.g., chewed tubes). To perform percutaneous rumenocentesis, a 16- to 18-gauge, 3-inch (7.6-cm) needle is inserted into the rumen fluid below the fiber mat. The site for rumenocentesis can be estimated by ballottement or percussion of the left flank (approximately 5–10 cm

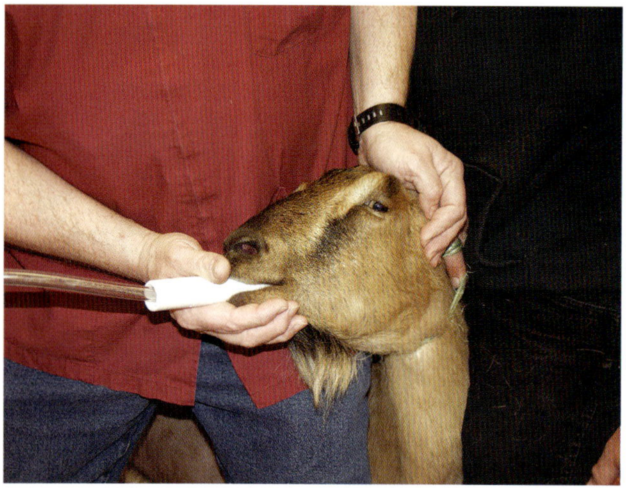

• **Fig. 5.1** Passage of an orogastric tube through a mouth speculum made from a polyvinylchloride (PVC) pipe. To avoid oral and esophageal trauma, the animal should be well restrained, and the tube should be lubricated and passed slowly down the esophagus.

caudal to the last rib along an imaginary line drawn at the level of the patella)[5] or, alternatively, at a ventral location caudal to the xiphoid and to the left of midline.[6] Use of sedation and/or a local block with 2% lidocaine may be necessary in fractious or patients likely to struggle. The site is clipped and aseptically prepared. The needle is introduced forcefully, in one swift motion. Once the rumen is entered, fluid is aspirated with a syringe. If the needle becomes obstructed with ingesta, a small amount of air or fluid should be forced backed through the needle. Rumenocentesis carries the advantage of avoiding salivary contamination of the sample, which can occur during orogastric intubation, as well as possibly being less stressful to the animal. The procedure does carry a slight risk of peritonitis, which is minimized through proper restraint. Rumenocentesis is contraindicated in pregnant females.[5,6]

Once collected, rumen fluid is analyzed for color, odor, pH, motility and types of protozoal species present, methylene blue reduction (MBR) time, Gram-staining characteristics, and chloride concentration. Normal rumen fluid characteristics are listed in Table 5.1. The pH of rumen fluid can be measured on pH strips with 0.5 increments or the use of sophisticated handheld meters. The sample pH will be falsely increased with salivary contamination.[7] Microscopic examination of a drop of fresh, warm fluid under a cover slip examined at 40× to 100× allows visualization of protozoa species, with no special staining required (Figure 5.2). Routine Gram staining is performed on a dried, fixed slide.[5] The MBR reflects the activity of bacterial fermentation in the rumen. It is performed by mixing 1 mL of 0.03% methylene blue with 20 mL of rumen fluid at normal body temperature and measuring the time required to return to the appearance of a control tube.[5] Rumen chloride concentrations can be determined from the supernatant of a centrifuged sample. Rumen chloride concentrations are minimally impacted by saliva contamination and a time lag between sample collection and analysis.[5] Normal rumen fluid is aromatic, olive to brownish-green, and has a pH between 6.5 to 7.5 depending on the diet fed. Microorganisms include a mixed population of large and small protozoal species with active motility and a predominance of gram-negative rods. Normal rumen chloride concentration is less than 30 mEq/L and MBR should be less than 6 minutes.[6] Changes observed in anorexic ruminants include thinner, darker

TABLE 5.1 Normal Rumen Fluid Characteristics of Sheep and Goats.

Characteristic	Normal Finding
Color	Green
Odor	Aromatic
pH[a]	6.5–7.5
Protozoa[b]	Mixed sizes and species rapidly moving
Methylene blue reduction time[c]	3–6 minutes
Gram stain	Gram-negative rods predominate
Rumen chloride	Less than 25–30 mEq/L

[a]Use pH paper with at least 0.5-unit gradations.
[b]Place a drop of fluid on a warm slide and cover with a coverslip. Examine under 100× magnification.
[c]Mix one part 0.03% methylene blue to 20 parts rumen fluid. Measure time for blue color to clear to match a control tube of fluid.
Data from Nordlund KV, Garrett EF: Rumenocentesis: a technique for collecting rumen fluid for diagnosis of subacute rumen acidosis in dairy herds. *Bovine Pract.* 28:109, 1994; Keefe GP, Ogilvie TH: Comparison of oro-ruminal probe and rumenocentesis for prediction of rumen pH in dairy cattle, Proceedings of the 30th Annual American Association of Bovine Practice Convention, 1997, 168; Smith MC, Sherman DM: *Goat medicine,* 2nd ed., Ames, Iowa: Wiley-Blackwell, 2009

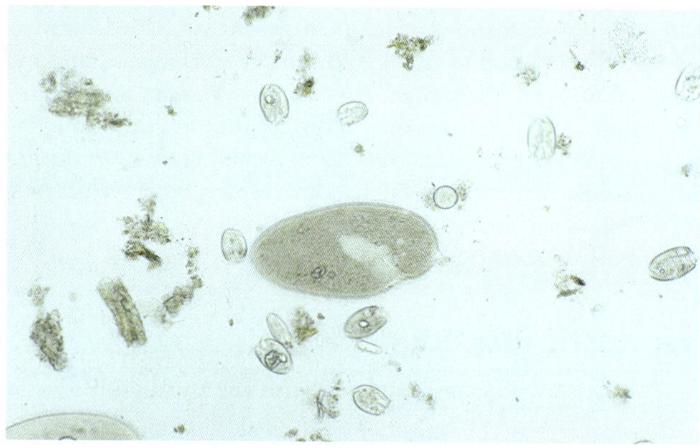

• **Fig. 5.2** Fluid obtained by rumenocentesis should be examined for both bacteria and protozoa. A drop of rumen fluid is placed on a microscopic slide and viewed under a coverslip. At low power (40×), normal rumen fluid will be observed to contain 35 to 40 organisms per field from several populations of protozoa, as seen here. Both low numbers and loss of motility signal a need for medical intervention or transfaunation.

fluid, with an increase in pH (7–7.5), and a reduction in the species and motility of protozoa present. In acute ruminal acidosis, the fluid is fetid, yellow to grey, with a low pH (< 5.2), and dead or no protozoa are present with a predominance of gram-positive rods (*Lactobacillus* species).[5,8] The MBR is prolonged with any type of indigestion/digestive disorder in which inactivity of the microflora is present. Increased rumen chloride concentrates indicate an abomasal or proximal small intestinal obstruction, either functional or mechanical, as a result of the internal reflux of hydrochloric acid from the abomasum into the reticulorumen.[9]

Abdominocentesis

Abdominocentesis is useful in the assessment of abdominal disease in ruminants and aids in the differentiation and diagnosis of ascites, peritonitis, strangulating intestinal lesions, enteritis, uroperitoneum, and abdominal neoplasia. There is normally a small amount of transudative fluid present in the peritoneal space. Characterization of peritoneal fluid as a transudate (low protein concentration and cell count), modified transudate (normal or mild increase in cell count with increased protein concentration), or exudate (increased protein concentration and cell count) is important from a pathophysiological standpoint and allows refinement of possible differentials for the abdominal disease present. Characteristics of peritoneal fluid from healthy sheep and goats are similar to cattle: transparent, colorless to slightly yellow, < 5 g/dL protein, and less than 5000 to 10,000 cells/mL.[10,11] Peritoneal fluid protein concentration can be measured using a refractometer. Other biochemical analyses may include determination of creatinine (e.g., to diagnose uroperitoneum), L-lactate, D-dimer, and glucose concentrations.[12,13] Cytologic examination is needed to characterize the types of cells present, the morphology of those cells, and to assess the presence of phagocytized bacteria. Typically, the cell population is made up of large mononuclear cells, lymphocytes, and non-degenerative neutrophils. Lymphocytes comprise < 20% of cells present, and a few mast cells or plasma cells may be seen.[10] Both the absolute number and proportion of cell types present need to be considered. Changes in peritoneal fluid cytology following exploratory laparotomy, rumenotomy, and enterotomy are reported in goats.[14–16] Two methods can be used. The first technique involves tapping the cranial abdomen at its lowest point cranial to the umbilicus and slightly to the right of midline (Figure 5.3). This technique is useful in conditions with a significant amount of free fluid such as uroperitoneum. When using the cranial abdominal site, one needs to avoid the prepuce in males and the mammary veins in females.[6] The second technique is a four-quadrant approach, as ruminants are very proficient at walling off inflammatory and infectious foci (e.g., peritonitis), which can hinder successful fluid collection. The two cranial sites are slightly caudal to the xiphoid and medial to the milk veins on both sides. The two caudal sites are slightly cranial to the mammary gland and to the left and right of midline.[5] For either technique, manual restraint with sedation is recommended; the use of real-time ultrasonography may help locate fluid pockets. Importantly, amniocentesis or allantocentesis can occur at these sites during gestation and caution is warranted.

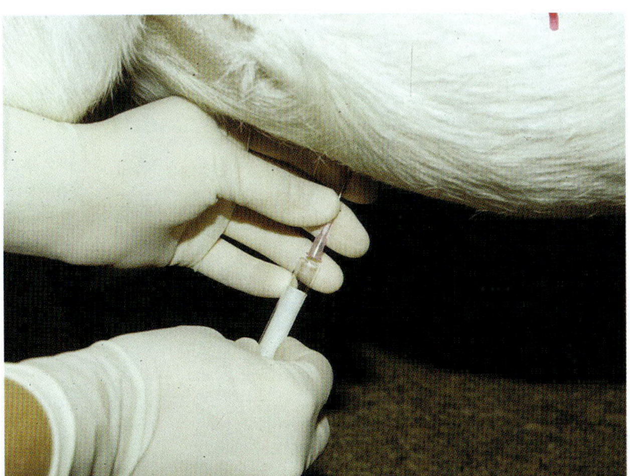

• **Fig. 5.3** Ventral and caudal sites for performing abdominocentesis. The needle indicates the ventral site. The caudal site is the clipped area below the flank.

An 18- to 20-gauge needle or teat cannula can be used for fluid collection. The site should be clipped and prepped using sterile technique and local anesthesia provided when a teat cannula is used. Fluid should be collected in an ethylenediaminetetraacetic acid (EDTA) tube for cytological analysis and a sterile red top tube or suitable inoculation vial for aerobic and anaerobic culture. Abdominal fluid can be difficult to obtain because of the small amounts normally present in both small ruminants. It is important to minimize the ratio of EDTA to fluid in the sample because EDTA can falsely increase the protein levels. Using EDTA tubes made for small animals, filling tubes to at least one-quarter full, or shaking excess EDTA out of large tubes resolves this problem. Air-dried, unstained slides should be prepared and shipped with EDTA tubes for samples shipped to an external laboratory for analysis.[10]

Radiography

Radiography of the abdomen can be performed in small ruminants using small animal techniques. In adult small ruminants, the rumen normally fills the entire abdomen. In cattle, radiography is a useful tool in demonstrating reticular metallic foreign bodies and changes suggestive of traumatic reticuloperitonitis.[17,18] Radiography of the abdomen may also demonstrate the displacement, distortion, distention, or superimposition of abdominal structures, as well as the presence of soft tissue opacities, gas-fluid interfaces, or abnormal gas inclusions.[19] Contrast techniques are useful for diagnosis of atresia of the rectum or colon. Unlike in small animals, contrast techniques are not possible for characterizing small intestinal problems in small ruminants because the rumen dilutes and slows passage of the contrast media.

Ultrasonography

Ultrasonography is well suited for examination of the ruminant GIT and other abdominal viscera. Ultrasonography allows the characterization of contour, dimensions, content, and motility patterns of the forestomach and intestines, as well as the presence of masses, intraluminal and free abdominal fluid, and lesions within the parenchyma of abdominal viscera. Ultrasonography also can be used to guide fluid and tissue sampling for abdominocentesis and biopsy of organs or masses, respectively.[20] Normal parameters for the forestomach compartments, small and large intestines, liver, and spleen have been described in small ruminants.[21,22] Imaging is best achieved using a linear or convex transducer with a frequency of 3.5 to 5.0 MHz. The reticulum is imaged in the cranioventral abdomen, bilaterally, as a crescent-shaped structure immediately adjacent to the diaphragm. Goats demonstrate monophasic, biphasic, and triphasic reticular contractions.[23] The rumen is visualized in the 8th through 12th intercostal spaces (ICS) and flank on the left, and from the 12th ICS and flank on the right. The rumen wall appears as a thick echoic line, and the ability to differentiate the gas cap, fiber mat, and fluid layer is variable. Rumen motility is discerned indirectly by changes seen in layering of the ruminal content. The dorsal and ventral rumen sacs are most easily distinguished caudally by the presence of the longitudinal groove.[24] The omasum is found on the right side from the 6th to 11th ICS (mainly in the 8th and 9th ICS), appears as a crescent-shaped echoic line medial to the liver, and moves passively with respiration due to its proximity to the diaphragm. Due to the gaseous nature of omasal content, the omasal leaves and omasal wall furthest from the transducer cannot be visualized.[25] The abomasum is visualized along the ventral midline and to the left and right paramedian areas as a heterogeneous, moderately echoic structure with echogenic stippling. Visualization of abomasal folds as prominent echoic bands is possible in approximately two-thirds of goats.[26] Examination of the small intestine takes place from the 8th to 12th ICS and the flank on the right side, from dorsal to ventral midline. Similarly, the large intestine (i.e., spiral colon and cecum) is visualized in the right flank. The descending duodenum can be differentiated based on proximity to abdominal wall and location between two serosal layers of greater omentum, whereas the jejunum and ileum cannot be differentiated from each other. Normal luminal diameters and wall thickness of the small intestine are described in normal goats.[27] The spiral colon and cecum are visible in the caudal right flank. The spiral colon often located medial to the small intestine, is garland-like in appearance, and visualization of only the wall closest to the transducer is possible due to intraluminal gas, which is also true of the cecum.[27] Ultrasonography of the liver for position, parenchymal and surface appearance, as well as visualization of the caudal vena cava, portal vein, and gall bladder are evaluated on the right side between the seventh and ninth ICS (largest visible extent of liver) and variably between the fifth to sixth and the 10th to 12th ICS. The parenchymal pattern of the normal liver consists of numerous fine, homogeneous echoes (Figure 5.4). On cross-section, the caudal vena cava is triangular in shape and is visualized in approximately 75% of goats in the 11th and 12th ICS. The portal vein always has a more ventral position and is closer to the liver surface compared with the caudal vena cava. It is circular to oval in cross section, with stellate ramifications into the liver parenchyma, and typically is visualized in all ICS in which liver is visible. The gall bladder is variable in shape and size, depending on amount of bile present and is visualized in most goats from the 9th to 10th ICS.[28] The spleen is visualized on the left side from the 11th and 12th ICS, situated between the rumen and abdominal wall. The parenchymal pattern consists of numerous, homogeneous, weak echogenic shadows.[29] Description of ultrasonography of the urinary and female and male genital tracts can be found in Chapters 12 and 8, respectively.[30]

Other Imaging Modalities

Although limited in its availability to referral centers, characterization of the thorax and abdomen in goats using computed tomography (CT) has been described.[31–34] Use of CT and magnetic resonance imaging (MRI) is of considerable expense and requires general anesthesia in most cases. However, given the use of sheep and goats as animal models for human medicine, as well as the growing popularity of goats as companion animals, the application of these imaging modalities will likely continue to increase.

Laparoscopy

Laparoscopy is more commonly used as a reproductive tool, but it also can be used diagnostically as an alternative to exploratory laparotomy in small ruminants.[17–21] General anesthesia is recommended to allow more inflation of the abdominal cavity and thus a more thorough examination, but laparoscopy can be done with sedation and local anesthesia at portal incision sites. The technique for laparoscopic exploration of the abdomen used for cattle and llamas can be modified for use in sheep, goats, and cervids.[18–21] Laparoscopic evaluation of the abdominal cavity is usually done via a ventral approach with the animal secured in dorsal recumbency. The abdominal cavity can be inflated with CO_2 by a needle, teat cannula, or after placement of a laparoscopic cannula. A time-saving method is to use suture to make a “bite” through the skin and into the external rectus sheath which can be used to tense the body wall. A stab incision can then be made in the skin and external rectus sheath before introducing a guarded trocar

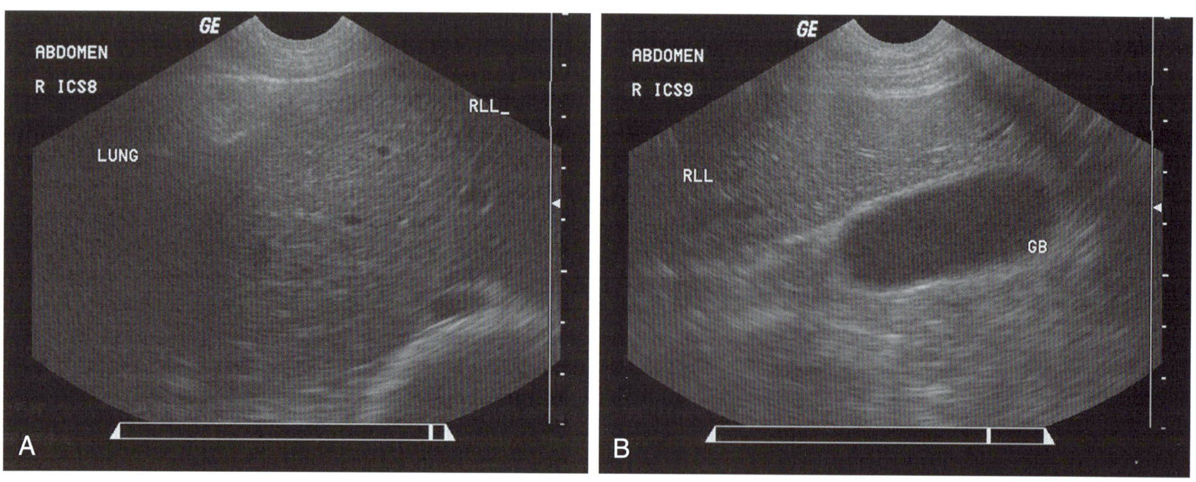

• **Fig. 5.4** **A.** Ultrasound image of the right abdomen obtained from the right eighth intercostal space in a 3-year-old La Mancha cross doe, showing the right liver lobe with the characteristic hepatic and portal veins represented by the small, tubular anechoic structures within the liver parenchyma. The ventral border of the lung is seen on the left side of the image. This ultrasound scan was obtained using a 7-MHz microconvex transducer. Dorsal is to the left of the image. **B.** Ultrasound image of the right abdomen obtained from the right ninth intercostal space of the same animal as in **A**, demonstrating normal right liver lobe and gallbladder. The gallbladder appears as an anechoic, fluid-filled structure directly adjacent to the right liver lobe. This ultrasound scan was obtained using a 7-MHz microconvex transducer. Dorsal is to the left of the image. (Courtesy Dr. Karine Pader, Purdue University.)

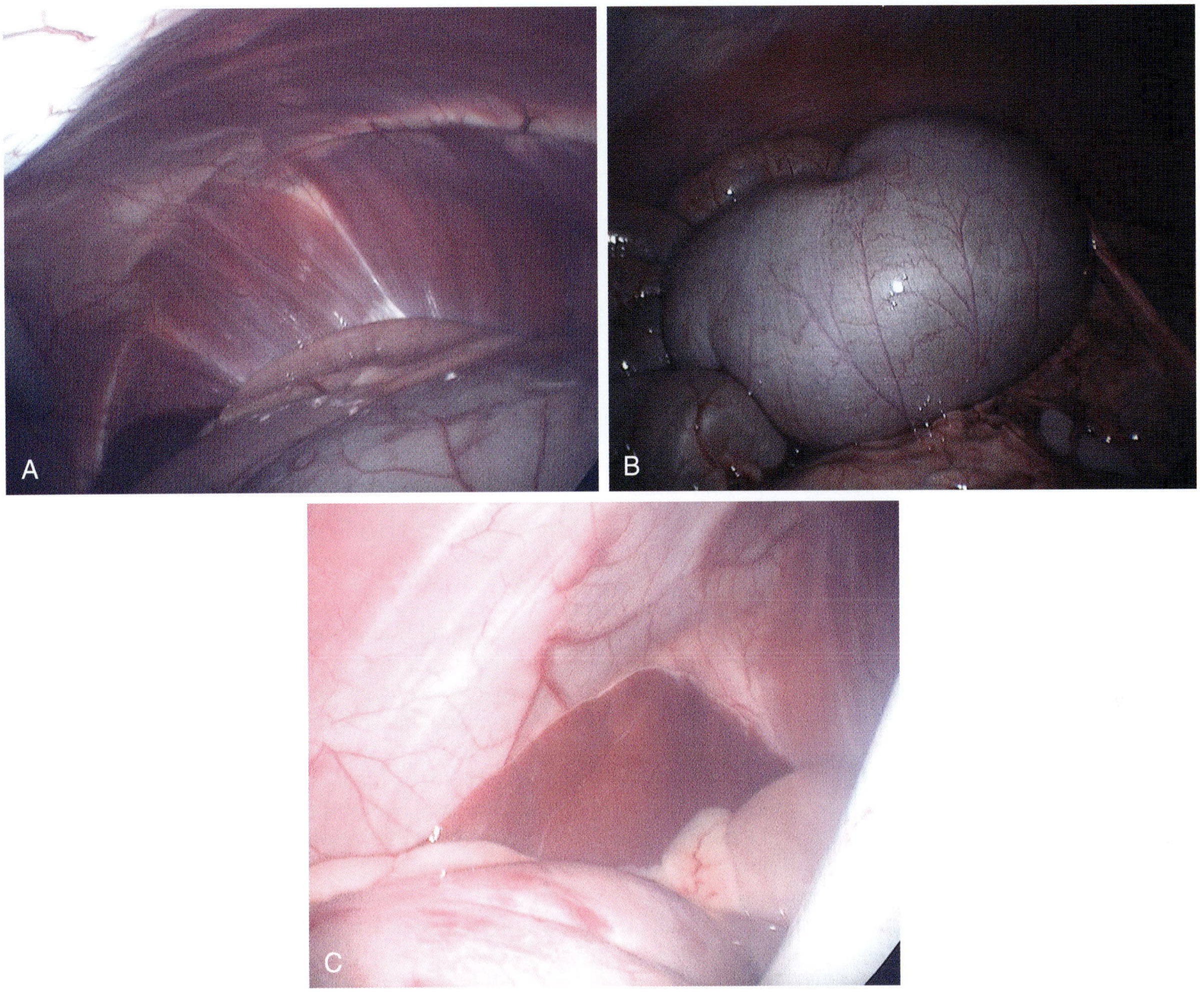

• **Fig. 5.5** A laparoscopic examination (performed using a 10-mm-diameter direct vision scope) of the abdomen in a 2-year-old Pygmy buck. **A.** The muscle fibers of the diaphragm are evident cranially in the center of this photograph. A small part of the liver is in the lower left of the image. **B.** The larger organ in the center of this photograph is the cecum. It normally appears darker in comparison with other portions of the intestine and contains ingesta of a doughy consistency. **C.** This photograph shows part of the liver on the right body wall.

into the abdominal cavity while tensing the abdominal wall with the previously placed suture. The laparoscope can then be placed through the trocar and the abdomen inflated while visualized through the scope. The clinician places the cannula in the inguinal area as described for laparoscopic insemination (see Chapter 8). This technique allows a more efficient use of time and minimizes the likelihood that the omentum will be "ballooned". Laparoscopic placement into the right side allows visualization of most of the abdominal organs (Figure 5.5 A, B, C). Obviously, the clinician should avoid the rumen when introducing the laparoscope into the abdomen. This procedure may be enhanced by lowering the head or rear of the animal, allowing better visualization of the entire abdomen. Visualization of the abdominal cavity and the ability to manipulate organs will be greatly improved by fasting the animal 24 to 48 h or at least decreasing the bulk in the diet. Respiration must be monitored closely, and assisted ventilation should be available during this procedure because inflation of the abdomen and lowering of the head can put pressure on the diaphragm.

Exploratory Laparotomy

Exploratory laparotomy can be a valuable diagnostic tool in evaluating gastrointestinal diseases when other tests indicate abdominal disease. It is often indicated in the ruminants presenting for acute abdomen. In some cases, therapeutic surgical procedures can be performed at the same time. The technique of exploratory laparotomy used in cattle can be adopted for small ruminants with the understanding that these animals are more likely to lie down during surgery. Therefore, standing surgery is the exception, with most performed with the patient in lateral or dorsal recumbency.

For this procedure, small ruminants should be heavily sedated or placed under general anesthesia. Use of a high-volume lumbosacral epidural can augment sedation and minimize the use of inhalant anesthetics needed. The use of perioperative antimicrobials and nonsteroidal antiinflammatories (NSAIDs) should be based on the clinical status of the animal, diagnostic findings found at surgery, as well as the environment in which the surgery takes place. Antimicrobial agents are not necessary for elective exploratory surgery performed aseptically, in a hospital setting, and without complications. However, antimicrobials are indicated under field conditions if infection is present, and if the forestomach or intestinal tract is opened (i.e., clean-contaminated surgery). A combination of ceftiofur (1.1–2.2 mg/kg intravenous/intramuscular/subcutaneous [IV/IM/SC] twice a day) and procaine penicillin G (22,000 IU/kg IM twice a day) or potassium penicillin (22,000 IU/kg, IV, every 6 h) can be administered until clinicopathological tests and bacterial culture results indicate an absence of infection. Use of NSAIDs (e.g., flunixin meglumine, 1.1 to 2.2 mg/kg, IV, every 12–24 h) for pain control and potential antiendotoxemia effects should be utilized when indicated. Other medications for control of pain may be required in some small ruminants, such as the short-term use of opioids (see Chapter 18). Postoperative care should include fluid therapy and rumen support (e.g., transfaunation, B-vitamins, highly palatable diet) in depressed and anorectic patients.

Liver Biopsy

Liver biopsy in sheep, goats, and cervids is performed using a similar technique used in cattle, but access to the liver in small ruminants is more limited. Therefore, whenever possible, ultrasound guidance is recommended. The biopsy is performed in the standing animal that is well restrained and sedation used as necessary. The recommended biopsy site is the ninth intercostal space slightly above an imaginary line drawn from the point of the elbow to the craniodorsal angle of the paralumbar fossa (Figure 5.6).[6] Other techniques, including laparoscopic liver biopsy are described.[35–39] The site should be surgically prepared and a local anesthetic (2% lidocaine) infused subcutaneously. A small scalpel blade is used to make a stab incision through the skin. A 14-gauge, 11.5-cm liver biopsy instrument (e.g., Tru-Cut biopsy needle) is inserted through the incision and the intercostal muscles and into the liver. The biopsy instrument is directed toward the opposite elbow, but the use of real-time ultrasonography greatly aids in determining the direction and depth needed (2 to 4 cm).[5] Perforation of the gall bladder as well as large vessels along the caudal border of the rib should be avoided. Samples can be submitted for culture (in a sterile plastic or glass tube), histopathologic study (in formalin, at a 10:1 ratio of formalin to tissue), or mineral analysis (in a trace element or plastic tube). The laboratory should be contacted for appropriateness of sample containers and specific instructions. When performing a liver biopsy for mineral analysis, the clinician should rinse the biopsy site with distilled and deionized water after sterile preparation to minimize sample contamination. Samples for mineral analysis should not be placed in formalin. Closure of the skin incision can be accomplished by suture or stapling, or if it is small enough, the wound can be left alone to heal by second intention. Fly repellent should be applied to the site as needed. Use of antimicrobials is at the discretion of the veterinarian, and should be considered in regions where *Clostridium novyi* or *Clostridium haemolyticum* are prevalent.[39] Vaccination status for clostridial diseases should be up-to-date, and if there is any doubt, a toxoid vaccine given before or at the time of biopsy.

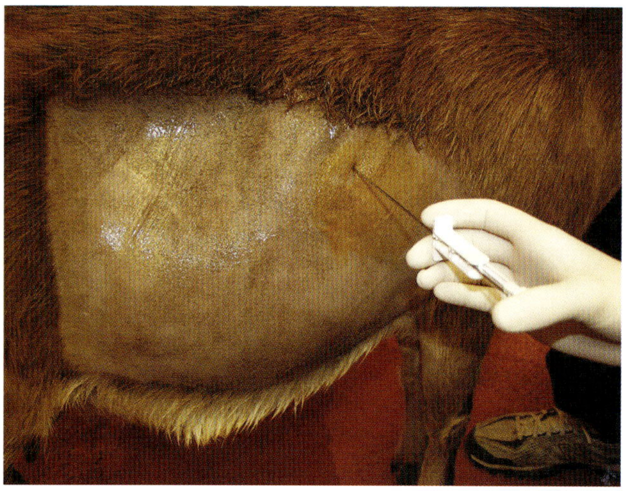

• **Fig. 5.6** Liver biopsy: after the skin is clipped, anesthetized, and aseptically prepared, the surgeon makes a stab incision in the skin and introduces a 14-gauge biopsy needle.

Diseases of the Forestomachs

Bloat

Bloat is less common in sheep compared with cattle, despite sheep having more selective eating habits (e.g., leaves over stems) and a tendency to select legumes over grasses which would promote the occurrence of bloat. Sheep are more tolerant than cattle to non-scabrous diets, as well as more tolerant of increases in intraruminal pressure. Dramatic increases in intraruminal pressure in sheep results in rapid changes in the frequency and type of ruminal contraction patterns responsible for eructation, promoting evacuation of intraruminal gas.[40] Goats are less commonly affected than sheep, and deer are remarkably resistant to bloat.

Bloat results as a failure in eructation of gases produced by microbial fermentation in the rumen. Most commonly, eructation fails because the gas remains trapped as tiny bubbles throughout the rumen ingesta (i.e., frothy bloat).[41] Other variations of this type of bloat include foamy or slime bloat, dependent on the class of animal and diet fed (e.g., high concentrate diets).[42,43] Another type of bloat is the build-up of free gas in the rumen with concurrent failure to eructate (e.g., free-gas bloat).[44] An example is the presence of an intraesophageal foreign body (e.g., potato, sugar beet) impairing eructation.

Pathogenesis. Acute, frothy bloat commonly occurs in animals grazing pastures of bloat-provoking forages. These include alfalfa, clovers (red, white, alsike, ladino, and sweet clover), and certain cereal grains, in contrast to forages relatively resistant to bloat such as sainfoin, birds-foot trefoil, and crown vetch.[45] Field conditions allowing rapid vegetative growth and ingestion of legumes during the vegetative (i.e., prebud) stage pose particular bloat risk, but bloat can occur on dry forage and at full bloom. Bloat-promoting forages are prone to rapid cell disruption and degradation with the release of soluble proteins and other constituents. The highly soluble plant protein ribulose-1,5-bisphosphate carboxylase/oxygenase is especially important in contributing to the formation of stable foam in the rumen.[46,47] This entrapment of gas within the rumen contents is the primary cause of frothy bloat. The stable foam prevents the coalescence of gas bubbles as well as the clearance of the cardia, impairing eructation. Frothy bloat can also occur on high-grain diets with limited roughage content. Plant factors that suppress bloat include condensed tannins, higher stem to leaf ratios, and plant lipids.

Reports of frothy or free-gas bloat are rare in farmed deer. A low incidence of frothy bloat likely reflects differences in forage browsing preferences, feedstuffs, pastures typically utilized on farmed deer operations, and an inherent ability of the rumen flora and physiology to consume and tolerate high tanniferous forages. For example, deer have a high concentration of proline-rich tannin-precipitating protein in their saliva, as well as alterations in rumen microflora that accommodate high tannin-containing diets. By forming insoluble complexes with plant proteins, tannins limit the production of stable foam in the rumen and prevent bloat in cattle, small ruminants, and deer species.[48,49]

The occurrence of slime (frothy) bloat under feedlot conditions (i.e., high grain diets) has a similar pathogenesis with the formation of a stable foam in the rumen, preventing eructation. When large amounts of corn or other cereal grains (e.g., barley) are fed, an excess release of mucopolysaccharides and other constituents from rumen bacteria and protozoa occurs. This alters the rumen fluid viscosity and allows a stable slime (or foam) to form.[42,43] Compounding the issue is a reduction in the amount of saliva contributing to the rumen liquor due to reduced rumination on diets lacking adequate fiber. Saliva normally acts as a buffer and limits the formation of a stable foam. Also, episodes of ruminal acidosis, commonly encountered on high-grain diets, can contribute to alterations in rumen motility patterns and the development of free-gas bloat.[43]

In the case of free-gas bloat, failure to eructate has a variety of causes. Physical obstruction of the esophagus with intraluminal foreign bodies (e.g., feedstuffs, masses) or extraluminal compression of the esophagus (e.g., enlarged mediastinal lymph nodes, thymoma) can result in bloat, ranging from mild to severe ruminal tympany, depending in the completeness of obstruction. Diseases of the rumen wall can result in mechanical disruption of normal motility patterns, impairing eructation. Systemic diseases, damage to the nerves innervating the esophagus and forestomach, electrolyte imbalances, endotoxemia, and pain can impair eructation.[50–52] Use of alpha2-agonists (e.g., xylazine) can impair reticulorumen motility, thereby altering eructation.[53,54]

Clinical Signs. Clinical signs of frothy bloat and free-gas bloat due to physical obstruction of the esophagus can be severe and life-threatening compared with bloat due to rumen wall or systemic diseases. Ruminal tympany is observed in the left paralumbar fossa which can extend above dorsal mid-line. The animal may appear anxious and demonstrate a tense abdominal wall and signs of colic. Changes in abdominal contour may be subtle and difficult to fully appreciate in heavily fleeced animals. The rumen may be either hypomotile or hypermotile. Due to compression of the diaphragm and lungs, respiratory distress with flaring of nostrils, open mouth breathing, and an altered stance are common. Death can be rapid if ruminal tympany is left untreated.[40,50]

Diagnosis and Treatment. Bloat is a medical emergency, necessitating decompression of the rumen and stabilizing the animal before a thorough workup is performed. If the animal is not in immediate danger of dying, an orogastric tube can be passed. Most cases of free-gas bloat are relieved with passage of the tube. A thorough history and complete physical examination are then indicated to find the cause of the free-gas bloat. If the bloat is not relieved with passage of an orogastric tube, the tube should be removed and examined for evidence of froth. Frothy bloat can be treated with poloxalene (44 mg/kg) or dioctyl sodium sulfosuccinate (DSS) (28 mL [1 oz]) delivered by orogastric tube. If frothy bloat is due to high-concentrate feeding, the pH is less than 5.5 and may be treated with mineral oil (100 mL, PO) and/or poloxalene. In emergency situations, other surfactants and detergents may be attempted, including peanut oil (20 to 50 mg/kg), vegetable oil (100 to 200 mL), and hand soap (10 mL).

If the animal is in severe respiratory distress, the clinician should insert a trocar or large needle into the rumen at the paralumbar fossa. If gas does not escape, or froth is seen coming out of the trocar, an emergency rumenotomy is indicated. With occurrence of bloat in multiple animals of a pastured group, the entire group should be removed from the pasture and reintroduced slowly after gradual acclimation. If only one or two cases of bloat are encountered, the healthy animals can remain on the offending pasture, but grazing should be limited to ensure gradual acclimation.

Prevention. Prevention of frothy bloat includes pasture management and use of antifoaming agents. Cultivated pastures should be seeded to grass-legume mixtures, with fertilizing and grazing management maintaining 50% or less of bloating legumes on pasture, depending on the incidence of bloat, as this percentage may need to be decreased to < 25 to 30%.[41] Use of non-bloating legumes in grass mixes may be used depending on geographic location as well as nutritive and carrying capacity of pastures required. Under intensive grazing conditions, management of exposure (e.g., creep, swath grazing with 24–48 h of wilting) and use of legume varieties engineered to possess less bloat risk can be utilized (e.g., AC Grazeland).[55,56] Grazing legumes with high leaf-tannin concentrations (e.g., arrowleaf clover, kudzu) usually are safer because tannins form insoluble complexes with legume proteins, which help break down stable foam in the rumen.[41] Monitoring of pasture conditions and recognizing weather events that impact the incidence of bloat should be viewed with respect to effects on plant growth. Examples are the avoidance of grazing during the presence of heavy dew (morning and evening), recent heavy rains, and frost. Important is the recognition that alfalfa still poses a bloat risk even after a killing frost and the observation of the predominant forage present on pastures in order to assess the bloat risk (e.g., regrowth of alfalfa faster than grasses in the fall or the selective grazing habits of the herd).[45]

Limiting access to offending pastures and feedstuffs, with slow introduction over the course of 2 to 3 weeks, should be carried out. Prior to introduction to offending pastures or feedstuffs (and when intermittently housed off pastures, e.g., overnight), sheep or goats should be fed to satiety with a coarse roughage. Offering supplemental roughage (e.g., grass or cereal hays) while on bloat-provoking pastures can be attempted but ensuring intake can be problematic and economically cost prohibitive.

Natural and synthetic surfactants are effective in preventing bloat when administered at the recommended levels. Use of poloxalene is widely used in cattle and appears to be efficacious in sheep, although the level required in sheep may be higher per unit of bodyweight (BW) compared with cattle and more variable in its control.[57] Inclusion of poloxalene in concentrate feed mixes as either a top-dressing or as pelleted premix can be fed twice daily at a rate of 2 to 4 g/100 kg BW. Water-soluble formulations delivered in metered-water sources have been found efficacious in grazing sheep and are available in other countries.[56,58] Inclusion in mineral supplements (e.g., salt molasses blocks, liquid molasses lick feeders) is another alternative. However, ensuring adequate intake of poloxalene from water sources and mineral blocks can be variable and should be monitored under extensive grazing conditions, with blocks most useful in small pastures. The efficacy and economic validity of these uses in small ruminants have not been critically evaluated under field conditions. Caution is warranted with respect to copper levels in minerals intended for cattle use when used in small ruminants. Use of poloxalene-containing products should be continued for 1 to 2 weeks prior to moving animals onto bloat-promoting pastures.

Oils (e.g., soybean, corn, peanut, olive) and emulsified tallow also exhibit good bloat control. However, disadvantages include rapid degradation in the rumen, requiring large doses. Mineral oil is effective but is problematic due to its laxative effect and impairment of vitamin A metabolism in the rumen.

Free-gas bloat from concentrate feeds can be controlled by slow introduction to these feeds to allow for rumen adaptation, proper balancing of a ration, type of grain and its processing, and bunk management, as well as the inclusion of ionophores in the diet.[43] Monensin (15 mg/head/day in sheep and 1 mg/kg/day in goats) and lasalocid (0.5 to 1 mg/kg/day in sheep and goats) both decrease the formation of free ruminal gas.[59] By enhancing propionic acid formation, these drugs not only reduce the amount of methane produced in the rumen but also improve the efficiency of nutrient assimilation from feedstuffs.[43]

Bloat in lambs and kids can have the same causes as in adults but also can be caused by improper milk feeding. Overfeeding, feeding of large infrequent meals, and feeding spoiled or cold milk have all been associated with bloat in lambs and kids. Rapid overdistention of the abomasum and improper chemical or physical composition of milk replacers both will inhibit rumen motility, leading to bloat. Even though the feeding of cold milk has been associated with bloat, the practice can be used effectively in orphan feeding programs. Lambs and kids tend to limit their intake of cold milk after they have become accustomed to a free-choice feeding system that delivers refrigerated milk. Milk usually is placed in the rumen when animals are tube-fed; this may result in milk spoilage.

Simple Indigestion

Simple indigestion is a mild form of upset of reticulorumen function caused most often by a change in feed. This can be the sudden addition of grain or other concentrates to the diet, or alteration of the energy provided, such as a change in grain processing. Changes in pasture and hay or ingestion of toxic plants or moldy hay or grain can also cause simple indigestion. Clinical signs include reduced feed intake to anorexia, diarrhea, and bloat, which are mild in their characteristics and short-lived, often resolving within 1 to 2 days. Minimal to no changes in rumen fluid characteristics may be observed depending on the cause. Most mild cases of simple indigestion resolve without therapy. Appropriate steps should be taken if the cause can be identified.

Rumen Acidosis

Ingestion of rapidly fermentable sugars and starches, such as corn and small cereal grains (e.g., barley, wheat, oats) as well as bread, candy, apples, and fruits can result in dramatic changes in ruminal fermentation and the development of ruminal acidosis. The common name for this condition is "grain overload". The type of grain processing (e.g., flaking, rolling) reduces the size of the feed particles and allows more rapid fermentation by rumen bacteria. Rumen acidosis commonly follows excessive consumption of offending feedstuffs (accidental or inappropriate ration formulation), abrupt changes in the diet not allowing for adaptation of the rumen microflora, inconsistent delivery of ration, or mixing errors. The severity of the disease depends on the composition of the feed, particle size, amount of feed consumed, and the period of adaptation to the diet.

Pathogenesis. Under normal conditions, a low concentration of lactate is found in the rumen and is rapidly metabolized by lactate utilizers such as *Selenomonas ruminantium* and *Megasphaera elsdenii*. The introduction of high-concentrate diets with rapidly fermentable sugars and starches leads to unbalanced ruminal fermentation and the accumulation of lactic acid.[60] Initially, the excess fermentable carbohydrates cause a general increase in the growth rate of all bacteria with a resultant increase in volatile fatty acid (VFA) production, which lowers ruminal pH. Bacterial species tolerant of lower ruminal pH, specifically *Streptococcus bovis*, outpace other bacterial species, resulting in increased lactate production. An increase in lactate concentration further decreases the rumen pH, and eventually it falls to a level where death of protozoa and gram-negative bacterial spp. occurs. In addition, the growth of *S. bovis* is inhibited and only very acid tolerant lactate-producing *Lactobacillus* spp. predominate. The rumen pH can decrease to 5, and in severe cases to less than 4.0. Lactate production (L- and D-isoforms) continues to increase.[61,62] The osmolality of the rumen fluid increases which pulls fluid from the systemic circulation and interstitium into the rumen. Stasis of reticulorumen motility, mucosal damage, and absorption of lactic acids, inflammatory mediators, as well as bacteria and endotoxins into the peripheral circulation results.[63–65] Clinically, dehydration, hypovolemic shock, acute inflammatory response, and metabolic acidosis result.[63] Depending on the severity of metabolic derangement, thiamine deficiency and the development of polioencephalomalacia (PEM) can occur.[66] Sequelae of severe ruminal acidosis or recurrent bouts of subacute ruminal acidosis may include laminitis, mycotic ruminitis, and occasionally liver abscessation; although, the latter is far more common in cattle than in small ruminants.[65,67–69]

Clinical Signs. Clinical manifestations vary with the amount and type of feed ingested and the time since ingestion. Clinical signs first appear 12 to 36 h after ingestion of the offending feed, ranging from anorexia, depression, reduced rumen motility, nasal discharge, and diarrhea. The presence of weakness, ataxia, or recumbency can develop in animals suffering from circulatory shock and severe metabolic derangements. Dehydration usually is severe, and evidence of toxemia is present (e.g., tachycardia, altered body temperature, infected mucous membranes, and scleral vessels). Rumen stasis, ventral abdominal distension, and a fluid-filled rumen are found on abdominal auscultation and percussion. Signs of abdominal pain, such as bruxism, stretching, and kicking at belly may be observed. Osmotic diarrhea commonly occurs, which can worsen the severity of dehydration. Diarrhea can range from pasty feces to soupy, watery diarrhea with the presence of whole grain/corn. Neurological deficits such as blindness, ataxia, head pressing, opisthotonus, seizures, and other abnormalities can develop due to thiamine deficiency PEM, as well as other metabolic derangements and endotoxemia.

Diagnosis. Examination of rumen fluid should be carried out in suspected cases of ruminal acidosis. Rumen fluid is milky colored, foul smelling with acidic odor, and has a reduced pH (below 5.5). Protozoa numbers and types are markedly reduced with poor to absent motility. Methylene blue reduction time is markedly prolonged ($>$ 9 minutes) in most cases. The normal 60:40 ratio of gram-negative to gram-positive bacteria is altered with a predominance of Gram-positive rods (*Lactobacillus* spp.). Rumen lactic acid concentration is increased.[62] Clinicopathologic laboratory data include hemoconcentration (increased PCV and total protein), prerenal azotemia, and metabolic acidosis, characterized by a low blood pH, low blood bicarbonate concentration, and a negative base excess.[62,70] Renal compensation results in acidic urine production after 12 h, along with an increase in urine-specific gravity.[70] Dehydration and impaired tissue perfusion, as well as an overwhelming delivery of inflammatory mediators and endotoxins to the liver can result in increased liver and muscle enzymes, depending on the severity of the disease. Changes in the leukogram and acute-phase proteins reflect an acute inflammatory response, ranging from normal to a degenerative left shift as well as increases in haptoglobin, ceruloplasmin, and reduced albumin concentration.[63] The transketolase test performed on peripheral blood can be used to determine the active thiamine status of the animal.[66] Increases in cerebrospinal fluid (CSF) leukocyte counts and total protein have been reported in sheep.[71]

Treatment. Treatment is aimed at correcting dehydration, metabolic acidosis, toxemia, and shock as well as the removal or neutralization of the offending feedstuff. Use of IV isotonic crystalloids supplemented with bicarbonate should be administered. Ideally, bicarbonate supplementation would be based on serum biochemistry analysis but can be empirically based on estimated base deficit. In certain instances, calcium may be indicated and can be added to the IV fluids (as calcium gluconate). The clinician should avoid mixing calcium salts and sodium bicarbonate. Administration of parenteral NSAIDs to alleviate pain and potentiate toxemia are indicated (e.g., flunixin meglumine 1.1 to 2.2 mg/kg, IV). Use of parenteral antibiotics is indicated in most cases, given a high likelihood of bacterial translocation and bacteremia. The systemic antimicrobial of choice is penicillin (procaine penicillin G, 22,000 IU/kg, IM, q12h, or potassium penicillin 22,000 IU/kg, IV, q6h) due to anaerobes being the most likely offending organisms. Use of oral fluids to restore hydration is contraindicated and counterproductive, as fluid absorption is impaired, and administration can worsen rumen distention and abdominal discomfort. Administration of agents to neutralize the rumen pH, such as magnesium hydroxide and magnesium oxide (1 g/kg, PO) can be sufficient in mild cases. However, if much of the feed is still in the rumen, these two alkalinizing agents will only work temporarily. The use of oral antibiotics is likely counterproductive, as their administration negatively impacts the regrowth of the healthy rumen microflora. Oral antibiotics are contraindicated as they have poor bioavailability (e.g., neomycin). If available, the animal should be transfaunated daily with rumen fluid from a healthy donor until rumen motility and appetite are restored. More effective, is the prompt removal of the offending feedstuff in order to curtail fermentation. Ruminal lavage is likely futile in most small ruminants, given the size limitation of orogastric tubes to allow sufficient bore diameter without becoming blocked with feed. Rumenotomy is indicated in severe cases of ruminal acidosis to remove the offending feed.

After the rumen pH is corrected, transfaunation of the sheep or goat with ½ to 1 L of rumen fluid from a donor animal (cow or small ruminant) is beneficial. Thiamine supplementation (vitamin B1, 10 mg/kg, SC, q6–8h) is indicated until rumen function is restored and is of utmost importance in animals demonstrating clinical signs suggestive of PEM. Supportive care should also include provision of grass hay and water when rumen motility returns in order to prevent excessive ruminal distention. With aggressive treatment, the prognosis for short-term survival is good. Delays in seeking medical treatment can result in poor outcomes and death in severe cases. Sequelae to ruminal acidosis (previously discussed), can significantly impact long-term survival and production.

Prevention. Prevention must involve addressing inappropriate management practices that put animals as risk for the development of ruminal acidosis, especially in classes of sheep and goats being fed high-grain rations (e.g., club lambs, feedlot lambs, dairy goats). A balanced diet with adequate forage and fiber should be formulated, properly mixed, and consistently delivered, along with adequate feeder/bunk space. The crude fiber content should constitute a minimum of 20% of the diet's total digestible nutrients (TDN). For example, if the TDN is 75%, the minimum acceptable crude fiber is 15%. Crude fiber levels lower than this can be fed for short periods if the rumen is properly adapted, but problems may nevertheless occur. In sheep and goats unaccustomed to high-concentrate rations, gradual introduction to increasing rates of inclusion should take place over several weeks, to allow for adaptation of the rumen microflora. In addition to a well-formulated ration, inclusion of rumen modifiers such as buffers, yeasts, and direct-fed microbials may also be utilized. Rumen buffers may improve milk production, increase feed intake, and increase rate of gain. Sodium bicarbonate probably is the most commonly used buffer; it can be offered on a free-choice basis or included in the diet as 1% of dry matter intake. Calcium carbonate or limestone (both of which have low rumen solubility) and magnesium oxide (which has poor palatability) also can be included in the feed. Magnesium oxide should be limited to 0.5 to 0.8% of the dry matter intake.

In the United States, direct-fed microbials refer to a source of live (viable), naturally occurring microorganisms which are used for supplementing microbes and modulation of the rumen microbiota, with the goals of maintaining a stable rumen pH, decreasing lactic acid, optimizing VFA production, and improving nutrient digestibility. Single or mixed bacterial cultures, as well as different species of yeasts can be found in commercial products, including *Lactobacillus acidophilus*, *Propionibacterium freudenreichii*, *Megasphaera elsdenii*, and *Saccharomyces cervisiae*.[72] Use of a yeast-based culture (*S. cerevisiae*) demonstrated a positive effect in the treatment and prevention of ruminal acidosis and potential sequelae in sheep under experimental conditions.[73,74] However, much research is needed as to the efficacy and proper use of pre- and probiotics in small ruminants.[75]

Reticulitis, Rumenitis, and Parakeratosis

Pathogenesis. Reticulitis and ruminitis can result from chemical or mechanical damage to the mucosal lining of the reticulorumen. The most common cause of chemical damage in sheep and goats is rumen acidosis. Rumenitis associated with a high carbohydrate supplemental feed has also been reported in white-tailed deer.[76] However, ingestion of caustic toxins also can damage the mucosa. Mechanical damage can occur from ingested foreign bodies or rumen bezoars. In cattle, viruses such as the agents of bovine virus diarrhea and infectious bovine rhinotracheitis can infect the rumen wall. Similar viruses have yet to be identified in sheep and goats.

After the mucosa has been damaged, secondary infection by bacteria or fungi can occur. Previous treatment with oral antibiotics may predispose animals to development of fungal infections of the rumen wall, especially if the mucosa is already damaged. Actinobacillosis, actinomycosis, and tuberculosis rarely affect the rumen wall. Tumors of the rumen wall also have been reported. Not all of these causes of reticulitis and ruminitis have been reported in sheep, goats, and cervids, but all are potential problems.

Clinical Signs. The clinical manifestations of these diseases are vague. Anorexia and forestomach hypomotility may be the only clinical signs.

Diagnosis. Confirming a diagnosis of these diseases also may prove difficult. Samples of rumen fluid may show only changes

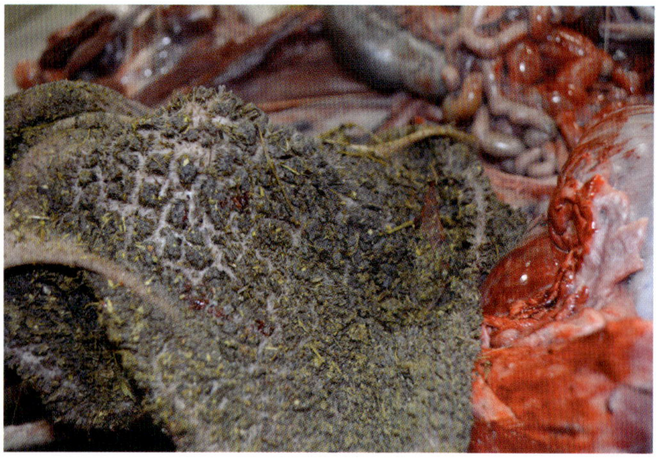

• **Fig. 5.7** An 8-year-old female white-tailed deer's rumen showing enlarged ruminal papillae. The pen-raised doe had signs of chronic acidosis/ruminitis prior to death. She was in a pen with other does being offered an ad lib grain/carbohydrate feed with minimal forage. The rumen had enlarged, hardened, and fused together papillae, and diffuse, severe ruminal hyperkeratosis. (Courtesy of Dr. Kelley Steury, ALVDL, Auburn, AL.)

associated with anorexia (alkaline pH, decreased numbers and motility of protozoa, prolonged MBR time; see Table 5.1 for normal values). Occasionally, fungal organisms may be seen on Romanowski (Diff-Quick)-stained slides of rumen fluid. In such cases, a diagnosis of fungal ruminitis should be made. An exploratory laparotomy and rumenotomy may be required to identify foreign bodies or masses. Rumen parakeratosis is characterized by dark, thickened, and clumped rumen papillae. It is seen mainly in feedlot lambs that consume finely ground or pelleted rations. The parakeratotic rumen papillae are fragile and vulnerable to damage which can increase the risk for development of rumenitis (Figure 5.7).

Treatment and Prevention. Treatment depends on the inciting cause. Dietary changes should be made to decrease energy density and increase fiber intake. Mild ruminitis may subside with time and supportive care (e.g., transfaunation, fluid support, high-quality feed). Fungal rumenitis can be treated with oral thiabendazole, 25–44 mg/kg, when available. Severe changes may lead to scarring and permanent impairment of rumen function.

Diseases of the Reticulorumen

Traumatic Reticuloperitonitis

Traumatic reticuloperitonitis (hardware disease) is an uncommonly reported condition in small ruminants, unlike cattle in which hardware disease is a primary cause of vagal indigestion. The selective grazing and browsing habits of sheep and goats, respectively, likely limit the intake of sharp, metallic objects such as wire, nails, and needles. Goats appear to be affected more commonly than sheep.[77] Penetration of a foreign body through the reticular wall can result in reticulitis, localized or diffuse peritonitis, abscessation and adhesion formation, as well as the development of pleuritis, pericarditis, or myocarditis if the foreign body penetrates the diaphragm into the thoracic cavity. Clinical signs include depression, anorexia, poor body condition, reluctance to ambulate, altered rumen motility (e.g., bloat, vagal indigestion), and abdominal pain.[78] Involvement of the pleura or pericardium can present with signs of respiratory distress and heart failure.[79] Abscessation and draining tracts of the thorax and forelimbs may be present.[77] A thorough workup is required to determine the cause of vagal indigestion and the potential internal sites involved. This may include the use of radiographs and ultrasound, as these imaging modalities will help determine the extent of infection and the most suitable approach to treatment. An exploratory laparotomy can be both diagnostic and therapeutic. Physical examination and diagnostics will direct the surgical approach used (e.g., left versus right flank), as well as the need for a rumenotomy. Most animals will require stabilization with fluid therapy as well as long-term antibiotics and supportive care. Reticuloperitonitis carries a guarded to poor prognosis.[78,80]

Rumen Impaction

Rumen impaction as the result of feeding inappropriate forages or feedstuffs (e.g., high fiber diets with low digestibility; *Ficus esquiroliana*), sand ingestion, or consumption of indigestible foreign material (e.g., plastic) can lead to the disruption of normal reticulorumen motility and function, as well as partial or complete blockage of the omasal orifice.[81,82] Malnutrition and unbalanced dietary habits results in pica and ingestion of indigestible foreign materials and is of growing concern worldwide. Goats reared in suburban and urban environments are particularly at risk.[83] Clinical manifestations are non-specific, such as depression, weakness, anorexia, and ruminal atony. A firm rumen can usually be palpated in the left flank. Signs of vagal ingestion such as ruminal tympany and scant dry feces may be present. Prolongation of methylene blue reduction time reflects poor anaerobic fermentation in the rumen.[82] Oral fluids containing magnesium sulfate (60 g), mineral oil, or DSS administered daily for a week may resolve fibrous and sand impactions, but a rumenotomy is required in severe cases and for impactions involving indigestible foreign materials. Prevention includes use of feed troughs and racks to elevate feedstuffs off the ground to minimize sand intake as well as ensuring a properly formulated diet, including the provision of a loose mineral source.[84]

Rumenotomy. Exploratory celiotomy is both a diagnostic and therapeutic intervention in ruminants with vagal indigestion. The decision to perform a standing left or the right flank, or use of other positions in recumbency, will be dictated by physical examination, clinicopathological tests, and the temperament and stability of the patient. A standing or recumbent left flank celiotomy and rumenotomy is suited for type II vagal indigestion (e.g., hardware disease, perireticular abscess). A right-sided approach (right flank, right paramedian, or right paracostal) for exploratory celiotomy is suitable for type III and IV vagal indigestion (e.g., abomasal impaction, pyloric obstruction). Many small ruminants may become recumbent during a standing flank approach. Recumbency can be facilitated by using a lumbosacral epidural anesthesia and sedation or by inhalant general anesthesia in very fractious animals. In nonemergent situations, the rumen fill should be minimized by withholding feed for 24 h. However, many cases present as an emergency. Perioperative antibiotics should be administered and be efficacious against anaerobes. Examples commonly used include procaine penicillin, ampicillin, and oxytetracycline. Use of nonsteroidal anti-inflammatories (e.g., flunixin meglumine, meloxicam) is indicated perioperatively. IV fluids should be used to correct dehydration and cardiovascular shock, both concurrent with and following surgery, as needed.

A brief description of a left flank celiotomy and rumenotomy is described herein.[78,85–87] In-depth review of other surgical and laparoscopic celiotomy approaches can be found elsewhere. The surgical site encompasses an area including the last two to three intercostal spaces cranially to the paralumbar fossa, extending caudally to the tuber coxae, and from dorsal midline to the lower abdomen. The surgical site is clipped and aseptically prepared.

A routine vertical incision is made through the skin and abdominal muscles in the middle of the left paralumbar fossa. Because the abdominal wall is relatively thin, and the rumen may be very distended, the surgeon should take care not to enter the rumen or bowel. To allow exploration and potential evaluation of the rumen, the body wall incision must be of adequate size to allow the surgeon's hand and forearm to comfortably enter the rumen without undue tension on the rumen wall. Once secured and incised, the rumen incision will be smaller than the body wall incision and should be considered. Thorough exploration of the abdomen should take place before the rumenotomy is performed (and is absolutely contraindicated after the rumenotomy is performed). Attention should be paid as to the presence of adhesions and perireticular abscesses while palpating the diaphragm and reticulum. After abdominal exploration, the rumen is secured to the skin by creating a watertight seal with continuous suture. The watertight seal is critical in preventing abdominal contamination. A monofilament (or coated) type of suture on a cutting needle should be used in a Cushing's pattern. It is important to exteriorize a generous part of the dorsal rumen sac to facilitate the creation of the rumenotomy without disrupting the rumen-to-skin seal. To prevent or minimize leakage, the rumen suture bites should be through the seromuscular layer but should not penetrate the mucosa, which could lead to leakage at closure. The suture line is started dorsally at the 12 o'clock position and continued ventrally until the 6 o'clock position is reached. A similar suture line is started on the other side dorsally and continued ventrally, overlapping with the initial suture line to prevent gapping and abdominal contamination at the 6 o'clock position. Two separate suture lines are used to limit the circumferential decrease in lumen size created by one suture line pulled tightly. Once the rumen is sutured to the skin, the rumen-skin suture line is carefully checked for a good seal (Figure 5.8). The rumenotomy incision is then made in the center of the exposed, secured rumen (Figure 5.9). The rumenotomy incision should be large enough to allow entry of the surgeon's hand into the rumen, but care must be taken to ensure inadvertent incision of the skin-rumen seal does not take place (e.g., 3-cm ventral to 12 o'clock position and extending to 3-cm dorsal to the 6 o'clock position). Once the rumen has been secured and opened, no other modifications should be made to the rumenotomy. Depending on the character of the rumen contents, the rumen can be evacuated by hand or by creating a siphon with a large-bore stomach tube. The surgeon then explores the reticulum and rumen in its entirety, ensuring palpation of the ruminoreticular fold, esophageal orifice, and omasal orifice. All foreign bodies should be removed, regardless of whether they are penetrating or nonpenetrating. To facilitate finding ferromagnetic foreign bodies, a magnet can be held in the surgeon's hand while sweeping the reticular wall. An ultrasound probe (5-MHz sector) within a rectal sleeve can also be taken into the rumen to help identify adhesions and abscesses. Advancement of a hand through the reticulo-omasal canal is not typically feasible in small ruminants but may cautiously be attempted in large sheep and goats. Confirmed perireticular abscesses tightly adherent to the reticulum can be opened into the reticulum using sharp incision.

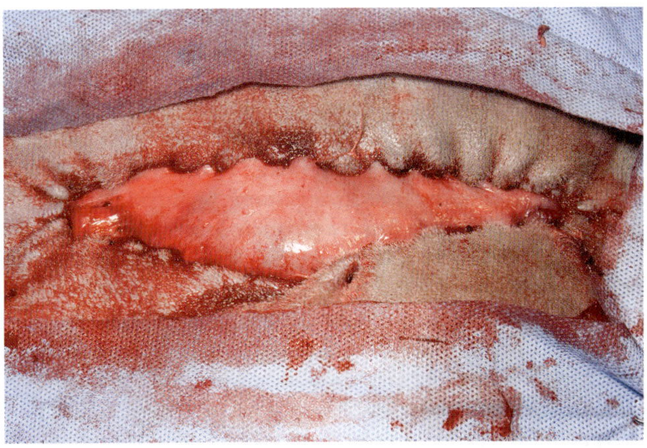

• **Fig. 5.8** Rumenotomy: the rumen is secured to the skin with a watertight seal, ready for the rumenotomy incision.

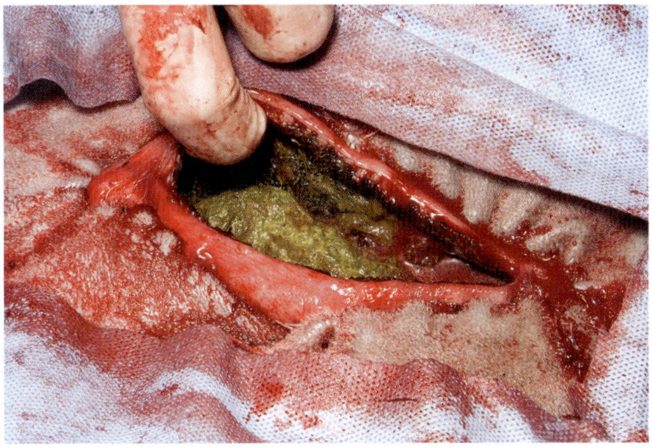

• **Fig. 5.9** Rumenotomy: rumen contents are visible through the rumenotomy incision.

Closure of the rumen is performed in two layers. Absorbable suture in a simple continuous pattern is used to close the rumen lumen for the first layer. Surgeon preference may dictate the use of a double-layer inverting pattern as described by Niehaus.[87] Once the initial layer of rumen closure is complete, the site is copiously lavaged with sterile saline. All soiled materials (e.g., gloves, gowns, drapes) are then removed and replaced, and sterile instruments used in the second part of closure. The second layer of the rumen closure is with absorbable suture in an inverting pattern (e.g., Cushing, Lembert). Suture of this second layer should start at the 12 o'clock position of the rumen incision, and retention sutures securing the rumen to the skin are removed as needed to free enough rumen for closure. When the second layer closure (Figure 5.10) is complete, the rumen is cleaned with moist sponges before being returned to the abdominal cavity. Again, it is emphasized that exploration of the abdominal cavity at this point is associated with an increased incidence of septic peritonitis and is contraindicated. The muscle and skin are inspected for gross contamination and cleansed with moist gauzes as needed. Routine closure of the muscle layers and skin are performed, based on surgeon's preference. Given that some contamination will occur during the procedure, incisional infections should be anticipated. The ventral aspect of the skin closure should include two to three interrupted sutures to allow drainage, if necessary, postoperatively.

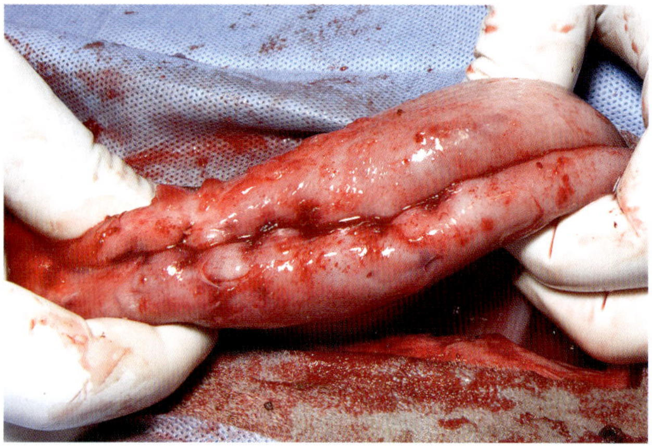

• **Fig. 5.10** Rumenotomy: the final inverted closure of the rumenotomy incision.

The sheep or goat should be observed closely by the clinician for signs of complications, including the major complication of peritonitis as well as incisional infection, abscessation, or dehiscence, and hernia formation. Given the nature of the procedure (i.e., clean-contaminated surgery), incisional infections can occur, and ventral drainage may need to be established by removing the most ventral two to three interrupted sutures of the skin closure. The skin sutures can be removed in 10 to 14 days after surgery. Antibiotic therapy (e.g., procaine penicillin at 22,000 IU/kg, IM, q12h or potassium penicillin 22,000 IU/kg, IV, q6h) should be continued for at least 5 days. The need for prolonged antibiotic use in uncomplicated cases may be of questionable value in cattle, but this has not been critically evaluated in small ruminants.[87,88] However, medical management of concurrent diseases may include long-term antibiotic therapy (e.g., treatment of local or generalized peritonitis). Postoperative antiinflammatory medication and pain control are indicated. Reestablishing rumen flora and rumen motility using rumen transfaunate as well as maintaining the patient's hydration with oral or IV fluids should be performed.

Diseases of the Abomasum

Abomasitis and Abomasal Ulcers

Several clostridial species are implicated as a cause of abomasitis in small ruminants. Sheep are more commonly reported compared with goats. Most cases present as sudden death, with the occasional observation of animals with severe abdominal pain, depression, and prostration early in the course of disease. Death can be within hours. Braxy is a necrotizing and hemorrhagic abomasitis of sheep caused by *Clostridium septicum*. Overgrowth of the clostridial species is proposed to be associated with recent frosts, snowfalls, or the feeding of frozen feedstuffs resulting in hemorrhagic, necrotic abomasitis with fatal enterotoxemia. Braxy is reported in Europe, Africa, and the Middle East and infrequently in the United States. Braxy-like lesions caused by *C. septicum* have been demonstrated in sheep under experimental conditions as well as naturally occurring disease in lambs, with evidence of suppurative abomasitis with extensive edema, emphysema, and necrosis of the abomasal wall on histopathology.[89,90]

Similar abomasal disease characterized by hemorrhage, necrosis, and potential ulcers is reported in pre-ruminant lambs caused by *Clostridium sordellii, Clostridium fallax,* and *Sarcina ventriculi.* A high incidence is observed in 3- to 10-week-old lambs and kids.[91–95] The presence of severe gaseous distention of the abomasum was often observed in cases with *Sarcina*-like bacteria, whereas hemorrhage and ulcer were more often observed with clostridial species.[92] *Sarcina* species are anaerobic, Gram-positive bacteria that occur in cubical packets, able to grow at very low pH conditions, and ferment sugars with significant gas production. The ability to tolerate low pH and the presence of sufficient fermentable carbohydrates in milk or milk-replacer fed lambs and kids may allow this bacterial species to overgrow in the abomasum.[95] Predisposing factors for abomasal bloat and hemorrhage in young lambs and kids may include free-choice milk replacer feeding regimens at inappropriate temperature and frequency as well as iron deficiency.[95–97] Iron deficiency may promote the ingestion of soil-containing clostridial and *Sarcina* species.

Abomasitis and abomasal ulcers in adult small ruminants, apart from clostridial diseases, are poorly documented and likely uncommon. Implicated risk factors include abrupt feed changes or inappropriately formulated rations (e.g., course feed, pelleted feed) with resultant rumenitis and ruminal acidosis. Heavy-metal intoxication can produce severe abomasitis and ulceration. Small ruminants with systemic illnesses, such as pasteurellosis or pregnancy toxemia, may develop abomasal ulcerations.[98] The potential role of a mineral deficiency (e.g., copper) has not been proven. Phycomycotic ulceration of the abomasum has been reported in sheep. Fungi species involved likely represent secondary invasion of disrupted and damaged mucosa due to an underlying digestive disturbance.[99] Abomasal ulcers have also been reported in white-tailed deer with ulceration occurring at the abomasal-pylorus and at the abomasal-duodenal junction. All deer reported had other concurrent disease.[100]

Clinical Signs and Diagnosis. The diagnosis of these conditions due to clostridial diseases is by postmortem examination. Overgrowth of clostridial species occurs quickly after death necessitating timely collection of samples for anaerobic culture and molecular diagnostics.

Abomasitis and abomasal ulcers may present with vague clinical signs or be asymptomatic. If abdominal pain is the main presenting sign, other causes of acute abdomen need to be ruled out. Bleeding abomasal ulcers may present with melena. No definitive antemortem diagnostic tests are available. Fecal occult blood test results can be negative in ulcerative disease, as well as confounded by the presence of gastrointestinal parasites.[101]

Treatment. Treatment in suspected antemortem cases of clostridial abomasitis is unsuccessful. Use of therapies for the treatment of stomach ulcers in monogastric animals can prove ineffective in ruminants, due to the rumen and the delay and dilution of medications before they reach the abomasum. Most research on oral antacid therapy in ruminants has been carried out in milk-fed calves, which presents suitable therapies in preweaned lambs and kids. These include coating agents (e.g., sucralfate), acid neutralizers (e.g., aluminum and magnesium hydroxide), histamine type-2 receptor antagonists (e.g., cimetidine, ranitidine), and proton pump inhibitors (e.g., omeprazole).[102–104] Use of intravenous formulations of H2-antagonists or proton-pump inhibitors (e.g., pantoprazole) may be attempted in sheep and goats but likely are cost prohibitive.[105,106] Diet formulations contributing to underlying mucosal damage should be addressed. Buffers can be added to the feed.

Prevention. Vaccinating against clostridial diseases may decrease the occurrence of abomasal hemorrhage. Ideally, ewes and does are vaccinated prior to parturition to maximize specific immunoglobulins in colostrum consumed by the neonate. Lambs or kids on farms where such disease has been a problem can be vaccinated with multivalent bacterins against clostridial infections during the first week of life.

Abomasal Impaction

Abomasal impaction can occur with the feeding of poor-quality roughage, but it can also be seen with foreign body obstruction of the pylorus. An example of the latter is the presence of abomasal phytobezoars as described in South African goats and sheep.[107] Goats appear to be more commonly affected than sheep, and Boer goats are more commonly affected than Angora goats. Pregnant animals may be more prone to impaction due to poor-quality roughage, whereas younger goats (6–12 months of age) appear to be at particular risk for the development of abomasal phytobezoars. In the South African condition, the composition of abomasal phytobezoars is made up of pappus hairs of certain Karoo bushes.[108]

Clinical Signs and Diagnosis. The onset of disease is insidious and affected animals usually are anorexic, depressed, and are in poor body condition. Distention of the ventral abdomen is characteristic, and in some cases the firm abomasum can be palpated through the abdominal wall on the right side. With deep abdominal palpation, the presence of phytobezoars may be appreciable. Sudden death is possible in the case of acute pyloric or intestinal obstruction with subsequent rupture of the intestinal or gastric wall. Clinicopathologic evaluation may be normal, or mild hypochloremic metabolic alkalosis may be present with increased rumen chloride concentration.

Treatment. Treatment of abomasal impaction due to poor quality forage most often requires dietary changes and oral administration of mineral oil. Abomasotomy can be attempted, although it has rarely been reported in small ruminants. For this procedure, the animal is positioned in dorsal recumbency and placed under general anesthesia. The abomasum can best be visualized through a right paramedian incision. The prognosis is poor for both conservative medical management and surgical intervention. The possibility of an underlying abomasal emptying defect should be considered. In the case of abomasal phytobezoars, the offending feedstuff should be removed from the diet. Surgical removal is the only treatment option.[107]

Prevention. Dietary manipulation to improve feed or forage quality is the best means of prevention.

Abomasal Emptying Defect

Abomasal emptying defect is a disease of predominantly Suffolk sheep, 2 to 6 years of age, which manifests as chronic, progressive weight loss and anorexia with abdominal distention. The duration ranges from several days to months. The disease is frequently reported in the post-lambing period (within 30 days), although it appears variable in onset relative to parturition and is reported in rams.[109,110] Although Suffolk is the predominant breed, cases in two Hampshire, one Dorset, and one Texel sheep are reported.[111–113] It is considered sporadic in occurrence, but herd outbreaks have been documented.[114] The underlying cause is unknown. Based on histological changes observed in the celiacomesenteric ganglion of affected sheep, a proposed pathophysiologic mechanism is alteration of autonomic innervation. Observed lesions, affecting only sympathetic nerves, suggest exposure to an excitotoxin resulting in an acquired dysautonomia.[114] Unlike abomasal impaction, this disease is due to increases in concentrate feeding associated with diet changes occurring at the time of lambing. The clinical signs are chronic weight loss, abdominal distention, and anorexia. Clinicopathologic laboratory findings reflect dehydration and metabolic alkalosis with hypochloremia. Rumen chloride concentration is increased due to abomasal reflux. Liver enzymes are increased in most cases, reflecting an increase in intra-abdominal pressure and impairment of the liver's vasculature which results in congestion, ischemia, and leakage of enzymes from damaged hepatocytes.[115] At necropsy, the abomasum is markedly distended, and the contents may be liquid or dry in character. Attempted treatment has included the use of laxatives, cathartics, motility modifiers (e.g., metoclopramide, neostigmine), and abomasotomy, with poor short- and long-term outcomes reported. The disorder carries a poor to grave prognosis.[109]

Azalea, Laurel, and Rhododendron Toxicity

Many plants of the Ericaceae family, including rhododendron, azalea, and laurel species contain diterpene grayanotoxins (also known as andromedotoxin). Ornamental and naturally occurring varieties are found in North America. All parts of the plant are potentially toxic. In cattle, *Rhododendron* has a toxic dose of 0.2% BW, while *Kalmia* has a toxic dose of 0.4% BW.[116] Toxic doses of 0.1% and 0.2 to 0.6% in goats and sheep, respectively, are reported.[117] The Japanese Pieris *(Pieris japonica)* is another broadleaf evergreen shrub that contains grayanotoxins and has resulted in small ruminant poisonings.[118–120] Grayanotoxin exerts its effects by binding to voltage-gated sodium channels of cells, especially neurons. Binding of the toxin modifies the configuration and prevents the inactivation of the sodium channel, thus rendering the neuron in a prolonged, depolarized (activated) state.[116] Cattle, sheep, and goats may present within hours of plant ingestion with evidence of GIT irritation (e.g., salivation, vomiting), cardiac arrhythmias, and neurological symptoms. Collapse and sudden death can occur in severe cases. Aspiration pneumonia of rumen contents is a significant sequela and common cause of death.

Clinical Signs. History may include the inadvertent feeding of plant clippings or access to stands of toxic plants, especially if alternative forage sources are scarce. Clinical signs include salivation, bruxism, vomiting, diarrhea, and colic. Other signs may include nasal discharge (with attempts to vomit), epiphora, and ataxia. Onset of clinical signs can be within 4 to 16 h of ingestion and occur with ingestion of only a few leaves. As severe intoxications progress, depression, collapse (bradycardia and hypotension), opisthotonus, and coma can occur.[117,121,123] Intoxicated sheep and goats are at a significant risk for aspiration pneumonia which can result in death.

Diagnosis. The diagnosis of this condition usually is based on clinical signs coupled with a history of ingestion of one of the offending plants. Identification of plant parts in ingesta is a diagnostic tool, as well as the identification of grayanotoxins in feces, urine, vomitus, and rumen contents using liquid chromatography-mass spectrometry analysis.[117]

Treatment. Intoxicated animals may recover in 1 to 2 days without any therapy if the offending plants are removed from the diet and ingestion was minimal. However, the administration of activated charcoal (2 to 9 g/kg orally), atropine (0.05 to 0.2 mg/kg, IV), antiarrhythmic drugs, thiamine (10 mg/kg, SC, q6–8h), laxatives, and IV fluids may be indicated. The risk of aspiration pneumonia is high in affected animals and should be treated with

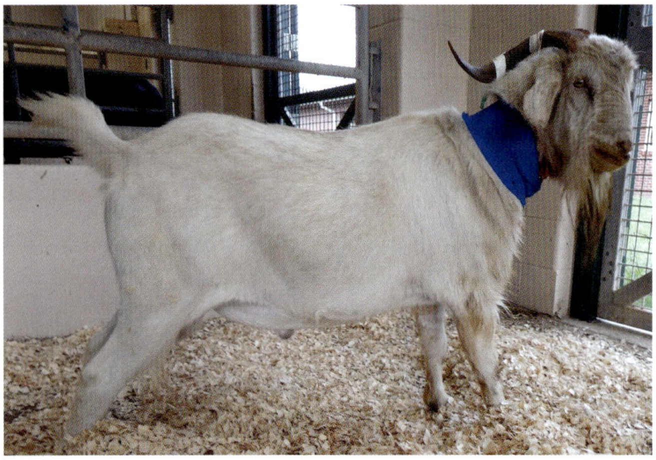

• **Fig. 5.11** Azalea Toxicity. A 3-year-old Kiko buck that presented for projectile vomiting (note beard stained from ruminal contents) and colic (note stretched out appearance due to abdominal pain).

appropriate antibiotics (e.g., procaine penicillin, oxytetracycline). The risk of aspirating orally administered medications should be heavily weighted against their use, especially when vomiting is frequent. IV lipid emulsion therapy has been used for *Pieris* ingestion in goats with recovery from severe clinical signs reported to occur within hours of administration[118] (Figure 5.11).

Prevention. Mountainous or hilly areas should be fenced to prevent animal access to toxic plants. Alternate forage sources should be offered during times when grazing or browsing is scarce to limit the intake of poisonous weeds. Feeding shrubbery clippings is discouraged.

Diseases of the Intestines

Diarrhea in Lambs and Kids: Overview

Diarrhea in lambs and kids is a complex, multifactorial disease involving the animal's susceptibilities, the environment, nutrition, infectious agents, and management. Decades of research have been devoted to the study of the pathophysiology of infectious diarrhea in calves; the pathophysiologic picture in lambs and kids is quite similar. Despite improvements in management practices and prevention and treatment strategies, diarrhea is still the most common and costly disease affecting neonatal ruminants.[124–128]

Some general preventive measures (e.g., improved sanitation) will decrease the risk of diarrheal disease from any cause. By contrast, specific control measures such as vaccination require the definition of a specific cause of diarrhea. Table 5.2 lists the agents most likely to cause diarrhea in lambs and kids, tissues or other samples required for diagnosis, and commonly used test methods. The color and consistency of the feces and any gross lesions can appear similar with numerous diseases. Laboratory identification of infectious agents and tissue histopathologic examination are therefore key to establishing a diagnosis (see Chapters 16 and 20). Because autolysis and secondary bacterial invasion of the gut begin within minutes of death, necropsy samples taken immediately from euthanized lambs and kids yield the most reliable diagnostic material. Mixed infections with two or more pathogens are common, and clinically important farm-specific pathogens change from year to year.[126–130] In some cases, an underlying nutritional deficiency or excess may be present, concurrently with infective disease. The clinician should therefore take a variety of samples to ensure identification of all pathogens and predisposing factors involved; continued reevaluation of the causes of diarrhea is

TABLE 5.2 Diagnostic Samples and Testing Methods Required for Differentiation of the Most Common Causes of Infectious Diarrhea in Lambs and Kids.

Causative Agent	Sample Required	Test Method[a]
Escherichia coli	2–3 g feces Formalin-fixed small intestine	Culture and serotyping for K99 and F41, PCR Histopathologic examination
Rotavirus	2–3 g feces or colonic contents Formalin-fixed small and large intestine Frozen small and large intestine	EM, ELISA, VI, CF tests, PCR assay Histopathologic examination VI, FA test, IP assay
Cryptosporidia	2–3 g feces Air-dried fecal smear Formalin-fixed small and large intestine	FA test, fecal flotation, PCR Acid-fast stain Histopathologic examination
Salmonella	2–3 g feces Formalin-fixed small and large intestine Frozen small and large intestine and mesenteric lymph nodes	Culture, PCR assay Histopathologic examination Culture
Giardia	Wet mount of feces Feces	Iodine staining ELISA, FA test, PCR
Clostridium perfringens	Frozen small intestinal contents and abomasum, small and large intestine Formalin-fixed abomasum and small and large intestine	Culture, toxin identification Histopathologic examination
Coccidia	2–3 g feces Formalin-fixed small and large intestine	Fecal flotation Histopathologic examination

[a]*EM,* Electron microscopy; *ELISA,* enzyme-linked immunosorbent assay; *VI,* virus isolation; *CF,* complement fixation; *PCR,* polymerase chain reaction; *FA,* fluorescent antibody; *IP,* immunoperoxidase

Data from Rings DM, Rings MB: Managing *Cryptosporidium* and *Giardia* infections in domestic ruminants. *Vet. Med.* 91:1125, 1996; Cohen ND, et al: Comparison of polymerase chain reaction and microbiological culture for detection of salmonella in equine feces and environmental samples. *Am. J. Vet. Res.*57:780, 1996; Drolet R, Fairbrother JM, Vaillancourt D: Attaching and effacing *Escherichia coli* in a goat with diarrhea. *Can. Vet. J.* 35:122, 1994.

crucial. Evaluation of material from multiple cases, with a focus on those in the acute phases, is important. Although examination of antemortem fecal samples can be diagnostic, laboratory testing of tissue samples may yield better results.

Treatment and preventive measures for specific diarrheal diseases are the focus of the remainder of this section, which is followed by sections on general supportive treatment and control measures for all infectious diarrheal diseases.

Causes of Diarrhea in Neonatal Lambs and Kids

Four major pathogens cause diarrhea in lambs and kids during the first month of life: enterotoxigenic *Escherichia coli* (ETEC), rotavirus, *Cryptosporidium* species, and *Salmonella* species. The relative prevalence of these infectious agents varies greatly among studies. This variability probably results from differences in location, season, and diagnostic techniques and the occurrence of mixed infections. Other, less common causes of diarrhea in neonates are *Giardia* infections and nutritional diarrhea.

Enterotoxigenic Escherichia Coli

Pathogenesis. ETEC employs two virulence factors to cause disease. The first is the ability to attach and colonize the intestinal villi, which is accomplished by means of fimbriae or pili. The most important fimbriae in lambs are K99 and F41.[131] The fimbrial antigens can be recognized from samples sent for analysis in most diagnostic laboratories and are important in identifying this agent as a cause of diarrhea. After the organism attaches to the villi, it produces the second virulence factor, enterotoxin. Enterotoxin interferes with the normal physiology of the gut, with resultant diarrhea.[131] Calves have an age-associated resistance that probably is related to the blocking of fimbrial attachment to the gut, so ETEC diarrheal disease occurs mainly in calves younger than 1 week of age.[132,133] The mode of infection is fecal-oral.

Clinical Signs. ETEC diarrhea is seen in lambs and kids younger than 10 days of age but is most common at 1 to 4 days, so age-related resistance also may be a factor in newborns of these species.[126,130] It usually manifests as an outbreak in lambs and kids between 12 and 48 h of age. Because ETEC causes a secretory-type diarrhea, bicarbonate loss in the diarrhea leads to severe acidosis, with lambs and kids quickly becoming dehydrated and recumbent. However, many infected animals die before developing diarrhea. Affected neonates are depressed, stop nursing, and may show excessive salivation. Fluid sequestration in the abomasum produces a splashing sound on movement. This condition is associated with high mortality if animals are not treated promptly.[130,131]

Diagnosis. Fecal culture and serotyping for the K99 and F41 fimbrial antigens constitute the basis for diagnosis. Because many nonpathogenic *E. coli* bacteria are normal gut inhabitants, growth of this organism on cultures usually is an insignificant finding.[131] Occasionally, the bacteria do not express the fimbrial antigens in culture, so ETEC cannot be ruled out if the culture is negative for K99 and F41.[134] Histopathologic evidence of colonization of the small intestine can support a diagnosis.

Treatment. Supportive care consisting of fluid therapy with either oral, IV, or SC administration of a polyionic solution is the mainstay of therapy. The use of oral antimicrobial agents is controversial. Although antibiotics may kill the ETEC, they also may interfere with normal gut flora. If fluid support is provided, the diarrhea usually subsides without antibiotic treatment. Nevertheless, oral neomycin (10 to 22 mg/kg twice daily) or trimethoprim-sulfa (30 mg/kg PO) and systemic ampicillin (10 to 20 mg/kg IM twice a day) or amoxicillin (10 to 20 mg/kg IM three times a day) may be beneficial. NSAIDs are indicated to decrease inflammation of the gut and provide some analgesia. The use of flunixin meglumine (1–2 mg/kg IM) has been shown to decrease fecal output in ETEC infections in calves[135] and appears to be beneficial in lambs.

Prevention. Vaccination of ewes and does with bovine ETEC vaccine before they give birth is recommended to increase passive immunity in the neonate.[126,127,131] Monoclonal and polyclonal antibody products for calves may be beneficial during an outbreak if administered to lambs or kids within the first 12 h of life. The use of neomycin (10 to 12 mg/kg PO twice daily) in lambs that appear clinically normal may help stop the progression of an outbreak. Shearing ewes prepartum to minimize fecal ingestion by neonates and ensuring that newborns ingest adequate colostrum both will help decrease the incidence of this disease. Making sure that ewes and does have a 2.5 to 3.5 BCS at parturition and are fed adequate diets in the final 2 months of gestation will increase the chance of adequate colostrum manufacture by the dam.

Rotavirus

Pathogenesis. Lambs and kids are infected with group B rotaviruses whereas most other animals, including cervids such as roe deer, and human beings are infected with group A rotaviruses.[136] Rotaviruses infect villus tip cells of the small intestine, which results in villus atrophy and malabsorptive diarrhea.[137]

Clinical Signs. Rotavirus generally causes diarrhea in lambs and kids 2 to 14 days of age, but older animals also can be affected. Young animals can become very depressed and dehydrated.[126,136,138,139]

Diagnosis. Detection of the organism by electron microscopy of fecal or colonic samples or by immunologic techniques applied to feces or tissue sections is the basis of diagnosis.[136,139] Because these organisms are sloughed with the villus tip cells they infect, and viral antigens are complexed with the animal's antibodies, tissue samples from acutely infected animals are of highest diagnostic value.[140] Rotavirus has been detected in animals without diarrhea, so other causes of diarrhea should be investigated as well.[127,129]

Treatment and Prevention. Rotavirus diarrhea is treated with supportive care. Prevention by vaccination of small ruminants with bovine rotavirus vaccines before they give birth is recommended to increase passive immunity in neonates.[126,127]

Cryptosporidium Species

Pathogenesis. *Cryptosporidium parvum* is a protozoan that can cause a malabsorptive diarrhea similar to that seen with rotavirus infection. Unlike other protozoal agents, such as the one that causes coccidiosis, cryptosporidia do not require fecal excretion for sporulation to infective stages.[141] They sporulate in the gut, whereupon approximately 20% become immediately infectious to other villus tip cells without leaving the intestines. This method of autoinfection can result in severe disease that may be sustained for long periods. Because some of the oocysts also are immediately infectious when they are shed in feces, spread of infection may be rapid.

Clinical Signs. Cryptosporidia can cause diarrhea in small ruminants at 5 to 10 days of age.[127,142,143] Affected animals often are active, alert, and nursing. The diarrheal stools usually are very liquid and yellow. Diarrhea can range from mild and self-limiting to severe, especially with mixed infections.[127,129,142,144] Relapses are quite common, and this organism usually occurs as a component of mixed infections.

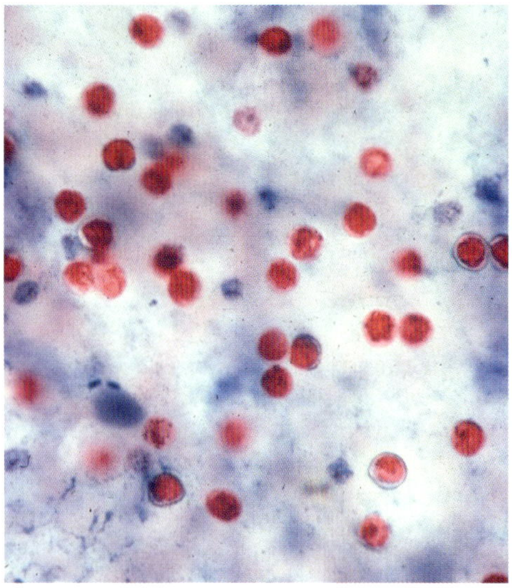

• **Fig. 5.12** Red-staining *Cryptosporidium* on a blue-green background in a fecal smear prepared with an acid-fast stain. This protozoal parasite induces villus atrophy and decreased digestion.

Diagnosis. Acid-fast staining of air-dried fecal smears is a quick and easy method of diagnosis. Examination under 40× to 100× magnification reveals round protozoa that have taken up the red color of the carbol fuchsin portions of the stain on a green background (Figure 5.12). Although cryptosporidial infection can be diagnosed by fecal flotation testing, the very small size (4 to 6 μm) of these organisms makes this method difficult and subject to false-negative results.[145,146] Both immunologic and polymerase chain reaction (PCR) techniques have been developed to improve detection limits.[145,147] Cryptosporidia also can be identified on histopathologic examination. Cryptosporidiosis is a zoonotic disease, and people can become infected from handling infected animals or feces.[141]

Prevention. No consistently effective treatment for cryptosporidiosis in ruminants has been identified. However, proper hydration and electrolyte balance should be maintained, along with other supportive care. Prevention through decreased exposure of neonates to organisms in the environment is critical, especially exposure of neonates at birth.[148] On farms endemic with coccidiosis or during an outbreak, improved hygiene may be of benefit (e.g., precolostral intake udder wash, feeding only low-heat-pasteurized colostrums, isolation of all exposed animals). Anecdotal reports suggest that decoquinate and monensin sodium may be useful in control of cryptosporidiosis. Decoquinate (2.5 mg/kg PO) fed to does and kids may be useful in decreasing morbidity and mortality associated with cryptosporidiosis in goat kids.[149] Treatment in all affected animals also should include fluid-electrolyte therapy.

During an outbreak, affected animals should be isolated from the rest of the flock. No new animals should be added to a pen in which the disease has been diagnosed. Keepers should depopulate pens in which the disease has been diagnosed and attempt to clean the environment. Cryptosporidiosis can be particularly difficult to control because of the organism's persistence in the environment and resistance to most chemical disinfectants. Ammonia (5–10%) and formalin (10%) seem to be the most effective agents, but, due to the potential for toxic effects, caution is indicated with the use of either chemical.[142,150] Feeders should be constructed to minimize fecal contamination. Early results are favorable for vaccine development in cattle, and vaccination may prove to be the best control method in the future.[151] Cryptosporidiosis is potentially a zoonotic disease; clinicians and keepers should therefore exercise great caution when handling affected animals, and well-planned biosecurity programs should be instituted (see Chapter 19).

Salmonella Species

Pathogenesis. The bacterial genus *Salmonella* has thousands of serotypes, all of which can potentially cause diarrhea in animals. Salmonellae can cause diarrhea in small ruminants of any age.[126,127] These microbes produce enterotoxins, are invasive, and cause severe inflammatory disease and necrosis of the lining of the small and large intestines.

Clinical Signs. Affected animals younger than 1 week of age are more likely to die acutely before onset of clinical signs, whereas animals older than 1 week are more likely to have diarrhea.[127,130,152] An acute onset of fever, depression, tenesmus, and shock occasionally is observed. *Salmonella*-induced diarrheal stool is more likely to contain blood.[127] Enteric salmonellosis also is a zoonotic disease that warrants implementation of protective measures.

Diagnosis. A diagnosis of *Salmonella* diarrhea is based on culture of the organism in feces or tissues and characteristic changes on histopathologic examination of the small and large intestine.[153] More sensitive PCR techniques for identifying *Salmonella* species in feces are being developed.[154] The diarrheal feces occasionally may contain fibrin, but many animals die before this development is observed. The clinician may note leukopenia or leukocytosis in the CBC results.

Treatment. Therapy for *Salmonella*-induced diarrhea involves supportive care and possibly parenteral antimicrobial therapy. The use of antimicrobial agents is controversial and probably does not influence the gastrointestinal infection. Nevertheless, because *Salmonella* is an invasive organism, parenteral use of antimicrobial agents may be beneficial in preventing septicemia. Antimicrobial susceptibility patterns are difficult to predict for *Salmonella* species, so antimicrobial therapy should be based on culture and sensitivity results. Ceftiofur sodium (1.1–2.2 mg/kg IM twice daily) or trimethoprim-sulfadiazine (15 mg/kg SC once a day) can be administered until antimicrobial sensitivity results are available.

Prevention. Latent carriers of *Salmonella* can potentially shed organisms to other animals, particularly when they are stressed.[127] Newly introduced animals should be isolated for 1 month, and fecal culture should be considered.[127] Bleach (sodium hypochlorite) and chlorhexidine are effective disinfectants to apply to the premises and animal handling/feeding equipment during an outbreak. Identification of carrier animals by fecal culture is recommended for herd problems. Vaccine efficacy is questionable, and to date its effects have not been thoroughly evaluated in sheep and goats.[155]

Giardia. *Giardia*-induced diarrhea is more commonly seen in, but not limited to, 2- to 4-week-old lambs, kids, and fawns.[127,156] The diarrhea usually is transient, but infected animals can continue to shed cysts for many weeks, even when they appear to be clinically normal.[145,157,158] Therefore, simply finding the pathogen in feces does not mean that it is the cause of the diarrhea, especially in older animals. *Giardia* can be found in herds without any history of neonatal diarrhea, so finding *Giardia* in herds in which newborn animals are experiencing diarrhea is of questionable relevance.[159] However, these animals may be a source of infection for others and possibly humans.[145,156] Identification of the organism on iodine-stained wet mounts of feces or tissue is the classic method of diagnosing giardiasis, but more sensitive immunologic techniques are now available.[145,156] Infected animals can be treated effectively with fenbendazole (5–10 mg/kg twice daily for 3 days or once daily for 5 days).[145] Giardiasis has historically been treated with oral metronidazole (50 mg/kg once a day for 5 days). However, use of this drug class in food animals is currently illegal in the United States. Giardiasis is potentially a zoonotic condition.

Nutritional Diarrhea. Infectious agents are not the only cause of diarrhea in neonates. Nutritional problems can result in diarrhea, but cases related to nutrition are underreported in the literature because the resulting diarrhea usually is mild and subsides without treatment. Nutritional diarrhea is most common in orphaned animals and usually is a result of improper management practices such as use of poor-quality milk replacers, mixing errors, or infrequent feeding of large amounts (see Chapter 2). Diarrhea resulting from consumption of lush pasture or high-energy rations also is commonly seen and usually is self-limiting. The incidence of this form of gastric upset can be minimized by a slow introduction (over 2–3 weeks) to energy-dense diets.

In calves with infectious diarrhea that develop maldigestion or malabsorption, secondary nutritional diarrhea may result from an inability to digest carbohydrates (lactose, xylose).[160,161] This digestive defect has been reported in goats and also is probably a cause of diarrhea in lambs.[162] Diarrhea resulting from primary lactose deficiency also has been reported in calves.[163] Calves on poor-quality milk replacers can develop an overgrowth of normal enteric *E. coli,* resulting in diarrhea.[164] If lactose intolerance is suspected, decreasing the amount of lactose fed and using commercially available lactose enzymes may alleviate clinical problems.

Causes of Diarrhea in Older Lambs, Kids, and Fawns

The most common cause of diarrhea in older lambs and kids is nematode infestation. Other major causes of diarrhea in older small ruminants are *Clostridium perfringens* infection and coccidiosis. Coccidiosis is covered in Chapter 6. *Giardia* has been reported to cause weight loss without diarrhea in 2- to 3-month-old lambs.[165]

Clostridium Perfringens. *C. perfringens* types A, B, C, and D all can cause diarrhea in lambs and kids, but type D is the most common etiologic agent in the United States.[127,130,166,167]

Pathogenesis. Clostridial diarrhea occurs in peracute, acute, and chronic forms and commonly is called *enterotoxemia* or *overeating disease.* In type C infection, a beta toxin can cause acute hemorrhagic enteritis. Type C infection is seen mostly in lambs or kids younger than 3 weeks of age. An epsilon toxin is responsible for pathologic findings in type D infections. Enterotoxemia usually is seen in rapidly growing feedlot lambs on high-concentrate rations. It also is associated with other feeding changes, including changes in type of pasture. However, it occasionally has been reported in the absence of any dietary changes, particularly in goats.[127,130,168] This disease commonly occurs in the fastest-growing and most well-conditioned animals. Even vaccinated herds (again, more usually goats) can be affected, so it should not be ruled out despite confirmation of previous vaccination.[127]

Clinical Signs. The *peracute* form of clostridial infection is characterized by the rapid onset of severe depression, abdominal pain, profuse and bloody diarrhea, and neurologic signs. Death occurs within hours of onset of clinical manifestations. Sudden death may occur without diarrhea. Sudden death following the onset of neurologic signs is more common in sheep, whereas goats are more likely to show signs of diarrhea before death.[127] Similar but less severe signs are seen in the *acute* form of the disease. The *chronic* form occurs more commonly in goats.[127,167]

Diagnosis. Antemortem diagnosis is based on clinical signs. At necropsy, *C. perfringens* can be cultured from intestinal tissue samples. The significance of a positive culture can be difficult to interpret, however, because these organisms can be a normal component of the gut flora but subsequently proliferate after death. This is true especially of type A, for which a role in actual disease is controversial.[169] Histopathologic examination of sections of the gut can be helpful. Identification of the toxins (namely, the epsilon toxin) in intestinal contents is required for a definitive diagnosis.[127,130] Because the toxin degrades within several hours of death, its absence does not preclude enterotoxemia as a diagnosis[166] (Figure 5.13).

Treatment. Treatment is rarely effective but consists mainly of aggressive supportive care. *C. perfringens* type D antitoxins (15–20 mL SC) can be administered to animals during an outbreak of enterotoxemia if clinical signs are noted. The antitoxin may be more effectively used as a preventive early in an outbreak of the disease. During an outbreak, any animals that have not been vaccinated should be given the antitoxin and vaccinated with the toxoid simultaneously; those previously vaccinated should receive a booster vaccination.

Prevention. Routine vaccination should start at 4 to 6 weeks of age and be followed by a booster 3 to 4 weeks later. In settings in which the disease has become endemic, lambs or kids can be vaccinated and given antitoxin during the first week of life. Yearly vaccination, preferably a few weeks before the ewes and dams give birth, increases colostral immunity in neonates and improves prevention programs. Goats may not respond as well to vaccination as sheep do, so biannual, triannual, or quarterly vaccination is recommended, especially in herds in disease-endemic areas.[127,162] Vaccination with only *C. perfringens* type C and type D vaccines and tetanus toxoid is superior to the use of more polyvalent clostridial vaccines.[127] Reducing the energy density of the diet and avoiding sudden dietary changes or alterations in the feeding routine are

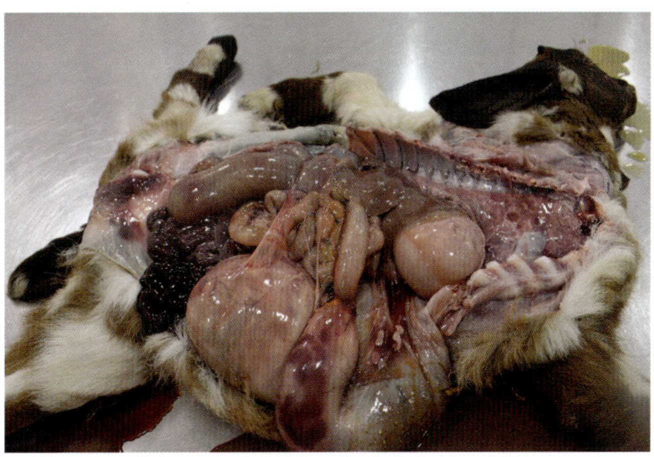

• **Fig. 5.13** A field necropsy of a 10-week-old intact, male Boer cross kid with watery diarrhea demonstrated necro-hemorrhagic enteritis. Laboratory diagnostics demonstrated *Clostridium perfringens* as the cause, and histologic examination of tissues was consistent with this diagnosis. The kid had no history of vaccination. (Courtesy of Dr. Kelley Steury, ALVDL, Auburn, AL.)

crucial to prevention. Control of internal parasites, particularly tapeworms, may further reduce the incidence of these disorders.

Miscellaneous Causes of Diarrhea in Kids, Lambs, and Fawns

Adenovirus, caprine herpesvirus, coronavirus, *Campylobacter jejuni, Escherichia fergusonii, Yersinia* species, and *Strongyloides papillosus* can cause diarrhea in lambs, kids, and fawns of various ages.[125,127,129,170] An adenovirus-induced hemorrhagic enteropathy has been seen in a captive, black-tailed deer herd.[171] Enterohemorrhagic *E. coli* (EHEC) and enteropathogenic *E. coli* (EPEC) also have been isolated from feces of both diarrheic and normal lambs and kids.[172–176] These *E. coli* serotypes are K99- and F41-negative. Culture and serotyping of these organisms from feces and tissue samples with typical histopathologic lesions are diagnostic. Although ETEC disease is not zoonotic, EHEC and EPEC can potentially affect humans and cause foodborne illness.

Treatment of Lambs and Kids With Diarrhea

Although specific therapies are available for some causes of diarrhea, many animals need to be treated for dehydration and metabolic acidosis regardless of the inciting cause. Animals with only mild diarrhea, especially mild nutritional diarrhea, may not require therapy unless they become dehydrated. If kids or lambs become less than 8% dehydrated and are only mildly depressed but still willing to nurse, they can be treated with oral electrolytes designed for calves. Fluids can be administered by bottle or by feeding tube (~ 18- to 24-inch, 3/8-inch diameter, catheter tip) if the animal will not nurse. The keeper or the clinician should carefully adjust the amount of fluids for lambs and kids (250–500 mL [8–16 oz], as opposed to 4 L in a calf). Because most electrolyte solutions designed for calves contain glucose, they should be refrigerated after they have been mixed and any leftovers discarded within 24 h. IV fluids may be needed to treat more severe dehydration. If the lamb or kid is too weak to stand, IV fluids are indicated. Isotonic fluids containing electrolytes should be given to replenish losses. Glucose can be added to make a 1 to 2.5% solution. Sodium bicarbonate also may be administered, especially if the dehydration is severe. A rule of thumb is to give one-fourth of the calculated fluid needed as isotonic bicarbonate (1.3%). Extra potassium (10–20 mEq/L) can be added to fluids, because most animals are severely dehydrated from diarrhea and depleted in potassium, even though their blood potassium levels may be elevated. If extra potassium is added, acidosis must be corrected concurrently. After correcting the dehydration, the keeper or the clinician can offer oral electrolyte-enriched fluids to replace ongoing losses caused by continued diarrhea (see also Chapter 3).

Removing milk or milk replacer from the diet is not recommended. Young animals need nutrients, and even high-energy, glucose-containing electrolyte solutions are no substitute for milk. Animals should continue to receive milk replacer in normal amounts or be allowed to nurse; oral electrolytes also can be given if necessary. Animals being hand-fed should be offered small amounts frequently to help minimize problems. Electrolytes should never be mixed with milk but should instead be given in separate feedings. If lactase deficiency is suspected, lactase drops or capsules (available in health food stores) can be added to milk or milk replacer.[162]

NSAIDs (e.g., flunixin meglumine, 1.1–2.2 mg/kg IV, or ketoprofen, 3 mg/kg IV) are beneficial, especially if toxemia is involved, as in ETEC, enterotoxemia, and salmonellosis. Antimicrobial agents should be reserved for proven outbreaks of salmonellosis and for animals with other causes of diarrhea that do not respond to fluid therapy and NSAIDs; these drugs should be administered only parenterally. Oral coating agents and antacids are popular, but such agents have not been shown to be beneficial, and their use is not therapeutically logical in light of the pathogenesis of these diseases. The therapeutic use of probiotics is questionable, but anecdotal reports suggest they may be beneficial in reestablishing the normal flora of the small intestine. Our own rule of thumb is that nothing should be given orally except milk, oral electrolytes, and possibly probiotics.

General Control Measures for Infectious Diarrhea

Ensuring adequate intake of high-quality colostrum and minimizing stress are important for prevention of all neonatal diseases. A normal lamb or kid will stand and nurse within 45 minutes to 1 h of birth. The ingestion of colostrum within 2 to 3 h is essential in preventing hypothermia and hypoglycemia and decreasing the incidence of various diseases. Lambs or kids born as twins or triplets, weak or injured neonates, those born during severe weather, those born from a dam with dystocia, and those delivered by cesarean section all are candidates for colostrum supplementation. Supplemental colostrum should be good-quality colostrum from females that have tested negative for Johne's disease, ovine progressive pneumonia (OPP), and caprine arthritis encephalitis (CAE). Mixing colostrum from several cows decreases the incidence of the "cow colostrum–associated" hemolytic disease sometimes seen in lambs. If the lamb or kid is unable to nurse, it should be tube fed 50 mL/kg of colostrum. The veterinarian or animal handler can sit comfortably holding the lamb or kid in sternal recumbency in the lap. A 12 to 14 French soft feeding tube is then lubricated, inserted into the side of the mouth, and passed slowly to the depth of the thoracic inlet. If the tube is placed in the trachea, the lamb or kid will show signs of discomfort and may shake and cough. The tube may be palpated on the left side of the throat. After correct placement of the tube, colostrum can be administered by gravity flow.

Antepartum shearing of the dam may decrease the likelihood of ingestion of feces by lambs. Good sanitation in lambing and kidding areas is paramount in management programs that stress prevention. The presence of organic matter interferes with the effectiveness of many disinfectants, so removal and proper disposal of feces, carcasses, and placentas are essential. When disposing of waste material containing either *Cryptosporidium* or *Giardia,* the keeper should be careful to avoid contaminating water sources. Infected animals should be isolated to prevent spread of the infection throughout the flock or herd. In general, infected animals should remain in the environment where the infection was first diagnosed, because it is already contaminated. Removing pregnant ewes or dams to a clean area before lambing or kidding helps minimize the continued spread of disease. If possible, lambs and kids already born but not showing clinical signs should be removed to a third area. If "safe" pastures are maintained for internal nematode control, they are ideal for use in an emergency situation to control these diseases (see also Chapter 6). Although some animals may appear normal, they may be incubating and possibly shedding the infective agents of disease. If such animals are moved with pregnant females, they can be a source of contamination in a clean area. If healthy lambs and kids cannot be moved to a third, relatively safe area, they should be left with the clinically infected animals because they have already been exposed.

Diarrhea in Adult Sheep and Goats

The list of considerations in the differential diagnosis for acute and chronic diarrhea in small ruminants is extensive.[1,2] The most common cause of diarrhea in adult sheep and goats is parasitism; another major cause is Johne's disease. Parasitism is discussed in Chapter 6. Other causes of acute diarrhea include rumen acidosis, peritonitis, endotoxemia, and ingestion of toxins. The list of toxins that cause diarrhea also is very long, and often diarrhea is not the primary clinical sign. Some of the more commonly encountered toxins that produce diarrhea are arsenic, salt in toxic amounts, levamisole, copper, oak, selenium, and pyrrolizidine alkaloids.[1] *Salmonella* infection and chronic enterotoxemia can cause diarrhea in adult animals. Coccidiosis can occur in adults under severe stress or in animals that possess limited immunity because of lack of exposure. Hepatic and renal disease and copper deficiency sometimes are accompanied by chronic diarrhea, but weight loss is a more common sign in adults.

Johne's Disease. Johne's disease, also called *paratuberculosis*, is a chronic wasting and diarrheal disease caused by the bacterium *Mycobacterium avium* subspecies *paratuberculosis.* All ruminants, including cervids, are thought to be susceptible to infection. While varying from each herd/flock, the prevalence of Johne's in most ruminants, including cervids, increases when animal density is higher.[3] Transmission of the organism is primarily by the fecal-oral route. Young animals are more susceptible to infection than adults. It can be transmitted through milk and the placenta.

Pathogenesis. Bacterial shedding in feces and milk and transplacental transmission are more common in animals showing clinical signs.[4–6] Therefore, the offspring of infected animals, and especially the offspring of animals showing clinical signs, are more likely to acquire the infection than other members of the flock/herd. After an animal is exposed, it will either clear the organism or acquire a chronic, persistent infection. The infection most commonly is isolated to the ileal regions of the small intestine where it causes granulomatous thickening of the intestinal wall and subsequent malabsorptive diarrhea. Infected animals may be asymptomatic for years.

Clinical Signs. Morbidity rates are low (approximately 5%), but for every infected animal with clinical signs, several are in the subclinical state and may be a source of both horizontal and vertical transmission.[4] Both sheep and goats appear to remain asymptomatic until they reach 2 to 7 years of age. The most consistent clinical sign in sheep, goats, and cervids is chronic weight loss. Chronic diarrhea occurs in approximately 20% of cases.[4] Signs may appear with or be exacerbated by stress, especially after parturition.[4,5] Hypoproteinemia and chronic mild anemia are the only consistent findings from clinicopathologic laboratory tests. Submandibular edema may develop as a consequence of low protein levels in infected animals, and because parasitism is ubiquitous, an accurate diagnosis may be difficult.

Diagnosis. Diagnosis is by culture of the organism from feces. Such testing unfortunately takes between 8 and 14 weeks but can identify 40 to 60% of clinically infected goats. Feces of noninfected sheep and goats within heavily infected herds can yield a positive culture from oral-fecal pass-through of the organism. Sheep strains of Johne's disease and some goat variant strains seem to be more difficult to culture in media used to identify cattle strains of the disease. Therefore, fecal culture in sheep and goats appears to be of limited benefit in a clinical setting.[5,6] A relatively inexpensive and easily performed method of identifying approximately 50% of all clinically infected animals is acid-fast staining of fecal smears.[4,5] A PCR fecal assay also is available, but its sensitivity is lower than that of fecal culture. Good diagnostic results can be obtained with serologic testing for antibodies (e.g., agar gel immunodiffusion [AGID] test, enzyme-linked immunospecific assay [ELISA], complement fixation test) in animals showing clinical signs. The specificity of all of the serologic tests is greater than 95% in sheep and goats with signs of clinical disease, although the sensitivity is not as high.[5–8] Therefore, a positive serologic test result in an animal showing clinical signs indicates that the animal has Johne's disease. However, the disease cannot be ruled out with a negative test result. Identification of subclinically infected animals using serologic tests is more problematic. A sensitivity of approximately 50% is all that should be expected. With the ELISA and complement fixation test, cross-reactivity with *Corynebacterium pseudotuberculosis* may occur, thereby limiting the value of such testing in flocks with caseous lymphadenitis infections.[5,9] ELISA performed on milk samples from goats had reduced sensitivity but increased specificity (less cross-reaction) compared with serum ELISA.[10] Sheep and goats appear to respond differently with regard to the formation of antibodies. In sheep, antibodies tend to develop in the later stages of the disease, whereas antibodies may be detected much earlier in the goat. Necropsy diagnosis is based on the finding of thickened, corrugated intestines, especially in the area of the ileum. Acid-fast staining of impression smears (taken from the ileum and ileocecal lymph nodes) can help yield a quick diagnosis. The staining of numerous clumps of acid-fast rods is highly suggestive of Johne's disease.

Prevention. Johne's disease has no effective treatment, so prevention and control are imperative. However, preventing the introduction of Johne's disease into a herd can be difficult. Because animals with subclinical infection may not shed the organism or shedding may occur in only small quantities, fecal culture is helpful only if a positive culture is obtained. The sensitivity of serologic tests of animals with subclinical disease is low and variable among flocks.[5,6] Negative test results in subclinically infected animals are common. However, the specificity of serologic tests remains high, so a positive test result is a valid reason to not purchase an animal.[5] Because Johne's disease also occurs in cattle, supplemental colostrum supplies should come only from dairy herds free of Johne's disease.

After Johne's disease is diagnosed in a herd, several control measures should be implemented. Sanitation is important, because the organism is highly resistant in the environment (i.e., capable of surviving longer than 1 year under most conditions).[6] Reduced stocking rates, frequent cleaning of pens, and use of automatic waterers will decrease fecal transmission. Keepers and herdsmen should cull the offspring of infected animals. Culling animals based on the results of flock/herd -wide AGID testing or ELISA and fecal culture is recommended. Animals should be tested at least once a year. More frequent testing as resources allow will speed the identification of infected animals. A vaccine for cattle is available only in some locales, and clinicians or keepers may require official permission for its (extra-label) use in sheep and goats. Vaccination for Johne's disease in cattle does not eliminate infection but can decrease herd prevalence, delay the onset of clinical signs, and decrease cross transmission by infective bacterial shedding in the feces.

Intestinal Obstruction

Any cause of intestinal obstruction that occurs in other ruminants may occur in sheep, goats, and cervids. Obstructive diseases of the intestinal tract may be divided into two general categories — strangulating and nonstrangulating (simple and functional). Examples of strangulating lesions include intussusception and torsion of the mesenteric root, whereas simple, nonstrangulating obstructions include enteroliths and phytobezoars. Functional, nonstrangulating lesions are most commonly associated with inflammation or infection, often presenting as intestinal ileus.[187] Most of these diseases produce abdominal pain and occasionally abdominal distention. Diagnosis is based on physical examination but distinguishing true obstruction from functional obstruction can be difficult. Abdominal radiographs and ultrasonography can help differentiate among differential diagnoses with further support given with the use of clinicopathological analyses (e.g., rumen fluid analysis, abdominal fluid analysis). On occasion, a "target-shape" lesion of an intussusception may be found via ultrasonography.[188] However, exploratory surgery may be required to obtain a definitive diagnosis and should be considered a reasonable diagnostic and therapeutic intervention in a small ruminant presenting for an acute abdomen. Clinical signs suggestive of obstructive intestinal diseases include vocalization, kicking at the abdomen, frequent lying bouts, and even recumbency with severe pain. The heart rate is increased due to hypovolemia and pain. Changes in the abdominal contour may become apparent with the development of low, bilateral abdominal distention, depending on the amount of fluid buildup in the intestinal tract proximal to the obstruction. Manure may be scant or absent with changes in appearance such as the presence of melena or mucus. The initial colic episode may be followed by chronic low-grade pain and signs suggestive of peritonitis.[187]

Intussusception

Intussusception is the telescoping of one segment of intestine into an adjacent segment. Any segment of the intestine can be affected, but the ileum and ileocecal junction are the most common areas involved. The condition is more commonly reported in young animals but can occur in mature animals. In this condition, one segment of the intestine telescopes into an adjacent segment (intussusceptum and intussuscipiens, respectively), resulting in narrowing of the intestinal lumen and blood supply compromise. The initiating cause is not always known, but suspected predisposing factors include segmental motility differences caused by enteritis (e.g., coccidiosis), intestinal parasitism (e.g., *Oesophagostomum* infestation), and intestinal masses.[189–193] Clinical signs and diagnosis are as described earlier. Treatment requires surgical correction, as well as fluid therapy and supportive therapy.

Torsion of the Root of the Mesentery and Cecal Volvulus

Torsion of the root of the mesentery and cecal volvulus can occur sporadically in small ruminants. Clinical signs include extreme abdominal pain, rapidly progressive abdominal distention, and circulatory collapse. Immediate surgical correction and circulatory support are needed.[187]

Foreign Body Obstruction

Ingested foreign bodies or bezoars can obstruct portions of the intestines.[194–198] The signs are similar to those of obstruction caused by other small intestinal accidents and depend on which part of the intestine is blocked. In some cases, the obstructing body can be seen with use of radiography or ultrasonography. Surgical removal is required for treatment.

Intestinal Atresia

Intestinal atresia can affect singly, or in combination, the segments of the small intestine, large colon, rectum, or anus, and are reported in common food animal species.[199–205] Apart from atresia anovaginalis (i.e., presence of a rectovaginal fistula), all cases are lethal if not surgically corrected. The clinical presentation of affected lambs and kids is progressive abdominal distention with failure to produce feces, as well as signs of abdominal pain, inappetence, weakness, and dehydration. In the case of atresia ani, lack of an anus is apparent, and bulging of the perineum may be observed when the animal strains or with abdominal palpation. A thorough physical examination is important for the discernment of other congenital abnormalities present.[205,206] Radiography (including contrast fistulogram) and ultrasonography of the abdomen, pelvis, and perineum may help classify the type of anorectal malformation present. Definitive diagnosis of atresia conditions of the colon and small intestine may require an exploratory celiotomy. The presence of other congenital abnormalities should be thoroughly evaluated on physical examination.

Surgical repair techniques are described for atresia ani and atresia coli in ruminants; however, based on economical and prognostic considerations, surgical correction of atresia ani is far more likely to be a viable option compared with atresia coli in small ruminants. A description of the surgical correction of atresia ani is reviewed later, whereas the reader is referred elsewhere for the detailed descriptions of creating a permanent colostomy and end-to-end anastomoses for the treatment of other intestinal atresia conditions.[207–209] Although not necessarily lethal, surgical correction of rectovaginal fistulas (as well as rectourethral and rectovesicular fistulas) should also be advocated, as the condition predisposes to urinary tract infections and can result in dilation of the rectum oral to the fistula, resulting in constipation and abdominal pain. Three basic classifications of intestinal atresia classification are described in animals. Type 1, membrane atresia, is caused by a membranous diaphragm occluding the lumen of the intestine. Type 2, cord atresia, is characterized by a fibrous band or muscular cord-like remnant of the gut connecting the two blind ends of oral and aboral intestinal segments. Type 3, blind end atresia, is caused by an absence of a segment of the intestine with unconnected ends and a corresponding gap in the mesentery. The etiopathogenesis of intestinal atresia conditions is likely multifactorial, including reported heritability in lambs. Affected animals should not be used for breeding purposes, ideally with neutering of the animal concurrently at the time of surgical correction of the atretic condition.[207]

Preparation of the animal for surgery should include stabilization including the administration of intravenous fluids where appropriate. Surgical correction of atresia ani is best achieved in animals in which a bulge in the perineal skin where the anus should be is appreciable. The procedure is performed using epidural anesthesia with or without light sedation, depending on the tractability of the animal. General anesthesia may be more appropriate in cases where extensive tissue dissection is anticipated. The animal is positioned in sternal recumbency with the perineal area clipped and aseptically prepared. A 1- to 1.5-cm diameter circular incision is made through the skin and subcutaneous tissues at the location of the bulge (or where the anus would normally be located). Blunt dissection is performed cranially to identify the rectal pouch. The pouch is gently retracted caudally with tissue forceps, and the rectum is sutured to the subcutaneous tissue with four to six interrupted sutures. The rectal pouch is incised, and the rectal mucosa sutured to the skin in a simple interrupted pattern or in a simple continuous pattern performed in quadrants. In females with rectovaginal fistulas, these should be located and transected prior to suturing the rectum to the perineal skin.[207,210]

In most cases, the absence of functional anal sphincter musculature is apparent during surgery and fecal incontinence is commonly encountered postoperatively. Postoperative care should include antibiotics and the use of laxatives (e.g., mineral oil) as indicated. Cases of atresia ani amenable to surgical correction carry a relatively good prognosis given the animal is not severely debilitated at the time of initial presentation.

Intestinal Ileus

Ileus of the small intestine is a functional, nonstrangulating obstruction most often secondary to abdominal pain, inflammation, or infection, resulting in the absence of intestinal motility. The animal's failure to pass ingesta leads to signs like those of other obstructive lesions discussed earlier. The cause of ileus may be unclear, but the condition is often secondary to systemic disease or as a complication of previous surgery (i.e., postoperative ileus). The same factors that can result in rumen stasis (e.g., abdominal inflammation, pain) may result in intestinal stasis and ileus. Treatment includes fluid therapy to address electrolyte derangements and dehydration, as well as the administration of NSAIDs for control of pain and inflammation. Administration of a lidocaine continuous-rate infusion, as commonly used in horses, may be considered with the caveat of potential lidocaine toxicity.[211,212] Use of prokinetic drugs is poorly described in small ruminants and should be used with caution, especially if the underlying cause is unknown (i.e., contraindicated in true obstructive disease).[213] If signs persist, however, surgical exploration is indicated.

Peritonitis

Pathogenesis

Anatomically, the peritoneum is divided into two continuous parts, the parietal and visceral peritoneum. The parietal peritoneum lines the diaphragm, abdominal wall, and pelvic cavity, whereas the visceral peritoneum encloses the intra-peritoneal organs and forms the omentum and mesentery. Normally, a small amount of fluid lies between the parietal and visceral peritoneum, which is transparent and straw-like in color with a total protein concentration less than 3 g/dL and a total nucleated cell count of less than 5000 cells/μL.[214–216] Inflammation of the peritoneum can be infectious or noninfectious (traumatic, chemical, or neoplastic) in etiology. Classifications of peritonitis include: cause (primary or secondary); onset and duration (peracute, acute, or chronic); location (localized or diffuse); and whether bacteria are present (i.e., septic or aseptic). Septic peritonitis is most common in ruminants. Common causes of septic peritonitis include rupture of gastrointestinal viscera (e.g., intestine secondary to obstruction; rupture of the abomasum secondary to abomasitis or abomasal ulcers), leakage of bacteria and intraluminal contents from ischemic or compromised viscera (e.g., ischemic intestine, uterine tears, urolithiasis), iatrogenic (e.g., trocarization of the rumen for bloat), and complications associated with surgical manipulation and entry into abdominal viscera (e.g., leakage at resection and anastomosis site).[217]

Clinical Signs

Signs of peritonitis are often nonspecific and are dependent on the stage, extent, and severity of the underlying condition. Clinical signs include altered body temperature, depression, anorexia, dehydration, and reduced gastrointestinal motility, including abdominal distention, reduced fecal output, and colic. The presence of fever is variable, and the systemic effects of dehydration, bacteremia, and endotoxemia typically manifest as tachycardia, tachypnea, and injection of mucous membranes. Peracute cases may present as sudden death, whereas chronic cases may include weight loss, poor body condition, intermittent diarrhea, or lack of fecal production with changes in abdominal contour.

Diagnosis

Abdominocentesis is important for the definitive diagnosis of peritonitis. Fluid should be collected in an EDTA tube for cytologic analysis, protein concentration, and Gram staining; in plain sterile tubes for aerobic and anaerobic culture; and in a lithium heparin tube if biochemical analysis is needed. The gross appearance of abdominal fluid can be suggestive of peritonitis, including an increase in the amount of fluid, and changes in the color, transparency, viscosity, and odor (e.g., cloudy, turbid, or red-tinged, to thick and purulent in character). Increases in total white blood cell counts, the percentage of neutrophils, and total protein concentration are observed.[218–221] In septic peritonitis, degenerative changes to neutrophils may be appreciable and, on occasion, intracellular bacteria are observed on cytologic examination.[215] Aerobic and anaerobic culture of abdominal fluid, including antimicrobial sensitivity testing, is indicated for proper treatment. A Gram- stain may aid identification of bacteria and assist in the choice of antimicrobial therapy before culture results are known (or in the absence of a positive culture). Failure to identify or culture bacteria should not rule out a diagnosis of septic peritonitis. Septic peritonitis usually involves a mixed bacterial population depending on the source of peritoneal contamination. Common bacterial isolates from exudative peritonitis include the Enterobacteriaceae, obligate anaerobic bacteria, and gram-positive organisms. Rumen bacteria are typically gram-negative anaerobes, whereas *E. coli* and other enteric species are common if the intestine is the source of infection.[218]

Use of ultrasonography may be useful in detecting increased amounts and changes in peritoneal fluid, as well as locating fluid pockets for abdominocentesis.[222] Hematologic and biochemical parameters reflect changes expectant of a systemic inflammatory response or sepsis (e.g., an inflammatory leukogram and, in severe cases, a degenerative left shift). Exploratory laparotomy may be required to identify the presence and source of abdominal infection.

Treatment

Treatment includes supportive, antibiotic, and surgical therapies. Supportive therapy includes crystalloid fluid administration to correct shock and electrolyte imbalances. Other supportive measures include NSAID medications (e.g., flunixin meglumine) for their pain control and anti-endotoxemia effects, as well as transfaunation. Systemic broad-spectrum antibiotic therapy is indicated with appropriate changes made when culture and susceptibility results are available. Surgical therapy includes peritoneal debridement, irrigation, and drainage. This may entail surgical correction of leaking abdominal viscera and physical removal of gross contamination. Use of abdominal drains can be problematic in ruminants, often readily becoming clogged with fibrin. The prognosis is guarded, especially if an intestinal rupture has occurred.[217]

Rectal Prolapse

Clinical Signs, Classification, and Pathogenesis

The typical presentation of a rectal prolapse is a mucosal mass (types I, II, and III) or tube (type IV) protruding beyond the anus with variability in the extent of edema, bruising, inflammation, and necrosis present. Type I rectal prolapse involves only the rectal mucosa and submucosa which can be symmetrical or asymmetrical in its protrusion from the anus. Type II rectal prolapse is a full thickness prolapse of all or part of the rectal ampulla. Type III rectal prolapse is a continuation of a type II rectal prolapse, with the addition of a variable amount of small colon intussuscepted into the rectum. Type IV rectal prolapse involves the intussusception of the peritoneal rectum and variable length of the small colon through the anus.[223] Types I to III palpate as a continuous protrusion from the mucocutaneous junction of the anus, whereas type IV is tube-like in appearance and forms a palpable trench inside the rectum on manual palpation. Rectal prolapse is more common in sheep than in goats and is often associated with short docked tails in lambs.[224] Producers should be encouraged to dock tails at the level of the attachment of the caudal tail fold rather than close to the body, as the latter is associated with an increased incidence of rectal prolapse. Other causes of rectal prolapse include excessive straining associated with diarrhea (e.g., coccidiosis, salmonellosis), chronic coughing, and tenesmus associated with dystocia or urolithiasis.[225] Over-conditioning (i.e., fat animals), grazing lush pastures or feeding of legumes (e.g., alfalfa, clover), and use of growth implants are also implicated as risk factors for the condition.[226] Regardless of the cause, eversion and exposure of the rectal mucosa results in irritation and inflammation, which causes further straining, which results in a vicious cycle of more and more tissue becoming prolapsed. Venous drainage of the prolapsed tissue may become compromised, further contributing to the swelling. Exposed tissue becomes edematous, inflamed, and eventually necrotic.

Treatment

Management of rectal prolapse includes the immediate resolution of the prolapse as well as addressing predisposing risk factors or causes for increased straining (e.g., treatment of coccidiosis). The type of rectal prolapse and severity of damage to the exposed tissue plays an important role in the type of treatment method selected. In general, the rectum recovers relatively well from injury and an attempt to salvage the prolapsed tissue should be made whenever possible, albeit within reason, as deep necrosis or extensive trauma to the tissue may necessitate surgical resection. A caudal epidural using 2% lidocaine should be performed to facilitate examination and cleansing of the prolapsed tissue while eliminating straining and providing adequate anesthesia for placement of a purse-string suture and surgical procedures, if necessary. Depending on the tractability of the animal, sedation may be required. In sheep with extremely short-docked tails, a lumbosacral epidural may be easier to perform and more likely successful in providing complete anesthesia of the perineum. In very mild, early type I cases, frequent topical application of hemorrhoidal ointment and replacement of the everted tissue may be successful and preclude the use of a purse-string suture. Another quick and inexpensive treatment option for mild cases is the injection of counterirritants (e.g., Lugol's iodine) in the retroperitoneal, perirectal space, either alone or in conjunction with a purse-string suturing.[227] The solution is injected using an 18-gauge needle, deeply (5 cm) within the soft tissues around the anus at the 12, 3, and 9 o'clock positions. Injection at the 6 o'clock position is avoided to prevent swelling and obstruction of the urethra.[228] Although the earlier suggestions are quick and inexpensive, resolution of a rectal prolapse often requires one of the following treatment options. These include: (1) replacement of the prolapse and placement of a purse-string suture, (2) amputation using a prolapse ring, (3) submucosal resection, or (4) resection and anastomosis.[223,225,229] In the case of type IV prolapses, an exploratory celiotomy with resection of affected tissue and an end-to-end anastomosis may be indicated. With all treatment options, restricted feeding for 24 to 48 h and the administration of mineral oil (or other appropriate laxatives) is recommended. Elimination of risk factors, such as the feeding of dusty hay, as well as the treatment of diarrhea or pneumonia should be carried out following replacement of the prolapse, as these conditions lead to increased abdominal pressures due to coughing or straining. In animals where correction of the rectal prolapse is cost-prohibitive, immediate harvest or euthanasia is recommended. Tetanus prophylaxis should be provided. Antibiotics used should be effective against anaerobes (e.g., penicillin), and their use is indicated when extensive necrosis and tissue damage is present (even if the prolapse is successfully replaced) or when surgical techniques are performed.

The use of an epidural anesthetic (e.g., 2% lidocaine, 0.5 mL/45 kg of BW) to decrease straining and ease pain associated with the procedure is required, regardless of treatment option used. The reader is referred to Chapter 18 for description of both caudal and lumbosacral epidural procedures. Combining xylazine (0.01–0.03 mg/kg) with 2% lidocaine may provide longer analgesia and reduced straining than that obtained by lidocaine anesthesia alone. In animals with irretractable straining, use of an alcohol epidural with either isopropyl alcohol or ethanol may be required to prevent straining for extended periods. This type of anesthesia is permanent and is not without risk, as its use causes demyelination of both sensory and motor nerves.[228] Potential complications include sciatic nerve damage, injection site necrosis, and the inability to pass feces. Therefore, it should be reserved for salvage purposes in animals intended for harvest. Because of the potential sciatic nerve damage, the clinician should perform a test injection of 2% lidocaine before using alcohol, to ensure the epidural is effective in eliminating straining with no apparent ataxia or muscle weakness in the hindlimbs. Following the test injection, a mixture of equal parts lidocaine and alcohol is used at the site previously injected.[228]

Replacement and Purse-String Suture. This technique is indicated for the treatment of salvageable rectal prolapses. Following epidural anesthesia, the prolapsed tissue is thoroughly evaluated, and the perineum and prolapsed tissue cleansed with a mild antiseptic. Edema can be reduced with the temporary topical application of hyperosmolar solution, such as granulated sugar or hypertonic saline. The prolapsed tissue is coated with lubricant (e.g., petroleum jelly) and gently manipulated back into its normal position. Placement of a purse-string suture is accomplished using appropriately sized nonabsorbable suture on a cutting needle, with tissue bites situated at the mucocutaneous junction of the anal sphincter. To minimize fecal contamination and allow easy adjustment, the bow-knot should be situated either dorsal or lateral to the anus. To facilitate tightening of the purse-string suture, an appropriately sized syringe case, tube, or the clinician's finger is placed in the rectum during suture tightening which is subsequently removed once the purse-string suture is secured. The purse-string suture is tightened sufficiently to prevent recurrence of the prolapse while allowing the passage of feces. Removal of the purse-string ideally should be within 1 week of placement to minimize suture-tract infection. If possible, topical application of petroleum jelly and hemorrhoidal gel daily will reduce inflammation and edema, facilitating earlier removal of the purse-string suture.[225,230]

Rectal Amputation Using a Prolapse Ring. Placement of a prolapse ring should be considered a salvage procedure. This procedure is often used under field conditions where surgical procedures are not economically or logistically possible. The prolapse ring is inserted into the rectum and an elastrator band placed. If a ligature is used in place of an elastrator band, it should be tightened sufficiently to allow purchase on the prolapse ring. Both the elastrator band or ligature serve to induce vascular compromise and necrosis of the aboral, prolapsed tissue eventually causing it to slough. A fibrotic band forms cranial to the elastrator band and mucosa subsequently grows across the area. Complications include failure due to premature dislodgement of the prolapse ring, rectal stricture, peritonitis, and abscess formation.[229]

Submucosal Resection. Submucosal resection involves the removal of necrotic or traumatized mucosa while salvaging healthy, underlying tissue. Advantages of submucosal resection compared with full-thickness resection (amputation) and anastomosis include: faster healing times, less postoperative straining, minimal constriction of lumen diameter, salvage of healthy tissue, the maintenance of the main blood supply thereby minimizing postoperative hemorrhage, and by not exposing the serosa, a reduction in the likelihood of peritonitis and perirectal abscess formation. However, submucosal resection requires more surgical time.

After surgical preparation of the perineum and prolapsed tissue, a piece of flexible tubing of appropriate diameter is inserted into the lumen of the prolapsed tissue and is fixed in place using two 18-gauge, 15-cm (6-inch) spinal needles placed at 90 degrees to each other in a cross-pinning fashion. Alternatively, stylets from similar in length catheters can be used if appropriate spinal needles are not available. The needles are placed through the external anal sphincter and approximately 2 to 4 mm cranial to the prolapse in healthy tissue in order to maintain the prolapse during dissection. Two complete circumferential incisions are made through the mucosa (of healthy tissue) on either side of the tissue to be removed. A longitudinal incision at the same tissue depth is made to connect these circumferential incisions. Deep dissection of the necrotic mucosa and submucosa is carried out, essentially elevating a strip of tissue to be removed but leaving a deep layer of healthy tissue. Hemorrhage is controlled by ligature of individual vessels. The mucosa is aligned with four simple interrupted sutures placed equidistant around the circumference of the prolapse, in order to prevent twisting of the closure. The four quadrants are then apposed separately in a simple continuous suture pattern, using 2-0 to 3-0 monofilament absorbable suture material on a taper needle. The spinal needles are removed, and the tissue replaced into the rectum.[225,229,231] A purse-string suture is placed as previously described to prevent prolapse of the surgical site. Postoperative management is as described earlier for all treatment options. The use of a nonsteroidal antiinflammatory postoperatively should be considered for control of pain and inflammation.

Resection and Anastomosis. Resection and anastomosis may be indicated in types III and IV prolapses if the prolapsed tissues are devitalized or the amount of tissue precludes the ability of reduction. The procedure can be performed as for submucosal resection, including the pinning technique for stabilizing the tissue during dissection. In contrast to the submucosal resection, full-thickness circumferential incisions are made through the inner and outer walls of the intussusceptum (in healthy tissue) with removal of all necrotic tissue. All mesenteric vessels within the prolapse are identified and ligated during resection. The proximal and distal edges are apposed with a monofilament absorbable suture (e.g., 1–2 polydioxanone suture (PDS)) using full-thickness, interrupted horizontal mattress sutures circumferentially. The mucosal edges are then apposed with a simple continuous pattern using 2-0 monofilament absorbable suture (e.g., PDS), divided into interrupted quadrants.[225] Alternatively, a stairstep amputation can be performed to maximize the length of the inner mucosal and submucosal layers, which facilitates easier adaptation of mucosal apposition of the respective segments.[230] Following resection and anastomosis, the cross-pins are removed and a routine purse-string suture is placed. Aftercare is as for the other techniques described. Antibiotics should be administered for 7 to 10 days postoperatively and the animal closely monitored for signs of peritonitis and sepsis. Potential complications include stricture formation, dehiscence of surgical site resulting in peritonitis, or evisceration of intestines, adhesion formation, and abscessation of the perirectal tissues.

Prevention

Preventative measures should address management practices that predispose to rectal prolapse. Importantly in sheep, this includes advising producers on the appropriate length of tail docking. Environmental factors should be addressed, including removal of dusty feeds and improvements in ventilation and air quality in intensively housed small ruminants to minimize coughing. Prevention and treatment of disease conditions, including diarrhea, pneumonia, and urinary calculi should be instituted. Other conditions such as over-stocked or unhygienic living conditions should be addressed. The producer should consider culling animals with a history of rectal prolapse from the breeding flock or herd. Sound nutrition and feeding practices, with frequent monitoring of BCS to avoid over-conditioned (excessively fat) animals will also aid in the prevention of rectal prolapse.

Diseases of the Liver

Liver Abscess

Formation of liver abscesses usually is the result of chronic rumenitis in cattle, but these lesions are rare in sheep and goats. They may occur in feedlot lambs and kids and other animals fed rations high in grain. In lambs and kids, septicemia or extension of an umbilical vein infection can lead to formation of liver abscesses.[232] In most cases, however, liver abscess is an incidental finding. Weight loss, anorexia, depression, and decreased production (e.g., growth, milk) may be noted in affected animals.

In adults, *C. pseudotuberculosis* is the most common pathogen. *Actinomyces pyogenes* and *Fusobacterium necrophorum* also are cultured from abscesses.[232,233] Liver enzymes may or may not be elevated. Diagnostic ultrasonography of the liver may help detect abscesses, especially if they are numerous and widespread. However, no specific treatment or control measure is available. Many of the preventive protocols used for feeder cattle can be applied to the control of abscesses in sheep and goats. Such strategies include slowly introducing concentrates into the diet, offering long-stemmed hay on a free-choice basis, and including rumen buffers (alkalizing agents) and antimicrobial agents in the feed.

Pregnancy Toxemia and Fatty Liver Syndrome

Pathogenesis. Fatty liver occurs in conjunction with pregnancy toxemia in ewes and does during the last month of gestation.[234,235] It is most common in both thin or obese ewes or does with a single large fetus, twins, or triplets.[235,234–236] During late gestation, particularly in obese females, the abdominal space is filled with accumulated fat and an ever-expanding uterus. Because of the lack of rumen space, these animals have difficulty consuming enough feedstuffs to satisfy energy requirements. In most management systems, late gestation occurs during the winter months when less pasture is available and poorer quality feedstuffs are offered. Energy requirements for ewes and does carrying twins or triplets are greatly increased during the final 2 months of gestation, because 70 to 80% of fetal growth occurs during this time. Ewes with twins require 180% more energy, and those with triplets need 200 to 250% more dietary energy. Glucose maintenance in ewes pregnant with twins is significantly more prone to disturbance resulting in hypoglycemia than in ewes bearing singletons.[235] Pregnancy toxemia also occurs in association with anorexia caused by other diseases (e.g., foot rot, OPP, CAE) or sudden stresses (e.g., feed or weather changes, predator attacks, hauling). A period of anorexia or lack of sufficient energy intake will result in a negative energy balance. Affected animals begin to mobilize body stores of fat and transport them to the liver. In the liver, fat is catabolized to glycerol and free fatty acids (FFAs). FFAs can be used in the citric acid cycle (Krebs cycle) as an energy source, but not in the direct formation of glucose. Anorexic animals have less ruminal substrate available for production of the glucose precursor, propionic acid. However, oxaloacetate, which is an integral part of the citric acid cycle, is removed from the cycle and converted into glucose. Depletion of oxaloacetate inhibits the normal function of the citric acid cycle, thereby inhibiting the use of FFAs. As the pool of FFAs increases, they are converted to ketone bodies or repackaged into lipoproteins. Because ruminants are not efficient at transporting lipoproteins out of the liver and back to the adipose stores, the lipoproteins overwhelm the liver's ability to handle fats, leading to a massive buildup, and resulting in a fatty liver. Because less substrate is available for glucose formation, more oxaloacetate is "cannibalized" from the citric acid cycle, further inhibiting the body's ability to use FFAs. This impairment in turn results in the continued accumulation of ketones. Hypoglycemia, hyperketonemia, and, potentially, uremia and death can occur.

Clinical Signs. Animals suffering from fatty liver or pregnancy toxemia become anorexic and depressed or dull, with altered behavior patterns, and may lag behind others in the group or become recumbent. Some are constipated, grind their teeth, have a ketone smell to the breath, demonstrate labored breathing or frequent urination, and suffer from dystocia. Neurologic signs include blindness, circling, incoordination, "star-gazing," tremors, and convulsions.[237–239] Death can occur if the condition is left untreated. In the case of fetal death in utero, maternal septicemia-endotoxemia and death are common sequelae.

Diagnosis. Diagnosis is based on clinical signs, the presence of multiple fetuses, and typical clinicopathologic findings.[234] CBC results may be normal or show an eosinophilia, neutropenia, and lymphocytosis. Affected animals may or may not be hypoglycemic, but ketoacidosis, hypocalcemia, and hypokalemia are common.[236–239] Liver enzymes usually are within normal limits but occasionally may be increased. Azotemia, both from dehydration and secondary to renal disease, is a common finding, and a fatal uremia may occur. Blood concentrations of β-hydroxybutyric acid greater than 7 mmol/L are consistent with pregnancy toxemia. Urinalysis will be positive for both ketones and protein.[234] Urine is collected from sheep by holding the nares and from does by frightening them and then allowing them a perceived escape, whereupon they stop, squat, and void.

Although not commonly performed, liver biopsy can help determine the extent of fatty infiltration. Serum protein pattern changes may become an available tool in the diagnosis of this condition in the future.[236] This syndrome must be differentiated from hypocalcemia, hypomagnesemia, PEM, encephalitis, lead toxicity, and cerebral abscesses.

Treatment. Very early cases (before onset of recumbency) may be treated with oral or intravenous glucose. A balanced electrolyte solution with extra calcium (25 mL of 23% calcium borogluconate/L), potassium (10–20 mEq/L), and 5% dextrose is needed.[234] In some cases, sodium bicarbonate is valuable in treating acidosis (see Chapter 3). Energy intake must be increased, and propylene glycol can be administered (15–30 mL every 12 h) as a glucose precursor. Rumen transfaunation and supplementation with vitamin B complex (including vitamin B_{12}, biotin, niacin, and thiamine) also are recommended.

After affected females become recumbent, treatment must be very aggressive. Flunixin meglumine (2.5 mg/kg once daily) appears to improve survivability, but should be used in conjunction with other therapies.[234] Flunixin meglumine can be given daily in depressed anorexic animals, and its use appears to improve feed intake.[234] Researchers using recombinant bovine somatotropin showed a response, but it was not significant in comparison with that in control animals.[240] Removal of the fetuses is crucial in these cases. Chemically inducing parturition (by administering 2.5–10 mg of prostaglandin $F_2\alpha$ or 0.75 μg/45 kg of cloprostenol in does and 15–20 mg of dexamethasone in ewes) and giving the ewe or doe medical support (fluids, B vitamins, glucose) while waiting is a useful protocol in some cases. Unfortunately, during the time before parturition, endotoxemia from dead fetuses further compromises the female's wellbeing. For this reason, we recommend immediate cesarean section in depressed moribund animals (see Chapter 8). The owner should be forewarned of the poor prognosis for animals already in a moribund state. Fluid support during and after surgery is crucial.

Regardless of the therapeutic plan, the animal should be offered a palatable, energy-rich, highly digestible feedstuff. The keeper and the clinician should take care to minimize the risk of a confounding disease during convalescence (e.g., lactic acidosis, PEM).

Prevention. Fatty liver and pregnancy toxemia can be prevented through proper management and nutrition. Maintaining animals in proper body condition throughout the year and making sure energy and protein levels are adequate in late gestation (see Chapter 2) are two key preventive measures.[234,237,238] The owner or manager should be taught to assess body condition in individual animals, avoid extremes in body condition, and maintain emergency stores of feed in case of severe weather or natural disasters. In over-conditioned females, the keeper should be encouraged to restrict institution of weight loss programs to early gestation (if at all) and to avoid abrupt feeding changes, while promoting exercise (e.g., by increasing walking distances from mineral access to shelter). The requirement for energy may be one and a half to two times maintenance for dams with single fetuses and two to three times maintenance for those with multiple fetuses. Prevention of concurrent disease, which may further increase energy demands or cause anorexia (e.g., intestinal parasitism, foot rot), is crucial. The keeper should take care to increase the grain portion of the diet slowly, and ensure the consistent availability of fresh, clean water, as anorexia from rumen upset can lead to pregnancy toxemia. Ewes should be offered 0.5 to 1 kg of a cereal grain (corn, oats, barley, or a combination) every day during the final months of gestation; does can be offered 1/2 to 1 kg of grain. Keepers should maintain ewes and does at a BCS of 2.5 to 3 (see Chapter 2) throughout gestation and evaluate the animals' energy intake every 2 to 4 weeks.

Ultrasonography can help identify females with multiple fetuses. These animals should be separated into groups and fed accordingly.[234] Ultrasonographic determination of fetal numbers is best accomplished between 35 and 90 days after breeding (see Chapter 8). Determination of fetal number may be enhanced with use of proper technique: shearing the hair or fiber in front of the udder; applying a coupling substance to the skin (e.g., alcohol, oil, lubricating gel); and interrogating (viewing) as much of the abdomen as possible while systematically moving from one side of the posterior abdomen to the other, to obtain an appreciation of the abdominal structures including any fetuses present.

Animal keepers and clinicians should ensure that ewes are healthy and free of chronic diseases (e.g., OPP, CAE, foot rot, chronic parasitism) and that a good-quality trace mineral salt mixture is available on a free-choice basis. The addition of lasalocid (0.5–1 mg/kg/day) or monensin (1 mg/kg/day) to the feed or mineral mixture will enhance the formation of the glucose precursor propionic acid and improve the efficiency of feed use. Monensin should be used with caution, however, because associated toxicity has been reported; the agent should be composed of no more than 30 ppm of the complete diet. The inclusion of niacin (1 g/head/day) in a feed supplement or mineral mixture will help prevent pregnancy toxemia. Supplementation with lasalocid, monensin, or niacin should begin 2 to 4 weeks before the animals give birth.

Shearing in the last trimester also is recommended in ewes.[238] Many sheep producers routinely clip the wool around the vulva. If complete body shearing is performed, the incidence of fatty liver or pregnancy toxemia may be decreased, by several mechanisms: sheared sheep require less energy to walk and graze. Sheared ewes also tend to shiver on cold days, exercising the enzyme systems that promote the more efficient use of FFAs as energy substrate. These ewes tend to seek shelter during cold weather, which may decrease lamb losses resulting from hypothermia. Obviously, if ewes are to be shorn, keepers should make adequate shelter available.

Keepers should avoid hauling or moving females during late gestation. Proper predator control measures should be maintained. Good hoof care programs should be in place on farms or ranches where grazing is the predominant form of nutrient intake. Sheep and goats should have their teeth checked to ensure good dentition before the breeding season. Animals with poor teeth should be culled.

Measuring serum β-hydroxybutyric acid concentrations is useful in assessing energy status in ewes. Values of 0.8 to 1.6 mmol/L suggest a negative energy balance. Keepers should take steps to correct the problem by feeding better-quality, more digestible feedstuffs.

White Liver Disease

White liver disease is a form of fatty liver disease reported only in Angora and Angora-cross goats and sheep. It is associated with cobalt deficiency.[241–245]

Pathogenesis. Cobalt is needed by rumen microflora to produce cyanocobalamin, or vitamin B_{12}, which is a coenzyme for methylmalonyl-coenzyme A (CoA) mutase. This enzyme is in turn needed to convert propionate to glucose through the Krebs cycle. Cobalt deficiency leads to the accumulation of methylmalonyl-CoA, or methylmalonic acid, which is converted to branched-chain fatty acids that accumulate in the liver. Diets high in grain, which is fermented to propionate, coupled with deficient or marginal cobalt intake, may predispose to this condition. White liver disease has not been reported in the United States, but ill thrift from cobalt deficiency has been observed. It is therefore possible that the disease goes unrecognized in some cases.[242–245]

Clinical Signs. Signs most commonly are seen in young animals and include ill thrift, anorexia, and diarrhea; sheep may exhibit photosensitivity. Clinical laboratory findings include a macrocytic-normochromic anemia and hypoproteinemia.[232,242,245]

Diagnosis. Abnormal serum or liver concentrations of vitamin B_{12} or liver cobalt levels are the basis for diagnosis. Liver cobalt concentrations of 0.08 ± 0.02 ppm determined on a dry matter basis were reported in goats with white liver disease, compared with 0.53 ± 0.11 ppm in control animals.[242,243]

Treatment and Prevention. Sheep can be treated with oral cobalt (1 mg/head/day) or vitamin B_{12} injections. The condition usually can be prevented by including cobalt in the ration by feeding a good-quality trace mineral salt; however, in areas in which cobalt is extremely deficient or absent from all feedstuffs, the oral administration of cobalt-containing "bullets" along with supplementation with a cobalt-containing salt-mineral mixture, may be required.[244]

Copper Toxicosis

Pathogenesis. Copper toxicosis is more common in sheep than in goats.[232,237,239] Goats appear to excrete copper more efficiently than sheep and are more cow-like in their ability to resist toxicosis, but nevertheless are susceptible.[232,237,246–248] The use of copper oxide wire particles to treat internal parasitism has been suggested as a cause of copper toxicity in goats. Toxicity results from chronic accumulation in the liver from the ingestion of excess copper in relation to molybdenum or sulfate in the diet. In sheep, a copper-to-molybdenum ratio greater than 10:1 leads to the accumulation of excess copper. The most common sources of excess copper in sheep and goats are trace mineral mixtures and feeds formulated for cattle or horses. Clinical signs often are absent during the chronic accumulation phase. Onset of acute disease is related to the sudden release of copper from the liver in large amounts. Stress usually precipitates this acute phase. Acute release of copper and subsequent high blood copper concentrations cause an acute hemolytic crisis, resulting in anemia, hemoglobinuria, and acute renal failure. Existing hepatic disease (such as that caused by liver flukes) may predispose animals to this condition. Some breeds (e.g., Merino sheep) seem to be prone to copper absorption and storage problems, whereas others (e.g., pygmy goats) tend to be more resistant and prone to deficiency (see Chapter 2).

Clinical Signs. Anorexia, depression, diarrhea, and weakness all are signs of copper toxicity. In many instances, affected animals are found dead with hemolysis and icterus. Abdominal pain and diarrhea sometimes are present. Port wine-colored urine is evidence of hemoglobinuria. Hemoglobinemia produces icterus of the mucosal membranes and fever.

Diagnosis. Findings on clinicopathologic examination include anemia, hemoglobinemia, hyperbilirubinemia, increased liver enzymes, and azotemia. Urinalysis reveals hemoglobinuria and isosthenuria. The combination of azotemia and isosthenuria indicates acute renal failure. Definitive diagnosis of acute disease requires measurement of copper concentrations in serum. Normal blood copper concentrations are approximately 50 to 200 μg/dL in sheep and goats.[249] These concentrations increase ten- to twentyfold with an acute hemolytic crisis.[237] On necropsy, kidney copper concentrations are the most diagnostic tissue, because liver concentrations may be normal after release into the bloodstream. Generally, kidney concentrations greater than 100 ppm and liver concentrations greater than 350 ppm on a dry matter basis are diagnostic. If tissue copper is reported in wet weight, the conversion to dry tissue weight can be estimated by multiplying the tissue concentration by a factor of 3.5.

Treatment. Treatment of acutely affected animals often is futile. Appropriate management consists of supportive therapy for the acute renal failure and anemia and attempts to lower liver copper stores. Fluid therapy for the acute renal failure (see Chapter 3) is of clinical benefit, and a blood transfusion may be needed if the PCV drops precipitously. Ammonium tetrathiomolybdate (1.7 mg/kg IV or 3.4 mg/kg SC on alternate days for three treatments) is the most economical agent for treatment in acute cases. In valuable animals, oral D-penicillamine (26–50 mg/kg twice daily or 52 mg/kg once daily for 6 days) increases urinary copper excretion. Trientine is used in human beings but has shown variable results in sheep. Treatment of the remainder of the flock should include the oral administration of ammonium molybdate (50–500 mg/head/day) and sodium thiosulfate (300–1000 mg/head/day) for 3 weeks. Stress should be minimized, so keepers and clinicians should delay routine maintenance procedures such as deworming and hoof trimming until after treatment. When applicable, spraying a combination of ammonium molybdate and sodium sulfate onto harvested forages low or deficient in copper to approximate the required therapeutic amount will decrease the stress required in daily oral dosing of chemicals. Allowing free access to grazing of forages high in sulfur (greater than 0.5% sulfur), if available, for all surviving ambulatory animals also may help to minimize death losses in a flock or herd. Overzealous attempts to clear excessive hepatic copper stores may potentially lead to deficiency, excessively stress the animal, and can be costly, thus should be avoided. The offending source of copper should be eliminated. Caution should be taken in such cases to remove ionophores from the diet, because these agents may contribute to copper absorption.[250]

Prevention. Avoiding high dietary copper (more than 10 ppm), a high copper-to-molybdenum ratio (greater than 10:1) in the feed, use of copper-containing foot baths, and other sources of copper is crucial. Including supplemental molybdenum in the diet to lower the copper-to-molybdenum ratio to 6:1 to 8:1 is beneficial. Addition of up to 2 to 6 ppm of molybdenum may be required in many instances.

Often too much emphasis is placed on the trace mineral component of the diet. The clinician should be aware that even if no copper is added to the trace mineral mixture and the element does not appear on the product label, the mineral mixture may nevertheless contain copper. Many components of mineral mixes are contaminated with copper (zinc sulfate may contain 400 ppm of copper, dicalcium phosphate may contain more than 30 ppm of copper). Therefore, the clinician needs to perform a dietary analysis to find and correct the problem.

Toxic Hepatitis

Pathogenesis. The liver is vulnerable to toxic insult because one of its major functions is detoxification. The most common plants that are gastrointestinal and liver toxins are shown in Table 5.3. Clinical signs will depend on the offending agent. Acute, severe toxicity is more common with chemical toxicosis, whereas plant toxins usually cause chronic disease. A thorough history is important, and in many cases, inspection of the animals' environment is required.

Clinical Signs. The clinical signs of toxic hepatitis can be subtle and nonspecific. Animals may exhibit only anorexia and depression. Icterus is more common with hemolytic diseases and is not always seen with liver disease. Photosensitivity is a common clinical feature in ruminants, and hepatoencephalopathy also can occur.

Diagnosis. Clinicopathologic data are more helpful in diagnosing acute toxicity. Serum aspartate aminotransferase (AST) and lactic acid dehydrogenase (LDH) levels can increase with hepatocellular necrosis, but such changes are not liver-specific, so muscle injury and disease must be ruled out. These enzymes also increase if serum is not separated from a blood clot in a timely fashion.[232] Increased levels of alkaline phosphatase (AP) and gamma-glutamyl transferase (GGT) indicate biliary stasis. AP concentrations also are not liver-specific, but increased serum levels of GGT are very specific for liver disease. GGT also increases in some hepatocellular diseases, so testing for normal concentrations is important.[249] Unfortunately, levels of all of these enzymes can be normal with liver disease, especially if it is chronic. Hyperbilirubinemia, hypoglycemia, low blood urea nitrogen (BUN), and hypoalbuminemia are not always evident, as is classically taught. If hepatoencephalopathy is suspected, blood ammonia concentrations may be elevated. Blood ammonia analysis may be impracticable in the field, because the blood should be kept on ice and the test should be performed within 30 minutes of collection. To enhance the accuracy of blood ammonia analysis, the clinician should collect blood from a normal control animal for comparison. Ammonia concentrations three times those in the control animal are diagnostic.[251] Liver biopsy remains the most valuable tool for diagnosing liver disease. Although clotting dysfunction may occur in liver disease, it is an uncommon complication in ruminants, and risk of bleeding should not discourage the clinician from performing a liver biopsy.

Treatment. If the intoxication is caught in the acute stage, activated charcoal (500 g in the adult animal) can be given. Supportive care, especially fluid support with dextrose solutions, is the mainstay of therapy. Low-protein diets may suppress ammonia production temporarily, but they can be detrimental over time, depending on the production status of the animal. Animals exhibiting photosensitivity should be housed indoors if possible, and broad-spectrum (systemic or topical) antibiotics may be necessary to control secondary bacterial dermatitis. Corticosteroids (e.g., dexamethasone 0.1 to 1 mg/kg IV or IM) may be indicated in early cases of photosensitization to decrease inflammation. Neurologic signs can be controlled with phenobarbital (initial dose: 10–20 mg/kg IV diluted in saline and administered over 30 minutes; subsequent doses: 1–9 mg/kg IV diluted in saline, as needed, up to three times daily). Diazepam (Valium) is contraindicated in hepatoencephalopathy because it may worsen deficits.[252]

TABLE 5.3 Plants That may Cause Gastrointestinal or Hepatic Disease.

Plant	Comments	Signs
Cocklebur	Erect annual herbage in sandy soils, flood plains, and overgrazed pastures; seeds are toxic	*Within hours to days of ingestion:* anorexia, vomiting, colic, dyspnea, gastroenteritis, chronic hepatitis, hepatic damage, death
Senecio (groundsel), *Crotalaria,* heliotrope, *Amsinckia* (fiddleneck), *Echium*	Pyrrolizidine alkaloids; excreted in milk and urine and can cross placenta; young more susceptible	Dullness, weakness, weight loss, icterus, fibrosis, hepatocytomegaly on histopathology, bile duct proliferation, photosensitivity, subcutaneous edema, diarrhea
Lantana	Found in sandy, tropical areas; berries, leaves, and hay are toxic	*Chronic toxicity:* slow hepatic failure, icterus, photosensitization, weakness, bloody diarrhea, cholestasis, hepatic failure
Sneezeweed, bitterweed, rubberweed	Grows in overgrazed pastures; all parts of plant are toxic	*Acute toxicity:* gastrointestinal upset, depression, serous nasal discharge, salivation, bloat; *chronic toxicity:* vomiting, hepatic and renal congestion, gastric edema, aspiration pneumonia, pulmonary edema
Cabbage, kale, rape, mustard, wild mushroom	Remove from diet; add iodine to diet (for goiter)	Gastroenteritis, hepatic necrosis, photosensitization, goiter, hemolysis
Horsebrush	Stop grazing, keep animals indoors	Itching, uneasiness, inflamed eyes, blindness, serum discharge from scabs; degenerative changes in liver and elevated liver enzymes
Clover (crimson, red, subterranean burclover)		Photosensitization
St. John's wort	Perennial herb; grows along roadsides and in overgrazed fields; remove from diet and keep animals in shade	Increased respiration, diarrhea, pruritus, dermatitis, death
Blue-green algae	Toxic after a bloom	Vomiting, diarrhea, liver failure, photosensitization; necropsy findings include swollen bloody liver, edema around gallbladder, centrolumbar apoptosis, necrosis
Pokeweed		Vomiting, cramps, diarrhea, weakness, dyspnea, prostration, tremors, convulsions
Gossypol (cottonseed)	Toxicity seen in younger pre-ruminants	Poor performance, convulsions, cardiac toxicity
Rhubarb	Contains oxalic acid	Gastrointestinal toxicity
Oak	Acorns and oak buds are most toxic	Abdominal pain, pseudomembranes in gastrointestinal tract, bloody diarrhea, depression, renal toxicity
Castor bean	Beans most toxic	Gastrointestinal irritation, bloody diarrhea, central nervous system disturbances
Mistletoe	Berries not toxic	Nausea, diarrhea
Other potentially pathogenic plants English ivy *Sesbania* Narcissus Elderberry Spurge Buckwheat Queen Anne's lace Milkweed Parsley, giant hogweed		

Miscellaneous Liver Diseases

Congenital hyperbilirubinemia, or black liver disease, occurs in certain mutant Corriedale sheep.[232] The underlying disorder, very similar to *Dubin-Johnson syndrome* in humans, is a genetically recessive condition characterized by an abnormality in the excretion of conjugated bilirubin and phylloerythrin. Appearance of disease manifestations in animals often is related to consumption of green forage. Clinical signs include anorexia, photodermatitis, and icterus. Liver biopsy in affected animals reveals dark pink to black granules in otherwise normal hepatocytes. The syndrome first manifests itself in lambs around 5 months of age.[253]

A similar condition, termed *Gilbert's syndrome* in people, occurs in Southdown lambs around 6 months of age. It appears to be a recessive condition characterized by decreased hepatic uptake of phylloerythrin and bilirubin, with concurrent renal failure.[253] Clinical signs include icterus, photodermatitis, and ulceration around the ears and mouth. Liver biopsy reveals normal hepatic tissue. In both of these conditions, affected animals should be kept out of sunlight and fed minimal amounts of green forage. Obviously, these animals should be neutered or culled.

Various tumors of the liver, including fibrosarcoma, lymphosarcoma, and cholangiocellular carcinoma, have been reported in sheep and goats.[252,253] The use of ultrasonography and ultrasound-guided liver biopsy may aid in diagnosis.

Pathological Conditions of the Umbilicus

The umbilicus consists of the urachus, umbilical vein, and paired umbilical arteries. These umbilical remnants normally regress after birth to become a vestigial part of the bladder apex, round (falciform) ligament of the liver, and lateral ligaments of the bladder, respectively. Umbilical masses can be uncomplicated umbilical hernias or involve infection of the umbilical remnants or subcutaneous tissues, with or without concurrent umbilical herniation.[254] Umbilical hernias are a common congenital defect in ruminants. Infection of the umbilicus is a common morbidity in neonates associated with partial or complete failure of passive transfer of immunity due to inadequate colostrum intake.[255] Infection can also be the result of environmental contamination or inappropriate human handling of the umbilical cord, with excessive tension or torsion. Dipping navels with antiseptic solutions shortly after birth is commonplace and proven to reduce umbilical infections under intensive rearing conditions.[256,257] However, the overzealous use of these solutions (i.e., not allowing the umbilical stalk to dry) or the use of caustic agents (strong tincture of iodine) can cause severe inflammation and infection of the umbilical structures. Physical examination of an animal with an umbilical mass should aim to distinguish between an uncomplicated umbilical hernia from infection of the umbilical remnants with or without the presence of an umbilical hernia. Visual inspection and palpation of the mass includes evaluation of its size, shape, temperature, discharge, pain on manipulation, reducibility and the presence of a hernial ring. Deep palpation of the abdomen in a calm animal (or under sedation) may allow discernment of the umbilical structures involved. Ultrasonography can be used to determine the umbilical structures involved (and extent) as well as the characteristics of hernial sac contents (e.g., omentum, abomasum, or small intestine).[258]

Uncomplicated Umbilical Hernia

Uncomplicated umbilical hernias are considered hereditary in cattle and are a common congenital defect in sheep.[259] Although a genetic predisposition has not been identified in goats, all sheep and goat breeding stock should be free of congenital defects.[260] Umbilical hernias can also be the result of infection of the umbilical remnants and body wall. Surgical correction of umbilical hernias should be considered for those having a diameter larger than 2 cm (1 finger in diameter) and persisting beyond 3 to 4 weeks in duration. Immediate surgical intervention is indicated in animals demonstrating signs of colic associated with hernias, regardless of size.

Pinning of Umbilical Hernias. Pinning techniques using umbilical clamps or elastrator bands may be considered for umbilical hernias which are small, nonpainful, display no evidence of infection, and are completely reducible (e.g., do not contain any abdominal viscera following reduction). Pinning is most useful in females and should be used with caution in males due to anatomical considerations and complications associated with urine scalding. The animal is lightly sedated, placed in dorsal recumbency, the skin infiltrated with local anesthetic (e.g., 2% lidocaine), and then followed by reduction of the hernial sac contents back into the abdomen. The skin is then tented away from the body wall and the clamp or elastrator band applied. Large safety pins can be placed in a crossing fashion distal to the elastrator band to keep the band immediately adjacent to the abdominal wall. The ensuing inflammation will cause the hernial ring to adhere to itself and heal within 7 to 14 days. The tissue distal to the elastrator band will undergo ischemic necrosis and will eventually slough. Tetanus prophylaxis should be provided at the time of pinning. The animal should be closely monitored for signs of colic and wound complications.[7]

Umbilical Hernia Surgical Resection. In large (greater than 2 cm), uncomplicated umbilical hernias, surgical resection is the treatment of choice. The procedure can be carried out using sedation and local anesthesia (including the use of a high epidural) or under general anesthesia, with the animal positioned in dorsal recumbency. The surgical site is clipped and aseptically prepared. A fusiform skin incision is made around the umbilicus, with sharp and blunt dissection of the subcutaneous tissues to expose the hernial ring at the external rectus sheath. In males, a semilunar skin incision and reflection of the sheath and prepuce may be required, depending on the hernia size. The abdominal cavity is opened just cranial (or caudal) to the hernial ring on the linea alba to allow digital palpation of intra-abdominal structures, including the presence of adhered viscera or infected umbilical remnants. The hernial sac is then carefully excised at the scarred edge of the hernial ring. Enlarged or infected umbilical remnants and adhesions are excised (see later) before closure of the defect in the abdominal wall. Closure of the hernial ring is performed by simple apposition of the incised edges of the external rectus sheath using an absorbable suture in a simple continuous or simple interrupted pattern. If significant tension on the body wall is present, a tension relieving pattern should be used (e.g., a near-far-far-near suture). The subcutaneous tissue is closed in a simple continuous pattern using an absorbable suture, and the skin is closed based on surgeon preference.[254,261] Alternatively, a closed herniorrhaphy technique, whereby the peritoneum is not incised, may be elected in uncomplicated umbilical hernias. Closure of the body wall is as described earlier. However, an open technique has the benefit of inspecting the umbilical remnants. Postoperative management includes tetanus prophylaxis, antibiotics where indicated (as in the case of infected umbilical remnants), exercise restriction for 1 to 2 weeks, and the monitoring for excessive swelling, discharge, surgical site dehiscence, and evidence of systemic illness (i.e., peritonitis, sepsis).

Umbilical Infections

Infection of the umbilical remnants includes omphalophlebitis, omphaloarteritis, and abscessation or persistent patency of the urachus. Involvement of multiple umbilical structures may occur. A concurrent umbilical hernia may also be present. Bacterial isolates from lambs and kids with omphalitis include *E. coli*, *Trueperella pyogenes*, *Pasteurella* sp., and *Streptococcus dysgalactiae*.[262,263] On physical examination, the umbilicus is enlarged, painful to palpation, and may be actively draining purulent discharge (or urine) or have a scab suggestive of drainage in the past. If an umbilical hernia is present concurrently, the hernia is typically only partially reducible or nonreducible, and the hernial ring is more difficult to fully discern on palpation compared with uncomplicated hernias. Deep abdominal palpation, effectively facilitated by proper restraint and sedation of the animal, may allow differentiation of the different umbilical structures. For example, the umbilical vein courses craniodorsally towards the liver, whereas the umbilical arteries and urachus course caudodorsally towards the bladder. However, ultrasonography of the ventral abdomen is the ideal method to document which umbilical structures are involved, as well as the presence of cellulitis, abscesses, or free abdominal fluid. Evidence of a patent urachus includes the presence of dermatitis, urine scalding of the ventral abdomen, and urine dribbling. The animal may have a history of poor weight gain, previous or concurrent infectious diseases (e.g., pneumonia, arthritis), and signs of systemic illness such as fever, depression, and anorexia. Use of clinicopathological analyses such as a complete blood cell count, blood culture, or cytology of the peritoneal fluid should be based on physical exam findings suggestive of sepsis or peritonitis.

Treatment

Medical Versus Surgical Management of Umbilical Remnant Infections. On occasion, some cases of omphalophlebitis-omphaloarteritis can be effectively treated medically with prolonged broad-spectrum antibiotic therapy.[7] However, if medical therapy is ineffective, the infected umbilical remnants should be surgically resected. The authors prefer timely surgical removal of the umbilical remnants over prolonged medical therapy, the latter of which may fail and still require surgical intervention.

Surgical Resection of Infected Umbilical Remnants. Anesthesia, positioning, and preparation of the surgical site is as described earlier for umbilical hernia repair. If extensive involvement of the umbilical remnants is present and prolonged or complex resection anticipated, general anesthesia should be considered. The surgical site should be of sufficient size to allow the abdominal incision to be extended cranially or caudally (depending on the umbilical structures involved), including the need to perform marsupialization of the umbilical vein or visualization of the bladder. Draining tracts should be sutured closed prior to surgery to prevent contamination of the abdomen. A fusiform skin incision is made around the infected umbilicus, with sharp and blunt dissection of the subcutaneous tissues to expose the fibrous ring. A small incision is made in the linea alba cranial or caudal (opposite to infected umbilical structure). Initially, digital palpation of the abdomen is performed through this small opening to identify involved structures and the presence of adhesions, followed by further opening of the abdominal wall in an elliptical fashion using scissors.[254,261] The infected umbilical structures are identified and resected as described later. Following resection of the umbilicus, the body wall is closed in three layers, as described earlier for umbilical hernia repair as well as based on surgeon's preference.

Omphalophlebitis

If the infection of the umbilical vein ends distally to the liver, the vein can be removed en bloc, with ligation prior to transection. If the infection extends to and involves the liver, marsupialization of the umbilical vein is needed. Marsupialization of the umbilical vein has been described in the cranial aspect of the midline surgical incision or using a separate incision lateral or cranial to the midline incision.[254,261] The former technique is associated with an increased risk of herniation of the marsupialization site. In the latter approach, the vein is dissected free from surrounding tissue, covered with a finger-tip of a sterile glove (or sutured closed), and exteriorized through a separate right paramedian, circular incision. The vein is sutured to the rectus sheath using multiple interrupted absorbable sutures, under minimal tension. In a similar fashion, a second layer of sutures between the vein and the skin is performed using either delayed absorbable or nonabsorbable suture.[254] The abdominal incision is then closed as described earlier. The venous stump end is then reopened and allowed to drain. Daily flushing with dilute antiseptic solution can be performed but should be done carefully without back pressure. The animal should be maintained on antibiotics until cessation of drainage, and healing of the venous stump is complete (typically more than 14 days). Rarely, a second operation may be required to resect the marsupialized umbilical vein.[254,261]

Patency or Abscessation of the Urachus

The urachus is identified and traced caudally to the urinary bladder. The body wall incision may need to be extended caudally to allow sufficient visualization and exteriorization of the bladder apex. The urachus and bladder apex are packed off from the abdomen using moist lap sponges or towels. Either stay sutures or use of Doyen forceps can be used to facilitate sharp resection of the urachus and tip of the bladder apex. The bladder is closed in two inverted layers in a continuous pattern (e.g., Cushing, Lembert) using 2-0 absorbable suture material, ensuring that the bladder lumen is not penetrated, and a water-tight seal is achieved.[254,261] The abdominal wall, subcutaneous tissue, and skin are closed as described for umbilical hernia repair.

Omphaloarteritis

En bloc resection is the treatment of choice for infection of the umbilical arteries. Visualization of the arteries can be difficult, and care must be taken not to exert excessive traction during manipulation, as this can lead to tearing of the internal iliac artery. The arteries are ligated with absorbable suture material as deep as safely possible, ideally using a three forceps technique for maximum safety.[254] Marsupialization of the umbilical artery is described, but fortunately is rarely necessary.[264]

Prevention. Prevention of umbilical infections is based on sound husbandry principles. This includes ensuring adequate intake of quality colostrum as well as clean lambing/kidding sheds and yards. Depending on the management scenario, dipping of the naval with noncaustic antiseptics may help reduce the incidence of infection.

References

1. Buczinski S, Dore E, Boulay G, et al: Validation of the handheld Lactate-Pro analyzer for measurement of blood L-lactate concentration in cattle, *Vet Clin Pathol* 43:567–572, 2014.
2. Hornig KJ, Byers SR, Callan RJ, Holt T, Field M, Han H: Evaluation of a point-of-care glucose and beta-hydroxybutyrate meter operated in various environmental conditions in prepartum and postpartum sheep, *Am J Vet Res* 74:1059–1065, 2013.
3. Karapinar T, Kaynar O, Hayirli A, et al: Evaluation of 4 point-of-care units for the determination of blood l-lactate concentration in cattle, *J. Vet. Intern Med* 27:1596–1603, 2013.
4. Pichler M, Damberger A, Arnholdt T, et al: Evaluation of 2 electronic handheld devices for diagnosis of ketonemia and glycemia in dairy goats, *J Dairy Sci* 97:7538–7546, 2014.

5. Smith BP: Collection and submission of samples for cytology and hematology. In Smith BP, editor: *Large animal internal medicine*, ed 4, St. Louis, MO, 2009, Mosby Elsevier, pp 836–839.
6. Smith MS, Sherman DM, editors: Digestive system. In *goat medicine*, ed 2, Ames, Iowa, 2009, Wiley-Blackwell, pp 377–500.
7. Constable PD, Hinchcliff, KW, Done, SH, et al: Perinatal diseases. In Constable PD, Hinchcliff KW, Done SH, Grünberg W, editors: *Veterinary medicine: a textbook of the disease of cattle, horses, sheep, pigs, and goat*, ed 11, St. Louis, MO, 2017, Elsevier, pp 1830–1903.
8. Snyder E, Credille B: Diagnosis and treatment of clinical rumen acidosis, *Vet Clin North Am Food Anim Pract* 33:451–461, 2017.
9. Foster D: Disorders of rumen distension and dysmotility, *Vet Clin North Am Food Anim Pract* 33:499–512, 2017.
10. Bohn AA, Callan RJ: Cytology in food animal practice, *Vet Clin North Am Food Anim Pract* 23:443–479, 2007.
11. Al-Rukibat RK, Ismail ZB, Al-Majali AM, et al: Peritoneal fluid analysis in adult, nonpregnant Awassi sheep, *Vet Clin Pathol* 35: 215–218, 2006.
12. Grosche A, Furll M, Wittek T: Peritoneal fluid analysis in dairy cows with left displaced abomasum and abomasal volvulus, *Vet Rec* 170:413, 2012.
13. Wittek T, Grosche A, Locher LF, et al: Diagnostic accuracy of d-dimer and other peritoneal fluid analysis measurements in dairy cows with peritonitis, *J Vet Intern Med* 24:1211–1217, 2010.
14. Adamu SS, Egwu GO, Malgwi JT: Biochemical changes in the peritoneal fluid following rumenotomy in goats, *Vet. Res Commun* 15:363–367, 1991.
15. Dehghani S, Nazifi S, Barzegar MR: Evaluation of cellular and biochemical parameters of blood and peritoneal fluid following exploratory laparotomy in the goat, *J Vet Med A Physiol Pathol Clin Med* 47:143–148, 2000.
16. Nazifi S, Dehghani S, Barzegar MR: Evaluation of cellular and biochemical parameters of blood and peritoneal fluid following enterectomy in the goat, *Small Rumin Res* 37:65–71, 2000.
17. Fubini SL, Yeager AE, Mohammed HO, et al: Accuracy of radiography of the reticulum for predicting surgical findings in adult dairy cattle with traumatic reticuloperitonitis: 123 cases (1981-1987), *J Am Vet Med Assoc* 197:1060–1064, 1990.
18. Braun U, Fluckiger M, Nageli F: Radiography as an aid in the diagnosis of traumatic reticuloperitonitis in cattle, *Vet Rec* 132:103–109, 1993.
19. Misk NA, Semieka MA: The radiographic appearance of reticular diaphragmatic herniation and traumatic pericarditis in buffaloes and cattle, *Vet Radiol Ultrasound* 42:426–430, 2001.
20. Braun U, Wild K, Merz M, et al: Percutaneous ultrasound-guided abomasocentesis in cows, *Vet Rec* 140:599–602, 1997.
21. Braun U, Jacquat D, Steininger K: Ultrasonographic examination of the abdomen of the goat. II. Liver, spleen, urinary tract and greater omentum, *Schweiz Arch Tierheilkd* 155:185–195, 2013.
22. Braun U, Jacquat D, Steininger K: Ultrasonographic examination of the abdomen of the goat. I. Reticulum, rumen, omasum, abomasum and intestines, *Schweiz Arch Tierheilkd* 155:173–184, 2013.
23. Braun U, Jacquat D: Ultrasonography of the reticulum in 30 healthy Saanen goats, *Acta Vet Scand* 53:19, 2011.
24. Braun U, Jacquat D, Hassig M: Ultrasonography of the rumen in 30 Saanen goats, *Schweiz Arch Tierheilkd* 153:393–399, 2011.
25. Braun U, Jacquat D: Ultrasonography of the omasum in 30 Saanen goats, *BMC Vet Res* 7:11, 2011.
26. Braun U, Jacquat D: Ultrasonography of the abomasum in 30 Saanen goats, *Res Vet Sci* 92:295–298, 2012.
27. Braun U, Steininger K, Tschuor, A, Hassig, M: Ultrasonographic examination of the small intestine, large intestine and greater omentum in 30 Saanen goats, *Vet J* 189:330–335, 2011.
28. Braun U, Steininger K: Ultrasonographic characterization of the liver, caudal vena cava, portal vein, and gallbladder in goats, *Am J Vet Res* 72:219–225, 2011.
29. Braun U, Steininger K: Ultrasonographic examination of the spleen in 30 goats, *Schweiz Arch Tierheilkd* 152:477–481, 2010.
30. Steininger K, Braun U: Ultrasonography of the urinary tract in 29 female Saanen goats, *Schweiz Arch Tierheilkd* 154:67–74, 2012.
31. Braun U, Irmer M, Augsburger H, et al: Computed tomography of the abdomen in Saanen goats: I. reticulum, rumen and omasum, *Schweiz. Arch Tierheilkd* 153:307–313, 2011.
32. Braun U, Irmer M, Augsburger H, Müller U, Jud R, Ohlerth S: Computed tomography of the abdomen in Saanen goats: II. Liver, spleen, abomasum, and intestine, *Schweiz Arch Tierheilkd* 153:314–320, 2011.
33. Braun U, Irmer M, Augsburger H, et al: Computed tomography of the abdomen in Saanen goats: III. Kidneys, ureters and urinary bladder, *Schweiz Arch Tierheilkd* 153:321–329, 2011.
34. Ohlerth S, Becker-Birck M, Augsburger H, Jud R, Makara M, Braun U: Computed tomography measurements of thoracic structures in 26 clinically normal goats, *Res Vet Sci* 92:7–12, 2012.
35. Humann-Ziehank, Riße R, Brügmann M, et al: Liver biopsy in sheep: experiences with two different techniques, *Tierärztliche Umschau* 54(3):151–157, 1999.
36. Donald GE, Paull DR, Langlands JP: Liver biopsy as a technique for assessing copper status of sheep, *Aust Vet J* 61:121–122, 1984.
37. Raoofi A, Asadi F, Mardjanmehr SH, et al: Blood parameters in female Zandi lambs as affected by liver biopsy methodology, *Trop Anim Health Prod* 43:1385–1388, 2011.
38. Kassem MM, el-Gendy SA, Abdel-Wahed RE, et al: Laparoscopic anatomy of caprine abdomen and laparoscopic liver biopsy, *Res Vet Sci* 90:9–15, 2011.
39. Swecker WS: Trace mineral feeding and assessment, *Vet. Clin North Am Food Anim Pract* 30:671–688, 2014.
40. Colvin HW, Backus RC: Bloat in sheep (*Ovis aries*), *Comp Biochem Physiol A Comp Physiol* 91:635–644, 1988.
41. Howarth RE: A review of bloat in cattle, *Can Vet J* 16:281–294, 1975.
42. Cheng KJ, McAllister TA, Popp JD, Hristov AN, Mir Z, Shin HT: A review of bloat in feedlot cattle, *J Anim Sci* 76:299–308, 1998.
43. Meyer NF, Bryant TC: Diagnosis and management of rumen acidosis and bloat in feedlots, *Vet Clin North Am Food Anim Pract* 33:481–498, 2017.
44. Dougherty RW: Eructation in ruminants, *Ann N Y Acad Sci* 150: 22–26, 1968.
45. Majak W, Hall JW, McCaughey WP: Pasture management strategies for reducing the risk of legume bloat in cattle, *J Anim Sci* 73(5):1493–1498, 1995.
46. Lean IJ, Golder HM, Hall MB: Feeding, evaluating, and controlling rumen function, *Vet Clin North Am Food Anim Pract* 30:539–575, 2014.
47. Jonker A, Yu P: The occurrence, biosynthesis, and molecular structure of proanthocyanidins and their effects on legume forage protein precipitation, digestion and absorption in the ruminant digestive tract, *Int J Mol Sci* 18:E1105, 2017.
48. Chapman GA, Bork EW, Donkor NT, et al: Performance and dietary preferences of white-tailed deer grazing chicory, birdsfoot trefoil or alfalfa in north central Alberta, *J Anim Physiol Anim Nutr (Berl)* 93:794–801, 2009.
49. Nelson KE, Thonney ML, Woolston TK, et al: Phenotypic and phylogenetic characterization of ruminal tannin-tolerant bacteria, *Appl Environ Microbiol* 64:3824–3830, 1998.
50. Constable PD, Hinchcliff KW, Done SH, Grunberg W: Diseases of the alimentary tract - ruminant. In Constable PD, Hinchcliff KW, Done SH, Grunberg W, editors: *Veterinary medicine a textbook of the diseases of cattle, horses, sheep, pigs, and goats*, ed 11, St. Louis, MO, 2017, Elsevier, pp 473–482.
51. Mills JH, Christian RG: Lesions of bovine ruminal tympany, *J Am Vet Med Assoc* 157:947–952, 1970.
52. Nishimura M, Toyota Y, Ishida Y, et al: Zygomycotic mediastinal lymphadenitis in beef cattle with ruminal tympany, *J Vet Med Sci* 76:123–127, 2014.
53. Hikasa Y, Takase K, Emi S, et al: Antagonistic effects of alpha-adrenoceptor blocking agents on reticuloruminal hypomotility induced by xylazine in cattle, *Can J Vet Res* 52:411–415, 1988.
54. Ruckebusch Y, Allal C: Depression of reticulo-ruminal motor functions through the stimulation of alpha 2-adrenoceptors, *J Vet Pharmacol Ther* 10:1–10, 1987.

55. Lei Y, Hannoufa A, Yu P: The use of gene modification and advanced molecular structure analyses towards improving alfalfa forage, *Int J Mol Sci* 18:E298, 2017.
56. Majak W, Hall J, McAllister T: Practical measures for reducing risk of alfalfa bloat in cattle, *J Range Manage* 54:490–493, 2001.
57. Lippke H, Vetter RL, Jacobson NL: Poloxalene for bloat prevention in lambs, *J Anim Sci* 28:819–821, 1969.
58. Stanford K, Wang Y, Berg BP, et al: Effects of alcohol ethoxylate and pluronic detergents on the development of pasture bloat in cattle and sheep, *J Dairy Sci* 84:167–176, 2001.
59. Katz MP, Nagaraja TG, Fina LR: Ruminal changes in monensin- and lasalocid-fed cattle grazing bloat-provocative alfalfa pasture, *J Anim Sci* 63:1246–1257, 1986.
60. Chen L, Luo Y, Wang H, Liu S, Shen Y, Wang M: Effects of glucose and starch on lactate production by newly isolated *streptococcus bovis* s1 from saanen goats, *Appl Environ Microbiol* 82:5982–5989, 2016.
61. Newbold CJ, Wallace RJ: Effects of the ionophores monensin and tetronasin on simulated development of ruminal lactic acidosis in vitro, *Appl Environ Microbiol* 54:2981–2985, 1988.
62. Braun U, Rihs T, Schefer U: Ruminal lactic acidosis in sheep and goats, *Vet Rec* 130:343–349, 1992.
63. Minuti A, Ahmed S, Trevisi E, et al: Experimental acute rumen acidosis in sheep: consequences on clinical, rumen, and gastrointestinal permeability conditions and blood chemistry, *J Anim Sci* 92:3966–3977, 2014.
64. Gregory PC: Inhibition of reticulo–ruminal motility by volatile fatty acids and lactic acid in sheep, *J Physiol* 382:355–371,1987.
65. Zhang RY, Jin W, Feng PF, et al: High-grain diet feeding altered the composition and functions of the rumen bacterial community and caused the damage to the laminar tissues of goats, *Animal* 12(12):2511–2520, 2018.
66. Karapinar T, Dabak M, Kizil O, et al: Severe thiamine deficiency in sheep with acute ruminal lactic acidosis, *J Vet Intern Med* 22: 662–665, 2008.
67. Chihaya Y, Matsukawa K, Mizushima S, et al: Ruminant forestomach and abomasal mucormycosis under rumen acidosis, *Vet Pathol* 25:119–123, 1988.
68. Nagaraja TG, Lechtenberg KF: Liver abscesses in feedlot cattle, *Vet Clin North Am Food Anim Pract* 23:351–369, 2007.
69. Li H, Liu J, Zhu W, et al: Intraruminal infusion of oligofructose alters ruminal microbiota and induces acute laminitis in sheep, *J Anim Sci* 95:5407–5419, 2017.
70. Cao GR, English PB, Filippich LJ, et al: Experimentally induced lactic acidosis in the goat, *Aust Vet J* 64:367–370, 1987.
71. Patra RC, Lal SB, Swarup D: Physicochemical alterations in blood, cerebrospinal fluid and urine in experimental lactic acidosis in sheep, *Res Vet Sci* 54:217–220, 1993.
72. McCann JC, Elolimy AA, Loor JJ: Rumen microbiome, probiotics, and fermentation additives, *Vet Clin North Am Food Anim Pract* 33:539–553, 2017.
73. Reis LF, Sousa RS, Oliveira FLC, et al: Comparative assessment of probiotics and monensin in the prophylaxis of acute ruminal lactic acidosis in sheep, *BMC Vet Res* 14:9, 2018.
74. Garcia Diaz T, Ferriani Branco A, Jacovaci FA, Cabreira Jobim C, Bolson DC, Pratti Daniel JL: Inclusion of live yeast and mannan-oligosaccharides in high grain-based diets for sheep: ruminal parameters, inflammatory response and rumen morphology, *PLoS One* 13:e0196184, 2018.
75. Basso FC, Adesogan AT, Lara EC, et al: Effects of feeding corn silage inoculated with microbial additives on the ruminal fermentation, microbial protein yield, and growth performance of lambs, *J Anim Sci* 92:5640–5650, 2014.
76. Woolf A, Kradel D: Occurrence of rumenitis in a supplementary fed white-tailed deer herd, *J Wildl Dis* 13(3):281–285, 1977.
77. Sharma KB, Ranka AK: Foreign body syndrome in goats — a report of five cases, *Indian Vet J* 55:413–414, 1978.
78. Miesner MD, Reppert EJ: Diagnosis and treatment of hardware disease, *Vet Clin North Am Food Anim Pract* 33:513–523, 2017.
79. Abo-Shehada MN, Al-Rawashdeh O, Al-Natour M: Traumatic pericarditis in an Awassi lamb, *Br Vet J* 147:78–81, 1991.
80. Hartnack AK, Niehaus AJ, Rousseau M, Pentecost RL, Miesner MD, Anderson DE: Indications for and factors relating to outcome after rumenotomy or rumenostomy in cattle: 95 cases (1999-2011), *J Am Vet Med Assoc* 247:659–664, 2015.
81. Zhai SL, Wen XH, Luo ML, et al: Ruminal impaction due to Ficus esquiroliana Levl. in Boer goats, *SpringerPlus* 2:608, 2013.
82. Abdelaal AM, El-Maghawry S: Selected studies on foreign body impaction in goats with special reference to ultrasonography, *Veterinary World* 7:522–527, 2014.
83. Otsyina HR, Nguhiu-Mwangi J, Mogoa EGM, et al: Prevalence of indigestible rumen foreign bodies in sheep and goats at Dagoretti andn Kiserian abattoirs, Kenya, *Int J Vet Sci* 4:75–80, 2015.
84. Smith MS Sherman DM, editors: *Digestive system, in goat medicine*, ed 2, Ames, Iowa, 2009, Wiley-Blackwell, pp 377–500.
85. Navarre CB, Baird AN, Pugh DG: *Sheep and goat medicine,* ed 2, Philadelphia, 2012, W.B. Saunders, pp 71–105.
86. Fubini SL, Ducharme NG: *Farm animal surgery*, Philadelphia, 2004, W.B. Saunders, pp 161–281.
87. Niehaus AJ: Rumenotomy, *Vet Clin North Am Food Anim Pract* 24:341–347, vii–viii, 2008.
88. Haven ML, Wichtel JJ, Bristol DG, et al: Effects of antibiotic prophylaxis on postoperative complications after rumenotomy in cattle, *J Am Vet Med Assoc* 200:1332–1335, 1992.
89. Ellis TM, Rowe JB, Lloyd JM: Acute abomasitis due to Clostridium septicum infection in experimental sheep, *Aust Vet J* 60: 308–309, 1983.
90. Eustis SL, Bergeland ME: Suppurative abomasitis associated with *Clostridium septicum* infection, *J Am Vet Med Assoc* 178:732–734, 1981.
91. Lewis CJ, Naylor RD: Sudden death in sheep associated with *Clostridium sordellii, Vet Rec* 142:417–421, 1998.
92. Vatn S, Tranulis MA, Hofshagen M: Sarcina-like bacteria, *Clostridium fallax* and *Clostridium sordellii* in lambs with abomasal bloat, haemorrhage and ulcers, *J Comp Pathol* 122:193–200, 2000.
93. Vatn S, Ulvund MJ: Abomasal bloat, haemorrhage and ulcers in young Norwegian lambs, *Vet. Rec* 146:35–39, 2000.
94. DeBey BM, Blanchard PC, Durfee PT: Abomasal bloat associated with Sarcina-like bacteria in goat kids, *J Am Vet Med Assoc* 209:1468–1469, 1996.
95. Edwards GT, Woodger NG, Barlow AM, et al: *Sarcina*-like bacteria associated with bloat in young lambs and calves, *Vet Rec* 163: 391–393, 2008.
96. Gorrill ADL, Nicholson JWG, Macintyre TM. Effects of formalin added to milk replacers on growth, feed intake, digestion and incidence of abomasal bloat in lambs, *Can J Anim Sci* 55:557–563, 1975.
97. Vatn S, Torsteinbo WO: Effects of iron dextran injections on the incidence of abomasal bloat, clinical pathology and growth rates in lambs, *Vet Rec,* 146:462–465, 2000.
98. Angus KW, Bannatyne CC: Abomasal ulceration in adult sheep: a report of two contrasting cases, *Vet Rec* 86:531–533, 1970.
99. Shirley AG: Two cases of phycomycotic ulceration in sheep, *Vet Rec* 77:675–677, 1965.
100. Palmer MV, Waters WR, Whipple DL: Abomasal ulcers in captive white-tailed deer (*Odocoileus virginianus), J Comp Pathol* 125(2-3): 224–247, 2001.
101. Colditz IG, Le Jambre LF: Development of a faecal occult blood test to determine the severity of Haemonchus contortus infections in sheep, *Vet Parasitol* 153:93–99, 2008.
102. Ahmed AE, Constable PD, Misk NA: Effect of an orally administered antacid agent containing aluminum hydroxide and magnesium hydroxide on abomasal luminal pH in clinically normal milk-fed calves, *J Am Vet Med Assoc* 220:74–79, 2002.
103. Ahmed AF, Constable PD, Misk NA: Effect of orally administered cimetidine and ranitidine on abomasal luminal pH in clinically normal milk-fed calves, *Am J Vet Res* 62:1531–1538, 2001.
104. Ahmed AF, Constable PD, Misk NA: Effect of orally administered omeprazole on abomasal luminal pH in dairy calves fed milk replacer, *J Vet Med A Physiol Pathol Clin Med* 52:238–243, 2005.

105. Balcomb CC, Heller MC, Chigerwe M, et al: Pharmacokinetics and efficacy of intravenous famotidine in adult cattle, *J Vet Intern Med* 32:1283–1289, 2018.
106. Smith GW, Davis JL, Smith SM, Gerard MP, Campbell NB, Foster DM: Efficacy and pharmacokinetics of pantoprazole in alpacas, *J Vet Intern Med* 24:949–955, 2010.
107. Bath GF, Bergh T: A specific form of abomasal phytobezoar in goats and sheep, *J S Afr Vet Assoc* 50:69–72, 1979.
108. Bath GF, Botha P, Vorster HJ, et al: Physical structure and chemical composition of abomasal phytobezoars of goats and sheep, *J S Afr Vet Assoc* 63:103–107, 1992.
109. Rings DM, Welker FH, Hull BL, et al: Abomasal emptying defect in Suffolk sheep, *J Am Vet Med Assoc* 185:1520–1522, 1984.
110. Ruegg PL, George LW, East NE: Abomasal dilatation and emptying defect in a flock of Suffolk ewes, *J Am Vet Med Assoc* 193:1534–1536, 1988.
111. Gabb K, Lofstedt J, Bildfell R: Abomasal emptying defect in a ewe of predominantly Dorset breeding, *Vet. Rec* 131:127–128, 1992.
112. Smith RM, Underwood WJ, Petersen GC, et al: Abomasal dilatation and impaction in two Hampshire rams, *Vet Rec* 130:468–470, 1992.
113. Sharp MW, Collings DF: Ovine abomasal enlargement and scrapie, *Vet Rec* 120:215, 1987.
114. Pruden SJ, McAllister MM, Schultheiss PC, et al: Abomasal emptying defect of sheep may be an acquired form of dysautonomia, *Vet Pathol* 41:164–169, 2004.
115. Kopcha M: Abomasal dilatation and emptying defect in a ewe, *J Am Vet Med Assoc* 192:783–784, 1988.
116. Jansen SA, Kleerekooper I, Hofman ZL, Kappen IF, Stary-Weinzinger A, van der Heyden MA: Grayanotoxin poisoning: 'mad honey disease' and beyond, *Cardiovasc Toxicol* 12:208–215, 2012.
117. Puschner B, Holstege DM, Lamberski N: Grayanotoxin poisoning in three goats, *J Am Vet Med Assoc* 218(4):527–578, 2001.
118. Bischoff K, Smith MC, Stump S: Treatment of pieris ingestion in goats with intravenous lipid emulsion, *J Med Toxicol* 10:411–414, 2014.
119. Plumlee KH, VanAlstine WG, Sullivan JM: Japanese pieris toxicosis of goats, *J Vet Diagn Invest* 4:363–364, 1992.
120. Power SB, O'Donnell PG, Quirk EG: Pieris poisoning in sheep, *Vet Rec* 128:599–600, 1991.
121. Black DH: Rhododendron poisoning in sheep, *Vet Rec* 128:363–364, 1991.
122. Hosie BD, Mullen CM, Gillespie ID, et al: Rhododendron poisoning in lambs, *Vet Rec* 118:110, 1986.
123. Humphreys DJ, Stodulski JB, Stocker JG: Rhododendron poisoning in goats, *Vet Rec* 113:503–504, 1983.
124. Sherman DM: *Causes of kid morbidity and mortality: an overview, in proceedings of the fourth International Conference on goats*, Brasilia, Brazil, 1987, EMBRAPA-DDT.
125. Vickers MC: Enteric infections in young goats and their control. In *Proceedings of the society of sheep and beef cattle veterinarians of the New Zealand Veterinary Association, Annual Seminar 1986, Volume*, Palmerston North, NZ, January 1986, The Society of Sheep and Beef Cattle Veterinarians of the New Zealand Veterinary Association.
126. Blackwell TE: Enteritis and diarrhea, *Vet Clin North Am Large Anim Pract* 5:557, 1983.
127. Smith MC, Sherman DM: *Goat medicine*, ed 2, Ames, Iowa, 2009, Wiley-Blackwell.
128. Nagy B, Palfi V, Nagy G, Hajtos I, Merenyi L: *Infectious gastrointestinal diseases of young goats.* In *Proceedings of the Fourth International Conference on goats*, Brasilia, Brazil, 1987, EMBRAPA-DDT.
129. Nagy B, et al: *Occurrence of cryptosporidia, rotaviruses, coronavirus-like particles and K99+ Escherichia coli in goat kids and lambs, in Proceedings of the Third International Symposium on Veterinary Laboratory Diagnostics,* Ames, Iowa, 1983.
130. Kimberling CV: *Jensen and Swift's diseases of sheep*, ed 3, Philadelphia, 1988, Lea & Febiger.
131. Hodgson JC: *Escherichia coli in domestic animals and humans*, Wallingford, UK, 1994, Cab International.
132. Runnels PL, Moon HW, Schneider RA: Development of resistance with host age to adhesion of K99+ *Escherichia coli* to isolated intestinal epithelial cells, *Infect Immun,* 28:298, 1980.
133. Zeman DH, Thomson JU, Francis DH: Diagnosis, treatment, and management of enteric colibacillosis, *Vet Med* 84:794, 1989.
134. Schultheiss P: Diarrheal disease in calves, *Large Anim Vet,* 47:24, 1992.
135. Roussel AJ, Sriranganathan N, Brown SA, Sweatt D: Effect of flunixin meglumine on *Escherichia coli* heat stable enterotoxin-induced diarrhea in calves, *Am J Vet Res* 49:1431–1433, 1988.
136. Theil KW, Grooms DL, McCloskey CM, Redman DR: Group B rotavirus associated with an outbreak of neonatal lamb diarrhea, *J Vet Diagn Invest* 7:148, 1995.
137. Babiuk LA, Sabara M, Hudson GR: Rotavirus and coronavirus infections in animals. In: *Infection and immunity in farm animals*, Basel, 1985, S. Karger, p 225.
138. Theil KW, Lance SE, McCloskey CM: Rotaviruses associated with neonatal lamb diarrhea in two Wyoming shed-lambing operations, *J Vet Diagn Invest* 8:245, 1996.
139. Munoz M, Lanza I, Alvarez M, Carmenes P: Rotavirus excretion by kids in a naturally infected goat herd, *Small Rum Res* 14:83, 1994.
140. Heath SE: Neonatal diarrhea in calves: diagnosis and intervention in problem herds, *Comp Cont Educ Pract Vet* 14:995, 1992.
141. Moore JA, Blagburn BL, Lindsay DS: Cryptosporidiosis in animals including humans, *Comp. Cont Educ Pract Vet* 10:275, 1988.
142. Foreyt WJ: Coccidiosis and cryptosporidiosis in sheep and goats, *Vet Clin North Am Food Anim Pract* 6:655, 1990.
143. Berg IE, Peterson AC, Freeman TP: Ovine cryptosporidiosis, *J Am Vet Med Assoc* 173:1586, 1978.
144. Sanford SE, Josephson GK, Rehmtulla AJ, Baker KC: Cryptosporidiosis, rotaviral, and combined cryptosporidial and rotaviral infections in goat kids, *Can Vet J* 32:626, 1991.
145. Rings DM, Rings MB: Managing *Cryptosporidium* and *Giardia* infections in domestic ruminants, *Vet Med* 91:1125, 1996.
146. Corwin RM: Cryptosporidiosis: a coccidiosis of calves, *Comp Cont Educ Pract Vet* 14:1005, 1992.
147. Webster KA, et al: Detection of *Cryptosporidium parvum* oocysts in feces: comparison of conventional coproscopical methods and the polymerase chain reaction, *Vet Parasitol* 61:5, 1996.
148. Delafosse A, Castro-Hermida JA, Baudry C, Ares-Mazás E, Chartier C: Herd-level risk factors for *Cryptosporidium* infection in dairy-goat kids in western France, *Prev Vet Med* 77:109–121, 2006.
149. Ferre I, Benito-Peña A, García U, Osoro K, Ortega-Mora LM: Effect of different decoquinate treatments on cryptosporidiosis in naturally infected cashmere goat kids, *Vet Rec* 157:261–262, 2005.
150. Campbell I, Tzipori AS, Hutchison G, Angus KW: Effect of disinfectants on survival of *Cryptosporidium* oocysts, *Vet Rec* 111: 414–415, 1982.
151. Perryman LE, Kapil SJ, Jones ML, Hunt EL: Protection of calves against cryptosporidiosis with immune bovine colostrum induced by a *Cryptosporidium parvum* recombinant protein, *Vaccine* 17: 2142, 1999.
152. Bulgin MS, Anderson BC: Salmonellosis in goats, *J Am Vet Med Assoc* 178:720, 1981.
153. House JD, Smith BP: Current strategies for managing salmonella infections in cattle, *Vet Med* 93:756, 1998.
154. Cohen ND, Martin LJ, Simpson RB, Wallis DE, Neibergs HL: Comparison of polymerase chain reaction and microbiological culture for detection of *Salmonella* in equine feces and environmental samples, *Am J Vet Res* 57:780, 1996.
155. Li H, McFarlane RG, Wagner J: Vaccination of pregnant ewes against infection with *Salmonella* Brandenburg, *N Z Vet J* 53:416, 2005.
156. Kirkpatrick CE: Giardiasis in large animals, *Comp Cont Educ Pract Vet* 11:80, 1989.
157. Koudela B, Vitovec J: Experimental giardiasis in goat kids, *Vet Parasitol* 74:9, 1998.
158. Olsen ME, McAllister TA, Deselliers L, et al: Effects of giardiasis on production in a domestic ruminant (lamb) model, *Am J Vet Res* 56:1470–1474, 1995.

159. Castro-Hermida JA, Delafosse A, Pors I, Ares-Mazás E, Chartier C: *Giardia duodenalis* and *Cryptosporidium parvum* infections in adult goats and their implications for neonatal kids, *Vet Rec* 157: 623–627, 2005.
160. Nappert G, Hamilton D, Petrie L, Naylor JM: Determination of lactose and xylose malabsorption in preruminant diarrheic calves, *Can J Vet Res* 57:152, 1993.
161. Gunn AA, Naylor JA, House JK: Diarrhea. In Smith BP, editor: *Large animal internal medicine*, ed 4, St. Louis, 2009, Mosby Elsevier, pp 340–363.
162. Weese JS, Kenney DG, O'Connor A: Secondary lactose intolerance in a neonatal goat, *J Am Vet Med Assoc* 217:372, 2000.
163. Olchowy TW, Linnabary RD, Andrews FM, Longshore RC: Lactose intolerance in a calf, *J Vet Intern Med* 7:12–15, 1993.
164. Roy JHB: *The calf*, ed 4, London, 1980, Butterworth.
165. Aloisio F, Filippini G, Antenucci P, et al: Severe weight loss in lambs infected with *Giardia duodenalis* assemblage B, *J Vet Parasitol* 142:154–158, 2006.
166. Uzal FA, Kelly WR: Enterotoxemia in goats, *Vet Res Commun* 20:481, 1996.
167. Miyakawa MF, Saputo J, Puschner B, et al: Necrotizing enterocolitis and death in a goat kid associated with enterotoxin E (CPE)-producing *Clostridium perfringens* type A, *Can Vet J* 48:1266–1269, 2007.
168. Songer JG: Clostridial diseases of small ruminants, *Vet Res* 29:219, 1998.
169. Uzal FA, Songer JG: Diagnosis of *Clostridium perfringens* intestinal infections in sheep and goats, *J Vet Diagn Invest* 20:253, 2008.
170. Seimiya YM, Sasaki K, Satoh C, Takahashi M, Yaegashi G, Iwane H: Caprine enteritis associated with *Yersinia pseudotuberculosis* infection, *J Vet Med Sci* 67:887, 2005.
171. Boyce WM, Woods LW, Keel MK, et al: An epizootic of adenovirus-induced hemorrhagic diseases in captive black-tailed deer (*Odocoileus hemionus*), *J. Zool Wildl Med* 31(3):370–373, 2000.
172. Hariharan H, López A, Conboy G, Coles M, Muirhead T: Isolation of *Escherichia fergusonii* from feces and internal organs of a goat with diarrhea, *Can Vet J* 48:630, 2007.
173. Duhamel GE, Moxley RA, Maddox CW: Enteric infection of a goat with enterohemorrhagic *Escherichia coli* (O103:H2), *J Vet Diagn Invest* 4:197, 1992.
174. Drolet R, Fairbrother JM, Vaillancourt D: Attaching and effacing *Escherichia coli* in a goat with diarrhea, *Can Vet J* 35:122, 1994.
175. Barlow AM, Wales AD, Burch AA, La Ragione RM, Woodward MJ, Pearson GR: Attaching and effacing lesions in the intestines of adult goats associated with natural infection with *Escherichia coli* O145, *Vet Rec* 155:807–808, 2004.
176. Caprioli A, Morabito S, Brugère H, Oswald E: Enterohaemorrhagic *Escherichia coli*: emerging issues on virulence and modes of transmission, *Vet Res* 36:289, 2005.
177. Smith BP, Magdesian KG: Alterations in alimentary and hepatic function. In Smith BP, editor: *Large animal internal medicine*, ed 4, St. Louis, 2009, Mosby Elsevier pp 92–116.
178. Smith MC, Sherman DM: *Goat medicine*, ed 2, Ames, Iowa, 2009, Wiley-Blackwell.
179. Manning EJB: Paratuberculosis in captive and free-ranging wildlife, *Vet Clin North Am Food Anim* 27:621–630, 2011.
180. Greig A: Johne's disease in sheep and goats, *In Pract* 22:146, 2000.
181. Smith MC: Paratuberculosis in small ruminants, In *Proceedings of the small ruminants for the mixed animal practitioner, Western Veterinary Conference*, Las Vegas, 1998.
182. Stehman SM: Paratuberculosis in small ruminants, deer, and South American camelids, *Vet Clin North Am Food Anim Pract* 12:441, 1996.
183. Manning EJ, Steinberg H, Krebs V, Collins MT: Diagnostic testing patterns of natural *Mycobacterium paratuberculosis infection* in pygmy goats, *Can Ve J* 67:213–218, 2003.
184. Clarke CJ, Patterson IA, Armstrong KE, Low JC, et al: Comparison of the absorbed ELISA and agar gel immunodiffusion test with clinicopathologic findings in ovine clinical paratuberculosis, *Vet Rec* 139:618–621, 1996.
185. Pepin M, Marly J, Pardon P: *Corynebacterium pseudotuberculosis* infection in sheep and the complement fixation test for paratuberculosis, *Vet Rec* 120:236, 1987.
186. Salgado M, Manning EJ, Collins MT: Performance of a Johne's disease enzyme-linked immunosorbent assay adapted for milk samples from goats, *J Vet Diagn Invest* 17:350, 2005.
187. Ducharme NG, Desrochers A, Fubini S, et al: Surgery of the bovine digestive system. In Fubini SL, Ducharme NG, editors: *Farm animal surgery*, ed 2, Philadelphia, 2017, W.B. Saunders, pp 223–343.
188. Braun U: Ultrasonography in gastrointestinal disease in cattle, *Vet J* 166:112–124, 2003.
189. Haibel GK: Intestinal adenocarcinoma in a goat, *J Am Vet Med Assoc* 196:326–328,1990.
190. Khodakaram Tafti A: Ileoileal intussusception associated with coccidiosis in sheep, *Zentralbl Veterinarmed B*, 46:659–663, 1999.
191. Milnes EL, McLachlan A: Surgical management of small intestinal intussusception associated with jejunal adenocarcinoma in a dairy cow, *N Z Vet J* 63:288–290, 2015.
192. Shakespeare A: Intussusception as a complication of rectal prolapse replacement in a ewe, *Vet Rec* 147:78–79, 2000.
193. Van Dresser WR, Ramirez MA: Surgical correction of intussusception in a lamb, *J Am Vet Med Assoc* 136:21–22, 1960.
194. Sherman DM: Duodenal obstruction by a phytobezoar in a goat, *J Am Vet Med Assoc* 178:139–140, 1981.
195. Sargison ND, Scott PR, Dun KA: Intestinal obstruction in a blue-faced Leicester ram associated with a phytobezoar lodged at the pelvic inlet, *Vet Rec* 137:222, 1995.
196. Bath GF, Botha P, Vorster HJ, et al: Physical structure and chemical composition of abomasal phytobezoars of goats and sheep, *J S Afr Vet Assoc* 63:103–107, 1992.
197. Bath GF, Smith FJ, Vorster HJ, et al: Experimental reproduction of phytobezoars, *J S Afr Vet Assoc* 63:108–112, 1992.
198. Hollins J: Multiple phytobezoars in sibling goats, *Vet Rec* 178: 323–324, 2016.
199. Constable PD, Rings DM, Hull BL, et al: Atresia coli in calves: 26 cases (1977-1987), *J Am Vet Med Assoc* 195:118–123, 1989.
200. Dreyfuss DJ, Tulleners EP: Intestinal atresia in calves: 22 cases (1978-1988), *J Am Vet Med Assoc* 195:508–513, 1989.
201. Dennis SM: Urogenital defects in sheep, *Vet Rec* 105:344–347, 1979.
202. Dennis SM, Leipold HW: Atresia ani in sheep, *Vet Rec* 91: 219–222, 1972.
203. Leipold HW, Dennis SM: Atresia jejuni in a lamb, *Vet Rec* 93: 644–645, 1973.
204. Littlejohn A: Atresia duodeni jejuni in a lamb *Vet Rec* 94:363, 1974.
205. Saperstein G, Leipold HW, Dennis SM: Congenital defects of sheep, *J Am Vet Med Assoc* 167:314–322, 1975.
206. Dennis SM: A survey of congenital defects of sheep, *Vet Rec* 95:488–490, 1974.
207. Meylan M: Surgery of the bovine large intestine, *Vet Clin North Am Food Anim Pract* 24:479–496, 2008.
208. Azizi S, Mohammadi R, Mohammadpour I: Surgical repair and management of congenital intestinal atresia in 68 calves, *Vet Surg* 39:115–120, 2010.
209. Cecen G, Salci H, Caliskan GU, Celimli N, Seyrek-Intas D, Gorgul OS: Modified colostomy technique for colonic atresia in calves, *Vet Surg* 39:722–728, 2010.
210. Trent, AM, Ducharme, NG, Fubini, SL, Steiner A: In Fubini SL, Ducharme NG, editors: *Farm animal surgery*, ed 2, Philadelphia, 2017, W.B. Saunders, pp 505–518.
211. Malavasi LM, Greene SA, Gay JM, et al: Cardiopulmonary effects of constant-rate infusion of lidocaine for anesthesia during abdominal surgery in goats, *J Am Assoc Lab Anim Sci* 55:431–435, 2016.
212. Malone E, Ensink J, Turner T, et al: Intravenous continuous infusion of lidocaine for treatment of equine ileus, *Vet Surg* 35: 60–66, 2006.
213. Constable PD, Nouri M, Sen I, Baird AN, Wittek T: Evidence-based use of prokinetic drugs for abomasal disorders in cattle, *Vet Clin North Am Food Anim Pract* 28:51–70, 2012.

214. House JK, Smith BP, VanMetre DC, Fecteau G, Craychee T, Neves J: Ancillary tests for assessment of the ruminant digestive system, *Vet Clin North Am Food Anim Pract* 8:203–232, 1992.
215. Bohn AA, Callan RJ: Cytology in food animal practice, *Vet Clin North Am Food Anim Pract* 23:443–479, 2007.
216. Al-Rukibat RK, Ismail ZB, Al-Majali AM, Al-Zghoul MB: Peritoneal fluid analysis in adult, nonpregnant Awassi sheep, *Vet Clin Pathol* 35:215–218, 2006.
217. Fecteau G: Management of peritonitis in cattle, *Vet Clin North Am Food Anim Pract* 21:155–171, 2005.
218. Wilson AD, Hirsch VM, Osborne AD: Abdominocentesis in cattle: technique and criteria for diagnosis of peritonitis, *Can Vet J* 26:74–80, 1985.
219. Dehghani S, Nazifi S, Barzegar MR: Evaluation of cellular and biochemical parameters of blood and peritoneal fluid following exploratory laparotomy in the goat, *J Vet Med A Physiol Pathol Clin Med* 47:143–148, 2000.
220. Nazifi S, Dehghani S, Barzegar MR: Evaluation of cellular and biochemical parameters of blood and peritoneal fluid following enterectomy in the goat, *Small Rumin Res* 37:65–71, 2000.
221. Wittek T, Grosche A, Locher LF, Fürll M: Diagnostic accuracy of d-dimer and other peritoneal fluid analysis measurements in dairy cows with peritonitis, *J Vet Intern Med* 24:1211–1217, 2010.
222. Braun U: Ascites in cattle: ultrasonographic findings and diagnosis, *Vet Clin North Am Food Anim Pract* 32:55–83, 2016.
223. Freeman DE: In Auer JA, Stick JA, editors: *Equine surgery*, ed 4, Philadelphia, 2012, W.B. Saunders, pp 494–505.
224. Thomas DL, Waldron DF, Lowe GD, et al: Length of docked tail and the incidence of rectal prolapse in lambs, *J Anim Sci,* 81:2725–2732, 2003.
225. Hartnack A, Jones M: Surgery of the sheep and goat digestive system. In Fubini SL, Ducharme NG, editors: *Farm animal surgery*, ed 2, Philadelphia, 2017, W.B. Saunders, pp 561–567,
226. Randles JL: Clinical, pathological and histopathological findings in lambs implanted with a growth promoting product containing progesterone and oestradiol, *J S Afr Vet Assoc* 61:126–127, 1990.
227. Parish SM: A method for nonsurgical correction of rectal prolapse in lambs, *Vet Med Small Anim Clin* 74:871–872, 1979 .
228. Navarre CB, Baird AN, Pugh DG: Diseases of the gastrointestinal system. In Pugh DG, Baird AN, editors: *Sheep and goat medicine*, ed 2, Philadelphia, 2012, W.B. Saunders, pp 71–105.
229. Anderson DE, Miesner MD: Rectal prolapse, *Vet Clin North Am Food Anim Pract* 24:403–408, 2008.
230. Ducharme NG, Desrochers A, Fubini SL, et al: Surgery of the bovine digestive system. In Fubini SL, Ducharme NG editors: *Farm animal surgery,* ed 2, Philadelphia, 2017, W.B. Saunders, pp 223–343.
231. Rakestraw PC, Hardy J: Large intestine. In Auer JA, Stick JA, editors: *Equine surgery,* ed 4, Philadelphia, 2012, W.B. Saunders, pp 454–494.
232. Fetcher A: Liver diseases of sheep and goats, *Vet Clin North Am Large Anim Pract* 5:525, 1983.
233. Rosa JS, Johnson EH, Alves FS, Santos LF: A retrospective study of hepatic abscesses in goats: pathological and microbiological findings, *Br Vet J* 145:73, 1989.
234. Zamir S, Rozov A, Gootwine E: Treatment of pregnancy toxaemia in sheep with flunixin meglumine, *Vet Rec* 165:265–266, 2009.
235. Schlumbohm C, Harmeyer J: Twin-pregnancy increases of ewes to hypoglycaemic stress and pregnancy toxaemia, *Res Vet Sci* 84:286–299, 2007.
236. Yarim GF, Ciftci G: Serum protein pattern in ewe with pregnancy toxemia, *Vet Res Commun* 33:431, 2009.
237. Smith MC, Sherman DM: *Goat medicine*, ed 2, Ames, Iowa, 2009, Wiley-Blackwell.
238. Maas J, Pearson EG: Hepatic lipidosis. In Smith BP, editor: *Large animal internal medicine*, ed 4, St Louis, 2009, Mosby Elsevier, pp 912–916.
239. Kimberling CV: *Jensen and swift's diseases of sheep*, ed 3, Philadelphia, 1988, Lea & Febiger.
240. Scott PR, Sargison ND, Penny CD: Evaluation of recombinant bovine somatotropin in the treatment of ovine pregnancy toxaemia, *Vet J* 155:197–199, 1998.
241. Johnson EH, Muirhead DE, Annamalai K, King GJ, Al-Busaidy R, Hameed MS: Hepatic lipidosis associated with cobalt deficiency in Omani goats, *Vet Res Commun* 23:215, 1999.
242. Black H, Hutton JB, Sutherland RJ, James MP: White liver disease in goats, *N Z Vet J* 36:15–17, 1988.
243. Kennedy S, McConnell S, Anderson H, Kennedy DG, Young PB, Blanchflower WJ: Histopathologic and ultrastructural alterations of white liver disease in sheep experimentally depleted of cobalt, *Vet Pathol* 34:575–584, 1997.
244. Mitchell PJ, McOrist S, Thomas KW, McCausland IP: White liver disease in sheep, *Aust Vet J* 58:181–184, 1982.
245. Sargison ND, Scott PR, Wilson DJ, Bell GJ, Mauchline S, Rhind S: Hepatic encephalopathy associated with cobalt deficiency and white liver disease in lambs, *Vet Rec* 149:770–772, 2001.
246. Adam SEI, Wasfi IA, Magzoub M: Chronic copper toxicity in Nubian goats, *J Comp Pathol* 87:623–627, 1977.
247. Belford CJ, Raven CR, Black H: Chronic copper poisoning in Angora kids, *N Z Vet J* 37:152–154, 1989.
248. Solaiman SG, Maloney MA, Qureshi MA, Davis G, D'Andrea G: Effects of high copper supplements on performance, health, plasma copper, and enzymes in goats, *Small Rumin Res* 41:127–139, 2001.
249. Kaneko JJ: *Clinical biochemistry of domestic animals*, ed 4, San Diego: Academic Press, 1989.
250. George LW: Copper toxicoses. In Smith B, editors: *Large animal internal medicine*, ed 4, St Louis, 2009, Mosby Elsevier, pp 1166–1169.
251. Roussel AJ, Whitney MS, Cole DJ: Interpreting a bovine serum chemistry profile: part I, *Vet Med* 92:553, 1997.
252. Divers TJ: Therapy of liver failure. In Smith BP, editor: *Large animal internal medicine*, ed 4, St. Louis, 2009, Mosby Elsevier, pp 921–923.
253. Ogilvie TH: *Large animal internal medicine*, Baltimore, 1998, Williams & Wilkins.
254. Mulon PY, Desrochers A: Surgical abdomen of the calf, *Vet Clin North Am Food Anim Pract* 21:101–132, 2005.
255. Sawyer M, Willadsen CH, Osburn BI, McGuire TC: Passive transfer of colostral immunoglobulins from ewe to lamb and its influence on neonatal lamb mortality, *J Am Vet Med Assoc* 171:1255–1259, 1977.
256. Robinson AL, Timms LL, Stalder KJ, Tyler HD: Short communication: the effect of 4 antiseptic compounds on umbilical cord healing and infection rates in the first 24 hours in dairy calves from a commercial herd, *J Dairy Sci* 98:5726–5728, 2015.
257. Fordyce AL, Timms LL, Stalder KJ, Tyler HD: Short communication: The effect of novel antiseptic compounds on umbilical cord healing and incidence of infection in dairy calves, *J Dairy Sci* 101:5444–5448, 2018.
258. Steiner A, Lejeune B: Ultrasonographic assessment of umbilical disorders, *Vet Clin North Am Food Anim Pract* 25:781–794, 2009.
259. Greber D, Doherr M, Drögemüller C, Steiner A: Occurrence of congenital disorders in Swiss sheep, *Acta Vet Scand* 55:27, 2013.
260. Smith MS, Sherman. Digestive system. In Smith MS, Sherman DM, editors: *Goat medicine*, ed 2, Ames, Iowa, 2009, Wiley-Blackwell, pp 377–500.
261. Baird AN: Surgery of the Umbilicus and related structures, *Vet Clin North Am Food Anim Pract* 32:673–685, 2016.
262. Watkins GH, Sharp MW: Bacteria isolated from arthritic and omphalatic lesions in lambs in England and Wales, *Vet J* 156:235–238, 1998.
263. Rutherford SJ, Rycroft AN, Ridler AL: Sources of Streptococcus dysgalactiae in English and Welsh sheep flocks affected by infectious arthritis (joint ill), *Vet Rec* 174:579, 2014.
264. Lopez MJ, Markel MD: Umbilical artery marsupialization in a calf, *Can Vet J* 37:170–171, 1996.

6

Internal Parasites of Sheep, Goats, and Cervids

LINDSAY A. STARKEY AND DAVID G. PUGH

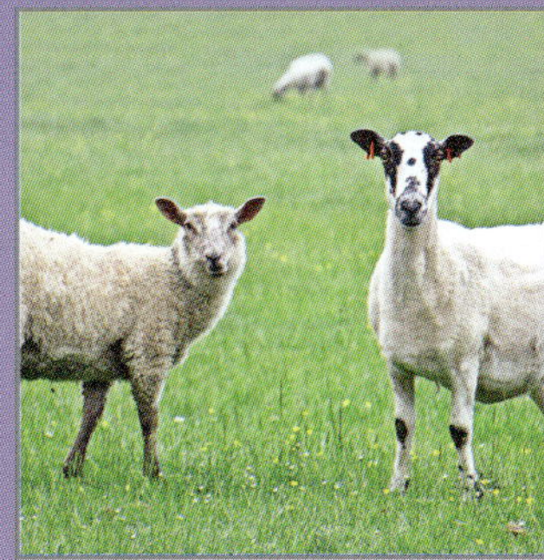

Introduction

A number of medical issues can result in decreased production and overt losses when it comes to rearing sheep, goats, and cervids. However, endoparasitism is of greatest concern when it comes to the health of sheep and goats and is also an important factor in cervid production systems.[1,2] Without proper management and control of internal parasites, fecundity, milk yield, antler size, and carcass value will all suffer. According to the most recent National Animal Health Monitoring System (NAHMS) survey looking at non–predator-related animal death, internal parasitism was the third most common cause of death in sheep, accounting for 9.6% of the nonpredator related losses; furthermore, it was the most common cause of non–predatory-related goat deaths (22.7%).[3,4]

Endoparasitism often results in anemia, weight loss, decreased immunity, decreased reproductive capacity, decreased meat, fiber, or milk production, and potentially death, any of which can be devastating to a producer.[1,2,5] To further complicate matters, historically effective anthelmintic regimens are no longer as efficacious, if effective at all, when it comes to treating internal parasites of sheep, goats, and cervids. Current recommendations to address endoparasitism focus on implementation of a sustainable integrated parasite management strategy, which can be difficult to put into practice.[1]

What follows in this chapter is a review of the relevant aspects of the different parasites that infect sheep, goats, and cervids including biology, clinical signs, diagnostics, treatment, and prevention measures.

Nematodes

Gastrointestinal Nematode Infections

Etiology and Life Cycle. Ruminant species share several of the same types of parasites, some with little host preference (e.g., *Haemonchus contortus*) and others with great host specificity (e.g., *Eimeria* spp.) Parasite variety will depend upon region, local climate, historical deworming practices, and variety of available ruminant hosts. The predominant gastrointestinal nematodes (GIN) that infect and can lead to clinical disease in sheep, goats, and cervids are *H. contortus*, *Teladorsagia circumcincta*, *Trichostrongylus* spp., *Ostertagia* spp., *Cooperia* spp., and *Oesophagostomum* spp. Additional parasite species such as *Trichuris* spp., *Nematodirus* spp., *Strongyloides papillosus*, and *Bunostomum* spp. may be identified, but are usually not of clinical importance.[1,2,5] See Table 6.1 for a more complete listing of GIN that have been described infecting sheep, goats, and cervids in the United States.[6] The majority of these parasites reside within the abomasum or small intestine of their host.

Disease resulting from gastrointestinal parasitism is usually of greatest concern in young, growing animals that are experiencing various stressors and have not yet had the opportunity to develop any immunity. Although infection with GIN does occur in adult animals (generally speaking, those > 18 months of age), the development of clinical signs of disease secondary to parasitism are uncommon in the absence of additional stressors. Stressors may include: pregnancy, parturition, and lactation; weaning; environmental extremes; overcrowding; improper nutrition, etc.[1,5]

The majority of the GIN are closely related and, therefore, so are their life cycles. In general, reproductively capable adult male and female parasites are present in their preferred site within the gastrointestinal tract (GIT). Females deposit eggs into the GIT which then exit the host via the feces. Egg hatching and larval maturation occur when the environmental temperatures (typically 10° C to 36° C) and moisture are favorable.[1] Extreme heat or freezing along with desiccation can be detrimental to larval growth or survival; nonetheless, irrigation systems even in arid climates may allow for parasite survival in the environment.[1] First-stage larvae (L1) and second-stage larvae (L2) feed on organic material in their environment for days to weeks prior to molting to the infective third-stage larvae (L3). The L3 retain their cuticle following the molt from L2; therefore, they are less susceptible to environmental extremes, but also cannot feed and acquire additional nutrients. The L3 stage may survive for protracted periods of time (several months) in the feces or on the pasture awaiting entry into an appropriate host via grazing. L3 require adequate moisture provided by rain, dew, or flooding in order to migrate from the feces and onto nearby graze-worthy forage.[1,2,5,7] Upon being ingested during grazing and entry into the rumen, the retained cuticle is lost and the L3 are free to move to the preferred location(s) within the GIT, penetrate the mucosa, molt to fourth-stage larvae (L4), leave the mucosa, and finish the maturation process into an adult. Some parasite species have gained the ability to utilize hypobiosis (a form of arrested

TABLE 6.1 **Nematode Parasites of Sheep, Goats, and Cervids in North America.**

Parasite Species	Superfamily	Predominant Host(s)	Anatomical Location	Life Cycle Stage[a]
Gastrointestinal Nematodes				
Gongylonema spp.	Spiruroidea	Ov, Ca, Ce, OU, *	Esophagus/rumen/reticulum	Larvated egg
Ostertagia spp.	Trichostrongyloidea	Ov, Ca, Ce, OU	Abomasum	Egg
Teladorsagia circumcincta	Trichostrongyloidea	Ov, Ca, Ce, OU	Abomasum	Egg
Haemonchus contortus	Trichostrongyloidea	Ov, Ca, Ce, OU	Abomasum	Egg
Trichostrongylus spp.	Trichostrongyloidea	Ov, Ca, Ce, OU, *	Abomasum/Small Intestine	Egg
Marshallagia spp.	Trichostrongyloidea	Ov, Ca	Abomasum	Egg
Spiculopteragia, Apteragia spp.	Trichostrongyloidea	Ce, OU	Abomasum	Egg
Nematodirus spp.	Trichostrongyloidea	Ov, Ca, Ce, OU	SI	Egg
Cooperia spp.	Trichostrongyloidea	Ov, Ca, Ce, OU	SI	Egg
Bunostomum spp.	Strongyloidea	Ov, Ca, Ce, OU	SI	Egg
Aonchotheca (*Capillaria*) *bovis*	Trichuroidea	Ov, Ca, Ce, OU	SI	Egg
Strongyloides spp.	Rhabditoidea	Ov, Ca, OU	SI	Larvated egg
Chabertia ovina	Strongyloidea	Ov, Ca, Ce, OU	Cecum/colon	Egg
Oesophagostomum spp.	Strongyloidea	Ov, Ca, Ce, OU	Cecum/colon	Egg
Skrjabinema spp.	Oxyuroidea	Ov, Ca, Ce	Cecum/colon	Egg
Trichuris spp.	Trichuroidea	Ov, Ca, Ce, OU	Cecum/colon	Egg
Nematodes of Other Organ Systems				
Mammomonogamus spp.	Strongyloidea	Ov, Ca, OU, *	Nasal cavity/larynx	Egg
Dictyocaulus spp.	Trichostrongyloidea	Ov, Ca, Ce, OU	Bronchi	Larvae
Protostrongylus spp.	Trichostrongyloidea	Ov, Ca, Ce	Bronchioles	Larvae
Muellerius capillaris	Trichostrongyloidea	Ov, Ca, Ce	Lung	Larvae
Parelaphostrongylus tenuis	Metastrongyloidea	Ov, Ca, Ce, OU	CNS	Larvae
Elaeophora schneideri	Filarioidea	Ov, Ca, Ce, OU	Blood vessels	MFF (tissue)

Ca, Caprine; *Ce*, cervid; *MFF*, microfilariae; *OU*, other ungulate species; *, zoonotic.
[a]Diagnostic stage from a patent host found in fresh feces unless otherwise stated.

development) to circumvent adverse environmental conditions outside of the host. The L4 may remain arrested in the mucosa for extended periods of time, and emergence from this 'hypobiotic' state in the mucosa, corresponds with the return of environmental conditions conducive for larval survival outside of the host animal.

A few notable exceptions to the aforementioned life cycle exist, including the adaptation seen with *Bunostomum* spp., which not only utilizes ingestion of L3 by the host via grazing, but may also be introduced to the host through percutaneous penetration by infectious L3. Additionally, *Nematodirus* spp. undergo delayed egg hatching until a fully mature L3 is present within the egg and environmental conditions are supportive for the hatched L3. *Trichuris* spp. are another exception, in that larval stages are never found free on pasture. They are retained until the egg is ingested by the host. Other nematodes, such as *S. papillosus*, can go dormant in the mammary tissues of the dam and may pass through the milk to the offspring.

The life cycles of GIN are direct, and thus rely predominantly upon grazing by the host in order for infection to occur. Implementing strategies to disrupt the life cycle (such as removal of feces or creating drier environmental conditions that would not support larval survival) may aid in decreasing the potential for reinfection.

Clinical Signs. Infection with GIN may or may not cause the infected host to exhibit clinical signs of disease, wherein many infected animals handle their parasite burden with no outward clinical abnormalities. However, some individual hosts—particularly those that are younger, experiencing stress or immune-compromise, or with high numbers of parasites present—exhibit clinical signs of disease. Clinical signs may include diarrhea, pale mucous membranes (anemia), edema (typically in the submandibular area [bottle jaw] or along the ventral midline), poor growth or weight loss, decreased milk or fiber production, and, in severe cases, death. Monospecific infections with one species of nematode is a rare phenomenon; parasitized hosts are usually infected with several different species of GIN which can lead to a complex manifestation of clinical signs depending upon the quantity and variety of GIN present.[1]

Diagnosis. The aforementioned clinical signs are consistent with, however, not confirmatory for, diagnosing intestinal parasitism, and achieving an accurate and meaningful antemortem diagnosis can be vital for appropriate individual animal and herd/flock management as it is no longer practical, from a drug efficacy and animal health standpoint, to deworm the entire group at timed intervals throughout the grazing season.[8,9]

Primary antemortem diagnostic options include fecal examination with quantification and FAMACHA scoring which are useful tools for determining which sheep or goats are most in need of treatment or are contributing most to pasture contamination (Boxes 6.1 and 6.2, Figures 6.1 and 6.2). FAMACHA scoring is more problematic in cervids, and other diagnostics should be utilized (e.g., fecal egg counts). More tertiary diagnostics (Box 6.3) include larval culture, differential egg-staining techniques, fecal PCR, and sero-diagnostics which are designed for determining the species of parasites present within an animal or group of animals and their proportion of the overall parasite population.[8,10] Additional diagnostics such as the in vitro assays to assess anthelmintic resistance allow for identification and determination of drug efficacy or resistance in the worm population.[9,10]

Examination of feces without employing any quantification technique provides little value leaving the producer with limited information regarding the types and numbers of parasites contributing to the overall parasite population. Benefits of performing a fecal egg count (FEC) technique are twofold: (1) it can provide the producer with information related to the overall number of parasites present within an animal, and (2) it can serve as a tool for monitoring drug efficacy following treatment. Use of the McMaster technique (Box 6.1, Figure 6.1) to determine FEC is widely accepted and practiced by many for determining FEC in sheep, goats, and cervids. Additional FEC techniques include

• BOX 6.1 McMaster Fecal Egg Count Technique

Required Materials

Compound microscope
Scale (measured in grams)
Fecal flotation solution (see note later)
50 mL centrifuge tube with screw cap
Tongue depressor
Tea strainer or cheesecloth (optional)
Pipette (or filter pipette [optional])
McMaster (chamber) slide
Fresh fecal sample (see note below)

Note: Fecal Flotation Solutions

Several recipes exist using table salt or sugar to create a solution with a specific gravity measuring approximately 1.20

Example recipe
- 1 pound table salt
- 3 quarts tap water
- Mix and heat to boiling while stirring
- Allow to cool (some precipitate may be present)
- Save the clear portion of the solution in a dispensing container at room temperature

Commercially available fecal solution preparations may also be purchased

Note: Collection of Fresh Feces

Use a glove to extract feces directly from the rectum if possible

Alternatively, a freshly deposited fecal sample may be collected from the ground

Feces should be placed in an air-tight container labeled with the date and any host identification information and refrigerated until testing is performed. If testing is delayed, eggs will ultimately mature and hatch, so it is important to have the feces tested as soon after collection as possible

McMaster Egg-Counting Procedure:

1. Weigh out 2 g of feces into a 50 mL centrifuge tube and fill to the 30 mL mark with your flotation solution
    - If a scale is not available, 28 mL of flotation solution may be added to the centrifuge tube and feces added until the total volume equals 30 mL (this will provide a close estimation of 2 g of feces but will not be as accurate as using a scale)
2. Break up fecal pellets with a tongue depressor
    - This may be facilitated by allowing the fecal sample to soak for a few minutes in the flotation solution or removing a large portion of the liquid and reserving it on the side, leaving only a small volume to initially begin homogenizing the pellets and later returning the full volume of flotation solution
3. Thoroughly mix the feces with the flotation solution (by vigorous stirring and/or replacing the screw cap and shaking the solution)
4. Once homogenized, the large debris may be strained out by using a tea strainer or cheesecloth. Removal of the large debris will make the slide easier to read
    - Alternatively, a filter pipette may be used to aspirate the solution while removing large debris
    - If no straining is desired, the solution may be aspirated with a standard pipette
5. Fill all chambers in the McMaster's slide completely with the homogenized mixture
    - It is important that the mixture is not allowed to sit as eggs will passively float in the solution. If more than a few seconds have elapsed between mixing and loading, rock the mixture in the capped tube to resuspend the eggs prior to pipetting
    - If the chambers to not fill completely or contain air bubbles, rinse the slide and chambers with water, shake or tap to remove excess water, and attempt filling the chambers again
    - Keep the slide on a flat surface or only slightly tilted while filling by gently squeezing the pipette to release the liquid
6. Allow the filled slide to sit for approximately 5 minutes prior to viewing to allow eggs to passively float within the chambers
    - Do not allow the slide to sit longer than 60 minutes as the liquid may begin to dry out or crystallize which will alter the results
7. View the slide using the 10× objective, focusing on any tiny air bubbles or the lines of the chamber (this will be the same plane of focus to find the eggs)
8. Count all trichostrongyle-type/HOTC-type eggs present within the lined portion of the chambers
9. Determine eggs per gram (EPG) by multiplying the total number of trichostrongyle-type/HOTC-type eggs by the multiplication factor
    - If using 2 g of feces, 28 mL of flotation solution, and a two-chamber slide that holds a total of 0.3 mL (0.15 mL per chamber), the multiplication factor is 50 and the sensitivity is 50 EPG
    - Alteration of the weight of feces, total volume of the flotation solution, or size/number of chambers will result in an altered sensitivity and multiplication factor
10. Once counting is complete, the chambers may be rinsed with water and used for additional testing in the future.

• BOX 6.2 FAMACHA Guidelines

1. Ensure that those performing the FAMACHA have been properly trained
2. Understand the limitation that the FAMACHA is designed to detect *Haemonchus* and that other diagnostic tools are necessary to detect other parasite species
3. Examine each host at 2- to 3-week intervals (and increase the frequency of exams during warm, humid weather when parasite transmission is at its peak)
   - Monitor young animals or those that exhibit any clinical signs or abnormalities more closely
4. Keep a record of each individual animal's results every time
5. Cull animals that need treated three times more often than the herd average
6. Use an integrated approach with attention to other management strategies to maximize health and minimize disease

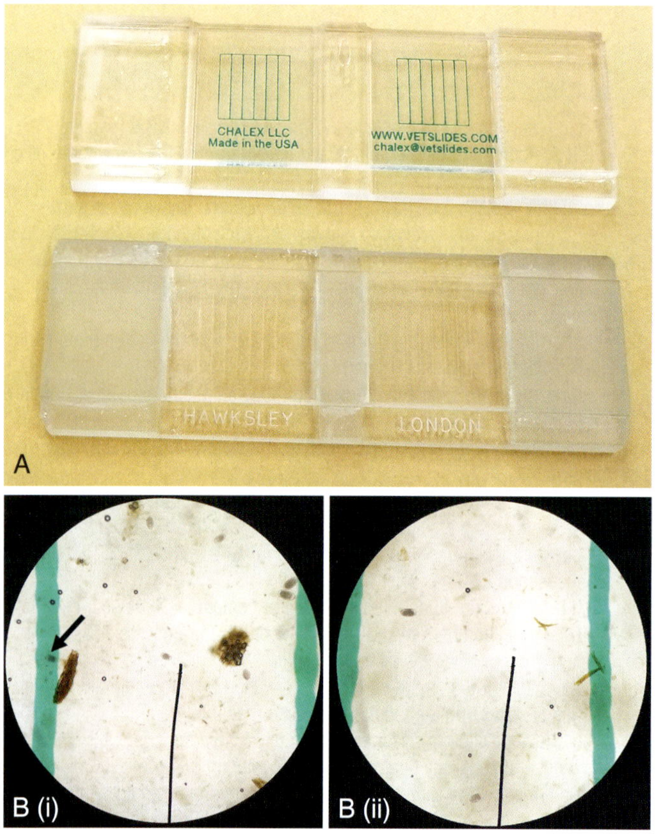

• Fig. 6.1 McMaster's Fecal Egg Count. **A.** Examples of two-chamber McMaster slides. **B.** View through the eyepiece of a McMaster's slide using the 10× objective. (i) Note the Haemonchus, Ostertagia, Trichostrongylus and Cooperia or other gastrointestinal strongyle 'type' eggs (HOTC Comples -type) in the field; an egg *(arrow)* is even under one of the lines. (ii) A small coccidia oocyst is located at the end of the pointer; coccidia are hard to see using McMaster slides due to their small size and the limitation of viewing only the 4× or 10× objectives (use of the 40× will scratch the top of the slide).

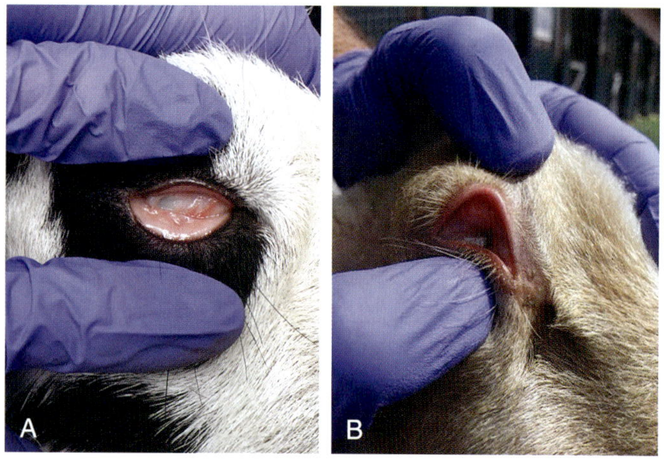

• Fig. 6.2 Examples of FAMACHA Scoring. **A.** A mixed breed goat with a FAMACHA score of 4 in the right eye. The left eye should also be evaluated prior to assigning the FAMACHA score. (Courtesy of Dr. Ricardo Stockler, Auburn University.) **B.** This mixed breed adult goat has a FAMACHA score of 2–3 when evaluating the right eye membranes. She had a packed-cell volume of 38. (Courtesy of Dr. Thomas Passler, Auburn University.)

• BOX 6.3 Summary of Tertiary Nematode Diagnostics

A. Larval culture
   Collection of eggs in a fecal sample that are propagated through the maturation process to identifiable larval stages which can be determined to species
   Available through several diagnostic laboratories
B. Pasture collection
   Grass samples collected and larvae present morphologically or molecularly determined to species
   Available through several diagnostic laboratories
C. Differential egg-staining techniques
   Haemonchus eggs can be stained with peanut lectin and viewed with fluorescent microscopy
   Research tool
   Research tool; not yet commercially available
D. PCR of feces
   A fecal sample can be analyzed by PCR to detect the different species present and their relative quantity to one another
   Research tool; not yet commercially available
E. Sero-diagnosis
   Saliva, serum, milk, or feces is submitted for the detection of either antibodies generated against specific parasites or antigens from the parasites
   Research tool; not yet commercially available for ruminants
F. In vitro assays for assessment of anthelmintic resistance
   Egg hatch, larval development, larval motility/migration, or larval feeding are measured in the presence of anthelmintic(s)
   Commercial assay (DrenchRite®) available through select diagnostic laboratories, other assays available through several diagnostic laboratories

modifications of the McMaster technique, the modified Stoll technique, the FLOTAC or mini-FLOTAC, FECPAK, or in hosts with suspected lower worm burdens, the Wisconsin or modified Wisconsin method.[8,11] Regardless of which quantification method is used, consistent use is paramount to allow for comparisons to be made and conclusions to be drawn over time.[1,10]

Results of an FEC are reported as number of eggs per gram (EPG). The number of eggs present can be impacted by several factors:[1]

- Species of parasites in the population (*Haemonchus* females generate higher numbers of eggs than *Teladorsagia* or *Trichostrongylus* females).

- Stages of parasites in the population (immature adults may be present and contributing to disease while not yet reproductively mature and contributing to the number of eggs).
- Consistency of the fecal sample (the number of eggs in a more liquid fecal sample will be diluted by the water present in the sample compared with a formed fecal sample).
- Recently used anthelmintic compound.

There are also two major drawbacks with FEC techniques. The first is their inability to determine the species of nematodes present in the fecal sample. This is where the tertiary diagnostics are of use (Box 6.3). Unfortunately, the eggs of many of the gastrointestinal nematode species lack any distinguishing morphologic characteristics unlike their adult counterparts. These eggs are typically classified as "trichostrongyle-type" or "HOTC-type" eggs due to their morphological similarities (Figures 6.1 and 6.3A). The acronym HOTC stands for four of the common GIN genera: *Haemonchus*, *Ostertagia*, *Trichostrongylus*, and *Cooperia*. Other genera with HOTC-type eggs include *Teladorsagia*, *Spiculopteragia*, *Apteragia*, *Bunostomum*, *Chabertia*, and *Oesophagostomum*. Other GIN species do have eggs that are distinct from one another (Figure 6.3B–D): *Nematodirus*, *Marshallagia*, *Aonchotheca*, *Strongyloides*, *Gongylonema*, *Skrjabinema*, and *Trichuris*. The second major drawback is the requirement of special equipment (e.g., microscope, technique-specific equipment, and centrifuge).

When evaluating the FEC results, it is important to not rely solely on the number of eggs counted to make treatment decisions. In general, sheep, goats, and cervids may have high FECs in the 1000 to 5000 EPG range and not exhibit any signs of disease, while other animals may be in poor body condition with other clinical signs and have lower EPG counts. If it is known that *H. contortus* is present in the population, FECs greater than 2000 to 3000 may indicate a more serious infection that may warrant treatment. If *H. contortus* is not present in the population, FECs ranging from 500 to 1000 may be significant. Clinical signs (if any), fecal consistency, body condition score, and FAMACHA results (if available) should always be taken into consideration prior to making a treatment decision for an animal.

Use of the FAMACHA card and scoring system is another primary diagnostic option that is practiced among sheep and goat producers, and it can be performed without any special equipment or a microscope (Box 6.2). According to the most recent NAHMS studies, 11.3% of sheep producers and 13.5% of goat producers utilize the FAMACHA with their animals.[12,13] The FAMACHA card was named after its creator, Professor Francois "Fafa" Malan). It is designed specifically to assist in detecting infection with anemia-inducing GIN, primarily *H. contortus*, and is of little use for detection of other GIN species. The FAMACHA card utilizes the coloration of the ocular mucous membranes of the host as a means to determine the relative packed-cell volume (PCV) of the host. The examiner compares the color of the lower eyelid conjunctiva to the five colors (ranging from red to white) represented on the FAMACHA card, while standing beside the

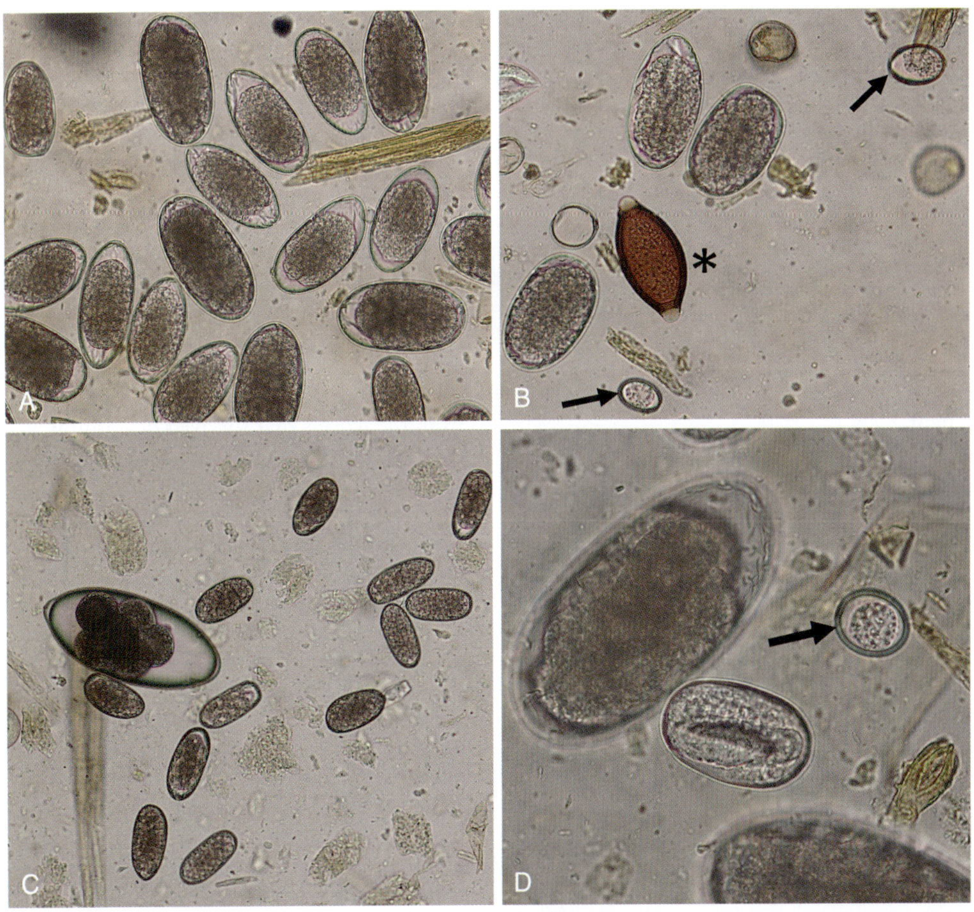

• **Fig. 6.3** Nematode eggs seen on fecal flotation. (Courtesy Jamie Butler, Auburn University.) **A.** Trichostrongyle-type or HOTC-type eggs. **B.** *Trichuris* spp. egg (*) with HOTC-type eggs and two *Eimeria* spp. oocysts *(arrows)*. **C.** Large *Nematodirus* spp. egg surrounded by HOTC-type eggs. **D.** *Strongyloides* spp. larvated egg with an HOTC-type egg and *Eimeria* spp. oocyst *(arrow)*.

sheep or goat, and using the index finger to slightly and gently "retropulse" the globe through the upper eyelid. This will help expose as much conjunctiva as possible, and assess color, comparing to the card for 2 to 3 seconds (see Figure 6.2). The associated color score (1–5) is reflective of the host's PCV and severity of disease associated with *H. contortus* infection.[14] (Alternatively, the PCV may be measured directly with a blood sample and the proper equipment.) Goats typically have a lower PCV than sheep, but a PCV of less than 20% (FAMACHA score = 3) may correlate with the development of clinical signs associated with anemia, and the lower the PCV (FAMACHA score = 4 or 5), the more severe the clinical signs. If large numbers of *Haemonchus* are present in the gastrointestinal tract (Figure 6.4), an animal may bleed to death quickly; however, blood transfusions can be life-saving in some situations.

Should an animal die from suspected parasite-related issues, postmortem may be of use for addressing the remainder of the herd or flock. A necropsy should be performed and GIT contents examined for presence of parasites. Many of the adult worms are small and may be intimately attached to the gut mucosa and easily missed if the examiner is not careful. Any worms recovered can be identified to species and the gut contents can be tested for presence and quantification of parasite eggs (see Chapter 19).

A "Five-Point Check" is also used to aid in parasite diagnosis and decision analysis to determine which sheep and goats should be dewormed. This program is described in great detail by Bath and van Wyk[14a], but may be very difficult to employ for cervid production units. The five categories of the Five-Point Check are:

1. EYE by employing the FAMACHA scoring system just described;
2. BACK by assigning a body condition score which is described in Chapter 1, Table 1.1 and Chapter 19;
3. TAIL or "Dag score" of 1–5, where 1 is an animal with no fecal soiling and a 5 is an animal with watery diarrhea extending to its hocks and possibly appearing to be sick. With a Dag score of 4 or 5, one should consider deworming or other methods of parasite control;
4. NOSE by examining for anything other than normally moist nostrils with very scant amounts of clear discharge (**Note:** large amounts of clear discharge, and animals rubbing their faces against walls or posts and stomping their feet may indicate Nasal Bots, see Chapter 7);
5. JAW by examination for evidence of bottle jaw or other dependent edema. The 5-point check in conjunction fecal egg counts will greatly aid in parasite and overall health monitoring.

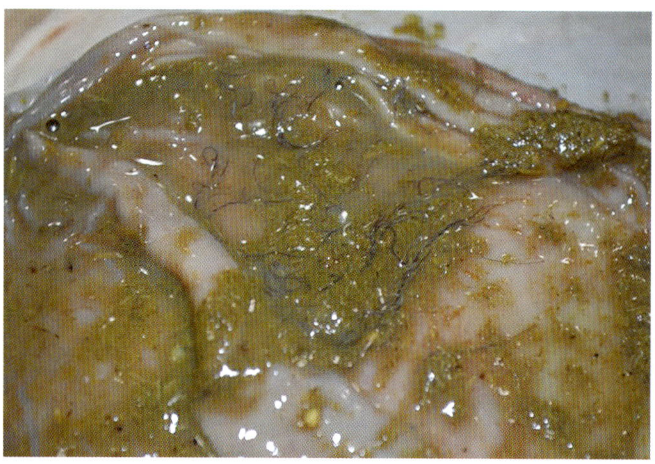

• **Fig. 6.4** *Haemonchus* seen in a necropsy of a ewe. Note the obvious "barber pole" pattern of the adult worms. (Courtesy Dr. Kelley Steury, Auburn University.)

Treatment and Control Programs. Traditional control programs for gastrointestinal nematodes have relied upon the use of broad-spectrum anthelmintic compounds in the entire herd or flock at timed intervals. This approach has been termed "suppressive deworming." This overuse of once highly effective drugs has led to a widespread development of parasites that are resistant to the available anthelmintics (discussed in further detail later).[10,15] Each administration of drugs would kill off the susceptible parasites within the host, but a small percentage of worms would survive the treatments. Those survivors would be the only worms left in the group of animals; therefore, the only eggs continuing to contaminate the pastures contained drug-resistant worms. With continued use of the same compounds, over time, the parasite population in the pasture transitioned to a larger proportion that could withstand the drugs. When those resistant parasites were subsequently ingested and could no longer be removed from the animals when dewormed, a vicious cycle ensued, resulting in increases in clinical disease that could not be fixed through routine deworming.

We have learned that the parasites are not evenly distributed amongst the animals in a group—in fact, a small portion of the animals contain the majority of the parasites.[1,14] This ultimately means that only a small portion of the animals are contributing to the majority of the pasture contamination. We also know that some animals are able to handle their parasite burden better than others. By targeting our anthelmintic treatments at those animals that are suffering from clinical disease associated with the parasitism or those animals contributing most to the pasture contamination, we can help to maintain refugia and decrease the overuse and misuse of anthelmintics. Refugia is defined as the portion of the parasite population that is not selected for through the use of anthelmintics. Sources of refugia include parasites within an animal host that is not dewormed, parasite stages within a treated host that were never susceptible to the anthelmintic being used (e.g., some dewormers are stage-specific), and all of the parasites on pasture at the time of deworming. This refugia population of susceptible parasites will help to dilute out any resistant genes from the worms that survived deworming in the treated subset of animals, thus helping to preserve the efficacy of the available anthelmintic compounds.[16]

The current recommended strategies for using anthelmintics are to utilize them with a *targeted selective treatment* (TST) approach, also known as *smart drenching*, of which there are many (e.g., FAMACHA or Fecal Egg Count/FEC), with varying benefits and disadvantages.[9] One disadvantage with the TST approaches is the increase in time and effort it takes to determine which specific parasites are present in the group and which hosts are the most heavily parasitized and in need of deworming. Historically, when all animals were treated, there was no additional effort required of the producer other than the time, effort, and cost to deworm all of the animals. Implementing a TST requires that the producer now employ different techniques, including consultation with the veterinarian and diagnostician initially, in order to make the TST effective, costing time and money. The benefits, however, are that there are now fewer animals will need to be treated, thus reducing the time and effort of the deworming process itself, less drug being used, saving the producer money, and the available anthelmintics remaining effective for longer, resulting in healthier animals. Developing an effective parasite control program involving the use of TST approaches is a continuous process that requires the evaluation of current strategies, the review of available approaches, and the updating of management practices.[1,5,9] Focusing on approaches that ensure adequate dosing of animals with proper dosing techniques and follow-up evaluation of drugs for evidence of continued efficacy, should be emphasized.

Strategic deworming works best when we remember the parasite's life cycle and epidemiology. Recall that animals are infected with GIN by grazing L3-infected pastures; therefore, we must focus on controlling infection during the grazing season when the majority of parasite transmission occurs. Using a routine parasite evaluation technique (e.g., FEC, FAMACHA, weight, or body condition score) at designated time intervals (typically 2 to 4 weeks) during the transmission season to determine the animals most in need of treatment is one way to implement a TST approach. By strategically deworming only the clinically ill animals or those responsible for the majority of pasture contamination during the transmission season, we will reduce pasture contamination and disease while maintaining refugia.[5]

One exception to the recommendation to strategically deworm is with animals imminently destined for slaughter. All of these animals should be dewormed prior to shipping which will enhance their condition without risking the contamination of pastures with resistant parasite genetics as all of these animals will be moved into confinement pens where grazing is not an option. This recommendation is not to be misconstrued as a blanket statement regarding all animals that are undergoing shipping or translocation; if the animals are destined for pastures elsewhere, it is still important to use a TST approach.[5]

Another exception involves pregnant animals in northern temperate climates in the winter. Strategically treating the animals with a drug that targets encysted (hypobiotic) and adult parasite stages as they are moved off pasture for the winter will keep the parasite burden low while also reducing the periparturient rise in FEC and pasture contamination the following spring. This strategy could prove problematic in farms already dealing with multidrug resistant parasites, and if that is the case, some animals should remain untreated to supply refugia to the pasture in the spring, typically those that have not had high FECs or clinical disease in the past. This strategy is less effective in warmer climates; monitoring animals as spring approaches to identify the problematic animals is a more fruitful use of time and resources.[5]

Safe pastures are another strategy. Safe pastures are those that have low levels of parasites present, including those that have been devoid of relevant animal hosts for several months during a season where the climate will eliminate larvae, pastures that have been used for hay or crops previously, pastures that have been burned, or pastures that have been recently grazed by hosts (e.g., horses or cattle) that largely shed parasite species of little or no concern to sheep, goats, and cervids. If safe pastures are used, it is crucial that TST also be used to preserve refugia on the new pasture. If all animals are treated just prior to or following movement to a safe pasture with a suppressive deworming program, all parasite stages present on that new safe pasture will be resistant after a single round of treatment.

Tactical deworming involves the removal of worms in the hosts before the worms can reproduce and contribute to pasture contamination, but situations where this strategy would be of best use can be hard to predict.[5]

Opportunistic deworming and *salvage deworming* are typically not very effective long-term. Opportunistic treatment involves deworming while the animals are already being handled or processed for some other purpose. Although convenient, it does not assist with animal health or overall productivity. A producer would be better off to schedule other procedures around when the animals are being handled for parasite monitoring and management reasons. Salvage deworming may save the lives of heavily parasitized animals, but if the animals must be so ill (bottle jaw, severe anemia, recumbency) in order to treat, productivity of the animal or herd/flock has already been compromised.[5]

With the current situation where many parasites have developed the ability to withstand treatment with multiple drug classes, it is imperative the producers and clinicians do all they can to maintain what efficacy remains and to minimize the further development of anthelmintic resistance. This involves employing one or more TST approaches, selecting the proper drugs, dosages, and routes of administration, keeping accurate records involving diagnostics and treatment, and implementing an integrated management approach which may involve alternative control methods (discussed in detail later). Additionally, valuable online resources for producers regarding parasite control are available (e.g., American Consortium for Small Ruminant Parasite Control [ACSRPC] [website www.wormx.info])[9] (see Chapter 19)

Many cervid producers attempt internal parasite control using a feed containing anthelmintic, or administration of a dewormer via topical application, drenching, or injection whenever the cervids are handled for other procedures. Necropsies of farmed white-tailed deer performed at the Alabama Veterinary Diagnostic Lab System (> 1000 from 2014 to 2018) revealed that internal parasites were not considered to be a significant problem. An exception may be with confinement-raised fawns reared in crowded conditions showing signs of poor growth and diarrhea; these animals in some instances have high *Strongyloides* FECs (> 1000 EPG). Overall, for farm raised cervids, the authors recommend the application of control programs that are useful for sheep and goats be employed when possible and practical (e.g., pasture rotation and management, browsing plant species with high condensed tannins, etc.), and to use fecal egg counts as part of a decision analysis for the need for using dewormers.

Anthelmintic Resistance

The broad-spectrum drug classes available for use against GIN in ruminants in the United States are listed in Table 6.2. Some of the listed products are approved for use in a single host species; when using these drugs in an extra-label fashion, particularly in food-producing ruminants including wild cervids, clinicians should consult the Animal Medicinal Drug Use Clarification Act (AMDUCA) and the Food Animal Drug Residue Avoidance and Databank (FARAD). Available anthelmintics include benzimidazoles, nicotinic membrane depolarizers, and macrocyclic lactones. Even though a product may have been labeled for a certain parasite when first approved, resistant GIN species have been documented with every single drug class available. Some drugs within a drug class are more potent than others, but once a parasite has become resistant (gained the ability to survive one drug in a drug class), even the more potent drugs within a drug class will ultimately fail. This is termed *side-resistance*.[1,5]

The benzimidazole (BZ) class includes the drugs thiabendazole, fenbendazole, and albendazole. They were among the first broad-spectrum anthelmintics introduced in the United States. The efficacy of the BZ anthelmintics is improved by increasing

TABLE 6.2 Commonly Used Anthelmintics Approved for Use in Sheep and/or Goats in the U.S.

				DOSAGE		WITHDRAWAL TIMES (DAYS)[a]		
Drug	Formulation	Parasite Spectrum	Approved Host(s)	Sheep	Goats	Meat (Ov, Ca)	Milk (Ca only)	Remarks
Fenbendazole (Safe-Guard)	Suspension	Nematodes	Ca	5 mg/kg (ELDU)	5 mg/kg	Ov: NE Ca: 6	NE	Approved in Bighorn sheep, not for use in domestic sheep In goats, 10 mg/kg is recommended but is considered ELDU and will require an extended WDT
Albendazole (Valbazen)	Suspension	Nematodes, trematodes, cestodes	Ov, Ca	7.5 mg/kg	10–15 mg/kg	Ov: 7 Ca: 7	NE	In goats, 10 mg/kg dose and WDT of 7 days in meat animals are approved for liver flukes only; 15 mg/kg for nematodes (ELDU) Do not use within 30 days of conception
Levamisole (LevaMed, Levasole bolus, Prohibit)	Soluble drench powder; bolus	Nematodes	Ov	8 mg/kg; 1 bolus/ 50 lb	12 mg/kg (ELDU)	Ov: 3 Ca: NE	NE	Weighing before treatment is recommended Dehydration increases risk of toxicity—caution when using in hot weather
Morantel tartrate (Rumatel 88, Mor-Max, Goat Care 2X)	Feed premix	Nematodes	Ca	10 mg/kg (ELDU)	10 mg/kg	Ov: NE Ca: 30	0	Approved for use in lactating dairy goats
Ivermectin (Ivomec, Ivermectin, Privermectin)	Oral drench	Nematodes, Arthropods (bots)	Ov	0.2 mg/kg	0.4 mg/kg (ELDU)	Ov: 11 Ca: NE	NE	Cattle injectable form not recommended
Moxidectin (Cydectin)	Oral drench	Nematodes	Ov	0.2 mg/kg	0.4 mg/kg (ELDU)	Ov: 7 Ca: NE	NE	Use of cattle pour-on formulation is discouraged
Decoquinate (Deccox)	Feed additive	Protozoa	Ov, Ca	0.5 mg/kg	0.5 mg/kg	Ov: 0 Ca: 0	NE	Feed for at least 28 days during periods of exposure For prepartum use 1 kg of 13% premix in 22 kg of trace mineralized salt
Lasalocid (Bovatec)	Feed additive	Protozoa	Ov	1 mg/kg	1 mg/kg (ELDU)	Ov: 0 Ca: NE	NE	Feed continuously For prepartum use 1 kg of 6% premix in 22 kg of trace mineralized salt
Monensin (Rumensin)	Feed additive	Protozoa	Ca	20 g/ton (ELDU)	20 g/ton	Ov: NE Ca: 0	NE	Feed continuously Do not allow horses or other equids access as ingestion may be fatal to those hosts

Ca, Caprine; *ELDU*, extra-label drug use; *NE*, not established; *Ov*, ovine; *WDT*, withdrawal time.

[a]This constitutes extra-label drug use, so a withdrawal time has not been established. Current recommendations are available on the Food Animal Residue Avoidance and Depletion (FARAD) program website (www.farad.org).

the dose, splitting the dose into two 12-hour treatments, giving the dose daily for 3 to 5 days, and fasting the animal (as long as it is not sick or reproductively stressed) prior to treatment in order to slow the transit rate of gut contents.[18] These adjustments, however, will not be effective long-term once the parasites have become resistant to this class of drugs, and once resistance has developed, susceptibility of the parasites to this class of anthelmintics is not regained, even if this drug class is not used for years.[1]

Nicotinic anthelmintics (imidazothiazoles [levamisole] and tetrahydropyrimidines [morantel tartrate]) were the next generation of broad-spectrum parasiticides. These drugs were not used as frequently as the BZs, and therefore, do not experience the high rates of anthelmintic resistance as is seen with the BZs. Even so, parasite populations have developed the ability to survive treatment with these classes of anthelmintics as well.[1]

The macrocyclic lactones (MCL) are the newest class of broad-spectrum anthelmintics available in the United States for ruminants.

Drugs within this class include ivermectin, moxidectin, eprinomectin, and others. Just like with the other drug classes, once resistance has been documented to one of the drugs in the class, side resistance will ultimately occur to the more potent drugs, especially if used frequently. Moxidectin is the more potent MCL available for use in the United States, and should be used judiciously to preserve its efficacy; it should be used only when all other anthelmintics have proven ineffective.[1,9]

One unique feature of the MCL drug class was the variety of ways in which they could be administered to the host, including oral drench, pour-on, and injectable, whereas oral formulations were the traditional means of administering other classes of anthelmintics. Data to support the efficacy of using pour-on formulations of cattle MCLs in sheep, goats, and cervids (with the possible exception of reindeer) is not available; it is recommended to use oral formulations in these hosts.[19] There are data to support the efficacious use of injectable moxidectin in goats, but not in sheep.[20]

A new anthelmintic class has been developed and is approved for use in countries outside of the United States, the amino-acetonitrile derivatives (monepantel).[21] Unfortunately, as with other drug classes, the parasites developed resistance to this novel drug class in record time.[22] This drug was used the same way the historic drugs were used, proving that suppressive deworming programs alone very quickly select for resistant parasites.

The only way to truly avoid the development of anthelmintic resistance is to never use the drugs at all, which is not a viable option. General guidelines for use of anthelmintics are provided in Table 6.2 and in Box 6.5.

- Sheep, goats, and cervids metabolize drugs at different rates.[23] When using cattle-approved drugs in these hosts, the cattle dose is usually effective for sheep and cervids, but a double dose is required for efficacy in goats. Levamisole is the exception, where a 1.5× dose is administered to goats rather than a 2× dose.
- Oral administration is preferred for sheep and goats; pour-on formulations lack efficacy when applied topically to sheep and goats.[19] Care should be taken to ensure that entire dose enters the rumen by using a dosing syringe to place the dose over the back of the tongue. Use of oral, pour-on, or injectable formulations has been successful in cervids, however, elevated doses (compared with the cattle dose) may be required for efficacy. Given the large variety of cervid hosts, specifics regarding choice of anthelmintic, route of administration, and dose should be researched for each cervid host and parasitic infection in question.
- Accurate weights should be obtained in order to provide an accurate drug dose.
- Withdrawal times are available through the FARAD databank.
- It is recommended to use one drug class until it fails before switching to a different drug class.[19] More frequent switching between drug classes may accelerate development of resistance.
- If multi-class resistance is present on a farm, using two anthelmintic classes simultaneously has been shown to improve efficacy (e.g., fenbendazole + levamisole or albendazole + ivermectin). It is important to note that the full dose of both components be administered.[19,24]
- Fecal egg count reduction tests (FECRTs) should be performed following treatment to ensure anthelmintic efficacy. The World Association for the Advancement of Veterinary Parasitology (WAAVP) recommends comparing the FEC of treated animals to the FEC of nontreated animals 1 to 2 weeks following treatment. If a group of nontreated animals is not available, it is possible to compare the pre- and posttreatment FEC among individual animals.[8,10,25]
- Fecal tests should be performed on a minimum of 10 individual animals within the group. Evaluation of composite samples is not recommended as it will decrease the overall accuracy of the test. Under the WAAVP guidelines, anything less than a 95% reduction in eggs is indicative of resistance, and changing anthelmintic class is warranted.[10,25]
- FECRTs should be performed every 2 to 3 years or whenever resistance is suspected.
- Some diagnostic laboratories provide highly accurate, yet expensive, in vitro methods to determine if anthelmintic resistance is present that can be used in lieu of FECRTs.
- Alternative control methods (described later) should be used in conjunction with judicious anthelmintic use to create a comprehensive parasite control program.
- Strict biosecurity programs should be in place for new additions. Animals should be confined for 3 to 4 weeks during which time they are treated with at least two (if not more) different drug classes. Efficacy should be confirmed and the resulting FEC should be as close to zero as possible prior to integrating the animal into the flock or herd. This will limit the potential introduction of anthelmintic-resistant parasites into the flock or herd (Box 6.5, and Chapter 19).[5,19]

• BOX 6.4 Summary of Additional Fecal Diagnostic Techniques

A. Baermann Technique

Used when looking for lungworm larvae

1. Several grams of feces are wrapped in a porous material (e.g., cheesecloth or chem-wipes)
2. Fecal pouch is suspended in warm water for several hours (overnight is preferred) in a funnel with clamped tubing, a cone-shaped collection vessel, or hollow stemware
   - The temperature of the water stimulates the larvae to migrate out of the feces, through the porous material, where they will sink to the bottom of the collection vessel and be concentrated in the narrow base
3. Larvae may be aspirated from the bottom with a pipette or dispensed in a few drops if using a funnel with clamped tubing
4. Sample should be placed on a microscope slide and viewed with a compound microscope

B. Sedimentation Technique

Used when looking for fluke eggs

1. Several grams of feces are mixed with tap water
2. Fecal slurry should be strained (cheesecloth or tea strainer) into a 50 mL centrifuge tube
3. Tube can be spun in a centrifuge or allowed to sit for 10 minutes, allowing the eggs and debris to settle
4. Supernatant should be poured off and the sediment resuspended with additional water
5. Repeat steps 3 and 4 several times to result in a cleaner sample, ending with pouring the supernatant off the final time
6. Optional: methylene blue stain may be added which will stain the debris while the fluke eggs will remain amber, brown in color
7. Eggs of *Fascioliasis hepatica* are large and may be seen by placing sediment into a petri dish on a dissecting scope or cover-slipped slide on a compound scope. Eggs of *Dicrocoelium dendriticum* are much smaller and should be observed using a compound microscope

• BOX 6.5 Guidelines for Use of Deworming Drugs

1. Only treat the animals in need (Smart)
2. Treat with an effective anthelmintic as determined by FECRT or other method of determining anthelmintic efficacy
3. Weigh animals prior to treating
4. Ensure full dose reaches rumen through proper drenching technique
5. Fast the animal 24 hours prior to dosing (as long as they are not sick or stressed) to increase efficacy
6. Split dose into two 12-hour doses
7. If anthelmintic resistance is present, use two classes of anthelmintics simultaneously

Note: use of alternative control methods to create an integrated parasite control program is highly recommended

FECRT, *Fecal egg count reduction test;* TST *targeted selective treatment.*

These guidelines outline the basic steps in optimizing a parasite control program with the goals of maintaining animal health and the efficacy of available anthelmintics. Even with these guidelines, implementation is lacking. Data in the most recent NAHMS studies revealed the following information regarding the methods used by producers to prolong or improve anthelmintic efficacy: rotation of dewormers (70.4% sheep), more frequent deworming (26.9% sheep) while strategic deworming (33% sheep), and monitoring drug efficacy with fecal testing (10.4% sheep).[12] Furthermore, when selecting the primary method to evaluate anthelmintic efficacy, producers were most likely to rely upon the subjective general appearance of the animal (67.2%) and the least likely to choose objective methods such as lab testing (3.3%) or improved eye score (4.0%).[12] Regarding treatment decisions, even though the majority of producers (sheep 69.1%, goat 64.0%, cervid 71.3%) valued the veterinarian as a source of deworming information, less than half (sheep 44.7%, goat 38.2%) included the veterinarian in the treatment decision (see Chapter 19).[12,26,27]

Alternative Control Methods

Nutrition. Perhaps the most important, yet easily overlooked, aspect regarding alternative parasite control strategies is nutrition.[28] Nutrients are absorbed via the gut and are partitioned to where they are most needed: growth, reproduction, immunity, etc. Animals that are adequately nourished can handle parasite infection better than animals that are malnourished or receiving an inadequate diet. Proper nutrition facilitates *resilience* and *resistance* of the animal. Resilience refers to the ability to cope with the parasite infection, while resistance, in this regard, refers to the host's ability to resist becoming infected. A properly nourished animal is better equipped to handle the negative physiologic effects caused by the parasite, while at the same time having a more sound immune system capable of keeping infections minimal (see Chapter 2 and Chapter 19).

Parasitism can impact appetite and interfere with the host's ability to absorb and utilize nutrients. Mucosal damage incited by some parasites can compromise the gut's ability to absorb nutrients leaving the host to rely upon body reserves. Parasites may also induce a protein-losing enteropathy due to the substantial damage to the intestinal cells. Decreased protein availability can lead to impaired immune function, as protein is an essential nutrient required for proper immune function. Impaired immunity leads to decreased host resistance to subsequent parasite infection. Supplementing the diet with proteins that can bypass the rumen appears to increase resilience and resistance. Additional supplementation with required vitamins, minerals, and energy may be beneficial, especially during times of increased nutrient demands (e.g., late gestation through early lactation). It is important to ensure host-appropriate supplementation for the specific animal host, as sheep, goats, and cervids all have different requirements. Taking care to ensure that nutrition is adequate will decrease the potential impact that parasitism may have on the host.

Genetic Selection. Animal selection is a helpful tool for internal parasite control. Certain breeds have demonstrated a genetic resistance to nematode infection: St. Croix, Gulf Coast Native, Katahdin, Red Maasai, and Santa Ines sheep and East African Dwarf and Saanen goats have expressed enhanced levels of innate resistance regarding nematode infection compared with other breeds.[31] The disadvantage of these breeds are that they may be less productive or produce fewer offspring, which may preclude their use in certain situations. The 2011 NAHMS study revealed that over half of sheep producers considered the selection for genetic resistance an important trait when selecting breeding stock.[32]

Outside of breed-specific resistance to parasites, individual animals within a herd or flock will experience increased levels of immunity and resistance to parasites compared with their cohorts. Parasite resistance is a heritable trait, therefore, producers can improve the ability of their herd or flock to genetically ward off parasitism by culling animals that routinely experience clinical illness or have high FECs or anemic FAMACHA scores. Recall that majority of the parasites are present in the minority of animals, therefore, retaining dams that rarely if ever experience clinical parasitism or need deworming will result in a herd or flock that is more innately resistant to parasites which can be highly beneficial in the changing landscape of anthelmintic resistance.[5,33] Additionally, identifying a ram or buck who has consistently low FAMACHA scores, low fecal egg counts, etc. in the spring has the potential to enhance overall herd or flock parasite resistance in one generation. One of the authors (DGP) includes FAMACHA scores, body condition score (BCS), Five Point Check, and FEC along with more routine breeding soundness evaluation techniques (e.g., physical examination, semen evaluation, testicular palpation and measurement, etc.) for routing Breeding Soundness Evaluation and/or sire selections for a herd or flock (see Chapter 8 and Chapter 19).

Co-Grazing (Mixing Livestock Species). In general, each animal species has its own variety of parasite fauna, and often the parasites that infect and cause disease in one type of animal do not infect a different type of animal. For example, very few parasites are shared between horses and cattle. Producers may exploit this phenomenon by grazing different groups of animals together on the same pasture or grazing them in sequence with one another. One species will consume the parasites of the other species, and vice versa, thus helping to clean up the pasture for one another. Sheep, goats, and camelids are an exception. These hosts do share many parasites, therefore, co-grazing of these species will not result in cleaner pastures.[1,5]

Pasture Rotation. The goal of pasture rotation is to allow the pasture to sit for a period of time after grazing in order for the forage to recuperate, thus providing more nutritious forage to the next set of grazing animals. It is common to use a 30-day period of rest, which unfortunately coincides with the developmental time required for many larval parasites. Placing a susceptible host species out on pasture that has been supporting larval development for the previous month may exacerbate infection rather than having a beneficial pasture-cleaning effect. Depending on the climate, pasture rest for 3 or more months would be indicated if there is to be any sort of larval parasite reduction, which isn't conducive to efficient forage utilization. Rotational systems also lend to increased stocking densities which may compound pasture contamination.[5] In general, pasture rotation is no longer recommended.[9] If rotational schemes are utilized, they must be combined with an appropriate TST approach to maintain levels of refugia in all of the pastures.

As mentioned previously in the co-grazing section, host rotation may benefit a pasture. Different hosts may not share the same types of parasites, therefore, a producer may consider grazing horses on a pasture that previously held sheep, goats, or cervids to assist in cleaning up the pasture by the new host(s) as long as forage quality and quantity are not of concern.

Copper Oxide Wire Particles. The use of copper oxide wire particles (COWP) has shown to have anthelmintic activity against *H. contortus* of sheep and goats, but COWP should be used with caution in sheep, with close monitoring, so as not to result in copper toxicity.[34,35] Doses of 0.5 to 2 g for lambs or kids and 2 g for ewes and does are effective as an aid or in some instances, the primary method of parasite control. It is still recommended to use COWP in a targeted or strategic manner by administering them to individual animals via gel caps or mixing into an individual animal's ration. Because of the potential of copper toxicity in sheep and occasionally goats, dietary evaluation with emphasis on molybdenum, copper, iron, and sulfur may be required.

Additionally, recent research has suggested that using COWP in conjunction with albendazole administration provides a synergistic effect, creating a greater reduction in the number of parasite eggs shed (reduced fecal egg counts) than with COWP or albendazole alone[36] (see Chapter 19).

Condensed Tannin-Containing Forages. Sericea lespedeza *(Lespedeza cuneata)* is a perennial condensed tannin-containing forage present in the United States which shows promise as a natural means of parasite control that can be used as an adjunct measure in a parasite control program. It grows during the warm season and can be grazed or processed as hay or pellets.[37] Benefits of condensed tannin-containing forages include reductions in FEC and *H. contortus* present in the abomasum. Indirect benefits include a decrease in larvae on pasture by hindering egg hatching or larval development. Additionally, since many condensed tannin-containing forages are browse or legumes, they grow above the ground, resulting in an overall reduction in parasite exposure with a simultaneous increase in protein and nutrient intake. Animals grazing sericea lespedeza may need 4 weeks to adjust to eating it, and if provided as hay or pellets, it needs to constitute at least 50% of the diet. Other forages that have exhibited some anti-parasite activity include chicory *(Cichorium intybus)* and sainfoin *(Onobrychis viciifolia)*[37] (see Chapter 19).

Nematode-Trapping Fungi. The use of fungi as a natural means of parasite control can also be exploited. Naturally occurring nematode-trapping fungi are found in soil throughout the world and feed on free-living nematodes by using hyphal traps. In order for fungi to be effective at killing parasitic larvae and ultimately decreasing pasture contamination, the fungi have to be present in high numbers within the feces.[38] This can be accomplished through the feeding of fungal spores to the ruminants which will subsequently pass out and germinate in the feces where they can trap the parasitic larvae. The fungi that has been most successful at surviving GIT in ruminant species is *Duddingtonia flagrans*.[39] The major disadvantages of nematode-trapping fungi are that a commercially available product containing the fungal spores does not yet exist, and the fungi have no known impact on adult parasites residing within the host. Should a commercial product become available, this biological parasite control method can be used in conjunction with other parasite treatment and control strategies to create a more comprehensive parasite control program.[39]

Vaccination. In the face of anthelmintic resistance, the development of GI nematode vaccines is increasingly enticing. The barber pole worm (*Haemonchus contortus*) vaccine is available in Australia and contains purified *H. contortus* antigen.[40] This vaccine is designed to reduce egg shedding and clinical disease associated with *H. contortus* infection. The antigens present in the vaccine are recovered from the gut cells of the worm. Antibodies generated by the sheep's immune system will then be ingested by the worms in the abomasum where they will interfere with the worm's ability to process nutrients, ultimately resulting in a dying or dead worm. The disadvantage to using antigens that are present only in the worm gut are that the host's immune system doesn't see these antigens during natural infection, therefore, there is no natural boosting of the immune response without additional vaccination which leads to vaccine administration four to five times each year.[31]

Additional vaccine targets include excretory/secretory compounds of *H. contortus*, but have yet to yield consistent protective results.[41]

Integrated Control. The use of any of the previously discussed alternative control strategies as an exclusive means for controlling parasites would result in disappointment. Yet, these techniques, when employed in combination with judicious and strategic use of anthelmintics and pasture management, will result in an effective and comprehensive parasite control program.

In addition to these strategies for controlling parasites in the animals and on the premises, a biosecurity program should be established to prevent the introduction of new parasites or anthelmintic-resistant parasites to the premises (see Box 6.5; Chapter 19).[5]

Nematodes of Other Body Systems

Lungworms

Etiology, Life Cycle, and Clinical Signs. Three major lungworm species can be found infecting ruminants in North America: *Muellerius capillaris* is found most commonly, followed by *Dictyocaulus* spp., then *Protostrongylus* spp.

The life cycle of *Dictyocaulus* is quite similar to the aforementioned life cycle of the gastrointestinal nematodes: larvae mature in the environment, L3 are ingested while grazing, and no intermediate host is required. Major distinguishing features of the life cycle are that the adult worms are present in the bronchi instead of the gut, larvae (Figure 6.5) are the diagnostic stage passed in the feces of the host rather than eggs, and the transmission season for this parasite in North America is more so in the fall and winter months.[2,6]

The life cycles of *Muellerius* and *Protostrongylus* are indirect, requiring the presence of a snail or slug intermediate host for the larvae to mature to the L3 stage. Adults reside in the small bronchioles or lungs of the ruminant host, and L1 are passed into the environment via the feces or potentially in respiratory secretions. Since completion of the life cycle is dependent upon the presence of snails and slugs, the transmission season is restricted to the seasons when the intermediate hosts are present: spring and summer.

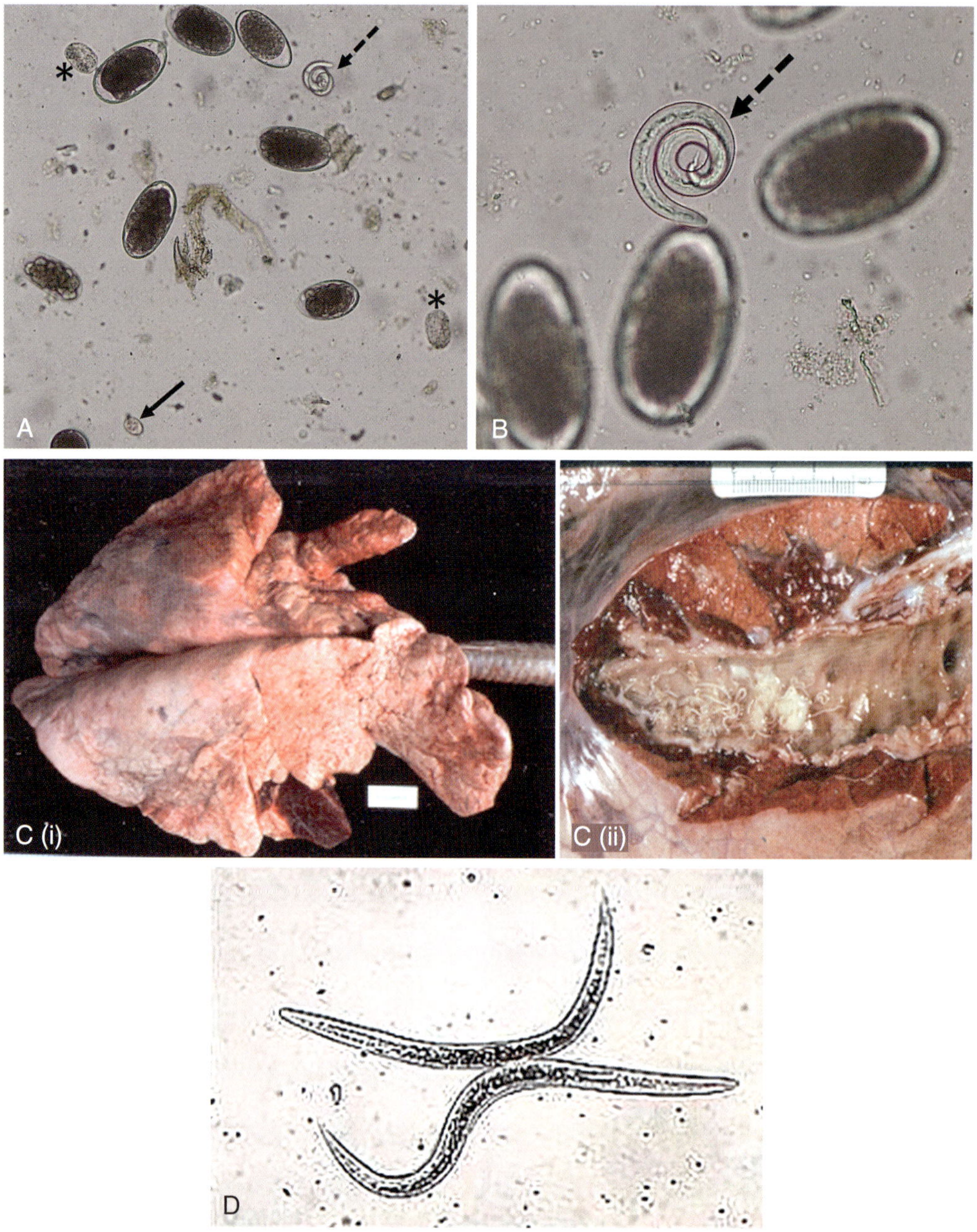

• **Fig. 6.5** Lungworms. **A.** A composite fecal examination showing 2 *Muellerius* larvae *(dashed arrow) larvae* with a coiled tails, HOTC-type eggs, two *Strongyloides* larvated eggs (*), and an *Eimeria* oocyst *(black arrow)*. **B.** Enlarged image of *Muellerius* larvae *(dashed arrow)* highlighting the detail of the kinked tail (HOTC-type eggs are in the background) (A and B, Courtesy of Jamie Butler, Auburn University.). **C.** Lungs from a sheep with *Dictyocaulus filaria* infection. (i) Atelectasis is evident in diaphragmatic lobes, and (ii) worms can be seen in the trachea. **D.** *Dictyocaulus* larvae recovered with the Baermann technique. (Ci and ii, and D, Courtesy of Dr. John Malone, Louisiana State University.)

Of the lungworms, *Dictyocaulus* are the most pathogenic, followed by *Protostrongylus*, then *Muellerius*. Clinical signs associated with *Dictyocaulus* infection are typically seen in younger animals and include coughing, difficulty breathing, increased respiratory rate, nasal discharge and unthriftiness. More severe cases may result in pulmonary edema, emphysema, and secondary bacterial or viral infection. Infection with *Protostrongylus* may be inapparent, but diarrhea, weight loss, or nasal discharge with increased respiratory sounds and rate may be observed. Adult animals may be the most heavily infected with *Protostrongylus* compared with younger animals. With *Muellerius* infection, clinical disease is usually absent unless numerous parasites are present, which may result in coughing.[2,6]

Diagnosis. Since larvae are the stage present in the feces, the Baermann technique (Box 6.4) is the preferred diagnostic strategy for enhanced larval recovery and parasite identification antemortem. Fecal flotation may have some limited utility for detecting lungworm infections as L1 will float in some flotation solutions, however, the specific gravity of the flotation solution may alter the appearance of the larvae making distinguishing morphologic

• BOX 6.6 Generic Biosecurity Program for Management of Internal Parasites

1. Place ALL new arrivals in a secure dry lot where they are sequestered from the rest of the herd/flock
2. Perform an FEC for presence of nematode eggs
3. Treat animal with all three drug classes in 1 day once acclimated to the property (within a few days of arrival)
4. Perform an FECRT 10–14 days after treating, and again 5–7 days later; results should be negative for both fecal exams. Animals with negative results on two separate tests may be placed with the flock/herd
   If results are not negative, repeat deworming; do not include animals shedding eggs into the herd/flock

FEC, *Fecal egg count;* FECRT, *fecal egg count reduction test.*

characteristics difficult or impossible to visualize. The L1 can be differentiated from one another using the structure of the tails and other features (see Figure 6.5).[2,6]

Adult parasites may also be found at necropsy. *Dictyocaulus* are typically found in the bronchi of the more caudal lung lobes (see Figure 6.5) and you may see emphysema, edema, or studding of the lung surface with purulent areas. *Protostrongylus* adults are present in the smaller bronchioles and you may notice small areas of greyish-yellow lobular pneumonia. *Muellerius* infection typically results in small, focal, nodules along the surface of the lungs.[2,6]

Treatment and Prevention. Parasite elimination in the host is usually achieved through the use of common anthelmintics: ivermectin (200 μg/kg), fenbendazole (7.5 mg/kg), or albendazole (10 mg/kg). Larval stages of *Muellerius* in the host are less responsive to the drugs, and using elevated doses more frequently (300 μg/kg of ivermectin or 15 mg/kg every 35 days to 30 mg/kg every 30 days of fenbendazole) might be required if the parasites are not cleared.[42,43]

Prevention is difficult as attempts to kill L3 on pasture or control the snail intermediate hosts are often unrewarding (see Chapter 7). A vaccine for *Dictyocaulus* infection in cattle is available, but not approved for use in other ruminant species.[44]

Brainworm

Etiology, Life Cycle, and Clinical Signs. White-tailed deer are the principle hosts for *Parelaphostrongylus tenuis*, the meningeal worm. However, other cervids as well as sheep and goats may be infected and often suffer serious complications from the infection.[2,6]

Adult worms are present in the central nervous system (CNS) in the venous sinuses of the meninges. Eggs make their way into the bloodstream, to the lungs, and ultimately to the GIT, maturing to the L1 stage along the way. The L1 in the feces must find its way into a snail or slug, the required intermediate host in the life cycle. Within the intermediate host, the L1 will mature to the infectious L3. Ungulates are infected following accidental ingestion of the snail or slug. The larvae then migrate through the gut wall and make their way to the CNS to finish maturing to the adult stages.[2,6]

Clinical disease in deer is rare; however, in sheep, goats, and other cervids, infection can result in devastating neurological signs: ataxia, circling, blindness, paresis, weight loss, and potentially death. In abnormal hosts, it is thought that the parasites become larger and more coiled than in white-tailed deer; variations in the host reaction to the parasite may also play a role in the severity of disease in abnormal hosts.[2,6] Acute colitis, peritonitis, and death have been reported in very young experimentally infected animals following the ingestion and initial migration of the L3.[2]

Diagnosis, Treatment, and Prevention. Antemortem diagnosis in deer involves detecting L1 in feces (Figure 6.6), which must be differentiated from other potential larvae that can be recovered in deer feces. Serologic and molecular-based detection methods are in varying stages of development.[2] It is difficult to confirm the diagnosis in other ungulate hosts as the infections are rarely patent (no L1 present in the feces). Often the diagnosis is made presumptively or postmortem when worms are found in different parts of the CNS.

Treatment is often not practical or attempted. Varying degrees of success have been obtained using multiple high doses of different anthelmintics alone or in combination; however, no controlled studies have documented treatment efficacy against *P. tenuis* aberrant migration.[45]

Prevention relies upon attempted snail control (via fencing off high-risk snail and slug environments or use of molluscicides) and controlling deer movement to decrease overlap in grazing areas with other potential hosts.[2,6] Prophylactic use of anthelmintics such as ivermectin or other macrocyclic lactones monthly, or daily pyrantel tartrate may prevent CNS signs by killing the larvae prior to arrival in the CNS, and may be advocated during the active snail season in areas where *P. tenuis* infection has historically been an issue.[45]

Filarial Dermatosis

Sheep, goats, and some cervid hosts may also suffer from a condition known as sorehead which is caused by infection with *Elaeophora schneideri*, slender worms that live in the blood vessels. The parasite is transmitted between hosts through the bite of an infected horsefly (*Tabanus* spp. or *Hybomitra* spp.) intermediate host. The fly ingests microfilaria while feeding on host blood. Those microfilaria will mature within the fly into L3, which are then transmitted to a naïve host when the horsefly feeds and will make their way to the circulatory system where they will reside as adult worms.[6,46]

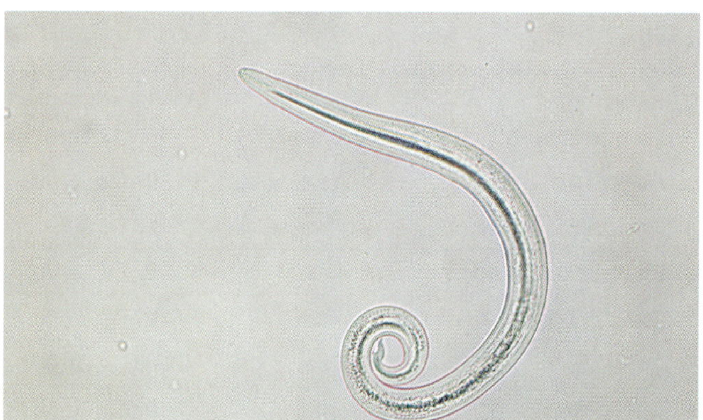

• Fig. 6.6 L1 larvae of *Parelaphostrongylus tenuis* recovered from white-tailed deer feces; notice the kinked tail. (Courtesy of Dr. Yoko Nagamori, Oklahoma State University.)

Certain deer species are thought to be the natural hosts of this parasite. Atypical hosts may suffer from elaeophorosis, usually caused by the presence of the adult worms in the arteries resulting in lost blood flow. Sheep experience pruritic dermatitis and wool loss which are usually more pronounced in the poll area or around the coronary bands of the feet. Elk have also been reported to suffer from facial damage, blindness, and potentially death secondary to thrombosis. Other atypical hosts that have been reported are red deer, sika deer, sambar, moose, goats, Barbary sheep, and bighorn sheep.[46]

Diagnosis is usually made based upon characteristic clinical signs, but biopsy of the affected area may allow for visualization of microfilariae. Detection of adults present in the arteries at necropsy is also diagnostic.[46]

No effective anthelmintics have been described, and control focuses on reducing the vector fly population or preventing fly bites.

Cestodes

Adult Cestode Infections

Etiology and Life Cycle. Having adult cestodes (tapeworms) in the intestinal tract sounds problematic for the host; however, the majority of tapeworm infections in ruminants are more of an aesthetic concern to the person who sees the tapeworm segments present in the feces rather than a cause of disease in the host. It has been noted that GIT tapeworm infection could lead to anorexia, impairment of gut motility, and in severe infections with many tapeworms present, possible rupture of the intestinal tract with subsequent peritonitis. In sheep, goats, and cervids in North America, the most common tapeworms inhabiting the GIT are *Moniezia* spp. with *Thysanosoma actinoides* a distant second.[6] Other tapeworm species may be present outside of the GIT and will be discussed later as they have much more potential to cause clinical signs of disease (Table 6.3).

The life cycle of tapeworms is more complex than that of most nematode species, as tapeworms require at least two different hosts to complete their life cycle. With *Moniezia*, the adult tapeworm is present in the small intestine and is anchored to the mucosa by the scolex. The strobila (chain of proglottids) dangles in the intestine and the worm absorbs nutrients through its cuticle. Each proglottid serves as an egg factory, and ultimately the most mature (gravid) proglottids at the terminal portion of the strobila are released from the worm and will pass out of the host in the feces. Tapeworm eggs can be present, both contained in the proglottid (which is visible to the naked eye), or free in the feces. Those tapeworm eggs are then ingested by a free-living pasture mite (oribatid mite) and develop within the mite to the intermediate tapeworm stage (cysticercoid). When a ruminant accidentally ingests the pasture mite while grazing, the cysticercoid is released and matures to the adult tapeworm in the small intestine.[6]

Diagnosis and Treatment. Visualization of proglottids in or on the fecal sample is often enough for a presumptive diagnosis, however, identification of the parasite eggs in a fecal flotation, or teasing eggs out of a proglottid can confirm the diagnosis (Figure 6.7).

A few drugs licensed for use in sheep and goats are effective at treating tapeworms (see Table 6-2); praziquantel (3.75 mg/kg) has been shown effective, but is not approved for use in ruminants in the United States.[47] Environmental control for this parasite is difficult to achieve as the intermediate mite host is free-living, and reinfection with tapeworms is likely.

Immature Cestode Infections

Etiology and Life Cycle. There are several tapeworm species that can use ruminant hosts as the intermediate host in the required two-host life cycle, namely *Taenia* and *Echinococcus* spp. (Table 6.3). Ruminants are infected with these immature tapeworm stages (cysticercus, coenurus, or hydatid cyst) following the accidental ingestion of tapeworm eggs from forage or feed contaminated with carnivore feces. Different carnivore species are the definitive hosts in these tapeworm life cycles, meaning the adult worms are present in the carnivore intestinal tract following the ingestion of the intermediate tapeworm stage present in the ruminant.[6,48]

Diagnosis and Treatment. Clinical disease is far more likely in ruminant hosts harboring the immature tapeworm stages which, depending on tapeworm species, can localize in different organs throughout the body. Infection with *Taenia ovis (Cysticercus ovis)* can lead to small, white nodules *(cysticerci)* in the muscles which often does not cause any clinical disease. More severe disease results from infection with *Taenia hydatigena (Cysticercus tenuicollis)*, *Taenia multiceps (Coenurus cerebralis)*, or *Echinococcus granulosus*. The immature tapeworms develop within the liver, lungs,

TABLE 6.3 Cestode Parasites of Sheep, Goats, and Cervids in North America.

Parasite Species	Superfamily	Predominant Host(s)[a]	Anatomical Location	Dx Stage[a]
Moniezia spp.	Anoplocephalidae	Ov, Ca, Ce, OU	SI	Egg
Thysanosoma actinoides	Anoplocephalidae	Ov, Ce, OU	SI/bile ducts/pancreatic ducts	Egg
Echinococcus granulosus	Taeniidae	Ov, Ca, Ce, OU, *	CNS/lung/liver	Unilocular hydatid cyst (tissues)
Taenia hydatigena	Taeniidae	Ov, Ca, Ce, OU, *	Lung/liver	Cysticercus (tissues)
Taenia ovis	Taeniidae	Ov, Ca, Ce, OU	Muscle	Cysticercus (tissues)
Taenia multiceps	Taeniidae	Ov, Ca, Ce, OU, *	CNS	Coenurus (tissues)

Ca, Caprine; *Ce*, cervid; *CNS*, central nervous system; *OU*, other ungulate species; *Ov*, ovine; *SI*, xxx; *, zoonotic.
[a]Diagnostic stage from a patent host found in fresh feces unless otherwise stated.

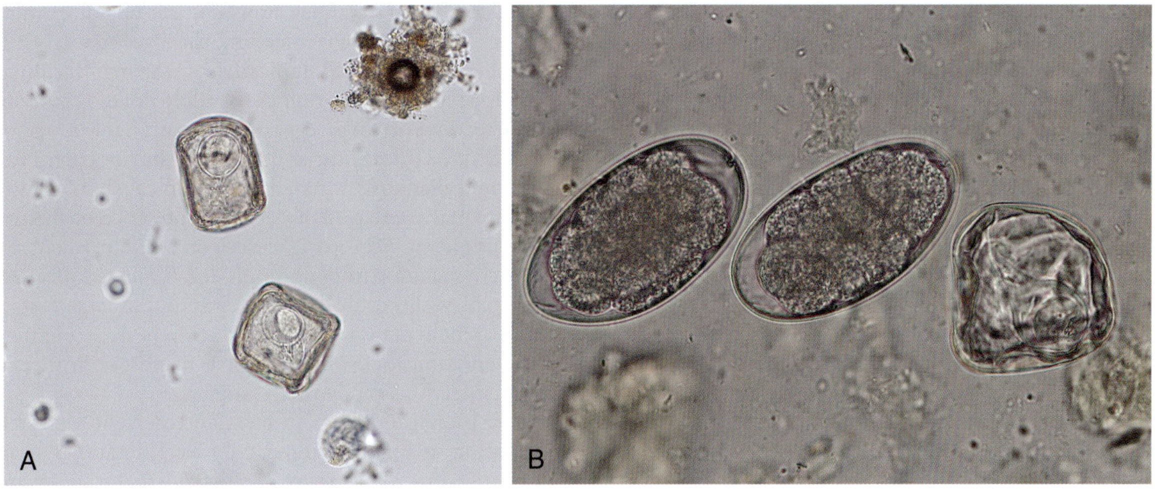

• **Fig. 6.7** *Moniezia* eggs. **A.** *Moniezia* spp. eggs recovered from white-tailed deer feces. (Courtesy of Dr. Mani Lejeune, Cornell University.) **B.** *Moniezia* spp. to the right of two HOTC-type eggs; note the pyriform apparatus within the egg containing hooks. (Courtesy of Jamie Butler, Auburn University.)

brain, or other tissues and clinical signs are highly dependent upon the organ system in which the immature tapeworm is developing. Even if clinical signs of infection are absent, the identification of these immature tapeworm stages at slaughter in the muscle or organs often leads to condemnation of the affected tissue or carcass resulting in an economic loss for the producer.

Detection of antibodies or antigen in serum, diagnostic imaging, or PCR of biopsy may assist in achieving an antemortem diagnosis, however, the majority of infections are identified at necropsy or slaughter.[8]

Treatment for the immature tapeworm stages in ruminants is often not effective or practical. Control measures rely on reducing environmental contamination by treating the carnivore definitive hosts with a product to kill the adult tapeworms along with trying to prevent fecal contamination of food sources by carnivores. It is also recommended to prevent carnivores from scavenging on ruminant carcasses. These practices will effectively break the parasite's life cycle. Development of reliable vaccines for ruminant hosts are underway, and these may soon be available to aid in the prevention of these tapeworm infections.[49–51]

Trematodes

Etiology and Life Cycle. Ruminants can be host to several trematode (fluke) species (Table 6.4), namely *Fasciola hepatica*, *Fascioloides magna*, and *Dicrocoelium dendriticum*. These parasites are geographically restricted in the United States based upon their need for the snail intermediate hosts and the particular environment that is suitable for those snail species. The majority of liver fluke infections occur in the Pacific Northwest, the Gulf Coast, and in the Great Lakes region.[2,6,52]

The indirect life cycle of these flukes are similar to one another. Sheep, goats, and cattle are the definitive hosts for *F. hepatica* while deer and other cervids are the definitive host for *F. magna*; any ruminant can serve as the definitive host for *D. dendriticum*. The definitive host passes operculated eggs in the feces. For *F. hepatica* and *F. magna*, an aquatic environment is required as the snail intermediate host is only present in and around water. The miracidium is present within the developed egg and hatches from the egg in water where it must find and penetrate a snail within the first 24 to 48 hours, otherwise the miracidium will die. Within the snail intermediate host, the parasite asexually replicates, and ultimately, cercariae are released. The cercariae are free in the water and will swim to and encyst upon aquatic vegetation as metacercariae to then be ingested by the ruminant definitive host while grazing.[2,6,52]

D. dendriticum has a terrestrial-based life cycle which includes two intermediate hosts: a terrestrial snail and then an ant. The developed egg of *D. dendriticum* awaits ingestion by the terrestrial snail, and these eggs are long-lived on pasture. Replication occurs

TABLE 6.4 Trematode Parasites of Sheep, Goats, and Cervids in North America.

Parasite Species	Superfamily	Predominant Host(s)	Anatomical location	Dx Stage[a]
Paramphistomum, Cotylophoron, Calicophoron spp.	Parmamphistomatidae	Ov, Ca, Ce, OU	Rumen/reticulum	Egg
Fasciola spp.	Fasciolidae	Ov, Ca, Ce, OU, *	Liver/bile ducts	Egg
Fascioloides magna	Fasciolidae	Ov, Ca, Ce, OU	Liver/bile ducts	Egg
Dicrocoelium dendriticum	Dicrocoeliidae	Ov, Ca, Ce, OU	Liver/bile ducts	Egg

Ca, Caprine; *Ce*, cervid; *OU*, other ungulate species; *Ov*, ovine; *, zoonotic.
[a]Diagnostic stage from a patent host found in fresh feces unless otherwise stated.

within the snail which will then release the cercariae in slime balls which are then ingested by the second intermediate host, the ant. *Dicrocoelium* utilizes the additional intermediate host to facilitate its transmission in the terrestrial environment. Within the ant, the cercariae mature to metacercariae. Ants infected with *Dicrocoelium* exhibit unusual behavior and they will migrate to the tops of the grass and stay there, thus increasing their chances of being ingested by the ruminant definitive host.[6]

Once the metacercariae is ingested by the ruminant definitive host, the parasite begins its migration to the final site of infection: the liver and/or bile ducts.

Clinical Signs. Disease with *F. hepatica* may be acute, subacute, or chronic. Acute disease is associated with ingestion of many metacercariae that simultaneously migrate throughout the liver parenchyma, leading to destruction and hemorrhage. Concurrent infection with *Clostridium novyi*, the causative agent of black disease, may also occur in nonvaccinated animals. Clinical signs of acute disease include sudden death, difficulty breathing with pale mucous membranes, weakness, ascites, and reluctance to move. Subacute disease is characterized by ingestion of metacercariae over a longer time frame where some are migrating through the liver parenchyma while others have matured to the point of residing and feeding within the bile ducts. You may see a combination of moderately severe liver lesions in conjunction with cholangitis. This disease manifestation may still be fatal if left untreated, but is not as rapidly fatal as acute disease. Subacutely, affected animals may exhibit reduced appetite, poor condition, edema, ascites, and pale mucous membranes. Chronic infection is the most common form of disease and is characterized by a decreased appetite with progressive loss of condition, weakness, and worsening hypoalbuminemia and anemia. Substantial scarring of the liver and thickening of the bile ducts (pipe-stem liver) are usually present.[2,6]

Clinical signs with *F. magna* infection are host dependent. In deer, the immune response results in flukes being walled-off into cystic structures within the liver parenchyma and clinical signs are usually mild or absent. However, in sheep and goats, there is no immune response and the *F. magna* flukes will migrate extensively throughout the liver parenchyma and infection can result in sudden death.[6,52]

Infection with *D. dendriticum* often does not cause any damage to the liver since there is no migratory phase, however, heavy infections may result in cirrhosis of the liver and distended bile ducts. Clinical signs are often absent, but anemia, edema, emaciation, and poor wool growth have been reported in severe infections.[6]

Diagnosis. Antemortem diagnosis of *F. hepatica* can be difficult as acute and subacute disease may occur in the absence of detectable parasite eggs in feces. Reliance upon clinical signs and bloodwork, in conjunction with the historic presence on that farm or in the area and seasonality, are more useful diagnostics early in infection. Eggs may be present in the feces during chronic infection and can be recovered through the use of a fecal sedimentation technique (see Box 6.6 and Figure 6.8a&b). Fluke eggs are too heavy to be recovered with standard fecal flotation solutions and would require the use of high specific-gravity flotation solutions.[2,8]

Postmortem identification of lesions consistent with *F. hepatica* and the presence of juvenile or adult flukes in the liver or bile ducts can confirm infection (Figure 6.8d&e). Lesions with acute fascioliasis typically include an enlarged, hemorrhagic liver with juvenile fluke migratory tracts. Subacute lesions are similar in that the liver is often enlarged; however, the migratory tracts may be necrotic. With chronic infection, the liver tissue is more irregularly shaped and firmed, indicative of scarring. Bile ducts are often distended and contain numerous adult flukes (Figure 6.8).[2,6]

Detection of fluke eggs is diagnostic for *F. magna* in deer (Figure 6.8). Infections with *F. magna* are not patent in sheep and goats and diagnosis is based upon clinical signs, a history of environmental overlap with deer, and presence of flukes or consistent lesions at necropsy. Streaks of black pigment in the liver parenchyma are pathognomonic for *F. magna* infection in sheep and goats while adult flukes often found in large cysts within the liver parenchyma is typical of infection in deer (Figure 6.8). Fecal sedimentation for *F. magna* eggs is of no use in sheep and goats as the infections rarely reach patency.[2,6]

The presence of eggs in feces antemortem (detected via sedimentation or high specific-gravity fecal flotation) or adult flukes in the bile ducts postmortem is diagnostic for *D. dendriticum.*

Evaluation of alternative methods for detection of trematode infections includes antigen or antibody detection in a variety of host samples, but these have yet to become routinely available.[2,8]

Treatment and Prevention. There are a few drugs that are effective at treating the younger stages of *F. hepatica* and *F. magna*, but none of them are currently approved in the United States. Triclabendazole is highly effective at killing young and old flukes but resistance to this drug is spreading.[6,53] Closantel will kill flukes greater than 4 to 6 weeks of age, but repeat treatments may be necessary. Albendazole and clorsulon (in a combination product with ivermectin) are available in the United States to treat adult flukes in cattle, however, the approval of these products for fluke control in sheep, goats, and cervids is complicated.[54] Albendazole at a flukicidal dose (10 mg/kg) is approved only in goats for *F. hepatica*. These drugs have some activity against *F. magna* as well, but are not 100% effective.[55] Thiabendazole has been shown effective for treating *D. dendriticum.*[54] Movement to a fluke-free/snail-free pasture is always recommended in combination with using effective drugs.[2,6,54]

Preventing pasture contamination with fluke eggs during the transmission season is one key for fluke control. This is achieved by proper timing of treatment and treating all animals in the flock or herd if *F. hepatica* is diagnosed. In the southern United States, peak snail activity and transmission occur in the winter months. It is recommended to treat animals in late summer or early fall to kill any adult parasites in the host to prevent contamination of the environment with eggs as the snail activity is increasing. In the cooler climates, transmission is opposite and the ideal treatment time to prevent environmental contamination is late winter or early spring.

For *F. magna*, attempts to reduce the presence of deer in areas where sheep and goats graze is essential, yet, oftentimes unobtainable.

Management of snail populations is also advisable but often impractical. For aquatic snails, draining the pastures or fencing off the contaminated areas may be pursued. Molluscicides are also available but come with some environmental concerns. Snail control for *D. dendriticum* is even more difficult and the eggs are long-lasting on pasture.[2,6]

Protozoa

Coccidiosis

Etiology and Life Cycle. Diarrhea in young animals can be associated with a protozoal infection with *Eimeria* spp., the causative

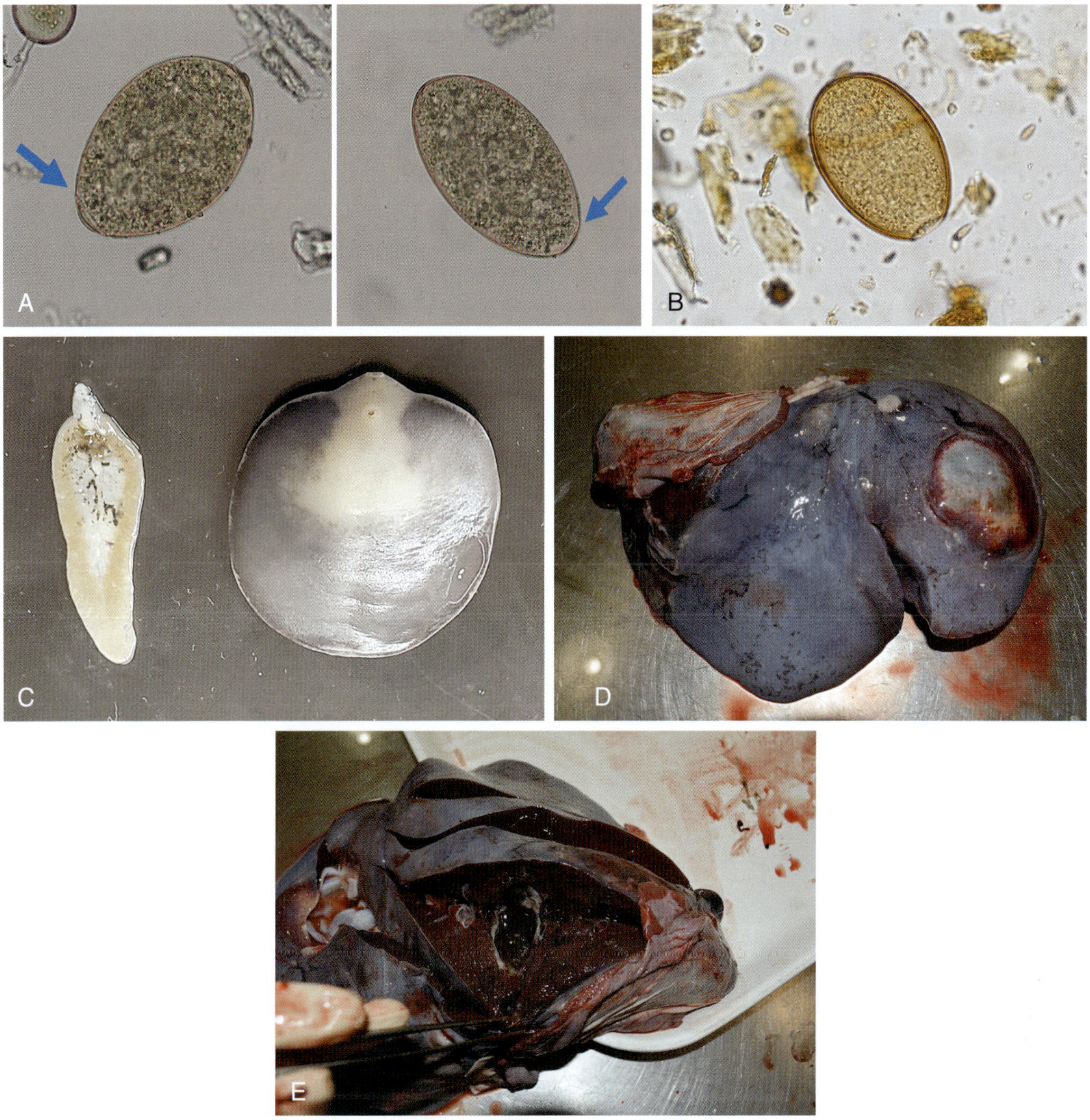

• **Fig. 6.8** Trematodes. **A.** Eggs of *Fasciola hepatica*; note the operculum which is more visible in the right image *(blue arrow)*. (Courtesy of Jamie Butler, Auburn University.) **B.** Egg of *Fascioloides magna* recovered from a white-tailed deer. (Courtesy of Dr. Mani Lejeune, Cornell University.) **C.** Adult *F. hepatica (left)* and *F. magna (right)*; notice the larger size and increased thickness of *F. magna* compared with the smaller, thinner *F. hepatica*. (Courtesy of Jamie Butler, Auburn University.) **D.** A large mass in the liver of a farm-raised, mature, white-tailed deer doe, with a large cyst containing clear fluid. Black tracts can be seen on the surface of the liver. (Courtesy of Dr. Kelley Steury, Auburn, AL.) **E.** After the small cyst is cut open shown in Figure 6.8D, black pigmented tissue from the flukes is readily identified. (Courtesy of Dr. Kelley Steury, Auburn, AL.)

agents of ruminant coccidiosis (Table 6.5). *Eimeria* spp. are incredibly host specific; therefore, they are not shared between different ruminant species. These parasites replicate within the cells lining the GIT leading to cellular destruction. The life cycle involves ingestion of sporulated oocysts from the environment. The parasite then undergoes asexual replication within the intestinal cells prior to the formation of gametocytes which will fuse to ultimately form an oocyst. Each round of asexual or sexual replication results in more destroyed cells. Ultimately oocysts rupture from the cell and pass from the host in the feces. Maturation to an infective sporulated oocyst can occur in as little as a couple of days in the environment and these infective oocysts may remain viable in the environment for months to years. Situations where the animals are crowded together and oocyst contamination in the environment is allowed to build up may predispose to heavier infections with the potential for more severe clinical disease.[6,56]

Clinical Signs. Animals of all ages can be infected with coccidia, however, disease is most severe in younger animals (i.e., lambs, kids, and fawns). Clinical signs are usually amplified if the animals are stressed by weaning, cold weather, or relocation. In general, the species that preferentially replicate within the crypt cells of the large intestine lead to more severe disease. In sheep,

TABLE 6.5 Protozoan Parasites of Sheep, Goats, and Cervids in North America.

Parasite Species	Superfamily	Predominant Host(s)	Anatomical Location	Dx Stage[a]
Eimeria spp.	Eimeriidae	Ov, Ca, Ce	Abomasum/SI/cecum/colon	Oocyst
Cryptosporidium spp.	Cryptosporidiidae	Ov, Ca, Ce, OU, *	SI	Oocyst
Giardia spp.	Giardiidae	Ov, Ca, OU, *	SI	Cyst or trophozoite
Toxoplasma gondii	Sarcocystidae	Ov, Ca, Ce, OU, *	Muscle, Reproductive, CNS	Cyst or tachyzoites (tissues)
Sarcocystis spp.	Sarcocystidae	Ov, Ca, Ce, OU, *	Muscle	Cyst (tissues)
Besnoitia spp.	Sarcocystidae	Ca, Ce, OU	Subcutaneous/skin/conjunctiva	Cyst (tissues)
Hammondia spp.	Sarcocystidae	Ov, Ca, Ce, OU	Muscle	Cyst (tissues)

Ca, Caprine; *Ce*, cervid; *CNS*, central nervous system; *SI*, xxx; *OU*, other ungulate species; *Ov*, ovine; *, zoonotic.
[a]Diagnostic stage from a patent host found in fresh feces unless otherwise stated

Eimeria crandallis and *Eimeria ovinoidalis* are considered the most pathogenic species. For goats, the most severe disease typically results from infection with *Eimeria christenseni*, *E hirci*, *E ninakohlyakimovae*, *E arloingi*, and *E caprina*. *Eimeria* spp. also cause infection in cervids. Clinical signs may be mild diarrhea with anorexia or reduced feed efficiency all the way to dehydration, hemorrhagic diarrhea, and death.[6,56]

Diagnosis. Fecal flotation can reveal high numbers of oocysts in patent infections; yet, it is important to note that animals may be clinically ill from coccidiosis before oocysts are ever shed in the feces (Figure 6.9). Also, clinically normal animals may shed small numbers of oocysts in the absence of clinical signs. Performing an FEC is not typically pursued for coccidia as the oocysts can be too small to appreciate in the standard McMaster's slide and the numbers of

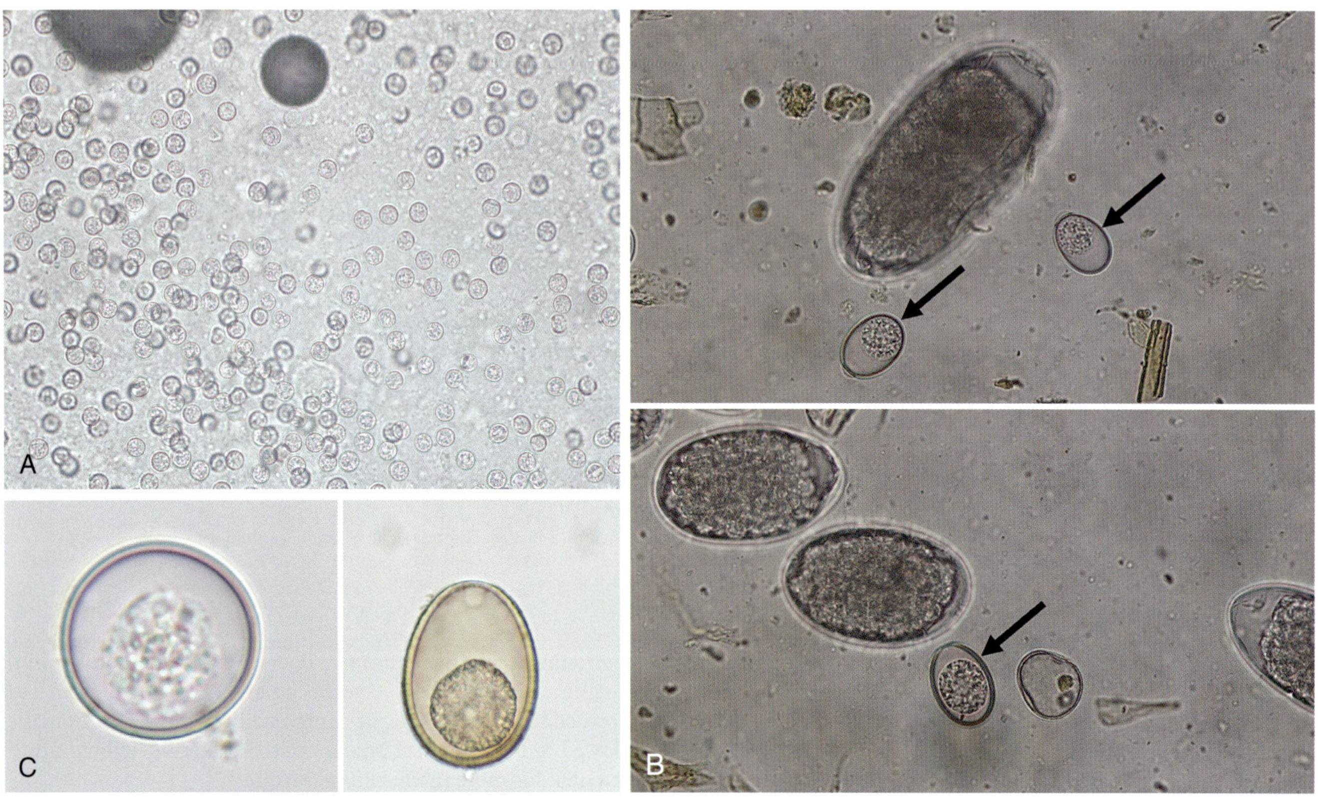

• **Fig. 6.9** Coccidia oocysts. **A.** Numerous *Eimeria* spp. recovered from a white-tailed deer. (Courtesy of Dr. Yoko Nagamori, Oklahoma State University.) **B.** *Eimeria* spp. oocysts *(arrows)* adjacent to HOTC-type eggs; note the presence of a micropyle (thinning) and micropyle cap on some of the oocysts. (Courtesy of Jamie Butler, Auburn University.) **C.** Enlarged images of *Eimeria* spp. recovered from white-tailed deer. (Courtesy of Dr. Mani Lejeune, Cornell University.)

oocysts don't necessarily correlate to clinical disease (Figure 6.9). At necropsy, a thickened, hyperemic GI mucosa may be present. Microscopic examination of mucosal scrapings or histologic tissue sections will reveal various stages of coccidia.[6,56,57]

Treatment and Prevention. Treatment for an animal suffering from clinical signs of coccidiosis includes anticoccidial therapy, ensuring proper supportive care, nutrition, and housing, and movement to an uncontaminated environment.[6,56] Several drugs have been shown effective in the treatment and control for *Eimeria* spp.; those approved for use in sheep and/or goats in the United States are listed (see Table 6.2).[56] Amprolium (25–40 mg/kg for 5 days) or sulfaquinoxaline (10–20 mg/kg for 3–7 days) has been used extra-label in sheep and goats, but should only be done so while following AMDUCA and consulting FARAD for withdrawal times.[55] Single doses of ponazuril (10 mg/kg) or toltrazuril (20 mg/kg) have also shown some efficacy when used extra-label.[58,59] The entire group of young animals may be treated in an outbreak situation as all are likely to be infected at some level. Diarrhea may continue following treatment as the intestinal mucosa may take days to weeks to heal.

Hand-raised fawns can be given a coccidiostat such as decoquinate daily, in milk. Fawns raised by their mothers are difficult to treat individually. Using a coccidiostat (e.g., decoquinate, rumensin, etc.) in a feed may be of value for fawn coccidia control, however, inadequate drug intake my compromise the useof such a system. Water medication with amprolium or sulfadimethoxine may be of value, and when used, the drug-containing water should be the only water source. Clean, dry areas with no standing water for the fawns to drink from are essential. (Personal Communication via email, Clifford F. Shipley, DVM.)

Good husbandry is crucial to preventing coccidiosis in the flock or herd. Avoiding overcrowding, decreasing stress, and raising food and water troughs off of the ground can all help to decrease the risk for coccidiosis. Use of a coccidiostat in the water or feed may also help to reduce clinical signs associated with infection, but should only be utilized in times of expected coccidiosis risk to reduce the potential development of drug-resistant *Eimeria* spp. Producers must also adjust the coccidiostat doses to account for increased intake as animals grow.[56] Of all sheep operations, 39.8% used a coccidiostat in the food or water in 2010; ionophores were used most common in feed, and amprolium was most common in water[12] (see Chapter 19, and Appendix l).

Toxoplasmosis

Etiology and Life Cycle. Any mammal can serve as an intermediate host for *Toxoplasma gondii*, ruminants included. Felines are the only definitive host for *T. gondii* and shed oocysts in their feces which will sporulate in the environment. Ruminants are infected following the ingestion of sporulated oocysts in the environment. The parasite will then spread to various tissues and organs throughout the body, where asexual replication during acute disease may result in local areas of inflammation and necrosis. Chronic infection is usually asymptomatic as the parasite is present in tissue cysts that enter a stage or dormancy awaiting ingestion by another host.[6,60,61]

Clinical Signs, Diagnosis, Treatment, and Prevention. Congenital infection is of concern as infection during gestation may lead to abortion in ewes or perinatal mortality in lambs.[6,62]

Diagnosis in intermediate hosts may be achieved by finding parasite stages present in tissue sections or aspirates. Techniques like immunohistochemistry (IHC) or PCR may assist in detection of the organism. The serum may also be tested for the presence of antibodies to *T. gondii.* [6,57,61]

Treatment is not indicated in ruminants. Prevention of infection involves avoiding feline fecal contamination of feed stuffs. There are commercially available Toxoplasmosis vaccines for sheep outside of the United States, and further development of additional vaccines to limit infection or reduce or eliminate cysts in the intermediate hosts are underway.[58,63,64]

Sarcocystosis

Etiology, Life Cycle, Clinical Signs, and Diagnosis. Ruminants can serve as the intermediate host for several *Sarcocystis* spp., leading to the development of muscle cysts termed "sarcocysts." Carnivores are the definitive hosts and shed infectious sporocysts into the environment through their feces. Following ingestion by the ruminant, asexual parasite replication occurs in the vascular endothelium followed by ultimate formation of sarcocysts in the muscles which will await ingestion by the carnivore definitive host. Clinical signs are rarely observed in either host; however, infected ruminants may exhibit fever, anorexia, myositis, encephalomyelitis, recumbency, or abortion. Diagnosis is usually made at slaughter, where the carcass may be condemned or downgraded if muscle cysts are present.[6,60]

Treatment and Prevention. The use of amprolium and halofuginone (0.66 mg/kg orally for 2 days) may be used in sheep to avoid clinical disease following infection. Prevention is difficult as it is based upon controlling carnivore defecation and predation/scavenging habits. [6,60]

References

1. Zajac AM: Gastrointestinal nematodes of small ruminants: life cycle, anthelmintics, and diagnosis, *Vet Clin Food Anim* 22:529–541, 2006.
2. Haigh JC, Mackintosh C, Griffin F: Viral, parasitic and prion diseases of farmed deer and bison, Rev *Sci Tech* 21:219–248, 2002.
3. NAHMS: *Sheep 2011 Part 2: reference of marketing and death loss on U.S*, 2012, Sheep Operations, 2012. https://www.aphis.usda.gov/animal_health/nahms/sheep/downloads/sheep11/Sheep11_dr_PartII.pdf. Accessed May 30, 2018.
4. NAHMS: *Goat and kid predator and nonpredator death loss in the United States*, 2015, 2017. https://www.aphis.usda.gov/animal_health/nahms/general/downloads/goat_kid_deathloss_2015.pdf. Accessed May 30, 2018.
5. Pugh DG, Navarre CB: Parasite control programs in sheep and goats, *Vet Clin North Am Food Anim Pract* 17:231–244, 2001.
6. Taylor MA, Coop RL, Wall RL: *Veterinary parasitology*, ed 4, West Sussex, United Kingdom, 2016, Wiley Blackwell.
7. Krecek RC, Hartman R, Groeneveld HT, Thorne A: Microclimatic effect on vertical migration of *Haemonchus contortus* and *Haemonchus placei* third-stage larvae on irrigated Kikuyu pasture, *Onderstepoort J Vet Res* 62:117–122, 1995.
8. Demeler J, Schein E, von Samson-Himmelstjerna G: Advances in laboratory diagnosis of parasitic infections of sheep, *Vet Parasitol* 189:52–64, 2012.
9. Kaplan RM: *Biology of anthelmintic resistance: these ain't your father's parasites*, Proceedings of the Annual Conference for the American Consortium for Small Ruminant Parasite Control, Fort Valley, Georgia, May 20–22, 2013.

10. Coles GC, Jackson F, Pomroy WE, et al: The detection of anthelmintic resistance in nematodes of veterinary importance, *Vet Parasitol* 136:167–185, 2006.
11. Rinaldi L, Coles GC, Maurelli MP, Musella V, Cringoli G: Calibration and diagnostic accuracy of simple flotation, McMaster and FLOTAC for parasite egg counts in sheep, *Vet Parasitol* 177: 345–352, 2011.
12. NAHMS: *Sheep 2011 part 3: health and management practiced on U.S.* sheep operations, 2011, 2013. https://www.aphis.usda.gov/animal_health/nahms/sheep/downloads/sheep11/Sheep11_dr_PartIII.pdf. Accessed May 30, 2018.
13. NAHMS: *Goat 2009 part II: reference of goat health and marketing practices in the United States*, 2009, 2011. https://www.aphis.usda.gov/animal_health/nahms/goats/downloads/goat09/Goat09_dr_PartII_rev.pdf. Accessed May 30, 2018.
14. Kaplan RM, Burke JM, Terrill TH, et al: Validation of the FAMACHA eye color chart for detecting clinical anemia on sheep and goat farms in the southern United States, *Vet Parasitol* 123:105–120, 2004.
14A. Bath GF, van Wyk JA: The Five Point Check© for targeted selective treatment of internal parasites in small ruminants, *Small Rumin Res* 86(1–3):6–13, 2009.
15. Howell SB, Burke JM, Miller JE, et al: Prevalence of anthelmintic resistance on sheep and goat farms in the southeastern United States, *J Am Vet Med Assoc* 233:1913–1919, 2008.
16. Kenyon F, Greer AW, Coles GC, et al: The role of targeted selective treatments in the development of refugia-based approaches to the control of gastrointestinal nematodes of small ruminants, *Vet Parasitol* 164:3–11, 2009.
17. U.S. Food & Drug Administration: *New antiparasitic drugs needed for sheep and goats*, 2018. http://www.wormboss.com.au/news/articles/drench-resistance/further-reports-of-monepantel-resistance.php. Accessed May 30, 2018.
18. Hennessy DR: Modifying the formulation or delivery mechanism to increase the activity of anthelmintic compounds, *Vet Parasitol* 72:367–390, 1997.
19. Craig TM: *Epidemiology of internal parasites: effects of climate and host reproductive cycles on parasite survival*, Proceedings of the Small Ruminant Mixed Animal Practitioner. Western Veterinary Conference, Las Vegas, February 1998.
20. Escudero E, Carceles CM, Diaz MS, Sutra JF, Galtier P, Alvinerie M: Pharmacokinetics of moxidectin and doramectin in goats, *Res Vet Sci* 67:177–181, 1999.
21. Kaminsky R, Ducray P, Jung M, et al: A new class of anthelmintics effective against drug-resistant nematodes, *Nature* 452(7184): 176–180, 2008.
22. Love S: *Further reports of monepantel resistance*, 2013. http://www.wormboss.com.au/news/articles/drench-resistance/further-reports-of-monepantel-resistance.php. Accessed May 30, 2018.
23. Hennessy D: The disposition of antiparasitic drugs in relation to the development of resistance by parasites of livestock, *Acta Trop* 56:125–141, 1994.
24. Miller DK, Craig TM: Use of anthelmintic combinations against multiple resistant *Haemonchus contortus* in Angora goats, *Small Rumin Res* 19:281–283, 1996.
25. Coles, GC, Bauer C, Borgsteede FH, et al: World Association for the Advancement of Veterinary Parasitology (WAAVP) methods for the detection of anthelmintic resistance in nematodes of veterinary importance, *Vet Parasitol* 44:35–44, 1992.
26. NAHMS: *Goat 2009 part III: biosecurity and disease-prevention practices on U.S.* goat operations, 2009, 2011. https://www.aphis.usda.gov/animal_health/nahms/goats/downloads/goat09/Goat09_dr_PartIIIa.pdf. Accessed May 30, 2018.
27. NAHMS: *Cervid 2014: health and management practices on U.S.* farmed cervid operations, 2014. 2016. https://www.aphis.usda.gov/animal_health/nahms/cervids/downloads/cervids14/Cervid14dr.pdf. Accessed May 30, 2018.
28. Coop R, Kyriazakis I: Influence of host nutrition on the development and consequences of nematode parasitism in ruminants, *Trends Parasitol* 17:325–330, 2001.
29. Torres-Acosta JFJ, Sandoval-Castro CA, Hoste H, Aguilar-Caballero AJ, Cámara-Sarmiento R, Alonso-Díaz MA: Nutritional manipulation of sheep and goats for the control of gastrointestinal nematodes under hot humid and subhumid tropical conditions, *Small Rumin Res* 103:28–40, 2012.
30. Steel, JW: Effects of protein supplementation of young sheep on resistance development and resilience to parasitic nematodes, *Anim Prod Sci* 43:1469–1476, 2004.
31. Zvinorova PI, Halimani TE, Muchadeyi FC, Matika O, Riggio V, Dzama K: Breeding for resistance to gastrointestinal nematodes – the potential in low-input/output small ruminant production systems, *Vet Parasitol* 225:19–28, 2016.
32. NAHMS: *Sheep 2011 part 1: reference of sheep management practiced in the United States*, 2011, 2012. https://www.aphis.usda.gov/animal_health/nahms/sheep/downloads/sheep11/Sheep11_dr_PartI.pdf. Accessed May 30, 2018.
33. Hunt PW, McEwan JC, Miller JE: Future perspectives for the implementation of genetic markers for parasite resistance in sheep, *Trop Biomed* 25:18–33, 2008.
34. Burke JM, Miller JE, Olcott DD, Olcott BM, Terrill TH: Effect of copper oxide wire particles dosage and feed supplement level on *Haemonchus contortus* infection in lambs, *Vet Parasitol* 123:235–243, 2004.
35. Burke JM, Terrill TH, Kallu RR, Miller JE, Mosjidis J: Use of copper oxide wire particles to control gastrointestinal nematodes in goats, *J Anim Sci* 85:2753–2761, 2007.
36. Burke JM, Miller JE, Terrill TH, Smyth E, Acharya M: Examination of commercially available copper oxide wire particles in combination with albendazole for control of gastrointestinal nematodes in lambs, *Vet Parasitol* 215:1–4, 2016.
37. Houdijk JGM, Kyriazakis I, Kidane A, Athanasiadou S: Manipulating small ruminant parasite epidemiology through the combination of nutritional strategies, *Vet Parasitol* 186:38–50, 2012.
38. Larsen M, Nansen P, Grønvold J, Wolstrup J, Henriksen SA: Biological control of gastro-intestinal nematodes — facts, future, or fiction? *Vet Parasitol* 72:479–485, 1997.
39. Terrill TH, Miller JE, Burke JM, Mosjidis JA, Kaplan RM: Experiences with integrated concepts for the control of *Haemonchus contortus* in sheep and goats in the United States, *Vet Parasitol* 186:28–37, 2012.
40. Maxwell D: *Barbervax*, 2015. http://www.wormboss.com.au/news/articles/nonchemical-management/barbervaxa-vaccine-to-protect-against-barbers-pole-worm.php. Accessed May 30, 2018.
41. Smith WD, Taylor S: Twists and turns en route to a vaccine for *Haemonchus contortus*, Proceedings of the 22nd International Conference of the World Association for the Advancement of Veterinary Parasitology, Calgary, Canada, August 8–13, 2009.
42. Helle O: The efficacy of fenbendazole and albendazole against the lungworm *Muellerius capillaris* in goats, *Vet Parasitol* 22:293, 1986.
43. McCraw BM, Mensies PI: Treatment of goats infected with the lungworm *Muellerius capillaris*, *Can Vet J* 27:287, 1986.
44. Holzhauer M, Holland WG, Ploeger HW: Preventive vaccination of lactating and pregnant heifers against lungworm: safety and protection in three dairy herds, *Tijdschr Diergeneeskd* 130(3):74–77, 2005.
45. Nagy DW: *Parelaphostrongylus tenuis* and other parasitic diseases of the ruminant nervous system, *Vet Clin Food Anim* 20:393–412, 2004.
46. Bernard J, Grunenwald C, Stalis IH, Varney M, Zuba J, Gerhold R: *Elaeophora* in the meninges of a Malayan sambar (*Rusa unicolor equina*), *J Vet Diagn Invest* 28(6):735–738, 2016.
47. Strobel H, de Ponte M, Knoppe TN, Bhushan C: Comparison of three different treatment schedules for praziquantel (Cestocur®, Bayer) in the treatment of tapeworm infections (*Moniezia* spp.) and their impact on body weight gains in a German Sheep flock, *Parasitol Res* 112(Suppl 1):139–147, 2013.

48. Cerda JR, Buttke DE, Ballweber LR: *Echinococcus* spp. tapeworms in North America, *Emerg Infect Dis* 24(2):230–235, 2018.
49. Lightowlers MW. Cestode vaccines: origins, current status and future prospects, *Parasitology* 133(Suppl):S27–S42, 2006.
50. Varcasia A, Tosciri G, Coccone GN, et al: Preliminary field trial of a vaccine against coenurosis caused by *Taenia multiceps*, *Vet Parasitol* 162(3–4):285–289, 2009.
51. Pourseif MM, Moghaddam G, Saeedi N, Barzegari A, Dehghani J, Omidi Y: Current status and future prospective of vaccine development against *Echinococcus granulosus*, *Biologicals* 51:1–11, 2018.
52. Malcicka M: Life history and biology of *Fascioloides magna* (Trematoda) and its native and exotic hosts, *Ecol Evol* 5:1381–1397, 2015.
53. Kelley JM, Elliot TP, Beddoe T, Anderson G, Skuce P, Spithill TW: Current threat of triclabendazole resistance in *Fasciola hepatica*, *Trends Parasitol* 32(6):458–469, 2016.
54. Rojo-Vázquez FA, Meana A, Valcárcel F, Martínez-Valladares M: Update on trematode infections in sheep, *Vet Parasitol* 189(1):15–38, 2012.
55. Pybus MJ: Liver Flukes. In Samuel WM, Pybus MJ, Kocan AA, editors: *Parasitic diseases of wild mammals,* ed 2, Ames, Iowa, 2001, Iowa State University Press, pp 121–149.
56. Keeton SNT, Navarre CB: Coccidiosis in large and small ruminants, *Vet Clin North Am Food Anim Pract* 34(1):201–208, 2018.
57. de Waal T: Advances in diagnosis of protozoan diseases, *Vet Parasitol* 189:65–74, 2012.
58. Gibbons P, Love D, Craig T, Budke C: Efficacy of treatment of elevated coccidial oocyst counts in goats using amprolium versus ponazuril, *Vet Parasitol* 218:1–4, 2016.
59. Stock ML, Elazab ST, Hsu WH: Review of triazine antiprotozoal drugs used in veterinary medicine, *J Vet Pharmacol Ther* 41:184–194, 2018.
60. Dubey JP, Lindsay DS: Neosporosis, toxoplasmosis, and sarcocystosis in ruminants, *Vet Clin North Am Food Anim Pract* 22(3): 645–671, 2006.
61. Wyrosdick HM, Schaefer JJ: *Toxoplasma gondii*: history and diagnostic test development, *Anim Health Res Rev* 16(2):150–162, 2015.
62. Benavides J, Fernández M, Castaño P, Ferreras MC, Ortega-Mora L, Pérez V: Ovine toxoplasmosis: a new look at its pathogenesis, *J Comp Pathol* 157(1):34–38, 2017.
63. Innes EA, Bartley PM, Maley S, Katzer F, Buxton D: Veterinary vaccines against *Toxoplasma gondii*, *Mem Inst Oswaldo Cruz* 104(2): 246–251, 2009.
64. Zhang NZ, Wang M, Xu Y, Petersen E, Zhu XQ: Recent advances in developing vaccines against *Toxoplasma gondii*: an update, *Expert Rev Vaccines* 14(12):1609–1621, 2015.

7

Diseases of the Respiratory System

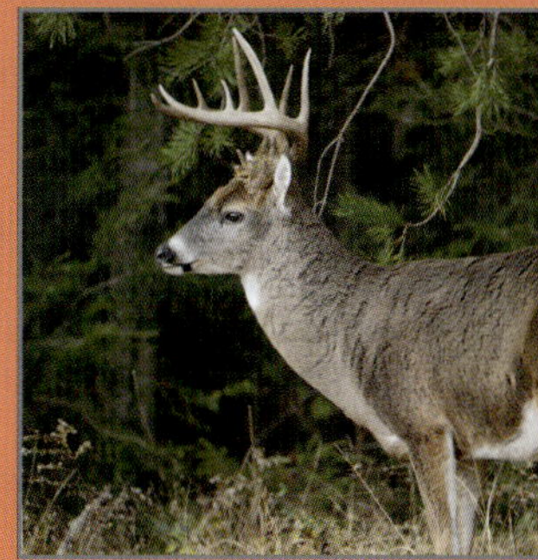

PAUL J. PLUMMER, KELLY M. STILL BROOKS, AND JENNA E. BAYNE

Anatomy

Clinically significant upper airway structures in the small ruminant include the frontal and maxillary sinuses, pharynx, larynx, and trachea. The nasopharynx is the primary path for respiration, but oral respirations are anatomically possible, and "panting" occurs under some fairly normal conditions such as high ambient temperature. The laryngeal structure is similar to that in other species, with small V-shaped vocal folds just caudal and ventral to the arytenoid cartilages.[1,2] The retropharyngeal lymph node is located dorsocaudally to the pharynx and can compress the larynx or trachea when enlarged or abscessed. The trachea runs down the ventromedial aspect of the neck from the larynx to the bronchial bifurcation in the thorax. It is composed of incomplete tracheal rings connected by a membranous wall. The tracheal diameter in small ruminants generally is smaller than might be expected and changes at the thoracic inlet. In goats the trachea narrows, whereas in sheep it enlarges.[2]

In the thorax, the trachea bifurcates into two main bronchi. Just cranial to this bifurcation a separate bronchus branches out to the right cranial lung lobe. The major lung divisions may exhibit some species-specific variations, but most commonly include left and right cranial lobes, each with a cranial and caudal part; the right middle (cardiac) lobe; the right accessory lobe; and the left and right caudal (diaphragmatic) lobes. When enlarged, the mediastinal lymph nodes and thymus may compress or shift the thoracic trachea or lung. The caudal lung border is demarcated by the sixth rib ventrally, by the seventh rib at the lateral midthorax, and by the eleventh rib dorsocaudally. The intercostal vessels and nerves run caudally along each rib, and care should be taken to avoid these structures during thoracocentesis or biopsy procedures.[2,3]

Physiology

The respiratory system permits reoxygenation of pulmonary venous blood and release of carbon dioxide formed by cellular respiration. Effective respiration requires both alveolar ventilation and gas diffusion across the respiratory membrane; together, these two processes can be quantified by the ventilation-perfusion ratio, which may be altered during disease. Alveolar ventilation occurs through movement of gas from the terminal bronchioles and depends on inspiratory tidal volume and expiratory functional reserve, in addition to respiratory rate. Anatomic dead space (e.g., nasal passages, pharynx, trachea, bronchi) does not contribute to alveolar ventilation. Once in the alveolus, respiratory gases must diffuse between the lung and capillaries. Gas movement across membranes is affected by the diffusion coefficient of the gas, the thickness of the septum, and the surface area available for diffusion. Because carbon dioxide diffuses much more readily than oxygen and is the direct stimulus for respiration, hypoxia may occur without significant increases in respiratory rate. Alveolar septum thickness can be increased by edema and fibrosis. Surface area can be physically decreased by consolidation and emphysema, or physiologically reduced by alteration in the ventilation-perfusion ratio stemming from increased physiologic dead space or shunting of blood away from ventilated alveoli.[4]

Significant innate immune defenses are present in the lung. The sneeze and cough reflexes forcibly expel large particles and irritants from the upper airway. Nasal hairs and air turbulence over the nasal concha filter out airborne particles as small as 6 μm. Gravitational precipitation filters smaller particles (1–5 μm) in the small bronchioles. Mucociliary clearance efficiently moves trapped particles to the pharynx, where they are either swallowed or coughed out. This system is formed by mucus-producing goblet cells and ciliated epithelial cells that line the respiratory tract from the nasal passages to the terminal bronchioles. Once in the alveoli, particles larger than 0.5 μm come to lie against the alveolar wall and are cleared by alveolar macrophages or the lung lymphatic system. Particles less than 0.5 μm in size remain suspended and are exhaled without consequence.[5]

Diagnostic Approaches

Physical Examination and Auscultation

A thorough and unbiased physical examination is the most important component of the diagnostic evaluation of small ruminants presented for abnormalities of the respiratory tract. Without a complete physical exam, important primary or secondary physiologic problems may be missed, and the diagnostic plan may be incomplete or result in failure to obtain a definitive diagnosis. However, complete diagnostic exams are often not a viable option on captive cervids. In these cases, careful observation with a spotting scope, over prolonged periods of time, may be the most viable option. Particular attention should be paid to nasal or ocular discharge, sneezing, coughing, general lethargy, an altered or increased abdominal component to the respiratory effort, and similar clinical signs in other animals should be considered. If deemed necessary, chemical restraint (darting) or evaluation of animals in a drop chute can be considered; however, the resulting stress and impact on respiratory effort and disease need to be considered in advance.

The physical exam should be conducted in a systematic manner and must include all aspects of the respiratory system. Before restraining the animal, the clinician should spend a few minutes observing its attitude, stance, respiratory rate, and respiratory pattern from a distance, because significant elevations in respiratory rate and pattern can occur after capture and restraint, particularly in animals that are less socialized. As a consequence of the flocking instincts of sheep, goats, and cervids, animals standing apart from the rest of the flock or herd are likely to be significantly ill. Once the animal is caught and restrained, the practitioner should begin by evaluating the respiratory system starting at the head (see Chapter 1). The nares should be examined for evidence of serous, mucopurulent, or hemorrhagic discharge from one or both nostrils (Figure 7.1). Unilateral nasal discharge may provide important information regarding the location of a lesion and should be noted on the examination form. Both nares should be accessed for patency by placing either a small cotton ball or a mirror in front of the nose and observing for movement or fogging, respectively. The remainder of the head should be evaluated for evidence of facial deformity or soft tissue swelling indicative of a localized lesion. The pharyngeal area should be palpated, with particular attention paid to the local lymph nodes. When possible, the palpation should include an attempt to feel the area lateral and dorsal to the pharynx by placing a hand alongside the trachea and palpating with gentle dorsal pressure. This area is a common site for retropharyngeal abscesses (often caused by *Corynebacterium pseudotuberculosis*), which may result in considerable respiratory stridor and effort. The extrathoracic trachea should be palpated from the pharynx down to the mediastinal entrance for any evidence of stricture, dilatation, or external compression. During this portion of the evaluation, occasional gentle squeezing pressure should be applied to the trachea, to determine how easily coughing can be induced. The mediastinal opening is another area that warrants palpation for evidence of space-occupying lesions or tracheal deviation associated with such findings.

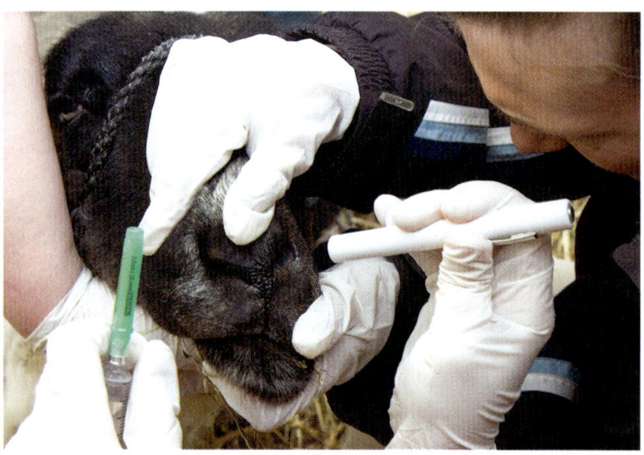

• **Fig. 7.1** The clinician is carefully examining the nares in this well-restrained ewe. (Note: Both a light source and saline are available to flush out any material that precludes proper evaluation.) (Courtesy Dr. A.N. Baird, Purdue University.)

Attention should then turn to performing a complete auscultatory examination of the thorax, when possible. Owing to the heavy wool cover on the thorax of sheep, this exam may be of limited usefulness without adequate shearing. At a minimum, the cranioventral aspect of the thorax of sheep can be auscultated in the nonwooled area located immediately behind the elbow. In sheared or haired sheep and lambs, goats, and restrained cervids, the entire thorax generally can be auscultated without further removal of fiber or hair. Attention should be paid to the intensity, duration, and character of the breath sounds, as well as the stage of respiration (i.e., inhalation or exhalation, early or late) during which they occur. In comparison with those in cattle, the normal airway sounds heard in sheep, goats, and cervids are much more obvious, owing to the thinner body wall. This perceived magnification often results in the erroneous impression of abnormal respiratory sounds.

Abnormal sounds should be classified as either of two different descriptive types: *wheezes* are high-pitched, continuous musical sounds associated with altered airflow through larger airways. They are indicative of either fluid in the airway or increased velocity of air movement in the airway. *Crackles* are noncontinuous brief "popping" sounds associated with sudden opening of small airways or alveoli. They most commonly are heard during inspiration, particularly late inspiration, and previously were described as "rales." If any abnormal breath sounds are auscultated, they should be localized and their anatomic location recorded on the examination form. In most instances, the use of a rebreathing bag, as is common in respiratory evaluation of horses, is not necessary for small ruminants, owing to their relatively thin body wall.

After completion of the auscultation exam, several additional pieces of information should be collected. The *rectal temperature* reveals whether the animal is febrile, normothermic, or hypothermic. The presence of fever may provide additional evidence of an inflammatory process that may warrant additional diagnostic effort. Additionally, the *nutritional status* of the animal should be evaluated, because immune dysfunction is more common in young animals with less than adequate reserves of body fat. This assessment is perhaps best performed by body condition scoring of multiple animals in the same management group. Finally, the practitioner should spend some time evaluating the *environment* in which the diseased animal is housed. Environments with poor ventilation, drafts, dust, or high stocking densities may predispose resident animals to the development of respiratory disease; in such instances, appropriate treatment may require addressing the environmental conditions.

With respiratory disease in preweaned animals, it also is worthwhile to consider the role of colostrum management and failure of passive transfer in the disease process. When warranted, serum samples from several animals can be collected and assayed for failure of passive transfer status. Our own preference is to test a group of 10 animals between 24 and 72 h of age; at least 8 of the 10 animals should demonstrate adequate evidence of passive transfer (serum total protein above 5.0 mg/dL). If increased rates of failure of passive transfer are identified, then herd- or flock-level changes are needed to improve immunity of this at-risk group.

After the physical exam has been completed, the clinician should use the findings to develop a comprehensive problem list that serves as a basis for development of a complete diagnostic plan and differential list. Although this step often is skipped in the interest of time, it is one of the few ways to ensure consideration of all possible clinical entities in the differential diagnosis.

Diagnostic Procedures

Once a complete list of diagnostic possibilities has been generated, the clinician can turn to the development of a useful and cost-effective diagnostic approach specific to the case. In this context, it is important to ascertain the expectations of the client with regard to desired outcome. For instance, the producer with 29 weaned kids in group-housing, of which 10 were lost to pneumonia in the past week, may have very different expectations and motivations to pursue diagnostic investigation from those for a producer with a single animal showing clinical signs. Many of the usual procedures for such investigation, as described next, may not be economically feasible or desirable if the producer perceives that the cost does not justify the return on investment. By contrast, if the results can be used to prevent disease in multiple animals, the motivation to pay for the diagnostics may be increased.

Blood Gas Analysis Blood gas analysis provides a rapid and useful assessment of hemoglobin oxygenation and alveolar diffusion of gases. Its usefulness is, however, limited by the need for rapid testing and appropriate sample handling to prevent erroneous results. The advent of portable blood gas analyzers that can be carried on the ambulatory care truck make this test feasible in the farm situation; in most instances, however, its application is limited to high-value cases in referral hospital settings. In our experience, an arterial blood gas sample is best collected from small ruminants using the brachial artery located on the medial aspect of the proximal portion of the front legs. Special blood-gas syringes are commercially available and should be used if accurate assessment of partial pressures is required, as would be the case in respiratory disease. While the animal is lying in lateral recumbency, the lower limb is extended and the pulsation of the artery is palpated between the index and middle fingers while the needle is inserted at a 90-degree angle to the skin. Once the artery is penetrated, the syringe is held steady and should self-fill. Negative pressure should not be applied to the syringe, because this alters gas partial pressures in the sample. Once the blood is collected, the needle should be rapidly sealed, typically with the rubber stopper supplied with blood-gas syringes. Care should be taken to not introduce any bubbles into the syringe during this process. Arterial partial pressures of O_2 (Pao_2) should be above 70 to 80 mmHg in an animal with normal oxygenation. Partial pressures below that level may be indicative of inappropriate ventilation, poor alveolar ventilation, or thickened alveolar walls that impair oxygen diffusion. Normal partial pressures of CO_2 in an arterial sample should be below 40 mm Hg, and if the sample yields a $Paco_2$ greater than that value in association with a very low oxygen partial pressure, the possibility that a venous sample has been obtained needs to be considered.

Radiography. Radiographs of the thorax, neck, or head often are required and can be of significant diagnostic benefit. Radiographs can easily be obtained using portable radiographic equipment commonly available to veterinary practitioners. When unilateral nasal discharge or facial deformities are observed during the physical exam, radiographic evaluation with both lateral and dorsoventral views of the head may elucidate the etiology. In many instances, nasal foreign bodies or sinusitis can be confirmed on the basis of the radiographic interpretation of the head views. Similarly, radiographs of the neck may provide additional evidence of tracheal compression or retropharyngeal masses that may be associated with coughing in affected animals. Thoracic radiographs can be obtained with the animal either standing or in lateral recumbency, depending on the facilities available to the practitioner (Figure 7.2A and B).

Lung field consolidation can be readily identified by observing radiographic opacities in the cranial ventral lung fields, and mediastinal masses, often associated with caseous lymphadenitis abscesses, generally are revealed as a line of masses of increased density coursing through the thorax at the level of the trachea. In rare instances, a thymoma may result in the appearance of a mass cranial to the heart that gives the appearance of the animal's having two hearts.

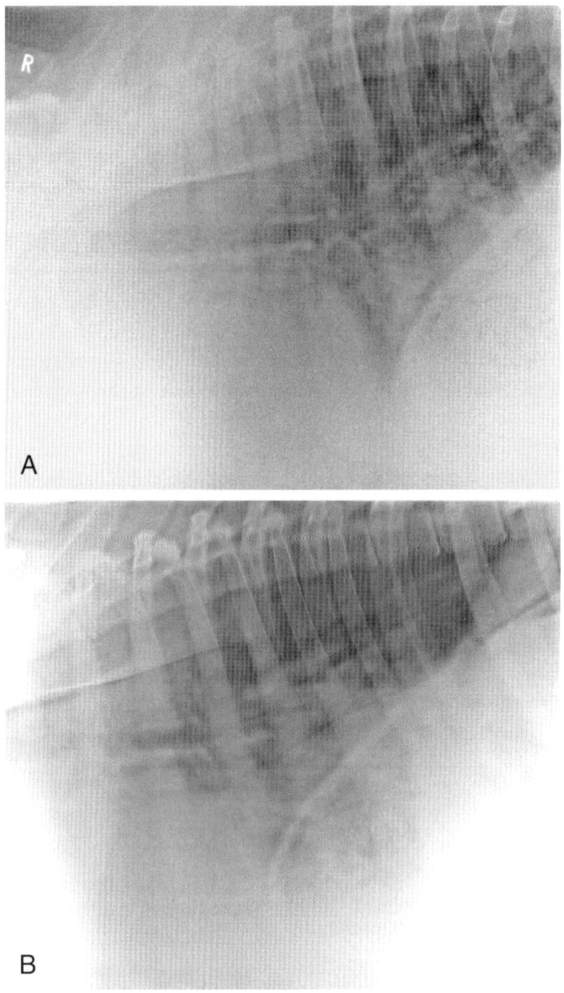

• **Fig. 7.2** Radiograph showing pulmonary edema related to a tracheal obstruction in a 6-year-old Suffolk ewe. **A.** Increased opacity is evident throughout the lungs, along with peribronchial cuffing and lack of visualization of the vascular markings. It is difficult to distinguish the borders of the caudal vena cava because of the increased interstitial opacity. Other considerations in the differential diagnosis for this pulmonary pattern would be pneumonia and pulmonary hemorrhage. **B.** Lateral view of the caudal thorax of the same patient 24 h after treatment with a tracheotomy, diuretics, and antibiotics. The vascular margins are better delineated, as are the borders of the caudal vena cava. Interstitial opacity within the lungs is less than on the previous radiograph. Although mild interstitial opacity persists, the pulmonary edema is resolving. (Courtesy Dr. Debra Baird, Purdue University.)

Ultrasound Imaging. Portable ultrasound units are becoming standard equipment in many large animal clinics, affording easy access to this imaging modality. Many units used for reproductive practice are equipped with a linear, 5- to 7.5-MHz transducer. This type of machine can provide reasonably good-quality images of the thorax and adjacent soft tissues. When available, a curvilinear probe provides superior image quality, but certainly is not required for diagnostic use. Appropriate patient preparation is paramount for obtaining a good-quality image. Wool or hair over the site of interest should be clipped, although the use of coupling agents (e.g., gel, vegetable oil, alcohol) can be helpful in some instances. Owing to the nature of the functioning, gas-filled lung, ultrasonography of the respiratory tract is more limited than that of other body systems. For example, ultrasound examination of the pharyngeal region may provide an easy means of identifying retropharyngeal abscesses when they are suspected from findings on palpation. In such cases, the probe should be placed parallel to the lateral aspect of the trachea and directed dorsomedially towards the opposite ear. Abscesses typically have a hyperechoic wall, with variable echotexture of the contents.

Ultrasound imaging also can provide useful information in evaluation of the thorax. The clinician should become familiar with the appearance of normal aerated lung, allowing rapid identification of areas that lack the normal appearance. Normal lung is recognizable by the bright hyperechoic line of the visceral pleura above a classic reverberation artifact induced by the aerated lung. The reverberation artifact is typical of ultrasound waves hitting a gas interface and consists of sequential hyperechoic lines spaced at regular intervals. It is important to realize that any images appearing on the screen deep to the start of the reverberation artifact are indeed artifacts and not images of the lung parenchyma (Figure 7.3). Once an appreciation for the normal appearance of lung has been achieved, the thoracic exam can be systematically performed. With use of a linear or a curvilinear probe, the probe should be oriented parallel to the ribs in the intercostal space. We prefer to start at the most dorsal aspect of each intercostal space and slowly move downwards to the ventral thorax observing the lung surface along the path. This is repeated in each intercostal space moving caudally. The image quality is maximized by following the natural "lay" of the wool or hair (in a dorsal-ventral direction). As the exam progresses caudally, the diaphragm comes into the image while moving ventrally, often with the adjacent liver filling the space below. With use of this method, the extent of the thoracic lung field can be determined. Focused examination of the cranioventral lung fields consistently identifies lesions associated with bronchopneumonia; this exam can be performed in the nonhaired axillary region without requiring clipping fleece and is facilitated by "flipping" the sheep and restraining them on their rump. The three primary lesions that may be observed are parenchymal masses in the lung that are adjacent to the visceral pleura, lung consolidation, and the characteristic "comet tail" lesions associated with pleural thickening and inflammation. The first of these lesions is readily identified by the observation of echo-dense masses interrupting the normal reverberation artifact of the lung. Such masses can be measured to allow for sequential ultrasonographic examination as a means of assessing treatment success or resolution of the lesion. In our experience, these lesions most commonly are associated with parenchymal abscesses. Consolidated lung is recognized on deeper imaging, beyond the normal lung reverberation. In many instances, the consolidated lung may have an appearance similar to that of liver ("hepatized lung") or may be seen to contain scattered gas shadows associated with presence of gas in the larger airways or in abscesses. "Comet tails" are recognizable as small, hyperechoic spots with a comet tail-shaped artifact located deep to the spot. These lesions are non-specific but often are associated with thickening or inflammation of the pleura.

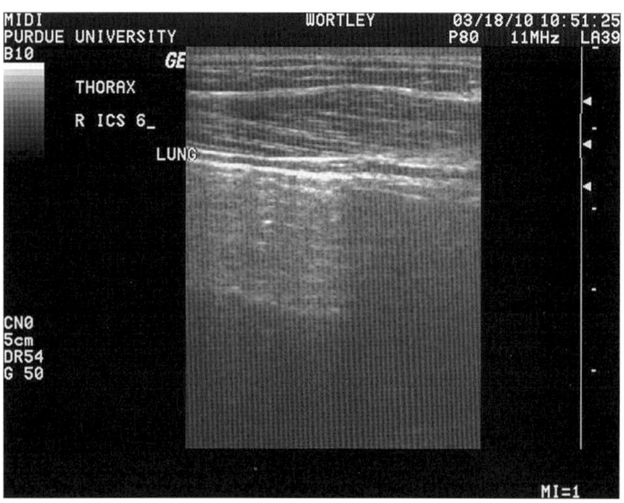

• **Fig. 7.3** Ultrasound image of the right cranioventral thorax obtained at the sixth intercostal space in a 3-year-old La Mancha cross doe with normal lungs. The linear hyperechoic structure with reflective echoes represents the normal, aerated pleural surface. This ultrasound image was obtained using a 10-MHz linear array transducer. Dorsal is to the *left* of the image. (Courtesy Dr. Karine Pader, Purdue University.)

If pleural fluid is present, it is imaged as an anechoic or hypoechoic area in the ventral thorax, with normal lung reverberation noted at the lung-fluid interface. Because the mediastinum is not always easily imaged, radiographs remain the preferred imaging modality for identification of mediastinal masses.

Nasal and Pharyngeal Swabs. Swabs are very useful as a means of obtaining material for microbiologic culture in cases of respiratory disease. The laboratory that will process the cultures should be contacted for recommendations on swab type and submission procedures. For instance, calcium alginate swabs and bleached cotton swabs have the potential to interfere with polymerase chain reaction (PCR) testing. Many swabs with wooden sticks have formaldehyde as a preservative in the wood, which can adversely affect bacterial growth. Similar considerations apply regarding the selection of transport media. The use of a guarded swab (i.e., mare uterine swabs), when available, should be considered to minimize contamination with oral flora. Use of an oral speculum (0.5- to 1.0-inch internal diameter [ID] polyvinylchloride [PVC] pipe, cut to length, with the ends sanded smooth), may help in obtaining a more reliable sample. Collection of the diagnostic sample involves simply rolling the swab surface on the pharyngeal mucosa around the palatine tonsil. Once prepared, the swab should be placed in the transport medium and refrigerated unless otherwise directed by the diagnostic laboratory. It is important to recognize that many lung pathogens (particularly *Pasteurella multocida* and *Mannheimia haemolytica*) can be found as normal commensal flora of the upper respiratory tract. If the clinician wishes to evaluate the swab for presence of *Mycoplasma* spp., the laboratory should be notified and a *Mycoplasma* culture requested. In most cases, pharyngeal swabs correlate better with clinical disease and should be preferred when feasible.

Sinus-Centesis. The technique of sinus-centesis provides the practitioner with an option for collecting representative culture material from a nasal sinus. Owing to the comparatively smaller nasal sinuses of sheep and goats, proper selection of a site for sampling is critical to ensure entry into the sinus cavity. Radiographic assistance in localizing the involved sinus cavity is recommended. If necessary, radiopaque markers can be placed on the skin before exposure to ensure appropriate site selection. Once the site is verified, the area should be clipped and surgically prepared. Raising a small bleb under the skin with lidocaine provides adequate anesthesia to the external surfaces but does not achieve anesthesia to the periosteum. Thus, the animal should be sedated or anesthetized (see Chapter 18 and Appendix 1). If the goal is to collect a small sample of material for culture, a small-diameter bone pin or heavy-gauge cerclage wire can be guided through a stab incision in the skin and used to drill a small hole through the bone. A hypodermic needle can then be introduced into the sinus and a sample aspirated. Samples should be submitted for aerobic bacterial and fungal culture. In cases in which drainage and lavage is needed, a small sinus trephine can be used to create a large-bore opening into the sinus.

After collection of the sample, the incision should be kept clean and allowed to heal by second intention. The operated animals should be fed low to the ground to help facilitate sinus drainage, and use of elevated hay racks should be avoided until the wound is fully healed.

Tracheal Wash. Faced with large herd outbreaks of respiratory disease or a high incidence of treatment failures, diagnostic sampling for determining the etiologic agent and antimicrobial susceptibility profile should be considered. Nasal swabs can be used in some circumstances but yield less reliable results than a tracheal wash. A tracheal wash provides the clinician with the opportunity to collect a sterile deep lung sample with minimal effort.

The animal should be standing and adequately restrained for this procedure. Sedation may be warranted. If a fiberoptic endoscope is available (8–9 mm diameter), it may be inserted through the nasal passage in some adult sheep, goats, or cervids. If this is not possible, the endoscope can be passed through an oral speculum. An endoscopic examination may allow visualization of the respiratory tract, identification of exudates, and enhancement of the sample collection. If an endoscope is unavailable, a percutaneous transtracheal wash (TTW) procedure can be performed. Use of a commercially available presterilized, complete kit designed for foals, when available, enhances the ease of this procedure (Figure 7.4A and B). Alternatively, a hypodermic needle of appropriate size to allow a sterile tube catheter (220 polyethylene) to pass through the bore may be used. If using the latter approach, care must be taken during manipulation of the catheter to prevent the needle bevel from cutting off the distal end of the catheter. On the ventral aspect of the neck, the hair or fiber should be removed over at least a 6-inch square of skin centered on the midline and located roughly one-third of the way down the neck from the throatlatch. The trachea should be identified and easily palpated at this level. The site should be disinfected using a standard surgical preparation, and a small bleb can be raised with lidocaine placed under the skin directly over the midline of the trachea in the center of the site. A stab incision should be made through the skin using a scalpel blade. The procedure should be performed using a sterile technique. If a commercial kit is to be used, the blunt-tipped needle and associated placement trocar should be identified in the kit, and the clinician should become familiar with their design and use before performing the procedure. The unit should be placed through the skin incision, and the tip of the trocar should be used to feel the tracheal rings while the operator's opposite hand is used to stabilize the trachea. The tip of the trocar should be positioned on midline between the tracheal rings while applying firm pressure to facilitate passage of the trocar into the trachea. A slight "pop" may be felt as the tip of the stylet enters the cavity. The trocar should be advanced until it can be felt to fully penetrate the trachea and can be slightly advanced in a

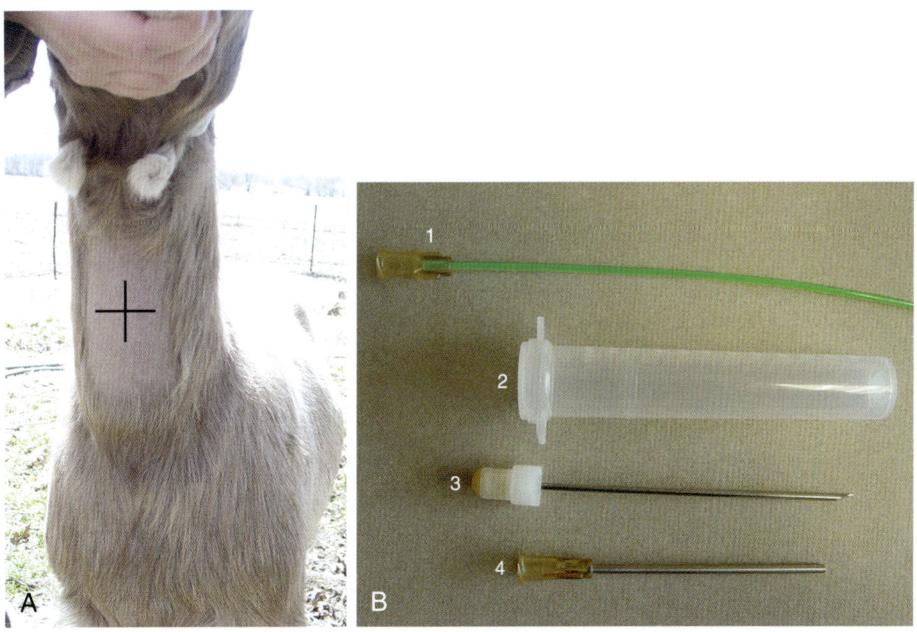

• **Fig. 7.4** Transtracheal Wash. **A.** Site of access for transtracheal wash on the ventral midline in the midcervical region. **B.** Supplies for transtracheal wash procedure: 18-inch flexible wash catheter *(1)*, sample vial *(2)*, trocar removed from cannula for visualization *(3)*, and wash cannula *(4)*.

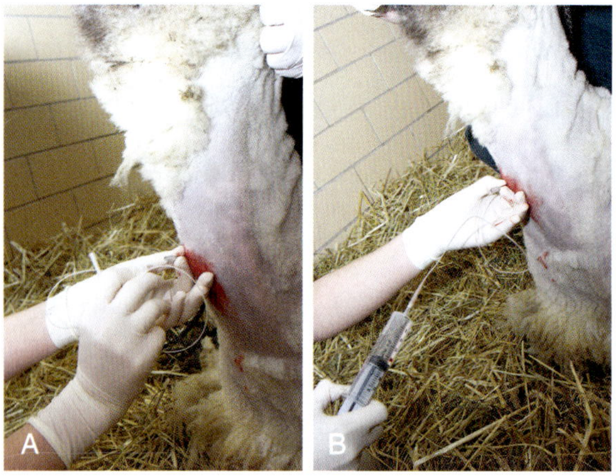

• **Fig. 7.5** **A.** The middle third of the neck is aseptically scrubbed, the skin and subcutaneous tissue are anesthetized, a stab incision is made through the skin and subcutaneous tissue, a 14-gauge needle or trocar is passed through the incision and into the trachea, and tubing is passed using sterile technique just beyond the tracheal bifurcation. **B.** The clinician injects sterile isotonic solution (12–30 mL) through the tubing and then immediately performs fluid retrieval by aspiration with the syringe. (Note: With this method, caution should be taken to avoid cutting off the tube in the trachea with the sharp needle.)

ventral direction (Figure 7.5A). The stylet should be removed, and the aspiration catheter passed (using sterile gloves) through the trocar to roughly the level of the tracheal bifurcation. For adult, full-sized small ruminants, 12 to 15 mL of sterile saline should be infused into the trachea and a sterile syringe used to apply gentle suction as the catheter is moved back and forth in the trachea (see Figure 7.5B). The goal is to move the catheter so that its tip is in the pool of fluid created just cranial to the tracheal carina. Although this cannot be visualized, it can be located with practice in a majority of cases. If needed, additional normal saline (another 5–10 mL as indicated) can be instilled to increase the recovery volume. Recovery volumes vary considerably; however, the larger the volume recovered, the higher the likelihood of success for culture and cytology. Generally, 1 to 2 mL would be considered the minimum for recovery to assure a higher quality sample. The catheter should be removed, followed by the trocar. In cases in which a needle and polypropylene catheter are used, the needle should be removed from the trachea before the catheter to minimize the risk of cutting off the distal tip of the catheter during its withdrawal.

Thoracocentesis. Thoracocentesis provides a reliable means of collecting a sample of pleural fluid for diagnostic submission. This is best performed in the cranioventral portion of the chest, where pleural fluid pools in the most dependent part of the thorax. While the animal is standing, this area can be evaluated by ultrasound imaging to identify an appropriate site as indicated by presence of fluid and absence of other viscera. The body wall thickness can be measured to assist in determining how deep to advance the needle to acquire the sample. Once collected, the sample should be evaluated for appearance, odor, and turbidity, in addition to being submitted for bacterial culture and cytologic study. The presence of a pungent foul odor often is associated with anaerobic infection, and treatment decisions should consider this possibility.

Upper Airway Disease

Stertor and stridor, sneezing, and nasal discharge are hallmark signs that suggest upper airway disease over pneumonia.

Rhinitis

Possible causes of rhinitis in small ruminants and cervids include foreign material such as from regurgitation, parasites, neoplasia, and other respiratory infections.

Nasal Bot Infestation

Pathogenesis. Nasal bot infestation is more common in sheep than in goats, and infected goats have a lower larval burden than that typical for sheep[6]; pharyngeal bot infestation is a common and potentially serious occurrence in North American deer populations. Clinical signs during the first spring infestation generally are mild, but disease severity markedly increases during subsequent infestations, probably owing to hypersensitization; goats may acquire immunity after repeated infections.[5] The adult *Oestrus ovis* fly deposits larvae at the animal's nostrils. The first instar larvae migrate up the nasal passages into the dorsal turbinates and sinuses. There, they develop over a 2- to 10-month-period to the third instar stage,[1,7] return to the nostril, and are sneezed out to pupate in the soil.[6] Both first instar larvae and pupae may overwinter.[7] Cervids are generally infected with a member of the *Cephenemyia* family of bots, of which at least five species have been associated with disease and all have a lifecycle that closely mirrors that of sheep bots.

Clinical Signs. Irritation from the adult flies induces avoidance activities such as head shaking, head rubbing, and feet stomping; if the animal's distress level is severe, grazing activity decreases.[7] Larval passage and development can cause inflammatory rhinitis characterized by sneezing, mucopurulent discharge, and decreased airflow through the nares. Sequelae can include bacterial rhinitis or sinusitis, and, infrequently, interstitial pneumonia secondary to antigen aspiration.[6]

Diagnosis. Sheep bot infection is associated with a profuse nasal discharge containing numerous eosinophils and mast cells, whereas deer bots often present with little to no external symptoms.[6,8] Direct visualization of the bots or mineralized remains may be possible with endoscopic or radiographic imaging. In commercial herds, clinical signs, cytologic examination of the discharge, and response to therapy usually are sufficient to make the diagnosis.

Therapy. Treatment usually is administered for heavy late summer infestations or to kill overwintering bots. Ivermectin (0.2 mg/kg subcutaneously [SC]) is effective in killing the *O. ovis* larvae[1,7,8] but requires an extended milk withdrawal period: 40 days if administered subcutaneously and 6 days if administered orally (if administered at a higher oral dose of 0.4 mg/kg, an 11-day milk withdrawal is recommended).[9] Pour-on eprinomectin (0.5 mg/kg) may be a better choice for commercial dairies because it has been shown to be effective in sheep against nasal bot infestation and has a zero-day milk withdrawal period.[10,11] Anecdotal evidence and experience suggest that treatment of nasal bots in deer can be effectively achieved by use of avermectins.

Once the bots are killed, secondary bacterial infections usually resolve without further intervention. If indicated, however, treatment is with broad-spectrum antimicrobials.[8]

Other Parasites

In the Himalayas, a nasal leech from standing water pools can cause similar clinical signs in sheep. Systemic ivermectin is ineffective, but direct application of ivermectin solution (0.1 mg/mL) to the leech kills it within a few hours. Wetting the animal's muzzle encourages the leech to migrate down to the nostril opening so that the ivermectin can be applied.[1]

On the Indian subcontinent, *Schistosoma nasale* infection ("snoring disease") has been reported as a cause of nasal obstruction in sheep from parasite-associated inflammation and tissue proliferation.[1,12]

Enzootic Nasal Tumor

Pathogenesis. ENTV belongs to the genus Betaretrovirus in the family Retroviridae, and exhibits genetic organization characteristic of type B and D oncoviruses.

Enzootic nasal tumors are transmissible, sporadically occurring tumors of the nasal passages of sheep and goats.[13,14] This condition has been reported in animals as young as 15 and 7 months, respectively,[15,16] and is believed to be caused by type D or B retrovirus infection.[13,17,18] These tumors can occur unilaterally or bilaterally and are locally invasive but not usually metastatic.[14,16] They originate from the olfactory mucosa and ethmoid or nasal turbinates and usually are classified as adenomas, adenopapillomas, or adenocarcinomas.[14–16] Other conditions on a differential diagnosis list for nasal masses include lymphosarcoma and fungal granuloma.[1]

Similar nasal tumors have been reported in roe deer *(Capreolus capreolus)*,[19] Eld's deer *(Cervus eldii)*,[20] Fallow deer *(Dama dama)*,[21] Persian fallow deer *(Dama dama mesopotamica)*,[22] Axis deer *(Axis axis)*,[23] and moose *(Alces alces)*.[19] Epidemiological characteristics of nasal tumors in wild ungulates suggest a similar etiology; however, a definitive retroviral etiology has not been confirmed in these species.

Clinical Signs. The tumor starts as small nodules that grow to form large nodular cystic masses, causing progressive inspiratory dyspnea and secondary emaciation.[14–16] Inflammatory polyps may be present near the tumor.[16,18] Primary clinical signs include unilateral or bilateral copious seromucous to mucopurulent nasal discharge with inspiratory stridor. Additional signs may include exercise intolerance, decreased airflow and open-mouth breathing, anorexia, head shaking and sneezing, exophthalmos, and bony facial asymmetry.[14–16]

Diagnosis. Antibody responses to ENTV-1 have been demonstrated in sheep.[24,25] However, only a moderate correlation exists between serum ENTV antibodies and the presence of a nasal adenocarcinoma, and the seropositivity of the animal should not be used as conclusive evidence for the presence of a tumor. Use of reverse transcription polymerase chain reaction (RT-PCR) for the detection of ENTV RNA from nasal swabs has been demonstrated a highly specific technique for the identification of preclinical and clinical ENT. However, appraisal of this antemortem diagnostic under extensive field conditions for the control or eradication of ENTV has not been performed to date.

A preliminary diagnosis can be made from the clinical signs and findings on sinus percussion. Radiographic or endoscopic imaging may be indicated. Definitive diagnosis requires surgical excisional biopsy.[15]

Treatment. If enzootic nasal tumor is untreated, death occurs within 90 days of appearance of clinical signs.[14,15] Surgical debulking is a palliative option,[15] but may not be curative.[26] The mass can be accessed for excision by creating an I-shaped incision in the skin and then the nasal bones along the dorsal facial midline axis, reflecting the cutaneous and bony flaps, and removing the nasal septum. Profuse hemorrhage is to be expected; epinephrine (1:100,000)-soaked gauze pads can help with hemostasis, and a blood donor should be readily available.[26] A temporary tracheostomy may be needed during the surgical procedure and the postsurgical period.[15] Herd or flock control of enzootic tumor is difficult in the absence of widely available commercial serologic tests to identify animals with preclinical disease. Enzootic nasal tumors can be spread by nasal discharge; infected animals should be isolated and culled.[18]

Other Causes of Rhinitis/Upper Airway Disease

Other respiratory pathogens involved in small ruminant rhinitis include herpesvirus and *P. multocida* infections. Herpesvirus infection causes fibronecrotic ulceration of the nasal septum with a marked catarrhal rhinitis, usually accompanied by additional severe systemic signs.[1] *P. multocida* infection causes nasal turbinate atrophy, which can be identified at necropsy by cross-sectioning the head at the level of the first premolar.[1] In tropical and subtropical regions, an important consideration in the differential diagnosis for bacterial rhinitis is nasal melioidosis (caused by *Burkholderia pseudomallei*).[1] Respiratory involvement is particularly common in small ruminant species and may include oculonasal discharge, coughing, lymphadenopathy, and pulmonary disease, all characterized by multiple caseous abscesses. Melioidosis is zoonotic and reportable in many parts of the world.[27]

Sinusitis

Pathogenesis. Sinusitis is a relatively rare condition in sheep and goats, and is usually related to dehorning infections (with consequent involvement of the frontal sinus) or dental abnormalities (with maxillary sinus involvement). Signs of frontal sinus infection may appear weeks to months after the dehorning process. Multi-sinus infection can result from nasal bot infestation, neoplasia, facial fractures, and horn injuries.[8] Facial deformities associated with *Fusobacterium necrophorum* may be commonly observed in cervids.

Clinical Signs. Indications of sinusitis include drainage from dehorning sites as well as swelling, softening, or deformities of the overlying facial bones. Malodor, unequal airflow, head shaking and rubbing, extension of the head and neck, or head resting or pressing also may be noted. Systemic signs such as pyrexia, anorexia, and lethargy may develop as well, and chronic sinusitis may lead to neurologic symptoms.[8]

Diagnosis. A presumptive diagnosis can be made from the clinical presentation and findings on percussion. Radiographic imaging is indicated for investigation of recurring or refractory cases. In one instance of chronic sinusitis in a pet goat, computed tomography was used to accurately characterize the lesion.[28] An oral exam with the animal under light sedation should be performed if dental abnormalities are suspected. Culture and sensitivity testing of the sinus exudate can help direct antimicrobial selection.

Treatment. Basic therapy involves daily lavage of the dehorning site and sinus with a dilute antiseptic such as 0.1% chlorhexidine. Lavage solution can be introduced through a teat cannula or 16–18 French catheter. Multiple trephination sites may be needed, especially in the highly compartmentalized ovine frontal sinus.[8] Trephine holes need to be large enough to establish drainage; 14-gauge needles commonly are used for diagnostic sampling but are too small for lavage. Placement and ease of trephination are facilitated by the softer bone and the bone deformity found in typical chronic sinusitis cases.[29] The caudal frontal sinus can be accessed 5 mm from the base of the horn while avoiding the frontal vein in the supraorbital groove; the rostral frontal sinus lies medial to the orbit. Trephination borders for the maxillary sinus are cranial to the orbit, caudal and dorsal to the facial tuberosity, and ventral to the infraorbital foramen.[30]

Complete resolution may require a couple weeks of daily treatment, because the sinus structure is complex and biofilm development is common. Sheep have been used in experimental models for antibiofilm approaches to sinusitis; early results are promising.[31] Animals showing systemic signs should be treated with antibiotics (penicillin, 22,000 IU/kg twice daily) and nonsteroidal antiinflammatories (NSAIDs) (e.g., flunixin meglumine, 1.1 mg/kg intravenously [IV] twice daily, ketoprofen, 3.0 mg/kg IV or intramuscularly [IM] once a day, or meloxicam, 1 mg/kg orally q72 h).

Sinusitis may be prevented by bandaging open dehorning sites for 5 to 7 days after the procedure and by gauze-packing extracted tooth sockets.[8]

Pharyngitis

Pathogenesis. In sheep, goats, and cervids, pharyngitis typically develops secondarily to traumatic injury, with subsequent bacterial colonization. Inciting trauma usually is caused by dosing equipment, rough feeds, or foreign objects. Plastic animal health devices (e.g., dosing and balling guns, stomach tubes, speculum), especially older devices that have been roughened from chewing, are notorious for traumatizing the pharynx. Commonly involved pathogens include *Trueperella pyogenes*, *F. necrophorum,* and *C. pseudotuberculosis*.[8] In deer, *F. necrophorum* is a leading cause of pharyngitis and is commonly referred to as diphtheria.

Clinical Signs. Coughing, painful swallowing, anorexia, and drooling are typical signs of pharyngitis. Oral malodor and dyspnea or stridor may be present, and the animal may stand with an extended head and neck. Systemic signs may include fever, dehydration, and aspiration pneumonia. Hyperemia, swelling, exudate, and foreign material may be identified on oral exam. Mild lesions may resolve spontaneously, but more severe infections can lead to cellulitis and formation of abscesses or granulomas in the pharynx or lung parenchyma.

Diagnosis. Cough and a pain response may occur on palpation of the pharyngeal region. An oral exam should be performed; light xylazine sedation facilitates this process. Radiographic and endoscopic imaging may be indicated in some cases. Bacterial culture and sensitivity testing may help with antimicrobial selection if uncontaminated samples can be obtained.

Treatment. Pharyngitis should be treated with parenteral broad-spectrum antibiotics and NSAIDs. Oral medications and forced tube feeding are contraindicated; a temporary rumen fistula can be placed if nutritional support is needed. Abscesses can be drained into the pharyngeal cavity and flushed with a dilute antiseptic, such as 0.1% or 0.2% povidone-iodine (Betadine).[8]

Retropharyngeal Abscesses

Although retropharyngeal abscesses can develop in association with pharyngitis and pharyngeal trauma, in sheep and goats they more commonly are due to *C. pseudotuberculosis* infection. Clinical signs result from pressure on the pharynx and trachea and include stridor, cough, and difficulty swallowing. Diagnosis is based on clinical signs, palpation, and, possibly, radiographic imaging. To avoid contamination of the environment, *C. pseudotuberculosis* abscesses should not be lanced. Surgical removal of the retropharyngeal lymph node is technically possible but difficult, owing to the presence of vital anatomic structures in the region. Closed-system lavage along with either intralesional or subcutaneous tulathromycin (2.5 mg/kg) is as effective as traditional methods of lancing, draining, and flushing subcutaneous caseous lymphadenitis abscesses,[32] and this approach may be an option if the retropharyngeal abscess can be accessed percutaneously.

Laryngitis and Tracheitis

Necrotic laryngitis (necrobacillosis, "calf diphtheria") is caused by invasion by the opportunistic anaerobe *F. necrophorum* through breaks or ulcers in the laryngeal mucosa. This condition is rare in sheep and goats but is seen more commonly with indoor housing systems and in feedlot environments. It is fairly common in deer, especially fawns. Clinical signs include a moist-sounding painful cough, inspiratory dyspnea, difficulty swallowing, and salivation. A presumptive diagnosis usually can be made on the basis of clinical signs, but laryngoscopic and endoscopic examinations are warranted with recurring or refractory cases. In cattle, most early cases respond well to broad-spectrum antimicrobial therapy[33] and NSAIDs. A temporary tracheostomy may be needed until medical therapy takes effect.

Laryngeal chondritis is characterized by edema, suppuration, necrosis, and abscessation of the arytenoid cartilages. This disease has been described in Texel sheep as well as in cattle and horses.[33–35] Breed predilections have been documented, but mode of inheritance is unknown.[35] Clinical signs may resemble those of necrotic laryngitis and include increased upper airway noise, dyspnea, cyanosis, and possibly halitosis; if the condition goes untreated, clinical progression and death are expected.[34,35] Diagnosis in live animals requires endoscopic evaluation of the arytenoids. Partial arytenoidectomy has been suggested as a treatment,[8,34] but subsequent aspiration pneumonia has been observed in cattle.[35] Goulding and associates reported a successful standing permanent tracheostomy in a heifer; the surgery was intended as a salvage procedure, but the heifer was retained and bred successfully.[33] If laryngeal chondritis is detected before cartilage necrosis, abscess formation, or granulation, early ovine and bovine cases have been successfully treated with broad-spectrum antibiotics (lincomycin) and dexamethasone.[34,35]

Laryngeal hemiplegia has been reported in an Alpine goat. No cause was identified on necropsy.[1]

Tracheitis most commonly is caused by pressure from collars and tethers or may result from airborne irritants such as dust and ammonia.[1]

Tracheal collapse is a rarely reported congenital condition in goats. In view of the surprisingly small diameter of goat tracheas, animals in which the condition is suspected should be evaluated by comparison with healthy peers. Clinical signs include stridor, exercise intolerance, and coughing. Affected animals may lag behind their peers in growth and performance.[36] One case has been reported in a previously asymptomatic adult goat; clinical onset presumably was triggered by increased respiratory effort secondary to pneumonia.[37] Diagnosis is based on recognition of clinical signs and tracheal palpation aided by radiologic or endoscopic examination. Successful treatment in cattle and one kid using surgically implanted prosthetic rings has been described.[36]

Cilia-associated respiratory bacillus (CAR) is a bacterium that causes tracheitis in laboratory rats and cattle. This bacillus also has been identified in tracheas from goats with chronic caprine tracheitis and in lungs from kids and adult animals with enzootic pneumonia.[38,39] The significance of CAR in small ruminant respiratory disease is not yet known.

The viral agent of infectious bovine rhinotracheitis (IBR), although rarely isolated from field cases, is capable of causing tracheitis, cough, and nasal discharge in experimentally infected goats. Goat isolates are indistinguishable from those from bovine cases, and some researchers theorize that goats may be latent carriers. IBR vaccination in goats is not recommended, because it is not clear that the causative organism has an actual role in caprine respiratory disease.[1]

Lower Respiratory Disease

General Approach to Respiratory Disease

Respiratory disease can affect small ruminant patients of all ages and breeds, although certain etiologic disorders are more common in specific age groups or management systems. In general, a ruminant with respiratory disease exhibits a variety of clinical signs associated with the respiratory system, including but not limited to nasal discharge, tachypnea, dyspnea, and coughing. Auscultation of the lungs may reveal increased respiratory sounds, crackles, wheezes, or loss of respiratory sounds. Many cases that involve the lower respiratory tract are of mixed etiology, with both bacterial and viral components. Although the disease initially may have started as a condition caused by a single agent, frequently, by the time of presentation to a veterinarian for examination, secondary infections have emerged, thereby complicating diagnostic interpretation.

Pathogens of Mixed Disease

Pasteurella and *Mannheimia* should be considered together in regards to pneumonia. In recent years, some of these organisms have undergone name changes, as pointed out when applicable. *P. multocida* and *M. haemolytica* (previously *Pasteurella haemolytica*) both cause pneumonia in goats, sheep, and cervids. *M. haemolytica* previously was divided into two biotypes, A and T. The biotype T organisms, named for their ability to utilize trehalose, subsequently were reclassified as *Pasteurella trehalosi* and then reassigned to a new genus named *Bibersteinia trehalosi*.[40] These organisms are Gram-negative coccobacilli that grow well on blood agar, forming 1- to 2-mm-diameter colonies. *M. haemolytica* type A2 has been isolated most commonly from goats and sheep, which is a different strain from that commonly isolated in cattle pneumonia cases, *M. haemolytica* type A1.

Pasteurella infections frequently are secondary infections that follow an initial infection with one of several different viral or bacterial agents such as parainfluenza type 3, adenovirus type 6, respiratory syncytial virus, *Bordetella parapertussis*, and *Mycoplasma ovipneumoniae*.[41] These predisposing pathogens interact with *Pasteurella* to overwhelm the immune system, allowing secondary infection to take hold. *Pasteurella* produces several virulence factors, including lipopolysaccharide and endotoxin, which are responsible for inducing physiologic changes in the respiratory tract that allow *Pasteurella* to grow and colonize.[41] Stress also is thought to play a role in predisposing animals to development of *Pasteurella* infections. Experimentally, combined infection with *Pasteurella* and other agents results in a more severe disease process with slower resolution of the lung lesions.

Pasteurella infections result in pneumonia along with septicemia, arthritis, and otitis media. Spring outbreaks are more likely in lambs 2 weeks to 2 months of age and frequently are seen in association with severe weather. Fall outbreaks are more likely to occur in 5- to 7-month-old lambs after shipment to feedlots. *Pasteurella* outbreaks are associated with morbidity rates of up to 50% of the flock or herd, but mortality rates typically are low.

Transmission of *Pasteurella* is through several routes. Inhalation of infectious droplets from carrier animals, direct contact with infected animals, and lambs nursing ewes with *Pasteurella* mastitis all are possible sources of infection. A wide range of signs may be observed in association with *Pasteurella* infections. In some cases, the clinical presentation may be sudden death.[41] In other cases, clinical signs may include fever (temperatures of 105° F to 108° F), depression, anorexia, weight loss, mucopurulent nasal discharge or lacrimation, tachypnea, coughing, and increased lung sounds. The affected animal also may self-isolate from the flock. The typical course of the disease lasts anywhere from 12 h up to 3 days. Full recovery usually requires 14 to 20 days. Chronic infections in lambs or kids can result in decreases in lung capacity, weight gain, and feed efficiency.[41]

Tentative diagnosis of *Pasteurella* infections can be made on the basis of a history of stress, presence of clinical signs of acute bronchopneumonia, and appropriate gross lesions observed at necropsy. Typical necropsy findings include pneumonitis with focal areas of acute fibrinopurulent bronchopneumonia, coagulative necrosis, and fibrinous pleuritis (Figure 7.6A and B). Isolation of *M. haemolytica* or *B. trehalosi* from tissues confirms a tentative diagnosis.

In cervids, mixed lung infections involving *Fusobacterium* spp. are commonly reported.[42–45] In a survey of 23 clinical isolates obtained from necropsy samples of deer, the majority (18/23) were identified as *Fusobacterium varium* and only 3 of the 23 isolates were *F. necrophorum* spp. *necrophorum*. Interestingly, the *F. varium* isolates were demonstrated to not contain a leukotoxin gene, the primary virulence factor recognized in *Fusobacterium*. As a consequence, the exact role that these organisms play in the actual pathogenesis of disease is unclear at present but they are widely isolated. It is likely that these organisms overgrow as part of a mixed bacterial disease process and treatment should be consistent with that described below for other mixed respiratory infections.

Treatment for *Pasteurella* consists of long-acting oxytetracycline. Sulfonamides can be given orally or added to the drinking water, but inconsistent dosing may result with delivery of medication in drinking water. A variety of other antibiotics have been reported to be efficacious in the treatment of pasteurellosis, including ampicillin or penicillin, tylosin, ceftiofur, tulathromycin, and florfenicol. Low levels of antibiotic resistance are seen within *Pasteurella* and *Mannheimia* species.[46] Tilmicosin should be avoided in goats on account of anecdotal reports of fatal toxicity. Treatment often involves extra-label drug use, and readers should refer to the section later in this chapter regarding therapeutics. Culture and sensitivity testing of a transtracheal wash sample or material obtained at necropsy can be used to direct antibiotic selection in herd outbreaks or chronic cases, or for very valuable animals (see Appendix I).

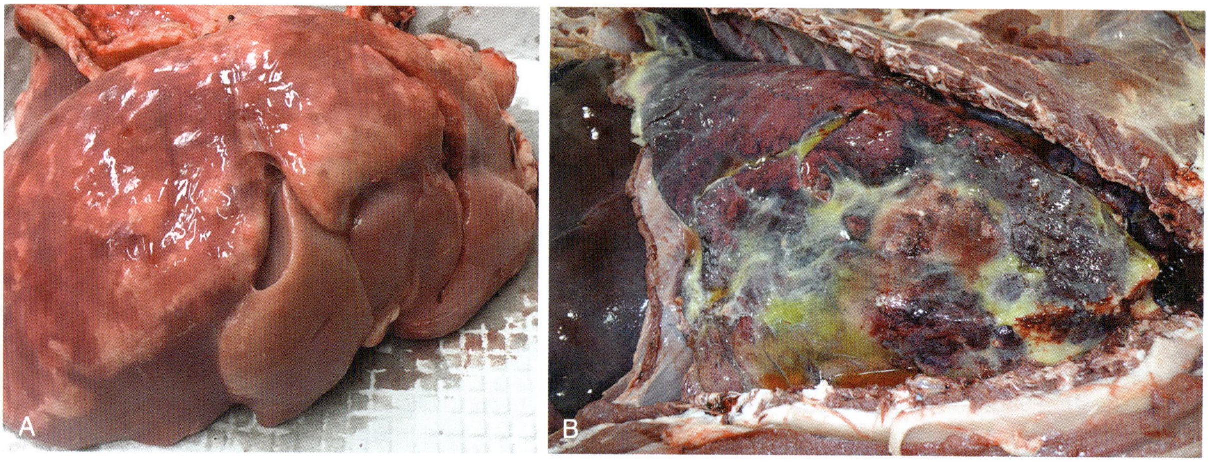

• **Fig. 7.6** **A.** Image of the right caudal lung lobe from an ovine with clinical pneumonia; dorsocaudal margin is oriented to the image left. Image demonstrates numerous disseminated dark abscesses near the parenchymal surface as well as focal areas of consolidation in the right middle lung lobe. **B.** Image of a lung of a white-tailed deer with severe fibrinous pneumonia. This lung was culture positive for *Pasteurella multocida.*

Prevention of pasteurellosis should be aimed at minimizing stress, an important factor in the development of the disease. At this time, no commercial vaccines are available for sheep and goats against *Pasteurella* or *Mannheimia* spp. Although commercial vaccines are available for cattle, they are aimed at a different strain from that typically detected in sheep and goats. Research has shown low efficacy of the commercial vaccine against *P. haemolytica* serotype A1 when used in goats.[47] Experimental intranasal vaccination produced elevated antibody levels in vaccinated goats but did not decrease disease in the vaccinated animals.[48] A study of vaccination of sheep in New Zealand with a commercially available vaccine did not show any difference in severity of disease or isolation of organism between vaccinated and unvaccinated animals.[49] Vaccination for predisposing infectious agents such as parainfluenza type 3, adenovirus type 6, respiratory syncytial virus, *Chlamydophila, B. parapertussis,* and *M. ovipneumoniae* could potentially be done using cattle vaccines when available. At present, no vaccines aimed at respiratory pathogens are labeled for use in small ruminants. Therefore, with institution of a vaccine program using cattle vaccines, a small sample group should be vaccinated first and monitored for potential reactions or side effects before vaccinating the entire herd or flock. Other management areas that should be evaluated in the face of a respiratory disease outbreak are ventilation and nutrition. Ventilation should be improved in barns to decrease the relative humidity and ensure adequate air exchange.

Mycoplasma Pneumonia

Mycoplasma pneumonia of sheep also is referred to as "enzootic pneumonia" or "atypical pneumonia." It is a chronic nonprogressive pneumonia of sheep caused by *M. ovipneumoniae.*[50,51] *P. haemolytica,* other *Mycoplasma* species, and *Chlamydophila psittaci ovis* all can act as secondary invaders after a mycoplasmal infection. In one study, *Mycoplasma* was isolated from 90% of animals with proven pneumonia in a slaughterhouse survey.[52] *Mycoplasma bovis* has been identified along with *T. pyogenes* as a cause of pneumonia in farmed white-tailed deer fawns.

Several predisposing factors may allow the development of *Mycoplasma* pneumonias. In addition to stress, minor viral pathogens also can predispose animals to *Mycoplasma* pneumonias. Intensively reared lambs in conditions of poor ventilation or assembled groups of lambs in feedlots are examples of groups in which *Mycoplasma* pneumonias are common. Older or convalescent animals can act as a reservoir for the other animals in the pen. Encapsulation of the organism allows it to evade the host immune system and is conducive to long-term colonization of the upper respiratory tract. Although pneumonia associated with *M. ovipneumoniae* is not common in goats, it has been reported occasionally.[53]

Transmission of *M. ovipneumoniae* is primarily through a respiratory route, either by direct contact or inhalation of an aerosol. *Mycoplasma* infections cause ciliostasis in the lungs and the production of exudate—factors that may predispose affected animals to secondary bacterial infections.[54] In some research trials, *Mycoplasma* infections appeared to limit the severity of *Pasteurella* infections.

Clinical Signs. *Mycoplasma* pneumonia in sheep usually is a mild disease. Typical clinical signs include chronic cough and dyspnea on exertion. When *Pasteurella* is involved, mucopurulent nasal discharge, fever, and depression also may be noted. Even in the presence of only mild clinical signs, *Mycoplasma* pneumonia causes a decrease in productivity in affected animals. Overall, *Mycoplasma* pneumonia is associated with high morbidity but low mortality, in keeping with the nonprogressive and subclinical nature of the infection.

Diagnosis. Diagnosis of mycoplasmal infection can be based on characteristic findings at necropsy. Such findings include consolidation of the cranial lung lobes and, occasionally, the anterior border of the caudal lobes. The consolidated areas appear gray to reddish-brown with red atelectatic areas. Gray-white nodules of a firm consistency also are visible on cut surfaces. Evidence of pleuritis may be seen as well. Histopathologic features are those of an interstitial, cuffing-type pneumonia, with nodular lymphoid hyperplasia and mononuclear lymphocytic cuffing around bronchioles and blood vessels. Exudate, composed mainly of macrophages and a few neutrophils, is observed within the alveoli. A characteristic feature of *Mycoplasma* infections is the presence of nodular hyaline "scars" in the bronchial walls. In recent research, however, these necropsy findings were present in only 60% of cases, and the remaining 40% of cases did not exhibit these pathologic features.[52] In addition to necropsy findings, culture of the organism in broth medium confirms the diagnosis. When samples are submitted for testing for *Mycoplasma,* it is important to specifically request this test from the diagnostic laboratory, because routine bacterial culture fails to grow this organism. Serologic studies can be performed to look for antibodies using the enzyme-linked immunosorbent assay (ELISA), but cross-reactivity is a possible concern.

Treatment. Treatment of *Mycoplasma* infections includes the use of oxytetracycline, tilmicosin, and florfenicol. Strategies for prevention of mycoplasmal disease include decreasing the stocking density of housed lambs, ensuring adequate ventilation in barns, and segregating lambs by age. No commercially approved vaccines against *M. ovipneumoniae* are currently available (see Appendix 1). Some laboratories are making autogenous vaccines, which have been anecdotally beneficial but to date no scientific evidence of benefit of use of these vaccines has been demonstrated.

Mycoplasma Infection in Goats

Several different but related *Mycoplasma* species are recognized to be associated with pneumonia in goats, with important differences in geographic distribution of the individual species. Collectively, these organisms are categorized as the *Mycoplasma mycoides* cluster of strains, including *M. mycoides* spp. *mycoides* Large Colony (MmmLC), *M. mycoides* spp. *capri* (Mmc), *Mycoplasma capricolum* spp. *capripneumoniae* (Mccp), and *M. capricolum* spp. *capricolum* (Mcc). Recently, this nomenclature has been slightly modified, with MmmLC being subsumed under the Mmc designation.[55] This change was based on a lack of ability to distinguish the two subspecies biochemically or by 16S sequencing.[56–60] This reclassification leaves three significant subspecies that are associated with disease in goats (and, in some cases, sheep). Both *M. mycoides* spp. *mycoides* and *M. capricolum* spp. *capricolum* are associated with mastitis, arthritis, keratitis, pneumonia, and septicemia in goats.[61] Both organisms have a worldwide distribution and have been documented in herds located within the United States[62–64] and elsewhere. One report found significant disease of dairy goat kids associated with *M. mycoides* spp. *mycoides* after apparent introduction of the organism into the herd by acquisition of a new group of animals that were found to be shedding these mycoplasmas in milk.[62] Significant morbidity and mortality were reported over a 1-year period, with necropsy demonstrating evidence of fibrinous arthritis, fibrinous pleuritis, interstitial pneumonia, and bronchopneumonia in some kids. Management changes associated with heat treatment of colostrum and feeding of pasteurized milk were successful at terminating the outbreak. In settings in which use of pasteurized milk is not practical, use of appropriately formulated milk replacer may be considered as an alternative intervention. This reported case also underscores the importance of biosecurity during herd introductions and inadequacy of colostrum management as a source of respiratory disease (see Chapters 16 and 19). Giaginis and co-workers reported the successful treatment of a herd-level outbreak of *M. capricolum* spp. *capricolum* disease with parenteral long-acting oxytetracycline therapy; however, other researchers in Jordan have demonstrated significant resistance of this organism to oxytetracycline.[61,65]

Mycoplasma spp. should be considered in any group of small ruminants demonstrating respiratory disease in conjunction with polyarthritis or mastitis. Because mycoplasmas do not grow well on routine media used for bacterial culture, it is important to notify the diagnostic laboratory that *Mycoplasma* culture is required in addition to routine procedures. To ensure accurate results, the laboratory's preferred methods for sample collection and transport should be confirmed. A variety of reports have demonstrated a role of the ear mite *Raillietia caprae* in transmission and maintenance of *Mycoplasma* spp. in goats.[66–68] The likelihood of *Mycoplasma* culture–positive earwax is increased in animals carrying the ear mite[67] compared with animals not infected with the ear mite; however, the exact role of the mites in transmission is still unclear. Sterile swabs can be collected from the ears of goats to test for the presence of subclinical carrier state. These swabs can be subjected to routine *Mycoplasma* culture or to newer PCR-based techniques that have a higher sensitivity and negative predictive value for the carrier state.[66] Clinical experience (specifically, of PJP) suggests that *Mycoplasma* culture is most effective when multiple types of *Mycoplasma* media are inoculated simultaneously, owing to differential growth on different media types.

Contagious caprine pleuropneumonia is a serious, highly transmissible respiratory disease of goats in Africa and Asia. It is caused by *M. capricolum* spp. *capripneumoniae* and is considered a foreign animal disease in the United States. Reports suggest that in many cases, entire herds of goats are affected, with mortality rates of 60 to 70%.[69,70] The clinical picture is that of an acute fulminant fibrinous pleuropneumonia, typically in the absence of polyarthritis or mastitis. Clinical suspicion of this disease process warrants contacting appropriate state health officials for further diagnostic input.

Chlamydophila Infection

Chlamydophila has been associated with cases of pneumonia in goats and sheep, but the clinical significance has not been fully determined. It has been theorized that *Chlamydophila* may cause a primary infection, with subsequent secondary invasion by *Pasteurella* or *Mannheimia,* but this possibility has not yet been proved. Clinical signs of *Chlamydophila* infection include depression, fever, dry, hacking cough, nasal discharge, dyspnea, and diarrhea. As suggested by our own experience, this organism should be considered when clinical respiratory disease appears simultaneously with herd or flock problems with septic arthritis, infertility, or abortions, since these are common signs of systemic chlamydial infection. Diagnosis includes identification of the organism on stained impression smears of the lung, immunofluorescence on fixed tissue sections, Gimenez staining, and yolk sac inoculation and isolation. Antibody titers using ELISA or complement fixation as well as real-time quantitative PCR assay are now commercially available and may provide more rapid and reproducible results. Available research data suggest that the PCR assay and ELISA show significant improvement in sensitivity over the complement fixation test.[71,72] Necropsy findings include consolidation of cranial lung lobes with interstitial changes. Histopathologic examination reveals intracytoplasmic elementary bodies within alveolar macrophages. Edematous septa and thickened bronchioles also are observed. Turgid exudate can be seen when the lungs are compressed. *Chlamydophila* infections usually are treatable with tetracycline antibiotics, although long-term therapy may be necessary. Tetracyclines also can be used during an outbreak in an attempt to slow or decrease spread of the disease. Published research in cattle and unpublished data in goats suggest that this organism may be more widespread than was previously believed and that disease outbreaks tend to be associated with changes in stress, environmental conditions, or immune status.[73] Further research is required; confirmation of these findings, however, would result in a situation in which management of stressors could provide the primary mechanism of disease control, as opposed to biosecurity.

Viral Pneumonias

Viral pneumonias generally are associated with fairly mild disease and clinical signs but can act as a predisposing factor for bacterial pneumonias. A number of viral agents have been identified as potential causes of viral pneumonia in sheep and goats.

Parainfluenza Type 3

Parainfluenza type 3 (PI3) is a member of the paramyxovirus family of RNA viruses. PI3 virus infections in sheep appear to be caused by a serotype other than those responsible for PI3 viral infections in cattle and humans. Seroprevalence rates for PI3 are reported at 24 to 87.2%.[74–77] The high end of this range suggests that many infections with PI3 are very mild, with few clinical disease manifestations.

Clinical signs associated with PI3 infections include frequent coughing, serous nasal discharge, and occasional ocular discharge. Fever is rare. Clinically apparent disease is more common in animals younger than 1 year of age. Diagnosis can be made using virus isolation, but infections should be less than 1 week in duration to permit a reasonable chance of isolating the virus. In herds or flocks in which PI3 infections are a problem, vaccination with a live intranasal vaccine aimed at PI3 may be attempted to decrease the incidence of disease. Live intranasal vaccine is available for cattle that could be used off-label in sheep and goats. One research trial showed protective effects of a commercial cattle vaccine in ewes and a decrease in the incidence of pneumonia in that flock.[78]

Adenovirus

Adenovirus is a DNA virus with multiple antigenic types. Depending on the serotype, seroprevalence ranges from 7 to 83%.[76,77] At this time, the clinical significance of adenovirus infection is not completely understood. Generally, adenovirus-associated disease is fairly mild, but the severity increases when a secondary bacterial infection is present. Adenovirus infections typically are seen in young lambs with both respiratory and enteric disease. Clinical signs of adenovirus infection include fever, anorexia, sneezing, and serous nasal discharge. Necropsy findings include atelectasis and hyperemia, mainly in the cranioventral portions of the lungs.[79] Histopathologic lesions include detachment and sloughing of foci of epithelial cells of the terminal bronchioles and alveoli.[79] Diagnosis of adenovirus infections is based on either virus isolation or paired serology samples. No vaccine for adenovirus is currently available in the United States.

Respiratory Syncytial Virus

Respiratory syncytial virus (RSV) is a pneumovirus that is a member of the paramyxovirus family. RSV infection is an important respiratory disease in cattle, but at present its importance in sheep and goats is unclear. As with the other viral agents, RSV is believed to predispose affected animals to secondary bacterial pneumonias. Studies have shown a range of seroprevalence rates from 27.5 to 84.5%.[74–77,80,81] Two different subgroups of RSV have been recognized, one in calves and goats and the other in sheep. Necropsy findings in experimentally infected lambs included bronchiolitis obliterans with destruction of the mucociliary apparatus, the presence of syncytial cells in alveoli, and a progressive interstitial reaction.[82]

Clinical Signs. Clinical signs of RSV infection include anorexia, fever, conjunctivitis, cough, tachypnea, and tachycardia. Thoracic auscultation reveals increased bronchial sounds and crackles in some cases. Friction rubs also may be auscultated in cases of mixed infection.

Diagnosis. Necropsy findings include a diffuse interstitial pneumonia, and the lungs are firm and edematous. Observation of syncytial cells on histopathologic examination is considered to be characteristic of RSV infection. Immunoperoxidase staining may reveal the presence of RSV antigen in epithelial cells of alveolar and bronchial walls and syncytial and alveolar lumens.

Prevention. Currently, no vaccine for RSV is available for use in sheep and goats. The use of a commercial cattle monovalent modified live virus vaccine against RSV has been recommended by some investigators in the face of an outbreak of RSV disease in a herd or flock, but no research has been done on the efficacy of this vaccine in sheep or goats. Furthermore, commercial monovalent vaccines for cattle are not yet available.

Herpesvirus

An ovine and caprine herpesvirus has been isolated from lung and nasal swabs during *Pasteurella* outbreaks. The role that this virus plays in the development of disease is unclear at this time. Ovine and caprine herpesvirus has been associated with rhinitis, vulvovaginitis, and, in some reports, abortions. After an experimental challenge with ovine-caprine herpesvirus, clinical rhinitis, along with histopathologic lesions of tracheitis, was observed. None of the animals in the study, however, exhibited severe clinical disease. Some reports have shown that the virus may go into a latent state. A PCR assay specific to caprine herpesvirus is now commercially available. Gammaherpesviruses including OHV-2 and a closely related but distinct strain have been implicated in cases of clinical malignant catarrhal fever (MCF) in deer.

Diagnostic Plan. Box 7.1 shows an approach to diagnosis of a respiratory disease outbreak.

Treatment. Treatment of lower respiratory disease in sheep and goats is aimed primarily at the bacterial infection. Viral infections may predispose affected animals to secondary bacterial infections, but viral infections alone do not typically cause severe clinical disease. Treatment of bacterial pneumonias should be based on culture and sensitivity testing of the organism in either tracheal or transtracheal wash samples or swabs obtained at necropsy. Until culture results are obtained, empirical antibiotic therapy should be initiated. Research has shown little antibiotic resistance in respiratory pathogens, most of which apparently are susceptible to commonly used antibiotics. However, some resistance to tetracyclines, which are readily available over the counter at the present time, has been reported. If no response is seen within 48 h after administration of a specific agent, then an alternative antibiotic should be tried. Evidence of clinical response may include improved appetite, decreased fever (unless antiinflammatories have been used), and return to the animal's usual attitude/demeanor. In addition to antibiotic therapy, fluid support and use of an antiinflammatory should be considered in the

• BOX 7.1 Approach to Respiratory Disease Outbreak Management

Outbreak Assessment

- Set case definition based on clinical signs.
- Determine morbidity and mortality data based on case definition.
- Identify age of animal affected.
- Monitor clinical progression of disease and response to treatment.

Diagnostic Sampling

Desired Samples With Acute Infections

- Select on basis of case definition above.
- Sample before treatment.
- Sample four to six animals minimum (ideally).
- Select appropriate test for suspected disease process.

Necropsy Results and Diagnostics

- Do these fit with the results for acute sampling?

Development of Standard Operating Procedures

Procedures must be established that support compliance with extra-label drug use requirements and ensure appropriate and consistent management. Protocol components include:

- Detailed case definition and selection criteria described in a manner understandable by all personnel
- Decision tree to determine if treatment is necessary
- Treatment instructions:
  - Drug to use
  - Frequency
  - Route
  - Withdrawal
- Assessment of treatment efficacy and retreatment algorithm
- Assessment and modification of vaccine protocols
- Assessment and modification of management (failure of passive transfer) and facilities

Record Keeping

- Record identification data and findings for all animals examined and treated.
- Maintain drug use and withdrawal paperwork.
- Assess disease outbreak progression and improvement.
- Generate evidence-based medicine data on response to therapy.

systemically ill patient. In valuable animals with severe respiratory disease, if severe dyspnea is present, oxygen therapy also may be of some benefit. All patients with respiratory disease should be separated from the rest of the flock or herd if possible and given easy access to food and water.

Control of Respiratory Disease

Control and prevention of respiratory disease in sheep, goats, and deer revolve primarily around environmental and stress management. Animals should be housed in well-ventilated but not drafty environments with an adequate number of air changes to prevent accumulation of noxious odors. Adequate transfer of passive immunity from dam to offspring through the colostrum is of utmost importance in the prevention and control of respiratory disease in young ruminants. On account of the lack of commercially available vaccines against all clinically important bacterial and viral small ruminant strains, most herd management programs do not include a vaccination plan for control of respiratory disease.

Other Acute Respiratory Disease

Verminous Pneumonia

Three primary lungworms of small ruminants are of clinical and economic importance: *Dictyocaulus* spp. filaria (including *Dictyocaulus viviparous* and *Dictyocaulus eckerti,* both of which have been demonstrated to cross infect multiple species including deer), *Muellerius capillaris,* and *Protostrongylus rufescens.* Of these, *M. capillaris* seems to be the most prevalent in the United States, with two studies performed in the eastern states showing prevalence rates upwards of 60% in goat herds.[83,84] In other parts of the world, prevalence rates of 100% in adult goats have been reported.[85] *D. filaria* has a direct life cycle, with a prepatent period of roughly 4 weeks after ingestion of infective larvae.[86] By contrast, both *M. capillaris* and *P. rufescens* have an indirect life cycle and require an intermediate molluscan host.[86] Goats appear to be more likely than sheep to demonstrate clinical disease after infection with *M. capillaris*, and the lesions more typically are interstitial in goats, whereas they more often are subpleural in sheep.[86]

Clinical signs are highly variable and are completely absent in some infected animals. The most common sign of disease is a cough, and in some cases, secondary bacterial infections may occur.[86] Diagnosis is made at necropsy; the diaphragmatic lung lobes are seen to be most affected, and nodular (*M. capillaris*) or lobular lesions that contain the worm may be present.[86] One study that evaluated severity of the lesions showed that an average of 35.1% (in kids) and 23.5% (in adults) of the lung surface was affected by parasite lesions.[85] Antemortem diagnosis traditionally has been obtained by means of a standard Baermann fecal exam; however, some evidence indicates that the Baermann procedure using the flask recovery method is more reliable than the funnel method commonly used in some laboratories.[87] In that study, 175% greater recovery rates were obtained with the flask method than with the funnel method. Therapy relies on traditional anthelmintics including moxidectin, fenbendazole, albendazole, oxfendazole, and ivermectin.[87–92] Research suggests that some immature stages of the worms may not be sensitive to all products, and that two or three doses administered at 35-day intervals may provide the greatest cure rates (see Chapter 6).[93]

Aspiration Pneumonia

Inhalation of significant amounts of feedstuffs or liquids leads to an intense inflammatory response and the development of aspiration pneumonia. This clinical scenario may be secondary to dysphagia or laryngeal paralysis. Aspiration pneumonia also may occur as an iatrogenic disorder secondary to forced delivery of liquids or application of drenches. The severity of the condition reflects the type of material present and the amount of material inhaled. Treatment consists of broad-spectrum antibiotics and antiinflammatory drugs. The prognosis for animals with this condition is guarded, and the condition often progresses until death or euthanasia supervenes.

Lentiviral Disease

Ovine Progressive Pneumonia

Ovine progressive pneumonia (OPP) is a chronic progressive pneumonia of sheep caused by a non-oncogenic, single-stranded RNA lentivirus of the Retroviridae family. OPP also is referred to as *maedi-visna* outside of North America. This disease plays an important economic role in the sheep industry in North America, causing economic losses related to decreased production and decreased sales. The magnitude of effect OPP has on the economics of sheep production varies with the reported study. One set of studies showed no negative effect on the number of lambs produced or on grease weight of fleece in a comparison of seropositive ewes with seronegative ewes within the same flocks.[94] On the other hand, research also has shown an estimated 10% decrease in milk production associated with indurative mastitis.[95] Additional research has shown that OPP infections can decrease weight gain and increase 30-day mortality rates in lambs.[95,96]

Once a sheep is infected with OPP, the virus persists in infected monocytes and macrophages and is capable of entering a latent stage for an undetermined period. OPP may occur in goats, but very infrequently.[97,98] Instances of cross-species transmission as well as recombination between the two viruses in vivo in mixed-species flocks have been reported.[99,100] OPP has a long incubation time, averaging 2 to 4 years. Owing to this prolonged incubation, clinical signs of OPP usually are seen in older animals. The seroprevalence of OPP varies depending on the region. One study showed a seroprevalence of 0.5% in a group of 2040 sheep in West Texas.[101] Another study showed a seroprevalence of 49% in sheep in the Rocky Mountain region.[101] Subsequent research showed a prevalence of 26.8% in cull ewes in Alberta, Canada and a seroprevalence rate of 44% in a slaughterhouse survey reported from Quebec.[102,103] In all published studies, seroprevalence increases with age.

Transmission. Transmission of OPP is through several routes. The most common route of transmission is through ingestion of infected colostrum or milk by a neonate.[104] Direct transmission, most likely through respiratory droplets, also has been reported. Vertical transmission has been rarely observed.[104] Close confinement and more than transient exposure of uninfected animals to infected ones both play an important role in transmission.

The OPP virus has a strong predilection to mutate and form new serovars. This antigenic drift, with continual production of new serovars, results in different patterns of disease. Some animals remain asymptomatic carriers for life, without ever developing clinical disease, but shed infective organisms into the environment. Once an animal is infected, it remains viremic for life.

After infection has occurred, the virus localizes to the lungs, central nervous system, and hematopoietic tissues. Within the lungs, the virus stimulates the reticular cells and lymphocytes to proliferate. This proliferative process leads to the thickening of the intraalveolar septa and produces adenomatosis of the alveolar lining.[105] OPP is a chronic degenerative condition with a slow, progressive nature.

Clinical Signs. Initial clinical signs may be subtle and may even go unnoticed, generally appearing only after periods of stress, exertion, or inclement weather. Initially, the producer may happen to observe an animal that just seems listless or dragging behind the flock. Regional lymphadenopathy is common in infected animals. Other disease manifestations may include indurative lymphocytic mastitis ("hardbag," see later), proliferative arthritis, and, less commonly, nonsuppurative encephalitis (Chapter 13).[93] The affected animal gradually becomes emaciated despite a good appetite. Dyspnea develops and is initially apparent only after exertion or exercise. In most cases, fever is absent unless a secondary bacterial pneumonia develops. Other findings may include nasal discharge and coughing, but lung auscultation reveals no abnormalities. As the disease progresses, open-mouth breathing, flaring of the nostrils, forced expirations, and worsening of coughing are noted. The clinical course may be as short as 3 to 6 months, but in some animals, the illness may persist for years. Although the primary clinical signs are respiratory in nature, arthritis, vasculitis, mastitis, encephalitis, and, rarely, posterior paresis also may be observed. The mastitis associated with OPP is described as an indurative mastitis in which a large, hard udder is palpated but no abnormal secretions are observed. This condition frequently is referred to as hardbag. Posterior neurologic manifestations frequently begin as ataxia, stumbling, and unilateral proprioceptive deficits, which progress over weeks to months to rear limb paralysis or occasionally quadriplegia.[105] Clinicopathologic studies occasionally reveal a moderate hypochromic anemia and leukocytosis; hypergammaglobulinemia is observed in advanced cases. Unfortunately, the case fatality rate is 100%, with most animals either dying or culled within 1 year of onset of clinical signs.

Diagnosis. Several options are available for diagnosis of OPP. Serologic testing includes both the ELISA and the agar gel immunodiffusion (AGID) test. Several ELISAs are available, and ELISA testing in general has been shown to be more sensitive than AGID testing.[95,106] PCR testing also is available and is more economical than virus isolation. PCR testing can be used for confirmation after a positive result on AGID or ELISA testing.[95] Current recommendations for testing and eradication are available at the OPP Concerned Sheep Breeders Society Website (http://www.oppsociety.org).

Necropsy of animals infected with OPP reveals large, heavy lungs, two to three times the normal weight. Occasionally, vertical rib impressions can be seen in the lungs owing to the degree of swelling of the lung tissue. The lungs are firm in consistency and gray-blue to gray-yellow and do not collapse.[105] In some instances, a secondary bacterial pneumonia may be observed. Tracheobronchial and mediastinal lymph nodes are enlarged, gray to white in appearance, and bulge on cut surface.[105] If evidence of arthritis is observed, it is generally the appendicular joints that are involved. Extensive proliferation of the synovium, fibrosis of the joint capsule, and degenerative changes of the articular cartilage and bone are observed.[105] Findings on gross examination of the spinal cord and brain are normal. Histopathologic lesions are those of a chronic, diffuse interstitial pneumonia. Hyperplasia of lymphoid cells around airways and blood vessels also are seen with an accumulation of mononuclear cells in the interstitium. Occasionally, characteristic changes of lymphocytic meningitis, choroiditis, or leukoencephalitis also may be observed.

Prevention. Prevention of OPP requires eliminating the virus from the flock. No vaccines are available for OPP. In order to eliminate OPP from a flock, the flock must be closed to new additions, and a rigorous testing and cull program must be instituted. The entire flock should be tested for OPP, and all seropositive animals along with any offspring that are younger than 1 year of age should be removed from the flock and raised at a separate facility.[107] All lambs should be fed OPP-negative colostrum (either from a negative ewe or heat-treated), milk, or milk replacer. The entire flock should be tested two times a year until two consecutive negative results are obtained. All seropositive animals must be removed from the herd. Once OPP has been eradicated from a flock, any new additions should be quarantined and tested for OPP before introduction into the flock.

Caprine Arthritis-Encephalitis

Caprine arthritis-encephalitis (CAE) is caused by a virus closely related to the agent of OPP (both are lentiviruses). Although respiratory disease is not the typical primary clinical manifestation of CAE, respiratory signs can be seen as a part of the disease process. Transmission of CAE is similar to that of OPP, primarily through ingestion of virus-infected colostrum or milk from an infected animal.[108] Horizontal transmission also is possible. Interstitial disease occurs with CAE and manifests as a chronic pneumonia with weight loss and dyspnea. The pulmonary lesions typically are distributed in the caudal or cranioventral lung lobes and closely resemble those seen in the lungs of animals affected with OPP. Diagnosis can be made through serologic testing or histopathologic examination (see Chapters 13 and 16).

Caseous Lymphadenitis

Caseous lymphadenitis is an abscess disease in sheep, goats, and, occasionally, deer caused by the bacterium *C. pseudotuberculosis*. This Gram-positive rod is found in manure, soil, and on the skin of infected herd or flock animals, and can be detected in infected organs upon necropsy examination. The organism is capable of surviving in the environment for long periods, so the environment can be a potential source of infection or reinfection. The organism enters the body through superficial wounds or mucous membranes or on contact with fomites such as shearing blades, feeders, grooming equipment, and bedding. Once *C. pseudotuberculosis* enters the body, it follows the lymphatics and migrates to the local lymph nodes; it then disseminates to the rest of the body, where it forms abscesses in lymph nodes.[109] These abscesses can be found in either peripheral or internal lymph nodes. The location of the affected lymph nodes affects the clinical presentation. With involvement of the retropharyngeal or thoracic lymph nodes, the affected animal may display clinical signs of respiratory disease such as dyspnea, tachypnea, and chronic cough, in addition to chronic weight loss.

Diagnosis. Diagnosis of caseous lymphadenitis can be based on identification of abscesses on radiographs (Figure 7.7) or culture of the organism from either a transtracheal wash sample or an abscess. Within the thoracic cavity, abscesses can be seen in the lung parenchyma, mediastinal lymph nodes, or the bronchial lymph nodes.[109] Abdominal and skeletal lymph nodes are less commonly affected. Internal involvement is seen more commonly in older animals.

Prevention. Prevention of caseous lymphadenitis is aimed at identifying all affected animals and removing them from the herd or flock. Serologic testing using the synergistic hemolysis inhibition (SHI) or ELISA test can be used to identify potential infected animals before the development of clinical signs or animals with internal involvement.[110] Animals that have been previously vaccinated test positive on the SHI test, so serologic testing is of little benefit in a vaccinated flock or herd.[110] Owing to the organism's ability to survive in the environment, it also is important to prevent contamination of the environment and transmission to other animals whenever possible. Good hygienic practices such as cleaning clipper and shearing blades can help to limit the spread of this disease. A vaccine is available and is labeled for use in sheep. The vaccine does not eliminate caseous lymphadenitis from a herd or flock but decreases the incidence of disease and reduces its severity.[110] Although use of the vaccine in goats constitutes an extra-label application, a vaccination program has been used successfully in goat herds to limit the spread of disease. Severe local reactions, anecdotally seen more commonly when the vaccine includes clostridial toxoids, consisting of large, firm swellings at the vaccination site have been reported; owners must be cautioned regarding the potential for such reactions before use of this vaccine in goats.

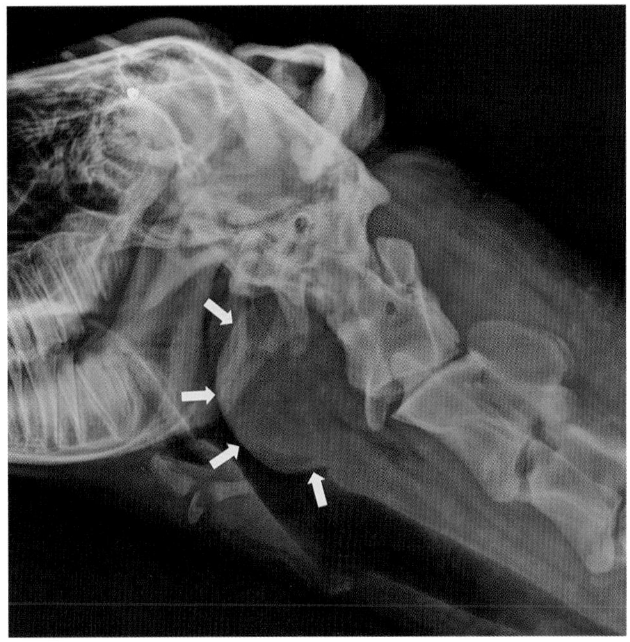

• **Fig. 7.7** Lateral radiograph of the pharyngeal region of a yearling ram with *Corynebacterium pseudotuberculosis* retropharyngeal lymph node abscess; cranial is to image left. The abscess (outlined by white arrows) can be seen as a 6-cm rounded mass caudal to the angle of the mandible. (Courtesy Dr. Jennifer Schleining).

Coccidioidomycosis

Coccidioidomycosis, caused by the soil fungus *Coccidioides immitis,* has been rarely reported in small ruminants. It is transmitted through inhalation, and possibly ingestion or cutaneous abrasions. This disease is enzootic in the southwestern United States.

Coccidioidomycosis is not a contagious disease. Clinical signs include chronic weight loss and a persistent cough. Occasionally fever and peripheral lymph node abscesses also are observed. On necropsy, granulomas containing creamy purulent material are seen and frequently are located in the bronchial or mediastinal lymph nodes. Diagnosis of coccidioidomycosis relies on the use of either an intradermal test or a complement fixation test. Culture of the organism or identification on microbiologic exam also can be diagnostic. No treatment or vaccination is available for coccidioidomycosis.

Tuberculosis

Tuberculosis in sheep, goats, and deer is caused by the bacterium *Mycobacterium bovis*. Goats are affected more commonly than sheep. Occasionally, *Mycobacterium avium* and *Mycobacterium tuberculosis* also have been reported to cause small ruminant disease. An increase in prevalence of tuberculosis has been seen in herds or flocks that are in close proximity to infected cattle or wildlife.

Transmission of tuberculosis generally is through the respiratory tract. Infectious organisms can be found in respiratory secretions, feces, milk, urine, vaginal secretions, semen, and draining lymph nodes. Once the tuberculosis bacillus enters through the respiratory tract, it invades the local lymph nodes and causes granuloma formation with central necrosis of the lymph node. Occasionally, abdominal involvement is observed, suggesting that ingestion may be a possible route of transmission.

Clinical Signs. Clinical signs of tuberculosis include weight loss and mild respiratory signs. Early in the course of the disease, affected animals exhibit a deep, moist-sounding, chronic cough. As the disease progresses, tachypnea, dyspnea, and abnormal lung sounds develop.

Diagnosis. Diagnosis in sheep and goats starts with the intradermal skin test at the caudal tail fold. False-positive results can occur with this test owing to cross-reactivity with *Mycobacterium paratuberculosis, M. avium,* or *M. tuberculosis.* In the United States, all positive or suspect test results must be reported to the state veterinarian, and tuberculosis itself is a reportable disease. In deer, the approved antemortem test for tuberculosis includes the cervical intradermal test and a relatively newer blood test offered through the National Veterinary Services Laboratory. Necropsy reveals granulomatous lymph nodes. The lymph nodes are encapsulated and contain yellow to orange, creamy to caseous purulent material and gritty foci. Respiratory lymph nodes are affected more frequently than liver or mesenteric lymph nodes and cervids often demonstrate involvement of the retropharyngeal lymph nodes. Histopathologic findings include presence of acid-fast organisms and central calcification and caseation surrounded by zones of epithelioid cells and Langerhans giant cells, all enclosed in fibrous capsules.[1]

Prevention. Prevention of tuberculosis is based on the identification and culling of all seropositive animals. All animals older than 12 months of age on the farm should be tested annually; with two consecutive all-negative results, the herd or flock can be considered to be free of tuberculosis. A national program is in place in the United States to eradicate tuberculosis from all livestock species and is based on an aggressive testing and cull program.

M. bovis is a zoonotic agent, and care should be taken in handling these animals.

Pneumocystis jirovecii (Pneumocystis carinii) Pneumonia

Pneumocystis jirovecii (formerly called *Pneumocystis carinii*) is a sporozoan more familiar as the cause of debilitating pneumonia in people with AIDS, although this fungus can cause infection in small ruminants as well. Affected animals usually have a history of chronic disease associated with some form of immunosuppression, allowing the pathogen to become established. Clinical signs include fever, weight loss, tachypnea, mucopurulent nasal discharge, chronic cough, weakness, and tachycardia, with progression to death. Necropsy of lungs from affected animals reveals diffuse and locally extensive interstitial pneumonia. Important diseases to rule out in making a diagnosis are tuberculosis and caseous lymphadenitis. No effective treatment is available for *Pneumocystis* pneumonia.

Ovine Pulmonary Carcinoma

Ovine pulmonary adenocarcinoma (OPA) also is known as sheep pulmonary carcinoma (SPA) or "jaagsiekte." Ovine pulmonary carcinoma is a slowly progressive, contagious viral infection caused by a retrovirus. An age-related susceptibility pattern has been observed, with neonates and lambs younger than 10 weeks of age being most susceptible to the disease. The natural occurrence rate is low in goats, but OPA has been experimentally transmitted in kids. OPA is seen worldwide (except for Australia) and may be either a sporadic occurrence or endemic within a region. High virus concentrations within lung fluids or nasal exudates are characteristic. The disease has been observed as a concomitant finding in some animals with OPP. Clinical signs typically are seen in 2- to 4-year-old animals and include progressive respiratory distress, tachypnea, and weight loss. Auscultation of the lungs after exertion reveals harsh lung sounds and sometimes crackles and wheezes. Coughing is only an occasional sign and is not a consistent finding. Fluid draining from the nostrils can be observed when the animal lowers its head or the rear end of the animal is elevated. Fever typically is absent, and most animals maintain their appetite unless a secondary bacterial pneumonia develops. OPA is a progressive disease, and death occurs within weeks to months of the development of clinical signs. Diagnosis is based on necropsy findings. On examination of the abnormally heavy lungs, a clear exudate is present on cut surfaces, and clear, foamy fluid is seen within the trachea. Large gray masses with a firm consistency are observed in the cranioventral lobes; smaller masses are present in the caudodorsal lung lobes. The tumors have been described as alveolar type II or nonciliated bronchiolar cells. Metastasis to the bronchial or mediastinal lymph nodes occurs in 10% of the cases. At present, no treatment or vaccine is available. Eradication programs have been based on extensive slaughtering, because no antemortem test is available at this time.

Extrapulmonary Disease

Pleuritis and Pleural Abscesses

Pathogenesis. Pleuritis is rare in the small ruminant, in which the condition usually is secondary to another pathologic process such as pneumonia, abscesses (pleural, pseudotuberculosis, liver, or sternal), trauma, hypoproteinemia, septicemia (including clostridial), and tumors.[1,8] *Mannheimia, Pasteurella,* and *Mycoplasma* are the most common bacterial causes of caprine pleuropneumonia[1]; *Helcococcus ovis* also has been reported to cause pleuritis and bronchopneumonia in sheep.[111] Pleural transudates result from hypoproteinemia, right heart failure, neoplasia, or acorn toxicity.[8]

Clinical Signs. Affected animals may present with weight loss, decreased production, fever, depression, pain and posturing, dyspnea, and restricted respiratory effort. Percussible fluid lines, friction rubs, and attenuated lung sounds may be present on auscultation; however, these clinical findings are not present in all cases, and normal findings on auscultation are possible with focal pleural abscesses.[112]

Diagnosis. Clinicopathologic findings may include an inflammatory leukogram, mild anemia of chronic disease, and hyperglobulinemia in chronic cases. An ultrasound exam is helpful and may be necessary to diagnose focal pleural abscesses.[112] Thoracocentesis, fluid analysis, and culture (when indicated) can help determine the cause of the effusion and guide the therapeutic plan.

Treatment. The underlying disease needs to be treated. Lavage through a chest tube with a commercially available lavage system is indicated in cases of pleuritis and can be performed as a standing procedure with use of local anesthesia. A large-bore chest tube should be inserted caudally in the fifth or sixth intercostal space, at the costochondral junction (level of the elbow). Use of ultrasound guidance, if available, is recommended. Generally, a single tube can be used for both lavage and drainage.[113] Focal pleural abscesses may respond to prolonged antibiotic therapy.[112]

Diaphragmatic Hernia

Diaphragmatic hernias may be congenital or acquired, usually secondary to parturition, breeding (in males), or trauma. The clinical signs vary, depending on which organ or organs herniate; in small ruminants, the reticulum most commonly is involved.[8] Dyspnea, weakness, cachexia, muffled lung sounds, and thoracic borborygmi may be noted.[113] Diagnosis is made by radiographic or ultrasound imaging. Surgical repair has been described in other species and should be applicable to sheep and goats. An important point in this context is that the relatively small size of sheep and goats makes the surgical exposure of the diaphragm more like that in a large dog than in other farm animals. The biggest challenge in repairing diaphragmatic hernias in adult cattle and horses is the considerable depth of the abdominal cavity and size of the diaphragm. Size considerations are why clinicians occasionally need to resort to paracostal, paramedian thoracotomy or some combination of incisions to repair diaphragmatic rents in those adult species. Adequate exposure of any diaphragmatic hernia in sheep and goats, however, should be possible through a cranially placed ventral midline laparotomy incision. Use of a tilt table for surgery and large visceral retractors also enhances the surgical exposure. The animal should be fasted for 48 h before the procedure to decrease rumen fill. A rumenotomy may be indicated for the same reason if the animal's condition dictates emergency surgery rather than waiting 48 h (see Chapter 5). The hernia can be repaired with large monofilament (absorbable or nonabsorbable) suture in a continuous mattress stitch pattern. Mesh should be used only when the hernia cannot be closed otherwise, and a clean surgical environment is imperative.[113]

Pneumothorax

Pneumothorax is uncommon in small ruminants. When it occurs, it generally is unilateral. Causes include trauma, predator attack, and rupture of emphysematous bulla. Animals present with inspiratory dyspnea, increased abdominal effort, and decreased lung sounds on the affected side. During percussion, a difference in resonance can be appreciated between the two sides. The diagnosis is confirmed with chest radiographs. A chest tube with a one-way valve should be placed dorsally in the caudal lung field on the affected side. The tube should be inserted in the caudal portion of the intercostal space, to avoid damaging the intercostal vessels running along the caudal rib margins. The skin incision should be placed 1 to 2 cm further caudally so that the tube then tunnels under the skin to penetrate the body wall, creating a seal. Prophylactic antibiotics are indicated to prevent pleuritis.[113]

Neoplasia

Parenchymal Tumors

Ovine pulmonary carcinoma has already been discussed in detail (under "Lentiviral Disease"). Other reported rare parenchymal tumors are rhabdomyosarcoma in lambs and multiple pulmonary papillae in Angora goats.[114]

Thoracic Cavity Tumors. The more common thoracic cavity tumors include thymomas, thymic lymphoma, mediastinal lymphoma, pleural mesothelioma, and squamous cell carcinoma. Thymomas are by far the most common tumor in goats[115,116] and are characterized as epithelial or lymphocytic origin tumors of adult goats and sheep.[115,117] By contrast, thymic lymphoma is a form of lymphoma that originates at the thymus and may metastasize to other organs and structures such as lymph nodes, liver, spleen, kidney, and lung. Thymic lymphoma is more common in young animals, although it has been reported in adult sheep.[117]

Clinical Signs. These thoracic tumors are space-occupying masses and as such may cause additional pleuritis and effusion.[114] Caseous lymphadenitis abscesses also may act as a space-occupying thoracic mass and should be included in the differential diagnosis. Animals may be asymptomatic (thymomas often are an incidental finding during slaughter[114]) or present with progressive dyspnea, a history of recurrent/intermittent mild to moderate bloat (type I vagal indigestion), cachexia, and exercise intolerance. An enlargement at the thoracic inlet may be palpated. Coughing secondary to tracheal displacement and congestive heart failure may occur.[115,116] Although myasthenia gravis is not associated with caprine thymomas,[115] one case of secondary megaesophagus has been reported in a goat.[118]

Diagnosis. Tumor margins, mineralization, and organ displacement may be seen on radiographic or ultrasound images.[115] Cytologic analysis of pleural fluid or tumor aspirate can be performed, but thymomas and thymic lymphomas often require a biopsy sample for diagnosis. Even ultrasound-guided biopsy may not provide sufficient tissue; the definitive diagnosis often is made at necropsy with histopathologic examination. In theory, thymomas may be surgically removed; thymic lymphomas and mesotheliomas frequently are metastatic or widespread in the pleural cavity and are not amenable to surgical excision.[114]

Plant Toxicity

Atypical Interstitial Pneumonia

Pathogenesis. Perilla mint *(Perilla frutescens)* contains a pneumotoxin in the leaves and seeds that when metabolized in the rumen produces toxic intermediaries. These substances damage type I pneumocytes and bronchiolar epithelial cells. The cellular injury results in formation of hyaline membranes, type II pneumocyte proliferation, and adenomatosis. The plant is most toxic during the flowering and seed stages of growth (August to October). Other similarly toxic plants include moldy sweet potato (the mold *Fusarium solani* produces the toxin 4-ipomeanol) and the *Brassica* genus of plants (e.g., rape, kale, turnip, and beet tops), which contain D,L-tryptophan. D,L-Tryptophan is converted in the rumen to the toxic 3-methyl indole intermediate.[1,8]

Clinical Signs. Clinical signs include acute dyspnea and tachypnea, open-mouth breathing, extended head and neck posturing, and acute death. Signs may be induced or exacerbated by exertion and stress.

Diagnosis. Diagnosis is based on clinical presentation and history. On necropsy, the lungs are wet, heavy, emphysematous, and noncollapsing; rib impressions may be observed. Histopathologic examination should confirm interstitial edema, emphysema, congestion, and alveolar epithelial hyperplasia.[8]

Treatment. Treatment should focus on minimizing stress and excitement and providing general supportive care. Of note, moving animals from pasture has been associated with increased mortalities, so fencing or confining them locally away from the toxic plants and providing appropriate shade should be considered.

Hydrogen Cyanide Toxicity

Pathogenesis. Under stress or in response to damage (such as from wilt, frost, or drought), cyanogenic glycoside plants produce hydrogen cyanide (HCN) (Table 7.1). Subsequent to ingestion of the offending plant, HCN blocks cellular respiration, resulting in tissue hypoxia. Under normal conditions, the liver can detoxify HCN; sheep can tolerate 22 mg of HCN/50 kg of body weight/hour.[119]

Clinical Signs. Clinical signs appear when the liver capacity is overwhelmed. Rapid intake of 2 to 4 mg HCN/kg of body weight is fatal. Sheep and cattle are more susceptible than goats.[8] Affected animals often are found dead. If HCN disease causing exposure is recognized early, permitting tracking of the clinical course, dyspnea, and other signs of cerebral anoxia such as anxiety, staggering, tremors, and terminal convulsions can be observed. The blood is bright red from hemoglobin-bound oxygen.[119]

Diagnosis. The rumen contents may have a characteristic "bitter almond" odor.[1] Liver and rumen contents can be tested for HCN concentrations; threshold values are 1.4 μg and 10 μg, respectively.[8] Samples should be quickly frozen or treated with 1 to 3% mercuric chloride to prevent postsampling loss of HCN.[119] Forage and plants also can be tested; HCN levels above 200 ppm are toxic.[119] The "picrate paper" test is easily performed in the

TABLE 7.1 Nitrate-Accumulating and Cyanogenic Glycoside–Producing Plants.

NITRATE-ACCUMULATING PLANTS		CYANOGENIC GLYCOSIDE–PRODUCING PLANTS	
Weeds			
Canada thistle	*Cirsium arvense*	Apple	*Pyrus malus*
Cheeseweed	*Malva parviflora*	Arrow grass	*Triglochin maritima*
Dock	*Rumex* spp.	Birdsfoot trefoil	*Lotus corniculatus*
Fireweed	*Kochia scoparia*	Cassava	*Manihot esculenta*
Jimsonweed	*Datura* spp.	Cherry, apricot, peach	*Prunus* spp.
Lambsquarters, goosefoot	*Chenopodium* spp.	Corn	*Zea mays*
Nightshades	*Solanum* spp.	Elderberry	*Sambucus canadensis*
Pigweed	*Amaranthus*	Flax	*Linum*
Russian thistle	*Salsola pestifer*	Hydrangea	*Hydrangea* spp.
Smartweed	*Polygonum* spp.	Lima Bean	*Phaseolus lunatus* L.
Sudan or Johnson grass	*Sorghum* spp.	Poison suckleya	*Suckleya suckleyana*
Sweet clover	*Melilotus officinalis*	Quick or star grass	*Cynodon* spp.
Wild sunflower	*Helianthus annuus*	Sudan or Johnson grass	*Sorghum* spp.
Crop Plants		Sugar gum	*Eucalyptus cladocalyx*
Alfalfa	*Medicago sativa*	Toyon, California holly	*Heteromeles arbutifolia*
Beet	*Beta vulgaris*	Velvet grass	*Hoecus lunatus*
Corn	*Zea mays*	Vetch seed	*Vicia sativa*
Flax	*Linum usitatissimum*	White clover	*Trifolium repens*
Oats	*Avena sativa*		
Rape	*Brassica napus*		
Rye	*Secale cereale*		
Soybean	*Glycine max*		
Sudan or Johnson grass	*Sorghum* spp.		
Wheat	*Triticum aestivum*		

Data from: Osweiler GD et al: *Clinical and Diagnostic Veterinary Toxicology,* 3rd ed., Dubuque, IA: Kendall/Hunt, 1985; Smith MC, Sherman DM: Respiratory system, in *Goat Medicine,* 2nd ed., Smith MC, Sherman DM, Eds., Ames, IA: Wiley-Blackwell, 2009; Galey, F.D. Disorders Caused by Toxicants, in Large Animal Internal Medicine, 4th ed., Smith, B.P., Ed., St. Louis, Mosby, 2009.

field, although less-than-toxic levels may generate a positive result. (Picrate paper is prepared by treating filter paper with a solution of 5 g of sodium bicarbonate and 0.5 g of picric acid in 100 mL of water.) The suspect plant material is crushed and infused in water. The picrate paper is wetted with that solution and heated to 86° F to 95° F. A positive test result consists of a change to a brick-red color after a few minutes.[119]

Treatment. Sodium nitrite (22 mg/kg) should be given by IV infusion as soon as possible.[119] In addition, sodium thiosulfate (67–660 mg/kg IV[119]) or methylene blue (4–15 mg/kg of a 1% solution IV[1]) should be given immediately and repeated if necessary. Methylene blue also may be given alone at the higher end of the dose range.[120] In goats, sodium thiosulfate also may be given orally every hour at 6 g per head to bind free HCN in the rumen.[1] Of note, these treatments fall outside the Animal Medicinal Drug Use Clarification Act (AMDUCA) guidelines in the United States. Withdrawal times vary, but the U.S. Department of Agriculture (UDSA)-sponsored Food Animal Residue Avoidance and Depletion (FARAD) Program has published recommendations of 48 h for milk and 24 h for meat after sodium nitrite and sodium thiosulfate use.[121] Because methylene blue may be carcinogenic, this drug should not be used in lactating animals, and an extended 180-day meat withdrawal protocol should be followed.[121]

Nitrate-Nitrite Toxicosis

Pathogenesis. Ingested nitrates from plants and water are converted to nitrite in the rumen. Nitrite then binds iron ions in the blood, converting hemoglobin to methemoglobin. Methemoglobin has a reduced ability to carry oxygen, resulting in hypoxia and death. Nitrate is accumulated during the vegetative state (see Table 7.1), especially after droughts, during rapid growth, and on highly fertilized soils; nitrates do not accumulate in the fruit or grains.[119] *Acacia nilotica* spp. *kraussiana* (the acacia tree) toxicity also can lead to methemoglobin formation.[1]

Clinical Signs. Clinical signs are consistent with generalized hypoxia and include dyspnea, tachycardia, cyanotic mucous membranes, exercise intolerance, and sudden death; abortions may occur days to a week after a sublethal exposure.[122] Clinical onset occurs once methemoglobin formation has reached the 30 to 40% threshold; death occurs once 80 to 90% of the hemoglobin has converted.[119]

Diagnosis. The clinical picture and history should be suggestive. Formation of methemoglobin causes the blood to appear dark brown; this change is concurrent with onset of clinical signs at the 30% methemoglobin threshold.[1] Toxicity can be confirmed by establishing definitive nitrite levels in the blood, urine, or aqueous humor; field samples should be frozen.[119] Feed nitrate levels should be below 1% of the diet, and water levels should be below 1500 ppm.[119]

Treatment. Animals with low levels of toxicity (as indicated by 40–50% methemoglobin concentrations) may recover spontaneously.[119] A 1% solution of methylene blue should be given intravenously at 4 to 15 mg/kg every 6 to 8 h; methylene blue overdose in ruminants (requires greater than 30 mg/kg in sheep) is difficult to achieve in a clinical setting.[119] This treatment falls outside of AMDUCA guidelines in the United States. Because methylene blue may be carcinogenic, this drug should not be used in lactating animals, and an extended 180-day meat withdrawal protocol should be followed.[121] Cold-water ruminal lavage and oral penicillin may be used to slow down nitrate conversion.[122]

References

1. Smith M, Sherman D: Respiratory system. In Smith M, Sherman D, editors: *Goat medicine,* ed 2, Ames, IA, 2009, Wiley-Blackwell.
2. Constantinescu G: *Guide to regional anatomy based on the dissection of the goat,* Ames, IA, 2001, Iowa State University Press.
3. Nakakuki S: The bronchial tree, lobular division and blood vessels of the Japanese deer (Cervus nippon) lung, *J Vet Med Sci* 55(3):443–447, 1993.
4. Guyton A, Hall J: Physical principles of gas exchange; diffusion of oxygen and carbon dioxide through the respiratory membrane. In Guyton A, Hall J, editors: *Textbook of Medical Physiology,* ed 9, Philadelphia, 1996, WB Saunders. [chapter 39].
5. Guyton A, Hall J: Pulmonary ventilation. In Guyton A, Hall J, editors: *Textbook of medical physiology* ed 9, Philadelphia, 1996, WB Saunders. [chapter 37].
6. Dorchies P, Duranton C, Jacquiet P: Pathophysiology of Oestrus ovis infection in sheep and goats: a review, *Vet Rec* 142(18):487–489, 1998.
7. Bowman D, editor: *Georgis' parasitology for veterinarians,* St. Louis, 2003, WB Saunders.
8. Belknap E: Diseases of the respiratory system. In Pugh D, editor: *Sheep and goat medicine,* ed 1, Philadelphia, 2002, WB Saunders.
9. Baynes RE, Payne M, Martin-Jimenez T, et al: Extralabel use of ivermectin and moxidectin in food animals, *J Am Vet Med Assoc* 217(5):668–671, 2000.
10. Hoste H, Lespine A, Lemercier P, Alvinerie M, Jacquiet P, Dorchies P: Efficacy of eprinomectin pour-on against gastrointestinal nematodes and the nasal bot fly (Oestrus ovis) in sheep, *Vet Rec* 154(25):782–785, 2004.
11. Habela M, Moreno A, Gragera-Slikker A, et al: Efficacy of eprinomectin pour-on in naturally Oestrus ovis infested merino sheep in Extremadura, South-West Spain, *Parasitol Res* 99(3):275–280, 2006.
12. Nithiuthai S, Anantaphruti MT, Waikagul J, Gajadhar A: Waterborne zoonotic helminthiases, *Vet Parasitol* 126(1–2):167–193, 2004.
13. De las Heras M: Experimental transmission of enzootic intranasal tumors of goats, *Vet Pathol* 32:19, 1995.
14. McKinnon AO, Thorsen J, Hayes MA, Misener CR: Enzootic Nasal adenocarcinoma of sheep in Canada, *Can Vet J* 23(3):88–94, 1982.
15. Rings DM, Rojko J: Naturally occurring nasal obstructions in 11 sheep, *Cornell Vet* 75(2):269–276, 1985.
16. De las Heras M, Garcia de Jalon J, Sharp J: Pathology of enzootic intranasal tumor in thirty-eight goats, *Vet Path* 28:474, 1991.
17. De las Heras M, Sharp JM, Ferrer LM, Garcia de Jalon JA, Cebrian LM: Evidence for a type D-like retrovirus in enzootic nasal tumour of sheep, *Vet Rec* 132(17):441, 1993.
18. DeMartini JC, York DF: Retrovirus-associated neoplasms of the respiratory system of sheep and goats. Ovine pulmonary carcinoma and enzootic nasal tumor, *Vet Clin North Am Food Anim Pract* 13(1):55–70, 1997.
19. Borg K, Nilsson PO: Ethmoid tumors in moose and roe deer, *Nord Vet Med* 37(3):145–160, 1985.
20. Brownstein DG, Montali RJ, Bush M, James AE: Nasal carcinoma in a captive Eld's deer, *J Am Vet Med Assoc* 167(7):569–571, 1975.
21. Steen M, Rehbinder C, Morner T: Nasal tumor in a fallow deer (Dama dama L). A case report, *Acta Vet Scand* 26(4):461–465, 1985.
22. Movassaghi AR, Davazdah Emami MR: Ethmoturbinate adenocarcinoma in a Persian fallow deer *(Cervus dama mesopotamica)*, *Vet Rec* 149(16):493–494, 2001.
23. Rajan A, Sreekumaran T, Sulochana S: Carcinoma of the mucosa of the ethmoid in the deer *(Axis axis)*, *Vet Pathol* 19(4):458–460, 1982.
24. Walsh SR, Stinson KJ, Menzies PI, Wootton SK: Development of an ante-mortem diagnostic test for enzootic nasal tumor virus and detection of neutralizing antibodies in host serum, *J Gen Virol* 95(Pt 8):1843–1854, 2014.
25. Walsh SR, Stinson KJ, Wootton SK: Seroconversion of sheep experimentally infected with enzootic nasal tumor virus, *BMC Res Notes* 9:15, 2016.
26. Trent A, Smart M, Fretz P: Surgical management of nasal adenocarcinomas in sheep, *JAVMA* 193:227, 1988.

27. Spickler A, Roth J: *Emerging and exotic diseases of animals*, ed 2, Ames, IA, 2004, Iowa State University Press.
28. Barrington G, Tucker R: Use of computed tomography to diagnose sinusitis in a goat, *Vet Radiol Ultrasound* 37(2):118, 2005.
29. Lakritz J, Rings D, Hull B: Disorders of the upper respiratory tract in food animals. In Anderson D, Rings D, editors: *Current veterinary therapy: food animal practice*, ed 5, Philadelphia, 2009, WB Saunders.
30. de Lahunta A, Habel R: Paranasal sinuses. In de Lahunta A, Habel R, editors: *Applied veterinary anatomy*, Philadelphia, 1986, WB Saunders.
31. Le T, Psaltis A, Tan LW, Wormald PJ: The efficacy of topical antibiofilm agents in a sheep model of rhinosinusitis, *Am J Rhinol* 22(6):560–567, 2008.
32. Washburn KE, Bissett WT, Fajt VR, et al: Comparison of three treatment regimens for sheep and goats with caseous lymphadenitis, *J Am Vet Med Assoc* 234(9):1162–1166, 2009.
33. Goulding R, Schumacher J, Barrett DC, Fitzpatrick JL: Use of a permanent tracheostomy to treat laryngeal chondritis and stenosis in a heifer, *Vet Rec* 152(26):809–811, 2003.
34. Lane JG, Brown PJ, Lancaster ML, Todd JN: Laryngeal chondritis in Texel sheep, *Vet Rec* 121(4):81–84, 1987.
35. Milne MH, Barrett DC, Sullivan M, Fitzpatrick JL: Successful medical treatment of laryngeal chondritis in cattle, *Vet Rec* 147(11):305–306, 2000.
36. Jackson PG, White RA, Dennis R, Gordon DF: Tracheal collapse in a goat, *Vet Rec* 119(7):160, 1986.
37. Belli CB, Benesi FJ, Leal ML, Nichi M: Trachael collapse in an adult goat, *Can Vet J* 44(10):835–836, 2003.
38. Fernandez A, Oros J, Rodriguez JL, King J, Poveda JB: Morphological evidence of a filamentous cilia-associated respiratory (CAR) bacillus in goats, *Vet Pathol* 33(4):445–447, 1996.
39. Oros J, Fernandez A, Rodriguez JL, Franklin CL, Matsushita S, Poveda JB: Association of cilia-associated respiratory (CAR) bacillus with natural chronic tracheitis in goats, *J Comp Pathol* 117(3): 289–294, 1997.
40. Blackall PJ, Bojesen AM, Christensen H, Bisgaard M: Reclassification of [Pasteurella] trehalosi as Bibersteinia trehalosi gen. nov., comb. nov, *Int J Syst Evol Microbiol* 57(Pt 4):666–674, 2007.
41. Brogden KA, Lehmkuhl HD, Cutlip RC: Pasteurella haemolytica complicated respiratory infections in sheep and goats, *Vet Res* 29(3–4):233–254, 1998.
42. Tell LA, Brooks JW, Lintner V, Matthews T, Kariyawasam S: Antimicrobial susceptibility of Arcanobacterium pyogenes isolated from the lungs of white-tailed deer *(Odocoileus virginianus)* with pneumonia, *J Vet Diagn Invest* 23(5):1009–1013, 2011.
43. Lawrence PK, Bey RF, Wiener B, Kittichotirat W, Bumgarner RE: Genome sequence of a presumptive Mannheimia haemolytica Ssrain with an A1/A6-cross-reactive serotype from a white-tailed deer *(Odocoileus virginianus)*, *Genome Announc* 2(2) e00114–14, 2014.
44. Brooks JW, Kumar A, Narayanan S, et al: Characterization of Fusobacterium isolates from the respiratory tract of white-tailed deer *(Odocoileus virginianus)*, *J Vet Diagn Invest* 26(2):213–220, 2014.
45. Hattel AL, Shaw DP, Love BC, Wagner DC, Drake TR, Brooks JW: A retrospective study of mortality in Pennsylvania captive white-tailed deer *(Odocoileus virginianus)*: 2000—2003, *J Vet Diagn Invest* 16(6):515–521, 2004.
46. Berge AC, Sischo WM, Craigmill AL: Antimicrobial susceptibility patterns of respiratory tract pathogens from sheep and goats, *J Am Vet Med Assoc* 229(8):1279–1281, 2006.
47. Ward AC, Weiser GC, DeLong WJ, Frank GH: Characterization of *Pasteurella* spp isolated from healthy domestic pack goats and evaluation of the effects of a commercial Pasteurella vaccine, *Am J Vet Res* 63(1):119–123, 2002.
48. Zamri-Saad M, Ernie ZA, Sabri MY: Protective effect following intranasal exposure of goats to live Pasteurella multocida B:2, *Trop Anim Health Prod* 38(7–8):541–546, 2006.
49. Goodwin-Ray KA, Stevenson MA, Heuer C: Effect of vaccinating lambs against pneumonic pasteurellosis under New Zealand field conditions on their weight gain and pneumonic lung lesions at slaughter, *Vet Rec* 162(1):9–11, 2008.
50. Ayling RD, Bashiruddin SE, Nicholas RA: Mycoplasma species and related organisms isolated from ruminants in Britain between 1990 and 2000, *Vet Rec* 155(14):413–416, 2004.
51. Lin YC, Miles RJ, Nicholas RA, Kelly DP, Wood AP: Isolation and immunological detection of Mycoplasma ovipneumoniae in sheep with atypical pneumonia, and lack of a role for Mycoplasma arginini, *Res Vet Sci* 84(3):367–373, 2008.
52. Sheehan M, Cassidy JP, Brady J, et al: An aetiopathological study of chronic bronchopneumonia in lambs in Ireland, *Vet J* 173(3): 630–637, 2007.
53. Goncalves R, Mariano I, Nunez A, Branco S, Fairfoul G, Nicholas R: Atypical non-progressive pneumonia in goats, *Vet J* 183(2):219–221, 2010.
54. Alley MR, Ionas G, Clarke JK: Chronic non-progressive pneumonia of sheep in New Zealand – a review of the role of *Mycoplasma ovipneumoniae*, *N Z Vet J* 47(5):155–160, 1999.
55. Manso-Silvan L, Vilei EM, Sachse K, Djordjevic SP, Thiaucourt F, Frey J: Mycoplasma leachii sp. nov. as a new species designation for Mycoplasma sp. bovine group 7 of Leach, and reclassification of Mycoplasma mycoides subsp. mycoides LC as a serovar of Mycoplasma mycoides subsp. capri, *Int J Syst Evol Microbiol* 59(6):1353–1358, 2009.
56. Abu-Groun EA, Taylor RR, Varsani H, Wadher BJ, Leach RH, Miles RJ: Biochemical diversity within the "Mycoplasma mycoides" cluster, *Microbiology* 140(Pt 8):2033–2042, 1994.
57. Harasawa R, Hotzel H, Sachse K: Comparison of the 16S-23S rRNA intergenic spacer regions among strains of the Mycoplasma mycoides cluster, and reassessment of the taxonomic position of Mycoplasma sp. bovine group 7, *Int J Syst Evol Microbiol* 50(Pt 3):1325–1329, 2000.
58. Manso-Silvan L, Perrier X, Thiaucourt F: Phylogeny of the Mycoplasma mycoides cluster based on analysis of five conserved protein-coding sequences and possible implications for the taxonomy of the group, *Int J Syst Evol Microbiol* 57(Pt 10):2247–2258, 2007.
59. Thiaucourt F, Lorenzon S, David A, Breard A: Phylogeny of the Mycoplasma mycoides cluster as shown by sequencing of a putative membrane protein gene, *Vet Microbiol* 72(3–4):251–268, 2007.
60. Vilei EM, Korczak BM, Frey J: Mycoplasma mycoides subsp. capri and Mycoplasma mycoides subsp. mycoides LC can be grouped into a single subspecies, *Vet Res* 37(6):779–790, 2006.
61. Giadinis ND, Petridou EJ, Sofianidis G, et al: Mortality in adult goats attributed to Mycoplasma capricolum subspecies capricolum, *Vet Rec* 163(9):278–279, 2008.
62. East NE, DaMassa AJ, Logan LL, Brooks DL, McGowan B: Milk-borne outbreak of Mycoplasma mycoides subspecies mycoides infection in a commercial goat dairy, *J Am Vet Med Assoc* 182(12):1338–1341, 1983.
63. DaMassa AJ, Brooks DL, Adler HE, Watt DE: Caprine mycoplasmosis: acute pulmonary disease in newborn kids given Mycoplasma capricolum orally, *Aust Vet J* 60(4):125–126, 1983.
64. DaMassa AJ, Brooks DL, Adler HE: Caprine mycoplasmosis: widespread infection in goats with Mycoplasma mycoides subsp mycoides (large-colony type), *Am J Vet Res* 44(2):322–325, 1983.
65. Jayaraman A, Wood TK: Bacterial quorum sensing: signals, circuits, and implications for biofilms and disease, *Annu Rev Biomed Eng* 10:145–167, 2008.
66. Amores J, Corrales JC, Martìn nG, Sanchez A, Contreras A, de la Fe C: Comparison of culture and PCR to detect Mycoplasma agalactiae and Mycoplasma mycoides subsp. capri in ear swabs taken from goats, *Vet Microbiol* 140(1–2):105–108, 2010.
67. Jimena ON, Laura JM, Elena MMR, Alonso NH, Teresa QM: Association of Raillietia caprae with the presence of Mycoplasmas in the external ear canal of goats, *Prev Vet Med* 92(1–2):150–153, 2009.
68. DaMassa AJ, Brooks DL: The external ear canal of goats and other animals as a mycoplasma habitat, *Small Rumin Res* 4:85–93, 1991.

69. Msami H, Kapaga A, Heldtander M, Bolske G: Contagious caprine pleuropneumonia in Tanzania, *Vet Rec* 148:22–23, 2001.
70. Kaliner G, MacOwan K: The pathology of experimental and natural contagious caprine pleuropneumonia in Kenya, *Zentralbl Veterinarmed B* 23:652–661, 1976.
71. Kaltenboeck B, Heard D, DeGraves FJ, Schmeer N: Use of synthetic antigens improves detection by enzyme-linked immunosorbent assay of antibodies against abortigenic Chlamydia psittaci in ruminants, *J Clin Microbiol* 35(9):2293–2298, 1997.
72. Huang J, DeGraves FJ, Gao D, Feng P, Schlapp T, Kaltenboeck B: Quantitative detection of Chlamydia spp. by fluorescent PCR in the LightCycler, *Biotechniques* 30(1):150–157, 2001.
73. DeGraves FJ, Gao D, Hehnen HR, Schlapp T, Kaltenboeck B: Quantitative detection of Chlamydia psittaci and C. pecorum by high-sensitivity real-time PCR reveals high prevalence of vaginal infection in cattle, *J Clin Microbiol* 41(4):1726–1729, 2003.
74. Lamontagne L, Descoteaux JP, Roy R: Epizootiological survey of parainfluenza-3, reovirus-3, respiratory syncytial and infectious bovine rhinotracheitis viral antibodies in sheep and goat flocks in Quebec, *Can J Comp Med* 49(4):424–428, 1985.
75. Lehmkuhl HD, Cutlip RC, Bolin SR, Brogden KA: Seroepidemiologic survey for antibodies to selected viruses in the respiratory tract of lambs, *Am J Vet Res* 46(12):2601–2604, 1985.
76. Goyal SM, Khan MA, McPherson SW, Robinson RA, Boylan WJ: Prevalence of antibodies to seven viruses in a flock of ewes in Minnesota, *Am J Vet Res* 49(4):464–467, 1988.
77. Giangaspero M, Vanopdenbosch E, Nishikawa H, Tabbaa D: Prevalence of antibodies against respiratory viruses (parainfluenza virus type 3, respiratory syncytial virus, reovirus and adenovirus) in relation to productivity in Syrian Awassi sheep, *Trop Anim Health Prod* 29(2):83–91, 1997.
78. Rodger JL: Parainfluenza 3 vaccination of sheep, *Vet Rec* 125(18):453–456, 1989.
79. Lehmkuhl HD, Cutlip RC, Meehan JT, DeBey BM: Pathogenesis of infection induced by an adenovirus isolated from a goat, *Am J Vet Res* 58(6):608–611, 1997.
80. Van der Poel WH, Langedijk JP, Kramps JA, Middel WG, Brand A, Van Oirschot JT: Bovine respiratory syncytial virus antibodies in non-bovine species, *Arch Virol* 140(9):1549–1555, 1995.
81. Gaffuri A, Giacometti M, Tranquillo VM, Magnino S, Cordioli P, Lanfranchi P: Serosurvey of roe deer, chamois and domestic sheep in the central Italian Alps, *J Wildl Dis* 42(3):685–690, 2006.
82. Masot AJ, Gazquez A, Regodon S, Franco A, Redondo E: Lesions in lambs experimentally infected with bovine respiratory syncytial virus, *Histol Histopathol* 10(1):71–77, 1995.
83. Ashraf M, Nepote KH: Prevalence of gastrointestinal nematodes, coccidia and lungworms in Maryland dairy goats, *Small Rumin Res* 3(3):291–298, 1990.
84. Anderson DL, Roberson EL: Gastrointestinal and respiratory parasitism in Georgia goats, *Agri-Practice* 17(9):20–24, 1996.
85. Berrag B, Cabaret J: Assessment of the severity of natural infections of kids and adult goats by small lungworms (Protostrongylidae, Nematoda) using macroscopic lesion scores, *Vet Res* 28(2):143–148, 1997.
86. Smith B: editor: *Large animal internal medicine*, St. Louis, 2007, Mosby.
87. McKenna PB: Comparative evaluation of two emigration/sedimentation techniques for the recovery of dictyocaulid and protostrongylid larvae from faeces, *Vet Parasitol* 80(4):345–351, 1999.
88. Bliss EL, Greiner EC: Efficacy of fenbendazole and cambendazole against Muellerius capillaris in dairy goats, *Am J Vet Res* 46(9):1923–1925, 1985.
89. Geurden T, Vercruysse J: Field efficacy of eprinomectin against a natural Muellerius capillaris infection in dairy goats, *Vety Parasitol* 147(1–2):190–193, 2007.
90. Helle O: The efficacy of fenbendazole and albendazole against the lungworm Muellerius capillaris in goats, *Vet Parasitol* 22(3–4):293–301, 1986.
91. McCraw BM, Menzies PI: Treatment of Goats infected with the lungworm Muellerius capillaris, *Can Vet J* 27(8):287–290, 1986.
92. Papadopoulos E, Sotiraki S, Himonas C, Fthenakis GC: Treatment of small lungworm infestation in sheep by using moxidectin, *Vet Parasitol* 121(3–4):329–336, 2004.
93. Smith M, Sherman D: editors: *Goat medicine*, Philadelphia, 1994, Lea & Febider.
94. Snowder GD, Gates NL, Glimp HA, Gorham JR: Prevalence and effect of subclinical ovine progressive pneumonia virus infection on ewe wool and lamb production, *J Am Vet Med Assoc* 197(4):475–479, 1990.
95. Peterhans E, Greenland T, Badiola J, et al: Routes of transmission and consequences of small ruminant lentiviruses (SRLVs) infection and eradication schemes, *Vet Res* 35(3):257–274, 2004.
96. Arsenault J, Dubreuil P, Girard C, Simard C, Belanger D: Maedi-visna impact on productivity in Quebec sheep flocks (Canada), *Prev Vet Med* 59(3):125–137, 2003.
97. Banks KL, Adams DS, McGuire TC, Carlson J: Experimental infection of sheep by caprine arthritis-encephalitis virus and goats by progressive pneumonia virus, *Am J Vet Res* 44(12):2307–2311, 1983.
98. Shah C, Huder JB, Boni J, et al: Direct evidence for natural transmission of small-ruminant lentiviruses of subtype A4 from goats to sheep and vice versa, *J Virol* 78(14):7518–7522, 2004.
99. Gjerset B, Jonassen CM, Rimstad E: Natural transmission and comparative analysis of small ruminant lentiviruses in the Norwegian sheep and goat populations, *Virus Res* 125(2):153–161, 2007.
100. Pisoni G, Bertoni G, Puricelli M, Maccalli M, Moroni P: Demonstration of coinfection with and recombination by caprine arthritis-encephalitis virus and maedi-visna virus in naturally infected goats, *J Virol* 81(10):4948–4955, 2007.
101. de la Concha-Bermejillo ASM, Magnus-Corral S: Seroprevalence of ovine progresive pneumonia in Texas sheep, *Texas Agric Exper Stn Res Rep* PR-5223:34–35, 1994.
102. Fournier D, Campbell JR, Middleton DM: Prevalence of maedi-visna infection in culled ewes in Alberta, *Can Vet J* 47(5):460–466, 2006.
103. Arsenault J, Girard C, Dubreuil P, et al: Prevalence of and carcass condemnation from maedi-visna, paratuberculosis and caseous lymphadenitis in culled sheep from Quebec, Canada, *Prev Vet Med* 59(1–2):67–81, 2003.
104. Leroux C, Mornex JF: Retroviral infections in sheep and the associated diseases, *Small Ruminant Res* 76(1–2):68–76, 2008.
105. de la Concha-Bermejillo A: Maedi-Visna and ovine progressive pneumonia, *Vet Clin North Am Food Anim Pract* 13(1):13–33, 1997.
106. de Andres D, Klein D, Watt NJ, et al: Diagnostic tests for small ruminant lentiviruses, *Vet Microbiol* 107(1–2):49–62, 2005.
107. Reina R, Berriatua E, Lujan L, et al: Prevention strategies against small ruminant lentiviruses: an update, *Vet J* 182(1):31–37, 2009.
108. Rowe JD, East NE: Risk factors for transmission and methods for control of caprine arthritis-encephalitis virus infection, *Vet Clin North Am-Food Anim Pract* 13(1):35–53, 1997.
109. Fontaine MC, Baird GJ: Caseous lymphadenitis, *Small Ruminant Res* 76(1–2):42–48, 2008.
110. Williamson LH: Caseous lymphadenitis in small ruminants, *Vet Clin North Am-Food Anim Pract* 17(2):359–371, 2001.
111. Zhang Y, Cui J, Parkinson A, Hayes J, Ott K, Byrum B: Isolation of Helcococcus ovis from sheep with pleuritis and bronchopneumonia, *J Vet Diagn Invest* 21(1):164–166, 2009.
112. Scott P, Collie D, McGorum B, Sargison N: Relationship between thoracic auscultation and lung pathology detected by ultrasonography in sheep, *Vet J* 186:53–57, 2010.
113. Gaughan E, Provo-Klimek J, Ducharme N: Surgery of the bovine respiratory and cardiovascular systems. In Fubini S, Ducharme N, editors: *Farm animal surgery,* ed 1, St. Louis, 2004, Elsevier.
114. Valentine B: Neoplasia. In Fubini S, Ducharme N, editors: *Farm animal surgery.* ed 1, St. Louis, 2004, Elsevier.

115. Olchowy TW, Toal RL, Brenneman KA, Slauson DO, McEntee MF: Metastatic thymoma in a goat, *Can Vet J* 37(3):165–167, 1996.
116. Rostkowski CM, Stirtzinger T, Baird JD: Congestive heart failure associated with thymoma in two Nubian goats, *Can Vet J* 26(9):267–269, 1985.
117. Sandison AT, Anderson LJ: Tumors of the thymus in cattle, sheep, and pigs, *Cancer Res* 29(5):1146–1150, 1969.
118. Parish SM, Middleton JR, Baldwin TJ: Clinical megaoesophagus in a goat with thymoma, *Vet Rec* 139(4):94, 1996.
119. Osweiler G: *Clinical and diagnostic veterinary toxicology*, ed 3, Dubuque, IA, 1985, Kendall/Hunt.
120. Pickerell J, Oehme F: Cyanogenic glycosides. In Plumlee K, editor: *Clinical veterinary toxicology*, St. Louis, 2004, Mosby.
121. Bright S, Post L: *Veterinary antidotes and availability: an update*, 2008. https://www.abvt.org/public/docs/antidoteupdate08.pdf. Accessed July 16, 2019
122. Casteel S, Evans T: Nitrate. In Plumlee K, editor: *Clinical veterinary toxicology*, St. Louis, 2004, Mosby.

8 Theriogenology of Sheep, Goats, and Cervids

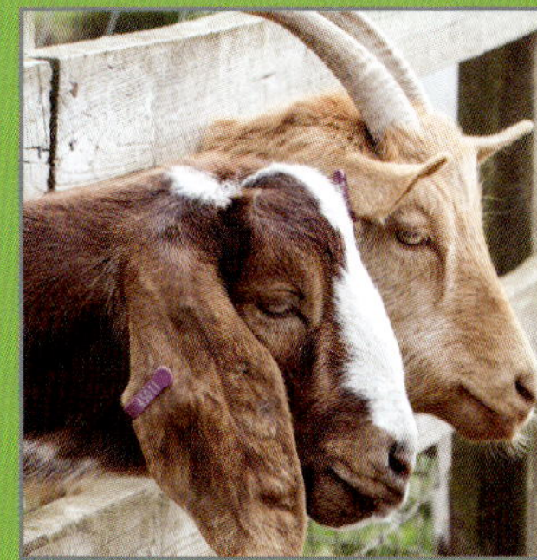

MISTY A. EDMONDSON AND CLIFFORD F. SHIPLEY

Theriogenology is the area of veterinary medicine concerned with reproductive physiology, pathology, surgery, and medicine. This chapter will attempt to cover the theriogenology of sheep, goats, and cervids. Each species is considered separately when relevant data are available, but when applicable, they are discussed together.

Sheep, goats, and cervids are very fertile animals with reproductive potentials far superior to that of most other domestic animals. Specific examination of the reproductive system should always be preceded by a complete physical examination to determine the general health status and to detect problems that warrant therapeutic or management intervention (see Chapter 1). Animals need to be productive (i.e., healthy) before they are able to be reproductive—in other words, sex is a luxury. A single-range ewe usually does not undergo the same sort of reproductive manipulation or physiologic stress as that of a donor used in an embryo transfer (ET) program.

Male Reproduction

Anatomy and Physiology of the Male

The anatomy of the reproductive organs of the ram and buck is similar to that of other ruminants. The penile urethra is surrounded by the corpus spongiosum penis (CSP) throughout its length. The urethra terminates as a vermiform appendage. Blood enters the CSP proximally and exits through two exhaust veins located on the free portion of the penis. Contractions of the urethralis and bulbospongiosus muscles force blood rhythmically through the CSP, producing the characteristic pulses of urine observed during normal micturition. The most prominent structure of the penis is the corpus cavernosum penis (CCP). It consists of cavernous space supported by fibrous trabeculae. This cavernous tissue is located on the dorsal surface and partially surrounds the CSP. At its origin in the pelvis, the CCP is composed of two crura that join before leaving the pelvis. The entire penis is surrounded by the tunica albuginea. The two paired retractor penis muscles arise from the coccygeal vertebrae and pass around the anus to become two distinct muscles that attach to the ventrolateral surface of the penis at the distal bend of the sigmoid flexure. The penis is normally held in an S-shaped bend (sigmoid flexure) except during erection and ejaculation by the retractor penis muscles.[1]

The testicles are suspended away from the body by the pendulous scrotum. The scrotum is composed of undulating epidermis that may or may not be covered by wool, depending on the breed and husbandry practices. A rich plexus of blood vessels, lymphatics, and sweat glands lies beneath the skin. The dartos, a smooth muscle layer, is connected to the vaginal tunics of the testicle by the scrotal fascia. The scrotal fascia is the connective tissue that is typically broken down when the clinician separates the skin from the testicle during routine castration. The vaginal tunics are outcroppings of the peritoneum and form a protective covering over the testicles. The space between the two layers of vaginal tunic (parietal and visceral) as it reflects around the testicle normally contains a small amount of peritoneal fluid. The scrotal septum, composed primarily of the dartos muscle, divides the scrotum into two halves.[2]

The testicle itself is surrounded by a thick fibrous connective tissue known as the *tunica albuginea.* The parenchyma of the testicle is composed of seminiferous tubules that contain the germ cells and their supporting cells (Sertoli cells). The seminiferous tubules drain into the rete testes, which in turn is drained by 10 to 12 efferent ducts. These ducts drain into the head of the epididymis, which is located on the dorsal craniolateral aspect of the testicle. The body of the epididymis curves around the lateral portion of the testes and ends caudomedially as the tail. The tubular structure is reflected dorsally and becomes the vas deferens.[2] Rams and bucks have a full complement of accessory sex glands. The small bulbourethral glands are located caudally in the pelvic cavity on either side of the pelvic urethra; they can be palpated rectally. They also have lobulated vesicular glands, disseminate prostates, and a widening of the vas deferens known as the ampulla.[3] Spermatogenesis requires about 49 to 60 days from the start of germ cell division until the sperm are released from the seminiferous tubules. Another 10 days to 2 weeks are required for the sperm to pass from the seminiferous tubules through the epididymis.[4]

Puberty and Seasonality

Ram. Puberty typically occurs in small ruminants at 4 to 6 months and at 60% of the mature body weight.[5] It is defined as the point at which the ram develops an interest in sexual activity and produces spermatozoa in sufficient numbers to achieve pregnancy in ewes. The exact age of puberty depends somewhat on breed and time of birth. Rams born early in the spring are older at puberty than late-born lambs. Moreover, rams that are periodically exposed to cycling ewes tend to reach puberty earlier.[6] Rams are seasonal breeders; the sperm quality, daily sperm output, and sexual activity are modulated by the increased periods of darkness that typically occur in the fall (Northern Hemisphere). This seasonality in the ram also is manifested by an increase in the testicular circumference (~1–2 cm increase). The increase in melatonin, which is secreted from the pineal gland during the dark hours as day length shortens, is responsible for many of the physiologic mechanisms associated with the ram in transition from the nonbreeding to the breeding season.[7] Manipulation of light-dark intervals and the use of melatonin can alter the breeding season of rams, but the practicality of these procedures is debatable.[8]

A change in the sexual attitude of the ram toward the ewe as day length decreases defines the onset of the breeding season. He becomes more sexually interested in the female, and courtship behavior occurs more frequently. Rams display a typical flehmen response to females in estrus after sniffing the vulva region and urine from the estrus female. He often strikes out at the female with one front leg before mounting her.[7] The physiologic changes in testicular size, mating behavior, and semen quality are caused by the activation of the hypothalamus and a decrease in the effectiveness of testosterone on the negative inhibition of gonadotropin-releasing hormone (GnRH). Significant differences are seen between the breeding and the nonbreeding season with respect to the pattern of GnRH and luteinizing hormone (LH) pulses and the response of the pituitary gland to GnRH.

Buck (Goat). Breed, age, and nutrition contribute to the onset of sexual maturity in the buck.[9] The age at puberty depends on the breed, varying from 2 to 3 months in pygmy breeds to 4 to 5 months in Nubian and Boer bucks. Most breeds of goats raised in the temperate environment of the Northern Hemisphere possess sperm in the ejaculate at 4 to 5 months. However, at this age, their semen quality is poor and they are not suitable for breeding.[10] Nubian and Boer bucks begin exhibiting libido at 10 to 12 weeks and start producing quality semen at about 8 months.[9,10] Natural adhesions of the urethral process and glans penis to the prepuce make the immature buck incapable of copulation. This attachment begins to separate at 3 months, and fertile mating is possible at 4 to 5 months.[9,10] Fast-growing, well-fed, and well-managed kids are able to breed sooner than starved males of equal age.

Many bucks have depressed libido, reduced pheromones, decreased scrotal circumference (SC), lower semen freezability, and a larger number of abnormal spermatozoa outside of the breeding season. All these changes reflect lower levels of LH and testosterone. LH and testosterone concentration, libido, and odor presence in the buck peak in the fall.[11,12] The sexual behavior of the buck includes actively seeking does in estrus, courtship (kicking, pawing, muzzling, grunting, and flehmen), mounting, intromission, and ejaculation. Ejaculation occurs spontaneously and is characterized by a strong pelvic thrust with a rapid backward movement of the head.[10] After ejaculation, the buck dismounts and shows no sexual arousal for a few minutes to several hours.

Buck (Cervid). Buck fawns born very early in the season and displaying hard antler "buttons" may be fertile in the fall of their birth year. Most buck fawns fed properly may be fertile by late breeding season or second or third rut. Yearling and older bucks "chase" does during the rut and display behavior of separating the doe from the rest of the animals during a 1- to 3-day estrus period. Fertile bucks can be expected to breed 10 to 25 does depending on age, pen size, and terrain.[13]

Breeding Soundness Examination in the Ram

A breeding soundness examination (BSE) should be performed on all rams before the beginning of the breeding season. With the ram being expected to breed as many as 100 ewes during a season, his individual worth far outweighs the cost of a BSE. A proper BSE consists of a thorough physical examination with special attention to the scrotum, testicles, and penis, as well as an evaluation of the semen quality. Most BSEs do not routinely include an evaluation of the ram's libido or his physical ability to make intromission. The veterinarian should communicate clearly with the client regarding the limitations of the BSE performed and the need for some sort of libido testing. This testing can often be accomplished by directly observing the animal in the first part of the breeding season. Large sheep producers may be encouraged to keep an extra 10% more rams that have been deemed satisfactory according to a veterinary examination to ensure adequate ram power.

Physical Examination. A complete physical examination should be performed on all rams, with emphasis on the eyes and feet. The ram can be restrained by placing him on his rump in a sitting position[14–24] (see Chapter 1).

Examination of Reproductive Tract. The scrotum should be palpated to ensure that both testicles are present, approximately equal in size, and of firm consistency; the clinician should note any localized swellings or areas of induration. The head and tail of the epididymis are palpated for swelling, pain, and signs of inflammation. Epididymitis is a relatively common problem in rams. Any ram exhibiting signs of epididymitis should be considered infected with *Brucella ovis* until proven otherwise. The clinician should examine the spermatic cord for deformities in the vascular plexus and vas deferens. The penis can usually be extended by pressing down around the external preputial orifice and grasping the protruding penis with a gauze pad (Figure 8.1). Occasionally, the sigmoid flexure may need to be straightened to assist in extending the penis. The clinician should carefully examine the penis for evidence of active lesions or old scars. The penis can be held in extension by wrapping a strip of gauze around the junction between the free portion of the penis and the prepuce.

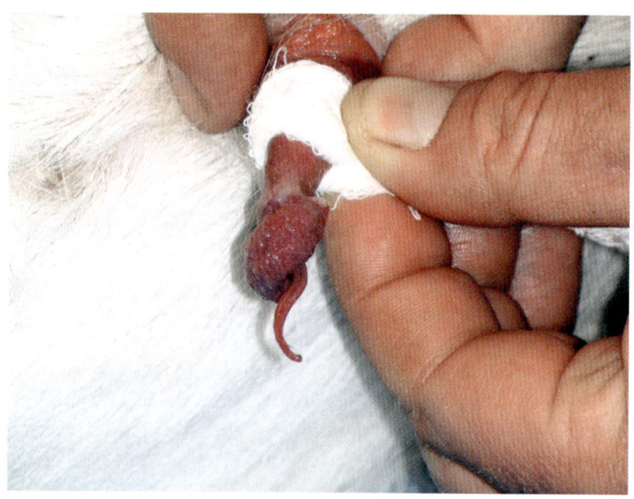

• **Fig. 8.1** A gauze strip is wrapped around the penis at the junction of the free portion of the penis and the prepuce to prevent retraction into the sheath. A prominent vermiform appendage can be seen in the 1-year-old goat pictured.

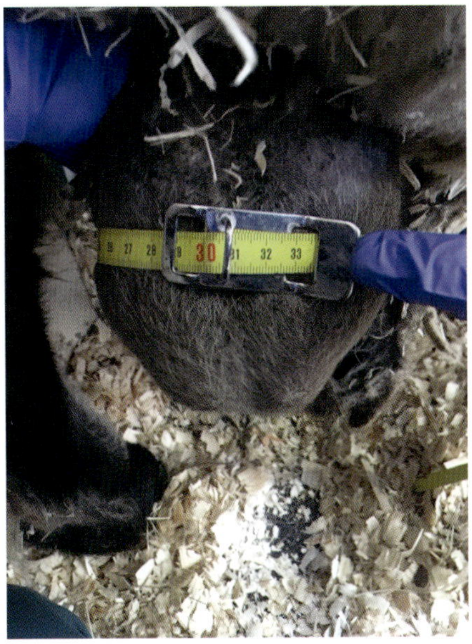

• **Fig. 8.2** Measuring the scrotal circumference of a ram. The procedure is the same for bucks. The tape measure should slightly indent the skin, and the examiner should firmly push the testicles into the scrotum with the free hand. Care should be taken to read the measurement at the correct location on the measuring tape.

This method also is helpful when collecting semen by electroejaculation (EEJ). The penis is generally easier to extend when the animal is being held up on his rump than when he is in lateral recumbency.

Scrotal Circumference. The clinician should pull both of the animal's testicles ventrally into the scrotum and measure it at its largest circumference using a tape measure marked in centimeters. Care must be taken with breeds that have heavy scrotal wool because wool may falsely enlarge the measured circumference. Taking the average of several measurements can increase the accuracy of the SC measurements. The tape should be snug on the scrotum and barely indent the skin so that the tape does not slide on the scrotum (Figure 8.2). SC in the ram is highly heritable and appears to be related to sperm output and age of puberty.[14,15] During the selection of ram lambs the testicular diameter at 170 days provides a long-range prediction of postpubertal testicular size and sperm output.[16–18] SC is a major criterion in selecting replacement rams. Minimum accepted SCs of 30 cm for ram lambs weighing more than 150 lb (68 kg), 33 cm for 12- to 18-month-old rams, and 36 cm for rams weighing more than 250 lbs (113 kg) have been suggested.[14] Based strictly on age, rams from 8 to 14 months should have 28 to 36 cm of SC to be classified as satisfactory and more than 36 cm to be classified as exceptional. Rams older than 14 months should have 32 to 40 cm of SC to be classified as satisfactory and more than 40 cm to be classified as exceptional[23] (Table 8.1). Scrotal size is usually greatest from August to October. Smaller testicular measurements (0.5 to 1.5 cm smaller) are to be expected when rams are tested outside of the normal breeding season (February to April) or during periods of extreme sexual activity.[14,15]

Semen Collection. The penis should always be extended prior to semen collection. Semen collected without the penis extended or while the penis is retained within the preputial cavity is more likely to have leukocytes in the ejaculate. These false results due to contamination from the prepuce could lead to the erroneous diagnosis of possible epidydimitis.[25] The penis should be extended as described previously. The ram is then placed in lateral recumbency to collect semen by EEJ. The same electroejaculators (EEs) described for use in bucks are used for rams (Figure 8.3). The clinician inserts the tip of the animal's penis and the urethral process into the warmed glass or plastic tube. Some rams ejaculate at this point of the examination. The rectum is cleared of feces and a lubricated electric rectal probe is carefully inserted. The clinician massages the accessory sex glands by moving the probe back and forth in a cranial to caudal direction 8 to 10 times while gently forcing the tip of the probe ventrally. Mild electrical stimulation is then applied for 5 seconds. The ram typically vocalizes during this procedure and attempts to escape. After the ram relaxes, the massage and electrical stimulation are repeated until the ram ejaculates into the tube. The spiraled urethral process straightens during the ejaculatory process. The collected semen is evaluated for motility, morphology, and the presence of inflammatory cells.[15,24]

TABLE 8.1 Scrotal Circumference by Age in Breeding Soundness Evaluation of Rams.

8–14 MONTHS		TYPE OF DIET (%)	
Size	**Rating**	**Size**	**Rating**
<28 cm	Questionable	<32 cm	Questionable
28–36 cm	Satisfactory	32–40 cm	Satisfactory
>36 cm	Exceptional	>40 cm	Exceptional

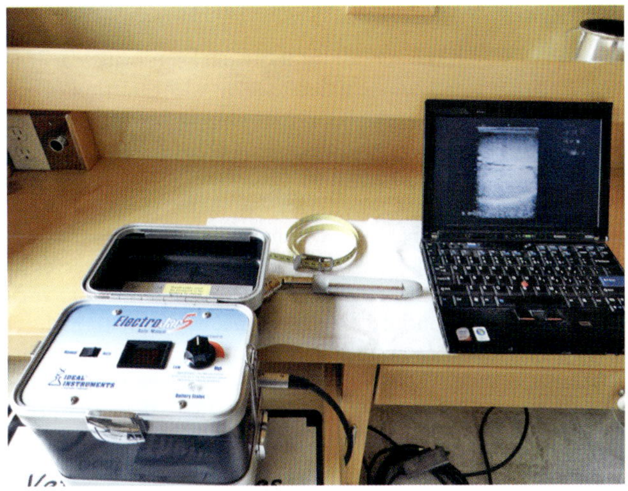

• **Fig. 8.3** There are many types and manufacturers of electroejaculators available. An electroejaculator that can draw power from a stationary source (e.g., truck battery) and has a built-in battery source is preferable. The ram probe shown in this picture may be too large for some goats but, with patience, is usable most of the time.

Semen Evaluation

Motility. A drop of raw semen is first examined under low power (100×) to estimate concentration and motility. A drop of warmed saline is placed on the slide. The clinician then dips the corner of a coverslip into the drop of raw semen and mixes it with the drop of warmed saline. The resultant mixture should allow the

TABLE 8.2 **Sperm Motility and Morphology Percentages Required for Classification of Reproduction Potential in Rams.**

	SPERM ATTRIBUTE	
	Motility	Morphology
Exceptional	>70%	>90%
Satisfactory	>30%	>50%
Unsatisfactory	<30%	<50%

examiner to watch the motion of individual spermatozoa. If the semen mixture is too concentrated to allow identification of individual spermatozoa, a new preparation should be made with less semen. With experience, the observer will be able to determine the amount of semen to place on the coverslip to make an adequate slide. The examiner should visually estimate the number of progressively motile sperm. A common error is to overestimate the percentage of progressively motile sperm. The observer can minimize errors by mentally "freezing" the microscopic image before making the motility estimate. One technique to make the estimate easier is to determine whether more or less than 50% of the spermatozoa are motile. After making that determination, the observer can try to arrive at the nearest 25%, then the nearest 10%. The observer also should record the number of round cells present in each image. If more than two round cells are seen in each medium power field, a smear of the semen should be made for cytologic evaluation (e.g., Wright's stain). The presence of white blood cells indicates inflammation and/or infection. The presence of early nucleated round germ cells indicates an aberration of spermatogenesis. Rams should have more than 30% progressively motile cells to obtain a satisfactory rating and more than 70% to have an exceptional rating[15,25,26] (Table 8.2). Motility is usually depressed outside the breeding season.

Morphology. A slide is next prepared for examination of spermatozoa morphology. A small drop of semen is placed on the edge of a slide, and a ribbon of eosin-nigrosin stain is placed slightly closer to the center of the slide. The corner of a second slide is dipped into the semen drop and the resultant "hanging drop" of semen is mixed with the ribbon of stain. The second slide is then pulled across the first slide in a manner similar to creating a blood smear. The amount of semen placed on the edge of the second slide is determined by experience. The resultant smear should have an even distribution of cells. Spermatozoa should be spaced so that individual cells are easily distinguished but each field should have approximately 10 cells. The slide is allowed to dry and then examined at 1000× with an oil-immersion lens. The observer should count at least 100 cells and determine a percentage of normal spermatozoa. Abnormalities are usually recorded as either primary or secondary. Primary abnormalities involve the head and midpiece of the spermatozoa, whereas secondary abnormalities involve the tail (Figure 8.4). The type of abnormality can be used to estimate the severity of problems in rams with an excessive number of abnormal cells. Abnormalities of the head and the acrosome are associated with severe testicular aberrations. Tail abnormalities are often associated with less severe problems or diseases of the epididymis. Round droplets of cytoplasm on the tail are usually seen in young rams and are associated with overuse, immaturity, or mild testicular degeneration. Droplets also can occur in samples taken from rams out of season. At least 50% to 70% of the observed spermatozoa should be morphologically normal for the ram to be considered a satisfactory breeder; more than 80% to 90% is considered exceptional[24] (see Table 8.2).

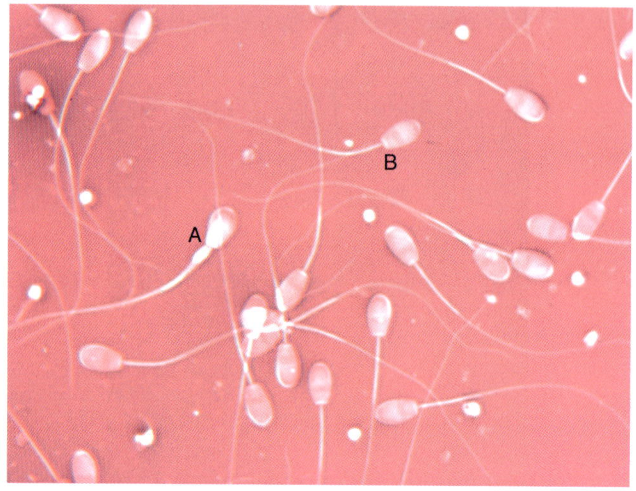

• **Fig. 8.4** Eosin-nigrosin stain of semen obtained from a 2-year-old mixed-breed goat. Abnormalities of the spermatozoa include an enlarged head and proximal droplet **A.** and other head/acrosome abnormalities. Normal spermatozoa **B.** are also present.

Breeding Soundness Prediction. The SC, progressive motility, and percentage of normal spermatozoa can be combined to classify rams into categories to help predict their usefulness in a breeding flock. Rams that are classified as satisfactory in all categories can be expected to impregnate about 50 ewes in a 60-day breeding season. Rams that receive exceptional ratings can be expected to impregnate 100 ewes during a 60-day breeding season. Any ram that does not receive at least a satisfactory rating in all categories should either be culled or retested in 60 days. The decision to cull or retest should be based on the severity of observed lesions and the economic value of the individual animal.[15,23–27]

Ancillary Tests

Ultrasonography can be used to evaluate the testicles of rams (or bucks). Changes from the normal homogeneous testicular parenchyma such as hyperechoic and hypoechoic areas are indicative of fibrotic changes or cystic structures. The examiner should not confuse the normal hyperechoic mediastinum that is found in the center of the testicle for a fibrotic lesion. The mediastinum appears as a distinct round area in the center of transverse images of the testicle and as a hyperechoic line on longitudinal images (Figure 8.5). The epididymis and spermatic cord also can be examined for fibrosis and cystic structures. Areas of fibrosis or degeneration and testicular abscesses can usually be visualized.[15]

Testicular biopsies using a 14-gauge biopsy needle can allow a direct examination of the testicular architecture. Testicular biopsies are useful in determining atrophy, degeneration, and hypoplasia. This technique is usually relegated to use in valuable animals. The clinician aseptically prepares the testicle and anesthetizes an area of skin. He or she then inserts the biopsy needle into the dorsum of the testicle, avoiding the epididymis and taking care not to penetrate the mediastinum. Tissue can be fixed in either Bouin's solution or 10% formalin for routine histopathologic analysis.[28]

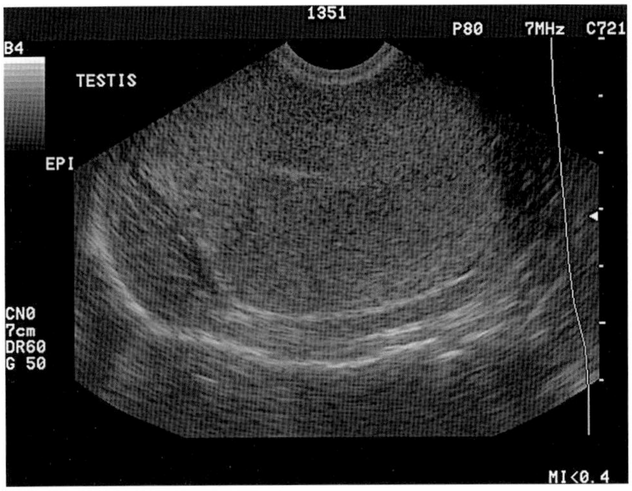

• **Fig. 8.5** Ultrasound of a normal testicle obtained from a 2-year-old crossbred ram demonstrating the normal echogenic, homogeneous appearance of the testicular parenchyma. The epididymis appears more hypoechoic compared to the testicular parenchyma, and the epididymal duct is seen running along the testicle. The parietal vaginal tunic is seen as a clearly defined hyperechoic linear structure surrounding the testicle. This ultrasound was obtained with a 7-MHz microconvex transducer. (Courtesy Dr. Karine Pader, Purdue University.)

Serologic screening in the form of an enzyme-linked immunosorbent assay (ELISA) for *B. ovis* should be performed annually on all rams at the time of the BSE.[15,27] *B. ovis* is a major cause of decreased fertility in flocks with multiple rams. *B. ovis* can have a significant impact on the production level of the flock by decreasing the number of multiple births, decreasing conception rates, and increasing the lambing interval. A study of rams in the western United States revealed a seroprevalence of *B. ovis* antibodies of 10%. Of the 10% that were seropositive, over half of the rams were subclinical.[25] Ram epididymitis due to *B. ovis* is a contagious venereal disease that generally affects mature rams. The bacterium is transmitted via homosexual activities or via the ewe during the breeding season. Ewes exposed to infected rams do not become permanently infected but serve as mechanical vectors for the spread of the disease. Thus, all rams that test positive for *B. ovis* should be culled immediately.[24]

BSE in the Buck (Goat)

All breeding bucks need to be evaluated for breeding soundness 3 to 4 weeks before mating season. As in the ram, the examination of the buck should include a physical examination, reproductive examination, measurement of SC, and semen collection and evaluation. BSEs are only able to evaluate the physical soundness and semen quality of the buck. A satisfactory finding cannot guarantee the buck's ability to produce live offspring.[15,29] Attempts to assess libido in the buck greatly aid in a complete reproductive evaluation. The libido measurement described for the ram can be adapted for the buck.[15]

Physical Examination. Physical examination of the buck must include a general examination for health, with particular attention to assessment of body condition and musculoskeletal condition (feet and legs). To be a satisfactory breeder, a buck should be in good body condition. Thin or excessively fat animals should be avoided (see Chapter 2).[29,30] The buck should be free of known genetic defects such as hernias, jaw malformation, cryptorchidism, supernumerary teats, and intersex condition. Bucks should not be phenotypically polled.

Examination of Reproductive Tract. Examination of the reproductive tract includes evaluation of the testes, epididymis, spermatic cord, and penis. Testis should be examined for size, symmetry, and consistency. A buck should have two large oval testes of equal size; they are firm during the breeding season and slightly softer during the nonbreeding season. If only one testicle is present, the male should be disqualified as a potential breeder. Ultrasonography may be useful in aiding detection or confirmation of abnormalities.[28–30] Gross changes in the epididymis are fairly rare in goats. The clinician should examine the penis for abnormalities when collecting a semen sample. The penis must be manually extended from the sheath so that a careful examination can be made. The urethra extends beyond the tip of the penis for about 2 to 3 cm, forming the urethral process. When bucks have a history of urinary calculi, the urethral process is usually removed during treatment because it is a common area of obstruction. The loss or removal of the urethral process appears to have no detrimental effect on the buck's fertility.[30]

Scrotal Circumference. Because of its high correlation of testicular size and capacity for sperm production, SC is important in the buck. However, its use in the evaluation of breeding soundness is not well defined. SC is measured in the buck as described in the ram. SC in 45-kg dairy goats has been reported to be 25 to 28 cm, with larger bucks having SCs of 34 to 36 cm.[29,30] In addition, the Western Regional Coordination Committee on Ram Epididymitis and Fertility recommends that ram lambs over 70 kg (150 lb) have a SC greater than 30 cm.[31] The SC of yearling rams (12–18 months) should measure greater than 33 cm.[32] In 1999, during the Georgia and Southeast Meat Goat Buck Performance Test, SCs in 45-kg, 7-month-old Kiko and Boer bucks averaged 26 to 29 cm.[33]

Semen Collection. Semen may be collected with an artificial vagina (AV) in a trained buck or by EEJ.[28] EEs should be 25 to 30 cm long and 2 to 3 cm in diameter. Many ram probes can be adapted for buck use. An AV can be built from a polyvinyl chloride (PVC) pipe or radiator hose with an inner liner made of a cut section of bicycle inner tube. An AV also can be purchased. The length of the AV should be 18 to 22 cm, and its outside diameter should be 6 cm. It should be filled with warm water to maintain proper turgor and warmth (38° to 40°C). A semen collection cone should be placed at one end. A nonspermicidal lubricant is placed in the open end. For EEJ, bucks are restrained in chutes or held against the wall. The rectum is cleaned of feces and a well-lubricated probe is inserted. The prostate is massaged five to six times, electrical current is applied through the probe for 4 to 6 seconds, and then the probe turned off for 3 to 4 seconds. This pattern is maintained until ejaculation occurs (usually four to five cycles). Libido cannot be assessed when collecting semen by an EE. During and after collection, semen should be protected from direct sunlight and temperature shock, and sperm motility should be evaluated within 10 minutes.[15]

Semen Evaluation. The volume of normal buck ejaculate is 0.5 to 1.5 mL (with an average of 1 mL). Semen is evaluated for color, gross and progressive mortality, morphology, and concentration.[30] Both semen quality and quantity may vary with age, season, temperature, breed, and even between individuals within the same breed. Normal semen values in the buck are as follows[30]:

Volume—1 mL (with a range of 0.5–1.5 mL)
Motility—80% (with a range of 70–90%)

• BOX 8-1 Minimum Acceptable Reproductive Criteria for a Satisfactory Potential Breeder Buck

Volume	0.5 mL
Motile sperm	70%
Concentration	2 billion
Morphology	80% normal

Concentration—4 billion (with a range of 2–5 billion) per milliliter

Normal morphology—80% (with a range of 70–90%)

Minimally acceptable values are shown in Box 8.1.

Volume is measured directly from the graduated collection vial. Volume is of some value in evaluating semen collected using an AV but of limited value when EEs are used. The color of semen depends on the number of spermatozoa per milliliter; it can vary from "whey-like" to "milky" to "creamy." Gross motility is measured as described for the ram. Even though concentration is not routinely assessed in field conditions, it is advisable to include it in the evaluation. Concentration can be easily assessed using a hemocytometer and a commercial Unopette system for white blood cell count.[30] Morphology can be determined by examination. An eosin-nigrosin–stained smear is evaluated using a 1000× objective; the examiner measures primary or secondary abnormalities in 100 to 200 spermatozoa per slide, as described for the ram (see Table 8.2). Normal values for a buck to be classified as a satisfactory potential breeder are shown in Box 8.1. A questionable potential breeder may require reevaluation after 8 weeks or need to be culled. The classification of unsatisfactory potential breeder may be given for reasons other than semen quality (e.g., cryptorchid, lameness). Bucks showing depressed libido, slightly decreased SC, and increased sperm abnormalities should be identified and culled.[28,29]

Buck (Cervid)

Previous comments for the ram and buck goat generally apply to cervidae. One exception would be SC, which is much smaller with normal ranges of from 15 to 23 cm depending on age and white-tailed versus mule deer. Yearling bucks tend to measure 15 to 18 cm and older and mature bucks measure 18 to 23 cm. Mule deer tend to have smaller SCs, in general, and have poorer semen quality and appear to be more seasonal than white-tailed deer. At the time of this writing, breeding soundness exams are unfortunately seldom performed on cervids, yet many bucks are infertile or have testicular damage from fighting and disease. Anesthesia is generally necessary for semen collection via EEJ. There are reports (Woodbury, personal communication, 2014) of semen collection in a cervid drop chute under haloperidol tranquilization. EEJ should be done carefully with a ram probe after cleaning out the rectum and palpating the internal genitalia, which can be easily reached with a finger. The penis is generally exteriorized by repelling the prepuce while applying pressure to the sigmoid flexure and pushing the penis out of the prepuce. A slow increase of power with 3–4-second pauses between stimulations has proven very effective in achieving ejaculation. The semen is very concentrated and usually of excellent quality (motility, morphology, and concentration). The male cervid does not have a urethral process, and the penis of the mule deer and white-tailed deer vary between each other as the mule deer has a blunter glans, versus the penis of the white-tailed deer, which has a rather long, narrow, pointed glans.

Selection and Management

Ram

A ram with good-quality semen, adequate testicular size, and good libido can breed 100 ewes in a 17-day breeding season.[15,20,24] However, most producers in North America use 3 to 3.5 rams per 100 ewes. Yearlings and mature rams can be expected to service 35 to 50 ewes, whereas ram lambs should only be expected to service 15 to 25 ewes.[15] Adjustments should be made for multiple sire breeding units. It is desirable to always have more than three rams to a multiple sire unit because this tends to alleviate some of the territorial fighting among rams.[15]

Libido serving capacity and testing can provide useful information regarding how many ewes a ram can be expected to service or even if a ram should be retained.[20–22] Serving capacity tests are performed to measure how many times a ram services ewes during a defined period. One report suggests that the test serving pen should be approximately 3 m × 5 m and in clear view of rams that are to be tested.[20–22] However, larger or smaller pens may be used. Typically, the ram is placed in a pen with two to four cycling, unrestrained ewes for a period of 20 to 40 minutes. The keeper monitors and records all sexual behavior with emphasis on the number of breedings. Such tests are the most reliable predictor of an animal's libido. Ewes used for libido tests may be synchronized to estrus. Compared with low-libido rams, rams that are identified as high-performing or having a high degree of libido have a higher lambing percentage and more live lambs born per exposed ewe. Serving capacity tests also may be used to determine proper ram-to-ewe stocking ratios. These tests of flock reproduction can produce a shorter, more uniform lambing season.[20–22] Adult rams achieving four to six or more breedings during a 30-minute period are preferred. Rams achieving two or three breedings in 30 minutes are acceptable. Rams that appear sexually inactive can be tested twice. If they still appear to be sexually inactive, the keeper can paint the rumps of the tested ewes with different colors of ink and leave the rams overnight in the pen with them. The next day, the keepers should examine the rams' chests for the colored ink.[15] Fertility is maximized if only acceptable groups of rams are kept for breeding.

Selection of rams from high-producing ewes as measured by the number of lambs born, the weight of lambs weaned, and a history of having lambs early in the season also may have a positive relationship with fertility.[15] It appears that rams born co-twin to male siblings have higher serving capacities than those born co-twin to females.[15,23] Rams also should be selected for structural soundness and for the genetics they can pass on to their offspring because they contribute approximately 60 to 80% of the genetics of the average flock.[16] Rams should be maintained on a good nutritional, vaccination, and deworming program. Their body condition scores before breeding season should be 3.5 to 4. Obesity minimizes willingness to breed. Rams should be sheared and their feet trimmed before breeding season. During breeding season, free access to shelter or shady areas should be provided to minimize heat stress–associated infertility. Special care should be taken during the initial examination of rams to eliminate those that have diseases of the reproductive tract.[15]

Buck (Goat)

Bucks are chosen based on individual performance or progeny testing for traits such as milk production, meat traits, adaptability, and twinning rate. Prolific bucks are preferred. Birth, weaning, and yearling information is valuable in establishing the superiority or inferiority of a potential sire. Selection for growth rate and meat production should be a high priority for meat goats. Bucks should have good conformation and be large and muscular. Selection based on testicle size is important; bucks with the largest testicles usually produce the highest-quality sperm.[15]

The same serving capacity tests used for rams are applicable to bucks. Bucks with apparent defects in posture and genital tract abnormalities should be avoided. Because the intersex condition has been linked to the polled gene, the use of phenotypic polled bucks should be avoided. Changing bucks every 2 years prevents loss of vigor and reduces inbreeding in the herd. Bucks should be kept separate from does in a group on pasture or in single housing. They should be introduced with females only during the established mating season, after which their job for the year is finished. Bucks require proper nutrition, routine foot care, vaccination, deworming, and exercise (see Chapter 19).

Bucks (Cervids)

In general, the previous information on buck (goats) and rams applies to cervids. The buck is generally chosen on antler size and conformation as well as genetic merit of dam and sire. At the time of this writing, very few other criteria are followed in the cervid industry and may lead to problems in the future.

Diseases of the Male: Testicular Abnormalities

Varicoceles

A varicocele is defined as a localized dilatation and thrombosis of the internal spermatic vein and is recognized as a fluctuant to hard swelling in the spermatic cord. Varicoceles are more common in rams than in bucks. This condition is often manifested as rear limb lameness and awkward posture as the ram tries to relieve pressure on the swollen cords. Affected animals may become weak and susceptible to other diseases as a result of debilitation brought on by an unwillingness to walk to obtain food and water. Varicoceles can be diagnosed by palpation and diagnostic ultrasound. Abnormalities such as decreased total sperm count, reduced sperm motility, and morphologic abnormalities of the sperm are often associated with varicoceles. The exact etiology of the condition is not known but a genetic predisposition is suspected. No easy treatment is available and affected rams or bucks should be culled.[34]

Epididymitis in Older Males

Epididymitis is a rare condition in the buck but a clinically important disease in rams. Epididymitis in rams should be considered to be caused by *B. ovis* until proven otherwise. This is especially true of older rams that have been actively breeding in multiple sire units. However, one case report involving an outbreak of *B. ovis* in a group of virgin ram lambs suggests that the disease may be spread in utero or neonatally, before any known sexual activity.[35] The primary means of spread is thought to be through contact with mucous membranes, which results in bacteremia. The organism localizes in the epididymis and secondary sex glands. Contact can occur among rams and from recently infected ewes; venereal and oral-nasal transmission also are possible.[36] Swelling of the epididymis is the primary presenting sign, occurring about 3 weeks after the initial exposure. Grossly, there is localized inflammation followed by hyperplasia and obstruction of the epididymal ducts. This obstruction causes a backup of spermatozoa, the development of sperm granulomas, and pressure necrosis. The seminal vesicles also are commonly affected, which may account for the large number of infected rams that show no palpable signs of epididymitis.[36] The quality of spermatozoa collected from infected rams, even without lesions present, is negatively impacted and usually contains a large number of detached heads and polymorphonuclear neutrophils that can be seen on the motility preparations or on Wright's stained specimens.[37] Microscopic evaluation of Stamp's modified Ziehl-Neelsen–stained semen can also be a useful tool in diagnosis. The coccobacilli *Brucella* will stain red against a blue background. Culture for the presence *Brucella* organism is a good diagnostic tool for suspects.

Serology for *B. ovis* should be considered a routine part of a BSE. The most commonly used serologic tests for diagnosis of *B. ovis* are the ELISA, gel diffusion tests (GDTs), and complement fixation tests (CFT). ELISA offers the best sensitivity (97.6%), followed by the GDT (96.4%) and the CFT (92.7%).[38] ELISA was also found to be able to detect infected rams earlier than the CFT does.[39] A minimum of two tests performed at 4- to 8-week intervals should be implemented because of test sensitivities below 100%.[40] Species-specific polymerase chain reaction (PCR) tests are in development and appear to show promise with similar results as semen culture.[36,41,42] Following experimental inoculation in rams, seroconversion is reported to occur between 2 and 5 weeks with shedding of the organism in semen occurring between 4 and 9 weeks.[40] Herd infections with *B. ovis* can result in a 15% to 30% reduction in lambing rate depending on the chronicity of the herd problem. This decrease in reproductive efficiency results from lowered fertility in the rams, failure of the ewes to conceive, reabsorption of embryos, abortions, stillbirths, and weak lambs.[43,44]

Recommendations outlined by Bulgin[39] include the following:

- Buying virgin rams that have been serologically tested for brucellosis and retested in 30 days
- Keeping newly purchased rams separate until all rams are tested free from *Brucella*
- Performing scrotal palpation and culling all rams with epididymitis before the breeding season
- Culling all *B. ovis*–positive rams
- Retesting all rams in the flock 60 days after any rams are found positive
- Performing annual BSEs on all rams

If a large number of serologically positive rams is found after a year of adherence to these guidelines, efforts should be made to determine whether a serologically negative carrier ram is present in the flock by culturing semen from all rams.

Antibiotic treatment has been attempted, but these cases often do not respond well to therapy. In addition, vaccination against *B. ovis* is not typically recommended due to interferences with the ELISA. A test-and-cull strategy is most often recommended.

Brucella in Cervids

Studies evaluating the spread of *Brucella abortus* among cattle, bison, and elk around the Greater Yellowstone Areas of Montana,

Wyoming, and Idaho suggest that Rocky Mountain elk *(Cervus elaphus nelsoni)* is the probable source for brucellosis outbreaks in cattle in Montana and Wyoming.[45] Male cervids can also become infected with *B. ovis*. Transmission from rams to red deer stags has been documented.[46]

Epididymitis in Young Males

In younger rams, and less commonly in bucks, epididymitis can be caused by a number of organisms such as *Histophilus*, *Actinobacillus*, and *Haemophilus* species; *Corynebacterium pseudotuberculosis*; and possibly other pathogens.[47–49] Lamb epididymitis can be spread from ram to ram by the oral or nasal route. The organisms responsible for lamb epididymitis can frequently be cultured from the preputial cavity of rams younger than 2 years of age and are commonly found in the mucous membranes of the prepuce, penis, mouth, and nasal cavity.[43] Colonization and subsequent disease of the reproductive tract may depend on the hormonal changes that occur during maturation and puberty, along with other unknown differentiating factors that allow most animals to eliminate the bacteria spontaneously while causing others to develop clinical signs.[50] Experimentally, supportive epididymitis and spermatic granulomas may be seen within 24 and 72 hours postinoculation with some pathogens, respectively.[51] Diagnosis of lamb epididymitis is made by palpation of the enlarged epididymis and by ruling out *B. ovis* infection. Semen from infected lambs is characterized by a large number of neutrophils and by the morphologically abnormal spermatozoa typical of epididymal disease. Although the signs of most cases of lamb epididymitis are restricted to the reproductive tract, occasionally, an associated fever and hindlimb lameness also occur. Lamb epididymitis can be treated with long-acting oxytetracycline (20 mg/kg intramuscularly [IM] or subcutaneously [SC]) injections for three treatments at 3-day intervals.[50,52] Inclusion of tetracycline (20 mg/kg by mouth [PO] daily) products in the ration may be appropriate in herds experiencing a high incidence of lamb epididymitis. Treatment should be reserved for valuable lambs and cases diagnosed in the early stages because most lambs develop scar tissue in the epididymis that prevents functional recovery.

Orchitis

Orchitis is a common occurrence in the ram and is occasionally seen in the buck.[53–55] Scrotal abscesses may be caused by trauma or may be an extension of epididymitis. Whenever testicular trauma or infection is encountered, it should be considered a medical emergency in breeding animals. Excessive heat from one testicle can result in possibly irreversible thermal injury to the germinal epithelium of the contralateral testicle.[47] All the organisms discussed in the section on epididymitis can cause orchitis. The signs include a hot, swollen scrotum (usually unilaterally), inability to move the affected testicle freely in the scrotum, and pain on manipulation of the affected testicle and the scrotum. Some animals may show signs of systemic disease, pain on walking, and decrease in libido.[55] In cases affecting valuable animals, hemicastration in the acute phase may prevent permanent infertility.

Sperm Granulomas

Although testicular tumors are rare in rams and bucks, granulomatous swellings are occasionally encountered. Sperm granulomas are more common in goats than in sheep, and unlike abscesses or other forms of orchitis, they usually occur bilaterally. Sperm granulomas are often caused by a partial or complete blockage of the efferent ducts draining into the epididymis.[55] As pressure builds, the ducts become distended and may rupture, resulting in a severe inflammation. As fluid accumulates, pressure continues to build, and testicular degeneration may occur. Some animals are initially fertile but lose fertility after the efferent ducts become completely occluded. Granulomas are firm swellings found in the head of the epididymis. On palpation, the testicles may be initially edematous, but they eventually become hard. The testicles may eventually become small and atrophic. Ultrasonographic evaluation may reveal mineralization of the testicles or the granuloma itself. No treatment is available for sperm granulomas, and the clinician should be cognizant of the potential association with the intersex condition.

Testicular Hypoplasia and Degeneration

Testicular hypoplasia and degeneration are difficult to differentiate during an initial examination.[53,55] In rams and bucks out of season, testicular size and palpation characteristics may be difficult to differentiate from subtle cases of testicular atrophy. More extreme differences are encountered in rams than in goats, but in general, the testicle in the nonbreeding season is smaller and lacks normal resiliency.[53] True hypoplasia can be associated with the intersex condition in bucks and a specific chromosomal abnormality in rams.[53,55]

Other causes of testicular atrophy include zinc deficiency, hypothyroidism (iodine deficiency, ingestion of goitrogenous plants), starvation diets, systemic disease, and heat and cold stress. Iodine-induced hypothyroidism has been associated with decreased testicular weight, depressed spermatogenesis, and decreased libido. Atrophic or degenerated testicles become elongated, small, and either softer or harder. Normal testicles usually have a homogenous echogenicity on ultrasound. Atrophic or degenerative testicles tend to have a heterogenous pattern and more hyperechoic areas.[56] Testicular biopsy can be of value in diagnosis. Many cases of atrophy and degeneration are not treatable; the exceptions are cases caused by diet or certain diseases. In treating diet-related atrophy, ensuring adequate protein-energy intake and free access to a good-quality trace mineral supplement is essential. If zinc deficiency is suspected, reducing the legume content of the diet and adding a chelated form of zinc (zinc methionine) to the diet or trace mineral mixture are useful. If iodine-induced hypothyroidism is diagnosed, the inclusion of iodine in a trace mineral mixture and the removal of goitrogenous plants from the diet should be undertaken; males should be kept off pastures with goitrogenous plants before and during breeding.[47]

Cryptorchidism

Cryptorchidism occurs when either one or both testes fail to descend from the abdominal cavity into the scrotum. The retained testicle may be located at any point along the normal path of descent. Among unilateral cryptorchids, the right testicle is retained in the abdomen in ~80 to 90% of the animals.[57,58] A higher incidence has also been reported in intersexes. However, cryptorchidism is not related to the intersex condition in Angora goats. In Angora bucks, cryptorchidism is a recessive trait.[59] The diagnosis is made by physical examination. Cryptorchidism is rare in ruminants, and cases are often complicated by a previous hemicastration. If either the history or physical examination suggests the presence of a testicle within the abdominal cavity, then an exploratory laparotomy should be performed to remove the retained testicle. As this condition is thought to be heritable, cryptorchid bucks should not be used for breeding and their sires and dams should also be culled.[60]

Intersex

Caprine intersexes are referred to as *male pseudohermaphrodites* because a majority of them have testes. True hermaphrodites have testicular and ovarian structures and generally constitute a much smaller proportion of intersexes.[61] Intersex is more prevalent in polled dairy goats (Saanen, Toggenburg, alpine, and Damascus breeds). The polled intersex condition is rare or not reported in some breeds (Nubian and Angora).[62] Cytogenetic evaluations of caprine intersexes clearly show that most polled intersexes are karyotypically female (XX), and the breeding histories of the parents indicate that intersexes are homozygous for the polled trait.[55]

Affected animals are genetically female but may exhibit male, female, or mixed external characteristics.[62] Generally, they are female-appearing at birth, but as they reach sexual maturity, they become larger than normal females, with masculine heads and erect hair on their necks.[50] An enlarged clitoris in a doe-like animal or a decreased anogenital distance in a more masculine individual is typical of intersex[62] (Figure 8.6). Intersexes may start to smell and may act aggressively toward other goats and people during the breeding season. Some dribble urine or stretch out with a concave back and urinate forward between the legs.[61] Whenever bilateral cryptorchidism is encountered, intersex should be suspected. The testes are generally intraabdominal (in the normal location of the ovaries), but they may be partially or totally descended.[47] Partially descended testes may be mistaken for udders, especially when they begin to enlarge during puberty.[61] Hypospadias (opening of the urethral orifice on the ventral aspect of the penis), sperm granulomas, and hypoplastic testicles should all be considered part of the intersex complex.[55,63]

The principal hormone produced by the gonads in caprine intersexes is testosterone, which accounts for masculine behavior. Intersex goats can be used as teaser animals because they do not produce sperm.[47] Gonadectomy is generally required if the animal is to be used as a pet. Identifying intersex animals with normal or nearly normal external genitalia is difficult. Failure to exhibit estrus, development of male behavior during the breeding season, a shortened vagina on speculum examination, and smaller-than-normal teats may be the first signs of the intersex condition.[62] The breeding of phenotypically polled bucks should be avoided.

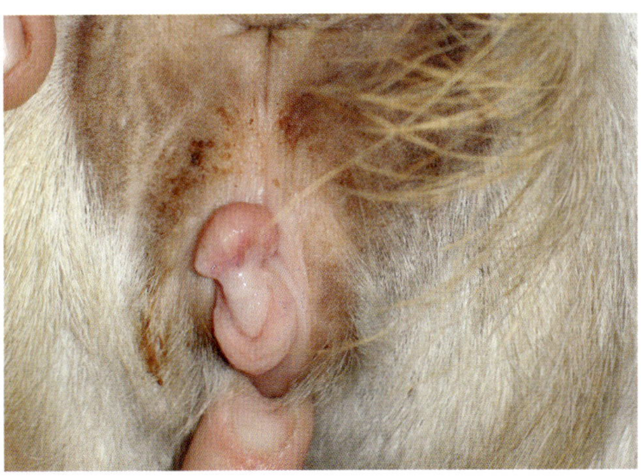

• Fig. 8.6 This intersex goat had two ovotestes in the inguinal region. The vulva joins to an enlarged clitoris at its termination.

Cervids. As a general rule, defects are rarely seen in bucks. Testicular damage is most often a result of fighting or systemic illness. However, there is no reason to believe that any or all of the previous conditions will not be found or reported in the future as deer farming continues and the incidence of inbreeding continues at the rate that is currently practiced.

Diseases of the Male: Penile Abnormalities

Hypospadias

Several penile abnormalities may occur, albeit rarely, in sheep and goats.[47,63–65] Both hypospadias and short penile length are associated with intersex in goats. Such animals should be culled. Careful examination of the penis in the fully extended state may reveal existing abnormalities. Occasionally, urethral rupture (as a sequela to urethral stones), balanoposthitis (see Chapter 12), injuries to the vermiform appendage, hair rings, and other abnormalities are identified.[47]

Ulcerative Posthitis

Ulcerative posthitis (enzootic posthitis, sheath rot, or pizzle rot) is an infectious, inflammatory condition of the penis, prepuce, and sheath of sheep and goats consuming high-protein diets.[47,66] The disease is caused by an interaction of the local bacterial flora (*Corynebacterium renale*) with excess urinary urea. Excess ammonia may damage the mucosal surfaces and result in ulcerative posthitis. Ulcerative posthitis is characterized by swelling of the prepuce, necrosis and ulceration of the preputial mucosa, and straining to urinate. Removing the animals from a high-protein diet and shearing the "prescrotal" wool/hair will clear most cases. Antibiotics, disinfectants, and antiinflammatory drugs may be needed in some cases (see Chapter 12).

Phimosis

Both phimosis (inability to extend the penis) and paraphimosis (inability to withdraw the penis into the prepuce) are occasionally seen in rams and bucks; both conditions can cause significant loss of libido and fertility. If they are not quickly diagnosed and treated, affected animals may be rendered infertile. These two conditions may be associated with hair ring, trauma, and balanoposthitis. In cases associated with a hair ring on the glans of the penis, inspecting the penis allows the clinician to identify the problem and remove the "ring" of hair.[47] Shearing the wool or mohair just anterior to the sheath can minimize the incidence of this problem.[53,55] Phimosis also may occur as a sequela to trauma, balanoposthitis, and congenital abnormalities. In cases of trauma, an adhesion may form in the sheath or in the sigmoid region, resulting in an inability to extend the penis. As a general rule, these cases may be difficult to treat. In cases in which inflammation and scarring result in posthitis, the treatment is the same as that described for balanoposthitis. The clinician can attempt to "break down" the adhesions manually. The use of nonsteroidal antiinflammatory drugs (NSAIDs; flunixin meglumine 1 to 2 mg/kg twice a day [BID]) or antibiotics (procaine penicillin 22,000 IU/kg BID) and lavage of the sheath with mild antiseptics may be of value. In cases of phimosis, most animals experience a loss of libido and should be culled because the prognosis is poor.[55]

Cervids. While undocumented, most of these conditions can be assumed to occur in cervids as their anatomy and physiology do not differ significantly from that of sheep and goats.

Paraphimosis

Paraphimosis also is associated with trauma, infection, and balanoposthitis. It is slightly more common in bucks than in rams, but it is rare in both. In cases of paraphimosis, applying antibiotic cream with or without corticosteroids, replacing the penis, and placing a purse-string suture into the preputial orifice may be of value. The inclusion of a tube in the sheath, exiting through the orifice, allows urine drainage. The clinician should take care to ensure proper urine flow. Flushing the sheath and penis with a mild antiseptic solution, providing penile hydrotherapy, and covering the penis with medicated ointments are valuable treatments for this condition. The penis should be extended at least every third day so the keeper or clinician can monitor healing. Sexual rest should be enforced throughout recovery. However, the prognosis in these cases is poor, particularly if the condition is more than 2 weeks old and the animal makes no attempt to retract the penis.[55]

Special Surgical Procedures

Castration

Castration of the normal young male is among the most commonly performed procedure in small ruminants. Kids and rams are castrated for management and production reasons. Mohair production is higher in castrated goats than intact ones.[67] Castration of kids fed to slaughter increases carcass weight, dressing percentage, and external fat score while reducing internal fat score.[68] There are volumes of publications on how castration age and techniques affect carcass quality and growth rates. This component of meat production management is beyond the scope of our discussion, which will concentrate on the description of different techniques of castration.[69–71] Some producers delay castration in animals that are intended to be used as a work or pet animal that will have an extended lifetime when compared to those used for meat. There is a trend to delay castration in some meat goats that are fed a very high concentrate diet and used for show before slaughter. This is often related to concerns of urolithiasis. While often debated, at least one study evaluating the effect of castration on penile length, diameter, and urethral diameter determined that lambs castrated prior to 3 months of age did not have the same penile development as intact lambs or ones castrated at 5 months of age.[72] Most importantly, relative to urolithiasis, the urethral cross-sectional diameter was also significantly smaller in the lambs castrated prior to 3 months of age when compared to the intact lambs. The lambs castrated at 5 months of age did not show a significant difference in penile or urethral diameter from the intact lambs.[72]

Most producers castrate their own animals although veterinarians may be called upon to perform routine castrations in small flocks or on older animals that were not castrated at an early age for whatever reason. The most frequently used techniques are the bloodless procedures using elastrator bands or the Burdizzo emasculatome. Alternatively, traditional surgical excision of the testes is done. Each method has advantages and disadvantages, but the method chosen often becomes a matter of individual operator bias. The elastrator band technique is frequently used in lambs and kids less than 1 week old in conjunction with tail docking and/or dehorning. It can be used up to 3 or 4 months of age depending on the size of the animal but is better done at an earlier age. The animal may be restrained with the rear end up by holding the hindlimbs or smaller animals may be held with the front and rear limbs of each side held together. The elastrator band should be placed in a disinfectant prior to use. Special pliers are used to place the band around the proximal scrotum, being sure that both testicles are distal to the band. Proper placement will have the band be distal to the rudimentary teats, making sure not to include the penis within the band (Figure 8.7). The elastrator band restricts blood flow to all tissues distal to the band and causes subsequent avascular necrosis and sloughing of the scrotum and testes. The tissue usually sloughs in 7 to 10 days. The sloughing tissue and subsequent wound are prime areas for infection with Clostridial organisms. Tetanus is not an uncommon sequela to castration, especially when elastrator bands are used (Figure 8.8). Therefore, any animal not previously vaccinated for

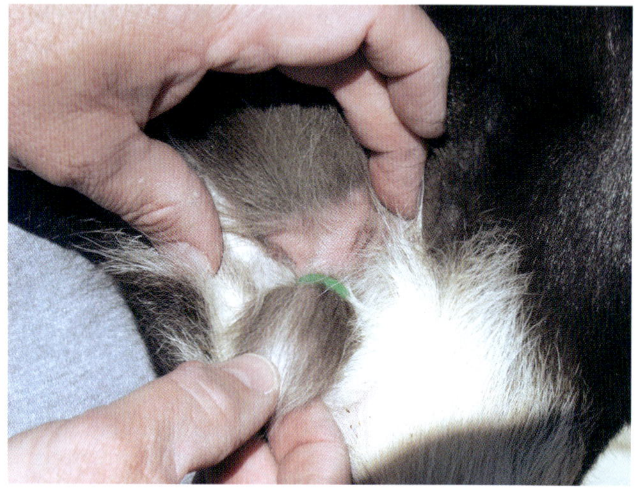

• **Fig. 8.7** A green elastrator band has been placed on the proximal scrotum of a 3-week-old Oberhasli-cross buck. Rudimentary teats can be seen proximal to the elastrator band in the nonhaired skin.

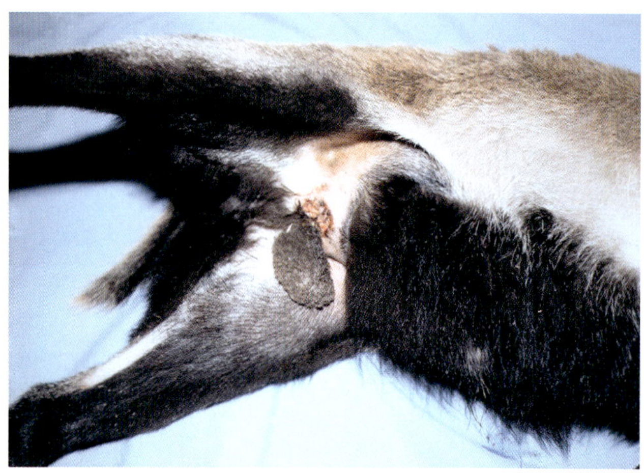

• **Fig. 8.8** The sloughing scrotum of a 5-week-old Barbados lamb approximately 1 week after application of an elastrator band for castration. The lamb, in lateral recumbency, exhibits the rigidity of tetanus. The owner performed the castration without providing any tetanus prophylaxis.

Clostridial diseases should be administered both tetanus antitoxin and tetanus toxoid at the time of castration. One may consider excising the tissue distal to the elastrator band 1 or 2 days after band application to lessen complications. If one (or both) testicle is proximal to the band, the animal will exhibit characteristics of an intact male. He will most likely be infertile because of improper thermoregulation of the testes displaced proximally near the external inguinal ring but surgical castration will be required to remove the remaining testes. The surgical castration in this case will be more difficult than a normal castration because of fibrous tissue and adhesions present. If the penis is included in the band, it is usually at the distal bend of the sigmoid flexure. This causes urethral obstruction and rupture subsequently leading to the euthanasia of the kid or ram, or at the very least an urethrostomy.

Another bloodless technique is the use of the Burdizzo emasculatome. The emasculatome crushes the spermatic cord within the scrotum, causing atrophy of the testicle while sparing the scrotal skin. The testicle should be gently pushed into the distal aspect of the scrotum and the spermatic cord held laterally within the scrotum. The Burdizzo should be applied twice (the second crush just distal to the first) to each respective spermatic cord and held about 10 seconds, without crossing the median raphe of the scrotum. If one crosses the median raphe of the scrotum with the Burdizzo crush, the scrotal skin is likely to become avascular and slough. The respective spermatic cords should be crushed at different levels, which helps maintain viability of the scrotum.

While both the elastrator band and the Burdizzo emasculatome are bloodless techniques, many still prefer surgical castration by excision of the distal half to one-third of the scrotum with a scalpel blade or using a Newberry knife to leave two flaps of scrotal skin (cranial and caudal). The testicles are exposed and removed after making the skin incision of choice (Figure 8.9). Many prefer to place ligatures on the spermatic cord or crush the cord with an emasculator to assure appropriate hemorrhage control. Care should be taken when using an emasculator routinely used for larger species such as horses in that an emasculator that functions well in equine castration may not adequately crush the smaller cord of the small ruminant. Therefore, the clinician may prefer to use ligatures that take very little time and do not add appreciable expense to the procedure. The spermatic cord is then transected distal to the ligature. The testicles may be removed by traction as is commonly done in calves, but this method has been associated with herniation almost immediately after the castration in some cases. If one chooses to pull the testicles, they should apply pressure over the respective external inguinal ring with fingers while pulling the testes with the other hand to minimize trauma to the ring and subsequent herniation. Animals less than 2 months old may be castrated this way using physical restraint but older animals should have local anesthesia and sedation if not general anesthesia. An alternative to traditional castration equipment is the Henderson Castration Tool.[73–75] The Henderson tool has been used successfully on bucks and rams over 30 to 40 lb depending on testicular size.

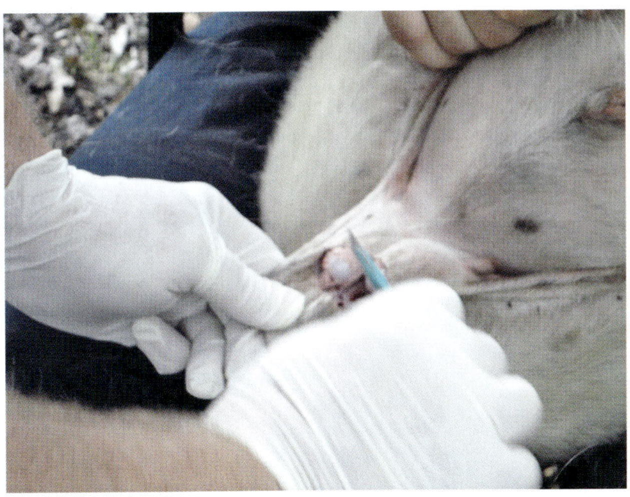

• **Fig. 8.9** In this picture, the ram lamb is being restrained by a sitting holder (as described in Chapter 1). The surgeon is removing the distal one half to one third of the scrotum, exposing the two testicles. The testicles were then separated from the surrounding tissues and removed by "pulling," and the goat was examined for inguinal hernia and given a tetanus toxoid inoculation. (NOTE: One of the authors—MAE—routinely sprays insect repellant around the scrotal area, post castration, regardless of the controversy surrounding this practice.)

Castrating 4- to 5-month-old lambs using the Burdizzo method was less stressful than conventional surgical castration.[76] Other workers suggest that both Burdizzo and elastrator band techniques caused less postoperative pain than traditional surgical castration in lambs over 10 weeks of age.[77] The Burdizzo method is subject to failure in some cases even when done by experienced practitioners. Histological sections of the testicles of 34 lambs castrated with the Burdizzo procedure showed failure of involution of testicular parenchyma in most of the samples.[78] Regardless of the method of castration used, local anesthesia in the spermatic cord reduces pain in the animals. Bupivacaine has been shown to be more effective than lidocaine in decreasing pain over time.[77]

A pinhole castration technique that entails a percutaneous stab incision in the proximal scrotum through which the spermatic cord is ligated has been reported.[79] The ligation leads to atrophy of the testis. The technique does not require any special instruments and the authors of the study believe that it is a simple, less painful, and cost-effective method of castration. Histopathologic evaluation of the testis 6 months after ligation showed seminiferous tubules with areas of calcification but no sperm.[79]

As an alternative to surgical castration, some report success with chemical castration. One effective method is to inject 88% lactic acid at a dose of 0.2 mL/kg of body weight into each testicle of adult goats. However, this may be more stressful than surgical castration because cortisol levels remained high for a longer time period in these animals than ones surgically castrated.[80] Another chemical castration technique involves injection of 10% formalin into the testicle. When done in 3-week-old goats, this method caused marked fibrosis and it was suggested to be a viable option for chemical castration in very young goats.[81]

Unilateral Castration

Rams and bucks can be rendered infertile by a number of unilateral scrotal conditions, including hydrocele, hematocele, orchitis, and tumors such as mesothelioma. Conditions such as those listed can have a detrimental effect on the thermoregulation of the unaffected testicle, thus causing infertility. If done early in the course of unilateral disease, the contralateral testicle frequently returns to normal sperm production and thus the male will be fertile.

Unilateral castration is done with the animal under general anesthesia in lateral recumbency with the affected testicle up and the upper leg abducted (see Chapter 18). One could probably do this surgery with sedation, epidural, and local anesthesia;

however, an aseptic technique is critical to avoid infection of the surgical site, which would have quite a negative impact on the return to fertility. The skin incision is made in an elliptical fashion longitudinally on the lateral aspect of the scrotum over the affected testicle. The incision is continued through the skin and subcutaneous tissues, leaving the vaginal tunic intact if possible. The testicle within the tunic is bluntly freed from the scrotum. Then double ligation of the cord is done with a circumferential suture proximal to a transfixation suture using absorbable #2 suture material. The elliptical incision allows resection of much of the scrotal skin, which in turn eliminates much of the potential dead space for closure. If the practitioner with limited experience performing this approach has concerns of removing too much skin, they can make the initial skin incision as a simple longitudinal incision then convert it to an elliptical one by resecting skin after removing the affected testicle when it is clear how much skin is needed for closure. Either way, the subcutaneous tissues should be closed in several layers to obliterate the dead space. The skin is closed in a continuous interlocking pattern. Some surgeons place a drain in the scrotum and/or leave the ventral most part of the skin incision open. One of the authors (MAE) prefers skin resection and complete closure to achieve primary healing of the skin incision (Figure 8.10A, B). Perioperative antibiotics and antiinflammatories are appropriate (see Appendix 1). If primary healing occurs without complications, the semen quality should no longer show negative effects of the unilateral disease by 90 days after surgery. Repeated semen evaluations of normal fertile goats after unilateral castration failed to show any detrimental effects on sperm motility compared to control, nonoperated bucks. There was no difference noted based on the particular testicle removed.[82]

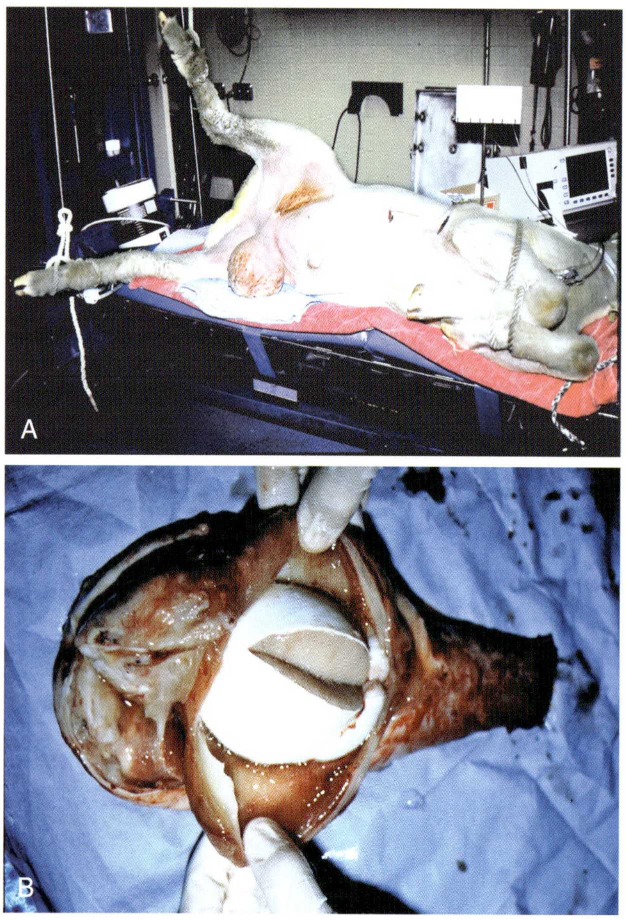

• **Fig. 8.10** **A.** A 3-year-old Rambouillet ram with right-sided scrotal swelling. The ram is positioned in left lateral recumbency under general anesthesia with the right hindlimb abducted for unilateral castration. **B.** The right testicle, which was removed from the ram, shows a thickened vaginal tunic, edema, and adhesions associated with the tail of the epididymis.

Cryptorchid Castration

Cryptorchidism is a rare condition in ruminants.[83] Cryptorchidism is an inherited recessive trait in at least the angora breed of goats.[84] It is most easily diagnosed when a reliable history tells that no attempts have been made to castrate (or hemicastrate) the animal in question. Frequently, male characteristics or behavior leads to an exploratory surgery to search for the retained testicle(s). If retained, the testicle is not usually located near the inguinal ring or easily retrievable via an inguinal extension of the gubernaculum testes as in the horse. The retained testicle is more likely within the abdomen and usually closer to the kidney than the inguinal ring, although it may also be found at the internal inguinal ring. The surgery can be done via a traditional laparotomy or laparoscopy. Laparoscopy allows better visualization of the abdomen and is preferred in most of these cases. The animal should be either sedated or under general anesthesia and in dorsal recumbency after having roughage withheld for 36 to 48 hours to decrease the visceral fill and allow better visualization within the abdominal cavity. Standard laparoscopic technique with a scope portal near the umbilicus and instrument portals between the scope portal and the caudal part of the fold of the flank is used (Figure 8.11). The retained testicle is often freed easily and exteriorized from the abdominal cavity for ligation. Other techniques such as cautery and intracorporeal ligation can be used at the preference of the surgeon.[85]

Alternatively, the animal can be placed in lateral recumbency for an exploratory surgery via a flank incision. The flank exploratory allows very limited visualization relying more on what the

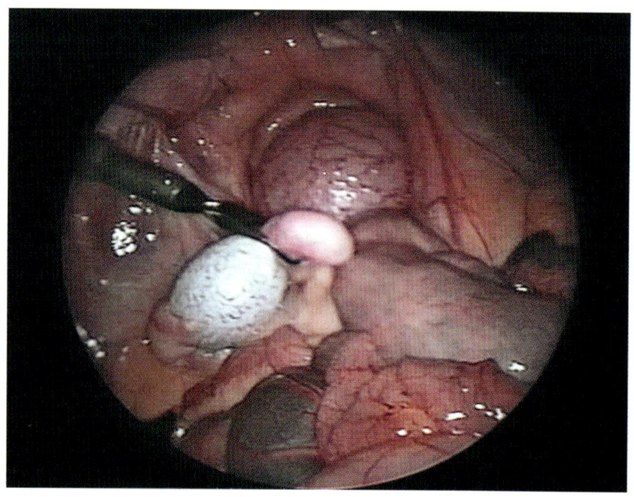

• **Fig. 8.11** Laparoscopic view of a left retained testicle in a 6-month-old Boer goat. The testicle is being held by laparoscopic forceps. The bladder is seen caudal and to the right of the testicle (top, center of the picture). This testicle was removed from the abdomen through the instrument portal after enlargement of the opening to allow extracorporeal ligation. A 10-mm diameter, direct-vision laparoscopic scope and camera was used for this procedure.

practitioner can palpate than see. The practitioner may find the retained testicle with a simple sweep of the abdominal cavity. If that fails, then attempts are made to locate the vas deferens as it crosses the ureter, then trace it to the testicle is the systematic approach to finding the retained testicle.

Teaser Ram/Buck

Male small ruminants are rendered infertile for use in estrus detection or more often to place with females prior to exposure to a fertile male as a management tool. The females will start cycling in response to the presence of the altered male before the fertile male is added to the flock. This system will lead to lambs being born in a shorter time period, which allows for more efficient labor, management, disease control, and a lamb crop of uniform age and size. Regardless of the intended use of the infertile male, we will describe common procedures to accomplish this goal.

The vasectomy is likely the most commonly used technique in small ruminants. The technique is described from a caudal incision in bulls,[86] but the vasectomy may be performed via a proximal-cranial incision located near the teats in sheep and goats where the vas deferens is easily palpable. This surgery can be performed with the ram either "sitting" on his hindquarters or in right lateral recumbency. The vasectomy can be done with local anesthesia in tractable animals, but sedation or general anesthesia makes the restraint more dependable. Lumbo-sacral epidural anesthesia is another option. The proximal scrotum is clipped and prepped for surgery. The vas deferens can be palpated as a firm structure within the spermatic cord. A 3- to 4-cm incision is made through the scrotal skin near the teat over the palpable vas deferens. The incision is continued through vaginal tunic to expose the vas, which is elevated with hemostats and isolated. Ligatures can be placed on the vas approximately 6 cm apart then the section of the vas between the ligatures is resected. The tunic and skin are closed in a routine fashion. The procedure is repeated on the other side. Some practitioners perform the vasectomy on one testicle then perform a unilateral castration to remove the opposite one to allow for easy identification of the teaser male in case ear tag or other identification is lost. Resecting, collecting, and fixing in formalin a section of the vas for histological examination are a good practice.[74] However, paternity can be diagnosed with DNA techniques in modern veterinary medicine. Expression of the contents of the removed section onto a slide and observation under a microscope for sperm is also diagnostic for diagnosis of the successful vasectomy (Shipley, personal experience).

The vasectomy may also be done laparoscopically using standard technique to visualize the vas as it enters the abdomen through the internal inguinal ring. The vas can be isolated and transected after ligation with suture or staples. Cautery is a useful tool to quickly perform the laparoscopic ligation. However, the laparoscopic procedure does not offer any real advantages over the conventional surgical technique so it is difficult to justify the added expense of the equipment required (Figure 8.12A–C).

About 80% of rams will develop sperm granulomas after vasectomy. Such granulomas are on clinical examination by palpation or ultrasound examination. The granulomas do not have any clinically significant detrimental effects.[87] Vasectomized bucks can be used for heat detection as early as 1 week after surgery.[88] Semen evaluations performed 14 days after vasectomy failed to show any viable, motile sperm in five rams.[89]

One may choose to perform an epididymectomy rather than a vasectomy to create the teaser male. The animal is restrained and

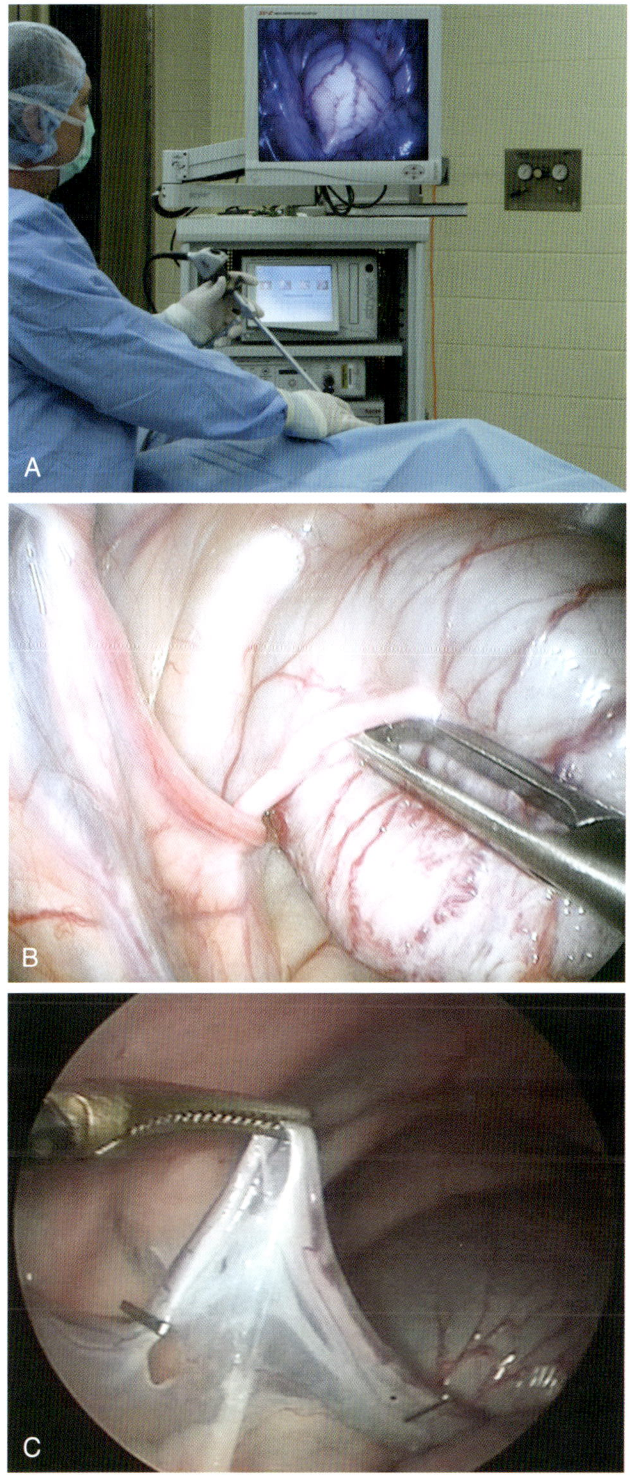

• **Fig. 8.12** Vasectomy in an anesthetized 2-year-old Pygmy buck. **A.** Laparoscopic evaluation of the internal inguinal ring, urinary bladder, and surrounding structures. The procedure was performed in a veterinary hospital, where a 10-mm-diameter, direct-vision laparoscopic viewing scope, camera, and TV monitor were available. **B.** The left internal inguinal ring is seen to the left of the bladder. The forceps are holding the vas deferens in the preferred location for occlusion by means of cautery or surgical staples before transaction for a laparoscopic vasectomy. **C.** Laparoscopic view of the vas deferens of a 1-year-old Alpine buck under general anesthesia. Laparoscopic staples are in place in the left vas deferens. The section of the vas deferens between the staples will be transected after being cauterized near the staples.

the distal third of the scrotum is prepared for aseptic surgery. Anesthesia can either be as an epidural or as a local infiltration of anesthetic in the ventral scrotum over the tail of the epididymis. The testicles are forced to the ventral aspect of the scrotum by grasping the neck of the scrotum. A caudal-to-cranial incision is made directly over the prominent tail of the epididymis about 2 to 3 cm long. The incision is extended through the skin and vaginal tunic until the epididymis bulges from the incision. Towel clamps placed on the epididymis help to retract the structure from the incision. When adequate tissue is exposed so as to assure complete removal of the tail of the epididymis, crushing forceps are placed across the tissue and a scalpel is used to excise the tissue. The excised tissue should be examined to ensure adequate resection. The skin can either be allowed to heal by second intention or a suture can be placed. The animal should be healed in 2 weeks and ready to use. Hemorrhage can be a problem with this technique, especially if the tunica albuginea of the testis is incised.[86] The blood and second intention wound healing may allow contamination and subsequently infection that can develop an abscess. Although both epididymectomy and vasectomy are applicable to both species, the clinician may find that the epididymectomy is more easily performed in the buck, while a vasectomy might be the best/easiest choice with the ram.

Cervid Castration

Cervids should not be castrated after pedicle development as they will grow "perruque" antlers.[90] Such "antlers" have abnormal conformation and do not "cast" as normal antlers will due to lack of rise and fall of testosterone levels. As such, they are in "velvet" constantly and are subject to freezing in cold weather and injury and infection to the velvet. If castrated prior to pedicle development, they will not grow antlers, so if castration is desired, it should be done early (probably less than 3 months in most cases). If castration must be done on a mature animal, then surgical removal of the pedicle may be attempted. Hormonal manipulation of the antler growth cycle may be a better choice in these situations. Using testosterone to harden the antler and shed velvet is followed by casting of the antler as testosterone wains. Antler growth is reinitiated, and the cycle starts over.

For sterilization, vasectomy or epididymectomy are easily done in the field under general anesthesia using the same techniques as described earlier for rams/buck goats. Most of the animals that are sterilized will have the hard antler cut just above the pedicle to render the buck safer during rut as they will fight and sometimes attack their handlers.

Penile Translocation

One method of preventing intromission is to "free" the penis and move it over to the left flank. This method is useful in some teaser systems. The surgery prevents intromission, but not ejaculation. Therefore, if penile translocation is attempted, a vasectomy (or epididymectomy) also should be performed. The clinician should give the buck or ram a systemic antimicrobial agent 2 or more hours before surgery. With the animal standing, the clinician marks an area 1 cm cranial to the flank fold.[67] The buck or ram is then heavily sedated, anesthetized with injectable anesthetics, intubated and maintained on gas anesthesia, or administered a lumbosacral epidural (see Chapter 18).[91] The animal is placed in right lateral recumbency, the ventral abdomen and left flank are clipped, and the surgical site is aseptically prepared.[86,91] The clinician excises a 4 to 7 cm circle of skin and cutaneous trunci muscle above the fold in the left flank. The lower edge of the circular incision should be 1 cm above the flank fold, just cranial to the mark made on the left flank. In mature rams with a large abdominal girth, some clinicians choose to graft the preputial orifice to a location medial to the fold of the flank rather than the further distance to the flank. Hemostasis is achieved, and the area is covered with saline-moistened gauze. The clinician then makes a circumferential incision, including 1 to 2 cm of haired skin around the preputial orifice. Then a ventral midline incision is made starting at the caudal aspect of the circumferential incision and extending two thirds of the way to the scrotum.[91] Care should be taken not to open the preputial cavity when making this incision. The penis is left inside the prepuce, and the two structures are freed of subcutaneous tissue by blunt dissection, avoiding large vessels. A single "reference" suture is placed in the skin at the most cranial aspect of the preputial orifice and a sterile glove is placed over the orifice.[86] From the circular incision in the flank to the most caudal aspect of the longitudinal incision, the clinician creates a tunnel using scissors and blunt dissection. The penis (along with the sterile glove covering the preputial orifice to maintain asepsis) is pulled through the tunnel. Alternatively, a sterile palpation sleeve with the hand cut off can be placed in the previously created tunnel and sponge forceps can be used to pull the freed skin surrounding the preputial orifice through the sleeve to the graft site. The penis should now be at a 45-degree angle to the long axis of the body.[86] The penis should not be restricted at any point through the tunnel, and the penis and prepuce should not be torsed. The reference suture should be used to align the cranial aspect of the preputial orifice to the dorsal portion of the circular flank incision.[86,91]

The preputial graft should be sutured to the circumferential incision with a two-layer simple interrupted pattern using absorbable material. The subcutaneous tissue of the transposed prepuce should be sutured to the cutaneous trunci and followed with closure of the skin. The clinician then closes the longitudinal incision, attempting to diminish all open dead space with absorbable material. The authors prefer either a simple interrupted or horizontal mattress type suture pattern. The skin over the longitudinal incision is closed by a simple interrupted pattern in all areas, except the most cranial aspect of the original preputial incision. To allow for ventral drainage, this area is not sutured.[86,91] Some clinicians routinely close the entire incision and achieve primary healing without drainage when good surgical technique is used. Fly control should be maintained, and tetanus prophylaxis should be provided (using tetanus toxoid or antitoxin). The clinician then performs a bilateral epididymectomy (or vasectomy), continues administering antibiotics for 5 to 7 days (procaine penicillin 22,000 IU/kg BID), and removes the sutures in 14 days. The male is ready for use in 1 month.

Semen Collection and Storage

Semen collection and storage from mature, healthy bucks and rams can used in many ways to maximize the overall fertility of a flock/herd and to enhance genetic progress in a breed and specie.[92–94] It appears that the semen of mature rams is of better quality and has higher fertility than that of young rams.[95] The two most common methods for semen collection employ either an EE or an AV. The AV is the preferred method for collecting semen as it is faster in trained males, is less stressful, and yields a more physiologically normal sample. The EE method may be considered for single collections and is generally the method of choice in cervids. EE-obtained samples tend to be inconsistent and often result in large amount of seminal fluid, lower concentration of spermatozoa than samples collected with an AV. In uncooperative or untrained males, an EE can be used with the male anesthetized.[92–94,96–98] Dairy bucks are handled more often and are more easily trained to use an AV. Semen from meat bucks is more commonly collected by EE, but they too can be trained to service an AV. Semen collected by EE is generally of larger volume but lower concentration than that collected by AV. Goat bucks can be collected two to three times daily on alternate days. Intervals of 30 minutes to 1 hour are advisable between daily collections to obtain good-quality semen.[96] White-tailed and mule deer bucks are generally collected after going hard antler (beginning of the rut) until antler drop (January to March). They may be collected two to three times 5 to 10 minutes apart under anesthesia to maximize semen collection. In general, the closer the cervid is collected to the "peak" rut, the better the semen output, quality, and probably freezability will be.

In sheep and goats, intervals of 30 minutes to 1 hour are advisable between collections in order to obtain good-quality samples and maintain adequate libido. The exact frequency at which semen may be collected will depend on the age, condition, and temperament of each animal. The quality of the semen collected is also very dependent upon the season of collection. The incidence of morphologically abnormal sperm is much higher under increasing day length conditions due to dropping LH-testosterone levels (spring/summer).

Upon collection, the ejaculate is placed in a water bath (37° C) and evaluated immediately. The initial examination consists of:

1. A macroscopic examination of the (i) volume, (ii) consistency, (iii) color, and (iv) foreign matter in the ejaculate; and
2. A microscopic examination of (i) gross motility, (ii) individual motility, (iii) morphology, and (iv) sperm concentration.

The parameters previously described for semen handling and evaluation for Breeding Soundness apply. The normal color of semen should be off-white/milky, with tinges of pink (blood contamination), brown (reproductive tract infection), yellow, and dilute (urine contamination) all indicating an inferior ejaculate[99] (see Figure 8.13).

Clean equipment and proper semen handling techniques are critical.

A 2-hour stress test should be performed. (Semen stress test: semen should be collected and immediately evaluated for progressive motility. The sample is then incubated at room temperature for 2 hours and progressive motility reevaluated. The incubated sample should maintain 20% of the motility of the initial sample.) (Figure 8.13)

The fertility potential of cryopreserved semen can be influenced by numerous factors. In addition to inherent variation in semen quality among males, management, nutrition, and environmental stressors can have a transient influence on spermatogenesis for weeks to months.

Semen from rams may be collected and used fresh or frozen for future use. Typically, rams are trained to service an AV in the presence of females in estrus or treated ovariectomized females (i.e., females that have been given 1 mg estradiol benzoate per week or prepared as described in the section on libido testing). The semen is collected into a warm (39° C) AV and handled carefully to avoid exposure to any contaminants or ultraviolet rays. Once it has been collected, semen can be used raw (undiluted), extended and chilled, or frozen and thawed. When raw (undiluted) semen is used, females can be inseminated with about 0.1 mL of normal, good-quality semen immediately after collection. Following evaluation, semen ejaculates are diluted with semen extenders to final semen-to-extender ratios ranging from 1:1 to 1:4 depending on the sperm concentration of the ejaculate. Where needed, semen can be diluted at 30° C with the extender and cooled to 4° C and kept at this temperature for up to 24 hours.

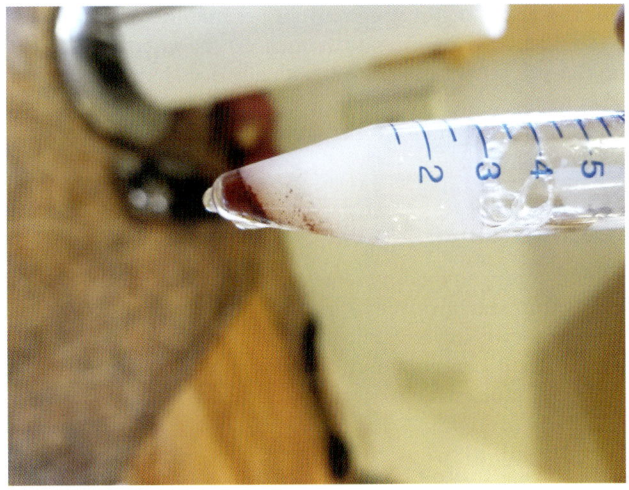

• **Fig. 8.13** The semen sample from a white-tailed deer buck, collected via electroejaculator, was placed in a warmed water bath prior to handling for freezing. In this case, blood/red blood cells can be seen to have settled at the tube's bottom. Blood in semen may be caused by inflammation, infection, or injury anywhere along the male small ruminant reproductive tract. Blood may reduce the fertility and possibly freezability of the semen in some cases. Evaluation, diagnosis, and treatment of the etiology of hematospermia should be pursued, if it appears to be clinically relevant. If required, methods of blood removal may include collecting different portions of the ejaculate in separate containers during the process, or by postejaculate "cushioned" or "layered" centrifugation.

Cooled Semen

Ram semen also may be collected and chilled for same- or next-day artificial insemination (AI). This provides producers with the opportunity to use semen shipped from other farms.[97,98] Prior to use, the collected-chilled semen should be maintained at or below 35° C. Temperatures above 37° C increase sperm metabolic rate and limit longevity.[99] Care should be taken to avoid cold shock while warming semen. The best method would be to allow the cooled semen to be "warmed" by the female's reproductive tract.

The diluents commonly used to dilute buck semen contain either tris or citrate as the buffer, glucose or fructose as the energy source, and egg yolk to protect the spermatozoal cell membranes against cold shock. The concentration of egg yolk should be reduced to 2% to avoid it reacting with the coagulating enzyme present in the seminal plasma.[96] This enzyme occurs in greater concentrations when semen is collected by EE. To overcome any problems with the coagulating enzyme, a low-concentration egg yolk diluent or skim milk can be used, or the seminal plasma can be removed by centrifugation immediately after collection.[96,106] Under field conditions, the most readily available semen diluent is skim milk. The ultra-heat-treated milk is sterile and may be used directly as a diluent without any further treatment.[94,96] When does are inseminated with fresh spermatozoa by laparoscopic technique, PBS with the addition of 1000 IU of sodium penicillin and 1 mg of streptomycin per milliliter can be used as an extender.[94,96] The extended semen can be inserted by pipette into 0.5-mL straws and cooled gradually over 1 to 2 hours from 30° C to the storage temperature of 5° C. This semen should be used within 6 to 8 hours.[96] The semen should be cooled gradually over 1 to 2 hours.

Freezing Semen

Ram. Many methods of semen freezing are used. The clinician is advised to search current scientific literature prior to engaging in this ever-evolving methodology.[94] Semen intended for freezing should have a concentration of more than 3×10^9/mL and a motility of more than 70% of the ejaculate. Normal concentrations range from 3.5×10^9 mL to 6.0×10^9 mL for rams and 2.5×10^9 mL to 5.0×10^9 mL for bucks. Semen extenders are commercially available (e.g., Minitube—http://www.minitube.com). The most commonly used semen extenders are formulated to enhance sperm cell maintenance. They provide energy, isotonic osmotic pressure, a buffering system, and protection from cold shock. Temperature control is of utmost importance in the successful freezing of semen. The semen should be placed in an incubator or water bath (30° C).[92] Semen intended for freezing should have a concentration of more than 3×10^9/mL and a motility of more than 70% of the ejaculate. Semen should be extended in a warmed extender (30° C).[96] This extender can be as simple as whole milk or Dulbecco's phosphate-buffered saline (PBS) with 10% fetal calf serum. Both synthetic and milk or egg yolk–based extenders are currently available. The three most common milk or egg yolk–based extenders include (i) egg yolk citrate-glycerol, (ii) egg yolk-tris-glycerol, and (iii) whole homogenized milk-glycerol. The most common extender is the egg yolk-tris-glycerol. For short-term storage, semen can be extended with the egg yolk-tris-glycerol extender and held at 5° C for up to 24 hours without a noticeable decrease in fertilizing capacity. Tris-based extenders also have satisfactory sperm survival on thawing when glycerol is added to semen kept at 30° C and slowly cooled to 4° C within 2 to 4 hours before freezing (a one-step method). Semen extended with milk diluents shows better survival rates during the freezing process if glycerol is added to the diluted semen after it is cooled to 4° C.

For freezing semen, several packaging systems have been developed for cryopreserving sperm (e.g., straws, pellets, and ampoules). Dilutions of extender and semen used in the cryopreservation process depend on what packaging system is employed.

Goat. Many of the same principles described for the storage of frozen ram semen are applicable to goats. Traditionally, goat semen has been centrifuged in order to remove the seminal plasma, enhancing freezability. However, if semen is adequately diluted, centrifugation might be omitted.[100] Goat semen can be placed in plastic straws and frozen in liquid nitrogen vapor by either slow or fast methods. Diluents for freezing goat semen should have similar properties to diluents used to extend fresh semen. In addition, they should contain an agent to protect the cell membrane during cooling (usually egg yolk) and a cryoprotective agent (usually glycerol) to protect the spermatozoa against membrane damage during freezing.[96,101,102] Dilution of semen can be performed in two ways. The two-step dilution method is similar to that used for bull semen. The semen is diluted at 30° C shortly after collection to half of the final diluted volume with a diluent containing no glycerol.[96] After cooling at 5° C for 1.5 to 2 hours, the semen is extended to the final volume with a diluent containing glycerol.[96] For one-step dilution, the semen is gradually diluted to the final prefreezing volume at 5° C in 1.5 to 2 hours in a refrigerator or cold room. The two-step dilution method has no advantage over the one-step method for goat semen. Therefore, the one-step method is preferred because it simplifies diluent preparation and reduces the handling of semen before freezing. Goat semen should be processed so the post thaw dose yields 50 to 100×10^9 progressively motile spermatozoa.[103]

Cervid. The same techniques for freezing bovine, ovine, and caprine semen appear to be of value for cervids. In a trial, OptiXcell (IMV) was found to be superior to other tested extenders; however, all were found to be acceptable.[104]

Straws. The most popular way of freezing semen today is to use plastic straws (0.25 or 0.5 mL). The ejaculate is normally diluted to a ratio between 1:1 and 1:4, with extenders added slowly by constant slow mixing.[92,96] The diluent is usually hypertonic; therefore, rapid mixing may cause osmotic shock in spermatozoa.[92] Box 8.2 is an example of a semen extender useful for freezing ram semen in straws. Extended semen is slowly cooled to around freezing (4–5° C) over a 1.5- to 2-hour period. The cooled, extended semen should be diluted (usually at a ratio of 1:1) with an additional freeze buffer containing an energy source, a protein, an antibiotic, and a cryoprotectant (glycerol) before being placed into labeled straws. The filled straws are placed (evenly and not touching each other) horizontally on a rack and then placed in a holding container in liquid nitrogen vapor, ~4 cm over the surface of liquid nitrogen for 10 minutes. The straws are then chilled to between –80° and –125° C.[92,105] The semen is then rapidly cooled to its final storage temperature of

• BOX 8-2 Semen Extender Formula for Cryopreservation in Straws

Ingredient	Amount
Tris (hydroxymethyl) amino methane	24.2 g
Citric acid	13.6 g
Fructose	10 g
Glycerol	64 mL
Egg yolk	200 mL
Total volume	1 L
Final pH	6.8

• BOX 8-3 Formula for Semen Cryopreservation in Pellets

Ingredient	Amount
Tris (hydroxymethyl) amino methane	3.63 g
Citric Acid	1.99 g
Glucose	0.5 g
Glycerol	5 mL
Egg yolk	15 mL
Distilled, deionized water	Sufficient to extend volume to 100 mL

–196° C by submersing the straws in liquid nitrogen. Formulas for mixing extenders and freeze buffers may be obtained by consulting the references and the current scientific literature.

Pellets. The pellet technique is simple and does not require sophisticated or expensive equipment. The disadvantages of freezing semen with this technique include difficulty of identification, poor sanitation control, and inconvenience of use in the field.[94]

Semen is frozen into pellets by dropping cooled semen into depressions drilled or scratched into dry ice. In this method, collected semen can be diluted by volume to contain 4% glycerol and 12% egg yolk in a slightly hypertonic, buffered solution.[92,96] Box 8.3 is an example of an extender useful for freezing ram semen in pellets. In a cooled, ventilated room, the examiner makes several small circular cuts (0.5–0.8 cm diameter) on a flat piece of solid carbon dioxide (dry ice). Cooled pipettes (4° C) are used to drop 0.1 to 0.3 mL into the cut surface of the dry ice. After 10 minutes, the frozen pellets are shaken into a pan of liquid nitrogen. The individual pellets can then be stored in labeled plastic goblets. For insemination pellets are put into thawing solutions (spare diluent, saline solution) prewarmed to 40° C until the pellets melt.

Thawing. The thawing and handling procedures must be consistent with on farm recommendations. Improper thawing procedure, lack of post-thaw thermoprotection, etc., can further corrupt semen quality. Proper semen handling techniques are of the highest importance. Proper handling of frozen semen is paramount in maximizing conception rates.[94]

Frozen Semen Handling

Frozen semen for bucks and rams is stored in liquid nitrogen (–196° C). Any changes in this storage temperature can alter semen quality.[107] The straw is placed in a holding goblet, with two goblets attached to a cane. Multiple canes are set inside a canister, which is immersed and maintained in a liquid nitrogen tank. The liquid nitrogen tank lid should be kept closed and the liquid nitrogen level checked and maintained at an adequate level. A schedule of tank maintenance should be planned, followed, and documented.[94] A record or "tank map" of where particular straws are stored (goblet, cane, and canister) helps expedite semen transfer and retrieval.[108] The tank should be kept in a cool, well-ventilated room. Straws should not be removed from the tank unless they are to be used; they should not be transferred from tank to tank unless the procedure takes less than 2 seconds.

To thaw the straws, the clinician should identify the canister holding the cane. The canister is raised until the cane tops can be seen (5 to 7 cm below the mouth of the tank). Straws should be maintained below the frost line in the neck of the tank at all times. Using a light source to identify the correct cane, the clinician removes the straw to be thawed with tweezers or forceps. The cane is immediately "dropped" back into the canister, and the canister is immersed in the liquid nitrogen. Straws should not be touched by the handler's hands.

The clinician should quickly identify whether it is the correct straw and then immerse it in a water bath (33–35° C). Straws should be thawed based on manufacturers' recommendations, but generally, thawing requires only 30 to 40 seconds for 0.5-mL straws and 20 to 30 seconds for 0.25-mL straws. Only as many straws as can be used in 10 to 15 minutes should be thawed at one time. If possible, the clinician should thaw no more than three straws at one time to avoid lowering the thaw water temperature.[107] The straw should be thoroughly dried, air bubble "shaken" to the crimp end, and the straw opened.

As goblets are emptied, they should be discarded to expedite the retrieval of straws in the lower goblets. However, if straws are to be retrieved from lower goblets, the cane is raised until the straws are even with the other cane tops, and then the straw to be used is removed.[107,108]

If pellets are used, the clinician removes the pellets from liquid nitrogen storage and places two or three directly in a dry, sterile tube. The tube is kept in a warm water bath (37° C). The thawed semen should be pulled into a pipette and used for AI immediately.[92] Alternatively, some processing techniques may require the addition of a warm diluent to the frozen pellets.

Evaluating Thawed Semen. When asked to evaluate frozen semen samples, guidelines on semen handling as listed above should be followed. The clinician should thaw the semen using the recommendations that were made by the company where it was originally processed/frozen. Generally, when evaluating frozen-thawed semen, the clinician should make all attempts to avoid post-thaw cold-shock, ensure that the straw was properly identified, thoroughly dry the straw, and examine the semen for motility (using prewarmed slides and coverslips), morphology, and a 2-hour motility test ("stress test"). The Society for Theriogenology has as minimally excepted standards for ram spermatozoa 70% normal, 50% intact acrosomes, initial motility of 25%, and a 2-hour percentage motility of 15%. They recommend a motile sperm dose (MSD) of 25 × 10^6.[106] These guidelines appear applicable for the buck (caprine and cervid).

Female Reproduction

Anatomy of the Ewe and Doe

The reproductive tract of the ewe and doe is similar to that of other domestic animals. It is composed of the external genitalia (vulva, clitoris), vagina, cervix, uterus, oviducts, and ovaries. The vulva has two labia, which are composed of adipose tissue and portions of constrictor vulvae muscle covered with skin. The labia are marked by dorsal and ventral commissures. On parting the vulva, the inner surface is easily visualized. The clitoris is homologous to the penis and has some erectile tissue. The vestibule is located cranial to the clitoris. It is lined with stratified squamous epithelium and is rich in mucous glands. The vestibule of the ewe contains paramedian glands that exist along the urethral orifice; the goat doe lacks these glands.

The tubular portion of the tract (vagina, cervix, uterus, and oviducts) is composed of an outer serosal surface, a double layer of muscular tissue, submucosa, and a mucosal layer. The vagina is located cranial to the vestibule. In the normal position, the vaginal walls are collapsed into folds. The vaginal lumen is composed of stratified squamous epithelium. The cervix is located at the most cranial portion of the vagina and is found in a subtle depression near the vaginal floor. The canal of the cervix has five to six and five to eight irregular overlapping rings in the ewe and goat, respectively. The white-tailed deer doe's cervix is less tortuous as it usually has only three rings, allowing for easier transcervical AI. However, this tortuous, narrow, cervical lumen causes great difficulty in transcervical AI, particularly in the ewe. The cervix of the ewe and doe, unlike the vagina, is not easily dilatable. The cervix opens cranially into the uterine body. The bicornate uterus is composed of a short body and two horns that, in the nongravid state, are slightly coiled and lie in the pelvic canal. The serosal surface of the uterus is held in the abdominal cavity by the highly vascular broad ligament. The endometrium is a pink-gray structure with folds that have convex caruncles. Melanin pigmentation is found in these caruncular regions in some breeds of sheep (Hampshire). This pigment is rare in goats and has not been reported in white-tailed deer.

The two oviducts attach the uterine horns to the ovarian bursa. The small (1.5 × 1–2 cm) oval ovaries are partially covered by the ovarian bursa. The ovarian surface is usually rough. During the breeding season or during gestation, the ovary can have two or more progesterone-secreting corpus lutea.

Ewe

Physiology. Age, nutritional status, and season of the year all play roles in the development of sexual maturity in the sheep.[109–112] The approach of the breeding season or artificial manipulation of light to mimic shorter days hastens the onset of estrus in ewe lambs. Melatonin implants can cause a similar effect.[113,114] Differing reports about the effect of light manipulation and melatonin implants can be found in the literature.[115–117] The sex of siblings in multiple-birth lambings does not seem to affect the age of puberty in the ewe[118]; however, exposure to intact rams can decrease the time required for the ewe lamb to achieve her first estrus.[112] The attainment of puberty depends on the interaction of the juvenile hypothalamus, the anterior pituitary, and the ovary. Estradiol secreted by developing follicles has a negative feedback on LH secretion. As puberty approaches, this inhibitory influence becomes less important and GnRH pulses from the hypothalamus and subsequent pituitary pulses of LH become more frequent. This stimulates further follicular development. As the follicle develops, it produces more estradiol until a threshold is reached, causing a positive feedback on LH secretion.[119] The resultant LH surge induces the luteinization of the follicle and usually ovulation. The lifespan of the resultant corpus luteum (CL) is usually shorter than that of subsequent cycles. This first ovulation in the sheep is not associated with behavioral estrus. The second and subsequent cycles of follicular growth, LH secretion, and CL development appear more normal and result in behavioral estrus. Follicle-stimulating hormone (FSH) also is released from the anterior pituitary gland in response to GnRH.[120]

Sheep are considered short-day breeders because their breeding season is regulated by the length of the day or, more specifically, by the increased duration of night.[121] Light duration and timing affect not only the induction of estrus, but short daylight regimens also can affect the length of the breeding season.[122] Seasonality is controlled by the visual perception of light that is transmitted by the superior cervical ganglion to the pineal gland. The pineal gland produces melatonin and secretes it during the night. Alteration in melatonin secretion provides cues to the hypothalamus in its pulse generations of GnRH.[120] The hypothalamus also changes in its sensitivity from a strictly negative feedback response to estrogen (from the developing follicles) to a positive feedback from increasing concentrations of estrogen.[123] The increased pulses of GnRH appear responsible for the induction of estrus during the breeding season.[124] In seasonally breeding animals, a similar scenario occurs during puberty as is observed in the yearly transition from anestrus to the seasonal cycle. However, much variation occurs among breeds with respect to the occurrence and length of the breeding season. Dorset, Merino, Rambouillet, and Finnish-Landrace sheep tend to have longer breeding seasons, whereas the Southdown, Shropshire, and Hampshire breeds respond to day length and adhere to the short-day breeding season. Sheep living near the equator (or breeds that originated there such as the Barbados) are usually less sensitive to the effects of the seasons.

Puberty. Suffolk ewe lambs show first signs of estrus at around 30 weeks of age. Much like an adult ewe in transition from anestrus to the breeding season, the first estrus in ewe lambs is usually a "silent" ovulation. The onset of sexual maturity in ewe lambs is dependent on nutrition, adequate growth, and photoperiod (long days followed by decreasing day length).[120]

Estrous Cycle. Estrus in the ewe lasts between 15 and 45 hours (with an average of 30 hours), and the interval between estrous activity is between 14 and 19 days (with an average of 17 days)—3 to 5 days of metestrus, 7 to 10 days of diestrus, and 2 days of proestrus). Ewe lambs, ewes cycling outside of the normal breeding season, and transitional ewes tend to have shorter estrus periods. As estrus approaches, the larger follicles of the FSH-induced follicular wave begin to produce more estradiol. This signals the hypothalamus to secrete GnRH, which results in the release of LH by the anterior pituitary gland. This LH surge typically occurs about 9 hours after the onset of estrus. The high estradiol concentration is partially responsible for the ewe showing signs of estrus. However, the sheep also must have been recently exposed to progesterone. Sheep ovulate toward the final third of estrus or occasionally after the end of behavioral estrus.[125] Ovulation typically occurs 14 to 26 hours after the LH surge. This coincides with about 21 to 45 hours after the beginning of estrus. The length of estrus may vary depending on the breed, with wool breeds generally having a longer estrus than meat breeds. Signs of estrus include vulvar swelling, anorexia in the ewe, seeking out, and standing for the ram. The ewe may secrete small amounts of thin mucus, much less than that secreted by the cow.

After ovulation, the follicle becomes luteinized and begins producing progesterone. The progesterone concentration remains elevated for about 12 to 13 days. In the absence of a conceptus, the ovaries produce oxytocin and the uterine endometrium begins to secrete prostaglandin $F_2\alpha$ ($PGF_{2\alpha}$). The $PGF_{2\alpha}$ is transported away from the uterus by the uterine veins and is transferred directly to the ovarian arteries that run adjacent to the veins. The increased concentration of $PGF_{2\alpha}$ in the ovarian arteries leads to the regression of the luteal tissue and diminished progesterone secretion. The cycle begins again with a decrease in serum progesterone, concurrent development of the follicle, and a subsequent increase in serum estrogen concentrations. Ovum transport to the uterus takes 2 to 4 days in ewes. Approximately 12 days after conception, signals are sent to the endometrium and ovaries to prevent lysis of the luteal tissue and to maintain the pregnancy. The substance that inhibits uterine production of estrogen receptors is interferon-τ; the decrease in estrogen receptors in turn inhibits oxytocin receptors. This breaks a link in the production of luteolytic amounts of $PGF_{2\alpha}$.[126] Attachment of the embryo to the uterine endometrium is a slow process, beginning around day 18.

Gestation. The normal gestation length of the ewe is 145 to 150 days. Sheep have a cotyledonary, epitheliochorial placenta. The placental cotyledon and the maternal caruncle together form a placentome. In the pregnant ewe, 90 to 100 cotyledons are dispersed over the chorionic membrane. Around day 16, the chorion begins attaching to the uterine caruncles. This type of placenta limits antibodies moving from the maternal to the fetal circulation, necessitating the ingestion of colostrum by the neonate for antibody transfer. After day 75, the concentration of progestin in the peripheral blood markedly increases. This increase results from the placental production of progestin and is of major clinical significance because luteolytic agents cannot guarantee abortion after day 75 of gestation. Parturition occurs as a result of a complex set of interactions involving the uterine musculature and fetus. As the fetal hypothalamus matures, it begins producing increasing amounts of corticotropin-releasing hormone, which stimulates the pituitary gland to produce and release corticotropin. This in turn stimulates the fetal adrenal glands to produce and release cortisol. Endogenous cortisol results in an increase in the estradiol, $PGF_2\alpha$, and prostaglandin-E2 concentrations. This in turn decreases progesterone production and relaxes the cervix. Uterine responsiveness to oxytocin also increases because of the estrogen-induced recruitment of oxytocin receptors. Normal parturition occurs over a period of 3 to 8 hours. The first stage of parturition (initiation of organized contractions) lasts from 1 to 4 hours. The second stage (active labor and delivery of the fetus) lasts as long as 2 hours. The final phase of parturition is the delivery of the placenta and should occur within 8 hours after the fetus is delivered.[120]

Goat Doe

Physiology. From a pure physiologic standpoint, small ruminants have many similarities. Nevertheless, they are dissimilar in length of the estrous cycle and maintenance of pregnancy. Goats in a temperate region are polyestrous and breed efficiently when day lengths are short (August to March), with a peak breeding season of October through December.[127] The transitional periods are approximately 2 months before and after breeding season, with deepest anestrus in April and May.[128,129] In cervids, anestrus in the northern hemisphere typically occur between midwinter to late fall. In tropical areas near the equator, native breeds show less seasonality and breed year-round (as do sheep). Variation in seasonality occurs among and within breeds of goats, which allows for selection of out-of-season breeders.[128,130] For example, pygmy and Tennessee stiff-legged meat goat breeds tend to cycle year-round in North America, whereas Nubian, Spanish, Boer, and Kiko goats show more seasonality.[129] Producers can use this seasonality to their advantage in a synchronization program by introducing bucks during the summer transitional period to induce estrus in does. This "buck effect" is lessened when males live year-round with does.

Puberty. Does reach sexual maturity and begin to cycle at 6 to 8 months.[127] In pygmy goats, puberty may occur as early as 3 months. Generally, a single-born doe has her first ovulation in the fall after her birth. Breeding should be delayed until a doe has attained 60% to 70% of her predicted adult weight (or 60–70 lb in meat goats and 70–90 lb in dairy breeds).[129]

Estrous Cycle. The length of the estrous cycle in the goat doe is 21 days (with a range of 18–22 days). White-tailed and mule deer does' estrous cycle tends to run longer still, with a range of 24 to 28 days. If they fail to become pregnant early in the breeding season, the estrous cycle tends to shorten until late winter, when anestrus occurs. Although variations exist, estrus tends to be longer in goat does than in ewes. Short cycles of 5 to 7 days are more common at the beginning and end of the breeding season in goat does and increases in frequency when ovulation in induced either just before or during the breeding season.[127,131] After midsummer, the decreasing day length causes increased melatonin release from the pineal gland, and the sequence of hormonal events is similar to that seen in the ewe. During estrus and seasonal anestrus, plasma progesterone concentrations are less than 1 ng/mL, whereas progesterone levels during the luteal phase are 4 to 8 ng/mL.[127,128]

Goat does in estrus are restless, seek out the buck, wag their tails, vocalize, and have swollen vulvas with clear mucous discharge that changes to cloudy toward the end of estrus. These behaviors may be pronounced in the presence of a buck. Milk production and appetite may decrease during estrus in dairy goats. Well-fed, healthy, mature does average two to three ovulations per cycle, which results in a high proportion of multiple births. Estrus varies from 24 to 72 hours, with most does exhibiting estrus for 36 hours. Ovulation is quite variable, as well, and ranges from 9 to 37 hours from the onset of estrus. However, ovulation typically occurs towards the end of standing estrus.[131]

White-tailed does are generally pursued by the buck and are "tended" by the buck for 1 to 3 days. Multiple matings occur over this period and conception rates are generally very high.

Gestation. Twins or triplets are more common than singletons. Oviductal transfer of the embryo(s) requires 3 to 4 days in goats. The average duration of gestation is 5 months, with a range of 147 to 155 days.[127] Similar to ewes, goat does have epitheliochorial, cotyledonary placentae. Pregnancy is maintained by progesterone, which is produced entirely by the CL of pregnant does and not by the placenta. This is different from ewes, which maintain sufficient progestogen output from their uteroplacental units. The plasma concentration of progesterone remains high until about 4 days before parturition.

Gestation length in white-tailed does generally runs about 192 to 200 days. That of mule deer tends to be a few days longer. Pregnancy can be terminated at any time by the use of prostaglandins. They have an epitheliochorial, cotyledonary placentae that is characterized by two very large cotyledons per horn as opposed to sheep and goats, which have 120 or so cotyledons total.

BSE of the Female

History. History is an essential component of a BSE of a doe or ewe because of the inaccessibility of the majority of the reproductive tract to palpation or visual inspection. Historical information of significance includes duration of heat, interestrous intervals, reaction to the male, and breeding and parturition history. A general physical examination emphasizing body condition, femininity, conformation of the mammary glands, and determination of whether the female is polled or horned (goats) is important in the evaluation of breeding soundness (see Chapter 1).

Physical Examination. External genital examination should include evaluation of the anogenital distance and whether the clitoris is visible without parting the lips of the vulva. The vulva should be examined for abnormalities. A clear AI speculum or an endoscope can be used to evaluate the vagina and cervix. The clinician should note any discharges from the cervix or vagina. A normal, clear mucous vaginal discharge in early standing estrus that turns into a cloudy or creamy mucous discharge late in standing estrus is common, particularly in goats.

Reproductive Ultrasonography. Transabdominal ultrasonography can be used to examine the uterus for pregnancy and pseudopregnancy. Pseudopregnancy is a more common problem in goats than in ewes. Transrectal probes often allow visualization of the nonpregnant uterus and ovaries and early pregnancy.

Breeding Management

Ewe

To maximize reproductive potential, ewes should be maintained in a healthy and disease-free state with a body condition score between 2.5 and 3.5 at the initiation of the breeding season (see Chapters 1 and 2). Ewe lambs should be bred so that they go through parturition earlier in the season than older ewes. In order to cycle, ewes require at least one cycle of increasing day length before the decreasing day length that signals the breeding season. Replacement lambs should be chosen from a pool of lambs born early in the previous lambing season. Ewe lambs should weigh approximately 70% of their projected mature weight at the time of breeding.

Doe (Goat)

Replacement doe kids should be selected at weaning (4–5 months). Selection of meat does should emphasize traits such as reproduction and soundness. Milking does are selected based on production traits such as soundness of the udder and teats, adequate body size, and good body condition. Female goats that were born as twins or triplets, those born early in the season, and those whose dams gave birth more than once each year are preferable replacement does. All females of breeding age should be maintained in a single group. Breeding should be delayed until a doe has attained 60% to 70% of its adult weight at a body condition score of 3 to 3.5. Does that do not kid by the time they are 2 years old should be culled. Breeding does should not be allowed to become too thin or too fat. Thin does may fail to conceive, have low twinning rates, and produce kids with low weaning rates. Obese does can suffer from pregnancy toxemia and/or decreased milk production if they are allowed to become fat before the onset of puberty.

Doe (Cervid)

Doe fawns that are born early in the year and that have attained 60 to 70% of their adult body weight will most likely cycle the fall of their first year. Selection criteria are generally based on genetic merit of the sire and dam (antler size and conformation) as well as disposition, phenotype, and other characteristics that are important to the producer. Does are generally best kept in breeding groups to diminish fighting and lower stress. This is especially true if using AI. Does will generally be productive for 10 or more years. Singletons are common in first parity, but older does will usually have twins with triplets or more not unusual.

Control of the Estrous Cycle

With the increasing use of AI and the desire of producers to concentrate their efforts around parturition, control of the estrous cycle of the female is necessary. Estrus synchronization programs useful in goats and sheep are shown in Table 8.3.[132–135] Producers often request estrus synchronization during the fall breeding season (cervids, sheep, and goats) and to induce estrus during the winter anestrus period (nonbreeding season) and summer transitional period (sheep and goats). To maintain a continuous milk supply from dairy goats and sheep, the flock should be divided into four equal breeding groups. This necessitates some form of estrus synchronization. In the Northern Hemisphere, these groups should be assigned to breedings in late August, mid-October, mid-November, and late December. Adequate nutrition, estrus detection, and adequate sire or insemination capabilities are essential components of a synchronization program. Because any form of stress can have a negative impact on the efficacy of a synchronization program, stress should be minimized as much as possible.

TABLE 8.3 Overview of the Methods of Estrous Cycle Manipulation in Sheep and Goats in the United States.

Sheep	
Breeding season	• Prostaglandins • Progestin source for 14 days ± gonadotropin
Transitional season	• Ram effect • Progestin source for 8–14 days + gonadotropin up to 48 hours before removal • Progestin source for 8–14 days + ram effect at removal
Out of breeding season	• Progestin source for 8–14 days + gonadotropin up to 48 hours before removal • Manipulation of lights • Melatonin administration
Goat	
Breeding season	• Prostaglandins • Progestin source for 14 days ± gonadotropin
Transitional season	• Buck effect • Progestin source for 14 days + gonadotropin + prostaglandin • Progestin source for 14 days + gonadotropin + buck effect
Out of breeding season	• Progestin source for 14 days + gonadotropin + prostaglandin • Manipulation of lights • Melatonin administration

Ram or Buck Effect. Introducing a buck or ram into a group of transitional period does or ewes is a powerful tool to induce estrus.[136–138] Introducing a ram into a ewe herd induces estrus in most ewes within 6 days. The females should have no contact with the males for 3 to 4 weeks before their introduction. Suddenly placing the male with females induces an LH surge and ovulation within a few days. Similarly, fence line contact by males can be used to achieve a ram or buck effect for hand mating. The use of high-performing rams, as defined by serving capacity tests, has been shown to be more effective in inducing early ovulation than the use of low-fertility rams.[137] One study indicated that the use of two high doses (1000 IU) of equine chorionic gonadotropin (eCG) administered to teaser rams increased the rams' ability to stimulate anestrous ewes. The ewes that were exposed to the eCG-treated rams experienced a significantly higher rate of estrus and pregnancy rates.[139] The response to male stimulation can be quite variable and is influenced by breed, previous isolation, depth of anestrus, nutrition, and length of time since parturition. This technique can be used in combination with pharmacologic out-of-season breeding programs and appears to enhance their efficacy. Males should be isolated from females for 30 to 60 days before introduction. When using the ram or buck effect in out-of-season breeding, producers should expose the male to a cycling female for 2 weeks before using him to breed. Males that have undergone vasectomy or epididymectomy and castrated males treated with testosterone (100 mg weekly for 3 weeks) may be used. Regardless of the type of teaser male used, he should be introduced to the females for 2 to 3 weeks to bring them into heat

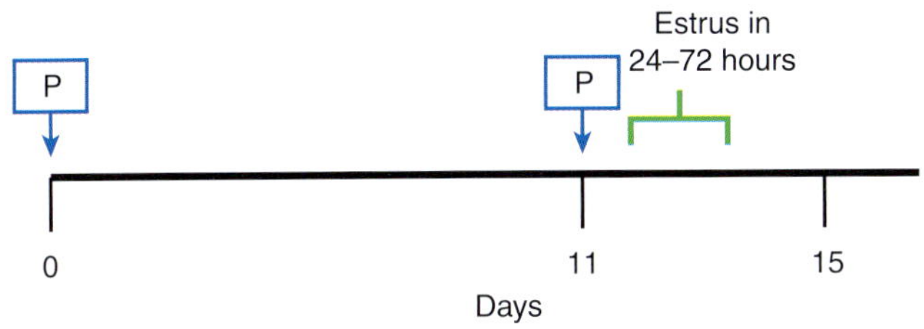

• **Fig. 8.14** Two doses of prostaglandin for estrous synchronization in small ruminants.

before the desired breeding male is brought in. The first estrus after introduction of the male is usually "silent."

Prostaglandins. $PGF_{2\alpha}$ can be used to lyse the CL and bring diestral females into heat. Ewes are generally susceptible to prostaglandin-induced luteolysis after days 5 to 6 of the estrous cycle while does are susceptible beginning at day 3 of the estrous cycle[140] (Figure 8.14). This method of estrus synchronization should be used if the producer is sure that a significant number of ewes and does are actively cycling; it is most effective during the middle to late fall (sheep and goats: October and November in North America; cervids November and December). One shot of $PGF_{2\alpha}$ can be expected to result in 60% to 70% of the females in the group to exhibit estrus within 30 to 60 hours. Ewes or does that do not show estrus after a properly administered prostaglandin injection have either been in estrus recently or are anestrus. A two-treatment method involving a second injection 9 to 11 days after the first results in tighter synchrony within the flock. An alternative is to observe the females actively for 4 days, breed all females that come into estrus during this time, administer $PGF_{2\alpha}$ on the fourth day, and breed all females that come into estrus during the next 3 days. This should result in most females being bred within a 7-day period. Both $PGF_2\alpha$ (10–20 mg) and cloprostenol (75 μg/45 kg of body weight) are used for estrus synchronization.[132] In addition, a two-dose prostaglandin regimen administered 7 days apart (Synchrovine) has been used for fixed-time AI at 42 hours after the last $PGF_{2\alpha}$ in ewes.[141] Producers should ensure that none of the ewes or does are pregnant at the time of administration of prostaglandins because abortion may be induced. Most of these methods are not conducive to the temperament of the cervid and cause much stress, leading to decreased conception rates. Generally, cervids are bred via TAI (timed artificial insemination) or natural service.

Progestins. Progestins are used to synchronize estrus by delaying its onset. Exogenous progestin can be used during the breeding season to artificially control the length of the luteal phase. The use of progestins is the most common method of estrus synchronization in goats for AI or ET. The most common route of application of progestin is transvaginal. After the progestin products are removed, estrus should occur within a few days. Placing devices that contain progesterone into the vagina (controlled intravaginal drug-releasing devices [CIDRs] or progesterone-soaked sponges) is becoming a popular method of estrus control.[133] Several progesterone concentrations are available in CIDRs. The new commercially available CIDRs contain 300 mg of progesterone (EAZI-BREED CIDR sheep insert, Zoetis Animal Health). Occasionally, CIDRs may be difficult to remove if the tail of the device is not visible from the vulva or the sponge has adhered to the vaginal wall. In both cases, the examiner should restrain the female, introduce a gloved finger into the vaginal vault, identify the CIDR or sponge, and carefully remove it after separating it from the vaginal wall (Figure 8.15). The use of norgestomet

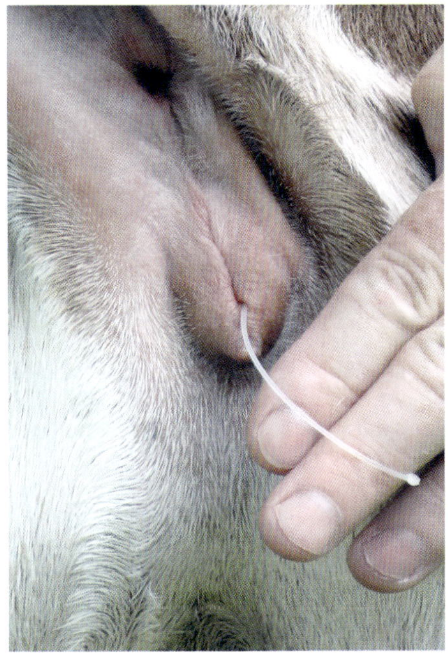

• **Fig. 8.15** A controlled intravaginal drug-releasing device (CIDR) has been placed in this ewe. The external plastic tail or string may need to be trimmed to prevent herd mates from pulling out the CIDR.

implants (half to one implant, or 3–6 mg) inserted between the skin and cartilage of the dorsal aspect of the ears' pinnae were used but are not currently available in North America. The feeding of oral melengestrol acetate (0.25 mg/ewe or doe for 14 days, or 0.125 mg/ewe or doe twice daily for 14 days) also is of value in controlling estrus. Synchronization rates after feeding melengestrol acetate are similar to those encountered with norgestomet implants.[135] However, it is generally recommended that breeding be delayed until the second heat after the melengestrol acetate feeding is discontinued as the first heat is usually nonfertile.[132] Also, if progesterone is added to the feed, a continuous adequate intake is imperative. This may be a problem in goats and some sheep, particularly if inadequate feeder or bunk space is available. All of these methods require the removal of the progestin after 9 to 14 days in the ewe and 12 to 14 days in the doe. The removal of the progestin source can be used to synchronize the entire flock at one time. The flock can be divided, and the progesterone source removed daily, so that one ram can be used for breeding or the AI program can be spread out. Estrus can be expected about 24 to 48 hours and 24 to 36 hours after the removal of the progesterone sources in ewes and does, respectively.

The introduction of a teaser male 24 hours after progestin removal enhances synchrony. Administering eCG (250 IU) or a combination of eCG and human chorionic gonadotropin (hCG) while removing the progestin can help tighten synchrony in the herd.[132] Administering prostaglandins 24 hours before progestin removal, followed by eCG 24 to 48 hours before or at the time of progestin removal, may further tighten estrus synchrony. The use and removal of these progestin products also may hasten estrus in the nonbreeding season.[134]

Seasonal Manipulation. Seasonal manipulation of the female cycle can be used to hasten the onset of estrus to obtain more than one breeding per year in sheep and goats. Seasonal manipulation also can change the time of lambing and kidding and lactation to better match forage availability. Dairy goats should be more than

120 days into the lactation period before the producer attempts an out-of-season breeding program.[142] All animals should be examined with real-time ultrasonography equipment to determine whether any reproductive abnormalities exist that may preclude the effectiveness of an out-of-season breeding program (e.g., pregnancy and hydrometra).[142] Artificial lighting, either by itself or in conjunction with exogenous melatonin can be used for effective manipulation of the breeding season. The sudden introduction of the male maximizes the efficacy of light-melatonin programs. Artificial lighting is mostly employed to mimic a long day. During the Northern Hemisphere winter, long days (approximately 20 hours of light) can be simulated for 2 months (in a barn) and then stopped on March 1. Animals are then exposed to natural daily sunlight. After 6 weeks of natural daylight exposure, males are introduced, and a fertile estrus occurs within 10 to 20 days. Does undergoing this type of estrus manipulation have a short breeding season of around 60 days. Bucks and rams also may benefit from this type of treatment to increase libido and quality of semen. Light manipulation, although effective, is rarely practical.

Some producers combine hormones and lighting for out-of-season breeding. Lighting manipulation is used successfully in many dairy goat operations. Exogenous melatonin can be administered to supplement the endogenous release and thereby mimic the short days associated with the onset of breeding season. Exogenous melatonin can be given as a slow-release implant, repeatedly as an injection, or orally over 30 to 60 days to accelerate the onset of breeding. After the cessation of melatonin administration, females begin to cycle in 40 to 70 days. The lack of availability of this drug limits its use. Exogenous melatonin should be combined with the introduction of the male. Melatonin works most efficiently in dairy goats when combined with artificial lighting for out-of-season breeding.

The most commonly used program for out-of-season breeding is a combination of progestin (delivered as an implant in the ear [norgestomet] or vaginally [CIDR]) and eCG. The progestin should be injected, fed, or implanted for 14 days. A gonadotropin, either FSH or eCG, is administered 48 hours before progestin removal. eCG (400 IU) is most commonly used because it requires only one injection. In areas where eCG is not available for use, a product containing both hCG and eCG (such as PG600) can be substituted. Variable results have been reported with the use of these products depending on the timing and dosage of administration. The introduction of a buck or ram enhances the synchronization of these programs.

Increasing Twinning Rates

Most successful sheep-rearing enterprises depend on the number of lambs raised and sold per ewe per year. Genetic selection for prolific ewes can be slow because of the low heritability of the trait (10%), but some breeds tend to have this predisposition (Finnish-Landrace sheep). However, large variation occurs among flocks with regard to this trait. This variation allows for the selection of superior animals with a good potential for genetic progress.[143] A review of several studies suggests that an annual improvement of 1.3 lambs per 100 ewes can be obtained. Although this number may seem small, when results are compiled over several years, a sizable influence on flock revenues is apparent. The ability to select prolific females depends highly on accurate records. The more information that is collected on each individual ewe or doe, the more accurate the selection becomes. Replacement females should be selected from lambs or kids born to females that consistently produce a larger than average number of young per year. The management practice of providing supplemental feeding to ewes 2 to 3 weeks before breeding (commonly known as *flushing*) can result in increased ovulation rates (see Chapter 2). The most demonstrative response to supplemental feeding is seen in flocks that are experiencing a low lambing rate and whose nutritional status is not adequate. Flushing has little benefit if the ewes are already in good body condition. Ewes can be flushed by feeding 1 lb of a high-energy supplement (e.g., corn, oats, barley, or a combination) per day. An increase in numbers of twins and triplets requires a concomitant increase in the ovulation rate; the embryos also must be in an acceptable environment for survival. Stressors that may be associated with decreased embryonic survival include the female's age, body temperature of both the male and the female, lactation status during breeding, and overall nutritional status.[143] Females bred outside of the normal breeding season may not be as prolific as those bred during it.

Cervids. With proper nutrition and management, most white-tailed and mule deer will twin normally, and little significance is given to selection for litter size. While having singles at first parity, subsequent parities will generally result in twins or even triplets.

Alternative Breeding Programs

Certain sheep breeds (Rambouillet, Dorset, and Finnish-Landrace) and goat breeds (pygmy and Tennessee stiff-legged) can be encouraged to breed outside of the traditional breeding season. This may be done to match forage sources, decrease some parasite burdens, and improve lamb or kid supplies for some seasonal markets. Sheep and goats can be selected to begin a fall lambing or kidding flock.[143] Selected females should be highly prolific and should have given birth early in the traditional lambing or kidding season. If they are normal, ewe lambs or doe kids from these reproductively efficient females should be saved as replacements. The producer should plan on retaining 30% to 40% more lambs or kids than are needed to select for out-of-season breeding potential.[143] This process should be repeated over several years to identify animals that will serve well in off-season breeding programs. Producers who do not have record systems to identify superior females should expose the flock to superior rams or bucks in the spring and retain any females that become pregnant to create a fall lambing flock. Females that do not lamb or kid can be exposed to males in the fall to follow traditional breeding programs. Males should be selected using a similar approach. Males born to the more prolific females should be selected as replacement males and older rams or bucks that have a proven history of superior fertility should be used. Good record-keeping systems and individual identification of females are essential in any selection program. Females born early in the lambing season as twins should be selected as replacements. With respect to growth traits, twins should be compared with other sets of twins because early selection based on size alone may discriminate against them compared with singletons. Ewe lambs of most meat breeds should weigh about 100 lb by the time they are 7 months old. Selected lambs should be bred at about 10 months so they will lamb at 15 months early in the spring. Ewes that bear twins early during lambing should be selected for the accelerated fall lambing flock.[144–146]

Sheep. A similar program for sheep, termed the *STAR management program*, has been developed at Cornell University. The STAR program's unique feature is that it allows for an almost continuous supply of market lambs. This is a good fit with the year-round niche market that many producers have developed.

A chart of the calendar year is made using a five-pointed star. The time lag between each point on the star is 73 days, which is also approximately half of the normal gestation length of the ewe. Therefore, an individual ewe exposed to the ram at the time corresponding to one point on the star will lamb at the time corresponding to the third point on the star (146 days later). She can then be exposed to the ram at the fourth point on the star (216 days after the first breeding). This spreads lambing throughout the year and provides five lambings in 3 years. The use of this system is contingent on the selection of highly prolific ewes that have the ability to cycle and conceive out of season. Accelerated breeding programs place demands on the producer to improve management of the flock's nutritional program and ensure that rams have excellent potential reproductive ability. These complex breeding schemes also demand the accurate identification of individual animals so that ewes capable of out-of-season breeding can be identified and replacement animals can be chosen from these females.[146]

Goats. In a controlled accelerated kidding program in which three kid crops every 2 years is desired, out-of-season breeding is necessary. This requires intense management, early weaning, and hormonal manipulation of does for induction and synchronization of estrus. Seasonal effects on reproductive characteristics also have been documented in bucks. Buck libido and ejaculate quality and quantity appear highest in the late summer and fall, which coincides with the seasonal breeding patterns of the does. Distinct behavior changes and odors also occur in the males in the fall to trigger the buck effect in bringing the female into heat. Bucks can be used successfully for out-of-season breeding without any additional treatment.[147] However, they will benefit from winter light treatment to increase libido and the quality of semen. Producers also can accomplish this by administering 50-mg GnRH injections three times daily for 4 days to boost testosterone production.[134]

Cervids. Due to the longer gestation length of cervids (200 days versus ~150 days for sheep and goats, respectively) and their life cycle (antler growth and strict seasonality), little manipulation of the reproductive cycle is possible. Some producers attempt to "move up" the breeding season 1 to 4 weeks, but fawning season can then occur during more inclement weather, resulting in increased fawn losses, especially in the far northern regions of the United States.

Natural Breeding Systems

Natural breeding is more commonly used in cervids, meat and fiber sheep or goat production systems, whereas AI or hand mating is the most common means in breeding stock producers. In a meat production system, productivity is largely a function of the number of offspring born and weaned and the frequency with which they are produced. The desired date of parturition in a given farm dictates the breeding date and the management of the breeding male. Females are usually bred in the fall for spring kidding, fawning, or lambing. Bucks should be kept separate from the females until they are to be used for breeding. After establishing a mating time, the producer should leave the bucks (goat) with the does for 32 days (1½ reproductive cycles) and the rams with the ewes for 27 days. This ensures that all kids or lambs are born within about 1 month of one another, reducing the amount of supervision required at parturition. The male-to-female mating ratio depends on the age and SC of the male, the size of the mating area, and whether one or more rams or bucks are to be used.

TABLE 8.4 Recommended Male-to-Female Ratios for Male Sheep and Goats.

Animal Age	Reproductive Practice/Use	Male-to-Female Ratio
1 year old	Paddock or confined pasture	1:20 to 1:25
	Paddock or confined pasture	1:40 to 1:50
Adults	Range	1:25 to 1:30
	Synchronized females in season	1:15 to 1:20
	Synchronized females out of season	1:5 to 1:10

Meat goat production systems should have one buck per 30 does. A buck may breed 50 to 200 does in a single breeding season, but three to four bucks should be put with 100 does.[148] Most sheep producers should keep 3 to 5.5 adult rams per 100 ewes. A marking harness should be used on the males to identify which females have been bred. In commercial flocks, males should be changed at least every 2 years to prevent inbreeding. Bucks or rams of high libido and good semen quality can be used in a staggered breeding program in which seven or eight synchronized ewes or does exhibiting estrus at the same time are placed with the male for breeding. Hand mating of males can be used as a modification of staggered breeding, with the same female ratio of 7:1 to 8:1. Table 8.4 outlines a proposed male-to-female ratio.

Artificial Insemination

The small ruminant industry has used AI commercially in North America for many years. The cervix of the cervid doe is less of an obstacle to insemination than the cervix of the goat doe, and the ewe cervix is the most complicated of all to traverse. As a result, commercial AI programs using fresh or frozen semen have been developed and are used most commonly in cervids and goats. Advantages of AI include the following[149]:

- Maximal use of superior sires
- Elimination of the need for rams and bucks on the farm
- Relatively inexpensive semen cost
- Decreased potential for venereally transmitted diseases
- Improved herd management

Disadvantages of AI include the following[149]:

- Cost for AI equipment and liquid nitrogen
- Increased labor for estrus detection and insemination
- Lack of standardization procedures for packing and quality control for goat semen
- Lack of suitable sire proofs for production traits
- Potential for spread of less desirable traits

The success of an AI program depends on many factors (fresh versus frozen semen, number and time of inseminations, insemination method, quality and quantity of semen, semen handling practices, and the management of the animals to be inseminated). The method of insemination (laparoscopic versus transcervical versus cervical versus vaginal), semen used (fresh, chilled, or frozen semen), and ability of the animal keeper (checking estrus, AI skill, etc.) will all greatly affect pregnancy rates. Females selected for AI should be in good health, have a body condition score of 2.5 to 3, and be put on an improved nutrition plan for 2 to 5 weeks before breeding (see Chapter 2). They also should be free of disease and have a history of giving birth to live, healthy young

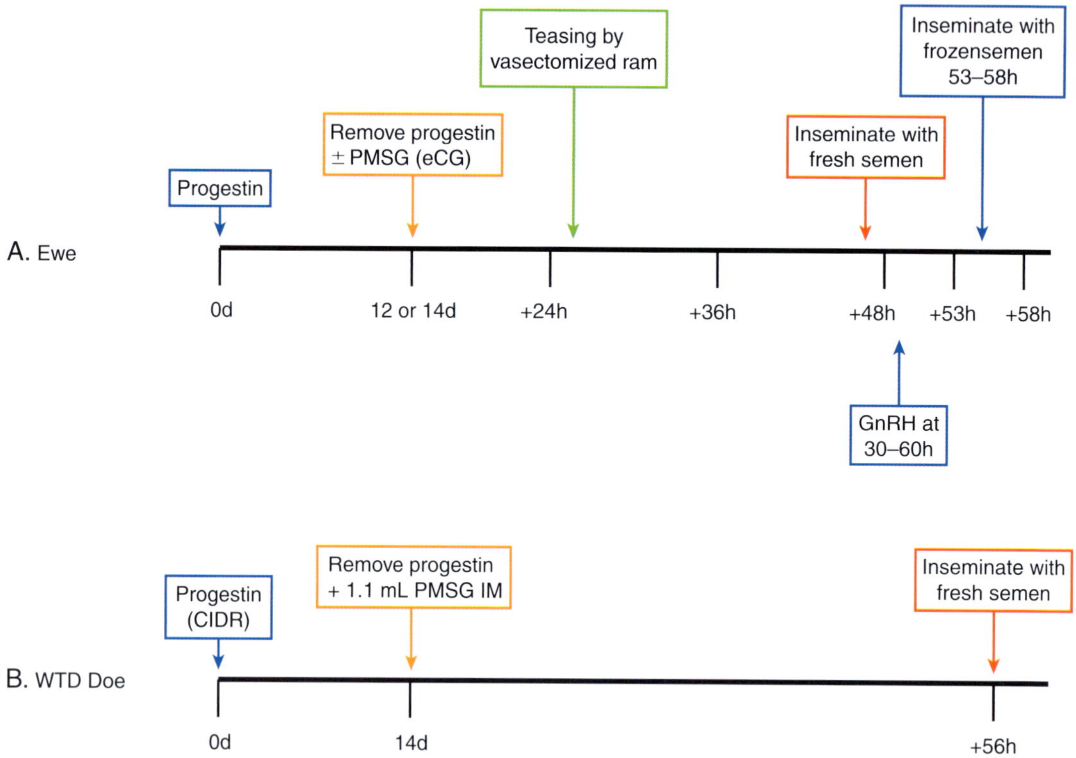

• **Fig. 8.16** Protocol for estrus synchronization in **(A)** ewes and **(B)** white-tailed deer (WTD) does for artificial insemination. *CIDR*, Controlled intravaginal drug-releasing device; *d*, day; GnRH, gonadotropin-releasing hormone; *H*, hour. Progestin: Implant, Vaginal Sponge, CIDR (Courtesy Dr. Jason Coe, Advanced Deer Genetics, LLC.)

and raising them to weaning. Preference should be given to females that conceive early in the breeding season, those that lambed or kidded during poor weather conditions, and those that gave birth to and raised multiple young.

AI is usually performed in conjunction with estrus synchronization. Although many protocols exist, most utilize either eCG, progestin, and $PGF_{2\alpha}$ singularly or in combinations.[149–151] A sample protocol for ewes and one for white-tailed deer are shown on Figure 8.16A, B. Combinations of GnRH and $PGF_{2\alpha}$ also appear to be of value in both sheep and goats.[152,153] This protocol could be implemented in sheep as follows:

Sheep:

GnRH → 5 d later administer $PGF_{2\alpha}$ → 36 h later administer GnRH → 12 to 14 h laparoscopic AI

Goat:

GnRH → 7 d later administer $PGF_{2\alpha}$ → 2 d later administer GnRH → 16 h transcervical AI

Because no uniform standards are available for cervid, goat, or sheep semen, any frozen semen to be used should be evaluated before an AI program is begun. Optimal timing of insemination is an important factor in the success of AI programs. Females do not ovulate until late estrus or shortly after the end of standing estrus. Therefore, recognizing the signs of standing heat is important. However, the optimal timing of insemination is best determined by changes in cervical mucus. As the goat doe progresses through estrus, the mucus turns from clear and thin at the beginning of standing heat to cloudy and stringy at middle to late heat. Insemination should be performed in goat does before or at the time the mucus turns cloudy, usually 12 to 15 hours after the onset of estrus.[154] If the doe continues to exhibit heat after insemination, she should be inseminated again after 12 hours, particularly if the program uses cooled or frozen semen.

Timed insemination of synchronized meat goats and ewes tends to work well. Fixed-time insemination using fresh semen 50 to 55 hours after removal of the progesterone source is an excellent labor-saving technique. If a laparoscopic AI is to be performed, sheep and goats should be inseminated 55 to 60 hours and 52 to 60 hours after progesterone removal for frozen and thawed or fresh semen, respectively.[155] Australian workers suggest that observation for estrus before breeding has no advantage over timed insemination (laparoscopy) in the ewe.[156] In dairy goats, does should be observed for heat using a teaser animal and inseminated accordingly, whereas meat goats are usually synchronized in groups. Techniques that place the semen into the uterus should be used for frozen semen.

Vaginal Insemination. The vulva is wiped clean with dry cotton or paper towels. The practitioner carefully advances a pipette into the cranial vagina by sliding it along the dorsal vaginal roof to avoid entering the urethral orifice. A cleaned, lubricated speculum may afford better visualization for pipette placement. Cassou guns made for cows can be effectively used in sheep and goats, but AI equipment for goats is readily available.[157] Insemination with 4×10^9 and 3×10^9 progressively motile, fresh spermatozoa close to the cervix maximizes fertility with vaginal insemination in ewes and goat does, respectively.[149,151,158–161] The conception rate with this method ranges from 15 to 30%. Results can be improved with experienced technicians, using well-conceived and implemented estrus synchronization detection programs in healthy, well-fed (body condition score 2.5–3 out of 5), disease-free animals.

Cervical Insemination. Cervical insemination is more time-consuming and requires greater skill but should yield superior results to vaginal methods.[149,151,162] In this method, the ewe's or doe's hindquarters (not its abdomen) are elevated and its legs are held over a table or, more commonly, a bale of hay. The cervid female is generally anesthetized or confined in a drop chute. The operator gently introduces a lubricated vaginal speculum approximately 12 cm through the cleaned vulva and into the vagina. With the help of a good light source such as a transilluminator, the cervix is visualized through the speculum. Alternatively, a small endoscope may be used to help visualize the cervix. The operator then introduces an insemination pipette through the speculum and attempts to atraumatically pass the pipette as far into the cervix as possible. The long (7–8 cm) cervix and the six to eight rear-directed cervical rings make completely traversing the cervix difficult in the ewe, resulting in semen deposition in the caudal cervix. A 12-gauge tube attached to the semen delivery system allows deeper penetration of the cervix. The goat doe's cervix has a smaller luminal size but is slightly easier to pass. Approximately 1×10^9 sperm cells from fresh semen are needed to ensure good lambing and kidding rates using this method.[149,157,158–161] If cooled or frozen and thawed semen is used, these numbers may need to be expanded by a factor of 1.5 and 2, respectively.[157–161] The cervid doe cervix generally has three rings and is easier to pass an insemination pipette through. The conception rate with this method ranges from 35 to 50% (and occasionally higher in skilled inseminators). Care should be taken to minimize trauma to the cervix, which, as might be expected, can reduce fertility.

Transcervical Insemination. The more invasive methods of insemination are designed to place semen directly into the uterus. With these methods, a much smaller number of progressively motile sperm are needed. Transcervical insemination (TCI) of dairy and meat goats is a relatively common procedure and one that can be easily mastered with some practice. The necessary speculum, light source, and insemination equipment are readily available through goat supply companies. All items that come into contact with the internal reproductive tract of the doe should be sterile. Dairy goats are usually restrained on a milking stand. Meat goats are not usually cooperative on stands and should be restrained by an assistant lifting the hindquarters and holding both hindlegs.

Ewes. There are several transcervical methods described for sheep.[151,163] The most popular is the Guelph system for transcervical AI.[151,157,159] The ewe is restrained on her back with the hindlimbs pulled forward. Special cradles designed for foot trimming or a V-shaped wooden trough can be used. A specially designed Plexiglas vaginal speculum that has a 1-cm opening running along its entire length is introduced into the vagina and the cervix is identified. A wand-type light source that can be partially introduced into the speculum with a retaining clip can be used to provide a light for this procedure. Alternatively, a small handheld endoscope may be used to visualize the cervix. The clinician inserts a pair of 25-cm Bozeman forceps into the speculum and grasps tissue near the cervical os. Any mucus preventing visualization of the cervical os can be aspirated with a syringe infusion pipette. The slit-like opening in the speculum allows the introduction of the forceps; after grasping the cervical tissue, the operator can retract the cervix caudally and slide the forceps partially through the slit to allow better visualization of the cervix. Holding the speculum and forceps with one hand, the clinician next introduces a special bent-tipped insemination rod into the cervical os and attempts to traverse the cervical rings. Manipulating the AI rod and the cervix with the grasping forceps facilitates the placement of semen directly into the uterus. The tip of the insemination gun can be used to locate the cervical canal. By turning the gun, most of the cervical rings can be traversed. Proper attachment of the forceps to the cervical os is crucial for maximal cervical penetration. If the AI pipette tip can be moved without resistance, it is in the cervical lumen or uterine body. The closer to the uterine body the semen is deposited, the higher the conception rate. This procedure requires 50 to 100 million progressively motile sperm cells. It also requires more experience and the reported results (40–70% lambing rates) are variable. Operators report a higher pregnancy rate when they can enter the uterus with the insemination pipette instead of depositing the semen into the cervix. Pregnancy rates may be similar to those achieved in laparoscopic methods when the semen is placed into the uterus.[164]

Goats. For AI of goats, the perineal area is washed with soapy water, rinsed, and dried with a paper towel. A lubricated clear AI speculum is inserted into the doe's vagina and directed dorsally first and then slightly ventrally to pass over the ischial arch. The AI light is inserted into the speculum and the cervix is visualized. Alternatively, a small handheld endoscope may be used to visualize the cervix. After locating the cervical opening, the clinician places pressure on the speculum to lock the cervix into the lumen of the speculum. An assistant should hold the speculum in the vagina while the inseminator prepares the semen. The frozen semen straw is placed in water based on the processor's recommendation (usually 30–60 seconds in 35° C water). The clinician dries the straw with a paper towel, cuts it, and places it in the AI gun. The insemination gun is manipulated through the cervical opening by gentle rotation and forward movement, slowly depositing the semen in the interior cervix or uterine body. After insemination, the doe is allowed to stand and relax for a few minutes. Conception rates between 50% and 85% have been reported, depending on the type of equipment used, the skill of the operator, and the quality of the semen.[149,165] Fresh extended semen produces better fertility than frozen semen.[149,160,161] In the doe, the desired number of motile sperm per insemination for fresh semen is 150 million; 200 million sperm are required for frozen semen.[157,160,161] Both fresh and frozen semen should be evaluated for quality before insemination.

Cervid. The technique for TCI in the cervid is the same as in goats. The cervix has fewer rings and is easier to pass a pipette through than goats or sheep. Most TCI is done in a drop chute or under anesthesia due to the temperament of the deer. Pregnancy rates vary from 30% to 80% depending on semen, operator, and management factors. TCI is much harder to perform on primiparous does than multiparous animals. Speculums of various sizes for females of different sizes should be available. Aspiration of vaginal and cervical secretions may need to be done to better visualize the cervical os using a pipette and syringe. A human proctoscope works very well for the procedure. Semen doses range from 10 to 50 million sperm.

Laparoscopic Insemination. Large animal laparoscopy (especially for abdominal exploration) is frequently performed using a 10-mm-diameter laparoscope with a 30-degree angled field of view. That diameter allows more light to view a large cavity and the angled field allows a more panoramic visualization of the abdominal cavity. However, laparoscopic insemination of small ruminants can be done very efficiently with smaller diameter laparoscopes (5–6.5 mm) that are direct (0 degrees) field of view instruments since the clinician can focus directly on the uterus and has no need to further examine the abdominal cavity. While conventional laparoscopic examinations are usually done via a scope portal near the umbilicus, insemination can quickly be done via more caudal portals for the laparoscope and the insemination gun.

The ewe (or doe) should be held off feed and water for 24 hours before laparoscopic insemination. The animal is sedated and placed in dorsal recumbency in Trendelenburg's position (head tilted down at a 45-degree angle or more) to allow good visualization and easy access to the uterus as the procedure proceeds. The abdomen should be clipped and prepared for aseptic surgery. Local anesthetics are infiltrated at the two sites of the portals for the laparoscope and the insemination pipette. The portals are located midway on a line between the cranial border of the udder on midline and the cranial aspect of the fold of the flank on each side. The clinician can decide based on comfort of instrument handling which side they prefer to use for the scope versus the insemination pipette. Conventional laparoscopic technique involves using a needle to inflate the abdominal cavity prior to inserting the trochar and cannula in the scope portal. Alternatively, the cannula can be efficiently and safely placed into the abdominal cavity and the scope inserted prior to inflation with 1 to 2 L of carbon dioxide. This also allows the clinician to make sure the cannula is not within the omentum. Filling the omentum with CO_2 inhibits visualization of the uterus and prolongs the procedure. After inflation of the abdominal cavity, the clinician watches the insertion of the opposite cannula via the laparoscope. The scope can be used to transluminate the site of the portal. The clinician makes a 6- to 10-mm incision through the skin and body wall into the abdominal cavity. The cannula is then placed through that incision (Figure 8.17A–D). The uterus is visualized, and the clinician inserts the insemination pipette (consisting of a special needle on the end of a pipette) into the second cannula to inseminate each horn. Alternatively, an insemination gun fitted with a brass injection tip or an aseptic needle (0.5–0.7 cm) is

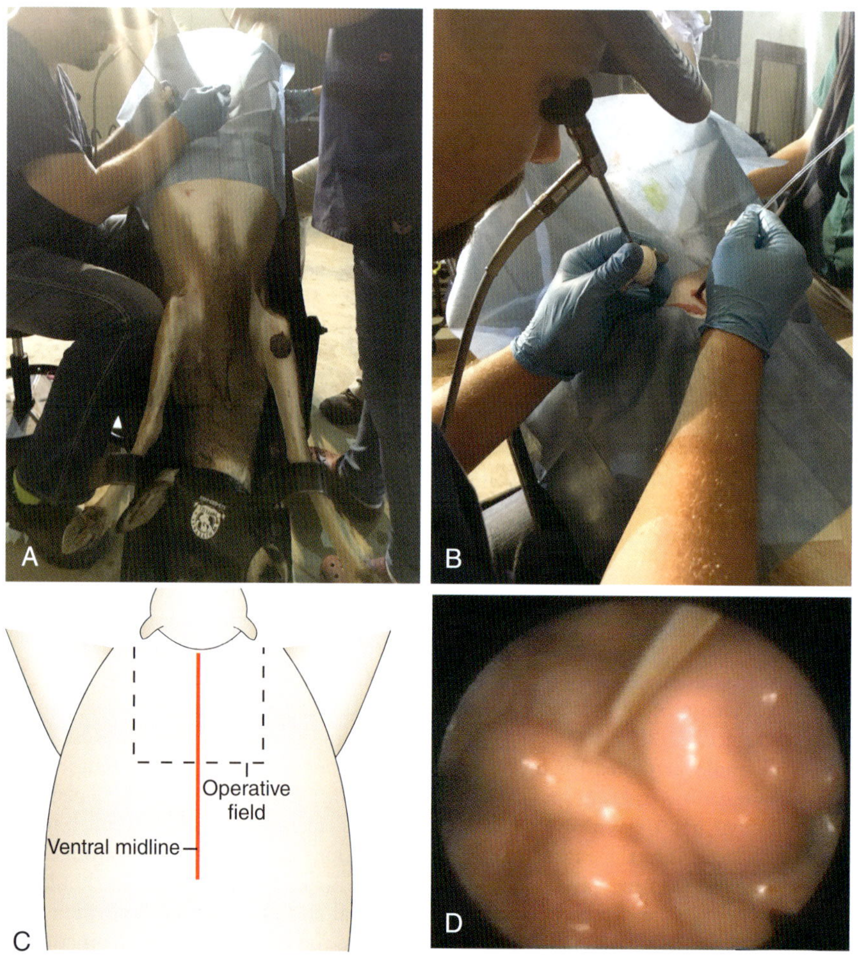

• **Fig. 8.17** Laparoscopic insemination in field conditions. **A.** The doe is secured on a reclining surgical table. The surgeon has placed both canula and is manipulating the laparoscope in order to visualize the uterus and judge the uterine tone. **B.** The left hand of the surgeon is operating a 5-mm laparoscope while visualizing the uterus. The right hand is manipulating the insemination gun through a canula. **C.** The skin incisions and canula placements should be inside the two marked operative fields. **D.** A laparoscopic view of the uterine horn being inseminated. Note that the insemination gun's needle (not seen) has penetrated the nonvascular curvature of the toned uterine horn and is depositing semen intra luminally. (A and B, Courtesy Dr. Jason Coe, Advanced Deer Genetics, LLC.)

inserted through the cannula into the abdominal cavity. The injection of the semen is done in an avascular area at the anterior uterine horn. The needle is inserted into the uterine lumen at a right angle to the uterine wall. The clinician should place the needle in the center of the horn, taking care to ensure that the needle is in the lumen of the uterus. The authors prefer to make a quick, controlled thrust into the uterine lumen. The semen should easily flow through the insemination device and into the uterus. If it does not, the needle is likely in the wall of the uterus and should be redirected. After insemination, the laparoscope and cannula are removed, and the puncture sites are sutured, stapled, or covered with an antibiotic ointment. Ewes and does should be moved to a recovery area and left undisturbed for 1 to 2 hours. The desired number of motile sperm injected into each uterine horn for laparoscopic AI using fresh or frozen semen is 20 million for goat does, 2 million to 50 million for cervid does, and 50 million for ewes.[159,160,166] Conception rates of 20% to 90% have been reported in small ruminants.[157] With a skilled laparoscopic surgeon and under good management conditions, use of a laparoscopic technique should yield the best results of all methods of AI.[157,167] The success of insemination depends largely on the quantity and motility of spermatozoa being inseminated. An experienced operator requires only 1.5 to 4 minutes to perform this procedure, and the females should recover uneventfully. Ewes and does may be laparoscopically inseminated many times throughout their lives.

Embryo Transfer

Traditional cross-breeding programs using AI focus on the male to produce many offspring. Breeding programs using multiple ovulation and ET use genetically superior females to contribute to this genetic diversity. The limited economic value of most sheep and goats precludes the widespread use of ET for the average production unit. Also, the invasive surgical procedure required makes ET less practical in goats than in cattle. Nevertheless, ET is an efficient method for moving genetics between flocks, across countries, and among continents.

ET is less practical in small ruminants than in cows because surgical collection and transfer are usually required. A successful ET program requires advanced planning and lots of attention to detail in donor and recipient selection, superovulation, synchronization of donor and recipient, and successful recovery and transfer of high-quality embryos. ET can be performed in or out of season, but the best response is attained during the breeding season when donors and recipients are cycling normally.[151,157,168–172]

Donor and Recipient Management. Donor and recipient selection and management are crucial to the success of an ET program. Recipient and donors must be synchronized to cycle together. Donors respond most successfully to estrus synchronization and superovulation when they are young, healthy, and cycling normally.[157,173] Does and ewes 2 to 5 years of age seem to respond best to synchronization and superovulation programs. Unfortunately, does and ewes presented as potential donors may often be older animals and therefore past their peak reproduction performance. Donors should be in good body condition (but not over conditioned) and good general health.[173] They should be vaccinated against any infectious diseases prevalent in the area and kept in separate groups for 2 to 4 months before the beginning of the ET program. This helps acclimate the donors and prevents stress.[170] Any changes in environment, feeding, and handling should occur well in advance of the initiation of an ET program. Premature luteal regression, a syndrome common in some breeds (Boer), appears to be caused by stress.

Recipients should be healthy animals with proven reproductive ability that are in good body condition (with a body condition score of 3–3.5) and cycling normally.[173] Females 2 to 4 years of age with good mothering characteristics and adequate potential for milk production are preferred. Recipients should also be current on their vaccinations against diseases prevalent in the area.

Synchronization. Most ET programs rely on exogenous hormones to induce and synchronize estrus in donors and recipients as described in the section on control of estrus cycle. Synchronization is commonly achieved using progestin sponges or CIDR. Accurate detection of estrus can be achieved using a teaser buck or ram. The method of estrus synchronization should be the same for both donor and recipient, with the exception that superior results are obtained if progestin sources are removed from recipients 12 hours before they are removed from donors. Figures 8.18 and 8.19 are generic synchronization/superovulation programs for goats and sheep, respectively (Johnson J: Personal communication, Lincoln Memorial University, Harrogate, TN 2010).

Superovulation. Superovulation of the donor is accomplished by injecting eCG and pituitary extracts of FSH. eCG has a longer half-life (about 72 hours). It is associated with overstimulation of the ovaries, resulting in the release of large numbers of eggs, an increased proportion of unfertilized embryos, and poorer-quality embryos. The eCG is administered in a single dose (1000 to 1500 IU) 48 hours before the progesterone source is removed. The donor also can be superovulated using an FSH product alone or in combination with eCG 2 days before the end of the artificially created luteal phase.[172] FSH has a half-life of about 6 hours and requires twice-daily injections beginning 48 hours before progestin removal. FSH is superior to eCG in ovulation and fertilization rates and production of good-quality embryos. Does and ewes generally exhibit estrus 24 to 36 hours after progestin removal. Frequent observation of does for estrus with the aid of a teaser animal is needed to ensure accurate recording of the time of estrus. Donors can be hand-mated 12 to 24 hours after estrus detection. Laparoscopic deposition of frozen and thawed semen into the uterine horns 24 hours after the animal is first seen in estrus yields optimal results. If donors are to be naturally bred, one buck or ram should be kept with one or two superovulated does or ewes.[171]

Embryo Recovery. Embryos (late morula to early blastocyst stage) are usually recovered from the donor's uterus on day 5 to 7 after breeding. In most instances, surgical collection may be employed. However, alternative techniques such as laparoscopic and nonsurgical embryo collection have been developed.[151,157,168–172,174–178]

Surgical. Does or ewes are held off feed and water 36 hours before surgical collection of embryos. Withholding feed and water decreases the chance of reflux and aspiration, decreases weight on the diaphragm, allowing easier respiration while under anesthesia, and decreases abdominal fill from ingesta, thus allowing easier manipulation and exteriorization of the uterus. After the female is placed under general anesthesia in dorsal recumbency, the caudal abdomen is clipped and prepared for aseptic surgery (see Chapter 18). A caudal ventral midline laparotomy incision approximately 8 to 10 cm in length extending cranially from the udder (or pelvic brim depending on udder development) is made. The uterus and ovaries are then carefully exteriorized. Some clinicians pour a physiologic solution (e.g., 250–500 mL physiologic saline with or without added ampicillin) into the abdominal cavity before

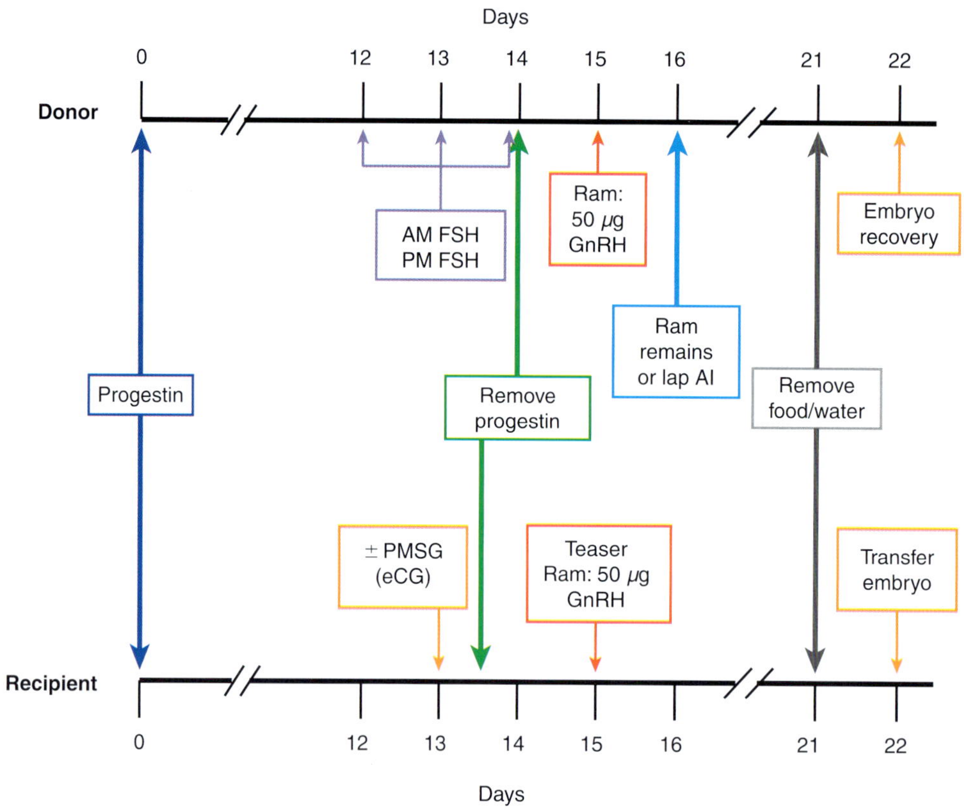

• **Fig. 8.18** Sample protocol for superovulation and estrous synchronization in the goat.
FSH: follicle stimulating hormone; PMSG: pregnant mare's serum gonadotropin; eCG: equine chorionic gonadotropin; GnRH: gonadotropin-releasing hormone

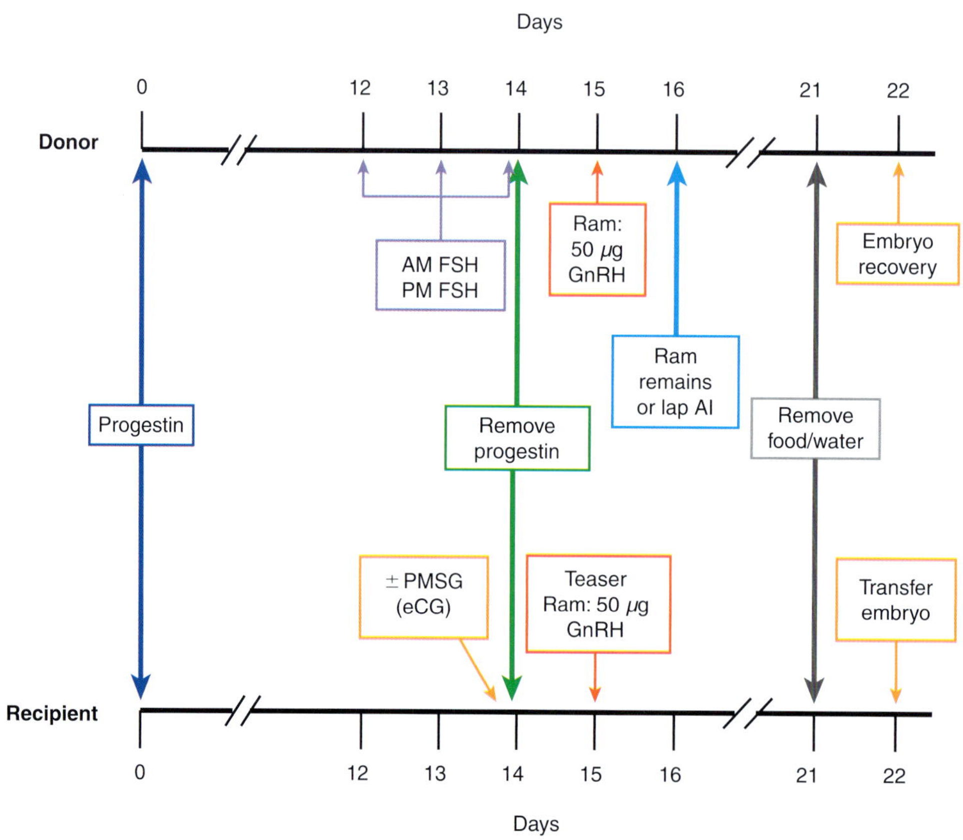

• **Fig. 8.19** Sample protocol for superovulation and estrous synchronization in the sheep.
FSH: follicle stimulating hormone; PMSG: pregnant mare's serum gonadotropin; eCG: equine chorionic gonadotropin; GnRH: gonadotropin-releasing hormone; lap AI: laparoscopic artificial insemination

exteriorizing the uterus. The clinician should carefully examine the ovaries to determine the response to superovulation. This examination of the ovaries can be accomplished laparoscopically before the laparotomy is performed to minimize ovarian handling. A blunt-tipped, 20-gauge needle is used to pierce the uterine wall near the uterotubal junction; an embryo or "tom cat" catheter is then inserted through the puncture site into the uterine horn. Tracing that uterine horn toward the body, a small artery forceps is used to "push-puncture" into the lumen of the horn near the bifurcation. An 8- to 10-French Foley catheter is placed through this "push-puncture" into the uterine body. The cuff is inflated with 3 to 5 cc of saline, and approximately 20 mL of flushing media (Dulbecco's PBS solution containing 100 IU/mL penicillin supplemented with 2% heat-activated goat serum) is infused through the embryo catheter to lavage the uterus. The lavage is followed by 10 to 15 cc of air. The fluid should drain through the Foley catheter and into a collection bowl or Petri dish. The dish operator monitors fluid flow and collection. The procedure is repeated on the opposite uterine horn. The uterine puncture sites can be left unsutured or closed with an inverting suture pattern using an absorbable 3-0 suture on a tapered needle. $PGF_{\alpha 2}$ should be administered postoperatively to lyse all luteal tissue. If embryos are to be collected before the fourth day after breeding, oviductal flushing (via cannulation of the oviduct near the fimbria) is necessary. The collection media is flushed in a retrograde direction through the oviduct using a catheter placed at the uterotubular junction.

The abdominal incision is then closed in a routine fashion according to clinician preference. The linea alba may be closed using no. 1 absorbable suture in a simple continuous pattern. The subcutaneous layer could be closed with 2-0 or 3-0 absorbable suture in a simple continuous pattern. The skin can then be closed with surgical staples or a suture material of choice using a simple continuous suture pattern.

Laparoscopic. Laparoscopic-assisted collection can be performed to exteriorize the tip of the uterine horn, with the flushing being performed in the same manner described for surgical collection. This method reduces the severity of adhesions that result from the handling required in a laparotomy approach.[169] Laparoscopy also can be used to collect the embryos within the abdomen without performing laparotomy. This technique requires considerable skill and is not practical for routine field use. A laparoscope-assisted procedure can be used to enhance this technique and decrease the risk of adhesion formation.[157,160] The laparoscopic method allows the operator to visualize the ovary, locate the CL, and more easily exteriorize the uterine horn. Advantages include reduced surgical time and a smaller abdominal incision.[160]

Nonsurgical. Nonsurgical or transcervical embryo collection techniques avoid the risk of postsurgical adhesions and maintain the value of genetically superior donors after multiple embryo collections. Several reports of successful nonsurgical collection in sheep and goats have been published.[175–178] Embryo recovery rate appears to be comparable to that achieved with surgical collection, but at present, most commercial embryo recovery procedures are still performed surgically.

Embryo Handling. The flush medium is searched under a dissecting microscope, and the embryos are retrieved and placed in a holding dish after washing. Before freezing or transfer, they are carefully assessed for quality and stage of development. Morula and blastocyst stages are expected when embryos are collected at day 5 or 6. Embryos should be held in Dulbecco's PBS with 5% to 20% fetal calf serum. The International Embryo Transfer Society has defined handling procedures to reduce the risk of disease transmission during ET.

Embryos are drawn-pulled into the tip of a small-bore intravenous (IV) catheter attached to a 1-mL syringe for immediate transfer into recipients. Alternatively, the embryos may be processed for freezing.

Embryo Transfer. Most transfers are performed surgically, with or without the aid of a laparoscope. Recipients are selected for transfer based on the greatest synchrony of estrus to the donor. This synchrony is one of the most important factors in the success of ET programs. The recipient is prepared as for surgical embryo collection, and a small ventral midline incision is made in front of the mammary gland. The ovaries are examined for a CL, and the uterine horn ipsilateral to the CL is exteriorized. Embryos are transferred to the oviducts via the fimbria using a "tom cat" catheter, Pasteur pipette, or embryo-specific pipettes if the embryos are in an early stage of development (earlier than day 4). Older embryos (those collected after day 4) are transferred to the uterine horns through a small stab incision made with a rounded 20-gauge needle or with the "eye" of a suture needle. Before closing the abdominal incision, the clinician should examine the catheter used to make the transfer microscopically to ensure that no embryos are retained in it. Most clinicians will transfer two embryos per recipient.

Recipient animals undergoing laparoscope-assisted transfer are prepared and placed on a surgical table or cradle as described for laparoscopic AI. Two cannulas are placed in the abdominal cavity, each 2 to 3 cm from the midline and approximately 10 cm cranial to the udder. The ovaries are examined through the laparoscope to identify the horn suitable for the ET. The tip of the uterus is grasped with forceps and gently elevated through the incision to the exterior. The tip of the uterus is punctured with a blunted needle and the embryos are introduced as previously described. The small incision in the midline is sutured.

Although the laparoscopic collection of embryos requires considerable expertise, laparoscopic transfer of embryos is relatively easy and recommended for large ET programs. However, laparoscopic-assisted transfer and surgical transfer are the techniques used most often for ET in goats.

For laparoscopic transfer, the recipient animals are prepared as described for laparoscopic-assisted ET. The clinician examines the ovaries through the laparoscope and identifies the horn ipsilateral to the CL for transfer of the embryos. The embryos are loaded in a 0.5-mL straw and inserted into an AI insemination gun fitted with a brass injection tip. The Cassou gun is inserted into the abdominal cavity through the cannula, an avascular area at the tip of the uterine horn is identified, and the needle is inserted into the uterine lumen at a right angle to the uterine wall. The clinician depresses the plunger of the AI gun gently to expel the embryos.

Many factors can affect the success of an ET program. An average of 8 to 10 transferable embryos can be expected per flush with expected pregnancy rates of 60 to 80% for the transfer of two fresh embryos per recipient.[179] Pregnancy rates from the transfer of frozen embryos are much lower.

Advanced Reproductive Techniques

Embryo freezing, in vitro fertilization, sexing semen, nuclear transfer (cloning), and other forms of assisted reproductive technology are useful in both research and propagating desired genetic traits. Information on specific areas of interest is widely available from the current scientific literature.[180–186]

Pregnancy Determination

Early pregnancy diagnosis and determination of the number of fetuses are of considerable value in goat and sheep reproductive herd health management. Goat owners frequently use clinical signs such as failure to return to estrus after breeding, enlarging abdomen, and developing mammary glands to make a presumptive diagnosis of pregnancy. However, pathologic conditions of the uterus and ovaries, physiologic anestrus late in the breeding season, and out-of-season breeding may cause postbreeding anestrus in nonpregnant goats.[187,188] Many goats and some ewes exhibit estrous behavior during pregnancy. Ultrasonography and hormonal assays are the most useful methods of pregnancy diagnosis. Abdominal palpation or ballottement, radiography, and rectal-abdominal palpation with a rod have limited use or have been abandoned.

The value of pregnancy determination lies in the identification of nonproductive females and ewes bearing multiple fetuses. Early identification allows appropriate nutritional and management programs to be implemented. The ability to divide the flock into groups of animals based on pregnancy status and fetal numbers not only improves the health care of these animals by reducing the incidence of some disease but also decreases production costs.

Diagnostic Techniques

Ultrasonography. Ultrasonographic techniques for pregnancy determination include amplitude modulation (A-mode), Doppler, and real-time (B-mode) imaging.[188] A-mode ultrasonography can be used to detect pregnancy between 60 and 100 days' gestation. Detection of a fluid density is interpreted as pregnancy. Accordingly, hydrometra or a large bladder may give a false-positive result. Therefore, A-mode ultrasound is an unreliable method for diagnosing pregnancy. Doppler ultrasonography can be used to detect movement that may indicate pregnancy (blood flow in the middle uterine artery or umbilical arteries, fetal heartbeat, and fetal movements). The external Doppler technique has an accuracy of 100% during the second half of gestation but is not as effective at 50 to 75 days or earlier. The transrectal technique for Doppler ultrasound may be attempted as early as 25 to 30 days after breeding but waiting until day 35 to 40 produces better results. False-negative and false-positive results are common and determining fetal numbers is difficult.

Pregnancy detection in small ruminants is now performed almost entirely with real-time ultrasonography. Linear array real-time ultrasound transducers can be used transrectally to diagnose pregnancy as early as 18 days and as late as 60 days.[189] A homemade plastic extension can easily be fashioned from PVC pipe to allow easy introduction of the transducer into the rectum. A 5- or a 7.5-MHz transducer is recommended for rectal scans. The doe or ewe should be prepared for transrectal ultrasonography by removing as much fecal material as possible from the rectum. The addition of 20 to 30 mL of methylcellulose into the rectum provides lubrication to facilitate the introduction of the transducer rectally. After 60 days, the gravid uterus is pulled down into the abdomen and may be difficult to visualize transrectally. Table 8.5 shows age of gestation and associated ultrasonographic findings for pregnant sheep and goats.

Transabdominal ultrasonography with a 3.5- or 5-MHz linear or sector scanner is used after 30 days of gestation. The transducer is placed on a fiberless area of the abdomen high in the inguinal region, preferably in the right flank.[187,188] A bland fluid (e.g., vegetable oil, methylcellulose, and alcohol) should be used to couple the ultrasound transducer to the skin. The clinician aims the transducer's beam toward the opposite side of the pelvis and scans the abdomen by slowly "sweeping" the transducer cranially. In goats, shearing the inguinal region increases the accuracy and speed of examination. Identification of the bladder (typically triangular in appearance) provides an excellent landmark. The uterus is normally located dorsal or cranial to the bladder. Pregnancy at this point can be diagnosed on the basis of finding a fetus, placentomes, or, less reliably, numerous fluid-filled uterine luminal sections. The placentomes appear as round "doughnuts" or C-shaped structures (Figure 8.20A, B) in sheep and goats, whereas in cervids, it will appear as a hyperechoic flat area on the uterine wall. Transabdominal ultrasonography can be used as early as 30 days and as late as 120 days. After day 90 to 120, reliable identification of the number of fetuses becomes difficult because their individual size fills the screen; one fetus may be mistaken for two, or two different fetuses may be mistaken for one.

Twin pregnancies can often be determined between 45 and 90 days of gestation. Sector scanning units provide a wider visual angle or view of the abdomen.[187] This allows more of the uterus to be seen in the visual field, improving the accurate identification of multiple fetuses. The clinician should shear the wool on the abdomen just cranial to the udder and scan the abdomen slowly to make a mental image of all abdominal contents. Generally, the C-shaped placentomes can be seen "pointing" their concave portions toward the fetus. The fetal bones form "shadows," and the fetal ribs produce a characteristic striated appearance. Careful attention to a complete and thorough examination helps minimize errors but viewing a single fetus too long can result in a false diagnosis of twins. After 120 days of gestation, the fetal bones can produce a distorted image, but a diagnosis can be made with some

TABLE 8.5 Ultrasound Findings in Pregnancy.

A. Ultrasound Findings at Various Stages of Gestation

Gestational Age (Days)	Ultrasound Findings
17–25	Transrectal: embryo visible after 24 days
26–35	Transabdominal: hypoechoic amnion and hyperechoic fetus
30–75	Transabdominal: doughnut-shaped to C-shaped placentomes
55–75	Transabdominal: visualization of genital tubercle
45–90	Transabdominal (midabdomen in front of udder): best time for twin detection
90 to term	Difficult to determine accurate number of fetuses as female gets closer to term

B. Fetal Age Determination Based on Crown-to-Rump Length for Saanen and Alpine Goats

Crown-to-Rump Length (mm)	Gestational Age (Days)
40 mm	45 days
100 mm	60 days
250 mm	90 days

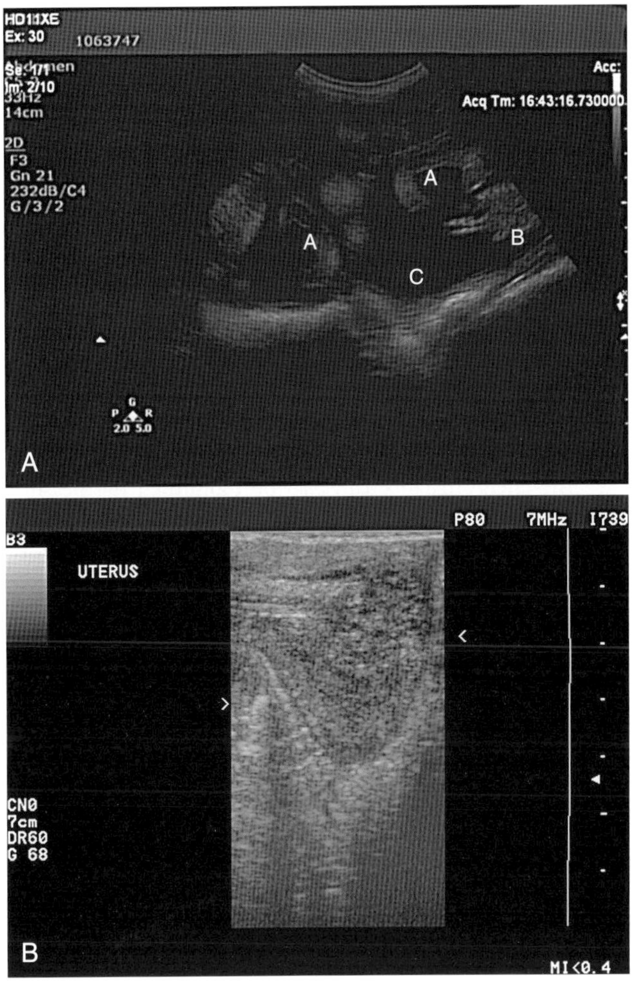

• **Fig. 8.20** These two ultrasound images contrast the transabdominally viewed gravid uterus with the rectally viewed nongravid uterus. **A.** Real-time, curvilinear array ultrasound using a 2.5-MHz transducer on a doe at 60 days in gestation. Notice the hyperechoic, "C-shaped" placentomes *(A)*, the hyperechoic fetal ribs *(B)*, and the hypoechoic amniotic fluid *(C)* from this transabdominal view. **B.** Ultrasound of a nongravid uterus obtained from a 3-year-old Cheviot ewe, 2 months after delivering twins, demonstrating an alternating echogenic and hypoechoic appearance. The lumen of the uterine horn is not visible of this picture. This long-axis view image was obtained transrectally with a 5-MHz linear array transducer. Cranial is to the right of the image. (Courtesy Dr. Misty Edmondson, Alabama Department of Agriculture and Industries, and Dr. Karine Pader, Purdue University, respectively.)

effort. To maximize the usefulness of ultrasound, ewes and does should be scanned between 45 and 60 days so producers can implement any management changes indicated by pregnancy status or number of fetuses. Clinicians also can use ultrasonography to stage pregnancies by measuring the biparietal diameter of the fetus.[188–190]

Abnormal ultrasonographic findings include hydrometra, pyometra, fetal mummy, and macerated fetus. Hydrometra appears as an anechoic, fluid-filled uterus, often with membranous strands visualized in the lumen of the uterus. The uterus also does not have the typical placentomes characteristic of pregnancy. Hydrometra is often seen in does with apparently normal reproductive histories.[188,189] Pyometra is also manifested as a fluid-filled uterus with more hyperechoic densities and a swirling appearance.

Assessment of fetal viability may be crucial in cases such as pregnancy toxemia.[1] Fetal mummification may be identified as hyperechoic areas without any identifiable body parts within a relatively fluid-free placentome-less uterus. The fetal heartbeat can be easily recognized by 30 to 35 days after breeding.[188] Early fetal death may be recognized by finding free-floating fetal masses along with ribbon-like placental membranes.[190] These ribbon-like membranes may be found contralateral to a normally developing fetus. Lack of fetal movement, amniotic fluid, heartbeat, and blood coursing through the umbilicus can easily differentiate a dead fetus from a living one with real-time ultrasonography. Soon after fetal death the placentomes lose their "crisp" margins.[187]

Abdominal Palpation and Ballottement. During the last half of gestation, the gravid uterus or fetus may be palpated through the abdominal wall. Ballottement may be useful in determining pregnancy status during late gestation. Ballottement is performed by gently pushing a fisted hand low in the right flank of the female. In a pregnant female in late gestation, the fetus should be pushed away from the fisted hand and then return in a fluid wave to "bump" the fist. Ballottement is unable to assess the viability of the fetus and false-positives have occurred when the ventral sac of the rumen was confused for a gravid uterus.

Hormone Assays. Measurement of hormones in blood, milk, or urine provides an alternative method of pregnancy diagnosis when ultrasound equipment is not available. The estrone sulfate test, pregnancy-specific protein B (PSPB), and progesterone measurement are examples.

Estrone Sulfate. Estrone sulfate is a pregnancy-specific hormone produced by the fetal placental unit. It can be detected in the urine, serum, or milk after day 50 of pregnancy. When performed 50 days or more after breeding, this test has been characterized as almost 100% accurate in the detection of pregnancy. A positive test indicates a viable fetus. False-positive results may occur if hemolyzed serum samples are assayed. False-negative results may occur if samples are collected before day 50 of gestation. Commercial laboratories offering this test are limited and expensive.[187]

Pregnancy-Specific Protein B. PSPB is produced by binucleate giant cells of the placenta throughout gestation. It can be used in small ruminants to detect pregnancy any time after day 30 postbreeding for sheep and goats and after 40 days postbreeding in elk, moose, deer, caribou, and African antelope. False-positive results can occur in the early postpartum period and false-negative results can occur if samples are collected prior to day 30 after breeding. An ELISA (BioPRYN, BioTracking, Inc., Moscow, Idaho) is presently commercially available for sheep, goats, cervids, as well as cattle and bison.[188] Multiple fetuses typically result in higher levels of PSPB.[187]

Progesterone. Progesterone analysis is not a test for pregnancy, and it more accurately detects nonpregnant rather than pregnant females. Goats and cervids depend on progesterone from the CL to maintain pregnancy throughout gestation. Plasma or serum progesterone concentrations below 1 to 2 ng/mL at 21 days and 18 to 19 days after breeding in the doe and ewe, respectively, indicate nonpregnancy based on the absence of a functional CL. Low progesterone concentrations after 24 days in cervids would indicate nonpregnancy. An elevated progesterone concentration at this time may indicate pregnancy, hydrometra, pyometra, early embryonic death, fetal mummification, or irregular estrous cycle. The accuracy of blood progesterone level analysis is reported as 80 to 100% for nonpregnancy and 67 to 100% for pregnancy. In some management scenarios, particularly in dairy goats, serum or milk progesterone is collected on day 19 to 22 after breeding. Serum or plasma progesterone concentrations more accurately reflect the true endocrine status of the goat doe and are more accurate than milk progesterone analysis. Commercial, on-farm cattle progesterone test kits can be used in goats with good accuracy.[187]

Radiography. Abdominal radiography is useful for detecting pregnancy and fetal numbers in the individual pet goat brought to a clinic. It also provides an accurate alternative when ultrasound equipment is not available. This procedure is applicable but rarely used in small ruminants. Radiography is not practical for examining large numbers of animals. The fetal skeleton may be seen as early as 58 days after breeding and may be radiopaque after day 65. Radiography is probably best performed 90 days or later after breeding in small ruminants to avoid false-negative results.

Fetal Age Determination

The size of the fetus can be used to estimate the gestational age of the fetus. The crown-rump length of the fetus in relation to gestational age has been estimated for Saanen and Alpine goat breeds. A crown-rump length of 40 mm is equivalent to 45 days of gestation, 100 mm to 60 days, and 250 mm to 90 days.[191] Fetal age has also been estimated for dairy goats and pygmy goats between 40 and 100 days of gestation by measuring the biparietal diameter with real-time ultrasonography. The formulas for calculating fetal age vary based on the breed.[192,193] Cervid fetal aging can be done, as well, by fetal crown-rump measurements.[194]

Fetal Sex Determination

Fetal sex can be determined through the use of real-time ultrasonography though visualization of the genital tubercle of the developing fetus between 55 and 75 days of gestation. Fetal sexing should be performed after 60 days in fetuses derived from fresh or frozen embryos.[195] The genital tubercle begins its development between the hindlimbs and moves back toward the tail in females or forward toward the umbilicus in males. Females should have two teats visible between the hind legs with the absence of a triangular-shaped scrotum. The penis and prepuce are located just caudal to the umbilical cord.[196,197] Visualization of the genital tubercle is more difficult with twins or triplets compared to a singleton fetus.[196,197]

General Female Management

Pregnant ewe and doe flocks should be intensely managed to control disease and lessen the chance of reproductive failure. A review of records provides the veterinarian with an opportunity to look at the reproductive performance of the flock over the past several years. This analysis can help in the implementation of management changes to enhance productivity. Particular attention should be given to lambing/kidding percentages and dystocia rates to determine whether more aggressive monitoring and intervention may be necessary around the time of parturition. Some basic guidelines should be followed with respect to control of infectious disease. Producers should attempt to keep flocks/herds closed during gestation and should be vigilant for potential fomite transmission among flocks/herds. Biosecurity should be extended to include pest and stray cat control (see Chapter 19).

Prepartum Care of the Small Ruminant

Females should be maintained at a body condition score of 2.5 to 3 and should be allowed free choice access to an acceptable mineral salt mixture (see Chapter 2) and clean water. All causes of stress should be avoided. Deworming, hoof trimming, shearing, vaccination, moving, and other stressful procedures should be minimized for 1 month prior to parturition.[198] Producers should determine the animals' pregnancy statuses and number of fetuses and sort and feed them accordingly, if appropriate. Females should be monitored and assessed for body condition score every 2 to 3 weeks throughout gestation. Basic feeding programs and herd health recommendations are covered elsewhere in this text (see Chapters 2 and 19).

A good herd health program should be planned and implemented to decrease the incidence of disease in the prepartum female. The energy balance can also be monitored by measuring beta-hydroxybutyrate concentrations in whole blood using a handheld monitoring system (Precision Xtra Blood Glucose and Ketone Monitoring System, Abbott, Columbus, Ohio). A clean, dry lambing area that is protected from severe cold and wind should be provided for the ewe or doe. She should be sheared before lambing and have her mammary glands examined to ensure that the lambs will be able to nurse and that no severe teat and udder lesions are present.[199]

Female dairy goats and ewes should be "dried off" 60 days before the expected due date. During the final 4 weeks of the dry period, females should be supplemented with concentrates or good-quality pasture. They should be watched closely for signs of ketosis, hypocalcemia, hypomagnesemia, or abortion diseases.[199] When possible, females should receive their annual vaccinations and be dewormed during the final month of pregnancy. Vaccination of females for enterotoxemia, tetanus, and other endemic diseases optimizes the presence of immunoglobulins in the colostrum. Dairy does should be brought into a kidding pen, and the hair around their udders, tails, and perineal areas should be clipped. Meat does should have access to a clean shelter for kidding and should be observed regularly. Cervid does should be kept as stress free as possible and in their normal/familiar groups. Clean, dry areas for fawning are important and providing some cover for the doe to fawn in and hide the fawns will improve success. One should leave the doe and fawn alone for several hours for bonding and colostrum consumption.

Parturition

Normal parturition requires the functional maturation of the fetal adrenal cortex. Parturition is triggered by activation of the fetal pituitary-adrenal axis. Adrenocorticotropic hormone is released by the fetal pituitary gland, stimulating the release of corticosteroids by the fetal adrenal glands. An increase in fetal corticosteroids stimulates placental estrogen biosynthesis, which in turn stimulates the synthesis and release of $PGF_{2\alpha}$ from the placenta and endometrium. $PGF_{2\alpha}$ causes luteolysis, which results in a decrease in progesterone. An increase in estrogen and a decrease in progesterone stimulate myometrial activity with subsequent oxytocin release.[198]

Birth is much more likely to occur during the daylight hours than at night; it is most frequent around midday. When the female is close to birthing, the udder fills up rapidly, the pelvic ligaments relax, and the vulva enlarges and shows small amounts of colorless mucous discharge. The cervical plug is often shed just before parturition, but it may be lost as much as 1 week prepartum. Parturition can be divided into three stages. The first stage is initiation of myometrial contraction, which lasts from 2 to 12 hours. The female may leave the group and act uncomfortable; she is restless, lies down and gets up, and urinates frequently. During this first stage, the cervix relaxes and releases the cervical seal. The second stage is delivery of the fetus, which is quick, lasting about 1 to 2 hours. Does and ewes may prefer lateral recumbency during this stage, but some older, more experienced females may remain standing for delivery. Initially, the amnion protrudes from the vulva, which should be followed shortly by the forefeet and the head. The fetus should be in a position such that the dorsum is aimed toward the sacrum of the female. NOTE: Any female that fails to continue progressing through parturition should be examined.

Some fetuses are born in posterior presentation, which is normal if both rear legs are extended and delivery occurs rapidly after the feet are delivered. In the case of multiple fetuses, the female may rest between deliveries or the deliveries may occur in quick succession. If a female strains, without producing any fetus for longer than an hour, intervention is indicated.

The third stage of labor is characterized by delivery of the placenta within 6 hours and involution of the uterus. In the absence of septicemia or toxic signs, failure to deliver the placenta should be of no cause for concern until 12 to 18 hours. Involution of the uterus is complete by day 28 after parturition. Lochia (a nonodorous, reddish-brown discharge) is normally discharged for as long as 3 weeks postpartum.

Induction of Parturition and Pregnancy Termination

Termination of pregnancy in the doe can be achieved at any time in gestation because she depends on progesterone from the CL to maintain pregnancy throughout gestation. Therefore, intentional or accidental administration of prostaglandins induces abortion or parturition at any stage of gestation. The typical reason for a client's request for early termination of pregnancy is mismating. The drug of choice to induce abortion or parturition in the doe is $PGF_{2\alpha}$ (5–10 mg) or cloprostenol (75–100 μg/45 kg). The ewe is similar to the cow in that $PGF_{2\alpha}$ may not induce abortion throughout gestation in all ewes. To allow the CL to mature and become receptive to the effect of prostaglandin, the doe or ewe should not be treated earlier than 5 to 7 days after breeding. Successfully aborted does typically show estrus in 3 to 5 days.[198]

Sheep. Farm personnel can use induction of lambing as a management technique to ensure proper attention to the delivery process. Lambing can be reliably induced in ewes after day 137 of gestation with dexamethasone (15–20 mg IM), but better lamb survival rates may be expected if induction is initiated within 1 week of the expected due date or after day 142 of gestation. Lambing can be expected within 36 to 48 hours after the administration of dexamethasone.[200,201] Aglepristone, a progesterone receptor blocker, has been suggested as another treatment for parturition induction in Europe, where it has been approved.[202]

Goat. The goat kid should be at least 144 days of gestation at the time of induction of parturition for the animal to be viable. Therefore, accurate breeding records are very important. Females with enlarged udders filled with colostrum are the best candidates for induction. A doe induced in the morning at the correct stage of gestation can be expected to kid by the next afternoon. Prostaglandins may be given all at once (5–10 mg of $PGF_{2\alpha}$ or 75–100 μg/45 kg of cloprostenol) or in a stepwise fashion (100 μg cloprostenol followed in 10 hours by 50 μg). This allows owners to plan the time and day of kidding so that assistance is available. Unlike cows, does seldom have problems with retained placentas after induced parturition. If does are to be induced because of pregnancy toxemia, administering a glucocorticosteroid (10–20 mg dexamethasone IM) 6 to 12 hours before induction may enhance fetal maturation and improve postinduction survivability.[203]

Cervid. As a general rule, cervids would not be induced unless the health of the dam is in question. Fetal-maternal disproportion issues almost never arise, and dystocia rates are small. But, if necessary, prostaglandin will usually induce parturition within 48 hours using sheep or goat dosages.

Dystocia Management

Dystocia can be a major cause of economic loss in sheep and goat flocks. The most common cause of dystocia is fetal postural abnormalities. Other causes include incomplete cervical dilation, simultaneous presentation of lambs or kids, cervicovaginal prolapse, uterine inertia, and occasionally fetal-maternal size disproportion. Cases of fetal-maternal size disproportion are usually associated with singleton births and overly finished ewes or does.[204] Most birthing problems are handled by owners, and only the more difficult cases are submitted for veterinary assistance. Most fetuses are born in cranial, longitudinal presentation. All manipulative procedures should follow general principles of veterinary obstetrics such as cleanliness, lubrication, and gentleness. Practitioners with small hands tend to have a technical advantage.

When a female is presented for dystocia management, the clinician should first assess her overall condition and rule out the presence of concurrent disease. The 3-30 rule is employed by many practitioners. That is, the ewe or doe should be examined 30 minutes after contractions begin or after the breaking of the chorioallantoic membrane. If the female is normal and parturition is progressing normally, the clinician should wait at least 30 minutes before beginning any treatments or manipulations. Females should be examined 30 minutes after delivery to determine whether another fetus is still in the uterus or birth canal. Some females with dystocia may have a complicating uterine inertia because they have become fatigued; signs of pain and panting may occur. Hypocalcemia (both primary or secondary to respiratory alkalosis) contributes to poor uterine contractility. Cervid does may have to be anesthetized or run into a chute system to examine. Preparation for anesthesia and reversal of such and support of the fetus are important.

Epidural Anesthesia. Administration of a caudal epidural analgesic facilitates corrections in fetal alignment and helps decrease the associated straining and pain. The area over the first two caudal vertebrae should be clipped and aseptically prepared. An 18- to 21-gauge, 4-cm needle is directed ventrally into the junction between the first two caudal vertebrae perpendicular to the slope of the tail head. In small goats, a 25- to 27-gauge needle may be required. After penetrating the skin, the clinician should use the "hanging drop technique" by filling the hub of the needle with 2% lidocaine (0.5 mL/45 kg body weight) and advancing the needle slowly in a ventral direction. When the needle is in the proper position, the lidocaine should flow into the space because of the negative pressure in the epidural space. The location of the site can be enhanced by moving the tail up and down to find the freely moveable vertebral space between the first two caudal vertebrae. Epidural administration provides approximately 1 hour of analgesia.

Physical Examination. Ideally, the area around the vulva should be clipped of wool and thoroughly cleansed before any obstetric maneuvers. The clinician should next attempt to palpate the fetus and determine the cause of the dystocia. The use of copious amounts of lubricant should be encouraged when performing obstetric maneuvers. Disposable gloves should be worn by all people participating in the birth process because of the potential for transmission of zoonotic diseases. Common causes of dystocia include deviations from normal presentation, position, or posture; flexion of the neck, carpus, and shoulder; fetal-maternal disproportion; and more than one fetus attempting to exit the vaginal canal at the same time.[203] However, not all cases of abnormal fetal presentation, position, or posture result in dystocia. Some does and ewes may give birth normally if only one forelimb is presented with the head. In dystocia caused by blockage of the vaginal canal by a relatively large head or fetus, one of the forelimbs may be repositioned into shoulder flexion, allowing room to pass the head and remaining forelimb; the kid can then be delivered by traction. In cases in which just the head is presented and both shoulders are in a flexed position, traction of the head with a snare may be sufficient for delivery if the vaginal canal has been well lubricated.

Carpal and shoulder flexions are corrected digitally by hooking a finger around the forelimbs below the flexed carpus and straightening the limb.

Breech Presentation. A true breech presentation implies that the fetus is in posterior presentation in a dorsosacral position with both back limbs retained beneath the fetal body. Breech fetuses are handled similar to those with carpal flexion by straightening each flexed hindlimb. In these cases, the rear quarters of the fetus and the tail are felt on vaginal examination. If the veterinarian's hands are small enough, manual correction of the dystocia may be possible. The fetus should be repelled or pushed cranially and to one side. Raising the female's hindquarters can make this maneuver much easier. The clinician should then try to pull a hock back into the pelvic canal. After one hock is in the pelvis, it should be rotated laterally in relation to the long axis of the fetus while the foot is pulled ventrally and medially out through the vulva. The veterinarian should take care not to injure the female's vagina with the fetal hooves. The same procedure is then repeated on the contralateral limb, and the fetus is extracted.

Head Malposition or Lateral Deviation of the Head. Repulsion should be attempted to gain enough room to pull the head back around in normal position. If this cannot be accomplished, the clinician can place a snare-type device over the laterally retained head and legs to keep the head of the fetus as tight against its body as possible and then extract the fetus by pulling on the forelimbs.

Front Leg Malposition. One or both front legs can be retained. If both front legs are retained, the head is usually in the pelvis or can be found protruding from the vulva. If the fetus is still viable, it should be repulsed into the pelvic canal to create the room necessary to extract both legs one at the time. Fetuses can be delivered with only one foot forward if repeated efforts to extend the second leg are unsuccessful. Care should be taken to ensure that the legs pulled into the pelvic canal are from the same fetus as the head. If no response is elicited from the fetus by pinching or pulling on the tongue and if the veterinarian is confident the fetus is dead, he or she can remove the head with a guarded wire saw or a fetotomy knife. This may allow for easier correction of the retained legs. The same basic procedure can be done if only one leg is retained. When both legs and the head present at the same time (i.e., the legs do not present before the head), the elbows often lodge against the inner entrance of the pelvic canal, creating an elbow lock. This can often be corrected by mild repulsion of the head followed by traction on one limb at a time.

Ringwomb. Failure of the cervix to dilate properly is encountered clinically in the ewe and, to a lesser extent, in the doe.[205] This condition is referred to as *ringwomb* and is considered to be a heritable condition. A similar clinical condition occurs when the natural birth process is disrupted, and the cervix is not properly stimulated for normal dilation to occur. If the veterinarian's hand can fit into the pelvis, he or she can attempt manual dilation of the cervix. Misoprostol applied topically to the cervix has been used to help ripen the cervix with some success in goats.[206] Oxytocin can be administered to induce uterine contractions; pushing against the closed cervix may aid in the dilation process. However, a cesarean section is usually required. A fetotomy knife can be used to open the cervix if the animal's value does not warrant surgery and the fetuses are still viable. Euthanasia should be considered after this procedure depending on the condition of the cervix and uterus.

Cesarean Section

Cesarean section is the most common abdominal surgery performed in small ruminants. While aseptic technique in a hospital setting is ideal for better results and fewer complications, the procedure can certainly be performed in the field with good results. In fact, if transportation to a clinic facility dramatically increases the time to delivery, the field procedure is often a better option than endangering survival by delaying delivery. Cesarean section can be performed in dorsal recumbency via a ventral midline approach, but more often, it is done with the animal in right lateral recumbency via a left paralumbar fossa incision. Local anesthesia via a paravertebral, inverted-L, or line block is adequate for sheep and goats, but general anesthesia will be necessary for the cervid. We suggest limiting the dose of lidocaine injected for local anesthesia to no more than 6 mg/kg of body weight. Diluting the 2% lidocaine from the bottle with an equal volume of saline to create a 1% solution will adequately anesthetize the surgical site without causing toxicity. Paravertebral nerve blocks can be performed in small ruminants as in cattle; however, it is frequently easier to achieve adequate anesthesia with an inverted-L block, line block, or local infiltration. The body wall of small ruminants is relatively thin, so the local infiltration does not need to go as deeply as in cattle. When paravertebral anesthesia is unsuccessful in achieving adequate anesthesia, one must be careful not to exceed the toxic dose of lidocaine with supplemental local infiltration (see Chapter 18).

The left paralumbar fossa approach allows the dam to remain in lateral recumbency, which leads to fewer respiratory complications than restraint in dorsal recumbency. The rumen is also oriented with the dorsal aspect up with this positioning, which serves to help retain abdominal viscera within the abdominal cavity. Should the dam bloat in right, lateral recumbency, the rumen has more room to dilate before causing respiratory compromise, and it can be decompressed if needed. Experience would suggest that this is not a frequent problem. When bloat does occur, the

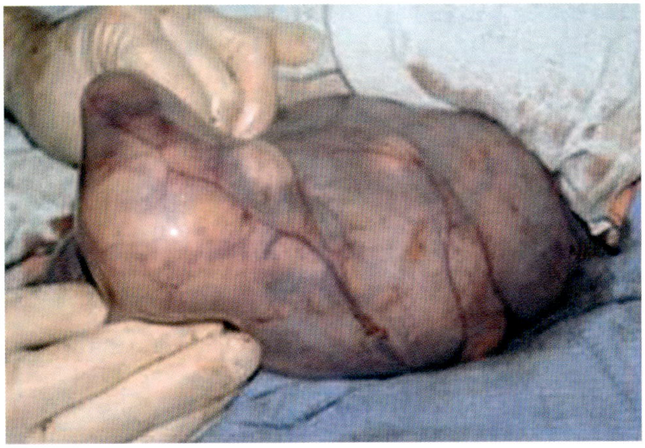

• **Fig. 8.21** The uterus of a ewe with pregnancy toxemia in left lateral recumbency with the uterus exteriorized and packed off. The uterine incision will be made over the head of the fetus with this exposure.

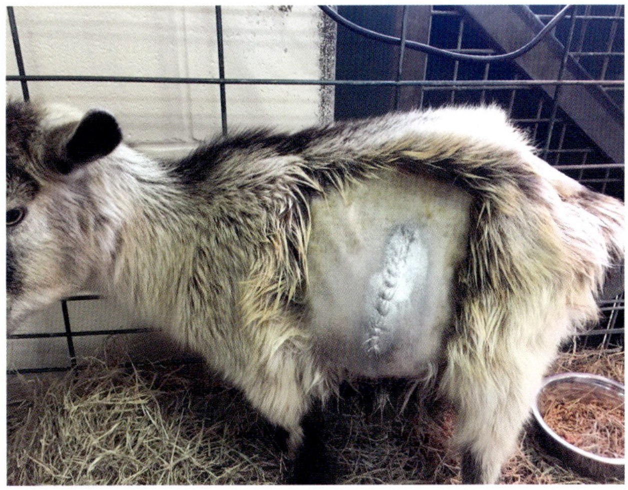

• **Fig. 8.22** Kid nursing a doe that had a Cesarean section performed via the left paralumbar fossa approach. Note the incision is away from the udder which allows for the kid to nurse sooner and more frequently.

practitioner is usually wise to quickly complete the surgery and return the dam to sternal recumbency rather than be overly concerned with rumen distention. The muscular body wall is relatively thin in small ruminants when compared to other large animal species. Therefore, utmost care is required when making the body wall incision to avoid inadvertently damaging deeper structures. Sheep, more so than goats, have a great deal of retroperitoneal fat that must be penetrated to reach the abdominal cavity. The gravid uterus usually can be well exteriorized in small ruminants to allow packing off of the uterus with sterile towels before incising into the uterus. If possible, both uterine horns should be exteriorized. The uterine incision is best made on the greater curvature of the uterus in an easily accessible area between the ovary and cervix. This incision can be made over the hindlimbs of the fetus; however, it is frequently easier to make the incision over the head, with care taken not to make a laceration in the fetus (Figure 8.21). The practitioner's needs are best served by making an incision over each respective fetus, but occasionally, two fetuses in the same uterine horn can be removed through one uterine incision. However, it is difficult to maneuver a fetus from one uterine horn into the other to permit removal through one incision. Therefore, it is usually best to make at least one uterine incision per uterine horn when fetuses are present in both uterine horns. Any placenta that is not firmly attached to the uterus should be removed before closure of the uterus. The uterine incision should be closed with absorbable suture in an inverting pattern (e.g., Utrecht, Cushing, and Lembert) to achieve a fluid-tight seal. The practitioner should be careful not to invert too much tissue as this may lead to a tunneling effect with subsequently leakage of uterine contents. One-layer closure is usually sufficient, although a second can be added if the integrity of the first layer is in question or if the uterine contents are severely contaminated. The uterus should then be cleaned of any blood or debris using a copious amount of fluid before it is replaced into the correct position in the abdominal cavity, being careful to limit any contamination of the abdominal cavity. Care should be taken to minimize contamination of the abdominal cavity. The muscular body wall is closed with absorbable suture in a manner chosen by the practitioner. Closure of each muscle layer separately is recommended, but, in the interest of time, layers may be combined without detriment. An approach via the left paralumbar fossa places the incision away from the udder which facilitates nursing of the dam sooner and more frequently than a midline or paramedian approach (Figure 8.22).

The most common reason for cesarean section in small ruminants is probably inadequate cervical dilation.[207] However, some consideration must be given to overdiagnosis of "ringwomb" when a time delay occurs before attention is given to the dystocia. The cervix in fact may have been adequately dilated during labor but does not maintain appropriate dilation for the duration of a prolonged dystocia. Other reasons to perform a cesarean section include pregnancy toxemia in the ewe or doe, relative fetal oversize, absolute fetal oversize and, less frequently, fetal malposition. Uterine torsion may occasionally lead to cesarean section in which case the practitioner will frequently encounter severe tissue damage to the avascular uterus. A torsed uterus may not be viable, and the dam could be very ill.

Retained placenta is the most common postoperative complication following cesarean section. In general, complications are decreased when dams receive perioperative antibiotics.

Pygmy goats, as a breed, are more at risk than others for dystocia.[203] The increased popularity of some meat breeds may lead to selective breeding of heavily muscled animals, which may become more prone to dystocia. Any delay in surgery after a dystocia occurs decreases fetal survival. Many owners will elect not to rebreed dams after a cesarean section. In one study, however, all ewes and does bred after cesarean section conceived and had uncomplicated vaginal deliveries.[207] Another experimental study comparing ewes experiencing natural delivery to those having elective cesarean sections did not find any significant difference in subsequent fertility.[208] It was found that bacterial cultures of deep cervical swabs were positive for a significantly longer period in does that underwent cesarean section than in does experiencing natural delivery.[209] The clinical significance of this finding would likely depend on the intensity of management systems. Lambs delivered prematurely by cesarean section from ewes pretreated with dexamethasone (16 mg) had better oxygen consumption and breathing frequency than control lambs. These lambs exposed to low temperatures also showed improved thermoregulation than control lambs.[210] These findings would support pretreatment of ewes with dexamethasone for all elective cesarean deliveries

Fetotomy

A complete fetotomy, such as that performed in cows, is rarely practiced in either goats or does. Before performing a fetotomy, the clinician should clean the animal's perineal area and lubricate the entire reproductive tract well; extreme caution is indicated during the procedure to avoid uterine rupture and cervical or vaginal damage. Partial fetotomy of the head, in most cases, is sufficient to allow enough room in the vagina for further manipulation or passage of the remaining fetal parts. In both sheep and goats, percutaneous fetotomy to remove the front legs may help reduce size so the fetus may be manipulated through the pelvic canal. If two fetuses are wedged into the pelvic canal and repulsion of one or both is not possible, partial fetotomy may be of benefit. Partial fetotomy is warranted when the fetus has been dead for some time and the female's uterus is very friable. In such cases, pretreatment with NSAIDs (e.g., flunixin meglumine) and antibiotics (e.g., penicillin) may be indicated.

NOTE: The clinician should be very careful when performing a fetotomy, as the uterus of small ruminants are quite friable as compared with that of the cow. Any full-thickness tear in the uterine wall that contaminates the abdominal cavity in an already physiologically or immunologically compromised animal can easily result in peritonitis, adhesions, long-term infertility, or death.

Neonatal Care

Lambs

After lambing, the ewes and lambs should be placed together in claiming pens for at least 24 hours. This allows the manager to observe the nursing behavior of the lamb and provides an opportunity for any indicated intervention. Newborn lambs should attempt to stand and nurse within 30 minutes of birth. Dipping the navel with an iodine solution (7% tincture), a weak iodine solution, or a chlorhexidine solution is recommended. The chlorhexidine solution appears to have a more residual antibacterial effect, and the strong iodine solutions may be associated with umbilical abscesses or patent urachus. In addition, the availability of 7% tincture of iodine is currently restricted in the United States due to the potential misuse for the production of methamphetamine drugs. Still, experience suggests that all of these solutions are safe and useful if used judiciously. Neonatal lambs are especially prone to hypoglycemia and hypothermia, so careful observation of newborns is mandatory. The newborn lamb should be up and nursing within the first 2 hours of life. If the lamb does not seem satiated after nursing or if the ewe has udder pathology with a potential for inadequate milk production, colostrum should be supplemented. Table 8.6 shows how to make and use a sodium sulfate solution that can be used to assess the success or failure of passive transfer of colostral antibodies. Recommendations for the supplementation of colostrum are 50 mL/kg in the first 2 hours after birth and a total of 200 mL/kg in the first day. Lambs can be supplemented with ovine or caprine colostrum. Fresh or frozen colostrum from animal sources is generally considered superior to commercial supplements. If possible, the colostrum donor should be from the same general geographic location as the dam and should be vaccinated against the clostridial diseases.[211]

Kids

At birth, kids should be observed for abnormal respiration and other evidence of fetal distress such as meconium staining. Mucus and fluids should be removed from the nose and mouth immediately. Normal kids attempt to stand within a few minutes of birth and nurse vigorously within the first few hours. Respiration in the newborn is stimulated by the doe's licking or by vigorous rubbing with a towel by the owner. The umbilicus should be inspected for hemorrhage or herniation, and the umbilical stump should be disinfected with 7% tincture of iodine or another suitable iodine or chlorhexidine solution. The way kids are raised and handled after birth depends on the type of goat and the owner's preference. Meat and fiber goats raise their kids on pasture, whereas dairy kids are typically removed before they have a chance to nurse. Kids need to receive adequate colostrum within the first 4 hours of birth. Dairy kids are bottle-fed heat-treated (at 56° C for 1 hour) goat colostrum to prevent caprine arthritis-encephalitis virus (CAEV) transmission. Weak kids should receive colostrum by an oral stomach tube or a lamb feeder. Kids should be fed 10% of

TABLE 8.6 A Method of Assessing Passive Transfer in the Neonate.

Sodium Sulfate Test for Passive Transfer

- Place 14, 16, and 18 g of powdered sodium sulfate with 100 mL of distilled water into three labeled containers.
- Place 1.9 mL of each of these solutions (14%, 16%, and 18%) into three separate sterile tubes.
- Add 0.1 mL of serum to each container, then mix thoroughly.
- Allow the mixture to stand undisturbed at room temperature for 1 hour to permit maximal precipitation. Assess the tubes for clarity. A cloudy appearance (manifested by the inability to read newsprint through the tube) is associated with immunoglobulin precipitation.

	Appearance of Sodium Sulfate Solution			
Immunoglobulin Concentration (mg/dL)	14%	16%	18%	Diagnosis
>1500	Cloudy	Cloudy	Cloudy	Successful passive transfer
>1000	Clear	Cloudy	Cloudy	Successful to partially successful passive transfer
500	Clear	Clear	Cloudy	Partial failure of passive transfer
<500	Clear	Clear	Clear	Failure of passive transfer

their body weight in colostrum the first day, divided into three or four feedings. Colostrum substitutes are not suitable for kids and do not increase their immunoglobulin levels. Delayed colostrum intake, inadequate colostrum ingestion, and ingestion of poor-quality colostrum are common reasons for failure of passive transfer.[199] In meat and fiber production herds, adequate colostrum intake can be assessed by observing kids nursing and palpating their abdomens.

Serum immunoglobulin levels can be assessed using a sodium sulfate test, zinc sulfate turbidity test, or other commercially available screening test. Levels higher than 1600 mg/dL are desirable; levels below 600 mg/dL may indicate failure or partial failure of passive transfer. Intravenous transfusion of 20 to 40 mL/kg of caprine plasma (preferred) or whole blood from the dam or another adult goat in the herd may be indicated for a valuable neonate exhibiting failure of passive transfer. Kids born in selenium-deficient areas should be injected with selenium at birth. (Note: Overdosing may result in death, so it is imperative to carefully calculate the dosage and properly administer all selenium-containing products.) Finally, kids are at greatest risk of hypothermia and hypoglycemia during the first few days of life. They should be protected from rain and cold weather and treated for hypoglycemia with glucose solution.

Fawns

Fawns are usually up and nursing within minutes of birth. Many will seek out the udder even while the dam is having another fawn. It is important that the fawn consumes colostrum as soon as possible but it is also important that the maternal-fetal bond be allowed to develop as does that are disturbed at fawning may abandon one or more fawns. This is especially true on first parity and dams that have had difficulty with parturition. Observing from a distance with binoculars and then examining the fawn in a few hours to ensure that it has a full abdomen, its mouth is warm to the touch, and its rectum is being cleaned by the mother is important. Usually, they are tagged, given vaccines, vitamins, minerals, probiotics, and antibiotics depending on the farm and region and vaccination status of the dam. If in a selenium-deficient area, it may be important to give to fawns, but the same precautions exist as they do for lambs and kids. If fawns are to be left with their dams, this may be the only time that they are handled until weaning. If they are to be bottle raised, they are generally "pulled" at 24 to 72 hours of age. Waiting any longer than that will make acceptance of a bottle very difficult. They are generally placed on a milk replacer specifically made for fawns, but many people will put them on whole cow's milk, lamb or kid replacer, or "multispecies" milk replacer. Fawns are generally weaned off dams at 3 to 5 months of age, while bottle fawns are generally weaned between 2 and 4 months of age. Fusobacteria can be a major fawn pathogen and vaccination and medication as well as management may need to be instituted on most farms. Clean, dry fawning areas and vaccination of the dam prior to fawning will usually help, as does judicious use of antibiotics at processing.

Postpartum Care of the Small Ruminant

Careful examination of the dam should be performed for the presence of additional fetuses by either ballottement of the abdomen or transabdominal ultrasonography. Vital signs and muscle tone should also be assessed as a means to detect hypocalcemia. After parturition, the placenta is passed rather quickly but is not considered retained until 6 to 12 hours postpartum. Dairy does should be milked soon after parturition. In meat and fiber production herds, the doe's or ewe's udder should be palpated for evidence of mastitis and to determine the quality and quantity of colostrum or milk production. Colostrum or milk should be expressed from each teat to ensure patency of the teat and detect any abnormal secretions.

Postpartum females should be monitored closely to ensure maternal bonding and to ensure that the neonate is nursing appropriately. This may be accomplished by placing the dam with her litter into a small pen for several days before transitioning into the main herd. Some less handled cervids may become extremely nervous if locked in a small pen, while others (especially dams bottle-fed as fawns) may be fine. Always observe the dam for mismothering and ensure that the offspring are satiated, warm, and clean. Does and ewes should also be monitored closely for signs of hypocalcemia or ketosis. Maximizing dry matter intake of fresh does and ewes will help prevent metabolic disease and ensure maximum production.

Periparturient Disease

A variety of periparturient conditions such as pregnancy toxemia, vaginal prolapse, milk fever, and uterine inertia may interfere with normal parturition or adversely affect the health and fertility of the ewe or doe after parturition. With the exception of pregnancy toxemia, these conditions are more frequently encountered in sheep than in goats or cervids.

Fetal Hydrops

Consumption of legumes with high concentrations of estrogenic compounds, hypothyroidism secondary to iodine deficiency, and ingestion of goitrogens are all associated with hydrops uteri. Hydrops also may result from placental or uterine disease. Retention of large quantities of fluid may result in rupture of the prepubic tendon. Induction of parturition or cesarean section should be considered in cases of fetal hydrops.

Rupture of the Prepubic Tendon

Rupture of the prepubic tendon is occasionally seen in females pregnant with multiple fetuses, pregnant females with fetal hydrops, and pregnant females that have experienced abdominal trauma. If the owner chooses to keep the female until parturition, applying a homemade canvas girdle (for added abdominal support), reducing rumen fill (increasing concentrate and decreasing forage intake), and reducing salt or trace mineral intake may all be effective treatments. Surgical correction may be cost-prohibitive and is often unsuccessful. If an accurate breeding date exists, the clinician may consider performing an elective cesarean section or inducing parturition. If parturition is induced, the clinician should closely observe the female in case she requires help to deliver. Preventing stress and trauma (e.g., deworming, shearing) in late-term females and selecting for animals that do not give birth to quadruplets may help prevent rupture of the prepubic tendon. Females that survive parturition should be culled.

Vaginal Prolapse

Vaginal prolapse is a relatively common problem in the ewe. It typically occurs during the last 3 weeks of gestation in multiparous ewes. Vaginal prolapse is relatively uncommon in goats but is occasionally encountered in dairy breeds. The ventral vaginal floor is usually the area that protrudes from the vulva. Many different theories have been advanced regarding the etiology of vaginal prolapse. The consumption of low-quality forage results in increased abdominal filling, which may lead to the vagina being forced out of the vulva. The estrogen content of some legumes also has been incriminated. Other nutrition-related problems include over- and under-conditioning and poor bunk management resulting in overcrowding. Other physical factors that have been implicated include obesity, persistent cough causing repeated episodes of high intraabdominal pressure, and improper or close tail docking in sheep. The tails of sheep should be docked beyond the sixth coccygeal vertebrae or left just long enough to cover the anus when pulled ventrally. Unfortunately, show animals are often docked closer than this to change the look of the rump area in the show ring.

Because of a possible genetic component, the offspring of ewes or does that have experienced vaginal prolapse should not be kept as breeding stock.[211] An epidural anesthetic (2% lidocaine, 0.5 mL/45 kg of body weight) helps prevent straining. Alternatively, a combination of xylazine (0.07 mg/kg) and lidocaine (0.5 mg/kg) can be used in an epidural to provide as much as 24 hours of relief from straining, although this may cause some pelvic limb ataxia.[212] The prolapsed vagina should be cleaned with a mild, soapy solution before replacement. Occasionally, the urinary bladder is found inside the prolapsed tissue. Real-time ultrasonography is beneficial in determining the location of the urinary bladder. If the bladder is within the prolapsed tissue, it can usually be drained by locating the urethral orifice beneath the prolapsed tissue (caudal to the vulvar commissures), inserting a finger into the orifice, and lifting the prolapse. A 12-French catheter can be inserted through the urethra and into the bladder if draining is required. The prolapsed tissue should be well lubricated with a water-soluble lubricant (methylcellulose), gently massaged, and carefully forced cranially to its natural position. Elevating the rear hindlegs of the ewe can facilitate the replacement of the prolapsed tissue. In the event of considerable swelling that makes replacement difficult or impossible, either a hydroscopic agent (e.g., Epsom salts, and sugar) or steady pressure can be applied to the prolapse to decrease edema and reduce size.

A popular method of retaining the prolapsed tissue is through the use of a specially designed plastic prolapse retainer. This retainer has a broad spoon-shaped end that pushes down on the replaced vaginal floor and two retention arms that are tied into the wool or sutured to the skin on either side of the rump. These devices can be successfully used in some goats.

Various types of purse-string and mattress-type sutures also have been used. Making a shoelace-pattern support across the vulva with soft rolled gauze, using small loops of umbilical tape placed lateral to each side of vulva, works well. The owner can loosen the lacing and check on the progress of parturition. If the female is 1 month from parturition, a Buhner suture can be used, with substitution of a standard cadaver needle for a Buhner needle. The Buhner method results in a suture that may last longer and will rarely tear out.

A retention harness has also been described. A rope or stout cord is placed over the back so that half of the rope is on either side of the body. The rope is then crossed under the front legs and then brought back dorsally to be crossed over the back legs. The rope is then passed ventrally and under the rear limbs on either side of the udder and crossed again as it is brought dorsally over the perineal area. The two ends are then tied to the rope that is crossed over the back. This configuration discourages straining and secures the perineum.

Uterine Prolapse

Uterine prolapse generally occurs within 12 to 18 hours after parturition and may be associated with any condition that weakens the dam or causes difficult delivery. Hypocalcemia may contribute to the flaccidity that predisposes to uterine prolapse. The prolapsed uterus is usually atonic and is slowly expelled through the vulva rather than being forcefully expelled by straining. The prolapsed tissue should be gently washed and well lubicated before replacement into the abdomen. The administration of a caudal epidural (lidocaine 2%, 0.05 mL/45 kg of body weight) before replacement decreases straining. The replacement procedure can be aided by raising the hindquarters off the ground. This allows the abdominal contents to fall away from the pelvic canal and promotes correct intraabdominal replacement of the prolapsed uterus.

Closure of the vulvar opening is accomplished using a Buhner or shoelace suture as described for vaginal prolapse. If hypocalcemia is suspected, the female should be given a calcium solution. Oxytocin is indicated to aid uterine contraction. The prognosis is normally good. Cases involving lacerated and heavy soiling of prolapsed tissue may be complicated by infection.

Retained Fetal Membranes

The placenta should be expelled by 6 hours after parturition. In the absence of toxemia, septicemia, or abnormal vaginal discharge, the clinician should take no action to remove the placenta until 12 to 18 hours postpartum. Retained fetal membranes (RFMs) may be caused by deficiency in selenium or vitamin A, infectious abortions (e.g., toxoplasmosis, chlamydiosis, and listeriosis), obesity of the dam, hypocalcemia, dystocia, and possibly other factors.[213,214] RFMs are uncommon in goats but appear to be a problem in some sheep flocks. A higher incidence of RFM has been reported in dairy goats and in does or ewes whose young have died or been removed. A retained placenta with no other concurrent clinical signs is of little significance, except that the condition may be associated with certain diseases or deficiencies. Occasionally, a vaginal examination can reveal the placenta if it is not visible externally. If the ewe or doe appears clinically normal, treatment should entail only the removal of the placenta. Manual removal should not be attempted. Instead, the doe or ewe can be given oxytocin (5–10 IU two to six times a day) or prostaglandins ($PGF_{\alpha 2}$, 5–10 mg; cloprostenol, 75 μg/45 kg body weight). Some practitioners prefer using $PGF_{2\alpha}$ or its analogues and avoid using oxytocin in females with nursing young.

Metritis and Endometritis

Metritis is uncommon in small ruminants but is encountered in dairy goat breeds and in association with RFM; dystocia; retained dead fetuses; abortion caused by toxoplasmosis, chlamydiosis, and listeriosis; and possibly other diseases.[213,214] A retained placenta may serve as a "wick" between the environment and the uterus.

Clinical Signs and Diagnosis. Clinical signs include a thin, watery, brown to red, possibly purulent, malodorous vaginal discharge. Infected females may be relatively normal or extremely ill and toxic. They may be febrile and exhibit decreased rumen motility, dehydration, increased scleral injection, and possibly

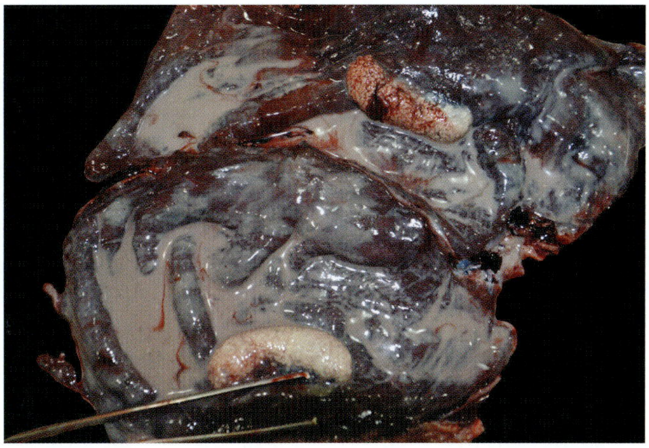

• **Fig. 8.23** The opened uterus from a postmortem examination of a 3-year-old, pen-raised white-tailed deer (WTD) doe. Portions of the diffusely reddened uterine mucosa are covered by tan fluid. The doe died of an acute postpartum uterine infection while still nursing a single fawn. A heavy growth of mixed species of bacteria including *Clostridium sordelli* was grown from necropsy collected uterine cultures. (Courtesy Dr. Kelley Steury, Alabama Veterinary Diagnostic Laboratory, Auburn, AL.)

depression. In severe cases, animals can become infected with *Clostridium tetani*, other *Clostridium* species, or other toxin-producing bacteria (Figure 8.23). Peritonitis may develop as a result of severe uterine infection or postpartum uterine tears or ruptures. Uterine tears are more common after dystocia, but they also may occur spontaneously.[215] As expected, a complete blood count (CBC) indicates toxemia or septicemia (see Appendix 2). Abdominocentesis may reveal increased protein, increased number of leukocytes, and possibly toxic leukocytes. Ultrasonographic examination usually reveals an enlarged fluid-filled uterus containing hyperechoic fluid. Females normally have a thick, nonodorous, brown to reddish brown vaginal discharge (lochia) for as long as 4 weeks after birth. This normal lochia requires no treatment. New, relatively inexperienced owners, particularly those with pet animals, may interpret this normal discharge as a sign of illness (e.g., metritis).

Treatment. Any underlying disease that results in metritis should be treated. Affected ewes or does should be given broad-spectrum antibiotics (oxytetracycline 10–20 mg/kg once or twice a day; ceftiofur sodium 1–2 mg/kg once a day) or antibiotics with good efficacy against anaerobic bacteria (penicillin 20,000 IU/kg twice daily). Uterine infusion of antibiotics is controversial, and clinicians performing it should take care not to damage the cervix, puncture the uterus, and cause greater uterine scarring or damage. Intrauterine infusions may damage the endometrium as well as decrease the function of the polymorphonuclear cells within the uterus. Uterine evacuation with prostaglandins ($PGF_{2\alpha}$, 5–10 mg; cloprostenol, 75–100 μg/45 kg of body weight) or oxytocin (5–10 IU), rehydration as needed, and NSAIDs (e.g., flunixin meglumine, 1 mg/kg) should be included in the therapeutic plan. If the placenta is retained, it should be removed, but not manually. Because of the potential for clostridial infections, particularly in animals with dystocia-induced uterine trauma, macerated fetuses, or uterine bacterial contamination, clostridial disease prophylaxis should be undertaken. Previously vaccinated females can be given a booster that includes *C. tetani*. In animals with no history of clostridial prophylaxis, antitoxin is indicated.[213,214]

Pyometra

Pyometra can occur as a sequela to cases of metritis in which the cervix has been damaged; it also occurs in females that cycle after parturition during the anestrus season (Nubians and dwarf goats). The late cycle can result in an ovulation and retention of the resultant CL for a prolonged period. Pyometra is a very uncommon disorder. Signs include anestrus, occasionally sustained elevated serum progesterone, ultrasonographic evidence of varying amounts of echogenic intrauterine fluid, and occasionally a purulent vaginal discharge.

Treatment should include prostaglandins ($PGF_{2\alpha}$, 5–10 mg; cloprostenol, 75–100 μg/45 kg body weight) and/or oxytocin (5–10 IU BID).[213,214]

Pregnancy Toxemia

Pregnancy toxemia (ketosis and hepatic lipidosis) typically occurs during the final trimester of gestation in ewes and does. The condition is usually seen in females carrying multiple fetuses and may result from their inability to consume adequate energy to match metabolic demands. Conditions that increase energy demands or decrease energy intake also can predispose to this disease.

In many instances, pregnancy toxemia can be prevented by balancing the nutritional demands of the dam and the increased requirements of the fetus during late gestation. Obese or extremely thin females may be more prone to developing the condition. Gestating ewes carrying twins require 180% more energy than those carrying singletons, and those carrying triplets require 240% more than ewes carrying singletons. Ewes and does may not be capable of consuming enough to meet these demands, resulting in a negative energy balance. More information on diagnosis, treatment and prevention of pregnancy toxemia can be found in Chapter 5. Lambs or kids born more than 7 days premature seldom survive. Fawns have a little more time and may still be viable as their gestation period is a little longer. If practical, glucocorticoids should be given 12 to 24 hours prior to cesarean section to help fetal lung development and survivability.

Hypocalcemia

Hypocalcemia is typically seen during the last 2 weeks of gestation. Twin-bearing ewes require as much as 8 g of calcium and 4 g of phosphorus daily.

Clinical Signs and Diagnosis. The clinical signs can overlap those of pregnancy toxemia because the two diseases are often seen concurrently. Hypocalcemic females are initially ataxic and hyperactive but soon become recumbent. Other clinical signs include bloat and failure of pupillary light responses. The initial hyperactivity results from a lack of membrane stabilization by calcium. The subsequent paralysis occurs because little to no calcium is available to release acetylcholine at the neuromuscular junction and influence muscle contractility. Calcium concentrations can be measured to confirm hypocalcemia. The serum calcium concentration is less than 7 mg/dL in clinically apparent cases.

Treatment. Clinical cases are treated with 1 g of calcium/45 kg body weight, and the response is dramatic. Females should have a good supply of calcium in their diets during the final 6 weeks of gestation. Alfalfa hay provides a good source of calcium, as does a mineral mix containing calcium.[213]

Reproductive Dysfunction

Reproductive Failure

During an investigation of reproductive failure in ruminants, the infectious causes always seem to garner the most attention. However, noninfectious causes can often be more problematic to diagnose but easier to treat. Deficiencies in iodine, copper, and other nutrients can result in reproductive failure in small ruminants. These and other nutritional problems are covered in more detail in Chapter 2.

Plant Toxicity

Veratrum Californicum

Members of the *Veratrum* genus are associated with numerous congenital abnormalities in lambs. *V. californicum*, commonly known as "false hellebore," contains a teratogenic alkaloid (cyclopamine) that is responsible for a number of congenital defects in lambs depending on the stage of gestation when they are consumed. Exposure to *V. californicum* during the first 10 days of gestation is associated with early embryonic death. The classic, demonstrable conditions associated with *V. californicum* ingestion—severe facial abnormalities such as a cyclops-like appearance (Figure 8.24), anophthalmos, and cleft palate—occur when exposure takes place between day 12 and 14, while exposure between day 25 and 36 results in hypoplasia of the metacarpals and metatarsals. Exposure has also been reported to cause inadequate development of the fetal pituitary glands. This can result in prolonged gestations, abnormally large fetuses, and an increased incidence of dystocia. *V. californicum* is an erect herb with an unbranched stem. Large, wide, alternate, clasping leaves with prominent spiraling parallel veins are characteristic (Table 8.7).

Locoweeds. Members of the genera *Astragalus* and *Oxytropis* are commonly referred to as "locoweeds"; they have been implicated as causing abortions, small weak lambs, and bent legs in newborns. The incidence of abortion and small weak lambs has been reported to be as high as 75% in exposed ewes. The toxin affects the fetal-placental unit, causing delayed placentation, decreased placental vascularization, fetal edema, and altered development of the cotyledons. It also is associated with decreased spermatogenesis in the ram.[216]

Broomweed. Broomweed *(Gutierrezia microcephala, Xanthocephalum lucidum)* ingestion can cause abortions and small, weak, premature lambs because of the toxic effects of an ecbolic toxin in these plants (triterpenoid saponin). Other clinical signs include gastrointestinal upset, hematuria, and death. Broomweed is a shrub found in arid regions of the western United States.[217]

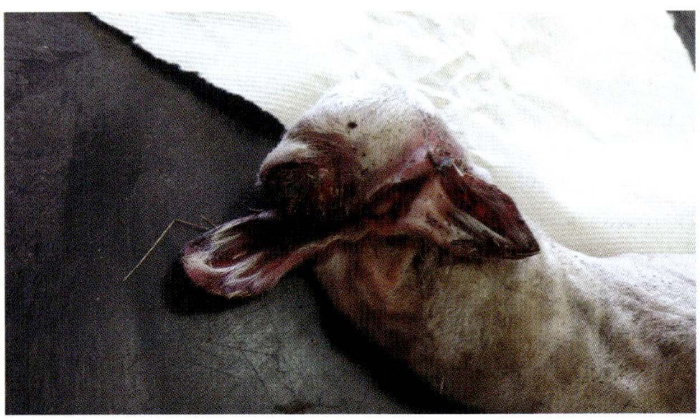

• Fig. 8.24 Lamb with cyclopia.

Ergot Alkaloids and Ergot. The consumption of fescue *(Festuca arundinacea)* infected with the fungus *Epichloe coenophialum* (formerly *Neotyphodium coenophialum*) is associated with decreased reproductive efficiency.[217] The ergot alkaloids produced by the fungus have been shown to affect prolactin production in ewes and increase the interval from introduction of the ram until conception.[218] Ergot concentrations greater than 0.1 to 0.7% of the diet can reduce the number of live births in sheep.[219] It has been reported that isoflavones produced by legumes can relax the persistent vasoconstriction in goats caused by consumption of ergot alkaloids.[220]

Estrogen-Producing Plants. Sheep appear to be sensitive to the effects of phytoestrogens from plants such as subterranean clover *(Trifolium subterraneum)*, white clover *(Trifolium repens)*, and alfalfa *(Medicago sativa)*. Clinical signs associated with phytoestrogen consumption include infertility, irregular and prolonged heat, vaginal prolapse, cystic glandular hyperplasia of the cervix and uterus, enlarged teats, and inappropriate lactation.[221] Dystocia and uterine inertia have also been reported.[219] Plants associated with depressed reproduction are shown in Table 8.7.

Pharmaceuticals

Some drugs have been associated with abortion and birth defects in sheep and goats when administered in mid to late gestation. The drugs implicated include chlorpromazine, phenylbutazone, phenothiazine anthelmintic, levamisole anthelmintic, and corticosteroids.[222]

Nutritional Abnormalities

Poor body condition, depressed energy intake, and decreased mineral and vitamin intake all suppress reproductive activity in ewes and does. Lower overall nutritional intake results in poor or weak signs of estrus, depressed ovulation, abnormal estrous cycle length, and delayed puberty. Deficiencies in energy, protein, vitamins A and E, phosphorus, and many trace minerals are most commonly seen. Deficiencies in vitamin A, copper, manganese, and iodine are associated with irregular estrous cycles (see Chapter 2).

Heat Stress

Heat stress depresses reproductive ability and causes fetal wastage. Causes of heat stress include decreased water intake, obesity, exercise, and fatigue during hot weather. Both very young and very old animals are susceptible to heat stress. High ambient temperatures and high humidity result in poor or compromised cooling. As the ambient temperature approaches body temperature, skin vasodilation no longer aids in heat dissipation. In sheep, the respiratory passages are important in cooling, so animals will pant when they are hot. Unsheared Angora goats and heavily woolled sheep, particularly young sheep, are especially susceptible to heat stress.

Clinical Signs. Common clinical signs include decreased fertility and depressed signs of estrus in females as well as an increased number of abnormal spermatozoa and depressed libido in males. Angora goats experience high embryonic mortality if the heat stress occurs during the first 3 to 6 weeks of pregnancy. However, all breeds and both sheep and goats can experience high embryonic losses. Other clinical signs include dullness, depression, rapid respiration, open-mouth breathing, congested conjunctiva, dilated

TABLE 8.7 Plants That Affect Reproduction.

<table>
<tr><th>Plant</th><th>Comment</th></tr>
<tr><td>Fusarium</td><td>• Found in moldy corn and wheat
• Produces estrogenic substance, zearalenone
• Clinical manifestations include decreased lambing and kidding percentage</td></tr>
<tr><td>Clovers (subterranean, crimson, red, white, alsike)</td><td>• Produce estrogen-like substances
• Clinical manifestations include cystic hyperplasia of the cervix and hydrops uteri
• White clover also contains cyanogenic ergot alkaloids
• Alsike also can cause photosensitization, liver disease, and stomatitis</td></tr>
<tr><td>Ponderosa pine</td><td>• Clinical manifestations include stillbirths, last-trimester abortions, renal tubular necrosis, pulmonary congestion, weak uterine contractions, and poor cervical dilation</td></tr>
<tr><td>Cottonseed</td><td>• Toxic substance is gossypol
• Clinical manifestations include testicular and spermatozoal abnormalities
• Toxic ingestions occur most often in young pre-ruminants</td></tr>
<tr><td>Broomweed, Monterey cypress, jumpweed</td><td>• Broomweed: toxic substances include mono- and diterpenes, saponins, oxygenated flavonolmethyl esters; clinical manifestations include abortion
• Monterey cypress: clinical manifestations include abortion
• Jumpweed: clinical manifestations include abortion</td></tr>
<tr><td>Veratrum californicum</td><td>• All parts of the plant are toxic
• Signs include salivation, diuresis, muscular weakness, and incoordination
• Preventive measures include delaying grazing until after the first frost and breeding ewes 5 weeks before putting on range containing V. californicum
<table>
<tr><th>Days of Gestation</th><th>Effect</th></tr>
<tr><td>0–10</td><td>Failure to implant</td></tr>
<tr><td>12–14</td><td>Cyclopia</td></tr>
<tr><td>12–34</td><td>Motor nerve paralysis</td></tr>
<tr><td>22–30</td><td>Cleft palate</td></tr>
<tr><td>25–36</td><td>Hypoplasia of metacarpals and tarsals</td></tr>
</table></td></tr>
<tr><td>Tobacco</td><td>Toxic effects more common in swine</td></tr>
<tr><td>Poison hemlock</td><td>Toxic effects more common in cattle</td></tr>
<tr><td>Lupine</td><td>Can cause arthrogryposis</td></tr>
<tr><td>Locoweed</td><td>Can cause arthrogryposis</td></tr>
<tr><td>Sudan grass</td><td>Can cause arthrogryposis and contracted tendons</td></tr>
</table>

pupils (early), constricted pupils (late), decreased feed intake, increased heart rate, weak rapid pulse, hyperthermia, acid-base alterations, dehydration, excessive loss of potassium and sodium from sweat, and increased packed cell volume (greater than 60% red blood cells). Angora goats have a decreased ability to respond to heat stress compared with other breeds of goats. Sheep can tolerate external temperatures higher than 110° F if the humidity is less than 65%, but they will pant if the rectal temperature is higher than 106° F. Secondary bloat and acidosis can occur if high-energy feed is made available at night or if a break in the weather occurs because animals may then gorge themselves.

Diagnosis. Diagnosis is based on recognition of the clinical signs. Necropsy findings include cerebral edema, rapid putrefaction, and large, distended veins. CBC results are unremarkable.

Treatment. Treatment should include lowering the body temperature with cold water submersion, cold water enemas, ice applications, or alcohol rubs. Affected animals should be sheared. Nonpregnant animals can be given glucocorticoids (dexamethasone 1–2 mg/kg IV). Normal hydration should be maintained. If animals are more than 10% dehydrated, IV fluids should be administered, but if animals are less than 10% dehydrated, fluids can be administered orally. Keepers should place affected animals in the shade and attempt to improve air circulation around them.

Bucks and rams should undergo a BSE after periods of heat stress. If spermatic abnormalities are noted, the examination should be repeated in 49 to 60 days.

Prevention. Prevention is aimed at keeping animals cool. Woolly or hairy animals should be sheared before periods of hot weather. Long scrotal wool also should be shorn. Animals should be maintained at a good body condition score. Providing shade at feed bunks and spraying water on the animals' backs around the lounging areas are helpful preventive strategies. Spraying or misting at the feed bunks can increase feed intake. On hot, humid days, animals should only be worked or handled in the early morning, late evening, or at night. Trace mineral salt and cool water should be provided free choice. Animals should be fed in the early morning or late afternoon. Toxins and plants that decrease peripheral vasodilation (e.g., fescue) should be avoided.

Providing ventilation across the animals' backs and housing in an open-ridge barn with a high ceiling helps keep animals cool.

For dairy goats or sheep, sprinklers and good ventilation in holding pens help minimize heat stress, but these measures may be contraindicated for the prevention of mastitis. Increasing the energy concentration of feed may improve production after a period of reduced intake. Feeding bypass protein (blood meal, fish meal, corn gluten meal, roasted soybeans, and extruded soybeans) improves production, particularly if fat has been added to the feed. The addition of sodium bicarbonate (0.85–1%) may enhance milk production in hot weather. Less heat is generated from good-quality forage than from poor-quality forage. The acid-detergent fiber content of the diet can be dropped to 21% of the dry matter intake for short periods. The addition of ionophores improves productivity and decreases intake for many animals but may not benefit lactating females. The feeding of long-stem hay should be implemented. If green or wet feeds are fed, the bunks should be checked for spoilage on a routine basis on hot days.

Pseudopregnancy

Pseudopregnancy (mucometra, hydrometra, "cloudburst") is caused by a prolonged luteal phase in goats. The incidence in dairy goats may be as high as 3 to 5% on some farms,[223] with the highest incidence occurring in November through December. It is much less common in fiber or meat breeds of goats and sheep. The cause of this condition is poorly understood, but possible modes of action that have been proposed include out-of-season breeding, sheep and goat hybrid pregnancy, and the overuse of hormonal manipulation of the reproductive cycle. Some cases probably occur as sequelae to abortion or early embryonic loss with a retained CL. Spontaneous CL retention outside of pregnancy, which may result from hormonal manipulation for superovulation or out-of-season breeding, also has been proposed as a cause of pseudopregnancy.[219,223] The condition may occur numerous times during the life of a doe, or it may occur only once. There may also be a genetic component, as well.[224]

Clinical Signs and Diagnosis. Some females may show signs of parturition, udder development, and a bloody vaginal discharge. Pseudopregnancy also is characterized by anestrus, occasionally increased abdominal size, and external and behavioral signs of pregnancy. Blood progesterone concentrations may be consistent with pregnancy and remain elevated for as long as 5 months. Real-time ultrasonography may reveal a uterus with varying amounts of fluid that is clear, slightly cloudy, or clear with some hyperechoic flecks. The uterus usually appears thin-walled, and no placenta or fetus can be visualized. In females that undergo ultrasound examination before placentomes are visible (before day 30 of gestation), this condition may be falsely diagnosed as pregnancy. Therefore, careful ultrasonographic examination with attention to the stage of pregnancy and positive signs of pregnancy (e.g., presence of fetus, placenta, umbilicus) is imperative.

Treatment. The most common treatment for pseudopregnancy is the injection of $PGF_{2\alpha}$ (10–20 mg) or cloprostenol (75–100 μg/45 kg of body weight).

Vaginitis

Vaginitis has several causes. Whenever either nonparturient or parturient vaginitis is encountered, particularly in sheep, contagious ecthyma should be ruled out. Other causes of vaginitis include caprine herpes vulvovaginitis (edema and cloudy gray discharge), granular vulvovaginitis caused by *Mycoplasma* and *Acholeplasma*, and *Actinomyces pyogenes* and *Staphylococcus* infections.[219] Lavaging the vagina with mild antiseptic solutions (commercial chlorhexidine) may be all that is required. If animals are in a lot of pain, NSAIDs are useful.

Ectopic mammary tissue on the vulva is occasionally encountered. It appears as vulvar swelling before parturition. Because outflow tracts for milk are rare, this glandular tissue usually undergoes pressure atrophy. The glandular tissue can be surgically removed, but this form of therapy is rarely required.

Cystic Ovarian Disease

Cystic ovaries appear to be more common in goats than in sheep. In one study, 2.4% of more than 1000 female goats examined at slaughterhouses had ovarian cysts.[225] Owners often make the diagnosis based on short cycles or nymphomania,[223] so cystic ovarian disease is probably overdiagnosed. Graafian follicles larger than 12 mm may be considered cystic, but few studies have been performed to document a standard size.[223] The normal follicle diameter size of sheep (15–19 mm) is larger than that reported in the goat.[219] The use of some superovulation protocols (eCG), possibly phosphorus deficiency, and the feeding of estrogenic compounds may be associated with the formation of cystic ovaries. Treatment with hCG (750–1000 IU) or GnRH (50–100 μg) may be effective.[223] Goats that have demonstrated repeated development of cystic ovaries can be treated with hCG or GnRH, watched for signs of estrus, bred, and then retreated with hCG or GnRH 24 hours after breeding.

Ovarian Tumors

Ovarian tumors are rarely reported in sheep and goats.[219,226,227] Granulosa cell tumor is the most common type of ovarian tumor occurring in ewes and does. Animals with these tumors may exhibit prolonged estrous cycles, nymphomania, virilism, and inappropriate lactation syndrome.[228,229] Ovarian ultrasonographic examination, either per rectum or transabdominal, usually reveals an enlarged ovary that is either solid or cystic. The contralateral ovary is devoid of structures and lacks a CL.

A tentative diagnosis can be based on elevated concentrations of testosterone or estradiol, diagnostic ultrasound findings, and clinical signs. The treatment is ovariectomy. The authors and others have suggested that females with granulosa cell tumors may have elevated concentrations of testosterone and estradiol.[226]

Ovariectomy

Ovariectomy is not a commonly performed procedure in small ruminants. Ovarian tumors or other ovarian diseases that are best treated by ovariectomy are uncommon. Practitioners may be called on to perform ovariectomies more frequently to render pet goats infertile. Ovariectomies should be considered in does that have had a mastectomy for chronic mastitis or inappropriate lactation syndrome to prevent unwanted pregnancy and the resultant need for hand-raising kids (see Chapters 9 and 15).

The ovaries in ewes and does are approximately 1.5 cm long and shaped like an almond. The uterine horns are coiled in a relatively small spiral.[230,231] This anatomic arrangement makes it somewhat difficult to exteriorize the ovaries for ligation and removal.

An ovariectomy may be performed via either a flank or midline incision. One may find the midline allows easier access if doing a bilateral ovariectomy rather than maneuvering the opposite ovary into the surgical field with a flank approach. With either approach, the incision should be made as caudal as possible for ease of exteriorization and ligation. The procedure may be performed with only local anesthesia; however, heavy sedation or even general anesthesia will be helpful as the tension placed on the ovarian pedicle to exteriorize the ovaries for ligation can cause the patient visceral discomfort, which is not alleviated with local anesthesia of the skin and body wall. The ovaries can be located by palpating the cervix in the pelvic canal and tracing the uterine horn to them. Once the ovary is located by palpation, gentle persistent traction on the ovary will allow visualization of the ovary at the incision site. Once the ovary is seen, hemostats should be placed on the vascular pedicle to allow double ligation before transection and removal. After transection of the ovary, the pedicle should be observed to determine if hemorrhage is controlled. With bilateral ovariectomy, the remaining ovary is removed in the same manner. The body wall is closed in routine fashion.

Alternatively, the practitioner choose to use a laparoscopic technique for ovariectomy. The laparoscopic procedure would be best used with the animal in dorsal recumbency with hind quarters elevated, to move the abdominal viscera cranially away from the pelvic canal (Trendelenburg position). The scope portal is located near the umbilicus with instrument portals lateral and caudal to the scope portal on the line from the umbilicus to the caudal part of the fold of the flank. The advantage of this technique is better visualization of the ovaries. Disadvantages include holding the animal off feed for up to 36 to 48 hours to empty the abdominal viscera as much as possible to allow better manipulation and visualization. It is also difficult to secure the ovaries and exteriorize them for extracorporeal ligation so intracorporeal ligation or cautery is needed. This aspect of the procedure requires more time and expertise with the laparoscope, which may ultimately outweigh any advantages to this technique over a conventional laparotomy.

Others

Freemartins are rare in sheep and goats compared with cattle because both sheep and goats are adapted to multiple births. However, the prevalence of freemartins in sheep may be increasing with an increase in high fecundity genes in flocks.[232]

Abortion and Perinatal Death

Abortion is the loss of the conceptus anytime during gestation but is most commonly detected during the final 2 months. Perinatal death may be associated with abortifacient etiologies but may also be caused by environmental or maternal factors. If an abortion is suspected, it is important to use caution when examining the female, the aborted fetus (if present), and placenta as many of the infectious causes of abortion may also be zoonotic. Embryonic loss is often influenced by failure to maintain progesterone levels that may be noninfectious or infectious.[233,234] Sheep are not luteal dependent during middle and late fetal development while does have prolonged luteal dependency.[233] Clinical signs of embryonic or early fetal loss may include return to estrus, unobserved abortion, or observation of a blood-tinged vaginal discharge.[235] Sheep and goats have a high incidence of abortion compared with other farm animals.[233,234] Abortion rates of 5% for these two species are commonplace; rates less than 5% are considered good, and a less than 2% abortion rate is considered excellent.[235–237] The majority of abortions are sporadic rather than epizootic and are caused by a number of "classic" abortifacient disease as well as maternal pyrogenic infectious disease, toxicities, or disruptive metabolic diseases.[233] "Abortion storms" result in loss up to and more than 20% of pregnancies and may also produce compromised neonates.[235]

An epidemiologic investigation may be the practitioner's strongest diagnostic tool. Information gathered should include percentage of the herd affected, calendar dates, gestational ages at time of abortion, age of ewes/does, information on recently introduced animals and vaccination, anthelmintic administration, and nutritional histories.[235] Environmental factors evaluated should include extremes in temperature, rain, wind, pasture composition, exposure to toxic plants, predation, and other causes of environmental stress. Additionally, events such as applications of nitrogen fertilizer or agrochemicals, changes in feed supplement, and rotation between pastures should be evaluated. During an "abortion storm," early epidemiologic data, collected before a definitive diagnosis is made, may greatly influence management decisions that can minimize loss. Pregnant animals should be moved out of the contaminated area and recently or imminently aborting females should be left in the contaminated areas.[235] Care should be taken not to distribute an infectious agent on fomites, clothing, boots, or skin. At-risk animals, such as new introductions or primiparous females, may benefit from being separated from older pregnant females with immunity. The use of feeders may limit exposure to discharged pathogens on the ground.[238] Infectious agents that can be quickly diagnosed by serology, clinical diagnosis, or necropsy should be ruled out early.

Clinical examination of aborting females and the flock or herd may yield information about systemic diseases or nutritional status. Unaffected ewes and does should be examined first.[235] Clinical signs produced by abortifacient agents in females could be mild such as diarrhea produced by campylobacteriosis or severe such as *Listeria* encephalitis. Evidence of vaginal discharge "lamb stain" may be detectable on clinically normal females.[239] Ultrasound is an excellent tool to evaluate in utero fetal viability as well as placental edema and character of amniotic fluid. Positive serology is not considered a confirmatory test for most agents, but comparison of data from multiple animals in a group, evaluation of past years results and taking acute versus convalescent titers may direct further diagnostics.[235]

Serology may be performed on fetal blood. The ovine fetus will begin to produce antibodies at the beginning of the second trimester and antibody production will increase with gestational age.[240] Sheep and goats have a similar time line of fetal development.[241]

Guidelines for judging gestational age include abdominal wall closure (both 5–6 weeks), visibility of the female genital tubercle and penile sheath (6 weeks), recognition of anterior fontanelle (both 7–8 weeks), eyelid hair (goat 10–11 weeks, sheep 11–12 weeks), hairs along dorsum of neck (goat 13–14 weeks, sheep 14–15 weeks), hardening of the calvarium (goat 13–14 weeks, sheep 15–16 weeks), eyelids separation (both 14–15 weeks), sparse coverage with wool or hair except limbs (both 16–17 weeks), dense coverage with wool or hair and teeth buds prominent (17–20 weeks), and one to three incisors erupted at birth (21–22 weeks)[241] (Figure 8.25). Crown-rump length and weight vary between individual fetuses and breeds, but these data may be useful for comparison between herd mates

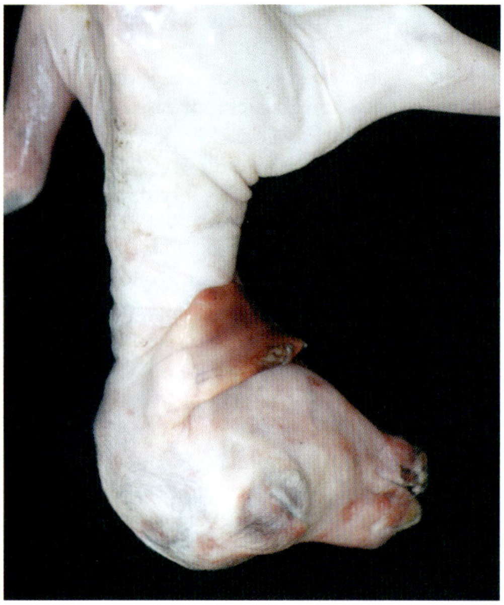

• **Fig. 8.25** This nonautolyzed goat fetus that aborted as a result of bacterial metritis has eyelid hair, hairs along dorsum of neck, hardening of the calvarium, but nonseparable eyelids. These characteristics place the gestational age at 15 weeks.

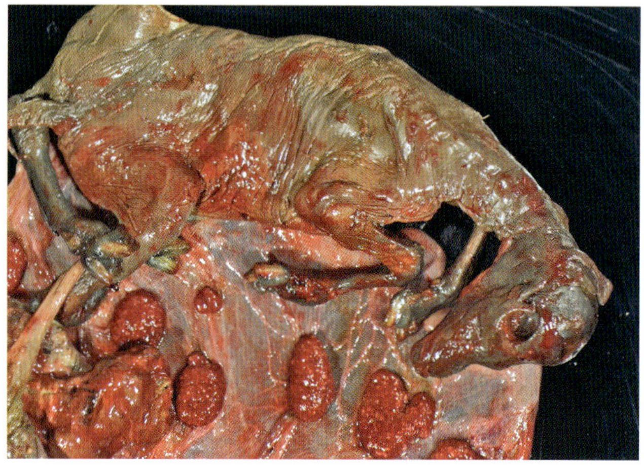

• **Fig. 8.26** The placenta and third-trimester fetus demonstrating characteristic gross lesions of *Toxoplasma gondii* infection. The cotyledons demonstrate areas of necrosis visible as small white foci. The fetus is mummified. (Courtesy Dr. John F. Edwards, College Station, Texas.)

and rough estimation of gestational age.[240,241] Fawn growth rates during gestation are well documented and may be used to age fetuses. Abortion is rarely in cervidae.

Good diagnostic labs achieve a definitive diagnosis rate of between 40 and 60% so multiple submissions are often necessary.[242,243] Reasons why a diagnosis may not be achieved from a necropsy include (1) etiologies that are difficult to quantitate such as a stress-producing induced prostaglandin level or corticosteroid surge, (2) maternal infections that produce fever or endotoxin release, (3) in utero autolysis and mummification that limit the diagnostic value of tissues, (4) exposure to unknown toxins or undescribed toxic plants, (5) septicemia by organisms that do not grow on routine culture, (6) failure to appreciate nutritional etiologies that produce a non-viable fetus, (7) failure to submit the proper sample, (8) local limitations of available diagnostic test, and (9) lack or experience or time limitations by diagnosticians and pathologists. If available for submission, the placenta usually contains the most diagnostic information. Organisms such as *Coxiella burnetii* (agent of Q-fever) cause severe placentitis but produce minimal fetal lesions.[242] It is important to determine if the abortion is an acute or chronic process and estimate the time line between fetal death and expulsion from the uterus. Abortion caused by fetal *Campylobacter* septicemia may produce a well-developed and minimally autolyzed fetus while *Salmonella* septicemia may produce a putrid fetus.[239,244] Fetuses with chronic placental insufficiency may appear emaciated. Fetal mummification is not a common finding in small ruminants. However, when fetal mummification occurs, toxoplasmosis, *Chlamydophila*, border disease, and *Coxiella* infection should be at the top of a differential list[242] (Figure 8.26). Skin lesions are often overlooked and may occur in some types of bacterial or mycotic abortions[242,245] (Figure 8.27A, B). Agents that produce pathognomonic teratogenic defects or developmental abnormalities such as bunyaviruses and specific toxic plants can be implicated from necropsy observations. Noninfectious heart defects, cleft palate, gastrointestinal

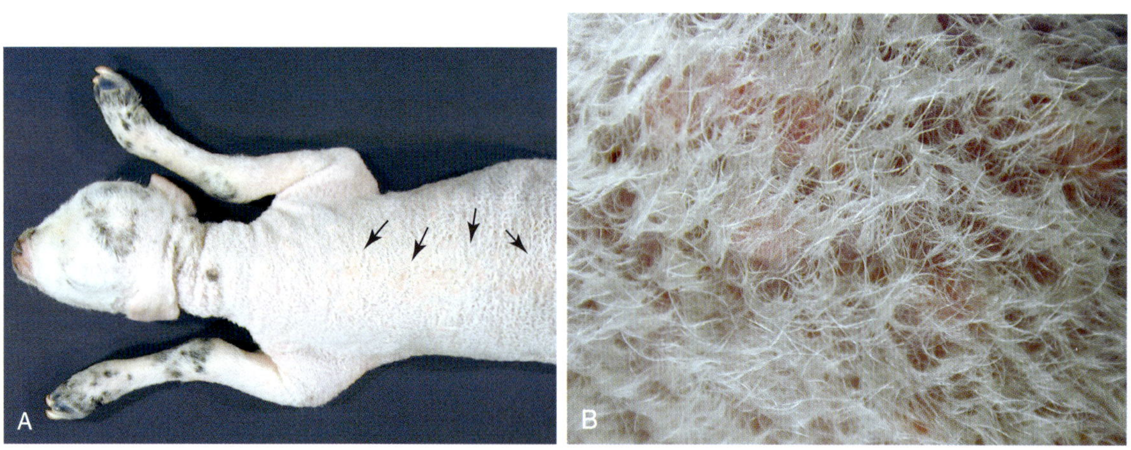

• **Fig. 8.27** Necrobacillosis along the dorsum of an ovine fetus **(A)** with multifocal suppurative dermatitis **(B)** caused by *Fusobacterium necrophorum*. (Courtesy Prof. Jørgen S. Agerholm, University of Copenhagen, Denmark.)

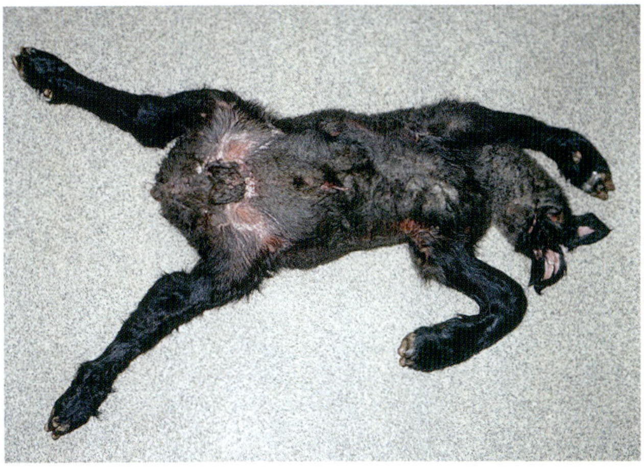

• **Fig. 8.28** Neural tube defect in a lamb resulting in anencephaly, the absence of a major portion of the brain and skull. (Courtesy Dr. Jim Cooley, Starkville, Michigan.)

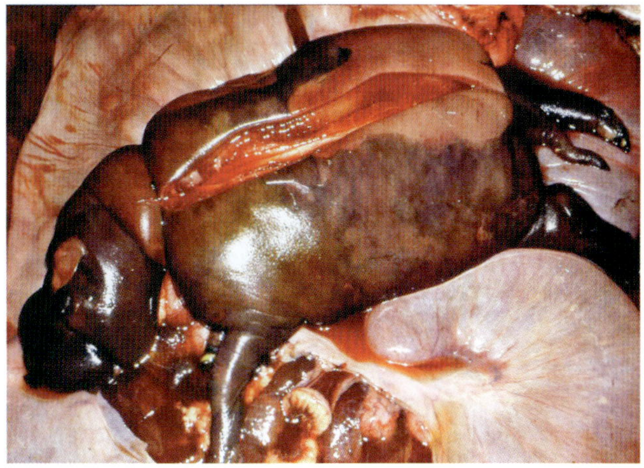

• **Fig. 8.30** Hydrops amnion and fetal anasarca resulted in an ovine fetus. The skin over the dorsum has been excised to demonstrate severe diffuse subcutaneous edema.

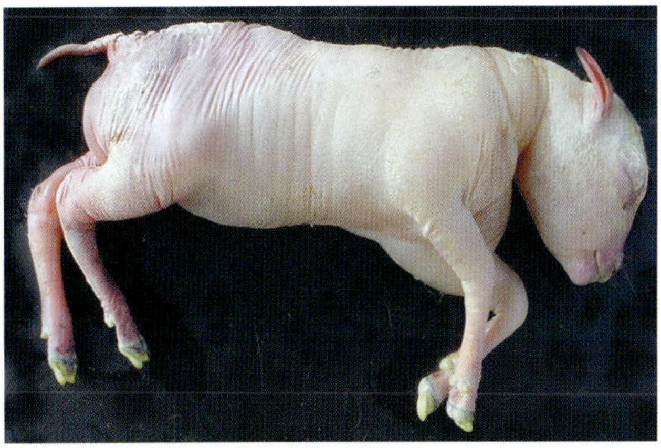

• **Fig. 8.29** Fetus that aborted as a result of toxic plant ingestion, *Tetrapterys multiglandulosa*, by the ewe at days 91 to 120 gestation, resulting in cardiac fibrosis, cardiac insufficiency, and anasarca. (Courtesy Dr. Gabriela Riet Correa Rivero, Castanhal, Pará, Brazil.)

atresia, neurologic defects, neural tube defects, and other random congenital abnormalities may contribute to sporadic abortions or postnatal death (Figure 8.28). Etiologies that cause fetal cardiac insufficiency may result in anasarca and hydrops amnion[246,247] (Figures 8.29 and 8.30). Many abortifacient microbial agents of sheep and goats are capable of causing disease in humans and this is addressed at the conclusion of the chapter.

Noninfectious Causes of Abortion

Noninfectious causes of abortion such as chromosomal rearrangement (Robertsonian translocation), creation of a sheep/goat hybrids, stress, nutritional deficiencies, pharmaceutical reactions and toxic plant ingestion can result in pregnancy loss.[6] Stress may trigger a higher percentage of abortions in goats versus sheep because of the goat's dependency on the CL for the maintenance of pregnancy.[233] Predator attack, severe weather, or shearing may all trigger early regression of the CL in the doe, resulting in abortion. Angora goats have an abortion etiology not typically seen in other breeds. Young Angora does are susceptible to stress abortions.[248] Some older Angora that typically are heavier than average and have very fine mohair may experience habitual abortions around gestation day 100 as a result of adrenal dysfunction.[238,248] This habitual, familial form of abortion usually starts when the doe is 4 or 5 years old and culling is indicated.[238] Heat stress also may result in early embryonic losses, abortions, stillbirths, or weak kids.[249]

Nutrition. Energy and protein deficiencies can result in embryonic loss, decreased fetal growth, depressed placental growth, fetal mummification, and the birth of weak young. Fetal wastage resulting from nutritional deficiencies often occurs between day 90 and 120 of gestation.[248] Increasing dietary protein supplementation of grass-fed goats by feeding leguminous tree leaves was shown to reduce abortions.[250] Deficiencies in a number of minerals and vitamins such as iodine, copper, magnesium, manganese, vitamin A, and selenium can cause abortion or the birth of weak fetuses.[238,248] High concentrations of dietary sulfur, particularly sulfate, may result in both selenium and copper deficiency.[249] Maintaining optimal body condition scores, ensuring adequate protein intake, and supplementing the diet with a good-quality, complete trace mineral mixture offered free choice are usually protective. Overweight does may be prone to hepatic lipidosis and pregnancy toxemia. Although death of the doe usually results, abortions may be observed in late stages of the disease.[248]

Iodine deficiency may be a problem in certain locations around the world. Affected neonates are born with enlarged thyroid glands, a condition commonly known as *goiter.* Late-term aborted fetuses with no wool and weak newborns are observed with iodine deficiency (see Chapter 2). Supplementation with iodine in iodine-deficient areas has been associated with increased lambing rates and decreased lamb mortality. Flocks grazing on plants that are members of the *Brassica* family (e.g., rape, kale, turnips, and flixweed) and animals of certain breeds (polled Dorset) are more susceptible to iodine deficiencies.[251] Iodine should be supplied at a rate of 0.10 to 0.80 mg/kg of dry matter of feed intake.

Copper deficiency causes a condition in newborns known as *enzootic swayback.* Neonates are typically normal at birth but develop rear-limb paresis or paralysis within a few weeks. The neurologic deficits are caused by a dystrophic demyelination of the white matter in the spinal cord. This lesion begins during gestation and cannot be corrected after diagnosis. Therefore, the focus of attention should be on the gestating ewes and does. Pygmy goats appear to be the most susceptible of the goat breeds. Infertility problems also have been blamed on copper deficiencies. Regions with sandy soils or years with increased rainfall may see increased cases of copper deficiency in sheep and goats on a diet high in pasture grasses. Copper supplementation in ewes should be done with caution because copper toxicity can result from over supplementation and also may cause abortions and other systemic disease. Copper should be fed to ewes at a rate of 5 ppm (mg/kg) of the diet on a dry-matter basis. Copper is commonly supplemented in salt mixtures. These salt mixtures should contain between 0.0625 to 0.13% copper in the form of copper sulfate, which would be between 0.25 to 0.50% copper sulfate in the salt mix. Important interactions occur between copper and molybdenum and copper and sulfur. High concentrations of molybdenum (1–2 ppm) and sulfur (more than 2000 ppm) in feed and water sources can decrease copper availability.[237] Interaction with other minerals such as iron (more than 400 ppm), cadmium (more than 3–7 ppm), and zinc (more than 100–400 ppm) also can negatively affect copper absorption and metabolism. The copper requirement in cervids is quite high, with some diets containing 25 to 75 ppm. Monitoring liver copper levels may be very helpful and should probably be done on a routine basis in most cervid herds (see Chapter 2).

Manganese deficiency during gestation can result in abortion or weak, small, paralyzed, or deformed neonates.[237] As with other deficiencies, the addition of a palatable trace mineral salt mixture offered free choice and year-round is usually preventative (see Chapter 2).

Vitamin E/Selenium deficiency Vitamin E/selenium deficiency has been implicated as a cause of abortion in Switzerland.[252]

Toxicologic Abortion

Heavy Metal Intoxication

Lead toxicity can cause fetal wastage in ewes.[249] Oversupplementation of copper may cause abortion. Excess selenium may cause abortion and failure of conception.

Rodenticide Environmental contamination with brodifacoum used for rat control resulted in abortions in sheep with clinical signs that mimicked Rift Valley fever virus infection.[253]

Toxic Plants. Teratogenic changes and/or altered fetal development have been associated with several plant species, including *Gutierrezia* (broomweed), *Nicotiana tabacum* (tobacco), *Nicotiana glauca* (wild tree tobacco), *V. californicum* (skunk cabbage), *Astragalus* (locoweed), *Lupinus. formosus,* (Lunara lupine), *Conium maculatum* (Poison-hemlock), *Lathyrus*, *Sophora*, and *Sorghum bicolor* (Sudan grass).[254] Toxicity induced by these plants must be differentiated from malformations caused by bunyavirus infections.[238] *Astragalus lentiginosus* (a locoweed) may also cause early fetal death in goats.[246] *Descurainia sophia* (flixweed) and other goitrogenic plants may cause decreased hair, large birth weights, and thyroid hyperplasia in fetuses.[251] *Ateleia glazioviana* has been shown to cause abortion, stillbirth, and perinatal death in sheep from Brazil.[255] Also reported from Brazil, *Tetrapterys multiglandulosa* causes ovine fetal death with anasarca and perinatal mortality proceeded by neurologic deficits.[247] Phytoestrogens found in legumes may reduce ovulation rates and have been implicated in increased embryonic mortality rate.[248]

Forage that accumulates nitrate such as sweet clover, Johnson grass, sorghum, lamb's quarter, Jimsonweed, sunflower, pigweed, and oat hay can cause abortion as a result of nitrate-nitrite toxicity.[248] Hay that was created from heavily fertilized pastures may also concentrate toxic levels of nitrate. If nitrate-nitrite toxicity is suspected, diluting the affected forage with other feedstuffs is a useful treatment. Cutting suspected forage 30 cm above the ground and avoiding the feeding of drought-stressed crops will help decrease nitrate concentrations in feeds to less than 1000 ppm nitrate as nitrogen, or less than 0.44% nitrate. Higher concentrations should be avoided or diluted with other feeds. Feeds containing more than 3500 ppm of nitrate nitrogen, or more than 1.76% nitrate, should not be fed to pregnant animals.[256] Elevated nitrate and nitrite levels in fetal ocular fluid can be used to confirm nitrate-induced abortion at necropsy.[257]

Pharmaceuticals Causing Abortion. Various pharmaceuticals are proven abortifacients, or at least their use has been associated with increased abortion incidence. Also, pharmaceuticals may be unfairly blamed for abortion when in fact it could have been rough handling during administration that may have caused the abortion.[248] Anthelmintics such as phenothiazine and levamisole given in the final months of gestation may cause abortion.[238,259] Use of anthelmintics in the benzimidazole class (netobimin, albendazole, parbendazole, and cambendazole) in pregnant females during the first trimester have been associated with fetal abnormalities.[238,260,261] Abortions were observed in 2 out of 27 mixed-breed dairy sheep 7 days after administration of artemether to treat liver flukes.[261] Anecdotal reports of abortion following the use of other dewormers (ivermectin, fenbendazole) are largely unsubstantiated. Xylazine and high doses of acepromazine in the first half of pregnancy may cause abortion because of their adverse effects on uterine contraction and placental perfusion.[248] Administration of corticosteroids in late gestation and estrogen and prostaglandins throughout most of gestation may induce abortion.[248]

Infectious Causes of Abortion

The most common microbial agents diagnosed as causes of abortion and placentitis in sheep and goats in North America are *Campylobacter fetus* subsp. *fetus*, *Campylobacter jejuni*, *Chlamydophila abortus, C. burnetii*, and *Toxoplasma gondii*.[235,238,242,243,262,263] Although sheep and goats are equally susceptible to many pathogens, exceptions to this rule, influenced by region, breed, and species of pathogen, have been recognized. For example, campylobacteriosis is more common in sheep in some locales, whereas herpesvirus infection is a goat disease.[249,264]

Definitive diagnosis of a specific infectious agent is dependent on collection of the appropriate sample, knowledge of available tests, and submission of properly prepared samples to a qualified laboratory. Most infectious abortions in sheep and goats have a primary bacterial etiology. As a general rule, abortions from bacteria or viruses are uncommonly reported in cervids.

Bacterial Abortion

***Chlamydophila Abortus* (Chlamydiosis, Enzootic Abortion).** *C. abortus* (previously *Chlamydia psittaci* serotype 1), a gram-negative intracellular bacterium and zoonotic agent, was recognized since 1950 as the species responsible for enzootic abortion. *C. abortus* was previously identified as *Chlamydia psittaci*, immunotype 1.[239,265] The term "Chlamydiosis" may still be relevant because *Chlamydophila* is a bacterial genus belonging to the family *Chlamydiaceae*, order *Chlamydiales*.[266] *C. abortus* is one of the most common causes of infectious abortion in sheep and goats in North America and the United Kingdom but also induces a persistent subclinical infection in nonpregnant and multiparous sheep and goats.[242,262,267–269] When introduced into naive flocks, 25 to 60% of ewes or does may abort.[267] In flocks in which the disease is epizootic, abortion rates tend to drop to between 1 and 15%, with abortions predominately occurring in flock additions or primiparous ewes and does.[235,270] *Chlamydophila pecorum* (previously *Chlamydia psittaci* immunotype 2) is commonly found in the gastrointestinal and reproductive tracts of healthy ruminants and has been implicated as a cause of sporadic abortion in small ruminants. *C. pecorum* is typically associated with polyarthritis, encephalomyelitis, pneumonia, diarrhea, and gastrointestinal disease. Although abortion may not occur commonly, fetal lesions associated with *C. pecorum* in a goat abortion included the following: severe suppurative and necrotizing placentitis with vasculitis and thrombosis, lymphohistiocytic and neutrophilic hepatitis, and fibrinosuppurative enterits.[235,249,268,271–273] *C. pecorum* may cross react on serologic test intended to diagnose *C. abortus* resulting in false-positives, but cross-protection does not occur.[239,274] Concomitant infections with *C. abortus* and *C. burnetii* are repeatedly reported.[275] Recently, utilization of species-specific real-time PCR has resulted in incidental discovery of *Chlamydophila psittaci*, an avian associated organism and a cause of human "psittacosis" in a fecal sample from a goat.[276]

Placentitis induced by *Parachlamydia acanthamoebae*, a zoonotic agent, has been confirmed by researchers in Switzerland.[277] *Parachlamydiaceae* are a family in the order *Chlamydiales* that also includes the families *Chlamydiaceae*, *Simkaniaceae*, and *Waddliaceae*.[266] Microscopic characteristics of necrotizing placentitis caused by *P. acanthamoebae* are similar to those of *C. abortus*.[277]

Transmission and Pathogenesis. The best documented transmission route of *C. abortus* is through oronasal contact with aborted tissues, vaginal discharges, or contaminated neonates.[233,269,278] Elementary bodies produced by *C. abortus* are resistant to many chemical and physical factors and will survive prolonged extracellular exposure.[279] Pigeons and sparrows may serve as reservoirs for the organism, and ticks or insects may play a role in the transmission of this disease.[280,281] The incidence of infection from environmental and wildlife sources is unknown. After entering at the tonsils, the intracellular bacteria become latent within an unknown population of cells.[269] The immunologic mechanisms of pathogenesis are not completely understood, but the progression of disease is remarkably consistent.[278] After experimental subcutaneous inoculation at day 70 of gestation, *C. abortus* can be detected in cotyledonary trophoblast at day 85 but does not begin rapid multiplication until around day 115.[278] This experiment parallels clinical observations of naturally occurring cases. At around day 115 of gestation, necrosis of the cotyledon, in response to massive proliferation of intracellular organism in trophoblast, prevents normal transfer of nutrients across the placentome, resulting in fetal death.[238] Aborting females initially shed large numbers of the organism in the uterine discharge and placenta for approximately 3 weeks after abortion. Ewes that have primiparous abortions from *C. abortus* may have subsequent normal pregnancies but continue to shed the organism in low numbers in vaginal secretions.[282] If infected between 5 and 6 weeks before parturition, ewes and does may develop clinical disease during the current pregnancy. If the ewe or doe is infected later in gestation, some animals will develop latent infections and will not have any problems until they experience abortion during the next gestation.[283] Although *Chlamydophila* has been isolated from the semen of experimentally infected rams for as long as 29 days after inoculation, this is not considered the primary mode of transmission.[280,281] Outbreaks of abortion among goats by dual infection with *Chlamydophila* and *C. burnetii* also have been reported.[284]

Clinical Signs and Pathology. When *C. abortus* is endemic to a farm, abortions caused by this organism are usually limited to primiparous females.[238] Abortions usually occur in the last 2 to 3 weeks of gestation or stillborn or weak lambs may be born after a normal gestation length.[283] After a transient fever and general malaise at initial infection, persistently infected ewes and does may have no clinical signs until the time of abortion.[249,262,285,286] Does and ewes develop a mild and transient pneumonia or hepatitis, become anorexic and febrile, and have a bloody vaginal discharge 2 to 3 days before aborting.[287] The fetus is usually delivered in a fresh state but can be retained in the uterus for 1 or 2 days, it which case it will be autolyzed. Some weak newborns may survive, and a few females may have a retained placenta.[262,267] Occasionally, pneumonia may be seen in young animals during an abortion storm. The placenta will have regional to generalized thickening, brownish exudate, opacity of the intercotyledonary space, and white gray foci on the chorionic surface of cotyledons[238,262,267] (Figure 8.31A). The severity of lesions will vary

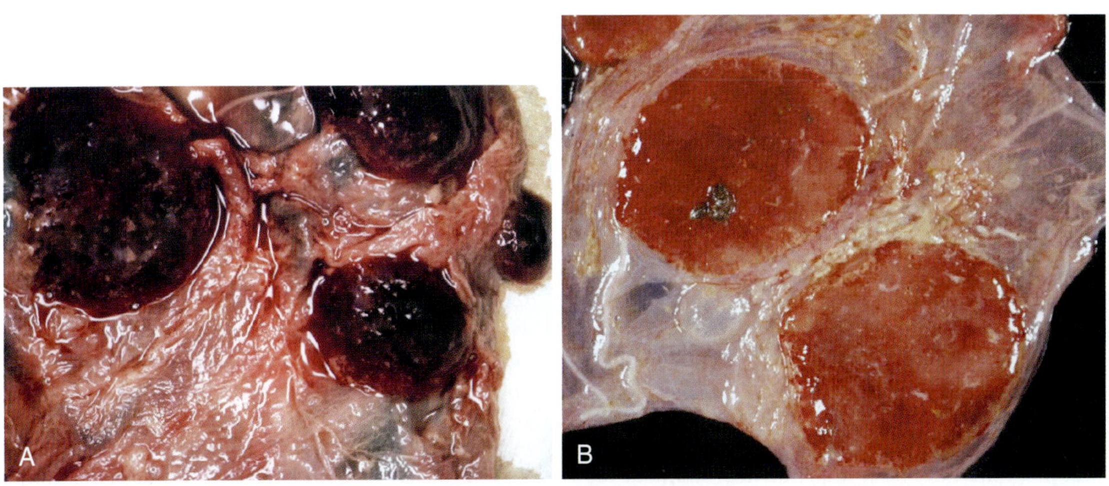

• **Fig. 8.31** Necrotizing placentitis in two different specimens, grossly similar in appearance, was caused by two different intracellular bacteria, respectively: **A.** *Chlamydophila abortus*. **B.** *Coxiella burnetii*. Pathologic changes include pinpoint white foci on cotyledons and thickened, opaque intercotyledonary areas. (Dr. Patricia Blanchard, DVM, PhD CAHFS-Tulare, University of California.)

between animals and between placentomes of the same placenta, and necrotizing vasculitis of placental vessels is observed microscopically.[242,287] Goat fetuses may occasionally have white spots on the liver identifiable grossly, but histologically, most fetuses have some combination of hepatitis, splenitis, bronchopneumonia, or encepahalitis.[242]

Diagnosis. Immediate diagnosis can be made by demonstration of the elementary bodies in impression smears in trophoblast made from cotyledons or uterine discharge. Gimenez or modified Ziehl-Neelsen special stains will improve cytologic detection.[235] Impression smears of cotyledons can be examined by florescent antibody techniques.[242] A definitive diagnosis is made by positive culture or PCR from fresh placenta, stomach content, or fetal tissue.[277,288] PCR assay conducted on vaginal swabs demonstrate high specificity and sensitivity.[289] Since *C. abortus* often only affects the placenta, histopathologic examination, culture, and PCR of fetal tissue can be unrewarding.[278] Examination of the placenta histologically with the use of special stains (Machiavelli, Giemsa, Gimenez, or modified Ziehl-Neelsen) should be diagnostic.[238,242] Immunohistochemistry or PCR performed on formalin-fixed paraffin-embedded placenta is a less sensitive back-up method if fresh tissues are not available.[290,291] The sensitivity of PCR decreases the longer tissues are stored in formalin.[292]

Ewes and does have significant increases in antibodies against *C. abortus* after abortion caused by this organism.[293] Paired serum samples taken 2 to 3 weeks apart from the aborting female or the presence of antibodies in fetal serum can aid in diagnosis.[262,265,272] CFT and various ELISA methods are useful tools to evaluate sera of *C. abortus* antibodies but may provide false-negative results because of cross-reaction with *C. pecorum* antigen. ELISA tests, developed recently, that target outer membrane protein fragments are more sensitive and do not cross react with *C. pecorum*.[294]

Treatment. Outbreak control in fiber-producing animals has been demonstrated by treating all females in the flock with tetracycline during the final 4 to 6 weeks of gestation.[262,267,272] Tetracycline (400–500 mg/head/day) mixed into the feed for 2 weeks can prevent the disease.[238,295] In dairy herds, it is customary to treat individual nonlactating does with injections of long-acting oxytetracycline (20 mg/kg of body weight SC) every 10 to 14 days.[238] An effective protocol may be one injection of long-acting oxytetracycline 6 to 8 weeks before parturition, followed by a second injection 3 weeks after parturition.[280] The authors prefer to include tetracycline in the feed or energy-protein supplement when possible, although practitioners in the United States should be sure to the follow the US Veterinary Feed Directive. Regardless of the route of administration, suppression of the organism with antibiotics may prevent additional placental damage and reduce shedding of *C. abortus.* Tylosin (20 mg/kg IM once or twice daily) also may be effective. *C. abortus* is also responsive to rifampicin and chloramphenicol, but use of these drugs is restricted in some countries, including the United States.[238]

Prevention. Culling of ewes and does that have previously aborted from *C. abortus* should be considered as a control measure.[281] Acquisition of replacement females from endemic herds into a naïve population should be avoided. ET from endemic farms into disease-free recipients has been proposed as a way to maintain the disease-free status of a farm.[238] Enzootic abortion is of such serious economic concern in some countries that compulsory vaccination programs have been implemented.[296] Killed vaccines for sheep are available in certain locales and live vaccines are available in Europe.[279] These vaccines may be used in goats but have been associated with local and systemic reactions (marked soreness and stiffness).[263,297] In the United States, vaccines are usually available only in combination with *Campylobacter* bacterin or *Campylobacter* and *Escherichia coli* bacterin.[263,297] Anecdotal evidence suggests that these three-way vaccines may result in fetal wastage if administered during the first month of pregnancy. If used, the vaccine should be given IM or SC 8 weeks before breeding and followed in 4 weeks with a booster.[297] Even though trials in sheep have demonstrated that protection against abortion lasts for about 3 years, annual revaccination is recommended.[298] Vaccination helps prevent abortion but may not eliminate infection and should therefore not be considered 100% effective.[238]

Aborting females should be removed from the herd for at least 3 weeks, and fetuses and placentas not submitted for diagnostics should be burned or buried. Producers should take care to prevent the contamination of feed and water. Supplemental feedstuffs should not be offered directly on the ground, and feeders should be designed to prevent animals from crawling into and contaminating feed.[238,296]

Coxiella Burnetii (Q Fever). *C. burnetii* is a zoonotic obligate, pleomorphic intracellular, rickettsial organism that can survive in a dried condition for extended periods.[235] Human infection known as "Q fever" was first recognized in abattoir workers in Queensland, Australia. *C. burnetii* can cause abortion in sheep and goats and has distribution in most parts of the world.[238,249,262,299,300]

Transmission and Pathogenesis. Cattle, sheep, goats, dogs, and birds may serve as carriers of *C. burnetii*, which is shed in placentas, uterine fluids, colostrum, milk, urine, feces, and possibly semen of ruminants.[233,238,300–302] Simultaneous abortion storms of cattle, sheep, and goats occurring on the same farm have been documented.[275] Multiple species of ticks are the primary natural reservoir for *C. burnetii* and likely responsible for disease transmission to domestic animals.[275,303] One study indicates a seasonal distribution in cold weather months (Northern Hemisphere) for *C. burnetii*–related abortions.[275] *C. burnetii* exist in a phase I virulent form and phase II less virulent form.[238] Sheep and goats may shed the organism for up to 4 months in vaginal secretion.[302,304] Sheep were shown to shed the organism in feces for 5 months and in milk for 4 months.[304] On farms experiencing epizootics, seronegative does that are kidding normally may shed *C. burnetii.*[305] Cattle have been implicated as the source of infection for sheep and goats when they share pastures, water, feed sources, and handling equipment. Contact with aborted material, vaginal discharge, and mucous membranes and sexual transmission are methods of transmission. *C. burnetii* may be aerosolized on contaminated particles and transmitted by inhalation.[305]

Clinical Signs and Pathology. Susceptible pregnant females develop placentitis, whereas nonpregnant ewes and does usually do not develop clinical signs of infection.[235] Stress, overcrowding, and poor nutrition likely influence of development of clinical signs.[238] Does may abort without apparent clinical signs or show anorexia and depression 1 to 2 days before aborting. Abortion or stillbirth usually occurs in the third trimester, but second-trimester abortions are possible.[242,262,300,306] Unlike *C. abortus, C. burnetii* may cause abortion in successive parturitions.[307] The placenta may have white areas of necrosis and mineralization on cotyledons that also involves intercotyledonary areas (Figure 8.31B). The chorionic surface may be covered by thick exudate (Figure 8.32). Fetuses usually have no gross lesions.[242]

Diagnosis. Diagnosis is based on placental findings, serology, isolation, and/or PCR detection of the organism in the place nta.[262,300,305] Submission of the fetus only is likely to result in no diagnosis.[242,308] Detection of *C. burnetii* by PCR does not necessarily

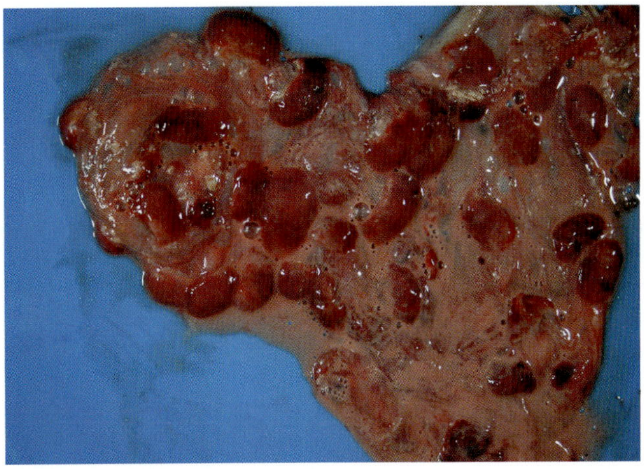

• **Fig. 8.32** *Coxiella burnetii* infection resulting in placentitis with intercotyledonary thickening, opacity, and exudate from a late-term goat abortion. (Courtesy Dr. J.A. Navarro, School of Veterinary Science, University of Murcia, Spain.)

translate to a diagnosis in cases of abortion because animals aborting from other causes may shed the organisms.[238] Although isolation of *C. burnetii* is the ideal means for diagnosis of the disease, it is usually not feasible because of the contagious and zoonotic potential of the organism. If *C. burnetii* is suspected, fresh tissues can be held frozen until the disease is ruled out with histology.[235] Fluorescent antibody test can be used to identify the organism in frozen placental sections. Some diagnostic laboratories, however, are unwilling to handle fresh tissues because of zoonotic transmission risk.[306] Gimenez or Wolbach's Giemsa stains of histologic sections of cotyledons or fetal abomasum are useful for observing organism.[242] PCR and or immunohistochemistry on paraffin-embedded tissue may provide a risk-free diagnostic technique.[291] Even though a variety of serologic tests have been described, a diagnosis of *C. burnetii* abortion cannot be given solely on the basis of positive serology results because infections without abortions are common.[309] Two commercially available ELISA tests were shown to be more sensitive than CFT but have the potential to miss animals that have not developed an immunoglobulin G response.[310] When the indirect immunofluorescence assay was used, titers above 1:32 were considered positive.[311] A four-fold increase in titers between acute and convalescent samples indicates recent infection.[306] A rapid presumptive diagnosis of infection with *C. burnetii* is possible by identifying a large number of characteristic organisms in the placental tissue and ruling out other causes of placentitis (*Brucella, Toxoplasma, Campylobacter,* and *Chlamydophila*).[263,298]

Treatment. Treatment with oxytetracycline did not significantly reduce shedding of *C. burnetii*.[304]

Prevention. After the infection is established, the female can carry the organism indefinitely, shedding it in milk and at parturition. Identification and removal of animals serving as permanent reservoirs should be considered.[312] Producers should burn or bury placentas and aborted fetuses promptly.[300] Prevention in sheep used in medical research is a major problem. Currently, available vaccines are unable to prevent infection but may reduce abortion and shedding of the bacterium.[302,313,314] Removing cattle, cats, and rodents may aid in control efforts.[263]

***Campylobacter* spp. (Campylobacteriosis, Vibriosis).** *C. jejuni* and *C. fetus* subsp. *fetus* (formerly *Vibrio* spp.) are zoonotic agents, gram-negative, microaerophilic rods that are a significant cause of abortion in sheep worldwide.[238,315,316] A United States Department of Agriculture (USDA)/Animal and Plant Health Inspection Service (APHIS) study sampling 87.4% of the US sheep industry identified *Campylobacter* as the number one cause of infectious abortion.[316] Campylobacteriosis is less documented as a cause of abortion in goats.[238] *C. jejuni* is the predominant species resulting in more sporadic abortions, while *C. fetus* subsp. *fetus* is more likely to be involved in abortion storms affecting large flocks in Western North America.[239] Most of the isolates of *C. fetus* belong to a single genetic clone.[316] *C. fetus* subsp. *fetus* has variation in serotypes that may affect response to vaccination or innate immunity.[239] *Campylobacter lari,* a species associated with birds of coastal habitat, has been recognized as a cause of sheep abortion in California.[317,318]

Transmission and Pathogenesis. *Campylobacter* can be commensal bacterium in the intestines and gall bladder of sheep, dogs, and some birds.[235] These organisms can be transmitted farm to farm by carrion-eating birds such as corvids (crows and jays). The organisms can be shed from the intestinal and biliary mucosa of carrier sheep and occasionally guard dogs that have ingested aborted fetuses. Infection occurs through ingestion of infected feces, aborted fetuses, placentas, and vaginal discharge by ewes.[235] Factors that suppress the asymptomatic intestinal infection from progression to diarrhea, bacteremia, and abortion are not known and may be associated with serotype.[239] The incubation period may range from 8 to 60 days.[239] In ewes experimentally inoculated with *C. jejuni,* abortion occurred 7 to 12 days after inoculation.[319] Ewes that become infected abort and then become immune. However, some become persistently infected and shed the organism in their feces.

Clinical Signs and Pathology. Late-gestation abortions, stillbirths, and weak lambs are common. Aborting does are usually asymptomatic but may have mild diarrhea and mucopurulent vaginal discharge.[320] Aborted fetuses and placentas are usually expelled with little or no autolysis. When fetuses are retained in utero, death of ewes may occur.[316] The placenta is often edematous and can have necrosis, resulting in mottled swollen cotyledons.[238] The fetuses may have some subcutaneous edema, pleuritis, hepatitis, and peritonitis. Necrotic areas on the livers of aborted lambs may occasionally look like "gray targets." Although abortion storms may occur in as much as 70 to 90% of a flock, they usually affect less than 20% of ewes in enzootically infected flocks.[237]

Diagnosis. Definitive diagnosis of *Campylobacter* abortion is through isolation of the bacterium and requires inoculation of special plates and use special microaerophilic culture technique.[242] Fetal lung, abomasal fluid, placenta, or vaginal discharge are preferred samples for culture.[242,321] Presumptive identification of organism by direct microscopic examination (dark field or contrast) of fresh cotyledonary smears is possible.[235,238,322] A serologic test can be done at a few specialized laboratories. Whenever the organism is isolated, culture and antibiotic sensitivity patterns are useful for guiding possible flock treatment. Fetal septicemia by *Helicobacter bilis* (previously *Flexispira rappini*) may cause gross lesions that mimic campylobacteriosis.[323,324]

Treatment. The antibiotic regimen of penicillin or streptomycin injections or tetracycline in feed (300 mg/head/day) may be useful in the face of a disease outbreak.[272,320] Tetracycline in the feed (200–300 mg/head/day) before and during lambing or kidding season appears to decrease the incidence of abortion, as does the use of injectable long-acting oxytetracycline (20 mg/kg every 48 hours) during an outbreak. Again, practitioners in the United

States should be sure to the follow the US Veterinary Feed Directive. Recently a tetracycline-resistant clone of *C. jejuni* has emerged as the predominant species in sheep abortion in the western United States.[316] In cases of apparent tetracycline resistance, sulfamethazine (110 mg/kg PO) or tylosin (30 mg/kg IM once daily) may be given.

Prevention. A combined killed *C. fetus-C. jejuni* bacterin is available for use in sheep. The vaccine is initially administered before breeding, with a booster in 2 to 3 months. Annual revaccination shortly before or just after breeding is recommended.[297] If a vaccine or immunologic agent for *E. coli* is combined with *C. fetus* or *C. jejuni*, it should be avoided in early gestation because it has been anecdotally associated with fetal wastage. On farms where *Campylobacter* is a confirmed cause of abortion, autogenous bacterins that are strain-specific are valuable. Because of the probable oral route of infection, maintaining sanitary conditions, avoiding fecal contamination of feedstuffs, and isolating aborting animals are recommended strategies.[320] The placentas and aborted fetuses should be burned or buried and kept away from hungry guard dogs.[238]

***Brucella* spp. (Brucellosis).** *Brucella* spp. are small, gram-negative coccobacilli that may cause abortion, weak kids, mastitis, epididymitis, and the formation of localized lesions in various tissue.[325,326] *Brucella melitensis* is a zoonotic agent that is widespread in goats in the Middle East, India, Pakistan, Africa, Mexico, and parts of South America.[237,262] *B. melitensis* is a cause of Malta fever in human beings.[237,262] The incidence of brucellosis caused by *B. melitensis* in goats has historically been extremely low in North America, but recent sporadic outbreaks have been reported in goats in Texas and Colorado.[326] Although considered goat specific, *B. melitensis* may cause abortion in sheep.[235] *B. ovis* is endemic in sheep throughout the western portions of North America and associated with epididymitis in rams and may cause abortion in rare incidences.[233] Occasionally, *B. abortus* infection occurs in goats living in close contact with infected cattle or as a result of inadvertent vaccination of goats with live strains of the organism.[325]

Transmission and Pathogenesis. The bacterium may be transmitted in contaminated feed or water, oral secretions, milk, urine, feces, semen, vaginal discharge, or placental membranes.[235,237,325] Crowded facilities are often implicated in Brucella outbreaks.[327] *Brucella* sp. enters through mucous membranes and becomes localized in the udder, uterus, testes, spleen, or lymph nodes.[235,237,325] In pregnant animals, localization in the placenta leads to the development of placentitis with subsequent abortion. Goats may excrete the organism for up to 2 to 3 months in vaginal discharge. If ewes become infected and abort, they usually clear the organism within 2 to 4 weeks.[235] Nonaborting infected females may give birth to infected kids or lambs that are capable of shedding the organism.[237,238,295]

Clinical Signs and Pathology. Sheep and goats with brucellosis often abort during the final trimester.[325,327] Substantial increases in initial farm abortions are followed by a period of resistance during which abortions are rare. Again, abortion appears to be more of a problem in goats than in sheep. In goats and rarely in sheep, a systemic disease with fever, depression, weight loss, diarrhea, mastitis, lameness, hygroma, and orchitis may occur.[237,325] Infected ewes are rarely ill. Mild placental lesions have been reported with *B. melitensis* infection in goats, whereas *B. ovis* infection in sheep is said to result in pronounced placental thickening and grossly visible necrosis of cotyledons.

Diagnosis. Identification of brucellosis as the cause of abortion is usually made by isolating the organism from the aborted fetus (abomasal contents), placenta (cotyledon), or vaginal discharge. Isolation is dependent on specialized culture, often utilizing increased CO_2 or less frequently used agars.[328] PCR may be used to diagnose *Brucella* in milk and blood samples.[329] Serologic testing alone may lead to a false diagnosis. Various agglutination, precipitation, and CFTs are available to detect carrier animals.[238] The milk ring test is an agglutination test conducted on milk samples.[330] PCR and or immunohistochemistry on paraffin embedded tissue may provide a risk-free diagnostic technique.[291,331]

Treatment and Prevention. No treatment is available for brucellosis in goats or sheep. Eradication of *Brucella* organisms is difficult because livestock populations can be reinfected from wildlife reservoirs.[327,332] Grazing in communal pastures places animals at increased risk.[333] In countries with a low prevalence of infection, slaughter of the entire flock is generally the control measure of choice.[237,238,327] In other situations, a test and slaughter program may be more appropriate.

Culling rams based on palpable signs of epididymitis, serologic testing, and vaccinating normal, nonaffected ram lambs may help control the disease.[235] In many countries in which caprine brucellosis is prevalent, the disease is controlled by an intensive vaccination program. Vaccination of goats is not permitted in the United States. The killed vaccine occasionally used in sheep *(B. ovis)* appears to have poor efficacy. Where permitted, a live attenuated strain of *B. melitensis* can be given subcutaneously in kids and lambs 3 to 8 months of age.[238,327] This vaccine causes abortion in goats and should therefore be avoided in pregnant animals or those within 1 month of breeding. Immunity from a single vaccination for *B. melitensis* is considered to be lifelong.[238]

All new animals should be serologically tested before introduction to the flock. Rams and bucks should be tested yearly before the start of the breeding season.[237] Placentas and aborted fetuses not used for diagnostic purposes should be burned or buried.

***Listeria* spp. (Listeriosis).** *Listeria monocytogenes* and *Listeria ivanovii* are zoonotic, gram-positive, non–acid-fast facultative microaerophilic bacteria that cause meningoencephalitis, abortion, and septicemia in goats and sheep. *L. monocytogenes* causes encephalitis, septicemia, and abortion in sheep and goats, whereas *L. ivanovii* is reported to cause abortion only in sheep.[3]

Transmission and Pathogenesis. *L. monocytogenes* can be found in soil, water, plant litter, silage, and the digestive tracts of ruminants and human beings.[238] The organism can survive in soil and feces for extended periods and grows in poorly fermented silage (with pH levels higher than 5.5).[237,238,249,262] Fecal shedding of *L. monocytogenes* peaks in the winter.[334] Abortion has been attributed to the feeding of contaminated silage. Abortions have also been observed in animals fed only hay or that browse on boggy, high-pH soils.[335] Experimentally infected does aborted 9 to 11 days after inoculation.[238]

Clinical Signs and Pathology. Infection in late gestation can result in stillbirth or weak neonates rather than abortion and is preceded by septicemia.[238,262] Signs of septicemia include fever, decreased appetite, and reduced milk production. Metritis may develop in sheep and occasionally in goats that abort. Kids grafted to the aborting female can contract listeriosis through the milk with subsequent fatal septicemia.[238] The abortifacient and encephalitic clinical presentations of listeriosis do not usually occur simultaneously in sheep but may occur in goat herds.[263] The uterus may have minimal lesions of metritis or be filled with necrotic, dark-colored putrid material.[336] Other findings may include a suppurative placentitis with necrotizing vasculitis (Figure 8.33). In chronically affected animals, the cotyledons may be thickened with

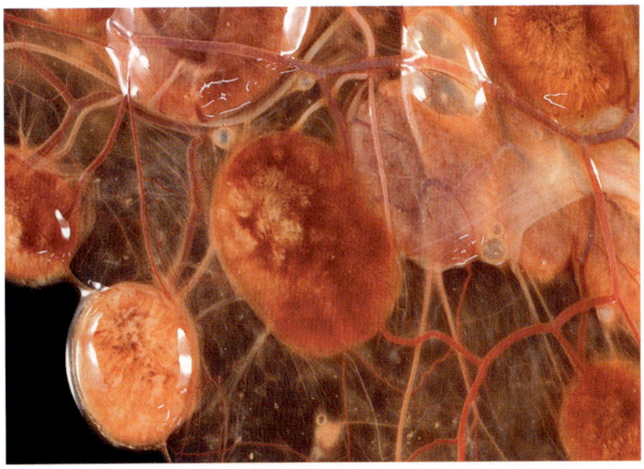

• **Fig. 8.33** Necrotizing placentitis caused by *Listeria monocytogenes* observed on the chorionic surface of a cotyledon, midterm goat abortion. The intercotyledonary space remains transparent and minimally affected. (Courtesy Dr. Jim Cooley, Starkville, Michigan.)

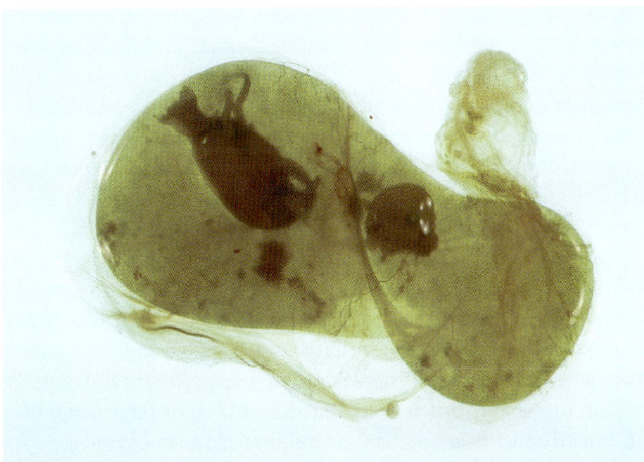

• **Fig. 8.34** *Listeria monocytogenes* infection resulting in a macerated fetus. (Courtesy Dr. Jim Cooley, Starkville, Michigan.)

a leathery texture.[238] In the aborted fetuses, microabscesses containing numerous bacteria may be seen in liver and other organs.[235] Fetuses may be severely autolyzed or macerated[235] (Figure 8.34).

Diagnosis. Culture of the organisms from the fetal stomach content, liver, placenta, or uterine discharge is diagnostic. Unfortunately, fetal autolysis can be so severe that culture may be difficult. The organism may be presumptively identified during histopathologic examination with the use of silver stains. PCR assay or immunohistochemistry studies of paraffin-embedded tissue may provide a risk-free diagnostic technique.[291]

Treatment. The addition of chlortetracycline (300 mg/head/day) to a grain supplement has been reported to stop abortions during a listeriosis outbreak.[335] Practitioners in the United States should be sure to the follow the US Veterinary Feed Directive. Long-acting oxytetracycline (20 mg/kg of body weight every 48 to 72 hours) is also of value.

Prevention. Feeding poor-quality or spoiled silage or grazing pastures linked with outbreaks or cases of listeriosis should be discouraged. Vaccination to produce cellular immunity has been investigated. The administration of two doses of reduced-virulence live vaccine before breeding is reported to have provided significant protection against experimental challenge in pregnant does.[238]

***Salmonella* spp. (Salmonellosis).** *Salmonella* are zoonotic, gram-negative bacteria that can cause abortion, metritis, and systemic illness in ewes and does. The genus has only two species, *Salmonella enterica*, divided into six subspecies and containing over 2500 serovars, and *Salmonella bongori*. The pathogenic species and subspecies of most interest in sheep and goats are *S. enterica* subsp. *enterica*. In the following discussion, therefore, *Salmonella* serotypes from this subspecies are identified by genus and serotype name, as is accepted in most literature. *Salmonella* Abortusovis, *Salmonella* Brandenburg, *Salmonella* Indiana, *Salmonella* Dublin, *Salmonella* Montevideo, *Salmonella* Schwarzengrund and *Salmonella* Typhimurium are associated with systemic disease and abortion in does and ewes.[235,238,337,338] *S. enterica* subsp. *arizonae* is a separate subspecies that has been implicated in small ruminant abortion. *S.* Abortusovis, which is uncommon in North America and mostly affects Europe and western Asia, was first implicated as a cause of sheep abortion in 1921. *S.* Abortusovis is unique among *Salmonella* species because it is more often associated with abortion rather than septicemia and enteritis.[339]

Transmission and Pathogenesis. Sources of infection include fecal contaminated feed, carrion feeding birds, cattle, dogs, cats, rodents, and some wildlife species.[239] An ovine abortifacient strain of *S.* Brandenburg was shown to be transmitted by seagulls in New Zealand.[338] *S.* Indiana was shown to be transmitted by pigeons and turtledoves in Spain.[337] Climatic changes, shipping, overcrowded conditions, feed deprivation, water deprivation, inappropriate use of antibiotics, and other factors all may predispose a flock to a *Salmonella* abortion storm.

The route of infection is by oral ingestion of the organism. In ewes infected with *S.* Abortusovis, PCR assay results may be positive up to 3 months after abortion.[338] Infections are often related to stressful situations and may not persist into the following season.[239,315]

Clinical Signs and Pathology. Abortion storms affecting as many as 70% of the females can occur. *S.* Brandenburg abortions are observed as early as 80 days but peak at 100 to 120 days gestation.[338] Infected females may become febrile and depressed and have diarrhea. Metritis and retained placenta are common findings. A high mortality rate among ewes after abortion has been described. Ewes that die may have an enlarged darkened uterus with foul-smelling fetal contents that have undergone rapid autolysis.[244] Salmonellae proliferating in the amniotic fluid may cause fetal pneumonia through amniotic inhalation or septicemia (Figure 8.35). Fetuses may become septic and develop a "cooked" appearance, with bruising and severe edema of subcutaneous tissues. Placental cotyledons may be pale and edematous.[338]

Diagnosis. A diagnosis can be made by isolating *Salmonella* organisms cultured on a selective broth inoculated from aborted fetuses, fetal abomasal contents, placentas, or uterine discharge. Identification of Salmonellae and specific serovars requires biochemical identification as well as sequencing of PCR-generated gene fragments from cultures. PCR analysis conducted on fecal and vaginal swabs has proved to be a more rapid and sensitive method for identification specific species and serovars in tissue.[340,341] PCR assay is also capable of detecting *S.* Abortusovis in samples that have been overgrown with other enteric bacteria.[340] Diagnostic immunohistochemistry studies and PCR assays may also be conducted on paraffin-embedded samples for *S.* Abortusovis.[291] Specific agglutinins can be demonstrated in the sera of adults and aborted fetuses.

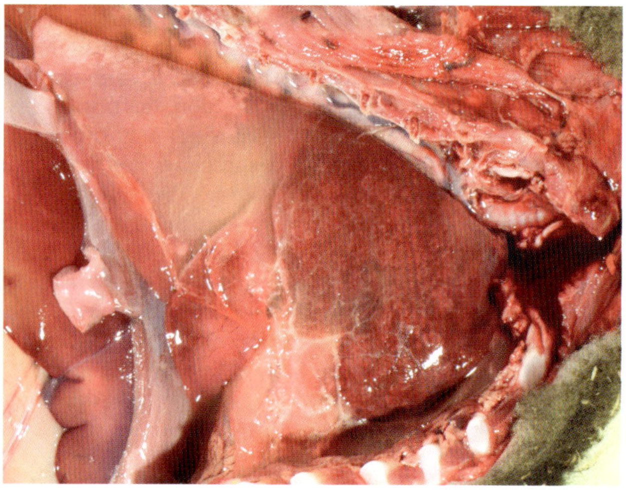

• **Fig. 8.35** Fetal pneumonia caused by *Salmonella* spp. infection. The lungs are firm and fill the thoracic cavity. (Courtesy Dr. John F. Edwards, College Station, Texas.)

Treatment. Prevention and control measures include treating pregnant females with appropriate antibiotics based on culture and antibiotic sensitivity. Once-daily intramuscular administration of enrofloxacin for 3 to 5 days reduced abortion losses during a *S.* Abortusovis outbreak.[337,339]

Prevention. Limiting contact to vectors by protecting drinking water with use of antibird meshes may be beneficial.[337] A vaccine constituted by inactivated *S.* Abortusovis was protective when challenged by fully virulent *S.* Abortusovis.[342] In a similar study, a vaccine constituted of an inactivated virulent *S.* Brandenburg isolate did not significantly protect sheep when experimentally challenged with *S.* Brandenburg.[343] Administering two doses of an autogenous vaccine followed by an annual booster and cleaning the environment may help minimize this disease.[238]

***Leptospira* spp. (Leptospirosis).** *Leptospira interrogans* is a zoonotic agent with worldwide distribution that causes a low percentage of abortions in goats and sheep.[242] Sheep are considered relatively resistant to *L. interrogans* infections and may serve as maintenance host while goats appear to be more susceptible to *L. interrogans*–induced abortion.[344–346] Serovars identified in sheep and goats include Hardjo, Pomona, Bratislava, Ballum, Icterohaemorrhagica, Grippotyphosa, Sejroe, and Wolffi.[235,300,346,347] In a study of goat abortion in Spain, 2.6% of abortions resulted from infection with *L. interrogans*, with the serovar Pomona being the most prevalent (75%), followed by the serovars Sejroe (12.5%) and Icterohaemorrhagica (12.5%).[271] In Brazil, serovar Hardjo was the most frequently identified.[347]

Transmission and Pathogenesis. Exposure to environments contaminated by urine from species other than sheep or goats appears to be the primary source of infection. Direct transmission from infected animals is rarely confirmed.[348]

Clinical Signs and Pathology. Clinical signs include anorexia, fever, jaundice, hemoglobinuria, anemia, nervous manifestations, abortion, and, occasionally, death.[238,346] Flaccid agalactia may occur in ewes.[235] Abortions have been reported during the final trimester of gestation in goats and to a lesser extent sheep.[346] Clinical signs and gross lesions in adult animals may mimic copper toxicosis.[239]

Diagnosis. Dark-field microscopy, florescent antibody techniques, and PCR of placenta, fetal tissue, and fluids are used to confirm the diagnosis.[238,346] Impression smears of the kidney can be examined by florescent antibody techniques.[242] The organism is difficult to isolate from contaminated specimens and difficult to find in silver-stained histologic sections. Aborted sheep fetuses may have a low positive titer but an abortifacient organism other than *L. interrogans* may be diagnosed in serum positive sheep.351 A single positive serum on an aborting ewe or doe is likely of no value, and evidence of raising titer in paired sera is needed to implicate *L. interrogans* in an abortion[238] (see Chapter 20).

Treatment and Prevention. Vaccination two to four times a year with multivalent cattle vaccines has been advocated in area of high leptospirosis activity. Other control measures include separating animal species, reducing the number of rodents, maintaining a clean water supply, and feeding tetracycline (300 to 500 mg/head/day) during middle to late gestation.[238]

Class Mollicutes: Mycoplasma spp. and Ureaplasma spp. Bacteria in class *Mollicutes* have the smallest genome of any free-living organisms and lack a cell wall and are enclosed in an outer cell membrane.[350] *Mycoplasma mycoides* species contains two taxa from a cluster that have been diagnosed as causes of abortion in sheep and goats.[351] *M. mycoides* subsp. *capri* is a collective designation for the former taxa *M. mycoides* subsp. *mycoides* LC and *M. mycoides* subsp. *capri*.[351,352] *M. mycoides* subsp. *capri* likely occurs worldwide but has been diagnosed as a cause of goat abortion in California and Hungary.[242,353] *Mycoplasma capricolum* subsp. *capricolum* occurs sporadically in the United States and has been reported as a cause of necrotizing placentitis and fetal septicemia in a goat.[354] Other species, *Mycoplasma agalactia* and *Mycoplasma putrefaciens*, have been reported as the species causing abortion in goats.[238,242,354] *M. mycoides* also causes septicemia and is capable of causing abortion. Changes in the surface proteins on the cells membrane allow the mycoplasma to elude the immune system of the host.[350] *Ureaplasma* ssp. has been isolated from ewes with a history of infertility and granular vulvitis.[355] *Ureaplasma parvum* causes altered lung development when experimentally given to sheep in utero and this is considered a model for fetal *Ureaplasma* spp. infection in humans.[356] Natural infection by *Ureoplasma* spp. as a cause of perinatal death and weak lambs is not routinely screened for and is minimally documented.

Clinical Signs and Pathology. Abortion is not the predominant clinical finding in an outbreak.

Abortion occurs in does (and rarely in ewes) in the final trimester of gestation. Females that abort generally shed the organism in their milk, amniotic fluids, and placenta.

Diagnosis. The organism also may be isolated from cotyledons, fetal abomasum content, liver, and spleen. Diagnosis of abortion caused by *Mycoplasma* species is by special culture and PCR of the isolate. Because mycoplasma are often difficult to culture and are not visible by routine histopathology, PCR techniques are rapidly evolving as the diagnostic method of choice.

Treatment and Prevention. Administration of tetracyclines or tylosin may be of benefit, but identification and culling of all infected animals are the best course of prevention.[357] No vaccines are currently available for use in sheep and goats.

Anaplasma Phagocytophila (Tick-Borne Fever) *Anaplasma phagocytophila* (formerly *Ehrlichia phagocytophila*) is a gram-negative, obligate intracellular bacterium that parasitize neutrophils in sheep and goats and also may infect humans.[358] Infected sheep have high fever, malaise, neutropenia, and thrombocytopenia.[358] Neutropenia may predispose infected sheep to other infectious agents.[358] *Ixodes ricinus* is the species of tick most recognized as a vector.[340] Infected sheep may have abortion and impaired spermatogenesis.[358,359] Microscopically, aborted sheep fetuses may have cerebral leucomalacia presumably caused from hypoxia.[360]

***Yersinia* spp. (Yersiniosis).** *Yersinia spp.* are zoonotic gram-negative enteric bacteria that have resulted in sheep abortion.[233] *Yersinia pseudotuberculosis* has been implicated as an abortifacient agent in sheep from United States, United Kingdom, Denmark, and Australia.[361] In a Nebraska flock outbreak, *Y. pseudotuberculosis* caused suppurative placentitis and abortion in ewes from 75 days' gestation, death of term lambs, and death of several ewes.[362] *Yersinia enterocolitica* (serotype O) was isolated from an aborted ovine fetus and then inoculated experimentally into a group of ewes, resulting in placentitis.[363]

Fusobacterium Necrophorum (Necrobacillosis). *Fusobacterium necrophorum*, a gram-negative anaerobic pleomorphic bacterium, present worldwide, has been reported to cause sporadic abortion in sheep. In a study of small flocks in Denmark, 4 of 24 ewes were found to have aborted from *F. necrophorum*.[361] The placenta may have purulent exudate on the chorionic surface, necrosis of cotyledons and intercotyledonary areas, edema, and hemorrhage.[245,364] The skin of the fetus may have severe multifocal dermatitis.[245] Because routine diagnostic procedures often exclude anaerobic culture, *F. necrophorum* infections may be an underrecognized cause of abortion in sheep and goats. Advanced techniques of laser capture micro dissection and fluorescent in situ hybridization were required in one instance to diagnose *F. necrophorum*.[361,365]

Escherichia Coli. Although usually sporadic, *E. coli* abortion is more common than abortion caused by "classic" abortifacient viruses and bacteria.[366] Diagnosis of *E. coli* abortion is usually based on obtaining a pure culture from lung or abomasum content and collaborating culture results with histopathology.[367] Epizootics are possible, however, and in one Scottish report, a verotoxigenic strain of *E. coli* resulted in 20% abortion in one flock. Infections are acquired hematogenously from a septic female or retrograde from an open cervix.[242] Fetuses commonly have bronchopneumonia but may also have no microscopic lesion, peritonitis, or epicarditis. Premature or weak lambs may die within 24 hours of birth.[367] Fetuses may be autolyzed or fresh.[367] In *E. coli* abortion storms, ewes may die with metritis and toxemia.[367] Results of culture and sensitivity can be used to select antibiotics if they are obtained promptly.

Helicobacter Bilis. *H. bilis* (previously identified as *F. rappini*, *Helicobacter rappini, Helicobacter* sp. flexispira taxa 2, 5, and 8) is a potentially zoonotic, weakly gram-negative, microaerophilic, motile, spiral, and flagellated enterohepatic bacterium that may colonize human, dog, cat, and rodent intestine.[243,324,368] The bacterium was identified in a significant number of sheep abortions in South Dakota.[369] Experimentally *H. bilis* may produce placental vasculitis, suppurative placentitis, and fetal septicemia that result in multifocal hepatic necrosis. Areas of hepatic necrosis may form grossly visible target lesions that are indistinguishable from lesions caused by *Campylobacter* spp.[369] Giemsa stain may provide the best visualization during histopathology, although it is considered gram-negative.

Miscellaneous Bacterial Agents. Any bacteria that cause septicemia, endotoxemia, or debilitation in sheep and goats is capable of causing abortion.[235] Bacteremia in a dam may result in a fever-related abortion.[233] Fetal septicemia may produce stillbirths, perinatal death, and week neonates. *Mannheimia hemolytica* and *Pasteurella multocida* may be isolated from sporadically aborted sheep.[243] *Arcanobacterium pyogenes* is consistently identified as cause of second- and third-trimester abortion in sheep and goats.[242,243] *Histophilus ovis* has been implicated as a cause of ascending placentitis, carried by asymptomatic rams or ewes, that may affected up to 50% of a sheep flock.[235] *Actinobacillus seminis* has been associated with abortion and metritis in ewes and may be transmitted from carrier rams.[370] *Francisella tularensis*, the agent responsible for tularemia, is a highly zoonotic bacterium that caused abortion in 396 of 840 coming 2-year-old ewes during a Wyoming outbreak.[371] Abortion from *Staphylococcus aureus* was reported in over 50% of ewes that underwent long-term venous catheterization and may also be an opportunistic pathogen.[243,372] *Burkholderia pseudomallei* is a zoonotic agent that causes goat abortion and is most frequently identified in Australia and Southeast Asia.[242] *B. pseudomallei* is rare in North America. *Erysipelothrix rhusiopathiae* was identified as the causative agent in an outbreak of ewe septicemia resulting in a 3.5% abortion rate in a Greek flock.[373] *Bacillus cereus* was identified as a bacterium causing sporadic abortion in sheep in a large survey and also confirmed as an abortifacient experimentally.[243,374]

Fungi. Mycotic abortion, although rare, may occur and is likely opportunistic. *Candida albicans* was reported as a cause of goat abortion in California.[242] *Aspergillus* spp. is often implicated in bovine abortion and is also a possible opportunistic pathogen in smaller ruminants.[375]

Protozoal Abortion

Toxoplasma Gondii (Toxoplasmosis). *T. gondii*, an apicomplexan protozoa, is a zoonotic agent with worldwide distribution and considered one of the primary causes of infective ovine abortion in Australia, United Kingdom, New Zealand, Norway, and United States.[376–378] *T. gondii* is capable of causing abortion, fetal mummification, stillbirth, and weak lambs and kids.[238,377] The percentage of toxoplasmosis abortions per region is difficult to estimate because submission of diagnostic samples to labs is limited, serologic test are not specific, infected females are usually asymptomatic, and the disease is sporadic.[377]

Transmission and Pathogenesis. Cats are the definitive host for *T. gondii* and are capable of shedding millions of oocysts within 4 to 12 days of initial infection.[239] Kittens infected in utero can shed *T. gondii* oocysts immediately at time of birth.[377] Ewes and does become infected by ingesting feed or water contaminated with low numbers of oocysts and the conceptus may become infected as soon as 14 days later.[377] In experimental studies of sheep, abortion occurs 4 weeks postinfection.[377] After ingestion, the organism enters the blood and spreads to the lymph nodes, where it undergoes asexual reproduction. Subsequently, it invades and multiplies in the placenta, causing a necrotizing placentitis that may invade the fetus.[379] Disruption of maternal nutrient and oxygen supply through disruption of placentomes results in fetal death, abortion, stillbirth, or weak neonates.[379] It is possible, however, for infected dams to give birth to nonaffected young.[379] It is also possible for ewes to have abortion in the acute phase of systemic infection and the pathogenesis is thought to be related to high fever and hormonal dysregulation.[379] Although *T. gondii* is found in goat semen, venereal transmission is an unlikely cause of transmission.[376] Ewes that are seropositive for *Toxoplasma* gain immune protection, but the organism persists in cysts in the brain and muscle of these animals.[380] A persistently infected ewe may transmit *T. gondii* infection to the placenta, but rates for vertical transmission are thought to be below 4%.[377,380] Goats that have been infected by *T. gondii* are likely to be resistant to reexposure and abortion of subsequent pregnancies.[381]

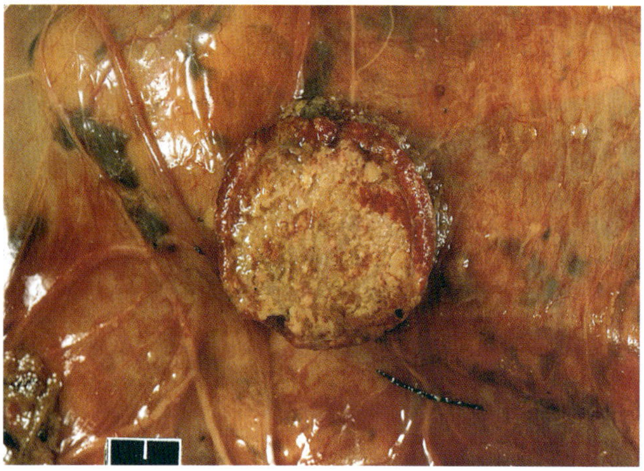

• **Fig. 8.36** *Toxoplasma gondii* infection resulting in cotyledonary necrosis and calcification with minimal intercotyledonary involvement. (Courtesy Dr. Jim Cooley, Starkville, Michigan.)

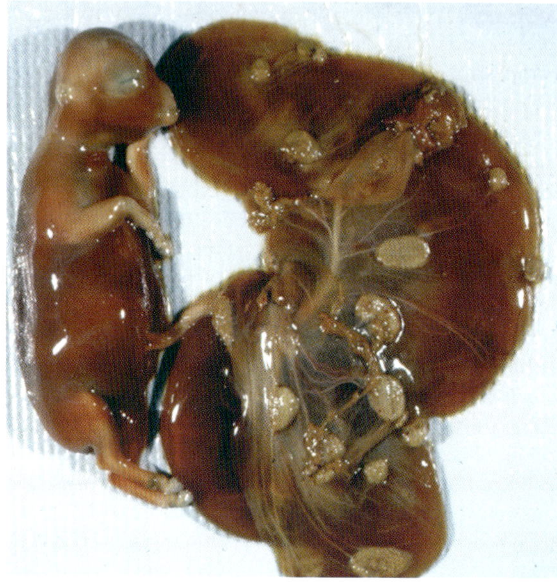

• **Fig. 8.37** *Neospora caninum* induced abortion caused by experimental inoculation in midgestation. The fetus and placenta are autolyzed. Mild multifocal necrosis in the brain is the only lesion detected microscopically. (Courtesy Dr. David Lindsay, Blacksburg, Virginia.)

Clinical Signs and Pathology. Goats appear to be more susceptible to *T. gondii* infection than sheep are.[376] Most abortions occur from infections during the latter half of gestation and fetuses within the same litter may be affected differently.[233,249] Does and ewes are often clinically normal at the time of abortion.[376] Rarely, the immunosuppressed pregnant female becomes febrile and may develop the neurologic form of the disease. Those infected in the first 40 days have embryonic resorption. Infections occurring between 40 and 120 days generally result in mummification, maceration, and abortion. Infection after 120 days' gestation may produce premature, stillborn, or weak lambs.[233] The intercotyledonary areas of the aborted placenta are usually normal, with the cotyledons having gray-white to yellow small focal areas of necrosis and calcification (1–3 mm in diameter)[379] (Figure 8.36). *Coxiella*, *Brucella*, and *Chlamydophila* species also can cause similar cotyledonary lesions, but the intercotyledonary region is more likely to be involved[275] (Figures 8.31A, B and 8.32). Microscopically, fetal brains may have leucomalacia caused by gradual loss of oxygen.[382]

Diagnosis. A presumptive diagnosis can be made from placental lesions alone, but rapid autolytic decomposition of the placenta may limit accuracy.[376] *T. gondii* isolation is a specialized procedure that requires a cooled, not frozen, sample of placenta cotyledon, fetal brain, lung, or muscles.[377] PCR detection is becoming more available and is often more practical because tissues can be frozen long-term prior to shipment.[383] PCR and or immunohistochemistry on paraffin embedded tissue may be an option if fresh tissue is not available.[291] The modified agglutination test can be used to detect antibodies in fetal and maternal serum and is more sensitive than other tests.[384] The ELISA and IFA tests also are used for fetal serologic diagnosis.[376] Thoracic fluid can be utilized to check *T. gondii* titers.[239] Identification of *T. gondii* antibodies in fetal fluids or presuckling blood is also diagnostic of transplacental *Toxoplasma* infection.[376] High antibody titer in the dam is not diagnostic of recent infection because titers may remain elevated from one season to the next. The absence of *T. gondii* antibodies in the blood of ewes and does within 7 days of an abortion, however, likely rules out the possibility of infection.[238,376]

Treatment. Feeding decoquinate (2 mg/kg body weight/day) or monensin (15–30 mg/head/day) throughout gestation may reduce the incidence of abortion. Lasalocid is less effective than monensin in toxoplasmosis control.[385]

Prevention. Control of toxoplasmosis is based on preventing the exposure of pregnant females to oocyst-contaminated pasture, food, water, and bedding. Fetal membranes and dead fetuses should be buried or incinerated so they do not serve as sources of infection for cats and other animals.[238] Cats should not be allowed near pregnant sheep and goats.[376] Older spayed cats can be kept on premises because this may help keep younger pregnant queens from occupying barns. Attempts should be made, such as placement of litter boxes, to prevent cats from defecating in feeders, hay, and other feedstuffs. A vaccine containing tachyzoites of a mildly infective strain of live *T. gondii* (S48 strain) is available in Europe and New Zealand. Ewes vaccinated with the S48 strain vaccine retain immunity for approximately 18 months.[386]

Other Protozoa Causing Abortion. *Neospora caninum*, an apicomplexan protozoon, similar to *T. gondii*, has been diagnosed with much less frequency in sheep and goat abortions.[387] When pygmy goats were experimentally inoculated at day 51 of gestation, fetal death was observed in two of six animals.[388] Fetuses and placentas were autolyzed with minimal gross lesions (Figure 8.37). Presumptive diagnosis is dependent on microscopic observation of mild multifocal necrosis in the brain. In a second experiment, a doe inoculated at 85 days produced a near-term mummified stillborn fetus with similar brain lesions.[388] Mummification of the fetus caused by prolonged in utero and retention of the dead fetus is also a characteristic of toxoplasmosis. A serological study of sheep in Slovakia revealed a low prevalence of *N. caninum*, suggesting a minor impact on sheep production in that region.[389]

Sarcocystis spp. has been implicated in experimental and natural abortion. Of the four species of sarcocyst that infect sheep, *Sarcocystis tennella* and *Sarcocystis arieticanis* are considered pathologic.[239] *S. tennella* abortion has been induced experimentally in sheep.[390] Abortion from *Sarcocystis* spp. has been reported in goats exposed to coyote feces.[391]

Trypanosoma congolense is associated with abortion of does and ewes in Africa.[392] Several studies indicated that sheep and goat infection with *Trypanosoma vivax* in South America and Africa has also been linked to an increased rate of abortion.[393]

Viruses

Family Bunyaviridae (Cache Valley Virus, Akabane Virus, Rift Valley Fever Virus, Nairobi Sheep Disease Virus). The family *Bunyaviridae* is composed of spherical negative-stranded RNA viruses that may infect a variety of animals, including man. Almost all bunyavirus infections are dependent on an arthropod vector.[394] The incidence of infection is linked to vector activity. Bunyaviruses in the genera Bunyavirus (Bunyamwera serogroup, Cache Valley virus; and Simbu serogroup, Akabane virus), Phlebovirus (Rift Valley fever virus), and Nairovirus (Nairobi sheep disease virus) are most commonly associated with epidemics of fetal loss in sheep and goats.[394,395] Other bunyaviruses associated with fetal disease in ruminants include Simbu serogroup, Aino and Peaton viruses, Bunyamwera serogroup, Main Drain virus, and California serogroup, LaCrosse, and San Angelo viruses.[396]

Pathology. At necropsy the fetuses may have a necrotizing nonsuppurative encephalomyelitis, polymyositis, hydrocephalus, axial skeletal deviations, anasarca, oligohydramnios.[394,396] Degeneration of the ventral horn of the spinal cord may result in muscle atrophy and tendon contracture (arthrogryposis). These viruses may also cause in utero death of the fetus. Rift valley fever virus and Nairobi sheep disease can cause fetal malformation but most often cause abortions without congenital deformities.

Diagnosis. The diagnosis is aided by the detection of antibodies in fetal fluids, heart blood or precolostrum serum, and development of characteristic congenital abnormalities.[397] Absence of titers from the dam also is significant, but absence from the lamb does not preclude diagnosis.[235]

Control and Prevention. Control and prevention measures for Bunyaviruses involve recognition of vector lifecycles. Natural immunity derived from infection may be for life.[235] Bunyavirus vaccines are not available in the United States. Reducing exposure to mosquitoes or other insects by killing larva in standing water, breeding during winter months, fencing off boggy low-lying areas, and using insect repellents are all potential preventative measures. Geographic distribution, host, and other specifics will be discussed individually for the most recognized bunyaviruses.

Cache Valley Virus. Cache valley virus, genus Bunyavirus, Bunyamwera serogroup, is endemic in parts of the Southwest and Northeast United States as well as Southern Canada.[397] The most common vectors are the mosquitoes, but *Culicoides* spp. may also be a vector.[394,395] Severe arthrogryposis with skeletal muscle hypoplasia may be observed in newborn lambs[396] (Figure 8.38). Sheep experimentally infected before 32 days gestation usually experienced fetal death. The greatest percentages of fetal abnormalities were observed in sheep infected between 32 and 45 days' gestation. The development of fetal abnormalities decreased as the gestation age increased, but experiments on fetuses infected after 50 days have not been reported and the effects of the virus on older fetuses are not known.[398] Cache Valley virus infects goats but has not been shown to cause fetal disease.[394]

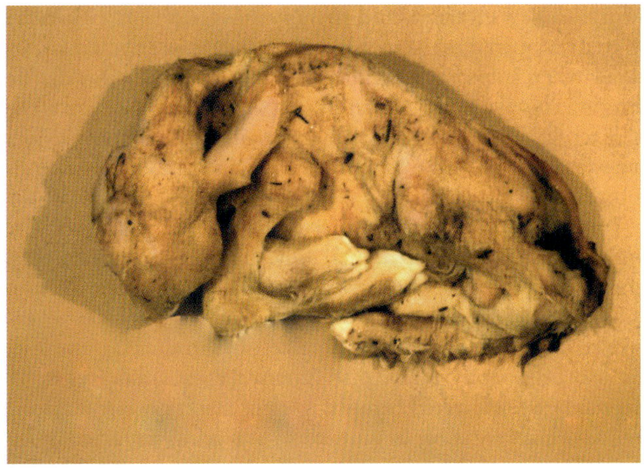

• **Fig. 8.38** Cache valley virus–induced stillbirth and malformation. The newborn lamb's limbs are fixed in flexion (arthrogryposis), as are the vertebra causing axial skeletal deviations (scoliosis and kyphosis). Muscle hypoplasia is visible. (Courtesy Dr. John F. Edwards, College Station, Texas.)

Akabane Virus. Akabane virus, genus Bunyavirus, Simbu serogroup, has been reported in Australia, Japan, South Africa, the Middle East, Argentina, Korea, and other parts of Asia. Akabane virus is rare in North America and may have *Culicoides* and mosquito vectors.[238,394] Like Cache Valley fever virus, gross lesions were most prevalent when sheep were infected during a certain period of fetal development (46–53 days' gestation).[399] Lesions may include skeletal muscle atrophy, degenerative disease of the cerebellum, porencephaly, hydranencephaly, brachygnathism, scoliosis, hypoplasia of lungs or spinal cord, and arthrogryposis.[394] An inactivated vaccine for Akabane virus is licensed for use in Australia and parts of Asia.[238]

Rift Valley Fever Virus. Rift Valley fever virus, genus Phlebovirus, is endemic to the African continent and causes large epizootics involving sheep, goats, cattle, horses, camels, numerous wildlife species, and humans.[400] In recent years, Rift Valley fever virus has jumped international borders into the Middle East and may possess a threat to North American and European agriculture industries.[400] A least six genera of mosquitoes are vectors for transmission.[400] Data from a 2006–2007 Kenyan outbreak indicate that the prevalence and clinical signs of Rift Valley fever in sheep and goats are similar.[400] Infection of naïve populations of sheep results in mortality of young lambs and abortion rates that can reach 100%.[400] Abortion is usually caused by maternal fever, with minimal evidence of fetal infection.[401] The virus less commonly causes multifocal necrosis of in numerous fetal organs, including extensive hepatic necrosis and necrotizing placentitis. Septic metritis may follow abortion.[401] The Smithburn strain of Rift Valley fever is reported to cause hydrops amnion, arthrogryposis, and hydranencephaly.[400] A modified live virus is available but may cause fetal malformations in sheep and goats.[238]

Nairobi Sheep Disease Virus. The Nairobi Sheep Disease virus, genus Nairovirus, family is a zoonotic tick transmitted agent endemic to East and Central Africa and elsewhere.[401] Ganjam virus historically endemic to India has been recently shown through S-RNA sequence to be an Asian variant of Nairobi Sheep Disease virus.[402] The virus causes acute gastritis, resulting in up to 90% mortality but may also cause abortions related to disease in the dam.[403]

Family Flaviviridae

Border Disease Virus. Border disease virus (BDV), genus Pestivirus, family *Flaviviridae*, is the causative agent of "hairy shaker disease" in lambs. It was originally described from the border region between England and Wales.[394] BDV causes abortion and congenital abnormalities of sheep in North America, Britain,

Australia, New Zealand, and possibly other areas.[235,315] Infection in goats is increasingly recognized and they appear equally affected when infected experimentally.[239,394] Bovine viral diarrhea virus is a closely related pestivirus that also causes "border disease" in sheep and goats. It has been estimated that economic losses caused by BDV can be as great as 20% in some flocks at initial outbreak.[404]

Pathogenesis. The ewe is infected by ingesting or inhaling the virus secreted from the placenta, saliva, urine, or feces of a persistently infected sheep or newborn. Persistently infected cattle, goats, and deer may also infect sheep.[394] Persistently infected ewes have reduced fertility but are capable of reproducing lambs that are also persistently infected.[394] Viremia ensues for 7 days. If a pregnant ewe is infected before day 85 of gestation, her fetuses are aborted, macerated, or mummified. Surviving lambs may have demyelination of the cerebellum and dysplasia of hair follicle epithelial cells and are termed "hairy shakers."[394] Lambs that survive in utero infection may be born persistently infected. Lambs infected after 85 days of gestation may be born normal, weak, or stillborn and be negative for the virus or have viral antibody titers.[235]

Clinical Signs and Pathology. Signs of infection include increased numbers of open females, mummified or macerated fetuses, stillbirths, and weak lambs with hairy fleece and tremors.[315] Fetal anomalies include cerebellar hypoplasia, hydranencephaly, porencephaly, and arthrogryposis.[394] The hairy fleece of affected lambs is usually darkly pigmented and most prominent around the head and shoulder.[235] These "hairy shaker" lambs tend to grow poorly and may develop polyarthritis and have shortened facial and long bones.[239] Cotyledons are small or dysmature, with area of pinpoint grayish necrosis.

Diagnosis. The virus can usually be isolated from fetal blood (buffy coat).[235] Antigen capture ELISA can be performed on serum of sheep over 2 months old.[239]

Prevention. All animals suspected of infection should be culled. Any replacement lambs should be screened (by BDV titers and/or viral isolation) before they are added to the flock.[235] Any flock additions should be quarantined for 30 days and tested for the presence of this and other diseases before being placed into the flock. Cattle and sheep should be separated, and the use of common water sources should be minimized. Modified live cattle vaccines should be avoided. The use of killed vaccines for BDV in cattle provides minimal cross-protection.[239]

Wesselsbron Virus. Wesselsbron virus, genus Flavivirus, family *Flaviviridae*, is a zoonotic agent that is endemic to the southern African continent, with serologic evidence of presence in Southeast Asia. Wesselsbron district is in South Africa. However, the primary vectors are mosquitoes of *Aedes* genus transmission from aerosols produced from infected tissues may occur.[405] Sheep appear to be the most sensitive ruminant to the virus, with death in newborn lambs and abortion.[406] Sick lambs may have neurologic signs and the placenta may have hydrops amnion. Antibodies may be detected with hemagglutination inhibition test but later developed ELISA test are more sensitive.[407] An attenuated live vaccine is available but may cause abortion if administered during pregnancy.[238,406]

Family Reoviridae; Bluetongue Virus. Blue tongue virus, genus Orbivirus, family *Reoviridae*, has at least 25 serotypes and occurs throughout tropical, subtropical, and some temperate regions of the world, where it causes disease in fine-wooled and mutton breeds of sheep.[408] The virus is noncontagious and seasonal epizootics are variable and controlled by environmental factors affecting populations or transport of the primary vector, *Culicoides* spp. gnat (or midge) and viral replication within reservoir host, cattle, and other ruminants.[408] This virus is noted for genetic variability caused by genetic drift of individual gene segments and reassortment of gene segments within a host or vectors infected with more than one strain.[394] Recently, the virus has had incursion into Northern latitudes and numerous authors speculate that this is associated with global climate change.[394]

Clinical Signs and Pathology. Infected ewes may become febrile; have vascular endothelial damage that results in a swollen tongue, ears or face; exhibit an ulcerated or crusting oral or nasal mucosa (catarrhal stomatitis and rhinitis); and develop dyspnea secondary to pulmonary edema and lameness secondary to myositis, laminitis, and coronitis.[235] In sheep that survive, loss of fleece may cause financial loss.[394] Ewes infected during pregnancy produces a wide variety of pathologic responses in the fetus that range from production of a viremic but normal live lamb to fetal death caused by hepatic necrosis and hydranencephaly.[394] Goats are frequently infected in endemic regions as evidenced by serology, but even when exposed to virulent serotypes rarely develop clinical signs.[408]

Diagnosis. Bluetongue viruses can be isolated from the blood, semen, brain, and spleen of aborted fetuses or detected by PCR from various organs. Viral isolation is enhanced if blood is collected during febrile periods. Serology on the dam and fetus may be useful to assess host response.

Prevention. Vaccination against bluetongue is of questionable value because of the large numbers of serovars. Vaccine regiments in endemic areas have been proven to be effective but include multiple injections with numerous serotypes.[394] Live attenuated vaccines may cause fetal deformity and embryonic death. *Culicoides* feed at night during cooler temperatures and breed around damp habitats. Some species reproduce in cattle dung.[394] Housing sheep away from low-lying or damp areas during gnat season and at night and separation of sheep from cattle may reduce risk. Other proven vectors that cause mechanically transmission include argasid ticks, sheep keds *(Melophagus ovinus)* and various mosquitoes but these vectors are thought to be of minor significance in epizootics.[394]

Caprine Herpesvirus 1 (CpHV 1). Caprine herpesvirus 1 (CpHV 1) is an α-herpesvirus that most commonly causes subclinical vulvovaginitis and balanoposthitis in goats.[234] The impact of the virus may be underestimated because of poor knowledge of the infection and difficulties making a diagnosis.[234] When experimentally challenged with CpHV 1, lambs developed minimal clinical signs and recovered while kids developed more severe disease.[264]

Transmission. The virus is likely spread to does by an infected buck.[409] Serologic studies proceeding a herpesvirus abortion storm in Wyoming indicate infection does not reduce reproduction in subsequent breedings.[410]

Clinical Signs and Pathology. Occasionally the virus may be more virulent or present in naïve populations, resulting in abortion storms and death in 1- to 2-week-old kids.[411] Experimental studies in naïve does confirm that CpHV 1 may cause abortion 10 to 60 days after inoculation.[234] Progression of the disease and gross and microscopic findings from the aborted fetus are similar to α-herpesvirus infection in other species. Aborted fetuses may be autolyzed, but placental lesions may be minimal.[411] Lungs, liver, kidneys, and adrenal glands of aborted fetuses may have pinpoint white foci that are represented by randomly distributed areas of coagulative necrosis[409,411] (Figure 8.39). Microscopically,

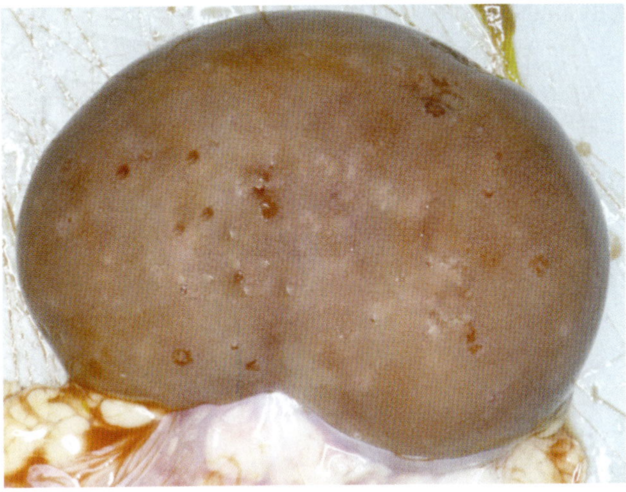

• **Fig. 8.39** Caprine Herpesvirus abortion. The pale white foci on the surface of the kidney are areas of necrosis. (Courtesy Dr. Francisco Uzal, San Bernardino, California.)

cells surrounding areas of necrosis may have intranuclear inclusion bodies.[409] Placental lesions may be mild or minimal.

Diagnosis. Virus isolation may be unsuccessful from vaginal swabs, aborted fetus, and weak kids.[234] Often, the virus is most detectable by PCR on fresh liver, lung, or spleen.[234] If fresh tissues are not available, PCR is possible but less sensitive on paraffin-embedded tissue.[411] Test validation is limited by the availability of positive controls.

Prevention. A noncommercial inactivated CpHV 1 vaccine has been shown to be protective.[412] Goats develop good humoral immunity and do not abort in the following kidding season.[412]

Zoonosis. Prior to initiating examination of an aborted fetus or placenta, the practitioner and farm owner should evaluate potential exposure to abortifacient zoonotic agents. While these agents may be ever-present in the environment or in animals, concentration of microorganisms in infected placental membranes of fetal tissues makes this an important time to be vigilant. Pregnant women, persons with cancer, and those who are immune-suppressed are at increased risk of zoonotic infection and should avoid handling aborted fetuses and placentas. Personal protective gear such as gloves, disposable rectal sleeves, respirators, and boots should be worn and appropriately cleansed or disposed of after necropsy.[239] Contaminated clothing and boots should be banned from human living quarters.[239] Although cytologic examination of fresh placental smears is widely discussed, these techniques are difficult to interpret and increase risk of human exposure to pathogens. Isolation of aborting animals will not only protect other sheep by may also limit human exposure to agents. Most bacterial diseases associated with abortion in sheep and goats have some potential for zoonotic transmission but vary widely in virulence to humans. Agents like *B. melitensis* and *Salmonella* Brandenburg are easily contracted from infected tissues while the risk of acquiring *L. interrogans* or *L. monocytogenes* at necropsy is minimal.[338,413,414] Knowledge of pathogens expected to cause abortion, their clinical signs and gross lesions, and potential risk to humans is probably the veterinarian's best defense.

B. melitensis, the causative agent of goat transmitted "Malta fever," is the most common species of *Brucella* infecting humans and is the most common zoonotic pathogen reemerging worldwide.[414] While France, Israel, and most of Latin America have gained control of brucellosis, the disease persists in the Mediterranean countries, North Africa, the Middle East and India.[415] It is an often unrecognized and uncontrolled public health problem in many developing countries.[415,416] Farmers face risk of clinical disease as well as economic impact from reproductive losses, eradication programs, and import/export restrictions. Clinical symptoms in humans include undulant fever, arthritis, hepatosplenomegaly, lymphadenopathy, epididymo-orchitis, liver abscesses, spondylitis, osteomyelitis, paravertebral abscess, and abortion.[417–420] Contact with placental and fetal tissues and consuming unpasteurized goat milk or cheese and under cooked meat are the most widely implicated in transmission to humans.[237,238,415] Crushing the umbilical cord of newborn lambs and kids with the teeth as practiced by some is implicated in transmission. *B. ovis* is not considered a zoonotic disease risk.[413]

Control measures to prevent human infection by *C. burnetii* causing "Q fever" are difficult to apply because ruminants may maintain a nonsymptomatic carrier state and the organism may be aerosolized on particles and is persistent in the environment.[305] Sheep manure used as garden fertilizer has been implicated as a source of human infection by *C. burnetii*.[312] Inhalation of aerosols and contaminated dust is the primary mode of human infection. The majority of human cases have a history of being in contact with epizootics in sheep, goats, or cattle.[308] *C. burnetii* may also be contracted by ingestion of nonpasteurized milk or consumption of goat cheese manufactured with nonpasteurized milk.[239,314] Clinical symptoms in humans includes influenza-like symptoms, undulant fever, myalgia, atypical pneumonia, hepatitis, endocarditis, premature delivery, repeated abortions, post–Q fever fatigue syndrome, and possible death in immunocompromised individuals.[235,300,302,312] People with heart valve lesions are at increased risk for developing Q fever, and endocarditis is the most common chronic form of the disease.[301] Abattoir workers in Australia are vaccinated, and vaccination may be the prevention method of choice for other high-risk groups such as farm workers, researchers, and veterinarians. In multiple surveys of the general population, farmers and stock breeders had the highest seropositivity.[421] In response to a human Q fever epidemic, the Netherlands enacted restrictions on manure spreading 3 months following detection of *C. burnetii* on a farm and mandatory vaccination of small ruminants.[301,305]

Infection by *C. abortus* in pregnant women may begin acute influenza-like symptoms and result in abortions or stillbirths.[279,422,423] *C. abortus* is capable of causing renal failure, hepatic dysfunction, disseminated intravascular coagulation, and death in humans.[279] Although most cases of zoonosis caused by bacteria in the order *Chlamydiales* are attributed to *C. abortus*, it should be noted that *P. acanthamoebae* and *Chlamydophila psittaci* are both zoonotic risks and have also been identified from small ruminants.[278]

C. jejuni is the most common cause of human bacterial gastroenteritis in the industrialized worldwide. Although disease may be caused by sheep strains, contaminated poultry produce is the major source of human infection.[424] Domestic animals and unpasteurized milk are thought to be sources of *C. jejuni* infection in human beings. Shepherds giving artificial resuscitation to infected lambs have reportedly acquired *C. jejuni*.[320] Although *C. fetus* subspecies *fetus* is rarely associated with human disease, most cases appear to involve direct contact with livestock.[425–427] At least 13 cases of *C. fetus* subsp. *fetus* abortion and fetal sepsis have been reported in humans.[428] *Salmonella* can cause abdominal pain, severe diarrhea, chronic enteritis, abortion, and death in human beings. During an outbreak of *Salmonella* Brandenburg in New Zealand, a spike in the numbers of human cases paralleled abortions observed in sheep. Agriculture workers, including two veterinarians, and families on affected farms were thought to have contracted the disease from aborted sheep.[338] *F. tularensis*, an agent endemic to North America and Eurasia, is capable of producing abortion storms in range sheep and may be contracted by contact with animal carcasses.[371,429] Clinical signs of Tularemia in humans include ulcerative dermatitis, lymphadenopathy, septicemia, and death. *Yersinia pseudotuberculosis* and *Y. enterocolitica* may cause mesenteric lymphadenitis, resulting in fever, anorexia, vomiting, and diarrhea in humans.[233] *T. gondii* can cause encephalitis or blindness in human fetuses infected in utero and death in AIDS patients. Approximately 30% of adults in the United States have antibodies to *T. gondii*.[235] Most cases of toxoplasmosis are contracted after drinking raw goat milk and undercooked meat.[377] Consumption of nonpasteurized goat and sheep milk is of particular concern in human infants.[377] *T. gondii* in aborted tissues probably possess the greatest risk for unborn children or immunosuppressed individuals.

Most viral diseases associated with abortions in sheep and goats are not zoonotic. Rift Valley fever virus, however, causes a limiting febrile illness in most infected people.[400] One to two percent of people who contract Rift Valley fever may develop hepatitis, encephalitis, retinitis, blindness, and hemorrhagic syndrome, resulting in death of 10 to 20% of hospitalized patients.[400] Zoonosis from Rift Valley fever was originally recognized in veterinarians and assistants who performed necropsies or obstetrics on infected animals. The 2000 epizootic in Saudi Arabia and Yemen resulted in thousands of human infections and at least 245 deaths.[400] Wesselsbron disease virus is endemic to the southern African continent and may be transmitted from aerosols produced from infected tissues handled during an abortion necropsy.[430]

Acknowledgments

The authors would like to acknowledge Dr. John Roberts (Auburn University College of Veterinary Medicine, Auburn, Alabama) for his significant contributions to the Theriogenology chapter, specifically the Abortion and Perinatal Death section.

References

1. Beckett SD, Wolfe DF: Anatomy of the penis, prepuce, and sheath. In Wolfe DF, Moll HD, editors: *Large animal urogenital surgery,* ed 2, Baltimore, 1998, Williams & Wilkins.
2. Heath AM, Purohit RC: Anatomy of the scrotum, testes, epididymis, and spermatic cord (bulls, rams, and bucks). In Wolfe DF, Moll HD, editors: *Large animal urogenital surgery,* ed 2, Baltimore, 1998, Williams & Wilkins.
3. Ashdown RR, Hancock JL: Functional anatomy of male reproduction. In Hafez ESE, editor: *Reproduction in farm animals,* ed 4, Philadelphia, 1980, Lea and Febiger.
4. Pineda MH, Faulkner LC: The biology of sex. In McDonald LE, editor: *Veterinary endocrinology and reproduction,* ed 3, Philadelphia, 1980, Lea and Febiger.
5. Jainudeen MR, H Wahid, ESE Hafez: Sheep and goats. In Hafez ESE, Hafez B, editors: *Reproduction in farm animals*, ed 7, Maryland, 2000, Lippincott, Williams, and Wilkins.
6. Price EO, Borgwardt R, Dally MR: Heterosexual experience differentially affects the expression of sexual behavior in 6- and 8-month old ram lambs, *Appl Anim Behav Sci* 46:193, 1996.
7. Fitzgerald J, Morgan G: Reproductive physiology of the ram. In Youngquist RS, editor: *Current therapy in large animal theriogenology,* Philadelphia, 2007, WB Saunders.
8. Nett TM: Controlling seasonal reproduction: emphasis on the male, *proceedings of the society for theriogenology,* 1991, Nashville, TN.
9. Smith MC, Sherman DM: *Goat medicine,* Philadelphia, 1994, Lea and Febiger.
10. Goyal HO, Memon MA: Clinical reproductive anatomy and physiology of the buck. In Youngquist RS, editor: *Current therapy in large animal theriogenology,* Philadelphia, 2007, WB Saunders.
11. Hill J: Goat reproductive management, *proceedings of the symposium on health and diseases of small ruminants,* Nashville, TN, 1996, American Association of Small Ruminant Practice.
12. Wilddeus S: Reproductive management for meat goat production, *proceedings of the southeast region meat goat producers symposium,* Tallahassee, FL, 1998, Florida A & M University.
13. Hewitt DG: *Biology and management of white-tailed deer*, Boca Raton, FL, 2011, CRC Press.
14. Burfening PJ, Rossi D: Serving capacity and scrotal circumference of ram lambs as affected by selection for reproductive rate, *Small Rumin Res* 9:61, 1992.
15. Goyal HO, Memon MA: Clinical reproductive anatomy and physiology of the buck. In Youngquist RS, Threllfall WR, editors: *Current therapy in large animal theriogenology*, ed 2, Philadelphia, 2007, WB Saunders, pp 511–514.
16. Fitzgerald JA, Perkins A, Hemenway K: Relationship of sex and number of siblings in utero with sexual behavior of mature rams, *Appl Anim Behav Sci* 38:283, 1993.
17. Grotelueschen DM, Doster AR: Reproductive problems in rams, *NebGuide* (http://www.ianr.unl.edu), Lincoln, NE, 2000, Cooperative Extension, University of Nebraska.
18. Fitzgerald J, Morgan M: Reproductive physiology of the ram. In Youngquist RS, editor: *Current therapy in large animal theriogenology,* Philadelphia, 2007, WB Saunders.
19. Katz LS: Sexual performance tests in sexually inexperienced rams. In Dziuk PJ, Wheeler M, editors: *Handbook of methods for study of reproductive physiology in domestic animals,* Urbana, IL, 1991, University of Illinois.
20. Fitzgerald J, Perkins A: Serving capacity tests for rams. In Dziuk PJ, Wheeler M, editors: *Handbook of methods for study of reproductive physiology in domestic animals,* Urbana, IL, 1991, University of Illinois.
21. Perkins A, Fitzgerald JA, Price EO: Sexual performance of rams in serving capacity tests predicts success in pen breeding, *J Anim Sci* 70(9):2722, 1992.
22. Fitzgerald JA, Perkins A: Ram sexual performance: a relationship with dam productivity, *Sheep Res J* 7(1):7, 1991.
23. Yarney TA, Sanford LM: Pubertal development of ram lambs: physical and endocrinological traits in combination as indices of postpubertal reproductive function, *Theriogenology* 40(4):735, 1993.
24. Kimberling CV, Marsh DJ: Breeding soundness evaluation and surgical sterilization of the ram. In Youngquist RS, editor: *Current therapy in large animal theriogenology,* Philadelphia, 2007, WB Saunders.
25. DC Van Metre, Rao S, Kimberling CV, Morley PS: Factors associated with failure in breeding soundness examination of Western USA rams, *Prev Vet Med* 105:118–126, 2012.
26. Bulgin MS: Ram breeding soundness examination and SFT form, Nashville, *proceedings of the society for theriogenology,* 1992, Nashville, TN.
27. Pugh DG: Examination of the ram for breeding soundness, *Proc Hudson-Walker Therio Conf* 7:19, 1996.
28. Carson RL, Powe TA, Pugh DG et al: Examination and special procedures of the scrotum and testes. In Wolfe D, Moll HD, editors: *Large animal urogenital surgery,* Baltimore, 1997, Williams & Wilkins.
29. Pugh DG: Breeding soundness examination in male goats, *Proc Hudson-Walker Therio Conf* 7:29, 1996.
30. Memon MA, Mickelsen WD, Goyal HO: Examination of the reproductive tract and evaluation of potential breeding soundness in the

buck. In Youngquist RS, editor: *Current therapy in large animal theriogenology,* Philadelphia, 2007, WB Saunders.

31. Kimberling CV, Parsons GA: Breeding soundness evaluation and surgical sterilization of the ram. In Youngquist RS, Threlfall WR, editors: *Current therapy in large animal theriogenology,* ed 2, St. Louis, MO, Saunders Elsevier, 2007.
32. Kimberling CV, Parsons GA: Breeding soundness evaluation and surgical sterilization of the ram. In Youngquist RS, editor: *Current therapy in large animal theriogenology,* Philadelphia, 2007, WB Saunders.
33. Mobini S: Reproductive management in goats, *Proceedings of the North American Veterinary Conference,* vol 14, 2000, Orlando, FL.
34. Kimberling CV: Disease of rams. In Kimberling CV, editor: *Diseases of sheep,* ed 3, Philadelphia, 1988, Lea and Febiger.
35. Bulgin MS: *Brucella ovis* epizootic in virgin ram lambs, *J Am Vet Med Assoc* 196(7):1120, 1990.
36. Saunders VF, Reddacliff LA, Berg T, Hornitzky M: Multiplex PCR for the detection of *Brucella ovis, Actinobacillus seminis* and *Histophilus somni* in ram semen, *Aust Vet J* 85:72–77, 2007.
37. Carrera-Chávez JM, Quezada-Casasola A, Pérez-Eguia E, et al: Sperm quality in naturally infected rams with *Brucella ovis, Small Rumin Res* 144:220–224, 2016.
38. Marín CM, Jiménez de Bagués MP, Blasco JM, Gamazo C, Moriyón I, Díaz R: Comparison of three serological tests for *Brucella ovis* infection of rams using different antigenic extracts, *Vet Rec* 125(20):504–508, 1989.
39. Ridler AL, Smith SL, West DM: Seroconversion and semen shedding in rams experimentally infected with *Brucella ovis, N Z Vet J* 62(1):47–50, 2014.
40. Ridler AL, West DM: Control of *Brucella ovis* infection in sheep, *Vet Clin North Am Food Anim Pract* 27(1):61–66, 2011.
41. Xavier MN, Silva TM, Costa EA, et al: Development and evaluation of a species-specific PCR assay for the detection of *Brucella ovis* infection in rams, *Vet Microbiol* 145:158–164, 2010.
42. Manterola L, Tejero-Garcés A, Ficapal A, et al: Evaluation of a PCR test for the diagnosis of *Brucella ovis* infection in semen samples from rams, *Vet Microbiol* 92:65–72, 2003.
43. Kimberling CV: Sheep flock fertility, *proceedings of the society for theriogenology,* 1990, Nashville, TN.
44. Bulgin MS: Epididymitis caused by *B. ovis, proceedings of the society for theriogenology,* 1991, Nashville, TN.
45. O'Brien MP, Beja-Pereira A, Anderson N, et al: Brucellosis transmission between wildlife and livestock in the Greater Yellowstone Ecosystem: inferences from DNA Genotyping, *J Wildlife Dis* 53(2): 339–343, 2017.
46. Ridler AL, West DM, Stafford KJ, Wilson PR, Fenwick SG: Transmission of *Brucella ovis* from rams to red deer stags, *N Z Vet J* 48:57–59, 2000.
47. Mobini S, Heath AA, Pugh DG: Chapter 6. Theriogenology of sheep and goats. In Pugh DG, editor: *Sheep and goat medicine,* ed 1, WB Saunders Co, Philadelphia, 2002, pp 129–196.
48. Ferreras MC, Muñioz M, Pérez V, et al: Unilateral orchitis and epididymitis caused by *Salmonella enterica* subspecies diarizonae infection in a ram, *J Vet Diagn Invest* 19(2):194–197, 2007.
49. Walker RL, Leamaster BR: Prevalence of *Histophilus ovis* and *Actinobacillus seminis* in the genital tract of sheep, *Am J Vet Res* 47:1928, 1986.
50. Bulgin MS: Ram lamb epididymitis, *proceedings of the society for theriogenology,* 1991, Nashville, TN.
51. Al-Katib WA, Dennis SM: Early sequential findings in the genitalia of rams experimentally infected with *Actinobacillus seminis, N Z Vet J* 56(2):50–54, 2008.
52. Ley WB: Ram epididymitis, *Agri-Pract* 14(5):34, 1993.
53. Bruer AN: Examination of the ram for breeding soundness. In Morrow DA, editor: *Current therapy in theriogenology,* ed 2, Philadelphia, 1986, WB Saunders.
54. Pugh DG: Breeding soundness evaluation in male goats, *Proc Hudson-Walker Therio Conf* 7:29, 1996.
55. Mickelsen WD, Memon MA: Infertility and diseases of the reproductive organs of bucks. In Youngquist RS, editor: *Current therapy in large animal theriogenology,* Philadelphia, 2007, WB Saunders.
56. Ahmad N, Noakes DE, Middleton DJ: Use of ultrasound to diagnose testicular degeneration in a goat, *Vet Rec* 132(17):436–439, 1993.
57. Ott RS, Memon MA: Breeding soundness examinations of rams and bucks, a review, *Theriogenology* 13:155, 1980.
58. Smith KC, Brown PJ, Morris J, Parkinson TJ: Cryptorchidism in North Ronaldsay sheep, *Vet Rec* 161:658–659, 2007.
59. Skinner JD, Van Heuden JAH, Goris EJ: A note on cryptorchidism in Angora goats, *S Afr J Anim Sci* 20:10, 1961.
60. Riddell MG: Developmental anomalies of the scrotum and testes. In Wolfe D, Moll HD, editors: *Large animal urogenital surgery,* Baltimore, 1997, Williams & Wilkins.
61. Basrur PK, Kochhar HS: Inherited sex abnormalities in goats. In Youngquist RS, Threlfall WR, editors: *Current therapy in large animal theriogenology,* Philadelphia, 2007, WB Saunders.
62. Smith MC, Sherman DM: *Goat medicine,* Philadelphia, 1994, Lea and Febiger.
63. King WW, Young ME, Fox ME: Multiple congenital genitourinary anomalies in a polled goat, *Contemp Top Lab Anim Sci* 41(5):39–42, 2002.
64. Smith KC, Brown P, Parkinson TJ: Hypospadias in rams, *Vet Rec* 158(23):789 795, 2006.
65. Fuller DT, Baird AN, Morris EL, Kraemer DC: What is your diagnosis? Hypospadias and urethral diverticulum, *J Am Vet Assoc* 201:1431–1432, 1992.
66. Loste A, Ramos JJ, García L, Ferrer LM, Verde MT: High prevalence of ulcerative posthitis in Rasa Aragonesa rams associated with a legume-rich diet, *J Vet Med A Physiol Pathol Clin Med* 52(4): 176–179, 2005.
67. Barina V, Kuchtik J: Evaluation of fibre diameter, length and mohair production in mohair goats and castrates, *Acta Univeritatis Agriculturae et Silviculturae Mendelianae Brunensis* 48(3):13–17, 2000.
68. Mourad M, Gbanamou G, Balde IB: Carcass characteristics of West African dwarf goats under extensive system, *Small Rumin Res* 42(1):83–86, 2001.
69. Tesfaye K, Tesfaye L, Hunduma D, Mieso G, Amsalu S: Growth performance and carcass characteristics of Arsi-Bale goats castrated at different ages, *J Cell Anim Biol* 2:(11):187–194, 2008.
70. Okeudo NJ, Moss BW: Production performance and meat quality characteristics of sheep comprising four sex-types over a range of slaughter weights produced following commercial practice, *Meat Sci* 80(2):522–528, 2008.
71. Koyuncu M, Duru S, Uzun SK, Ozis S, Tuncel E: Effect of castration on growth and carcass traits in hair goat kids under a semi-intensive system in the south-Marmara region of Turkey, *Small Rumin Res* 72(1):38–44, 2007.
72. Bani Ismail ZA, Al-Zghoul MF, Al-Majali AM, Khraim NM: Effects of castration on penile and urethral development in Awassi lambs, *Bulg J Vet Med* 10(1):29–34, 2007.
73. Baird AN, Wolfe DF: Castration of the normal male. In Wolfe DF, Moll HD, editors: *Large animal urogenital surgery,* ed 2, Baltimore, 1999, Williams & Wilkins.
74. Scott PR: Husbandry. In Scott PR, editor: *Sheep medicine,* London, 2007, Manson Publishing Ltd.
75. Matthews J: Surgical techniques. In Matthews J: *Diseases of the goat,* ed 3, Chelmsford, 2009, Blackwell Publishing Ltd.
76. Bonelli P, Dimauro C, Pau S, Dattena M, Mollica A, Nicolussi PS: Stress responses in lambs castrated with three different methods, *Ital J Anim Sci* 7(2):207–217, 2008.
77. Melches S, Mellema SC, Doherr MG, Wechsler B, Steiner A: Castration of lambs: a welfare comparison of different castration techniques in lambs over 10 weeks of age, *Vet J* 173(3):554–563, 2007.
78. Stoffel MH, Rotz A von, Kocher M, Merkli M, Boesch D, Steiner A: Histologic assessment of testicular residues in lambs and calves after Burdizzo castration, *Vet Rec* 164(17):523–528, 2009

79. Fazili MR, Bhattacharyya HK, Buchoo BA, Kirmani MA, Darzi MM, Khan I: Evaluation of pinhole castration technique in rams, *Small Rumin Res* 84(1-3):61–64, 2009.
80. Okwee-Acai J, Olet S, Ojok L, Acon J: An evaluation of non-surgical castration by single intratesticular injection of lactic acid in adult Mubende goats, *Bull Anim Health Prod Africa* 56(2): 116–124, 2008.
81. Awal MA, Rahman MM, Das SK, Siddiki NH, Kurohmaru M, Bibin AB: Formalin affects the male reproduction of black Bengal goats during prepubertal stage even at low concentration, *J Med Sci (Pakistan)* 4(1):84–89, 2004.
82. Oyeymi MO, Akusu MO: Short-term effect of hemi-orchectomy on testicular and ejaculate characteristics of West African Dwarf bucks, *Small Rumin Res* 31(1):75–78, 1999.
83. Riddell MG: Developmental anomalies of the scrotum. In Wolfe DF, Moll HD, editors: *Large animal urogenital surgery*, ed 2, Baltimore, 1999, Williams & Wilkins.
84. Matthews J: Male infertility. In Matthews J, editor: *Diseases of the goat*, ed 3, Chelmsford, 2009, Blackwell Publishing Ltd.
85. Rutherford DJ, Fnding E: Laparoscopic castration in a cryptorchid pygmy goat, *Vet Rec* 165(1):27–28, 2009.
86. Wolfe DF: Surgical preparation of estrus-detector males. In Wolfe DF, Moll HD, editors: *Large animal urogenital surgery*, ed 2, Baltimore, 1999, Williams & Wilkins.
87. Gouletsou PG, Galatos AD, Fthenakis GC: Clinical, ultrasonographic and pathologic features following unilateral vasectomy in rams, *Anim Reprod Sci* 103(1-2):52–68, 2008.
88. Batista M, Prats N, Calero P, et al: Semen characteristics and plasma levels of testosterone after bilateral vasectomy in bucks, *Reprod Domest Anim* 37(6):375–378, 2002.
89. Janett F, Hüssy D, Lischer C, Hässig M, Thun R: Semen characteristics after vasectomy in the ram, *Theriogenology* 56(3):485–491, 2001.
90. Goodard PJ: Castration. In Alexander TL, Buxton D, editors: *Management and diseases of deer*, ed 2, London, 1994, The Veterinary Deer Society.
91. Heath AM, Pugh DG, Edens MS: Urogenital surgery in goats, In Youngquist RS, Threlfall WR, editors: *Current therapy in large animal theriogenology*, ed 2, Philadelphia, 2007, WB Saunders.
92. Evans G: Freezing sheep semen. In Dziuk PJ, Wheeler M, editors: *Handbook of methods for study of reproductive physiology in domestic animals,* Urbana, IL, 1991, University of Illinois Press.
93. Buckrell, BC, et al: Artificial insemination of small ruminants. American College of Theriogenologi and Society for Theriogenology—Short Ruminant Course 87–94, 1994.
94. Mobini S, Heath AM, Pugh DG: Chapter 6. Theriogenology in Sheep and Goats. In Pugh DG, editor: *Sheep and goat medicine*, Philadelphia, 2002, WB Saunders, pp 129–186.
95. Lymberopoulos AG, Tsakmakidis IA, Khalifa TA: Effect of ram age on structural and functional competence of frozen-thawed spermatozoa in dairy sheep, *Reprod Domest Anim* 45(4):572–578, 2010.
96. Evans G, Maxwell WMC: *Salmon's artificial insemination of sheep and goats,* Sydney, 1987, Butterworth Publishing.
97. Buckrell BC, et al: Reproductive technologies in commercial use for sheep, goats, and farmed deer, *Proceedings of the Society for Theriogenology,* 1997, Nashville, TN.
98. Mylne MJA, Hunton JR, Buckrell BC: Artificial insemination of sheep. In Youngquist RS, editor: *Current therapy in large animal theriogenology,* Philadelphia, 1997, WB Saunders.
99. Shipley CFB, Buckrell BC, Mylne MJA, et al: Artificial insemination and embryo transfer in sheep, Youngquist RS, Threlfall WR, editors: *Current therapy in large animal theriogenology*, Philadelphia, 2007, WB Saunders, pp 629–641.
100. Xu CL, Zhou JB, Zhao BT, et al: Liquid storage of goat semen in chemically defined extenders, *Reprod Domest Anim* 44:771–778, 2009.
101. Cehmineau P, Caignie Y, Guerin Y, et al: *Training manual on artificial insemination in sheep and goats*, Rome, 1991, FAO of the United Nations.
102. Leboeuf B, Restall B, Salamon S: Production and storage of goat semen for artificial insemination, *Anim Reprod Sci* 62:113–141, 2000.
103. Nuti L: Techniques for artificial insemination of goats. In Youngquist RS, Threlfall WR, editors: *Current therapy in large animal theriogenology*. Philadelphia, 2007, WB Saunders, pp 529–534.
104. Bag S, Joshi A, Naqvi SM, Rawat PS, Mittal JP: Effect of freezing temperature, at which straws were plunged into liquid nitrogen, on the post-thaw motility and acrosomal status of ram spermatozoa, *Anim Reprod Sci* 72:175–183, 2002.
105. Chenoweth PJ, Pretzer S, Samper J, Shipley C: *Committee report: proposed minimum standards for frozen semen.* Society for Theriogenology.
106. Buckrell BC: *Guelph system for transcervical AI (user manual),* Georgetown, Ontario, Canada, Small Ruminant Genetics.
107. Marshall CE: Handling of frozen semen straws. In Dziuk PJ, Wheeler M, editors: *Handbook of methods for study of reproductive physiology in domestic animals,* Urbana, IL, 1991, University of Illinois Press.
108. Stewart JL, Shipley CF, Katich AS, et al: Cryopreservation of white-tailed deer (*Odocoileus verginianus)* semen using soybean-, liposome-, and egg yolk-based extenders, *Anim Reprod Sci* 171: 7–16, 2016.
109. Mukasa-Mugerwa E, Kasali OB, Said AN: Effect of nutrition and endoparasitic treatment on growth, onset of puberty and reproductive activity in Menz ewe lambs, *Theriogenology* 36:319, 1991.
110. Forcada F, Abecia JA, Zarazaga L: A note on attainment of puberty of September-born early-maturing lambs in relation to level of nutrition, *Anim Prod* 53:407, 1991.
111. McCann MA, Goode L, Harvey RW, Caruolo EV, Mann DL: Effect of rapid weight gain to puberty on reproduction, mammary development and lactation in ewe lambs, *Theriogenology* 32:55, 1989.
112. Kassem R, Owen JB, Fadel I: The effect of pre-mating nutrition and exposure to the presence of rams on the onset of puberty in Awassi ewe lambs under semi-arid condition, *Anim Prod* 48:393, 1989.
113. Rajkumar RR, Argo CM, Rodway RG: Effect of melatonin on pulsatilla release of luteinizing hormone in female lambs, *Horm Metab Res* 24:229, 1992.
114. Fitzgerald JA, Butler WR: Sexual maturation of ewes raised without ram exposure in a controlled lighting environment, *Theriogenology* 29:811, 1988.
115. Kennaway DJ et al: Pituitary response to LHRH, LH pulsability and plasma melatonin and prolactin changes in ewe lambs treated with melatonin implants to delay puberty, *J Repro Fert* 78:137, 1986.
116. Nowak R, Rodway RG: Effect of intravaginal implants of melatonin on the onset of ovarian activity in adult and prepubertal ewes, *J Reprod Fertil* 74:287, 1985.
117. Sunderland SJ, O'Callaghan D, Boland MP, Roche JF: Effect of photoperiod before and after birth on puberty in ewe lambs, *Biol Reprod* 53:1178, 1995.
118. Meridith S, Kiesling DO: Age of puberty in ewes which developed prenatally with either a ram or a ewe fetus, *Small Rumin Res* 20:137, 1996.
119. Kinder JE, Bergfeld EG, Wehrman ME, Peters KE, Kojima FN: Endocrine basis for puberty in heifers and ewes, *J Reprod Fertil Suppl* 49:393, 1995.
120. Rawlings NC, Bartlewski PM: Clinical reproductive physiology in ewes. In Youngquist RS, editor: *Current therapy in large animal theriogenology,* Philadelphia, 2007, WB Saunders.
121. Sweeny T, O'Callaghan D: Physiology of seasonal reproductive transitions in the ewe—regulation by photo period and other environmental cues, *Repro Domestic Anim* 30:178, 1995.
122. O'Callaghan D, et al: Role of short days in timing of onset and duration of reproductive activity in ewes under artificial photoperiods, *Bio Repro* 44:23, 1991.

123. Karsch FJ, Dahl GE, Evans NP, et al: Seasonal changes in gonadotropin-releasing hormone secretion in the ewe: alteration in response to the negative feedback action of estradiol, *Bio Repro* 49:1377, 1993.
124. Barrell GK, Moenter SM, Cahaty A, Karsch FJ: Seasonal changes of gonadotropin-releasing hormone secretion in the ewe, *Bio Reprod* 46:1130, 1992.
125. Keisler DH: Endocrine control of reproduction in the ewe and ram: a review. Small ruminant short course, *Proceedings of the Society for Theriogenology,* 1994, Nashville, TN, p 2.
126. Spencer TE, Becker WC, George P, Mirando MA, Ogle TF, Bazer FW: Ovine interferon-tau regulates expression of endometrial receptors for estrogen and oxytocin but not progesterone, *Bio Reprod* 53:732, 1995.
127. Smith MC: Clinical reproductive physiology and endocrinology of does. In Youngquist RS, editor: *Current therapy in large animal theriogenology,* Philadelphia, 2007, WB Saunders.
128. Hill J: Goat reproductive management, *proceedings of the symposium on health and disease of small ruminants, American association of small ruminant practice,* 1996, Nashville, TN, p 114.
129. Mobini S: Reproductive management in goats, *Proceedings of the North American Veterinary Conference,* vol 14, 2000, Orlando, FL, p 219.
130. Wilddeus S: Reproductive management for meat goat production, *proceedings of the southeast region meat goat production symposium,* Tallahassee, FL, 1996, Florida A & M University.
131. Fetet A, Pellicer-Rubio M, Leboeuf B: Reproductive cycle of goats, *Ani Reprod Sci* 124:211–219, 2011.
132. Rowe JD: Reproductive management of sheep and goats, *proceedings of the annual meeting of the American veterinary medicine association,* 1998, Schaumburg, IL, p 616.
133. Wheaton JE, Carlson KM, Windels HF, Johnston LJ: CIDR: a new progesterone releasing intravaginal device for induction of estrous and cycle control in sheep and goats, *Anim Reprod Sci* 33:127, 1993.
134. Bulgin MS: Increasing reproductive performance of the ewe flock, *Proceedings of the society for theriogenology,* 1990, Nashville, TN, p 244.
135. Quispe T, Zarco L, Valencia J, Ortíz A: Estrus synchronization with melengestrol acetate in cyclic ewes. Insemination with fresh or frozen semen during the first or second estrus post treatment, *Theriogenology* 41:1385, 1994.
136. Cushwa WT, Bradford GE, Stabenfeldt GH, Berger YM, Dally MR: Ram influence on ovarian and sexual activity in anestrous ewes: effects of isolation of ewes from rams before joining and date of ram introduction, *J Anim Sci* 70:1195, 1992.
137. Perkins A, Fitzgerald JA: The behavioral component of the ram effect: the influence of ram sexual behavior on the induction of estrus in anovulatory ewes, *J Anim Sci* 72:51, 1994.
138. Haresign W: Manipulation of reproduction in sheep, *J Reprod Fertil Suppl* 45:127, 1992.
139. Unferfeld R, Clemente N, Bonjour L, Orihuela A: Equine chorionic gonadotrophin administration to rams improves their effectiveness to stimulate anoestrous ewes (the "ram effect"), *Anim Reprod Sci* 149:194–198, 2014.
140. Romano JE, Alkar A, Amstalden M: Onset of luteolytic action of exogenous prostaglandinF-2α during estrous cycle in goats, *Theriogenology* 92:45–50, 2017.
141. Vilariño M, Cuadro F, Dos Santos-Neto PC, García-Pintos C, Menchaca A. Time of ovulation and pregnancy outcomes obtained with the prostaglandin-based protocol Synchrovine for FTAI in sheep, *Theriogenology* 90:163–168, 2017.
142. Rowe JD, East NE: Reproductive management—estrous cycles, synchronization, artificial insemination, pregnancy diagnosis: small ruminants for the mixed practitioner, *proceedings of the western veterinary conference,* 1998, Las Vegas, NV, p 137.
143. Thomas DL: Improving reproductive performance of sheep through selection, *proceedings of the society for theriogenology,* 1996, Nashville, TN, p 178.
144. Robinson JJ: Embryo survival in the sheep, *proceedings of the society for theriogenology,* 1995, Nashville, TN, p 270.
145. Fitch GQ: *A breeding program for fall lambing,* OSU extension facts, no. 3801, Stillwater, OK, 2000, Cooperative Extension Service, Oklahoma State University.
146. Keisler DH: Sheep breeding strategies. In Youngquist RS, editor: *Current therapy in large animal theriogenology,* Philadelphia, 2007, WB Saunders.
147. Goyal HO, Memon MA: Clinical reproductive anatomy and physiology of the buck. In Youngquist RS, Threlfall WR, editors: *Current therapy in large animal theriogenology,* ed 2, Philadelphia, 2007, WB Saunders, pp 511–514.
148. Alford A, Strickland J: *Meat goat production in Georgia,* Athens, GA, 1998, UGA Extension Bulletin.
149. Nuti L: Chapter 68. Techniques for artificial insemination of goats. In Youngquist RS, Threfall WR, editors: *Current therapy in large animal theriogenology,* ed 2, Philadelphia, 2007, WB Saunders, pp 529–534.
150. Karaca F, Tasal I, Alan M: Preliminary report on induction of estrus with multiple eCG injections in colored Mohair goats during the anestrus season, *Anim Reprod Sci* 114:306–310, 2009.
151. Shipley CF, Buckrell BC, Mylne MJA, et al: Chapter 86. Artificial insemination and embryo transfer in sheep. In Youngquist RS, Threfall WR, editors: *Current therapy in large animal theriogenology,* ed 2, Philadelphia, 2007, WB Saunders, pp 629–641.
152. Deligiannis C, Valasi I, Rekkas CA, et al: Synchronization of ovulation and fixed time intrauterine insemination in ewes, *Reprod Domest Anim* 40:6–10, 2005.
153. Holtz W, Sohnrey B, Gerland M, Driancourt MA: Ovsynch synchronization and fixed-time insemination in goats, *Theriogenology* 69:785–792, 2008.
154. Mobini, S: Reproductive management in goats, *proceedings of the North American veterinary conference,* vol 14, 2000, Orlando, FL, p 219.
155. Karatzas G, Karagiannidis A, Varsakeli K, Brikas P: Fertility of fresh and frozen-thawed goat semen during the nonbreeding season, *Theriogenology* 48:1049, 1997.
156. Moses D, Martínez AG, Iorio G, et al: A large-scale program in laparoscopic intrauterine insemination with frozen-thawed semen in Australian Merino sheep in Argentine Patagonia, *Theriogenology* 48:651, 1997.
157. Mobini S, Heath AM, Pugh DG: Chapter 6. Theriogenology in sheep and goats, In Pugh DG, editor: *Sheep and goat medicine,* Philadelphia, 2002, WB Saunders, pp 129–186.
158. Mylne MJA, Hunton JR, Buckrell BC: Artificial insemination of sheep. In Youngquist RS, editor: *Current therapy in large animal theriogenology,* Philadelphia, 1997, WB Saunders.
159. Buckrell B, et al: Reproductive technologies in commercial use for sheep, goats, and farmed deer, *proceedings of the society for theriogenology,* 1997, Nashville, TN, p 185.
160. Evans G, Maxwell WMC: *Salmon's artificial insemination of sheep and goats,* Sydney, 1987, Butterworth Publishers.
161. Chemineau P, Caignie Y, Guerin Y, et al: *Training manual on artificial insemination in sheep and goats,* Rome, 1991, FAO of the United Nations.
162. Paulenz H, Söderquist L, Adnøy K, et al: Effect of cervical and vaginal insemination with liquid semen stored at room temperature on fertility of goats, *Anim Reprod Sci* 86:109–117, 2005.
163. Wulster-Radcliffe MC, Lewis GS: Development of a new transcervical artificial insemination method for sheep: effects of a new transcervical artificial insemination catheter and traversing the cervix on semen quality and fertility, *Theriogenology* 58:1361–1371, 2002.
164. Halbert GW, Walton JS, Buckrell BC: Evaluation of a technique for transcervical artificial insemination of sheep, *proceedings of the society for theriogenology,* 1990, Nashville, TN, p 293.
165. Sohnrey B, Holtz W: Technical note: transcervical deep cornual insemination of goats, *J Anim Sci* 83:1543–1548, 2005.

166. Eppleston J, Maxwell WM: Sources of variation in the reproductive performance of ewes inseminated with frozen-thawed ram semen by laparoscopy, *Theriogenology* 43:777, 1995.
167. Anel L, Kaabi B, Alvarez M, et al: Factors influencing the success of vaginal and laparoscopic artificial insemination in churra ewes: a field assay, *Theriogenology* 63:1235–1247, 2005.
168. Buckrell BC, Pollard J: Embryo transfer in sheep. In Youngquist RS, editor: *Current therapy in large animal theriogenology,* Philadelphia, 1997, WB Saunders.
169. Scudamore CL, Robinson JJ, Aitken RP, Kennedy DJ, Ireland S, Robertson IS: Laparoscopy for intrauterine insemination and embryo recovery in superovulated ewes at a commercial embryo transfer unit, *Theriogenology* 35:329, 1991.
170. Ishwa AK, Memon MA: Embryo transfer in sheep and goats: a review, *Small Rumin Res* 19:35, 1996.
171. Hill J: Maximizing the results of goat embryo transfer programs, *proceedings of the American association of small ruminant practitioners, research symposium on health and disease,* 1996, Nashville, TN, p 120.
172. Husein MQ, Bailey MT, Ababneh MM, Romano JE, Crabo BG, Wheaton JE: Effect of eCG on the pregnancy rate of ewes transcervically inseminated with frozen-thawed semen outside the breeding season, *Theriogenology* 49:997, 1998.
173. Wallace JM, Milne, Aitken RP: Effect of weight and adiposity at conception and wide variations in gestational dietary intake on pregnancy outcome and early postnatal performance in young adolescent sheep, *Biol Reprod* 82:320–330, 2010.
174. Li QY, Guan H, An XR, Chen YF: Technical note: transfer of ovine embryos through a simplified mini-laparotomy technique, *J Anim Sci* 86:3224–3227, 2008.
175. Pereira RJ, Sohnrey B, Holtz W: Nonsurgical embryo collection in goats treated with prostaglandin F2alpha and oxytocin, *J Anim Sci* 76:360, 1998.
176. Melican D, Gavin W: Repeat superovulation, non-surgical embryo recovery, and surgical embryo transfer in transgenic dairy goats, *Theriogenology* 69:197–203, 2008.
177. Flohr SF, Wulster-Radcliffe MC, Lewis GS: Technical note: development of a transcervical oocyte recovery procedure for sheep, *J Anim Sci* 77:2583–2586, 1999.
178. Agrawal KP, Goel AK, Tyagi S: Successful non-surgical embryo recovery from a goat, *Indian J Exp Biol* 29:1144, 1991.
179. Rowe JD: Reproductive management in sheep and goats, *proceedings of the American association of small ruminant practitioners, research symposium on health and disease,* 1998, Nashville, TN, p 39.
180. Keskintepe L, Darwish GM, Kenimer AT, Brackett BG: Term development of caprine embryos derived from immature oocytes in vitro, *Theriogenology* 42:527, 1994.
181. Samake S, Amoah EA, Mobini S, et al: In vitro fertilization of goat oocyte during the nonbreeding season, *Small Rumin Res* 35:49, 2000.
182. Keskintepe L, Simplicio AA, Brackett BG: Caprine blastocyst development after in vitro fertilization with spermatozoa frozen in different extenders, *Theriogenology* 49:1265, 1998.
183. Leoni GG, Berlinguer F, Succu S, et al: A new selection criterion to assess good quality ovine blastocysts after vitrication and to predict their transfer into recipients, *Mol Reprod Dev* 75:373–382, 2008.
184. Cognié Y, Baril G, Poulin N, Mermillod P: Current status embryo techniques in sheep and goats, *Theriogenology* 59:171–188, 2003.
185. Baldassarre H, Karatzas CN: Advanced assisted reproduction technologies (ART) in goats, *Anim Reprod Sci* 82–83:255–266, 2004.
186. Cran DG: XY sperm separation and use in artificial insemination and other ARTs, *Soc Reprod Fertil Suppl* 65:475–491, 2007.
187. Rowe JD, East NE: Reproductive management—Part I: estrous cycles, synchronization, artificial insemination, pregnancy diagnosis, *small ruminants for the mixed animal practitioner western veterinary conference,* 1998, Las Vegas, NV, p 137.
188. Mastas D: Pregnancy diagnosis in goats. In Youngquist RS, Threlfall WR, editors: *Current therapy in large animal theriogenology,* ed 2, Philadelphia, 2007, WB Saunders, pp 547–554.
189. Amer HA: Ultrasonographic assessment of early pregnancy diagnosis, fetometry and sex determination in goats, *Anim Reprod Sci* 117:226–231, 2010.
190. Haibel GK: Use of ultrasonography in reproductive management of sheep and goat herds, *Vet Clin North Am: Food Anim Pract* 6:597, 1990.
191. Mialot, JP, Levy I, Emery P: Echographie et gestion des troupeaux, *Rec Med Vet* 168:399–406, 1991.
192. Haibel GK: Real-time ultrasonic fetal head measurement and gestational age in dairy goats, *Theriogenology* 30:1053–1057, 1988.
193. Haibel GK, Perkins NR, Lidl GM: Breed differences in biparietal diameters of second trimester Toggenbubrg, Nubian and Angora goat fetuses, *Theriogenology* 32:827–834, 1989.
194. Hamilton RJ, Tobin ML, Moore WG: Aging fetal white-tailed deer, *Proc Annu Conf, SE Assn Fish Wildl Agen* 39:389–395, 1985.
195. Neto LM, Santos MH, Filho CR, et al: Reliability of ultrasound for early sexing of goat fetuses derived from natural mating and from fresh, frozen and vitrified embryo transfer, *Reprod Fertil Dev* 22(2):489–493, 2010.
196. Santos MH, Moraes EP, Bezerra FQ, et al: Early fetal sexing of Saanen goats by use of transrectal ultrasonography to identify the genital tubercle and external genitalia, *Am J Vet Res* 68:561–564, 2007.
197. Bürstel D, Meinecke-Tillman S, Meinecke B: Ultrasonographic diagnosis of fetal sex in small ruminants bearing multiple fetuses, *Vet Rec* 151:635–636, 2002.
198. Thomas JO: Survey of the causes of dystocia in sheep, *Vet Rec* 127:574, 1990.
199. Menzies PI: Lambing management and neonatal care. In Youngquist RS, Threlfall WR, editors: *Current therapy in large animal theriogenology,* Philadelphia, 2007, WB Saunders.
200. Peters AR, Dent CN: Induction of parturition in sheep using dexamethasone, *Vet Rec* 131:128, 1992.
201. Owens JL, Bindon BM, Edey TN, Piper LR: A note on the effects of dexamethasone-induced parturition on ewe behavior and lamb survival in prolific Booroola Merino ewes, *Anim Sci* 41:417, 1985.
202. Özalp RG, Yavuz A, Orman A, et al: Parturition induction in ewes by a progesterone receptor blocker, aglepristone, and subsequent neonatal survival: preliminary results, *Theriogenology* 87:141–147, 2017.
203. Rowe JD: Reproductive management of sheep and goats. *Proceedings of the American association of small ruminant practitioners, research symposium on health and disease,* 1998, Nashville, TN, p 39.
204. Brawn W: Parturition and dystocia in the goat. In Youngquist RS Threllfall WR, editors: *Current therapy in large animal theriogenology,* Philadelphia, 2007, WB Saunders.
205. Majeed AF, Taha MB: Preliminary study on treatment of ringwomb in Iraqi goats, *Anim Repro Soc* 18:1999, 1989.
206. Alan M, Taşal I: Efficacy of prostaglandin F2alpha and misoprostol in the induction of parturition in goats, *Vet Rec* 150:788–789, 2002.
207. Brounts SH, Hawkins F, Baird AN, Glickman LT: Outcome and subsequent fertility of sheep and goats undergoing cesarean section because of dystocia: 110 cases (1981–2001), *J Am Vet Med Assoc* 224(2):275–279, 2004.
208. Veksler Hess J, Decaminada E, Carcagno A, et al: Post caesarian reproductive performance of ewes, *Revista Brasileira de Reproducao Animal* 25(3):343–344, 2001.
209. Makawi SA, Badawi ME: Effect of Caesarean section (C.S) on uterine aerobic bacteria and post-partum period in Nubian goats, *J Anim Vet Adv* 6(3):375–378, 2007.
210. Clarke I, Heasman L, Symonds ME: Influence of maternal dexamethasone administration on thermoregulation in lambs delivered by caesarean section, *J Endocrinol* 156(2):307–314, 1998.
211. Bulgin M: Diseases of the periparturient ewe. In Youngquist RS, Threlfall WR, editors: *Current therapy in large animal theriogenology,* Philadelphia, 2007, WB Saunders.
212. Scott PR, Sargison ND, Penny CD, Strachan WD: The use of combined xylazine and lignocaine epidural injection in ewes with vaginal or uterine prolapses, *Theriogenology* 43:1175, 1995.

213. Rowe JD: Reproductive management—Part III. Small ruminants for the mixed animal practitioner, *small ruminants for the mixed animal practitioner western veterinary conference,* 1998, Las Vegas, NV, p 147.
214. Braun W: Periparturient infection and structural abnormality. In Youngquist RS, Threlfall WR, editors: *Current therapy in large animal theriogenology,* Philadelphia, 2007, WB Saunders.
215. Pugh DG, Hardin DK: Ovine uterine rupture, *Agri-Pract* 7:15, 1986.
216. Kampen KR, Ellis LC: Prolonged gestation in ewes ingesting *Veratrum californicum: morphological changes and steroid biosynthesis in the endocrine organs of cyclopic lambs, J Endocrin* 52:549, 1972.
217. James LF: Teratological research at the USDA-ARS poisonous plant research laboratory, *J Nat Toxins* 8:63, 1999.
218. James LF: Effect of locoweed feeding on fetal lamb development, *Can J Comp Med* 40:380, 1976.
219. Putman MR: Toxicologic problems in livestock affecting reproduction, *Vet Clin North Am: Food Anim Pract* 5:325, 1989.
220. Porter JK, Thompson FN: Effects of fescue toxicosis on reproduction in livestock, *J Anim Sci* 70:1594, 1992.
221. Roberts SJ: *Veterinary obstetrics and genital diseases (theriogenology),* North Pomfret, VT, 1986, David and Charles.
222. Aiken GE, Flythe MD, Kagan IA, Ji H, Bush LP: Mitigation of ergot vasoconstriction by clover isoflavones in goats (*Capra hircus*), *Front Vet Sci* 3:17, 2016.
223. Adams NR: Organizational and activational effects of phytoestrogens on the reproductive tract of the ewe, *Proc Soc Exp Biol Med* 208:87, 1995.
224. Smith MC, Sherman DM. Reproductive system. In Smith MC, Sherman DM, editors: *Goat medicine,* Ames, IA, 2009, Wiley-Blackwell.
225. Braun W: Noninfectious infertility in the doe. In Youngquist RS, Threlfall WR, editors: *Current therapy in large animal theriogenology,* Philadelphia, 2007, WB Saunders.
226. Hesselink JW: Hydrometra in dairy goats: reproductive performance after treatment with prostaglandins, *Vet Rec* 133(8):186–187, 1993.
227. Lyngset O: Studies on reproduction in the goat. V. Pathological conditions and malformations of the genital organs of the goat, *Acta Vet Scand* 9:364, 1968.
228. DeWalque J: Tumeur ovarienne et masculinization chez une chamoisee de Alpas, *Annales de Med Vet* 322, 1963.
229. Lofstedt RM, Williams R: Granulosa cell tumor in a goat, *J Am Vet Med Assoc* 189:206, 1986.
230. Gardner RB, Alcaraz A, Porter BF, Divers TJ: Udder development, lactation and ascites in a ewe with an ovarian granulosa cell tumour, *Aust Vet J* 83(8):486–488, 2005.
231. "Deleted in review as the 232 reference was repeated in 233"
232. Riddell MG: Ovariectomy. In Wolfe DF, Moll HD, editors: *Large animal urogenital surgery,* Baltimore, 1999, Williams & Wilkins.
233. Heath AM, Pugh DG, Edens MS: Urogenital surgery in goats, In Youngquist RS, Threlfall WR, editors: *Current therapy in large animal theriogenology,* ed 2, Philadelphia, 2007, WB Saunders.
234. Padula AM: The freemartin syndrome: an update, *Anim Reprod Sci* 87(1–2):93–109, 2005.
235. Givens MD, Marley MS: Infectious causes of embryonic and fetal mortality, *Theriogenology* 70:270, 2008.
236. Tempesta M, Camero M, Sciorsci RL, et al: Experimental infection of goats at different stages of pregnancy with Caprine herpes virus 1, *Comp Immunol Microbiol Infect Dis* 27:25, 2004.
237. Menzies PI, Miller R: Abortion in sheep: diagnosis and control. In Youngquist RS, Threlfall WR editors: *Current therapy in large animal theriogenology,* ed 2, St. Louis, 2007, WB Saunders.
238. Smith MC: Some clinical aspects of caprine reproduction, *Cornell Vet* 68(Suppl 7):200, 1978.
239. Smith MC: Causes and diagnosis of abortion in goats. In Morrow DA, editor: *Current therapy in theriogenology,* ed 2, Philadelphia, 1986, WB Saunders.
240. Smith MC, Sherman DM: Reproductive system. In Smith MC, Sherman DM editors: *Goat medicine,* ed 2, Ames, 2009, Wiley-Blackwell.
241. Menzies PI: Control of abortion in sheep and goats, *world veterinary congress,* Vancouver, 2008, British Columbia.
242. Kirkbride CA: Examination of Bovine and Ovine Fetuses, *Vet Clin North Am Food Anim Pract* 2:61, 1986.
243. Sivachelvan MN, Ali MG, Chibuzo GA: Foetal age estimation in sheep and goats, *Small Rumin Res* 19:69, 1996.
244. Moeller RB: Causes of caprine abortion: diagnostic assessment of 211 cases (1991–1998), *J Vet Diagn Invest* 13:265, 2001.
245. Kirkbride CA: Diagnoses in 1,784 ovine abortions and stillbirths, *J Vet Diagn Invest* 5:398, 1993.
246. Clark RG, Gill JM, Fairley RA, Smart JA: Abortions in sheep caused by *Salmonella* Brandenburg: pathological findings, *N Z Vet J* 55:356, 2007.
247. Agerholm JS, Boye M, Aalbaek B: Ovine fetal necrobacillosis, *J Comp Pathol* 136:213, 2007.
248. Furlan S, Panter KE, Pfister JA, et al: Fetotoxic effects of locoweed (*Astragalus lentiginosus*) in pregnant goats, In Panter KE, Wierenga TL, Pfister JA editors: *Poisonous plants: global research and solutions,* Wallingford, Oxfordshire, 2007, CABI International.
249. Riet-Correa G, Riet-Correa F, Schild AL, Barros SS, Soares MP: Abortion and neonatal mortality in sheep poisoned with *Tetrapterys multiglandulosa, Vet Path* 46:960, 2009.
250. Braun Jr. WF: Noninfectious prenatal pregnancy loss in the doe, In Youngquist RS, Threlfall WR, editors: *Current therapy in large animal theriogenology,* ed 2, St. Louis, 2007, WB Saunders.
251. Roberts SJ: *Veterinary obstetrics and genital diseases (theriogenology),* ed 3, Woodstock, VT, 1986, David and Charles.
252. Pamo ET, Fernand T, Nanda AS, et al: Effects of *Calliandra calothyrsus* and *Leucaena leucocephala* supplementary feeding on goat production in Cameroon, *Small Rumin Res* 65:31, 2006.
253. Knight AP, Stegelmeier BL: Flixweed (*Descurainia sophia*): a goitrogenic plant, In Panter KE, Wierenga TL, Pfister JA editors: *Poisonous plants: global research and solutions,* Wallingford, Oxfordshire, 2007, CABI International.
254. Chanton-Greutmann H, Thoma R, Corboz L, Borel N, Pospischil A: Abortion in small ruminants in Switzerland: investigations during two lambing seasons (1996–1998) with special regard to chlamydial abortions, *Schweiz Arch Tierheilkd* 144:483, 2002.
255. Feinsod FM, Allam I, Ragai A, Saah AJ: Rodenticide-induced signs simulating Rift valley fever in sheep and goats in Egypt, *Vet Rec* 118:270, 1986.
256. Bunch TD, Panter KE, James LF: Ultrasound studies of the effects of certain poisonous plants on uterine function and fetal development in livestock, *J Anim Sci* 70:1639, 1992.
257. Raffi MB, Barros RR, Bragança JF, Rech RR, Oliveira FN, Barros CS: The pathogenesis of reproductive failure induced in sheep by the ingestion of *Ateleia glazioviana, Vet Hum Toxicol* 46:233, 2004.
258. *Pioneer forage manual—a nutritional guide,* Des Moines, 1995, Pioneer Hi-Bred International.
259. Anderson ML, Blanchard PC, Barr BC, Hoffman RL: A survey of causes of bovine abortion occurring in the San Joaquin Valley, California, *J Vet Diagn Invest* 2:283, 1990.
260. East NE: Common infectious conditions, *Small ruminants for the mixed animal practitioner western veterinary conference,* 1998, Las Vegas, NV.
261. Navarro M, Cristofol C, Carretero A, Arboix M, Ruberte J: Anthelmintic induced congenital malformations in sheep embryos using netobimin, *Vet Rec* 142:86, 1998.
262. Middleton HD, Plant JW, Walker CE, Dixon RT, Johns DR: The effects of methyl-5(6)-butyl-2-benzimidazole carbamate (parbendazole) on reproduction in sheep and other animals. 3. Teratological study in ewes in Australia, *Cornell Vet,* 64(Suppl 4):56, 1974.
263. Keiser J, Rinaldi L, Veneziano V, et al: Efficacy and safety of artemether against a natural *Fasciola hepatica* infection in sheep, *Parasitol Res* 103:517, 2008.

264. Braun WF: Manifestations and aberrations of caprine pregnancy, *proceedings of the society for theriogenology,* 1986, Nashville, TN.
265. Bretzlaff K: Problems of reproduction of goats, *proceedings of the small ruminant short course, society for theriogenology,* 1994, Nashville, TN.
266. Berrios PE, McKercher DG, Knight HD: Pathogenicity of a caprine herpesvirus, *Am J Vet Res* 36:1763, 1975.
267. Gatewood DM, Spire MF: *Chlamydial abortion in domestic ruminants, theriogenology fact sheet B-5,* Hastings, NE, 1990, Society for Theriogenology.
268. Everett KD: Chlamydia and Chlamydiales: more than meets the eye, *Vet Microbiol* 75:109, 2000.
269. East NE: Chlamydiosis. In Morrow DA, editor: *Current therapy in theriogenology,* ed 2, Philadelphia, 1986, WB Saunders.
270. Souriau A, Le Rouzic E, Bernard F, Rodolakis A: Differentiation of abortion-inducing and intestinal strains of *Chlamydia psittaci* isolated from ruminants by the microimmunofluorescence test, *Vet Rec* 132:217, 1993.
271. Rocchi MS, Wattegedera S, Meridiani I, Entrican G: Protective adaptive immunity to *Chlamydophila abortus* infection and control of ovine enzootic abortion (OEA), *Vet Microbiol* 135:112, 2009.
272. Bagdonas J, Petkevicius S, Russo P, Pepin M, Salomskas A: Prevalence and epidemiological features of ovine enzootic abortion in Lithuania, *Pol J Vet Sci* 10:239, 2007.
273. Carter GR: *Veterinarian's guide to the laboratory diagnosis of infectious diseases,* Lenexa, KS, 1986, Veterinary Medicine Publishing.
274. Kimberling CV: Diseases of reproduction, *proceedings of the first national sheep reproduction symposium,* Fort Collins, CO, 1989, Colorado State University Press.
275. Schachter J, Banks J, Sugg N, Sung M, Storz J, Meyer KF: Serotyping of *Chlamydia.* I. isolates of ovine origin, *Infect Immun* 9:92, 1974.
276. Parisi A, Fraccalvieri R, Cafiero M, et al: Diagnosis of *Coxiella burnetii*–related abortion in Italian domestic ruminants using single-tube nested PCR, *Vet Microbiol* 118:101, 2006.
277. Pantchev A, Sting R, Bauerfeind R, Tyczka J, Sachse K: Detection of all *Chlamydophila* and *Chlamydia* spp. of veterinary interest using species-specific real-time PCR assays, *Comp Immunol Microbiol Infect Dis* (article in press), 33(6):473–484, 2010.
278. Ruhl S, Goy G, Casson N, et al: *Parachlamydia acanthamoebae* infection and abortion in small ruminants, *Emerg Infect Dis* 14:1966, 2008.
279. Maley SW, Livingstone M, Rodger SM, Longbottom D, Buxton D: Identification of *Chlamydophila abortus* and the development of lesions in placental tissues of experimentally infected sheep, *Vet Microbiol* 135:122, 2009.
280. Longbottom D, Livingstone M: Vaccination against chlamydial infections of man and animals, *Vet J* 171:263, 2006.
281. Timoney JF, Gillespie JA, Scott FW, et al: Chlamydiaceae. In Timoney JF, et al, editors: *Hogan and Bruner's microbiology and infectious diseases of domestic animals,* ed 8, Ithaca, NY, 1988, Comstock Publishing Associates.
282. Storz J: *Chlamydia*-induced diseases of sheep and goats. In Howard JL, editor: *Current veterinary therapy food animal practice,* ed 2, Philadelphia, 1986, WB Saunders.
283. Papp JR, Shewen PE, Thorn CE, Andersen AA: Immunocytologic detection of *Chlamydia psittaci* from cervical and vaginal samples of chronically infected ewes, *Can J Vet Res* 62:72, 1998.
284. Schopf K, Khaschabi D, Dackau T: Outbreak of abortion among goats caused by dual infection with *Coxiella burnetii* and *Chlamydia psittaci, Tierarzll Prax* 19:630, 1991.
285. Hall RF: Infectious abortions in ewes, *Comp Cont Ed Pract Vet* 4:S216, 1982.
286. Storz J: *Chlamydia and Chlamydia induced diseases,* Springfield, IL, 1971, Charles C Thomas.
287. Navarro JA, García de la Fuente JN, Sánchez J, et al: Kinetics of infection and effects on the placenta of *Chlamydophila abortus* in experimentally infected pregnant ewes, *Vet Pathol* 41:498, 2004.
288. Güler L, Hadimli HH, Ergani̇ş O, Ateş M, Ok U, Gündüz K: Field evaluation of a PCR for the diagnosis of chlamydial abortion in sheep, *Vet Rec* 159:742, 2006.
289. Marsilio F, Di Martino B, Di Francesco CE, Meridiani I: Diagnosis of ovine chlamydial abortions by PCR-RFLP performed on vaginal swabs, *Vet Res Commun* 29(Suppl 1):99, 2005.
290. Szeredi L, Bacsadi A: Detection of *Chlamydophila* (*Chlamydia*) *abortus* and *Toxoplasma gondii* in smears from cases of ovine and caprine abortion by the streptavidin-biotin method, *J Comp Pathol* 127:257, 2002.
291. Navarro JA, Ortega N, Buendia AJ, et al: Diagnosis of placental pathogens in small ruminants by immunohistochemistry and PCR on paraffin-embedded samples, *Vet Rec* 165:175, 2009.
292. Ortega N, Navarro JA, Nicolás L, et al: Evaluation of *Chlamydophila abortus* DNA extraction protocols for polymerase chain reaction diagnosis in paraffin-embedded tissues, *J Vet Diagn Invest* 19:421, 2007.
293. Storz J: Chlamydial absorption. In Kirkbride CA, editor: *Laboratory diagnosis of livestock abortion,* ed 3, Ames, IA, 1990, Iowa State University Press.
294. Wilson K, Livingstone M, Longbottom D: Comparative evaluation of eight serological assays for diagnosing *Chlamydophila abortus* infection in sheep, *Vet Microbiol* 135:38, 2009.
295. Hungerford TG: *Diseases of livestock,* ed 9, Sydney, 1990, McGraw-Hill.
296. Mobini S: Infectious causes of abortion in the goat, *proceedings of the international goat producers symposium,* Tallahassee, FL, 1990, Florida, A & M University Press.
297. Council on Biologics and Therapeutics: Vaccination guidelines for small ruminants, *J Am Vet Med Assoc* 205:1539, 1994.
298. Watson WA: Clinical problems of preventive medicine. The prevention and control of infectious ovine abortion, *Br Vet J* 129:309, 1973.
299. Behymer D, Riemann HP: *Coxiella burnetii* infection (Q fever), *J Am Vet Med Assoc* 194:764, 1989.
300. Miller RB, et al: *Coxiella burnetii* infection in goats. In Morrow DA, editor: *Current therapy in theriogenology,* ed 2, Philadelphia, 1986, WB Saunders.
301. Schimmer B, Dijkstra F, Vellema P, et al: Sustained intensive transmission of Q-fever in the south of the Netherlands, 2009, *Euro surveill* 14(19):19210, 2009.
302. Arricau-Bouvery N, Souriau A, Bodier C, Dufour P, Rousset E, Rodolakis A: Effect of vaccination with phase I and phase II *Coxiella burnetii* vaccines in pregnant goats, *Vaccine* 23:4392, 2005.
303. Sanders DM, Parker JE, Walker WW, Buchholz MW, Blount K, Kiel JL: Field collection and genetic classification of tick-borne Rickettsiae and Rickettsiae-like pathogens from South Texas: *Coxiella burnetii* isolated from field-collected *Amblyomma cajennense, Ann N Y Acad Sci* 1149:208, 2008.
304. Astobiza I, Barandika JF, Hurtado A, Juste RA, García-Pérez AL: Vet J 2010 May; 184(2): 172-175. of *Coxiella burnetii* excretion in a commercial dairy sheep flock after treatment with oxytetracycline, *Vet J* (Article in press) 184(2):172–175, 2010.
305. Rousset E, Berri M, Durand B, et al: *Coxiella burnetii* Shedding routes and antibody response after outbreaks of Q fever-induced abortion in dairy goat herds, *Appl Environ Microbiol* 75:428, 2009.
306. Moore JD, Barr BC, Daft BM, O'Connor MT: Pathology and diagnosis of *Coxiella burnetii* infection in a goat herd, *Vet Pathol* 28:81, 1991.
307. Berri M, Rousset E, Champion JL, Russo P, Rodolakis A: Goats may experience reproductive failures and shed *Coxiella burnetii* at two successive parturitions after a Q fever infection, *Res Vet Sci* 83:47, 2007.
308. Masala G, Porcu R, Sanna G, et al: Occurrence, distribution, and role in abortion of *Coxiella burnetii* in sheep and goats in Sardinia, Italy, *Vet Microbiol* 99:301, 2004.
309. Zeman DH, Steen PL, Peacock MG: Ovine abortion caused by *Coxiella burnetii.* In Kirkbride CA, editor: *Laboratory diagnosis of*

livestock abortion, ed 3, Ames, IA, 1990, Iowa State University Press.

310. Kittelberger R, Mars J, Wibberley G, et al: Comparison of the Q-fever complement fixation test and two commercial enzyme-linked immunosorbent assays for the detection of serum antibodies against *Coxiella burnetii* (Q fever) in ruminants: recommendation for use of serological tests on imported animals in New Zealand, *N Z Vet J* 57:262, 2009.
311. Pape M, Bouzalas EG, Koptopoulos GS, et al: The serological prevalence of *Coxiella burnetii* antibodies in sheep and goats in northern Greece, *Clin Microbiol Infect,* 15(Suppl 2), 146–147, 2009.
312. Berri M, Rousset E, Champion JL, et al: Ovine manure used as a garden fertilizer as a suspected source of human Q fever, *Vet Rec* 153:269, 2003.
313. Rousset E, Durand B, Champion JL, et al: Efficiency of a phase 1 vaccine for the reduction of vaginal *Coxiella burnetii* shedding in a clinically affected goat herd, *Clin Microbiol Infect* 15(Suppl 2):188–189, 2009.
314. Rodolakis A: Q Fever in dairy animals, *Ann N Y Acad Sci* 1166:90, 2009.
315. Fielden ED: Infectious ovine abortion. In Morrow DA, editor: *Current therapy in theriogenology,* Philadelphia, 1986, WB Saunders.
316. Sahin O, Plummer PJ, Jordan DM, et al: Emergence of a tetracycline-resistant *Campylobacter jejuni* clone associated with outbreaks of ovine abortion in the United States, *J Clin Microbiol* 46:1663, 2008.
317. Campero CM, Anderson ML, Walker RL, et al: Immunohistochemical identification of *Campylobacter fetus* in natural cases of bovine and ovine abortions, *J Vet Med B Infect Dis Vet Public Health* 52:138, 2005.
318. Hughes LA, Bennett M, Coffey P, et al: Molecular epidemiology and characterization of *Campylobacter* spp. isolated from wild bird populations in northern England, *Appl Environ Microbiol* 75:3007, 2009.
319. Hedstrom OR, Sonn RJ, Lassen ED, et al: Pathology of *Campylobacter jejuni* abortion in sheep, *Vet Pathol* 24:419, 1987.
320. Anderson KL: Campylobacteriosis. In Morrow DA, editor: *Current therapy in theriogenology,* ed 2, Philadelphia, 1986, WB Saunders.
321. Hirsh DC: Spiral-curved organisms III: *Campylobacter, Arcobacter, Lawsonia.* In Hirsh DA, MacLachlan NJ, Walker RL, editors: *Veterinary microbiology,* ed 2, Awes, Iowa, 2004, Blackwell Publishing.
322. Dennis SM: *Campylobacter* abortion in sheep. In Kirkbride CA, editor: *Laboratory diagnosis of livestock abortion,* ed 3, Ames, IA, 1990, Iowa State University Press.
323. Crawshaw TR, Fuller HE: *Flexispira rappini* suspected in ovine abortion, *Vet Rec* 134:507, 1994.
324. Hänninen ML, Kärenlampi RI, Koort JM, et al: Extension of the species *Helicobacter bilis* to include the reference strains of *Helicobacter* sp. Flexispira taxa 2,3 and 8 and Finnish canine and feline Flexispira strains, *Int J Syst Bacteriol* 55:891, 2005.
325. Meinershagen WA, Frank FW, Waldhalm DG: *Brucella ovis* as a cause of abortion in ewes, *Am J Vet Res* 35:723, 1974.
326. Kahler SC: *Brucella melitensis* infection discovered in cattle for first time, goats also infected, *J Am Vet Med Assoc* 216:648, 2000.
327. Elzer PH, Hagius SD, Davis DS, DelVecchio VG, Enright FM: Characterization of the Caprine model for ruminant brucellosis, *Vet Microbiol* 90:425, 2002.
328. Walker RL: *Brucella.* In Hirsh DA, MacLachlan NJ, Walker RL, editors: *Veterinary microbiology,* ed 2, Awes, Iowa, 2004, Blackwell Publishing.
329. Leal-Klevezas DS, Martínez-Vázquez IO, García-Cantú J, López-Merino A, Martínez-Soriano JP: Use of polymerase chain reaction to detect *Brucella abortus* biovar 1 in infected goats, *Vet Microbiol* 75:91, 2000.
330. Ocholi RA, Kwaga JK, Ajogi I, Bale JO: Abortion due to *Brucella abortus* in sheep in Nigeria, *Rev Sci Tech* 24:973, 2005.
331. Ilhan F, Yener Z: Immunohistochemical detection of *Brucella melitensis* antigens in cases of naturally occurring abortions in sheep, *J Vet Diagn Invest* 20:803, 2008.
332. Muma JB, Samui KL, Siamudaala VM, et al: Prevalence of antibodies to *Brucella* spp. and individual risk factors of infection in traditional cattle, goats and sheep reared in livestock-wildlife interface areas of Zambia, *Trop Anim Health Prod* 38:195, 2006.
333. Al-Talafhah AH, Lafi SQ, Al-Tarazi Y: Epidemiology of ovine brucellosis in Awassi sheep in Northern Jordan, *Prev Vet Med* 60:297, 2003.
334. Nightingale KK, Fortes ED, Ho AJ, Schukken YH, Grohn YT, Wiedmann M: Evaluation of farm management practices as risk factors for clinical listeriosis and fecal shedding of *Listeria monocytogenes* in ruminants, *J Am Vet Med Assoc* 227:1808, 2005.
335. Wiedmann M, Mobini S, Cole JR Jr, Watson CK, Jeffers GT, Boor KJ: Molecular investigation of a listeriosis outbreak in goats caused by an unusual strain of *Listeria monocytogenes, J Am Vet Med Assoc* 215:369, 1999.
336. Gray ML, Singh C, Thorp F Jr: Abortion and pre- or postnatal death of young due to *Listeria monocytogenes.* III. Studies in ruminants, *Am J Vet Res* 17(64):510, 1956.
337. Luque I, Echeita A, León J, et al: Salmonella Indiana as a cause of abortion in ewes: genetic diversity and resistance patterns, *Vet Microbiol* 134:396, 2009.
338. Clark RG, Fenwick SG, Nicol CM, et al: *Salmonella* Brandenburg emergence of a new strain affecting stock and humans in the South Island of New Zealand, *N Z Vet J* 52:26, 2004.
339. Habrun B, Listes E, Spicic S, et al: An outbreak of *Salmonella* Abortusovis abortions in sheep in South Croatia, *J Vet Med B Infect Dis Vet Public Health* 53:286, 2006.
340. Belloy L, Decrausaz L, Boujon P, Hachler H, Waldvogel AS. Vet Microbio. 2009 Sep 18; 138(3-4):373-377.
341. Masala G, Porcu R, Daga C, et al: Detection of pathogens in ovine and Caprine abortion samples from Sardinia, Italy, by PCR, *J Vet Diagn Invest* 19:96, 2007.
342. Cagiola M, Severi G, Forti K, et al: Abortion due to *Salmonella enterica* serovar Abortusovis (*S.* Abortusovis) in ewes is associated to a lack of production of IFN-gamma and can be prevented by immunization with inactivated *S.* Abortusovis vaccine, *Vet Microbiol* 121:330, 2007.
343. Li H, McFarlane RG, Wagner J: Vaccination of pregnant ewes against infection with *Salmonella* Brandenburg, *N Z Vet J* 2005 Dec; 53(6):416-422.
344. Farina R, Cerri D, Renzoni G, et al: *Leptospira interrogans* in the genital tract of sheep. Research on ewes and rams experimentally infected with serovar hardjo (Hardjobovis), *New Microbiol* 19:235, 1996.
345. Dorjee S, Heuer C, Jackson R, et al: Prevalence of pathogenic *Leptospira* spp. in sheep in a sheep-only abattoir in New Zealand, *N Z Vet J* 56:164, 2008.
346. Leon-Vizcaino L, Hermoso de Mendoza M, Garrido F: Incidence of abortions caused by leptospirosis in sheep and goats in Spain, *Comp Immunol Microbiol Infect Dis* 10:149, 1987.
347. Lilenbaum W, de Souza GN, Ristow P, et al: A serological study on *Brucella abortus,* caprine arthritis-encephalitis virus and *Leptospira* in dairy goats in Rio de Janeiro, Brazil, *Vet J* 173:408, 2007.
348. Ellis WA: Leptospirosis as a cause of reproductive failure, *Vet Clin North Am Food Anim Pract* 10:463, 1994.
349. Kirkbride CA, Johnson MW: Serologic examination of aborted ovine and bovine fetal fluids for the diagnosis of border disease, bluetongue, bovine viral diarrhea, and leptospiral infections, *J Vet Diagn Invest* 1:132, 1989.
350. Ruffin DC: Mycoplasma infections in small ruminants, *Vet Clin North Am Food Anim Pract* 17:315, 2001.
351. Manso-Silván L, Vilei EM, Sachse K, Djordjevic SP, Thiaucourt F, Frey J: *Mycoplasma leachii* sp. nov as a new species designation for *Mycoplasma* sp. bovine group 7 of leach, and reclassification of *Mycoplasma mycoides* subsp. *mycoides* LC as a serovar of *Mycoplasma mycoides* subsp. *capri, Int j Syst Evol Microbiol* 59:1353, 2009.

352. Shahram M, Nicholas RA, Wood AP, Kelly DP: Further evidence to justify reassignment of *Mycoplasma mycoides* subspecies *mycoides* large colony type to *Mycoplasma mycoides* subspecies capri, *Syst Appl Microbiol* 33(1):20–24, 2010.
353. Szeredi L, Tenk M, Dán A: 2003. Infection of two goatherds with *Mycoplasma mycoides* subsp. *Capri* in Hungary, evidence of a possible faecal excretion, *J Vet Med B Infect Dis Vet Public Health* 50:172, 2003.
354. Rodriguez JL, Damassa J, Brooks DL: Caprine abortion following exposure to *Mycoplasma capricolum* subsp. *capricolum*, *J Vet Diagn Invest* 8:492, 1996.
355. Doig PA, Ruhnke HL: Isolation of *ureaplasma* from sheep with granular vulvitis, *Vet Rec* 100:179, 1977.
356. Moss TJ, Knox CL, Kallapur SG, et al: Experimental amniotic fluid infection in sheep: effects of *Ureaplasma parvum* serovars 3 and 6 on preterm or term fetal sheep, *Am J Obstet Gynecol* 198:122e1-8, 2008.
357. East NE: Mycoplasmosis. In Morrow DA, editor: *Current therapy in theriogenology*, ed 2, Philadelphia, 1986, WB Saunders.
358. Stuen S: *Anaplasma phagocytophilum*—the most widespread tick-born infection in animal in Europe, *Vet Res Commun* 31(Suppl 1):79, 2007.
359. Garcia-Perez AL, Barandika J, Oporto B, Povedano I, Juste RA: *Anaplasma phagocytophila* as an abortifacient agent in sheep farms from Northern Spain, *Ann N Y Acad Sci* 990:429, 2003.
360. Chianini F, Adams C, Buxton D: Neuropathological changes in ovine fetuse caused by tickborne fever, *Vet Rec* 155:805, 2004.
361. Agerholm JS, Aalbaek B, Fog-Larsen AM, et al: Veterinary and medical aspects of abortion in Danish sheep, *APMIS* 114:146, 2006.
362. Karbe E, Erickson ED: Ovine abortion and stillbirth due to purulent placentitis caused by *Yersinia pseudotuberculosis*, *Vet Pathol* 21:601, 1984.
363. Corbel MJ, Ellis B, Richardson C, Bradley R: Experimental *Yersinia enterocolitica* placentitis in sheep, *Br Vet J* 148:339, 1992.
364. Kirkbride CA, Gates CE, Libal MC: Ovine and bovine abortion associated with *Fusobacterium nucleatum*, *J Vet Diagn Invest* 1:272, 1989.
365. Boye M, Aalbaek B, Agerholm JS: *Fusobacterium necrophorum* determined as abortifacient in sheep by laser capture microdissection and fluorescence in situ hybridization, *Mol Cell Probes* 20:330, 2006.
366. Sargison ND, Howie F, Thomson JR, Dun K, Penny CD: Ovine placentitis and abortion associated with a verotoxigenic strain of *Escherichia coli*, *Vet Rec* 149:711, 2001.
367. Sargison ND, Howie F, Mearns R, Penny CD, Foster G: Shiga toxin-producing *Escherichia coli* as a perennial cause of abortion in a closed flock of Suffolk ewes, *Vet Rec* 160:875, 2007.
368. Dewhirst FE, Fox JG, Mendes EN, et al: '*Flexispira rappini*' strains represent at least 10 Helicobacter taxa, *Int J Syst Evol Microbiol* 50:1781, 2000.
369. Kirkbride CA, Gates CE, Collins JE: Abortion in sheep caused by a nonclassified, anaerobic, flagellated bacterium, *Am J Vet Res* 47:259, 1986.
370. Foster G, Collins MD, Lawson PA, Buxton D, Murray FJ, Sime A: *Actinobacillus seminis* as a cause of abortion in a UK sheep flock, *Vet Rec* 144:479, 1999.
371. O'Toole DO, Williams ES, Woods LW, et al: Tularemia in range sheep: an overlooked syndrome? *J Vet Diagn Invest* 20:508, 2008.
372. Edwards JF, Lassala AL, Spencer TE: *Staphylococcus*-associated abortions in ewes with long-term central venous catheterization, *Vet Pathol* 45:881, 2008.
373. Fthenakis GC, Christodoulopoulos G, Leontides L, Tzora A: Abortion in ewes associated with *Erysipelothrix rhusiopathiae*, *Small Rumin Res* 63:183, 2006.
374. Wohlgemuth K, Kirkbride CA, Bicknell EJ, Ellis RP: Pathogenicity of *Bacillus cereus* for pregnant ewes and heifers, *J Am Vet Med Assoc* 161:1691, 1972.
375. Pier AC, Cysewski SJ, Richard JL: Mycotic abortion in ewes produced by *Aspergillus fumigatus*: intravascular and intrauterine inoculation, *Am J Vet Res* 33:349, 1972.
376. Dubey JP: Toxoplasmosis in goats, *Agri-Pract* 8:43, 1987.
377. Dubey JP: Toxoplasmosis in sheep—the last 20 years, *Vet Parasitol* 163:1, 2009.
378. Morley EK, Williams RH, Hughes JM, et al: Evidence that primary infection of Charollais sheep with *Toxoplasma gondii* may not prevent foetal infection and abortion in subsequent lambings, *Parasitology* 135:169, 2008.
379. Dubey JP: Transplacental toxoplasmosis in goats. In Morrow DA, editor: *Current therapy in theriogenology*, ed 2, Philadelphia, 1986, WB Saunders.
380. Buxton D, Maley SW, Wright SE, Rodger S, Bartley P, Innes EA: *Toxoplasma gondii* and ovine toxoplasmosis: new aspects of an old story, *Vet Parasitol* 149:25, 2007.
381. Obendorf DL, Statham P, Munday BL: Resistance to *Toxoplasma* abortion in female goats previously exposed to *Toxoplasma* infection, *Aust Vet J* 67:233, 1990.
382. Buxton D, Gilmour JS, Angus KW, Blewett DA, Miller JK: Perinatal changes in lambs infected with *Toxoplasma gondii*, *Res Vet Sci* 32:170, 1982.
383. Masala G, Porcu R, Madau L, et al: Survey of ovine and caprine toxoplasmosis by IFAT and PCR assays in Sardinia, Italy, *Vet Parasitol* 117:15, 2003.
384. Dubey JP: Diagnosis of livestock abortion due to *Toxoplasma gondii*. In Kirkbride CA, editor: *Laboratory diagnosis of livestock abortion*, ed 3, Ames, IA, 1990, Iowa State University Press.
385. Kirkbride CA, Dubey JP, Libal MC: Effect of feeding lasalocid to pregnant ewes experimentally infected with *Toxoplasma gondii*, *Vet Parasitol* 44:299, 1992.
386. Dubey JP: Toxoplasmosis, *J Am Vet Med Assoc* 205:1593, 1994.
387. Eleni C, Crotti S, Manuali E, et al: Detection of *Neospora caninum* in an aborted goat foetus, *Vet Parasitol* 123:271, 2004.
388. Lindsay DS, Rippey NS, Powe TA, Sartin EA, Dubey JP, Blagburn BL: Abortions, fetal death, and stillbirths in pregnant pygmy goats inoculated with tachyzoites of *Neospora caninum*, *Am J Vet Res* 56:1176, 1995.
389. Spilovská S, Reiterová K, Kovácová D, Bobáková M, Dubinský P: The first finding of *Neospora caninum* and the occurrence of other abortifacient agents in sheep in Slovakia, *Vet Parasitol* 164:320, 2009.
390. Dubey JP, Speer CA, Fayer R: Sarcocystosis in sheep. In *Sarcocystosis of animals and man*, Boca Raton, Florida, 1989, CRC Press, Inc.
391. Dubey JP: Abortion and death in goats inoculated with *Sarcocystis sporocysts* from coyote feces, *J Am Med Vet Assoc* 178:700, 1981.
392. Goossens B, Osaer S, Kora S: Long-term effects of an experimental infection with *Trypanosoma congolense* on reproductive performance of trypanotolerant Djallonké ewes and West African Dwarf does, *Research in Veterinary Sci* 63:169, 1997.
393. Batista JS, Oliveira AF, Rodrigues CM, et al: Infection by *Trypanosoma vivax* in goats and sheep in the Brazilian semiarid region: from acute disease outbreak to chronic cryptic infection, *Vet Parasitol* 165:131, 2009.
394. Radostits OM, Gay CC, Hinchcliff KW, Constable PC, editors: Diseases associated with viruses and Chlamydia, viral diseases characterized by alimentary tract signs, In: *Veterinary medicine*, ed 10, Philadelphia, 2007, Saunders Elsevier.
395. Campbell GL, Reisdorf ES, Powell JM, et al: Second human case of cache valley virus disease, *Emerg Infect Dis* 12:854, 2006.
396. Edwards JF, Karabatsos N, Collisson EW, de la Concha Bermejillo A: Ovine fetal malformations induced by in utero inoculation with main drain, San Angelo, and LaCrosse viruses, *Am J Trop Med Hyg* 56:171, 1997.
397. Edwards JF, Livingston CW, Chung SI, Collisson EC: Ovine arthrogryposis and central nervous system malformations associated with in utero Cache Valley virus infection: spontaneous disease, *Vet Pathol* 26:33, 1989.
398. Chung SI, Livingston CW Jr, Edwards JF, Gauer BB, Collisson EW: Congenital malformations in sheep resulting from in utero inoculation of Cache Valley virus, *Am J Vet Res* 51:1645, 1990.

399. Parsonson IM, McPhee DA, Della-Porta AJ, McClure S, McCullagh P: Transmission of Akabane virus from the ewe to the early fetus (32 to 53 days), *J Comp Pathol* 99:215, 1988.
400. Bird BH, Ksiazek TG, Nichol ST, Maclachlan NJ: Rift valley fever virus, *J Am Vet Med Assoc* 234:883, 2009.
401. Swanepoel R, Coetzer JAW, Rift Valley fever, In Coetzer JAW, Tustin RC editors: *Infectious diseases of livestock,* ed 2, Cape Town, 2004, Oxford University Press.
402. Marczinke BI, Nichol ST: Nairobi sheep disease virus, an important tick-borne pathogen of sheep and goats in Africa, is also present in Asia, *Virology* 303:146, 2002.
403. Davies FG: Nairobi sheep disease, *Parassitologia* 39:95, 1997.
404. Sharp MW, Rawson BC: The Cost of Border disease infection in a commercial flock, *Vet Rec* 119:128, 1986.
405. Jupp PG, Kemp A: Studies on an outbreak of Wesselsbron virus in the Free State Province, South Africa, *J Am Mosq Control Assoc* 14:40, 1998.
406. Mushi EZ, Binta MG, Raborokgwe M: Wesselsbron disease virus associated with abortions in goats in Botswana, *J Vet Diagn Invest* 10:191, 1998.
407. Williams R, Schoeman M, Van Wyk A, Roos K, Josemans EJ: Comparison of ELISA and HI for detection of antibodies against Wesselsbron disease virus, *Onderstepoort J Vet Res* 64:245, 1997.
408. Maclachan NJ, Drew CP, Darpel KE, Worwa G: The pathology and pathogenesis of Bluetongue, *J Comp Pathol* 141:1, 2009.
409. Uzal FA, Woods L, Stillian M, et al: Abortion and ulcerative posthitis associated with Caprine herpesvirus-1 infection in goats in California, *J Vet Diagn Invest* 16:478, 2004.
410. McCoy MH, Montgomery DL, Bratanich AC, Cavender J, Scharko PB, Vickers ML: Serologic and reproductive findings after a herpesvirus-1 abortion storm in goats, *J Am Vet Med Assoc* 231:1236, 2007.
411. Chénier S, Montpetit C, Hélie P: Caprine herpesvirus- 1 abortion storm in a goat herd in Quebec, *Can Vet J* 45:241, 2004.
412. Tempesta M, Camero M, Greco G, Pratelli A, Martella V, Buonavoglia C: A classical inactivated vaccine induces protection against Caprine herpesvirus 1 infection in goats, *Vaccine* 19:3860, 2001.
413. Acha PN, Szyfres B: Bacterioses. In Acha PN, Szyfres B editors: *Zoonoses and communicable diseases common to man and animals,* ed 2, Washington DC, 1987, Pan American Health Organization.
414. Pappas G, Papadimitriou P, Akritidis N, Christou L, Tsianos EV: The new global map of human brucellosis, *Lancet Infect Dis* 6:91, 2006.
415. Mantur BG, Amarnath SK: Brucellosis in India—a review, *J Biosci* 33:539, 2008.
416. Refai M: Incidence and control of brucellosis in the Near East region, *Vet Microbiol* 90:81, 2002.
417. Chourmouzi D, Boulogianni G, Kalomenopoulou M, Kanellos I, Drevelegas A: Brucella liver abscess; imaging approach, differential diagnosis, and therapeutic management: a case report, *Cases J* 25:7143, 2009.
418. Akritidis N, Tzivras M, Delladetsima I, Stefanaki S, Moutsopoulos HM, Pappas G: The liver in brucellosis, *Clin Gastroenterol Hepatol* 5:1109, 2007.
419. Malavolta N, Frigato M, Zanardi M, et al: Brucella spondylitis with paravertebral abscess due to *Brucella melitensis* infection: a case report, *Drugs Exp Clin Res* 28:95, 2002.
420. Memish ZA, Venkatesh S: Brucellar epididymo-orchitis in Saudi Arabia: a retrospective study of 26 cases and review of the literature, *BJU Int* 88:72, 2001.
421. Pape M, Mandraveli K, Nikolaidis P, Alexiou-Daniel S, Arvanitidou-Vagiona M: Seroprevalence of *Coxiella burnetii* in a healthy population from northern Greece, *Clin Microbiol Infect* 15(Suppl 2): 148–149, 2009.
422. Pospischil A, Thoma R, Hilbe M, Grest P, Gebbers JO: Abortion in woman caused by caprine *Chlamydophila abortus* (*Chlamydia psittaci* serovar 1), *Swiss Med Wkly* 132(5–6):64–66, 2002.
423. Walder G, Hotzel H, Brezinka C, et al: An unusual cause of sepsis during pregnancy: recognizing infection with *Chlamydophila abortus, Obstet Gynecol* 106(5 Pt 2):1215–1217, 2005.
424. Sheppard SK, Dallas JF, MacRae M, et al: Campylobacter genotypes from food animals, environmental sources and clinical disease in Scotland 2005/6, *Int J Food Microbiol* 134:96–103, 2009.
425. Wong PL, Fedder G, Heilmann FG: A man with Campylobacter endocarditis, treatable as *Campylobacter fetus* following identification, *Ned Tijdschr Geneeskd* 147(9):399–403, 2003.
426. Zonios DI, Panayiotakopoulos GD, Kabletsas EO, Tzima EL, Stefanou I, Archimandritis AJ: *Campylobacter fetus* bacteraemia in a healthy individual: clinical and therapeutical implications, *J Infect* 51(4):329–332, 2005.
427. Nadir A, Wright HI, Nadir F, Van Thiel DH: *Campylobacter fetus* presenting as a septic pleural effusion: a case report, *J Okla State Med Assoc* 87(6):267–269, 1994.
428. Fujihara N, Takakura S, Saito T, Iinuma Y, Ichiyama S: A case of perinatal sepsis by *Campylobacter fetus* subsp. fetus infection successfully treated with carbapenem—case report and literature review, *J Infect* 53:e199–e202, 2006.
429. Sjöstedt A: Tularemia: history, epidemiology, pathogen physiology, and clinical manifestations, *Ann N Y Acad Sci* 1105:1–29, 2007.
430. Swanepoel R, Coetzer JAW: Wesselsbron disease, In Coetzer JAW, Tustin RC editors: *Infectious diseases of livestock,* ed 2, Cape Town, 2004, Oxford University Press.

9

Diseases of the Endocrine System

BENJAMIN W. NEWCOMER AND MANUEL F. CHAMORRO

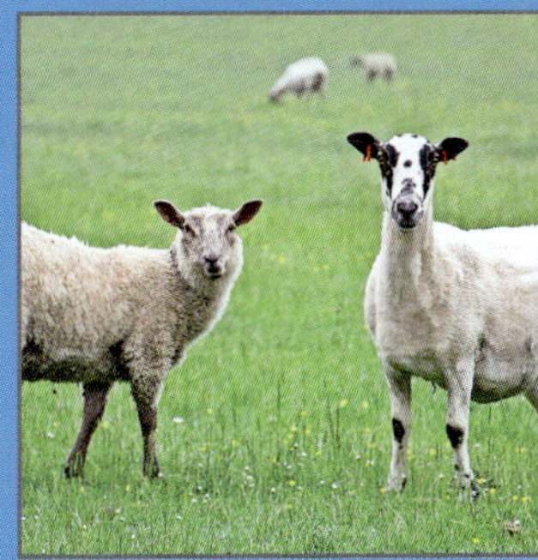

Introduction

The endocrine system facilitates the coordination and regulation of homeostatic and physiologic processes and is integral for normal growth, development, and reproduction. Hormones, the chemical messengers of the body, are generally produced and secreted by the glands of the exocrine system, namely the hypothalamus, pituitary gland, thyroid gland, parathyroid glands, adrenal glands, and pancreas. Endocrinopathies are uncommonly diagnosed in small ruminants (sheep, goats, and cervids) but may be underreported due to their infrequent occurrence and the economic and diagnostic constraints of confirming a presumptive diagnosis. This chapter will review the normal structure, function, and pathology of the major endocrine organs in small ruminants and discuss other common endocrine abnormalities in these species with the aim of assisting the veterinary practitioner in identifying and managing endocrinopathies.

Hypothalamus

The hypothalamus is composed of several nuclei that impart several distinct functions. The hypothalamus lies just ventral to the thalamus at the base of the brain and together they form the diencephalon region of the central nervous system. The functions of the hypothalamus include the regulation of the autonomic nervous system, the control of several physiologic and metabolic processes involved in homeostasis, and the synthesis and secretion of several neurohormones that act on the anterior pituitary gland to inhibit or stimulate the secretion of the pituitary hormones. The hypothalamic neuropeptides are transported to the posterior pituitary gland by axoplasmic flow and then released into the circulatory system. Certain hormones are transported directly from the hypothalamus to the anterior pituitary gland via the hypophyseal portal system.

The primary hypothalamic neuropeptides that act on the anterior pituitary are thyrotropin-releasing hormone (TRH), corticotropin-releasing hormone (CRH), dopamine, growth hormone-releasing hormone (GHRH), gonadotropin-releasing hormone (GnRH), and somatostatin (SS), which is also called growth hormone-inhibiting hormone (Table 9.1). Vasopressin, or antidiuretic hormone, and oxytocin are produced in the hypothalamus and released from the posterior pituitary gland, which is functionally an extension of the hypothalamus. The median eminence forms part of the ventral boundary of the hypothalamus and is the area from which hypothalamic peptides are secreted. The median eminence is connected to the posterior pituitary through the pituitary stalk, alternatively called the infundibulum.

Regulation of the pituitary-hypothalamic unit is complex and involves both central and peripheral regulatory systems. Formation and maturation of the unit begins early in gestation with the median eminence becoming observable as early as on day 48 of gestation in sheep.[1] Likewise, the hypophyseal portal system, the vascular connection between the hypothalamus and anterior pituitary is fully formed by the end of the first trimester of gestation. It is believed that this enables endocrine regulation of development during gestation through direct transport of hypothalamic neuropeptides to the anterior pituitary.

While hypothalamic disorders are rarely diagnosed in small ruminants, a growing understanding of the importance of hypothalamic regulation in the seasonality of reproduction has the potential to influence management procedures in the future.[2,3] Limited understanding of the regulation of reproductive seasonality has prevented the development of therapeutics to influence hypothalamic function, but ongoing research will assist in the development of practical applications to improve reproductive efficiency in sheep, goats, and cervid species.

Pituitary Gland

Structure and Function

The pituitary gland is composed of two distinct parts: the adenohypophysis (anterior pituitary gland) and the neurohypophysis (posterior pituitary). Both parts act as independent organs with different endocrine functions. Embryologically, the adenohypophysis is derived from the invagination of the pharyngeal epithelium *(Rathke's pouch)*, and the neurohypophysis is an extension of the neural tissue from the hypothalamus. Diseases affecting the pituitary gland in small ruminants might result in varied clinical syndromes characterized by generalized endocrine dysfunction and neurological abnormalities.

Anterior Pituitary Gland. The hypothalamic-hypophyseal portal system connects the anterior pituitary gland with the central nervous system (hypothalamus). This network of blood vessels serves as the mechanism by which the hypothalamus regulates the

TABLE 9.1 Hypothalamic Neuropeptides.

Hormone	Abbreviation	Main Function
Corticotropin-releasing hormone	CRH	Stimulation of adrenocorticotropic hormone (ACTH) release from the anterior pituitary
Dopamine	DA	Inhibition of prolactin release from the anterior pituitary
Gonadotropin-releasing hormone	GnRH	Stimulation of luteinizing hormone (LH) and follicle-stimulating hormone (FSH) release from the anterior pituitary
Growth-hormone-releasing hormone	GHRH	Stimulation of growth hormone (GH) release from the anterior pituitary
Oxytocin	OXY	Stimulation of uterine contractions and milk letdown
Somatostatin	SS	Inhibition of growth hormone (GH) release from the anterior pituitary
Thyrotropin-releasing hormone	TRH	Stimulation of thyroid-stimulating hormone (TSH) from the anterior pituitary
Vasopressin (antidiuretic hormone)	ADH, AVP	Increase reabsorption of free water in the renal tubules

function of the anterior pituitary gland. Inhibitory or releasing hypothalamic peptides control the synthesis and release of hormones produced by the anterior pituitary gland. A variety of different glandular cells with different functions composes the anterior pituitary gland. These heterologous populations of cells can synthesize and release the following hormones: thyroid-stimulating hormone (TSH), adrenocorticotropic hormone (ACTH), growth hormone (GH), luteinizing hormone (LH), follicle-stimulating hormone (FSH), and prolactin (PRL).

Thyrotropes in the adenohypophysis secrete TSH, a glycoprotein with two structural subunits, α and β, that stimulates the secretion of the thyroid hormones thyroxine (T_4) and triiodothyronine (T_3). Diseases that affect the pituitary gland can result in secondary hypothyroidism due to reduced secretion of TSH. In contrast, diseases affecting the thyroid gland may result in primary hypothyroidism resulting in inadequate plasma levels of T_3 and T_4 in the presence of high levels of TSH. Excessive TSH release might result in enlargement of the thyroid gland (goiter). Corticotropes secrete ACTH, which stimulates the secretion of glucocorticoids and aldosterone by the adrenal glands. The hypothalamic hormones CRH and arginine vasopressin (AVP) are responsible for the secretion of ACTH by the pituitary gland in cattle and sheep.[4] Stress and painful stimuli increase CRH, AVP, and ACTH secretion. Inadequate function of the hypothalamic/pituitary/adrenal axis has been associated with poor survival rates in systemically ill neonates due to the inability to regulate severe inflammatory responses.[5]

Somatotropes release GH, which is important not only for normal growth and body development in young animals, but also for milk production, fiber production, and reproductive functions in adults. The action of GH is mediated by the somatomedins insulin growth factor I (IGF-I) and insulin growth factor II (IGF-II). These factors play important roles in cell proliferation and prevention of apoptosis. The gonadotropins, FSH and LH, are synthesized by gonadotropes and are responsible for the control of the reproductive cycle in small ruminants.[6] PRL stimulates udder development and lactation and has luteotropic effects. Different from other hormones produced in the adenohypophysis, the regulation of PRL production is not exerted by positive or negative feedback to the hypothalamus, but by dopamine secretion. Plasma levels of PRL vary in photoperiodic seasonal breeders such as small ruminants.[7] PRL levels tend to be greater during the anestrous season of the year and during longest days (May to September). In contrast, during the breeding season (October to February), PRL levels tend to be lower. De novo synthesis of PRL has been reported in mammary gland tissue of sheep and goats during lactation and it has been suggested as a potential cause of inappropriate lactation syndrome in small ruminants.[8]

Posterior Pituitary Gland. Neuronal cell bodies from hypothalamic supraoptic and paraventricular nuclei are neurosecretory and synthetize oxytocin and arginine vasopressin (AVP), also known as antidiuretic hormone (ADH). These hormones migrate from the cell bodies through the neuronal axons (hypothalamic-hypophyseal tract) to the distal nerve endings of the neurohypophysis, where they are stored and ultimately released into general circulation.

The function of ADH is to decrease the excretion of water by the kidneys in cases of plasma hyperosmolarity, hypovolemia, and hypotension. In the distal collecting ducts of the kidneys, ADH increases the permeability to water and allows water to be reabsorbed by expression of aquaporin 2 in the cell membrane, thus increasing plasma volume and decreasing overall osmolarity. Conversely, when the osmolarity of the extracellular fluid decreases, water moves in the opposite direction by osmosis and ADH secretion stops. Other potent stimuli for ADH secretion are hypovolemia and hypotension. Higher levels of ADH have a potent vasoconstrictor effect on peripheral vasculature throughout the body and therefore can increase arterial pressure. In goats, low blood volume due to hemorrhage or severe dehydration can increase the secretion rate of ADH by as high as 100-fold.[9,10] Dysfunction of the neurohypophysis that results in inadequate secretion of ADH leads to neurogenic diabetes insipidus (DI). In contrast, decreased sensitivity of epithelial cells of collecting ducts to ADH is known as nephrogenic DI. This disease is well characterized in humans, dogs, and horses; however, clinical reports of DI in small ruminants are scarce. Clinical signs of neurogenic DI in sheep include marked diuresis, polyuria, and hyposthenuria. Treatment with AVP restores the ability to concentrate the urine. Another report described a case of acquired neurogenic DI in a 7-month-old Suffolk ram with a history of polydipsia and polyuria that failed to concentrate urine in response to water deprivation.[11] The water deprivation test is the diagnostic method of choice for

DI in animals with history of polyuria/polydipsia in absence of dehydration or azotemia. Failure to concentrate urine after water deprivation in well-hydrated animals suggest DI. Nephrogenic DI should be suspected in animals that are still unable to concentrate the urine after treatment with exogenous AVP (desmopressin nasal drops applied topically to the eyes; one drop per eye equivalent to 10 μg/dose from a 0.1 mg/mL solution).[12] Neurogenic DI is rare in large animals, and most cases have been attributed to pituitary neoplasia or encephalitis. Compression of the neurohypophysis by a chromophobe adenocarcinoma of the adenohypophysis was believed to be the cause of neurogenic DI in a 4.5-year-old Black Brown Mountain ram euthanized due to severe DI.[13]

One function of oxytocin is to cause contraction of the myometrium of the uterus during parturition by direct action of the hormone on myoepithelial cells. Additionally, oxytocin plays an important role in lactation by stimulating contraction of myoepithelial cells of the mammary ducts and causing milk ejection. Distention of the reproductive tract during parturition or manipulation of the mammary gland by milking or suckling/nursing activate sensory neurons, inducing release of oxytocin by the neurohypophysis. The induction of uterine contractions by oxytocin aids in the normal expulsion of the fetal membranes and uterine involution. Therefore, pharmacological application of exogenous oxytocin as an ecbolic agent in the treatment of retained fetal membranes and other reproductive diseases is common.

Pituitary Abnormalities

Although diseases affecting the pituitary gland in ruminants are rare, pituitary tumors, including adenomas and carcinomas, and pituitary abscesses have been described.[13-19]

Pituitary Adenoma. The most common pituitary gland neoplasia in domestic animals are adenomas. In sheep and goats, acidophilic adenomas of the anterior pituitary gland have been reported.[14,15] Reports of pituitary neoplasia in cervids currently do not exist. Due to the presence of a restrictive diaphragma sellae around the infundibular stalk in small ruminant species, pituitary adenomas do not grow toward the hypothalamus and remain extradural, compressing adjacent pituitary tissue.[16,17] Some pituitary adenomas in small ruminants might protrude dorsally toward the optic chiasm, erode the sphenoid bone, and cause enlargement of the sella turcica ventrally. Based on current reports of pituitary adenomas in sheep and goats, affected animals are usually adults from 3 to 8 years of age with no apparent breed predisposition. History and clinical signs associated with pituitary adenomas are variable. Abnormal hormone production and/or compression of pituitary tissue can disrupt the regulatory axis between hypothalamus and hypophysis leading to hormonal imbalances and subsequently, to clinical and metabolic abnormalities. While some affected animals may be clinically normal, possible clinical signs include a lack of response to prostaglandin ($PGF2\alpha$) treatment, abnormal mammary development, inappropriate lactation syndrome (ILS), refractory abdominal distention, and neurologic signs. Clinicopathological abnormalities include persistent hypoglycemia, decreased insulin levels, and increased serum PRL concentrations. Acidophil-type cells of pituitary adenomas produce GH and PRL, both of which are lactogenic and can influence glucose metabolism; however, endocrinologically inactive tumors have also been reported.[20] In humans, pituitary adenomas or other pituitary tumors usually result in hypopituitarism. Definitive antemortem diagnostic tests for pituitary neoplasia in small ruminants are currently unavailable, and necropsy and histopathology are necessary to obtain a final diagnosis. However, noninvasive imaging techniques have been used for diagnosis and monitoring of pituitary neoplastic disease in dogs.[21] The pituitary gland can be visualized by contrast-enhanced computer tomography (CT) and magnetic resonance imaging (MRI). Treatment for pituitary adenomas in small ruminants has not been reported. In horses with Cushing disease due to microadenoma or macroadenoma formation in the pituitary pars intermedia, treatment is aimed to reverse or retard hyperplastic growth with dopamine agonists (e.g., pergolide).[22] Functional (disease-inducing) sellar tumors in dogs and cats, including pituitary adenomas, are usually treated medically with radiation therapy, or by surgical excision.

Pituitary Carcinoma. Pituitary carcinomas are rare in small ruminants. Two literature reports have described the clinical presentation of pituitary adenocarcinomas in sheep.[13,19] However, scientific reports of pituitary adenocarcinomas in goats and cervids are currently lacking. In both reports, affected sheep were adults (a 14-year-old ewe and a 4.5-year old ram). The history in both cases included lethargy, decreased appetite, "dog sitting," and neurological signs. Neurologic abnormalities detected during physical examination of both sheep included depression, head pressing, reduced conscious proprioception, wide-based stance, tendency to pace and circle, moderate tetraparesis, hypometria, and absent or reduced pupillary light reflexes (PLRs). One of the sheep had a coexistent intraocular melanoma in addition to the pituitary adenocarcinoma. One sheep had slow spinal reflexes and the other had normal spinal reflexes. Polyuria and polydipsia (PU/PD) in addition to hyposthenuria noticed in one affected sheep indicated neurogenic or nephrogenic DI.[13] Other clinicopathological abnormalities reported in one of the cases included a stress leukogram, azotemia attributed to dehydration, decreased serum calcium and potassium concentrations attributed to decreased food intake, and decreased urine-specific gravity attributed to PU/PD. Compression of the adjacent neural tissue by an expanding and infiltrating pituitary adenocarcinoma leads to a variety of neurological signs such as the signs observed in the affected sheep. The compression of the mass on the posterior pituitary, infundibular stalk, and hypothalamus in one of the cases led to interruption of production, transport, and normal release of ADH, resulting in neurogenic DI and consequently, in signs of PU/PD. The modified water-deprivation test, which could include an additional ADH response test, is the diagnostic method of choice to differentiate neurogenic versus nephrogenic DI. However, rapid deterioration of the small ruminant patients in both reported cases prevented a complete diagnostic workup. Noninvasive imaging techniques such as CT and MRI could be used to evaluate suspected pituitary neoplastic disease as previously mentioned. Definitive diagnosis of pituitary adenocarcinoma in these cases was achieved after postmortem examination and histopathology. Macroscopically, both cases presented as large neoplastic masses replacing the pituitary tissue and compressing adjacent brain structures including the hypothalamus.[13,19] Histopathologically, the masses were composed of pleomorphic cells with variable amounts of eosinophilic cytoplasm and variable nuclei shapes. Areas of necrosis, hemorrhage, and calcified foci were observed internally in both masses. Both masses were diagnosed as pituitary chromophobe adenocarcinomas based on histopathology. Hepatic and intracranial metastasis were reported in one case[13] and no metastases were reported in the other,[19] although coexistence with other primary tumors (ocular melanoma and ovine pulmonary adenocarcinoma) was found in that case. Treatment of pituitary adenocarcinomas in ruminants including cervids has not been reported. In small animals, medical, radiation therapy, and surgical excision of pituitary masses including pituitary adenocarcinomas has been reported.

Pituitary Abscess Syndrome. Abscesses in the pituitary gland of ruminants occur sporadically and have been reported in cattle, sheep, and goats but not cervids.[23-26] This condition results in progressive cerebral and brainstem neurological deficits in affected animals and is usually fatal. In 11 of 20 cases in one study, pituitary abscessation was associated with the presence of another septic process at a distinct location of the body.[24] Bacteria commonly isolated from cases of pituitary abscessation in ruminants include *Trueperella pyogenes*, *Staphylococcus* spp., *Streptococcus* spp., *Fusobacterium necrophorum*, *Corynebacterium pseudotuberculosis*, and *Mycoplasma arginine*. Previous studies suggest that hematogenous or lymphatic spread of bacteria in the rete mirabile, an extensive capillary network surrounding the pituitary gland in ruminants, from initial pyogenic foci (i.e., sinusitis, osteomyelitis, tooth abscess, mastitis, etc.) serves as the most common pathway for pituitary abscessation. One retrospective study of 20 cases of pituitary abscess in cattle reported that 55% of the cases had sites of chronic infection separate from the pituitary gland.[27]

The reported age of affected ruminants with this condition was between 9 months to 12 years of age, although animals between 2 and 5 years of age were more commonly affected.[24,28] A history of anorexia, incoordination, lethargy, inability to chew or swallow, and drooling from the mouth are commonly described by producers or owners. Clinical signs vary depending on the extent of the abscess but typically are associated with cerebral and brainstem dysfunction. Depression, recumbency, opisthotonus, convulsions, and asymmetrical cranial nerve deficits such as facial paralysis, blindness, abnormal pupillary light reflexes, nystagmus, ventrolateral strabismus, dysphagia, jaw and tongue hypotonia, and head tilt are commonly reported in affected animals.[24,25,29] Some affected animals present with exophthalmos due to extension of inflammation to the orbit.[30] Hypothalamic compression by pituitary abscessation may result in bradycardia in one-half of affected animals.[24] A presumptive diagnosis of a pituitary abscess is based on the clinical signs of cerebral and brainstem dysfunction, cerebrospinal fluid (CSF) abnormalities, and advanced diagnostic imaging. Increased concentrations of CSF protein between 70 to 502 mg/dL in addition to mild to marked neutrophilic or mononuclear pleocytosis with cell counts between 6 to 12,640 cells/μL have been reported in affected animals.[24,27] Complete blood count changes are consistent with infection and inflammation with leukocytosis, neutrophilia, and hyperfibrinogenemia.

While the use of CT for the diagnosis of intracranial abscesses in ruminants has been reported, reports on the use of this technique to diagnose a pituitary abscess are unavailable.[31] Measuring pituitary hormone levels might be of some value for the diagnosis of pituitary abscessation in small ruminants. One report indicated that TSH, FSH, and LH levels were decreased below the reference range in a sheep with pituitary abscessation.[26] Definitive diagnosis of pituitary abscessation typically occurs at necropsy. Typically, a 3- to 5-cm encapsulated abscess in the area of the pituitary gland and compressed surrounding nervous tissue is detected. Differential diagnosis of pituitary abscessation in small ruminants should include conditions that result in cerebral and brainstem dysfunction such as encephalitic listeriosis, otitis media/interna, and rabies (see Chapter 13). Treatment for pituitary abscessation is usually unrewarding due to inaccessibility of the lesion, which usually results in treatment failure.

Thyroid Gland

Structure and Function

The thyroid gland is a bilobed gland located just caudally to the trachea at the level of the first tracheal rings. The gland consists of two lobes that lie laterally to the trachea and are connected by an isthmus, which is relatively thin and can be difficult to identify in the surrounding connective tissues. The thyroid gland is important in the regulation of metabolism and homeostasis. Histologically, the thyroid gland is composed of follicles. Thyroid follicles consist of a layer of cuboidal epithelial cells surrounding the colloid, an eosinophilic secretion. The homogenous-staining colloid is the reservoir for the thyroid hormones produced by the cuboidal cells. The parafollicular cells, or C cells, are located outside of the thyroid follicles and secrete calcitonin, which functions in calcium metabolism (discussed elsewhere in this chapter).

T_4 and T_3 are produced by the thyroid gland in response to the secretion of TSH by the anterior pituitary. Secretion of TSH is stimulated by TRH released from the hypothalamus. In sheep, over 90% of the secretory output from the thyroid gland is in the form of T_4, while approximately 9% of the output is in the form of the more biologically active T_3 form.[32] Conversion of T_4 to T_3 by monodeiodinase can occur in peripheral tissues, particularly the liver and kidneys. The thyroid hormones are major determinants of basal metabolism. Among others, the effects of T_3 include increasing cardiac output, upregulating the basal metabolic rate and the effects of catecholamines, and boosting catabolism of carbohydrates and proteins.

Thyroid Enlargement

Pathophysiology. Goiter is an alternative term for enlargement of the thyroid gland and, though not common, is the most frequent abnormality of the thyroid gland in small ruminants. Goiters are noninflammatory and non-neoplastic. Decreased blood concentrations of T_4 and T_3, regardless of etiology, stimulate increased TSH output from the anterior pituitary and TRH from the hypothalamus. Elevated concentrations of TRH and TSH lead to a hyperplastic response by the thyroid follicular cells in an attempt to upregulate and normalize blood concentrations of the thyroid hormones. Gland enlargement may produce an adequate compensatory response resulting in normal blood concentrations of thyroid hormones. However, when the underlying cause is severe or ongoing, the animal remains hypothyroid, resulting in further TRH and TSH production and stimulation.

The most common causes for hypothyroidism in small ruminants include consumption of an iodine-deficient diet or consumption of plant-based goitrogens, substances that disrupt thyroid hormone production by inhibiting thyroid uptake of iodine. Primary iodine deficiency is more commonly observed in neonates,[33] but is relatively rare in well-managed flocks due to the widespread inclusion of iodine in trace-mineral salt mixtures. Heavy rainfall may leach iodine from the soil, and low iodine levels are often found in areas with sandy soils. Consequently, animals grazing forages grown on sandy soils, or in areas known to be iodine deficient, may be susceptible to iodine deficiency if iodine is not supplemented. Thiocyanate and goitrin are the most commonly encountered goitrogens in grazed forages; these compounds can decrease iodine uptake by the thyroid gland and inhibit iodination steps in the production of thyroxine. The plants most commonly found to contain

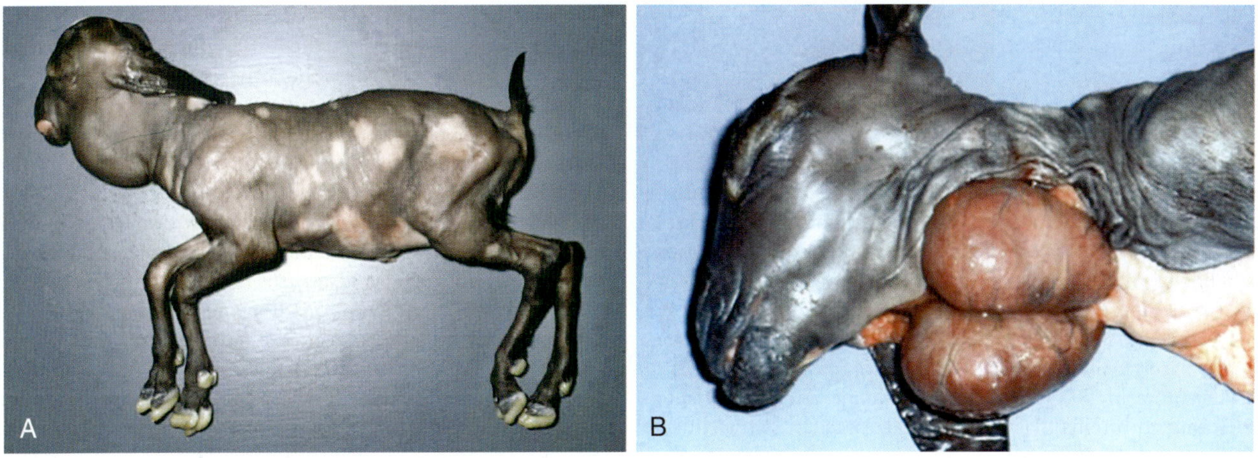

• **Fig. 9.1** **A.** and **B.** Congenital goiter in a neonatal goat. Congenital goiter often results from nutritional deficiencies during gestation. (From: *Noah's Arkive: Hedstrom*. F03304 and F03305. https://noahsarkive.cldavis.org/index.html Accessed August 20, 2018)

goitrogens include *Brassica* species (e.g., kale, rapeseed, mustard), legumes (e.g., soybeans, white clover), and some grains (e.g., sorghum, pearl millet).[34,35] Nutritional deficiency in dams during gestation may result in the development of congenital goiters in the offspring (Figure 9.1A and B).

Dorset sheep, Boer goats, and Angora goats are suspected to have increased susceptibility to iodine deficiency-induced hypothyroidism. Genetic congenital goiter has been described in both sheep and goats. An autosomal recessive mode of inheritance for goiters was demonstrated in Merino sheep suffering from defective thyroglobulin synthesis.[36,37] A similar mechanism has been proposed for hereditary congenital goiter seen in Dutch, Pygmy, and Nubian goats.[38,39]

Clinical Signs. Goiter is more commonly reported in goats than in sheep.[40] Thyroid enlargement is palpable just caudal to the larynx. Pathologic enlargement must be distinguished from the normal thymic gland, which is easily palpable in neonates and young lambs and kids. Palpation is generally not painful, nor is the mass inflamed. Additional signs of hypothyroidism reflect the multitude of effects the thyroid hormones play in basal metabolism and development.[41] Clinical signs are generally most pronounced in young growing animals, geriatric patients, or females in heavy production. Poor quality of hair or wool, alopecia, dry skin, tendon laxity, and other musculoskeletal abnormalities are seen in young lambs and kids. Affected kids fail to thrive and exhibit poor growth rates.[33] Poor fertility is seen in older animals as a result of depressed libido and poor semen quality in males. Females may suffer from irregular cyclicity, decreased conception rates, abortion, and birth of stillborn or weak offspring. Poor milk production may also been seen in affected ewes and does and contributes to growth retardation in the offspring.

Diagnosis. Hypothyroidism in sheep or goats is suspected based on compatible clinical signs, particularly in animals grazing in areas known to be iodine deficient. Thyroid enlargement (goiter) may be easily palpated on physical exam as a firm, noninflammatory, nonpainful mass caudal to the larynx at the level of the first tracheal rings. Supportive hematologic changes include decreased serum triglyceride, phospholipid, and cholesterol concentrations. Definitive diagnosis is achieved through demonstration of thyroid hormone concentrations below defined reference ranges. In goats, normal serum thyroxine concentrations have been reported to be 38.6 to 54.4 nmol/L[42] or 64 to 107 nmol/L.[33,43] A similar range of 38.0 to 100.5 nmol/L has been reported in sheep.[42] Normal T_3 levels in sheep and goats are reported to be 1.0 to 2.3 and 1.3 to 3.0 nmol/L, respectively. Thyroid hormone levels vary seasonally in many deer species, particularly T_3 levels.[44,45] Hormone levels are relatively decreased in the fall and levels may also be affected by nutritional quality. Reported ranges for T_3 and T_4 levels throughout the year are 2.3 to 6.1 and 80 to 230 nmol/L, respectively.[45] Normal serum iodine levels are reported to be between 2.1 and 9.3 µg/dL.[39,43] However, practitioners are encouraged to consult with their reference laboratory for reference ranges specific for the assay used in testing. Hormone response tests using either TSH or TRH are routinely used diagnostically in horses and small animals and are also used in small ruminants, albeit less commonly.[46] Thyroxine concentrations are expected to double and reach physiologic levels by 4 h following exogenous TSH or TRH administration; failure to do so confirms a diagnosis of hypothyroidism. Response tests should also stimulate a rapid increase in T_3 concentrations.

Treatment and Prevention. Most commonly, dietary iodine supplementation is used for treatment and prevention, as nutritional deficiency is the most common cause of hypothyroidism in small ruminants. Dietary iodine requirement is approximately 0.5 mg/kg dry matter weight for most goats and 0.8 mg/kg dry matter weight for lactating does. When goitrogenic plants are extensively consumed, the dietary requirement increases correspondingly. Iodized trace mineral mixtures should be provided for herds and flocks in deficient areas, particularly for gestating and lactating does. Mixtures containing 0.007 to 0.01% iodine are considered to be sufficient to prevent hypothyroidism, assuming adequate consumption. To ensure consumption, the iodized salt mixture should be the only salt source provided. Alternatively, susceptible does and ewes can be drenched orally with 200 to 300 mg potassium iodide or 2 mL of Lugol's iodine weekly during late gestation and heavy lactation. A long-acting parenteral formulation has also been used effectively to treat sheep in areas of endemic iodine deficiency.[47] Oral treatment of affected kids is achieved with 20 mg of potassium iodine or 3 to 5 drops of Lugol's iodine daily in the milk over the course of a week. When supplementing iodine, the iodate form is more biologically available than the iodide form.

Parathyroid Gland

Structure and Function

The parathyroid glands are in close association with thyroid tissue and are responsible for secreting parathyroid hormone (PTH). This hormone is the primary regulator of calcium (Ca) homeostasis in the body. When levels of ionized calcium in plasma are low, Ca-sensitive receptors located in the surface of parathyroid glands release PTH from the principal (chief) cells into circulation. Receptors of PTH present in bone, kidney, and indirectly in the gastrointestinal tract, are activated, and ultimately increase the levels of ionized calcium in plasma.[48]

The receptors of PTH in target cells (bone and kidney) are transmembrane proteins that are in contact with the extracellular fluid where binding of PTH occurs. The internal portion of the receptor is linked to a G-stimulatory protein that changes to its tertiary structure when PTH binds to the receptor. A second messenger reaction mediated by magnesium and cyclic adenosine monophosphate ultimately helps increase extracellular Ca concentrations.[49] Three major mechanisms for increasing plasma Ca levels have been attributed to PTH. The first mechanism increases renal reabsorption of Ca from proximal renal tubular fluids while reducing phosphorus (P) reabsorption at the same time. The second mechanism increases Ca resorption from bone, and the third mechanism indirectly increases the dietary Ca absorption in the intestines.[50]

Normally, only a small amount of Ca is excreted in the urine so when the Ca deficit in plasma is small, increasing renal absorption of Ca is sufficient to restore Ca plasma to normal levels. However, at the onset of lactation in dairy sheep or goats, the Ca demands for colostrum and milk production can be much greater and additional mechanisms must be used to maintain normocalcemia. Calcium stored in bone constitutes the body's major Ca reserve, and when Ca deficits are of greater magnitude, mobilizing Ca from the bone can result in a larger amount of Ca delivered to circulation. The majority (99%) of Ca in bone is stored as hydroxyapatite crystals and can only be released by osteoclastic activation. Receptors of PTH are not present in osteoclasts but in osteoblasts that line all bone surfaces.[50,51] When PTH stimulates receptors on the bone surface, a second messenger reaction results in the secretion of cytokines such as nuclear factor κβ and macrophage colony-stimulating factor (M-CSF) that consequently activate osteoclastic activity releasing Ca and P into circulation. A secondary mechanism of resorption of Ca from the bone is the PTH-mediated release of Ca from intercellular fluid of osteocytes. A minority of bone Ca is in this soluble form within lacunae and canaliculi systems in the intercellular space of osteocytes. Once PTH receptors on osteocytes are activated, pumping of the Ca-containing intercellular fluid into circulation occurs very rapidly.[52]

Active intestinal absorption of Ca occurs in the small intestine by stimulation of intestinal epithelial cells by vitamin D_3 (1,25[OH]$_2$D). Receptors for PTH in the kidney induce conversion of vitamin D_2 to vitamin D_3, which is released into the blood and travels to the intestine.[53] Vitamin D_3 receptors in the nucleus of intestinal epithelial cells induce the synthesis of Ca channel proteins that promote active transport of dietary Ca and P across the cell into the blood. Additionally, Ca is acquired by a mechanism of paracellular intestinal absorption, which occurs independently of vitamin D_3 but requires a concentration gradient across intestinal epithelial cells. When the concentration of ionized Ca in the intestinal lumen is greater than the ionized Ca present in the extracellular fluid (ECF), Ca is transported by gradient by the tight intercellular junctions into ECF and blood.[53] This mechanism is more active when the concentration of dietary Ca is greater than normal.

In contrast to PTH, calcitonin, a 32-amino-acid peptide hormone secreted by C cells of the thyroid gland, is secreted when significant elevation of Ca levels are detected by receptors on the surface of C cells. Calcitonin has the opposite effect of PTH in bone, kidney, and intestines. Disturbances of the Ca homeostasis are usually attributed to PTH dysfunction due to its primary role in regulation of blood Ca. Based on etiology, hyperparathyroidism is classified as either primary or secondary. Primary hyperparathyroidism is associated with hyperplasia or neoplasia of the parathyroid gland, but reports of this condition in small ruminants do not exist. Secondary hyperparathyroidism results from an excessive secretion of PTH in response to other physiological or pathological processes and is usually classified as nutritional secondary hyperparathyroidism or renal secondary hyperparathyroidism.

Nutritional Secondary Hyperparathyroidism

This condition affects animals fed a diet low in Ca, high in P, or with an imbalanced Ca to P ratio ($\leq$ 1:3).[54,55] Additionally, vitamin D deficiency can result in nutritional secondary hyperparathyroidism due to continuous reduction on intestinal absorption of Ca.[54] Low dietary Ca, high P, or vitamin D deficiency results in hypocalcemia, which upregulates PTH secretion to maintain normal Ca concentrations in plasma. However, in cases of a very low Ca and high phosphate diets, the effect of PTH on the synthesis of vitamin D_3 is limited and therefore intestinal absorption of Ca is compromised. In contrast, the PTH-induced bone resorption of Ca becomes the only meaningful mechanism by which plasma Ca levels can be regulated, resulting in a marked osteoclastic activity, Ca resorption from the bone, bone loss, and replacement of bone with unmineralized connective tissue.[55-57] This condition is known as osteodystrophia fibrosa and occurs sporadically in goats while is rarely observed in sheep and cattle.[56] Goats affected with osteodystrophia fibrosa usually present with facial bone enlargement/swelling particularly in the mandibular and maxillary bones (big head), difficulties in apprehension and mastication of fiber, long bone fractures, and intermittent shifting lameness. In one report, seven goats fed a diet with a Ca:P ratio of 1:6 developed severe secondary nutritional hyperparathyroidism that resulted in mandibular and maxillar enlargements in addition to different degrees of dyspnea, protruding of the tongue, and apprehension and mastication abnormalities.[57] Typical laboratory abnormalities in animals affected with nutritional secondary hyperparathyroidism and osteodystrophia fibrosa might include hyperphosphatemia, hypocalcemia or normocalcemia, increased intact PTH levels, increased alkaline phosphatase activity, decreased urinary fractional excretion of Ca (hypocalciuria), and increased urinary fractional excretion of P (hyperphosphaturia). However, if the animal is eating a normal balanced diet at the time of evaluation, these values might be normal. Radiologic findings demonstrate decreased bone mass (if bone loss is greater than 30%), decreased facial bone density, and fibrous proliferation.[55] Diagnosis is based on a combination of history, clinical signs, laboratory abnormalities, and radiologic findings in affected animals. Necropsy findings include increased bone resorption, bone fragility and incomplete fractures (ribs), obstruction of nasal passages, and parathyroid gland hyperplasia.

Risk factors for nutritional secondary hyperparathyroidism include high-grain low-fiber diets with a high content of P, pastures and toxic plants with high oxalate content that interfere with Ca absorption in the intestine such as Bermuda grass, dallisgrass, foxtail grass, pokeberry, red-rooted pigweed, and sugar beet.[54,58,59] Additionally, the use of anionic salts to acidify the urine and prevent struvite formation to control urolithiasis could result in excessive PTH secretion and response and, consequently, in greater bone resorption and remodeling.[58] Treatment and prevention of nutritional secondary hyperparathyroidism and osteodystrophia fibrosa are focused on correction of the diet and re-establishing a normal to increased Ca:P ratio ($\geq$ 3–4:1 ratio).[55] Avoiding high-grain diets and feeds containing high levels of oxalates also aids in the prevention of this condition. The addition of feedstuffs and forages containing high levels of Ca, such as alfalfa, and supplementation with calcium carbonate ($CaCO_3$) or di-calcium phosphate may be helpful.

Renal Secondary Hyperparathyroidism

Renal secondary hyperparathyroidism is secondary to renal failure and consequent hyperphosphatemia. In ruminants, several hemodynamic, toxic, and infectious conditions can lead to acute or chronic renal failure and loss of renal function. Once the functional renal tissue is less than 25%, renal function is compromised, and accumulation of phosphates in blood leads to hyperphosphatemia.[55] As a consequence of renal failure and hyperphosphatemia, hypocalcemia arises as a result of precipitation of Ca in the blood and reduction of vitamin D_3 synthesis in the kidneys. Reduction of Ca absorption in the intestines further reduces the blood Ca concentrations and induces a marked PTH response that eventually causes continuous Ca resorption from the bone resulting in bone loss and fibrous osteodystrophy. Clinical pathology and electrolyte abnormalities are typical of acute or chronic renal failure in addition to those described for nutritional secondary hyperparathyroidism. When indicated, treatment is directed at reducing the effects of acute or chronic renal failure as described elsewhere (see Chapter 12).

Adrenal Glands

The adrenal glands are bilaterally symmetric endocrine organs located near the cranial pole of each kidney. Histologically, the adrenal gland is characterized by an outer cortex and the inner medulla (Table 9.2). The adrenal cortex has three distinct zones; from outward to inward, the layers are the *zona glomerulosa*, *zona fasciculata*, and *zona reticularis*. In ruminants, the zona fasciculata can be further divided into inner and outer zonal layers. The adrenal cortex functions primarily in the production of mineralocorticoid and glucocorticoid steroid hormones. The mineralocorticoids, of which aldosterone is the main example, are produced in the zona fasciculata. Glucocorticoids, including cortisol, are produced primarily in the zona fasciculata, the largest cortical zone, and the zona reticularis serves to produce several androgens. The chromaffin cells of the adrenal medulla produce the catecholamines epinephrine and norepinephrine.

As in any species, normal values for hormone levels vary according to the reporting laboratory and the assay used for hormone level determination. Consequently, clinicians are encouraged to use reference values provided by the laboratory performing the assay when available. However, because the caseload of small ruminants at many veterinary diagnostic laboratories is relatively low, reference values may not be provided. For aldosterone levels in sheep, a baseline value of 1.01 $\pm$ 0.32 ng/dL has been reported.[60] Assay results vary based on the hydration status of the patient with levels in goats ranging from 5.5 to 13.9 ng/dL in one study.[61] Accurate measurement of cortisol levels can be difficult as levels are also subject to external factors including season, breed, and sex. Normal levels for sheep and goats have been reported as 62 $\pm$ 10 and 65 $\pm$ 8 nmol/L, respectively.[62] In deer, baseline levels have been reported as 28 to 55 nmol/L.[63] Hormone concentrations in individual deer may vary based on seasonality and reproductive status.[44,64,65]

Disorders of the adrenal gland in small ruminants are infrequently but sporadically described. Most reported adrenal lesions are neoplastic (either primary or metastatic) in origin. In one necropsy study of 2500 (mostly Angora) goats, 500 cortical adenomas were found in 316 individual goats, although many lesions were small and only diagnosed microscopically.[66] The presence or absence of clinical signs in affected goats was not described and most lesions are presumed to be incidental findings. The study detected a significant overrepresentation of wethers compared to intact male or female goats. Elsewhere, adrenal cortical neoplasia has been reported in association with lactation in a castrated male goat.[67] Pheochromocytomas are sporadically documented in goats, including in two does with inappropriate lactation and in three generations of related does in Finland.[18,68,69] Other reported primary neoplasms in the adrenal gland of small ruminants include an undifferentiated ganglioneuroblastoma[70] and cortical carcinoma.[71] Metastasis to the adrenal glands from other primary neoplasms, including ovine pulmonary adenocarcinoma, also occurs.[72-74]

A syndrome of habitual abortion was described in Angora goats believed to be suffering from hypoadrenocorticism and decreased adrenocortical responsiveness.[75] Does appear healthy through their initial kiddings but begin to abort habitually at the

TABLE 9.2 Adrenal Gland Organization.

Layer	Zone	Hormone Class	Example	Function
Cortex	Zona glomerulosa	Mineralocorticoids	Aldosterone	Blood pressure regulation
	Zona fasciculata	Glucocorticoids	Cortisol	Stress response
	Zona reticularis	Androgens	Androstenedione	Testosterone precursor
Medulla		Catecholamines	Epinephrine	Fight-or-flight response
			Norepinephrine	Fight-or-flight response

age of 4 to 5 years. Abortion general occurs around 100 days of gestation following a stressful incident. Dams suffering from the syndrome have small adrenal glands and low blood cortisol levels.[76] Premature parturition is induced by the resultant fetal adrenal hyperplasia and increased fetal cortisol levels.

Pancreas

The pancreas serves as the interface of the digestive and endocrine systems through its endocrine and exocrine functions. In ruminants, the pancreas is located in the craniodorsal abdomen in close proximity to the descending duodenum. The bilobed gland is loosely structured, lobulated, and of irregular form that is pink to yellow in appearance. The primary endocrine functions of the pancreas are the production of glucagon and insulin from the alpha- and beta-cells, respectively, of the pancreatic islets. Other cells within the pancreatic islets secrete somatostatin and pancreatic polypeptide.

Diabetes mellitus (DM) is characterized by a persistent elevation in blood glucose and glucosuria. Primary DM is caused by damage to the pancreatic beta-cells resulting in decreased insulin levels and hyperglycemia. Secondary DM is defined as an elevation in glucose levels despite normal or elevated plasma insulin concentrations secondary to insulin resistance. Spontaneous cases of either primary or secondary DM are rare in small ruminants.[77-79] Clinical signs of DM in small ruminants include lethargy, anorexia, and weight loss. Polyuria and polydipsia are consistent findings. Severe depression of milk production may be seen in lactating goats.[80] Insulin treatment of both spontaneous and experimental DM in small ruminants generally results in improvement in clinical signs and normalization of glucose levels within 4 days of treatment onset.[78,81] Anecdotally, low doses (0.25 IU/kg) of human ultralente recombinant insulin have been administered to ruminants every 24 to 48 h to increase tissue glucose uptake and stimulate hepatic glycolysis.[82] Discontinuation of therapy results in a recurrence of clinical signs. However, successful control of clinical signs was achieved over a nearly 4-year-period in one goat with primary DM.[79] Attention to the proper insulin dosage is important to avoid the potential for life-threatening hypoglycemia. Pancreatic neoplasias are rare in small ruminants.[74]

Inappropriate Lactation Syndrome (Aberrant Lactation, Precocious Udder) and Pseudopregnancy

Pseudopregnancy or hydrometra (mucometra) is a condition in which aseptic fluid accumulates in the uterus of does and ewes in the absence of a fetus and/or placentomes, resulting in anestrous.[83] In some geographic areas, pseudopregnancy is the most common noninfectious uterine pathology of goats.[84] This condition usually results from a persistent corpus luteum (CL) and prolonged luteal phase. Initially, serum progesterone (P4) levels are similar to those of pregnant does. However, concentrations return to basal levels after day 100.[85] Affected does/ewes do not return to estrus and suffer temporary infertility that results in economic losses for producers. The incidence of the disease varies between 3.0 and 20.8%.[86] The prevalence is also variable at 10.4 to 30.4% depending on the geographic location.[87] There is some evidence that pseudopregnancy could have a genetic/hereditary component in goats. One study suggested that the frequency of this condition was greater in daughters and mothers of pseudopregnant does.[87] Another study demonstrated that pseudopregnancy was genetically associated with a longer productive lifespan but not with milk production in dairy goats.[88] Induction of ovulation (estrus synchronization) with exogenous hormones (i.e., progestogens and equine chorionic gonadotropin) has also been implicated in the development of pseudopregnancy in goats.[86,89]

Clinical signs of animals affected with pseudopregnancy are variable and might include anestrous, hydrometra (presence of fluid in the uterus), teat swelling and udder development, reduction in milk production, and distention of the abdomen.[83,90,91] Complete blood count and serum biochemistry parameters of affected animals are usually within normal limits. The pathophysiology of pseudopregnancy is associated with abnormal luteolytic activity that causes a persistent CL and prolonged luteal phase and leads to fluid accumulation in the uterus.[89] The disease can occur after early embryonic death or without history of previous mating. Serum progesterone levels of goats with pseudopregnancy are usually lower than those of pregnant goats; however, when progesterone levels rise above 2 ng/mL, fluid accumulation in the uterus can occur and prostaglandin production might be disrupted.[89,92] Although serum levels of p PRL, LH, growth hormone GH, and GnRH have been associated with the pathophysiology of this condition in goats, reported serum hormonal levels in affected animals have been inconsistent and are not always reliable in diagnosis of the condition.[93-95]

Transabdominal ultrasound examination of the uterus and ovaries confirms the diagnosis of pseudopregnancy. Usually, the diagnosis of this condition is an incidental finding when pregnancy checking does 30 days or more after insemination. The presence of hypoechoic fluid in the uterus in the absence of a fetus or caruncles is indicative of the disease.[87] Spontaneous expulsion of the accumulated uterine fluid might occur after natural aging of the retained CL but can take several weeks or months prolonging the anestrous and infertility.[85,89] Treatment of pseudopregnancy involves inducing drainage of the retained uterine fluid and promoting return to estrus. Two to three intramuscular injections of PGF2α (5–10 mg of dinoprost or 125–250 μg of cloprostenol) administered 10 to 12 days apart are usually efficient in inducing draining of uterine fluid and return to estrus.[83,96] Goats that do not respond well to the prostaglandin therapy can be treated with oxytocin (50 IU BID intramuscularly [IM] for 4 days).[94]

Inappropriate lactation syndrome (ILS) is defined as an abnormal development of the mammary gland tissue and lactogenic synthesis without history of breeding or artificial insemination. Although the condition has been described primarily in females (does and ewes), reports of this condition in male goats exist.[97,98] Pseudopregnancy has been identified as one of the possible causes of ILS in female goats.[99] Dairy and pygmy goats are more commonly affected by ILS and pseudopregnancy. In male goats, ILS has been associated with development of mammary glands (gynecomastia) and lactation that can result in reduced libido and reduced semen quality.[97]

Physical examination parameters of affected animals are usually normal. The mammary gland (one or both halves) of does and ewes with ILS is enlarged, soft, with no signs of mastitis or inflammation. Although history of being nursed or milked in affected goats is rare in cases of ILS, milk secretions usually remain in the teat cisterns, which become abnormally large (bottle teats). The udder secretions of animals affected with ILS consist of a milk-like secretion that becomes clearer and translucent with subsequent milkings.[19] Duration of signs of ILS may persist for long periods. A variety of factors has been involved in the etiology of ILS. Feeding estrogenic forage or grains (i.e., clover, moldy grains), increased serum and mammary gland PRL- and PTH-related protein (PTHrP) production, and pituitary adenomas may stimulate lactation and cause ILS. Increased autocrine PRL and PTHrP production in sheep and goats has been associated with ILS. Pituitary adenomas were associated with ILS in two goats in one study. One of the affected goats demonstrated persistently high serum levels of PRL and the authors suggested this as a possible cause of ILS in this goat.[19] Masculine behavior (virilism) and ILS have been described in two does and a ewe with granulosa cell tumors.[100,101] Increased serum levels of testosterone and estradiol and inconsistent serum levels of progesterone found in these animals were identified as possible contributor causes of ILS in these studies.

Diagnosis of ILS is based on history and clinical signs. Elevated serum levels of PRL, progesterone, testosterone, and estradiol can be of help in the diagnosis of pituitary adenomas and granulosa cell tumors in small ruminants with ILS; however, the practitioner should exert caution when using hormonal testing for the diagnosis of ILS, as hormonal values have been inconsistent in some studies.[17,19,101] In cases of a granulosa cell tumor-associated ILS, ultrasonographic evaluation of the ovaries and hormonal profiles for testosterone and estradiol are diagnostic.[102] The treatment of choice for ILS for dairy goats in the absence of pseudopregnancy is with dopamine agonist (antiprolactin) agents such as bromocriptine mesylate and cabergoline with limited efficacy.[93,95] Bromocriptine mesylate is administered at a total dose of 5 mg/day for 14 days and cabergoline at 5 μg/kg or 0.1 mL/kg orally or 5.6 mg IM.[103-105] Surgical removal of the mammary gland (mastectomy) remains the treatment of choice for pet small ruminants with ILS. In one study of five pet goats with ILS in which previous medical treatment with cabergoline had not been successful, complete mastectomy was effective in resolving clinical signs.[106] In cases of ILS associated with a granulosa cell tumor, treatment consists of surgical removal of the affected ovary.[102] Prevention strategies for pseudopregnancy include selenium supplementation and breeding in the first heat of the season.[90]

Antler Growth in Cervids

Antler growth in cervids represents a regenerative response unique in mammals. Deer antlers are the only mammalian appendages that undergo serial regeneration, which has led to intense study of antler growth and development as a potential model of organ regeneration, bone development, and growth control. However, antler growth is a complex and multifaceted process influenced by both intrinsic and extrinsic factors; the molecular mechanisms are still not completely understood.

Antlers are a secondary sexual characteristic that, except in members of the *Rangifer* genus (reindeer), are present only in male deer. Antlers are bony organs that develop from pedicles that are extensions of the frontal bone. Pedicle development begins around the time of puberty after the deer has attained a species-specific threshold of body weight.[107] Experimentally, resection of the antlerogenic periosteum prevents antler development, and transplantation to other sites on the frontal bone or even the legs leads to antler development at the transplantation site and not at the original location.[108] As antler development begins, the skin over the pedicles transitions to a characteristic "velvet" that contains fewer hair follicles than normal skin. Almost all types of deer integument can be induced into velvet skin by the antlerogenic periosteum. Following initiation, antlers enter a rapid growth period that generally occurs in the spring. Growth occurs as a modified endochondral process and generally yields unbranched spikes. In this phase, antlers are not yet calcified and may be painful or bleed when damaged. Antler growth ceases in the fall as breeding season approaches and is replaced by a period of calcification. Calcification begins at the base and proceeds upwards, terminating at the distal ends of the antlers.[107] Following calcification, the velvet skin covering the antlers is shed and the antler remains firmly attached to the underlying bone throughout the winter in most species. Initiation of antler regeneration begins again almost immediately.[109] In white-tailed deer, the initial set of antlers is cast in late autumn or early winter with antler regeneration beginning in the spring. Removal of the antlers from captive breeder bucks may be desirable in certain management schemes to prevent injury. When this is desired, the antlerogenic pedicle should be left intact, unlike dehorning in cattle and small ruminants where the entire horn base is often removed. The antlers should be cut off after formation of the hard horn, leaving approximately one inch of antler above the pedicle.

Hormonal control of antler growth, casting, and regeneration has yet to be fully elucidated. The primary hormones associated with antler growth and development are testosterone and insulin-like growth factor 1 (IGF-1), although other hormones and local factors are also involved throughout the growth process. Testosterone levels are important internal regulators for the seasonal pattern of antler growth, calcification, and casting seen in most species of deer.[108] Initiation of antler growth in the spring takes place as day length is increasing. Testosterone levels are relatively low in most male deer throughout much of the spring but it has been postulated that a short testosterone pulse in the spring is responsible for antler growth initiation.[110] In castrated males, antler development could be stimulated by the administration of exogenous testosterone.[111] However, high testosterone levels prevent antler initiation and pedicle activity. Elongation continues throughout the summer while hormone levels remain low. Antler bone development and elongation are completed in a low testosterone environment.[112] Then, as testosterone levels surpass 1 ng/mL in the fall, mineralization and calcification of the antlers occur. The velvet skin dries and is shed as the mating season approaches. Following the breeding season, testosterone levels fall to prebreeding levels. Antler casting is associated with serum testosterone levels falling below 1 ng/mL.[113] For most species, this occurs in the following spring, although in some cervid species, this will occur in early winter. Antler casting is prevented by exogenous administration of testosterone.[111,114] Conversely, surgical or chemical castration of antlered deer results in premature casting of the antlers.[108] Castration of bucks does not prevent future antlerogenesis but does preclude calcification of the velvet horns.[115] Thus, antlers of normal shape develop during the species' appropriate time period but remain covered in velvet and are susceptible to trauma.

Though changes in testosterone concentrations are considered to be the main stimuli associated with steps in antler growth dynamics, elongation of the antlers occurs when testosterone levels are low. Once initiation has occurred, IGF-1 has been proposed as the main endocrine player stimulating antler growth. Produced primarily in the liver in response to GH released from the anterior pituitary, IGF-1 stimulates systemic body growth in multiple cell types, but especially, skeletal muscle, cartilage, and bone. It regulates proliferation and differentiation of osteocytes and chondrocytes through multiple signaling pathways and often has stage-specific effects on the same cell types. In male deer, circulating IGF-1 concentrations are positively correlated with antler growth.[116] Both IGF-1 and IGF-1 receptors are located in antler tissues and in vitro proliferation of antler progenitor cells is seen when incubated in the presence of IGF-1.[117] However, because IGF-1 is known to be involved in the regulation of bone density and proliferation, and antler is composed of true bone, it is not fully understood if IGF-1 is the driving stimulus behind antler growth or is just an active player in the process once initiated.

References

1. Matwijiw I, Thliveris JA, Faiman C: Hypothalamo-pituitary portal development in the ovine fetus, *Biol Reprod* 40(5):1127–1130, 1989.
2. Barrell GK, Ridgway MJ, Wellby M, et al: Expression of regulatory neuropeptides in the hypothalamus of red deer *(Cervus elaphus)* reveals anomalous relationships in the seasonal control of appetite and reproduction, *Gen Comp Endocrinol* 229:1–7, 2016.
3. Batailler M, Chesneau D, Derouet L, et al: Pineal-dependent increase of hypothalamic neurogenesis contributes to the timing of seasonal reproduction in sheep, *Sci Rep* 8(1):6188, 2018.
4. Senn M, Maier PM, Langhans W: ACTH, cortisol and glucose responses after administration of vasopressin in cattle and sheep, *J Comp Physiol B* 164(7):570–578, 1995.
5. Hart KA, Slovis NM, Barton MH: Hypothalamic-pituitary-adrenal axis dysfunction in hospitalized neonatal foals, *J Vet Intern Med* 23(4):901–912, 2009.
6. Adams GP: Comparative patterns of follicle development and selection in ruminants, *J Reprod Fertil Suppl* 54:17–32, 1999.
7. Santiago-Moreno J, Gonzalez-Bulnes A, Gomez BA, et al: Nocturnal variation of prolactin secretion in the Mouflon *(Ovis gmelini musimon)* and domestic sheep *(Ovis aries)*: seasonal changes, *Anim Reprod Sci* 64(3-4):211–219, 2000.
8. Le PF, Leroux C, Martin P, et al: Prolactin gene expression in ovine and caprine mammary gland, *Neuroendocrinology* 60(3):305–313, 1994.
9. Rundgren M, Olsson K, Appelgren B, et al: Effects of hemorrhage on vasopressin secretion and arterial blood pressure during experimental diabetes insipidus in goats, *Acta Physiol Scand* 116(1):57–65, 1982.
10. Lohmeier TE: Neurohypophysial hormones, *Am J Physiol Regul Integr Comp Physiol* 285(4):R715–R717, 2003.
11. Thomson JR, Anderson DH, Gilmour JS: Neurogenic diabetes insipidus in a sheep, *J Comp Pathol* 96(1):119–124, 1986.
12. Kranenburg LC, Thelen MH, Westermann CM, et al: Use of desmopressin eye drops in the treatment of equine congenital central diabetes insipidus, *Vet Rec* 167(20):790–791, 2010.
13. Zanolari P, Botteron C, Jaggy A, et al: Chromophobe adenocarcinoma of the pituitary gland in a ram, *J Vet Intern Med* 18(5): 748–752, 2004.
14. Olson DP, Ohlson DL, Davis SL, et al: Acidophil adenoma in the pituitary gland of a sheep, *Vet Pathol* 18(1):132–135, 1981.
15. Reed SD, Bauer RW: Pituitary acidophil macroadenoma in a pygmy goat *(Capra hircus hircus)*, *J Vet Diagn Invest* 21(2):262–266, 2009.
16. Oda S, Wada Y, Kondo H, et al: Pituitary adenoma with prolactin and growth hormone production in a sheep, *J Comp Pathol* 1997:117(2);171–175.
17. Gonzalez L, Balaguer L, Romano J, et al: Prolactinoma in a sheep, *J Comp Pathol* 111(3):321–326, 1994.
18. Miller CC, Williamson LH, Miller-Liebl DM, et al: Lactation associated with acidophilic pituitary adenoma, pheochromocytoma, and cystic endometrial hyperplasia in two goats, *J Am Vet Med Assoc* 210(3):378–381, 1997.
19. Ortin A, Ferrer LM, Loste A, et al: Coexistence of pituitary adenocarcinoma and intraocular melanoma in a sheep, *Vet Rec* 159(21):718–719, 2006.
20. Capen CC: Tumors of the endocrine glands. In Moulton JE, editor: *Tumors in domestic animals*, Berkeley, CA, 1990, University of California Press, pp 553–639.
21. Goldstein EJ, Burnett KR, Wolf GL, et al: Contrast enhancement of spontaneous animal CNS tumors with gadolinium DTPA: a correlation of MRI with x-ray CT, *Physiol Chem Phys Med NMR* 17(1): 113–122, 1985.
22. Donaldson MT, LaMonte BH, Morresey P, et al: Treatment with pergolide or cyproheptadine of pituitary pars intermedia dysfunction (equine Cushing's disease), *J Vet Intern Med* 16(6):742–746, 2002.
23. Morin DE: Brainstem and cranial nerve abnormalities: listeriosis, otitis media/interna, and pituitary abscess syndrome, *Vet Clin North Am Food Anim Pract* 20(2):243–273, vi, 2004.
24. Perdrizet JA, Dinsmore P: Pituitary abscess syndrome, *Comp Cont Educ Pract* 8(6):S311–S318, 1986.
25. Lomas ST, Hazell SL: The isolation of *Mycoplasma arginini* from a pituitary abscess in a goat, *Aust Vet J* 60(9):281–282, 1983.
26. Dabak M, Eroksuz Y, Baydar E, et al: Decreased pituitary hormone levels in a sheep with pituitary abscess, *J Appl Anim Res* 44(1):5–8, 2016.
27. Stokol T, Divers TJ, Arrigan JW, et al: Cerebrospinal fluid findings in cattle with central nervous system disorders: a retrospective study of 102 cases (1990–2008), *Vet Clin Pathol* 38(1):103–112, 2009.
28. Taylor PA, Meads EB: Pituitary abscessation, and a "farcy-like" condition in cattle due to *Cornebacterium pyogenes*, *Can Vet J* 4(8): 208–213, 1963.
29. Fernandes CG, Schild AL, Riet-Correa F, et al: Pituitary abscess in young calves associated with the use of a controlled suckling device, *J Vet Diagn Invest* 12(1):70–71, 2000.
30. Moriwaki M, Watase H, Fukumoto M, et al: Exophthalmos due to rete mirabile abscess caused by infection with *Corynebacterium pyogenes* in cattle, *Natl Inst Anim Health Q (Tokyo)* 13(1):14–22, 1973.
31. El-Khodery S, Yamada K, Aoki D, et al: Brain abscess in a Japanese black calf: utility of computed tomography (CT), *J Vet Med Sci* 70(7):727–730, 2008.
32. Chopra IJ, Sack J, Fisher DA: 3,3',5'-Triiodothyronine (reverse T3) and 3,3',5-triiodothyronine (T3) in fetal and adult sheep: studies of metabolic clearance rates, production rates, serum binding, and thyroidal content relative to thyroxine, *Endocrinology* 97(5):1080–1088, 1975.
33. Bath GF, Wentzel D, van Tonder EM: Cretinism in Angora goats, *J S Afr Vet Assoc* 50(4):237–239, 1979.
34. Abel Gadir WS, Adam SE: Development of goitre and enterohepatonephropathy in Nubian Goats fed with pearl millet *(Pennisetum typhoides)*, *Vet J* 157(2):178–185, 1999.
35. Knowles SO, Grace ND: Serum total iodine concentrations in pasture-fed pregnant ewes and newborn lambs challenged by iodine supplementation and goitrogenic kale, *J Anim Sci* 93(1):425–432, 2015.
36. Rac R, Hill GN, Pain RW, et al: Congenital goitre in Merino sheep due to an inherited defect in the biosynthesis of thyroid hormone, *Res Vet Sci* 9(3):209–223, 1968.
37. Falconer IR. Studies of the congenitally goitrous sheep. Composition and metabolism of goitrous thyroid tissue, *Biochem J* 100(1):197–203, 1966.
38. De Vijlder JJ, van Voorthuizen WF, Van Dijk JE, et al: Hereditary congenital goiter with thyroglobulin deficiency in a breed of goats, *Endocrinology* 102(4):1214–1222, 1978.
39. Rijnberk A, De Vijlder JJ, Van Dijk JE, et al: Congenital defect in iodothyronine synthesis. Clinical aspects of iodine metabolism in goats with congenital goitre and hypothyroidism, *Br Vet J* 133(5): 495–503, 1977.
40. Saiyari M, Mandavi H, Mayahi M, et al: Spontaneous lesions in the thyroid of sheep and goats in Iran, *Rev Elev Med Vet Pays Trop* 48(3):231–232, 1995.

41. Campbell AJ, Croser EL, Milne ME, et al: An outbreak of severe iodine-deficiency goitre in a sheep flock in north-east Victoria, *Aust Vet J* 90(6):235–239, 2012.
42. Capen CC, Martin SL: The thyroid gland. In Pineda MH, Dooley MP, editors: *McDonald's veterinary endocrinology and reproduction*, Ames, IA, 2003, Iowa State Press, pp 35–70.
43. Reap M, Cass C, Hightower D: Thyroxine and triiodothyronine levels in 10 species of animals, *Southwestern Vet* 31:31–34,1978.
44. Bubenik GA, Schams D, White RG, et al: Seasonal levels of metabolic hormones and substrates in male and female reindeer *(Rangifer tarandus)*, *Comp Biochem Physiol C Pharmacol Toxicol Endocrinol* 120(2):307–315, 1998.
45. Hamr J, Bubenik GA: Seasonal thyroid hormone levels of free-ranging white-tailed deer *(Odocoileus virginianus)* in Ontario, *Can J Zool* 62(5):2174–2180, 1990.
46. Sipos W, Miller I, Fountoulakis M, et al: Hypothyroid goitre in a ram: chemical analysis gives indirect evidence for a structurally altered type of ovine thyroglobulin, *J Vet Med A Physiol Pathol Clin Med* 51(2):90–96, 2004.
47. Ferri N, Ulisse S, Aghini-Lombardi F, et al: Iodine supplementation restores fertility of sheep exposed to iodine deficiency, *J Endocrinol Invest* 26(11):1081–1087, 2003.
48. Brown EM: Clinical lessons from the calcium-sensing receptor, *Nat Clin Pract Endocrinol Metab,* 3(2):122–133, 2007.
49. Potts JT, Gardella TJ: Progress, paradox, and potential: parathyroid hormone research over five decades, *Ann N Y Acad Sci* 1117: 196–208, 2007.
50. Goff JP: Calcium and magnesium disorders, *Vet Clin North Am Food Anim Pract* 30(2):359–381, vi, 2014.
51. Hoorn EJ, Zietse R. Disorders of calcium and magnesium balance: a physiology-based approach, *Pediatr Nephrol* 28(8):1195–1206, 2013.
52. Teti A, Zallone A: Do osteocytes contribute to bone mineral homeostasis? Osteocytic osteolysis revisited, *Bone* 44(1):11–16, 2009.
53. Christakos S: Recent advances in our understanding of 1,25-dihydroxyvitamin D(3) regulation of intestinal calcium absorption, *Arch Biochem Biophys* 523(1):73–76, 2012.
54. Wan ZM, Scott D, Loveridge N, et al: The effect of high phosphorus intake on calcium and phosphorus retention and bone turnover in growing lambs, *Exp Physiol* 79(2):175–181, 1994.
55. Goff JP: Calcium, magnesium, and phosphorous. In Smith BP, editor: *Large animal internal medicine,* St. Louis, 2015, Mosby, pp 1258–1266.
56. Andrews AH, Ingram PL, Longstaffe JA: Osteodystrophia fibrosa in young goats, *Vet Rec* 112(17):404–406, 1983.
57. Bandarra PM, Pavarini SP, Santos AS, et al: Nutritional fibrous osteodystrophy in goats, *Pesqui Vet Brasil* 31(10):875–878, 2011.
58. Espino L, Guerrero F, Suarez ML, et al: Long-term effects of dietary anion-cation balance on acid-base status and bone morphology in reproducing ewes, *J Vet Med A Physiol Pathol Clin Med* 50(10): 488–495, 2003.
59. Abu DH, Scott D, Loveridge N, et al: The effects of feeding diets containing either $NaHCO_3$ or NH_4Cl on indices of bone formation and resorption and on mineral balance in the lamb, *Exp Physiol* 76(5):725–732, 1991.
60. Pradier P, Davicco MJ, Safwate A, et al: Plasma adrenocorticotrophin, cortisol and aldosterone responses to ovine corticotrophin-releasing factor and vasopressin in sheep, *Acta Endocrinol (Copenh)* 111(1):93–100, 1986.
61. Wittenberg C, Choshniak I, Shkolnik A, et al: Effect of dehydration and rapid rehydration on renal function and on plasma renin and aldosterone levels in the black Bedouin goat, *Pflugers Arch* 406(4):405–408, 1986.
62. Kaneko JJ, Harvey JW, Bruss M: *Clinical biochemistry of domestic animals,* ed 6, Amsterdam, 2008, Academic Press.
63. Bubenik GA, Bartos L. Cortisol levels in red deer *(Cervus elaphus)* and fallow deer *(Dama dama)* after an acute ACTH administration, *Can J Zool* 71(11):2258–2261, 1993.
64. Pavitt AT, Pemberton JM, Kruuk LE, et al: Testosterone and cortisol concentrations vary with reproductive status in wild female red deer, *Ecol Evol* 6(4):1163–1172, 2016.
65. Pavitt AT, Walling CA, Mostl E, et al: Cortisol but not testosterone is repeatable and varies with reproductive effort in wild red deer stags, *Gen Comp Endocrinol* 222:62–68, 2015.
66. Altman NH, Streett CS, Terner JY: Castration and its relationship to tumors of the adrenal gland in the goat, *Am J Vet Res* 30(4):583–589, 1969.
67. Lofstedt RM, Laarveld B, Ihle SL: Adrenal neoplasia causing lactation in a castrated male goat, *J Vet Intern Med* 8(5):382–384, 1994.
68. Lairmore MD, Knight AP, DeMartini JC: Three primary neoplasms in a goat: hepatocellular carcinoma, phaeochromocytoma and leiomyoma, *J Comp Pathol* 97(3):267–271, 1987.
69. de Gritz BG: Hereditary caprine phaeochromocytoma, *Zentralbl Veterinarmed A* 44(5):313–316, 1997.
70. Yener Z, Kiran MM: Undifferentiated ganglioneuroblastoma in a sheep, *J Comp Pathol* 126(2-3):216–219, 2002.
71. Marco-Sanchez I, Vilafranca M, Lavin S: Adrenal cortical carcinoma in a free-ranging mouflon *(Ovis musimon)*, *Vet Rec* 139(10): 236–237, 1996.
72. Minguijon E, Gonzalez L, De las HM, et al: Pathological and aetiological studies in sheep exhibiting extrathoracic metastasis of ovine pulmonary adenocarcinoma (Jaagsiekte), *J Comp Pathol* 148 (2 3):139–147, 2013.
73. Ruby RE, Daverio H, Barrell EA, et al: Pathology in practice. Peritoneal mesothelioma with metastasis to adrenal glands, heart, and lungs, *J Am Vet Med Assoc* 248(1):63–65, 2016.
74. Yau W, Rissi DR: Cholecystic adenocarcinoma and pancreatic insulinomas in a goat, *J Vet Diagn Invest* 26(6):827–831, 2014.
75. Braun JR: Noninfectious prenatal pregnancy loss in the doe. In Youngquist RS, Threlfall WR, editors: *Current therapy in large animal theriogenology,* ed 2, Philadelphia, 2007, WB Saunders, pp 585–587.
76. van Rensburg SJ: Reproductive physiology and endocrinology of normal and habitually aborting angora goats, *Onderstepoort J Vet Res* 38(1):1–62, 1971.
77. Mattheeuws D, Derijcke J, Rottiers R, et al: Diabetes mellitus in two twin male lambs, *Vet Q* 4(3):135–138, 1982.
78. Lutz TA, Rossi R, Caplazi P, et al: Secondary diabetes mellitus in a pygmy goat, *Vet Rec* 135(4):93, 1994.
79. Braun U, Gansohr B, Seidel M, et al: Diabetes mellitus type 1 in a goat, *Schweiz Arch Tierheilkd* 150(12):608–612, 2008.
80. Nowak J, Dzialoszynski L: Effect of alloxan diabetes in goats on the production and composition of milk, *Acta Physiol Pol* 18(4): 595–606, 1967.
81. Nowak J, Dzialoszynski L: Effect of alloxan diabetes in goats on the production and composition of milk, *Acta Physiol Pol* 18(4): 595–606, 1967.
82. Fleming SA. Endocrine and metabolic diseases. In Smith BP, editor: Large animal internal medicine, ed 3, St. Louis, 2002, Mosby, pp 1241–1247.
83. Maia ALRS, Brandao FZ, Souza-Fabjan JMG, et al: Hydrometra in dairy goats: ultrasonic variables and therapeutic protocols evaluated during the reproductive season, *Anim Reprod Sci* 197:203–211, 2018.
84. Freitas VJ, Rondina D, Lopes ES, Jr., et al: Hormonal treatments for the synchronisation of oestrus in dairy goats raised in the tropics, *Reprod Fertil Dev* 16(4):415–420, 2004.
85. Llewelyn CA, Ogaa JS, Obwolo MJ: Plasma progesterone concentrations during pregnancy and pseudopregnancy and onset of ovarian activity post partum in indigenous goats in Zimbabwe, *Trop Anim Health Prod* 24(4):242–250, 1992.
86. Hesselink JW: Incidence of hydrometra in dairy goats, *Vet Rec* 132(5):110–112, 1993.
87. Hesselink JW, Elving L: Pedigree analysis in a herd of dairy goats with respect to the incidence of hydrometra, *Vet Q* 18(1):24–25, 1996.

88. Desire S, Mucha S, Coffey M, et al: Pseudopregnancy and a seasonal breeding in dairy goats: genetic basis of fertility and impact on lifetime productivity, *Animal* 12(9):1799–1806, 2018.
89. Lopes Junior ES, Cruz JF, Teixeira DI, et al: Pseudopregnancy in Saanen goats *(Capra hircus)* raised in Northeast Brazil, *Vet Res Commun* 28(2):119–125, 2004.
90. Srivastava KK, Waldridge BM, Shofner-Stewart D, et al: What's your diagnosis? Bilateral teat swelling in a female goat. Pseudopregnancy with hydrometra, *Lab Anim (NY)* 30(1):19–20, 2001.
91. Yotov S, Dimitrov D, Fasulkov I: Hydrometra in a sheep after oestrus synchronization and insemination in the anoestral season, *Slov Vet Res* 46:143–147, 2009.
92. Kornalijnslijper JE, Bevers MM, van Oord HA, et al: Induction of hydrometra in goats by means of active immunization against prostaglandin F2 alpha, *Anim Reprod Sci* 46(1-2):109–122, 1997.
93. Hesselink JW, Taverne MA, Bevers MM, et al: Serum prolactin concentration in pseudopregnant and normally reproducing goats, *Vet Rec* 137(7):166–168, 1995.
94. Taverne MA, Lavoir MC, Bevers MM, et al: Peripheral plasma prolactin and progesterone levels in pseudopregnant goats during bromocryptine treatment, *Theriogenology* 30(4):777–783, 1988.
95. Kornalijnslijper JE, Kemp B, Bevers MM, et al: Plasma prolactin, growth hormone and progesterone concentrations in pseudopregnant, hysterectomized and pregnant goats, *Anim Reprod Sci* 49(2-3):169–178, 1997.
96. Hesselink JW: Hydrometra in dairy goats: reproductive performance after treatment with prostaglandins, *Vet Rec* 133(8):186–187, 1993.
97. Dafalla EA, Ramadan RO, Gameel AA, et al: A functioning udder in a male goat, *Zentralbl Veterinarmed A* 37(9):686–691, 1990.
98. al Jassim RA, Khamas WA: Gynaecomastia and galactorrhea in a goat buck, *Aust Vet J* 75(9):669–670, 1997.
99. Troedsson MH, Christensen BW: Hydrometra (pseudopregnancy in goats). In Smith BP, editor: *Large animal internal medicine,* St. Louis, 2015, Mosby, pp 1335.
100. Gardner RB, Alcaraz A, Porter BF, et al: Udder development, lactation and ascites in a ewe with an ovarian granulosa cell tumour, *Aust Vet J* 83(8):486–488, 2005.
101. Lofstedt RM, Williams R: Granulosa cell tumor in a goat, *J Am Vet Med Assoc* 189(2):206–208, 1986.
102. McEntee K: *Reproductive pathology of domestic animals,* San Diego, CA, 1990, Academic Press.
103. Matthews J: *Diseases of the goat,* ed 2, Oxford, 1999, Blackwell Science.
104. Forsyth IA, Lee PD: Bromocriptine treatment of periparturient goats: long-term suppression of prolactin and lack of effect on lactation, *J Dairy Res* 60(3):307–317, 1993.
105. Bertulat S, Isaka N, de PA, et al: Effect of a single injection of cabergoline at dry off on udder characteristics in high-yielding dairy cows, *J Dairy Sci* 100(4):3220–3232, 2017.
106. Arlt S, Reinecke A, Drillich M, et al: Inappropriate lactation syndrome in goats—case collection and experiences with mastectomy, *Tierarztl Prax Ausg G Grosstiere Nutztiere* 39(1):27–32, 2011.
107. Li C, Suttie J: Morphogenetic aspects of deer antler development, *Front Biosci (Elite Ed)* 4:1836–1842, 2012.
108. Price J, Faucheux C, Allen S: Deer antlers as a model of mammalian regeneration, *Curr Top Dev Biol* 67:1–48, 2005.
109. Li C: Histogenetic aspects of deer antler development, *Front Biosci (Elite Ed)* 5:479–489, 2013.
110. Bartos L, Bubenik GA, Kuzmova E: Endocrine relationships between rank-related behavior and antler growth in deer, *Front Biosci (Elite Ed)* 4:1111–1126, 2012.
111. Wislocki GB, Aub JC, Waldo CM: The effects of gonadectomy and the administration of testosterone propionate on the growth of antlers in male and female deer, *Endocrinology* 40(3):202–226, 1947.
112. Gaspar-Lopez E, Landete-Castillejos T, Estevez JA, et al: Biometrics, testosterone, cortisol and antler growth cycle in Iberian red deer stags *(Cervus elaphus hispanicus)*, *Reprod Domest Anim* 45(2):243–249, 2010.
113. Muir PD, Sykes AR, Barrell GK: Changes in blood content and histology during growth of antlers in red deer *(Cervus elaphus)* and their relationship to plasma testosterone levels, *J Anat* 158:31–42, 1988.
114. Fletcher TJ: The induction of male sexual behavior in red deer *(Cervus elaphus)* by the administration of testosterone to hinds and estradiol-17beta to stags, *Horm Behav* 11(1):74–88, 1978.
115. Kierdorf U, Kierdorf H, Knuth S: Effects of castration on antler growth in fallow deer *(Dama dama L.)*, *J Exp Zool* 273(1):33–43, 1995.
116. Suttie JM, Gluckman PD, Butler JH, et al: Insulin-like growth factor 1 (IGF-1) antler-stimulating hormone? *Endocrinology,* 116(2):846–848, 1985.
117. Sadighi M, Haines SR, Skottner A, et al: Effects of insulin-like growth factor-I (IGF-I) and IGF-II on the growth of antler cells in vitro, *J Endocrinol* 143(3):461–469, 1994.

10 Diseases of the Integumentary System

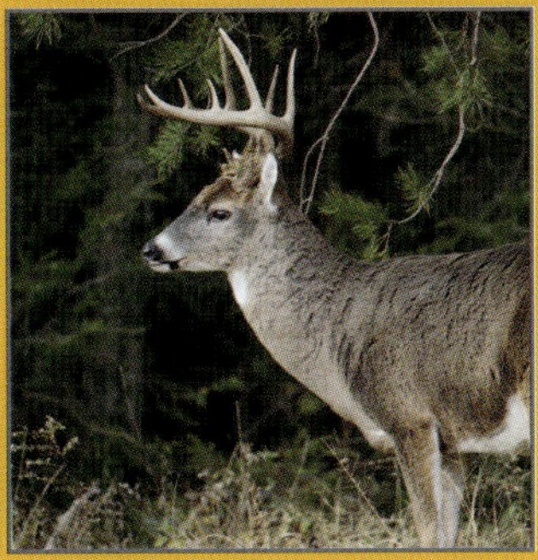

A.N. BAIRD AND CLIFFORD F. SHIPLEY

Dermatologic lesions, which tend to be more common among goats than sheep and cervids, constitute a relatively major reason for examination of small ruminants. Although small ruminant production has historically been an economic enterprise, an increasing number of owners keep these animals as pets and therefore have animals examined more frequently for cosmetic reasons. Diseases of the integumentary system include those that affect skin, hair, and wool. International trade in small ruminants has increased the need to be diligent in watching for previously undiagnosed skin diseases.[1] This chapter will focus on both presumptive and definitive diagnoses and conservative as well as optimum treatments.

Anatomy

A complete discussion on the anatomy and physiology of the skin is beyond the scope of this book. This section will include the unique anatomy and physiology that is pertinent to managing small ruminant diseases and conditions. The skin functions as a protective barrier from the environment. It also aids in thermoregulation, acts as a sensory organ, and communicates through the secretion of chemicals.[2,3] Small ruminants have relatively thin skin with sheep skin averaging 2.6 mm and goat skin 2.9 mm.[2] Hair is important for thermoregulation. The short thick hair coat is best for regulating body temperature during high environmental temperatures, and long, fine hair coats are most efficient at low environmental temperatures. Shearing sheep when environmental temperatures are low is not without risk. Likewise, not having sheep shorn by the time that hot weather arrives might predispose to heat exhaustion. Secondary hairs are more common in goats and sheep than primary or guard hairs. In Angora goats and sheep, three types of wool are described: true wool, Kemp fibers, and hair fibers. True wool fibers are fine and tightly crimped. Kemp fibers are coarse, relatively short, and poorly crimped. Hair fibers are somewhere in between wool and Kemp fibers. Guard hairs are undesirable in wooled breeds because the medulla makes the hairs brittle and these hairs do not take up dye well. Small secondary hairs of goats are nonmedullated. Cervids have hollow hair that insulates them from low temperatures and a summer coat that is very light and allows cooling. The coats are different colors as well, with the summer coat being more reddish and winter coat gray.

Hair grows in a cycle. The growing period is called anagen and the resting period is called telogen. The hair cycle is controlled by various influences, including photoperiod, temperature, nutrition, hormones, health, and genetics, among other things. Wool follicles are an exception in that there is no established cycle. Interestingly, hair growth is most active during summer months, and during winter months nearly all primary hair follicles and about half of secondary hair follicles are in the telogen phase. During periods of ill-health or stress, the anagen phase may be considerably shorter resulting in "hair break" or "wool break" (also known as telogen defluxion) due to growth stoppage. Hairs are more easily lost or pulled out during the telogen phase.

Specialized cells such as the sweat gland allow cooling. The lanolin glands of sheep provide protection from drying out. The lanolin glands are located near the medial canthus of the eye, between the toes, and caudal to the udder in the inner flank.

The epidermis is composed of five layers (from outermost): stratum corneum, stratum lucidum, stratum granulosum, stratum spinosum, and stratum basale. The stratum basale produces new cells that continuously move up to replace the sloughing cells of the stratum corneum. The melanocytes of the stratum basale and hair follicles are primarily responsible for the color of the animal. All melanins arise from a common metabolic pathway that is catalyzed by a copper-containing enzyme. Thus, one of the signs of copper deficiency is a lighter than normal color. Besides the obvious physical barrier presented by the epidermis and hair/wool, there are also chemical and microbial barriers to infection. The secretion produced by the sweat and sebaceous glands has antimicrobial properties. Included within this secretion are fatty acids, inorganic salts, interferon, transferrin, complement, and immunoglobulins. Increased hydration of the skin greatly increases microbial populations. Normal skin flora can inhibit colonization of other potential pathogens. However, some skin pathogens may also be considered normal flora. For example, dermatophytes and *Staphylococcus aureus* can be recovered from clinically normal mammals that do not develop clinical disease.

The dermis contains the arrector pili muscles, blood, and lymph vessels and nerves. The dermis functions as the major source of tensile strength and elasticity of the skin. Most of the dermal fibers are collagen. Collagen defects may arise from genetic disorders, vitamin C deficiency, iron deficiency, copper deficiency, and beta-aminoproprionitrite poisoning.

Hair (and wool) follicles are divided into the innermost medulla, the cortex, and the outmost layer, the cuticle. The color of the hair is primarily due to pigment in the cortex. With simple hair follicle arrangements (bovine and equine), each hair follicle is accompanied by sebaceous and sweat glands and an arrector pili muscle. Sheep and goats have a compound hair follicle arrangement in which hair follicles occur in clusters with two to five primary hairs surrounded by smaller secondary hairs. Each primary hair has sebaceous and sweat glands and an arrector pili muscle, whereas secondary hairs have sebaceous glands only. The wool of sheep becomes finer with a higher secondary to primary hair ratio. Merinos, known for fine wool, have a ratio of 20:1, whereas the wool of meat breeds tends to be 5:1.

In goats, wattles may be present—typically along the ventral neck caudal to the angle of the mandible. Although the function of wattles is unknown, they contain extensive neurovascular structures and cartilage. The presence of wattles is controlled by an autosomal dominant gene.

Sebaceous glands (holocrine) produce an oily secretion that keeps the skin soft and pliable and helps to retain moisture, thereby helping to maintain hydration. This oily substance also covers the hair, yielding a glossy hair coat. In times of stress or illness, the hair coat may appear dull and dry, in part due to inadequate sebaceous gland function. The dull hair coat may occur due to the fact that estrogen and glucocorticoids cause involution of the sebaceous glands. Sebaceous glands increase in size in intact male goats at the beginning of rut. Sebaceous scent glands are located caudal and medial to the base of the horn tissues on the head of goats. In male goats, these glands produce a pungent odor. Surgical procedures to remove the scent glands of goats (descenting) involve excising the sebaceous glands caudal and medial to the horn base. This procedure is easily done in young buck kids at the time of dehorning. In sheep, scent glands are present rostral and medial to the eye and may produce a pungent odor in rams. Scent glands in cervids are located in the infraorbital area, forehead, interdigital space, tarsal, and metatarsal areas. These glands are used for scent marking of territory and communication purposes. During the rut (and other times), bucks and sometimes does will urinate on the tarsal glands with the bucks developing a very pungent odor.

Sweat glands are present in small ruminants. Although sweat production increases in response to heat and exposure to a hot environment, sweat glands are not thought to be major means of thermoregulation in these species.

Approach to Diagnosis

The approach to diagnosis will certainly vary from clinician to clinician depending on previous experience, knowledge of herd or flock disease history, economics, and availability of diagnostic centers. With experience, many veterinarians will be able to diagnose the disease with reasonable accuracy based on history and reported clinical signs alone. The confidence and competence of the veterinarian will be enhanced by definitively confirming the diagnosis early in one's career. The diagnosis of skin disease is confirmed in the same way as that of diseases affecting other body systems: complete historical data, including environment and commingling risk assessment; detailed clinical signs; thorough physical examination; and diagnostic testing based on differential diagnosis lists. Specific diagnostic tests may be performed when diseases fail to respond to seemingly appropriate therapy or when animals are scheduled for sale or show activities.

Historical data should include the signalment of the animal: species, breed, age, gender, weight, and color. Some breeds have a higher likelihood of developing specific disease conditions. Therefore, breed information is useful to assess for susceptibility. The clinician should note details concerning the origin of and exposure risks to the animals. Origin of the animal includes whether the animal was born and raised on the farm, purchased by farm contracts, purchased through sale barns, or imported from another state or country. Exposure risks include transportation to another farm; commingling in sales, shows, or fairs; farm tours involving children or livestock owners; and diseases that are endemic to the particular farm. In the latter case, the clinician should also note when the last outbreak occurred. Chronologic data are important in making a differential diagnosis. The date of the first observation of clinical signs should be determined, the duration of clinical signs should be evaluated, and details regarding the progression of the disease within the affected animals should be described. The region of the body affected and the spread of disease to other regions of the body also are important. Often, the current state of disease is so severe that the point of origin cannot be determined by physical examination. Assessment of whether the disease has spread from one animal to another within the flock or herd is particularly important. Finally, the veterinarian may assemble a detailed chronology of any treatments applied, the dosage and route used for administration, and the duration of treatment.

Clinical signs are important in the development of a differential diagnosis. They can vary widely and depend on the tissues involved in the disease process. Differential diagnoses are most easily determined early in the course of disease, when the primary lesions are abundant (Table 10.1). As the disease progresses, secondary lesions such as infection, thickening, crusting, and hair loss may overwhelm the primary disease and make assessment of skin disease extremely difficult. Therefore, animals with newly emerging disease should be selected for examination.

Erythema refers to reddening of the skin. It is not a disease-specific change but usually indicates the presence of inflammation. Papules are solid masses, small in diameter (less than 1 cm), that are reddened, raised from the surface of the skin, and may be painful to palpation. They are consistent with infection, allergic reaction, and ectoparasites. When the papule is centered on a hair follicle, bacterial or fungal folliculitis and ectoparasites such as demodectic mange should be suspected. When papules occur independent of hair follicles, allergic skin reactions and ectoparasites such as scabies mites should be suspected.

Scratching associated with skin disease is termed pruritus. Assessment of the severity of pruritus can aid in the formulation of an accurate differential diagnosis. Severe pruritus typically is seen with ectoparasitism. Mild pruritus is more often associated with nutritional deficiency, allergic skin disease, bacterial or fungal skin disease, and autoimmune disease. It is a common clinical sign associated with scrapie that also is seen in pseudorabies virus and rabies virus infections.

Vesicles are similar in size and shape to papules, but these masses are filled with a serous fluid and are fluctuant. Vesicle formation may be preceded by a papule. Vesicles are most often associated with viral skin diseases such as poxvirus infections, contact allergies, and autoimmune diseases such as pemphigus. Pustules are similar to vesicles but are purulent in nature. Purulent exudate is formed because of migration of neutrophils either in response to infection or because of an autoimmune disease. Vesicles and pustules are ruptured by abrasion or spontaneous

TABLE 10.1 Typical Distribution of Lesions Associated With Selected Diseases of the Skin.

Area Involved	Disease	Primary Lesion Type
Head and neck	Dermatophytosis	Papulocrustous
	Dermatophilosis	Pustolocrustous
	Demodicosis	Papulonodular
	Elaeophoriasis	Ulcerative
	Fly bites	Papulocrustous
	Actinobacillosis	Nodular
	Clostridiosis	Edematous
	Sarcoptic mange	Papulocrustous
	Contagious viral pustular dermatitis	Pustolocrustous
	Ovine viral ulcerative dermatitis	Ulcerative
	Goat pox	Pustolocrustous
	Sheep pox	Pustolocrustous
	Pemphigus foliaceous	Vesiculopustular, crusts
	Zinc deficiency	Crusts
	Contact dermatitis	Variable
	Viral papillomatosis	Papulonodular
	Squamous cell carcinoma	Nodular, ulcerative
Ears	Dermatophytosis	Papulocrustous
	Dermatophilosis	Pustolocrustous
	Sarcoptic mange	Papulocrustous
	Fly bites	Papulocrustous
	Pemphigus foliaceous	Vesiculopustular, crusts
	Ergotism	Necrotizing
	Fescue toxicosis	Necrotizing
	Frostbite	Necrotizing
	Photodermatitis	Edematous, necroulcerative
	Squamous cell carcinoma	Nodular, ulcerative
Mucocutaneous	Contagious viral pustular dermatitis	Pustolocrustous
	Goat pox	Pustolocrustous
	Sheep pox	Pustolocrustous
	Bluetongue	Erythema, edema
	Zinc deficiency	Crusts
	Bullous pemphigus	Vesiculoulcerative
	Pemphigus foliaceous	Vesiculopustular, crusts
	Dermatophytosis	Papulocrustous
	Dermatophilosis	Pustolocrustous
	Squamous cell carcinoma	Nodular, ulcerative
Dorsum	Dermatophilosis	Pustolocrustous
	Fly bites	Papulocrustous
	Psoroptic mange	Papulocrustous
	Contact dermatitis	Variable
Ventrum	Dermatophilosis	Pustolocrustous
	Fly bites	Papulocrustous
	Sarcoptic mange	Papulocrustous
	Contact dermatitis	Variable
	Goat pox	Pustolocrustous
	Sheep pox	Pustolocrustous
	Contagious viral pustular dermatitis	Pustolocrustous
	Zinc deficiency	Crusts
	Corynebacterium pseudotuberculosis	Abscesses infection
Trunk	Dermatophytosis	Papulocrustous
	Dermatophilosis	Pustolocrustous
	Psoroptic mange	Papulocrustous
	Psorergatic mange	Alopecia, pruritus
	Keds	Alopecia, pruritus
	Ovine fleece rot	Moist dermatitis
	Pemphigus foliaceous	Vesiculopustular, crusts
	Demodicosis	Papulonodular
	Caprine viral dermatitis	Papulonodular
	Scrapie	Excoriation, pruritus
	Vitamin A deficiency	Hyperkeratosis
	Iodine deficiency	Alopecia, scaling
	Biotin, niacin, riboflavin, pantothenic acid deficiency	Alopecia, scaling, crusts
	Vitamin C–responsive dermatosis	Alopecia, erythema, purpurea
	Copper deficiency	Depigmentation
Hindquarters	Dermatophilosis	Pustolocrustous
	Chorioptic mange	Papulocrustous
Legs and feet	Dermatophytosis	Papulocrustous
	Dermatophilosis	Pustolocrustous
	Chorioptic mange	Papulocrustous
	Contact dermatitis	Variable
	Elaeophoriasis	Necroulcerative
	Clostridiosis	Edema

Continued

TABLE 10.1 Typical Distribution of Lesions Associated With Selected Diseases of the Skin.—cont'd

Area Involved	Disease	Primary Lesion Type
	Sarcoptic mange	Papulocrustous
	Zinc deficiency	Crusts
	Vitamin C–responsive dermatosis	Alopecia, erythema, purpurea
	Ovine viral ulcerative dermatitis	Ulcerative
	Pemphigus foliaceous	Vesiculopustular, crusts
Tail	Psoroptic mange	Scales, pruritus
	Selenosis	Alopecia
Coronary band	Pemphigus foliaceous	Vesiculopustular, crusts
	Bluetongue	Erythema
	Contagious viral pustular dermatitis	Pustolocrustous
	Ergotism	Edema
	Fescue toxicosis	Edema
	Dermatophilosis	Pustolocrustous
	Zinc deficiency	Crusts

Adapted from Scott DW: *Large animal dermatology,* Philadelphia, 1988, WB Saunders.

disruption of the overlying membrane. The fluids accumulated on the skin surface form crusts, and the underlying skin becomes thickened in response to the injury. Crusts are firm, adherent amalgamations of serum, pus, blood, cellular debris, and associated organisms. The presence of crusts indicates an exudative process but is not disease specific. Microscopic examination of crusts may reveal infectious organisms such as fungi, bacteria, or cells. The term scale simply refers to desquamated stratum corneum and is not disease specific. Thickening of the skin (specifically, thickening of the stratum corneum) often is referred to as hyperkeratosis. The term orthokeratosis is used to describe hyperkeratosis without the presence of nuclei. Parakeratosis is hyperkeratosis with nuclei present in the keratinized skin. Unfortunately, these findings are consistent with chronic dermatopathy and are not disease specific. The distribution of lesions may be more important than the actual histologic description in this scenario.

Alopecia is hair loss. It may be associated with disease or other stressors, producing a stress-induced telogen phase. This "stress break" in the hair shaft may result in generalized hair loss. Stress alopecia usually is associated with normal skin and normally growing hair. Systemic disease causing prolonged pyrexia also can disrupt normal hair and fiber growth and result in easily epilated hair. In sheep, this is referred to as wool break. Nutritional deficiencies in zinc, selenium, and vitamin E may cause hair loss.

Changes in skin and hair pigmentation are uncommon in most ruminant diseases. Exceptions to this include the hair pigment lightening seen in cattle with chronic copper deficiency and molybdenosis and the black wool pigment that develops in blackface sheep after skin injury (abrasions, laceration, chronic irritation). The development of dark pigmentation also has been observed in Saanen goats exposed to excessive sunlight.

Lesion location can be useful in establishing a differential diagnosis (see Table 10.1). Regions commonly affected in the early stages of skin disease include the face, ears, feet, udder, and perineal region. Fungal skin infections more commonly occur on the face, neck, and ears, whereas bacterial skin diseases also affect the feet, udder, and perineum. Nutritional deficiencies typically involve all regions to various degrees. Photosensitization is more severe in areas that receive little protection by the hair coat and areas with slight or no pigmentation. Ectoparasite lesions are most severe around the feet, face, and ears.

Diagnostic Tests

Although many skin diseases are diagnosed based on clinical signs and intuition, specific diagnosis requires confirmation by laboratory tests (Table 10.2).

TABLE 10.2 Tests Used for Diagnosis of Skin Disease.

Cause of Skin Disease	Tests used
Parasites	Acetate tape
	Skin scraping
	Fecal flotation
Fungi	Potassium hydroxide
	Mineral oil mount
	Wood's lamp
	Fungal culture
	Cytology
Bacteria	Direct smear
	Bacterial culture
Viruses	Viral isolation
	Electron microscopy
	Serology
Allergy	Intradermal skin tests
Miscellaneous pathology	Histopathologic tests—biopsy sections, immunofluorescent tests, antinuclear antibody tests, special stains

Adapted from Scott DW: *Large animal dermatology,* Philadelphia, 1988, WB Saunders.

Skin Scraping. Skin scraping and cytology are easily performed under field conditions and may be diagnostic of certain diseases. Observation of bacteria on cytology is not diagnostic because bacteria are ubiquitous on the surface of the skin. Bacteria observed in pustule fluid are more diagnostic. The contents of skin pustules or abscesses may be aspirated and cultured for identification. A direct smear should be done and a Gram stain performed for immediate identification of infectious bacteria. The presence of phagocytized bacteria supports a diagnosis of bacterial infection. Bacteria in the absence of neutrophils or macrophages suggests that the bacteria are contaminants rather than causes of disease.[1]

Description of the morphology of groups of bacteria may be helpful. For example, *Dermatophilus congolensis* is a gram-positive filamentous branching bacterial colony. Scales and crusts also can be examined under a microscope. Direct examination is usually not rewarding, but softening the material with sodium nitrate solution may allow for visualization of ectoparasites or fungal hyphae. These organisms often float to the top of the solution; a slide placed on top of the solution aids in identification because mites often are carried with the water adhesion onto the slide.

Skin scrapings can be frustrating to interpret. The scraping should be done firmly and deeply into the skin surface. The presence of blood at the site of scraping indicates that the depth is adequate to collect any infesting ectoparasites. Careful microscopic examination of the debris is useful to identify mites or their eggs. Potassium hydroxide solution may be used to clear the sample for examination.

Microbial Culture. Bacterial and fungal cultures can be used to determine the presence of pathogenic organisms. Culture results may be challenging to interpret because some cultured microbes may be part of the normal resident flora of the skin of small ruminants. Bacterial cultures may be obtained by aspirating pustules, abscesses, and other nodules. If a skin biopsy is to be performed, bacterial culture may be obtained from a sample of skin tissue. The clinician cleanses the desired sample area with alcohol and obtains a hair sample from the periphery of an active lesion. Cultures for dermatomycotic agents must be set up on special media. Fungal cultures may require weeks in a favorable environment before a positive or negative result can be reported.

Impression Smear. Impression smears may be of some (albeit limited) value, particularly in the diagnosis of very exudative or very dry lesions. A moist lesion or an area from which a scab has just been removed is selected. A clean glass microscope slide is carefully pressed against the lesion and is allowed to air dry or is fixed. The slide is then suitably stained, and the cytological evaluation is performed.

Biopsy. Skin biopsy is most useful to identify lesions consistent with ectoparasites and allergic and autoimmune disease. Skin biopsy is indicated when a lesion is unusual, has failed to respond to treatment, is suspected to be neoplastic, or is persistently ulcerative or exudative. It also can be used to rule out various pathologies during differential diagnosis. Biopsy specimens should be obtained from primary lesions and ideally should include the junction of normal and abnormal skin. Commercial skin biopsy instruments (with internal diameters of 4–8 mm) provide the best-quality samples for pathologists. Areas with minimal skin tension should be chosen. A needle and scalpel blade can be used to harvest a skin sample, or the entire lesion may be submitted if surgical excision is performed. Full-thickness skin biopsy is recommended to allow examination of all layers of the epidermis and dermis. Sedation or tranquilization of the patient may be required. The clinician may clip the hair surrounding the area of skin biopsy; however, hair emerging from the skin sample is desirable to enhance the pathologist's evaluation. Therefore, only minimal clipping should be performed, and a razor blade should not be used. A small amount of lidocaine hydrochloride 2% is deposited in the subcutaneous tissue deep within the specimen. This should be done carefully and immediately before biopsy because the side effects of lidocaine include vascular dilatation and edema, both of which may confuse histologic evaluation. Many pathologists prefer that skin specimens be preserved attached to a wooden plank such as a piece of a tongue depressor. Fixatives for skin samples include 10% neutral buffered formalin for routine light microscopy and glutaraldehyde for electron microscopy. Skin biopsies may be fixed with Michel's fixative or fresh-frozen without fixative if immunohistochemistry or other such tests are desired. In one study, shrinkage was similar for formalin-fixed and fresh-frozen specimens (approximately 20%).[4] Skin biopsy specimens should be submitted to a veterinary pathologist experienced in the interpretation of skin histology. Because skin histology varies dramatically among species, a pathologist experienced in the evaluation of the skin of small ruminants is preferable. If preferred by the clinician or owner, the biopsy site can be closed (using a simple interrupted or cruciate pattern) with either absorbable or nonabsorbable material.

Viral Diseases

Contagious Ecthyma (Sore Mouth/Orf/ Contagious Pustular Dermatitis)

This unique viral skin disease is caused by a parapoxvirus. It is seen primarily in sheep and goats but has also been reported in farmed and wild cervids, domestic ruminants, and humans.[5] The morbidity in naïve herds or flocks will approach 100%, but mortality rarely exceeds 1%. Mortality is not usually due to the infection itself but rather secondary complications such as pneumonia or starvation. The virus can persist in the soil for years and has survived in a laboratory environment at room temperature for 20 years.[2] A conflicting report indicated that the virus was undetectable in scabs shed naturally from healed lesions.[6] However, once on the farm, it is considered on the farm forever. Outbreaks tend to occur around lambing, fawning, or kidding time when newly susceptible offspring are present. Colostrum does not have antibodies protective against Orf, which leaves newborn kids susceptible to the disease.[1] Transmission may be through direct contact with the clinically affected, via fomites contaminated by the clinically affected, or indirectly via viral contaminated soil or shed scabs, and there is some evidence for spread via nonclinical carriers.[7] This transmission is likely more of a fomite transmission by animals not clinically infected than by animals positive for the virus yet clinically normal. "ORFV does not cause latent infections in animals that recover from clinical disease, but clinically healthy animals that are moved from infected to noninfected premises or transported in contaminated vehicles can act as mechanical carriers."[8] Asymptomatic carriers of Orf may contribute to the development of clinical disease.[9] The virus typically infects via a break in the skin. Thus, the disease tends to be most prevalent in young stock sometimes associated with teeth eruption.[10] The incubation period is 3 to 14 days. It is one of the more significant zoonotic skin diseases of sheep and goats and is considered to be extremely painful to the affected human. Veterinarians and producers should take precautions to avoid exposure by wearing disposable gloves when treating or examining suspect cases.

Clinical Signs. Clinical signs are relatively unique with scab-like lesions appearing most often on the lips, muzzle, and in the oral cavity. Lesions appear as crusty proliferations at mucocutaneous junctions similar to fever blisters. Initial lesions appear as papules, followed by vesicles, pustules, and scab formation. Scabs heal over and drop off in 1 to 4 weeks. The typical mild course of the disease in 10- to 21-day old lambs has been reported with resolution occurring beginning at 7 days.[10] Lesions may also develop on the teats and udders of nursing dams often due to suckling of affected young. Udder and teat lesions appear to be more painful, leading to dams refusing to nurse their offspring. This in turn may result in neonatal starvation. Lesions have also been reported on the ears, face, periorbital region, poll, scrotum, perianal region, and distal extremities. Rare cases of body (trunk and flanks) have been reported in both sheep and goats.[1,11,12] More severe forms described as malignant, persistent, and or chronic have been reported. In rare cases, there are extension of lesions down the respiratory tract predisposing to pneumonia and extension down the alimentary tract leading to gastroenteritis. Ten percent mortality was reported among 550 5-month-old lambs in which severe facial edema and extensive proliferative necrotic lesions developed in the anterior two thirds of the buccal cavity, including the tongue.[13] The stress of transportation may have increased the clinical severity of the disease in the aforementioned report.

Diagnosis. Diagnosis is most commonly based on clinical signs. In many countries, there are few other differentials that have an appearance and history of contagious ecthyma (typically mild disease with a high morbidity); other differentials include bluetongue, ulcerative dermatosis, sheep pox, capripox, and foot and mouth disease. A skin biopsy and histopathology can be confirmatory. Histopathology reveals ballooning and degeneration of keratinocytes and eosinophilic intracytoplasmic viral inclusions. Electron microscopy has been used to detect the virus in scabs. More viral particles are present in early scabs than aged scabs; thus, "fresh" scabs, rather than old ones, should be submitted for electron microscopy. Samples for diagnosis can be submitted refrigerated or at room temperature but should be packaged to prevent human contact. One drawback to electron microscopy is that all parapoxviruses (e.g., bovine papular stomatitis and pseudocowpox) are morphologically indistinguishable. Serology can be used to determine exposure status and gives presumptive evidence for the disease. Polymerase chain reaction (PCR) tests have been developed and may become the preferred method of diagnosis.

Treatment. Treatment is seldom attempted as the disease is self-limiting and should resolve within 3 weeks. At that time, the scab will fall off, contaminating the environment. The disease is really of little consequence in weaned and older stock, but neonates may need supplemental feedings. Secondary bacterial infection may occur and if suspected may be treated with topical or systemic antibiotics (see Appendix 1). In some parts of the world, blowfly strike can complicate contagious ecthyma and thus should be observed for and treated as necessary. Cases with greater economic or sentimental value that result in anorexia due to painful oral lesions may be treated with electrocautery and debridement after first using spray cryotherapy with good results.[14] Ointments and astringent lotions may actually delay healing.[15]

Prevention. Prevention is best performed by preventing the disease from entering the farm by use of quarantine and physical examination of stock entering the farm and or by purchasing new stock from contagious ecthyma free herds or flocks. Special efforts should be made to prevent contact of suspect animals at livestock shows and sales and avoiding using common feed, water, and grooming equipment. In an outbreak situation, the affected stock should be isolated and the remainder vaccinated. This method should help control production losses due to control of the location of the disease. Once the disease is on the farm, vaccines are available that can help control the disease. Vaccines are live and should not be used unless the disease is known to be present in a herd or flock. Most commercial vaccines are labeled for sheep but not goats. Although use of these vaccines in goats has at times appeared anecdotally efficacious, research has indicated that sheep vaccines were not effective in protecting goats from the wild-type contagious ecthyma virus found in goats.[16] A goat strain vaccine for contagious ecthyma was found to be protective against experimental challenge.[17] Vaccines are typically placed on scarified skin of the medial thigh. Other sites should be used, such as inside the ear pinna or under the tail, when vaccinating lactating females. Scabs should be present by 3 to 4 days if the vaccination is successful. If vaccination is used, its use should be tailored for the particular herd or flock management. One example of vaccine use is to begin with vaccination of all stock that have not been previously exposed and then vaccinate only the new naïve stock (new births and new additions) annually. Immunity is reported to occur 3 weeks after vaccination but is not considered to be lifelong.[18] Naturally exposed stock that have recovered are usually solidly immune for 2 to 3 years.[15] It has been stated that colostrum immunity does not occur as antibodies do not appear to be passed in the colostrum.[2,15] Yet a study by Perez demonstrated that kids of vaccinated does when challenged at < 45 days of age did not develop lesions whereas kids > 45 days of age did develop lesions.[19] Some farms, in which the disease is endemic, chose to simply live with the disease. The disease has a shorter course and is less severe in reinfected stock.

Malignant Contagious Ecthyma

A persistent form of contagious ecthyma known as *malignant contagious ecthyma* has been recognized in a limited number of sheep within infected flocks. Proliferative lesions develop, especially on the distal legs and feet and less commonly on the head. However, unlike ordinary contagious ecthyma, the lesions fail to regress and may continually enlarge. Secondary bacterial infections, fly strike, and hemorrhage are major complications. Although a poxvirus morphologically similar to the contagious ecthyma virus has been identified by electron microscopy in typical lesions, the disease has a different course. Affected sheep do not pass the infection to commingling animals. Preliminary studies of the cellular immune systems of affected sheep have failed to demonstrate any deviation from normal.[20]

Ulcerative Dermatosis

Ulcerative dermatosis is a disease of sheep caused by a virus similar to but distinct from the contagious ecthyma parapoxvirus.

Infection typically follows a break in the skin, such as shearing injuries and breeding injuries. The virus may be spread via physical contact during breeding season. This may be one reason why the disease is most common in the fall and winter. The incubation period is 2 to 7 days. Healing occurs in 2 to 6 weeks. In the United States, the disease is most common in the west and morbidity is usually 15 to 20% but may be as high as 60%.

Clinical Signs. Lesions develop as ulcers and develop a thin but very adherent scab. Lesions associated with the initial viral infection may become infected with *Fusobacterium necrophorum*. Lesions may occur on the face, eyes, lips, and nostrils but also occur in the interdigital space, legs, penis, and vulva. Lesions of the lower limb may lead to septic arthritis. Lesions of the penis may result in phimosis or paraphimosis. The facial and lip lesions are not typically associated with the mucous membranes, which helps differentiate them from contagious ecthyma lesions.

Diagnosis. The most likely differential is contagious ecthyma, but the morbidity is lower and the lesions are ulcerative rather than proliferative like contagious ecthyma. Confirmation is based on histopathology of biopsied lesions.

Treatment. The disease is self-limiting, but antibiotics are justified for secondary bacterial infections and severe cases. Otherwise, treatment is symptomatic.

Prevention. Prevention is best carried out by examination of breeding stock during breeding season and isolation of affected animals. When the disease is a common occurrence, efforts should be made to decrease skin trauma via reduction of shearing injuries, removing stock from areas that are abrasive to the feet and legs, and utilizing feeds that are nonabrasive. No vaccine is available and immunity is short-lived (~5 months).

Sheep Pox and Goat Pox

The agents of sheep pox and goat pox are closely related viruses of the Capripox genus in the family Poxviridae. Although the viruses tend to be species specific, cross-species infection has been known to occur. Practitioners must be careful in conversation with laypeople that may refer to a staphylococcal dermatitis as "goat pox."[1] True sheep pox and goat pox mortality is low in endemic regions but may be high when naïve sheep or goats are exposed. Transmission (thought to be aerosol and contact with lesions) increases with close contact with infected herds or flocks. These diseases are currently endemic in northern Africa, the Middle East, and southeastern Asia, with occasional outbreaks in southeastern Europe. There is one report of goat pox in the United States,[21] but the U.S. Department of Agriculture–Animal and Plant Health Inspection Service website states that neither disease has occurred in the United States. Contagious ecthyma is the primary differential of sheep and goat pox. However, sheep and goat pox lesions tend to occur over the entire body skin surfaces. The two viral agents (contagious ecthyma and sheep or goat pox) are easily differentiated via electron microscopy. A protein-based enzyme-linked immunosorbent assay (ELISA) has been tested and shown effective in detecting serum levels of virus for both sheep and goats.[22] A thorough review of sheep pox has been published.[23]

Scrapie and Chronic Wasting Disease

A discussion of scrapie is beyond the scope of this chapter. However, due to the intense pruritus, (although pruritus is much less common in goats than in sheep) scrapie-infected sheep or goats may present with hair or wool loss due to mechanical excoriations. Scrapie does not directly affect the skin; skin lesions are simply a result of the intense pruritus and subsequent aggressive itching. There may be a breed predilection for Suffolk sheep. Chronic wasting disease affects at least six species of cervidae (white-tailed deer, mule deer, moose, wapiti, red deer, and reindeer). The disease is beyond the scope of this chapter and cervids do not exhibit the pruritus seen in sheep or goats.

Bluetongue and Epizootic Hemorrhagic Disease (EHD)/Hemorrhagic Disease (in Cervids HD)

A discussion of bluetongue is beyond the scope of this chapter. However, skin lesions suggestive of bluetongue include coronitis, ulcerations of the oral mucosa, and muzzle edema. Goats are relatively resistant to clinical bluetongue. Easily the most costly disease to the cervid industry in morbidity and mortality, HD does not commonly cause skin lesions, but hoof lesions are very common due to coronitis. Those that survive may slough hooves.[24]

Vesicular Stomatitis

Vesicular stomatitis (VS) is a viral disease that creates ulcerations of the oral mucosa of cattle, swine, and horses. Although both goats and sheep may be experimentally infected with VS virus, natural clinical disease is quite rare and no case reports could be found that documented clinical disease. Sheep and goats never show clinical signs of VS.[23] A 1995 outbreak of VS in the western United States did not identify a single sheep or goat positive for VS.[25] However, unpublished reports of VS in goats indicated that vesicles may occur at the commissures of the lips.[26] Although experimentally infected with VS, no cases have been reported in the United States in wild cervids.[24]

Bacterial Diseases

Dermatophilosis (Streptothricosis, Lumpy Wool Disease, Rain Scald, Rain Rot)

This is a disease of all ruminants caused by the gram-positive, filamentous bacterium *D. congolensis* (Figure 10.1). The bacterium appears to be maintained within herds or flocks via carrier animals. The organism is considered an obligate parasite of ruminant skin and was not thought to survive for very long in the soil, but later research indicates that it may survive for several months, especially within cast-off crusts.[27,28] Predisposing factors for clinical disease include skin damage (e.g., biting insects and physical abrasion), excessive moisture (hence the common name Rain Rot), and concurrent diseases and stresses that compromise the host's immune systems. The loss of the sebaceous film layer on skin is thought to predispose the animal to the disease. Thus, excessively rainy conditions without appropriate shelter can lead to dilution of this sebaceous layer, increasing the chance of clinical disease. The incubation period averages 2 weeks. The infective form of the organism is the motile zoospore that germinates, penetrates the epidermis, and invades hair or wool follicles. Neutrophils migrate to the affected areas and a serous exudate accumulates and seeps to the epidermal surface. The older epidermal skin deteriorates while a new layer of epidermis forms below. This new layer

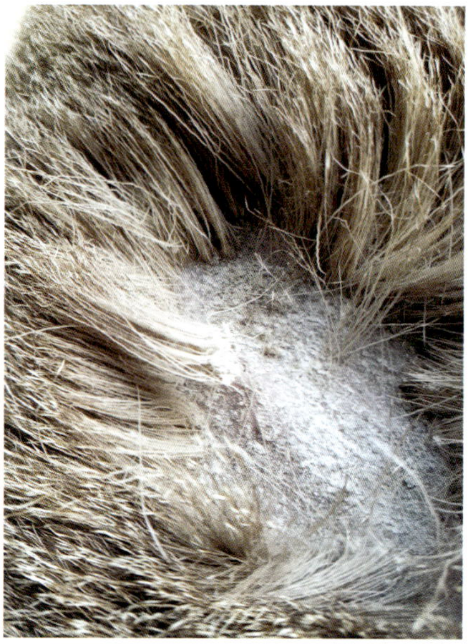

• **Fig. 10.1** A dermatophilosis lesion on the dorsum of a mule deer.

also becomes infected with hyphal branches. Eventually, thick scabs are formed. Early signs of clinical disease are characterized by small, raised, and circumscribed crusts of epidermal cells and serous exudates with embedded hairs or wool. The disease follows a similar pattern in sheep, but the serous exudates may not be adhered to the epidermis. It does have a negative impact on the quality of the wool.[29] It is also responsible for "strawberry foot rot" of sheep and appears as dry scabs on the lower legs.[30] The removal of the dry scabs leaves a mass of granulation tissue that has the appearance of a strawberry (hence the name). Although it can be spread from acutely infected animals, outbreaks are rare but have been reported.[31] Young goats appear to be more susceptible to clinical disease than adults.[31,32] Likewise, young sheep are more susceptible than adult sheep.[33] Fawns are the most commonly affected age group in cervids, especially bottle-reared fawns, due to milk spilling on the faces as fawns aggressively nurse bottles. These wet areas are perfect media sites for the bacteria. Dermatophilosis has been shown to temporarily decrease fertility in bulls during an active clinical case.[34]

Clinical Signs. Follicular and nonfollicular papules and pustules develop and rapidly coalesce and rupture, resulting in groups of hairs or wool being matted together. These are classically described as "paintbrush lesions" in haired ruminants. Lesions may be painful but are not pruritic. In sheep, crusts occurring at the coronary band (called strawberry foot rot) may also extend to the carpi or tarsi. Lesions may also be present on other parts of the body. In goat kids, lesions tend to be on the ears and tails; in adults, lesions tend to be on the muzzle, dorsal midline, scrotum, or distal legs.[32] Lesions have been reported in the ears of kids at 5 days of age.[35] Fawns typically get lesions around the face or legs. Usually, the lesions are circular and well circumscribed. Although relatively rare, in livestock debilitated by other diseases and poor nutrition, death can occur.

Diagnosis. Staining (Gram stain or methylene blue) of direct smears of lesions should reveal branching hyphae with cuboidal packets of coccoid cells arranged in parallel rows (similar to railroad tracks) within the filaments. Skin biopsy and histopathology may also be helpful. Culture can be confirmatory, although possible subsequent infestation by other bacterial and fungal organisms may complicate the diagnosis in chronic cases.[36]

Treatment. Topical treatment includes iodophors, 2 to 5% lime sulfur, 0.2% copper sulfate, 0.5% zinc sulfate, and 1% potassium aluminum sulfate. Treatments may be applied as total body washes, sprays, or dips for 3 to 5 consecutive days then weekly until healing has occurred. Systemic antibiotics such as procaine penicillin G (5000 IU/kg BID for 4–5 days), oxytetracycline (one or two doses at 20 mg/kg at a 72-hour interval), or ceftiofur (1 ml/23 kg SID for 4–5 days) may be effective. The organism is reported to be resistant to polymyxin B, bacitracin, and sulfonamides. Lesions of kids tend to heal without treatment within 2 to 3 months.[37] Most fawns respond to topical and systemic treatment as done for lambs and kids. They tend to resent daily treatment and it is suggested that they be treated with long-acting antibiotics to reduce stress of daily handling if possible. Dermatophilus is potentially zoonotic to humans.

Prevention. Where the disease is prevalent, removal and disposal of crusts, keeping stock dry (providing shelter from wet weather), providing good-quality nutrition, and control of ectoparasites may limit clinical cases. Vaccines have been studied but do not appear to offer significant protection.[33]

Fleece Rot (Water Rot, Weather Stain)

Fleece rot is an exudative bacterial dermatitis of sheep that is characterized by a greenish-discolored, matted wool. This disease reduces the quality of the wool but is most important as a predisposing factor for fly-strike. Although other fleece bacteria may play a significant role in the disease, *Pseudomonas aeruginosa* is considered the primary etiologic agent.[38] The disease was first recognized in Australia in the latter part of the 1800s.[33] Bacteria cultured from the skin of affected sheep, when applied to unaffected sheep, resulted in the disease.[39] The necessity of moisture for disease symptoms was noted by Seddon and McGrath in 1929.[40] Both wool traits and body conformation traits predispose sheep to fleece rot and this susceptibility is reportedly heritable.[40] The disease appears to be most prevalent in Australia with reports averaging 24%.[33] The disease does not appear to be significant in the United States but has been reported.[41] The reason that young sheep are more susceptible than older stock is not known but may be due to the maturity of wool and skin characteristics or could be that a certain level of immunity develops after exposure.[33] Fleece rot predisposes sheep to blowfly strike.

Clinical Signs. The most characteristic clinical sign is the greenish discoloration of wool. A copious serous exudation may also be evident and this exudation is likely the attraction that leads to associated fly-strike.[33] The inflammatory reaction can result in grayish matted wool. Pruritus has also been reported, but not all affected sheep demonstrate this.[42] Lesions are most common on the back and withers.

Diagnosis. Culture of the skin and wool is the definitive method to diagnose fleece rot (would be especially definitive for greenish-discolored wool). *P. aeruginosa* may be found in pure culture. It produces the green pigment, pyocyanin.[43] Fleece rot may be distinguished from dermatophilosis in that no scab is associated with the infection

Treatment. Antibiotics may be helpful, but studies have shown *P. aeruginosa* to be quite resistant to many antibiotics.[44,45]

Practically speaking, shearing and allowing the lesion to dry are the most effective means of treatment.

Prevention. Vaccines have and are being developed, but efficacy to date has been disappointing.[33] Some prevention is afforded by producing more resistant sheep by breeding for characteristics of wool and body conformation that are less predisposing. Perhaps the most practical control measure is to shear the sheep prior to the onset of the rainy season.

Malignant Edema (Swelled Head, Bighead)

Malignant edema is a rapidly fatal disease caused by Clostridial species, most commonly *Clostridium sordellii*, *Clostridium novyi*, *Clostridium septicum*, and/or *Clostridium chauvoei* and is seen most commonly in young rams. Although swelled head of bucks (goats) is listed in many textbooks, no studies or case reports could be found for goats. Blackleg and malignant edema have both been reported as individual cases and herd outbreaks.[46] One of the authors (CFS) has seen clostridial infection in velvet antler in a white-tailed buck. The organisms typically exist as spores in the soil but appear to predominate in humid soils that are rich in organic matter.[46] The organisms usually enter the body through breaks in the skin or mucosa. When the anaerobic conditions arise in body tissues, the organisms proliferate and release several exotoxins that react locally and systemically. The spores of clostridial organisms are thought to survive in the environment for several years. The disease is most common in Montana in the United States but also occurs in South Africa, South America, and Australia.[18]

Clinical Signs. The disease is usually sporadic in nature but can occur as outbreaks. A Brazilian outbreak likely occurred through the use of a single common needle to vaccinate a 1000-head flock of sheep with a commercial clostridial vaccine.[46] There is another report of a herd outbreak after vaccination with a multivalent vaccine. The vaccine was administered intramuscularly in the hindlimb using new needles and syringes for each animal.[47] Several sheep died in that outbreak. All affected sheep died within 1 to 3 days of vaccination. Clinical signs seen prior to death included severe depression, swelling around the vaccination site, lameness, subcutaneous edema, and crepitation. The classic epidemiology of bighead in sheep is due to butting of rams that leads to breaks in the skin, allowing bacterial spores access to the bruised subcutaneous tissues. Once infection occurs, there are swelling and edema of the face, head, and neck.

Diagnosis. An aseptically collected aspirate of the subcutaneous swelling followed by staining of an impression smear and subsequent anaerobic culture can be definitive. Clostridial organisms stain as large gram-positive rods. The fluorescent antibody test can differentiate between the different clostridial species.

Treatment. If treatment is not initiated immediately, the fatality rate will be high. Treatment primarily consists of high doses of penicillin products that should be administered both locally and systemically. Additional treatment is primarily symptomatic.

Prevention. Vaccination can be preventative as long as administered after the period of passive transfer and prior to traumatic events. Hygiene is also emphasized as some cases have been documented to occur after a simple blood draw.[48]

Actinobacillosis

Actinobacillus lignieresii, a non–spore-forming, gram-negative rod, causes a pyogranulomatous bacterial infection of the soft tissues of the head of sheep (not documented in goats[3] and rarely reported in cervids). These bacteria usually are inoculated into the tissues by grass awns or stemmy forage. A local granulomatous reaction occurs, but these bacteria also may spread to regional lymph nodes or the bloodstream. They can produce chains of small nodules leading to the lymph nodes.

Clinical Signs. Purulent material may be observed draining from lymph nodes. Caseous lymphadenitis (CL) is a differential diagnosis for this condition.[49] Severe enlargement of submaxillary or parotid lymph nodes may cause difficulty in breathing or eating; sheep may die from malnutrition. Nasal exudate may be noted if the infection drains into the nasopharynx.

Diagnosis. The diagnosis is made by performing cytology and a Gram stain on the exudate. The gram-negative rods are filamentous and form sulfur granules in the pus that can be seen without the aid of a microscope.

Treatment. Therapy includes surgical drainage, antibiotics (procaine penicillin G, 22,000–66,000 units/kg body weight subcutaneously [SC] every 24 hours for 7 days), and iodine therapy. Sodium iodide can be administered (80 mg/kg body weight) intravenously (IV) and repeated once or twice at 7-day intervals. Alternatively, organic iodides can be added to the feed (7.5–15 g/head/day) for 14 to 21 days.

Staphylococcal Dermatitis (Eye Scab, Impetigo)

Staphylococcus dermatitis is a typically nonfatal skin disease of sheep and goats that affects predominately the head and face or mammary gland and is caused by *S. aureus* but occasionally other staphylococcal species are involved. The condition appears more commonly during warm seasons of the year. Transmission appears to be social contact with clinical or nonclinical carriers.[50] Sporadic cases may occur but outbreaks have been reported.[51]

Clinical Signs. Facial signs may present as nonpruritic lesions above the upper eyelid that expand to other parts of the face and in extreme cases the lower limbs.[51] The skin lesions were characterized by alopecia, papules, crusts, erosions or ulcers, exudation, erythema, hyperpigmentation, and thickening of the skin.[51] The lesions bleed easily.[49] Overall, the dermatitis did not appear to adversely affect the health of the affected sheep. *S. aureus* dermatitis of a ewe has been described as a dermatitis and hyperkeratosis on the skin of the udder and teats with accompanying pustules.[52] *Staphylococcus hyicus* was determined to be the causative agent in a case of seborrheic dermatitis that proved fatal in an 18-month-old pygmy goat.[53] The clinical signs of the aforementioned case were similar to greasy pig disease in that there was a generalized seborrheic dermatitis with alopecia; the skin was greasy and had a severe scaly to scabby appearance.

Diagnosis. The differential diagnosis should include ectoparasites, zinc deficiency, elaeophoriasis, and mycotic infections. Definitive diagnostics require culture and absence of other causes. Histopathological lesions have been well documented.[51]

Treatment. Antibiotics may be required in severe cases and may hasten resolution in any case. Oxytetracycline and enrofloxacin were minimally effective while a lincomycin/spectinomycin combination was effective in one case report.[51] Penicillin has been reported to be efficacious.[54] However, facial staphylococcus dermatitis tends to resolve within 2 months.[55] Other treatments consist of washing with an iodophor or chlorhexidine shampoo, drying, and then coating with an antiseptic or antibiotic ointment.[3]

Prevention. Feeding and housing in an environment that lessens the chance of facial injuries and close head-to-head contact should reduce the incidence of the disease. Fly control may be important in transmission reduction. Isolation of the affected stock and care to avoid fomite transmission is important to limit new staphylococcal intramammary infections.

Abscesses

Abscesses of the soft tissues are not uncommon in small ruminants. Abscesses usually begin when wounds allow entry of surface bacteria through the epidermis. Therefore, *Staphylococcus* species, *Corynebacterium* species, *Arcanobacterium pyogenes*, and streptococcal bacteria are expected on culture. *Fusobacteria* sp. and *Trueperella pyogenes* are commonly found in cervid abscesses. Noncontagious abscesses may be treated by lancing after infiltration of local anesthesia. The interior capsule of the abscess is debrided and flushed with a dilute iodine solution (1%). For large abscesses, roll bandages soaked in dilute iodine solutions may be stuffed into the capsule of the abscess with removal of a portion of the bandage daily over the next 3 to 5 days. Systemic antimicrobial agents are not indicated in most cases but may be administered if numerous abscesses or deeply seeded abscesses are present.

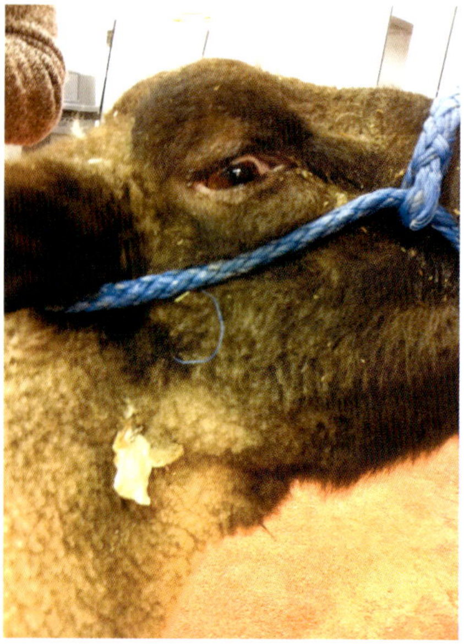

• **Fig. 10.2** A sheep with rupture and drainage of purulent exudate from the caseous lymphadenitis abscess of the parotid lymph node. Notice the thickness of the discharge. (Photo courtesy of Dr. Sandra Taylor, Purdue University)

Caseous Lymphadenitis

CL is a common, contagious, suppurative bacterial disease of sheep and goats worldwide that most frequently infects the lymph nodes and lymphatic system. A study of cull sheep in the western United States reported a prevalence of 42%.[56] The agent of the disease, *Corynebacterium pseudotuberculosis*, creates chronic infections that can eventually be fatal. The agent enters the body through broken or intact skin or mucous membranes, via inhalation and ingestion.[57] Once a lymph node becomes infected, an abscess then develops and spreads to other lymph nodes and internal organs via the lymphatic and hematogenous routes. Abscesses tend to be caseous and the classic CL abscess on cut surface has an onion-ring-layered appearance, which is only rarely present in goats.[58] The organism survives for months in the environment, and environmental exposure, especially fomites, plays a key role in transmission. The disease is considered zoonotic. At the current time, this disease is not considered to be significant in cervids.

Clinical Signs. The most obvious clinical signs are enlargement of external lymph nodes especially the parotid, submandibular, and supramammary, but the prescapular and prefemoral may also be enlarged.[59] (Figure 10.2). Although abscesses typically develop during a period of 2 to 6 months,[60] abscess development and lymph node enlargement have occurred within 2 weeks of shearing with apparently contaminated clippers.

Enlargement of the external lymph nodes does not usually result in other clinical signs, but enlargement of the internal lymph nodes and major organ infection can lead to eventual death. Approximately 25% of sheep with overt abscesses are predicted to develop respiratory abscesses.[60] The predominate clinical sign seen in goats and sheep with internal abscessation is a history of chronic weight loss, but coughing and respiratory symptoms may be present, as well as chronic bloat. Less frequently, affected animals may show mastitis, cellulitis, or orchitis. Thus, clinical signs vary according to the organ affected. Affected organs may include the liver, kidneys, mediastinal lymph nodes (Figure 10.3), gastrointestinal lymph nodes, the central nervous system, and the mammary gland (mastitis). Hormonal imbalances have been shown to occur in chronically infected does, which may lead to a decrease in reproductive efficiency.[61]

Diagnosis. Although other bacteria may occasionally be isolated from enlarged external lymph nodes, the primary differential should be *C. pseudotuberculosis* until proven otherwise. Another differential is tuberculosis more often in the United Kingdom than the United States, as tuberculosis is present in parts of the United Kingdom.[49] Because the abscess material is so potentially contagious, special care should be taken to avoid allowing the pustular material from reaching the environment. A positive culture of the material is definitive for CL, which appears as small gram-positive rods of variable length. Occasionally, a coccoid form of *C. pseudotuberculosis* may be seen so do not automatically

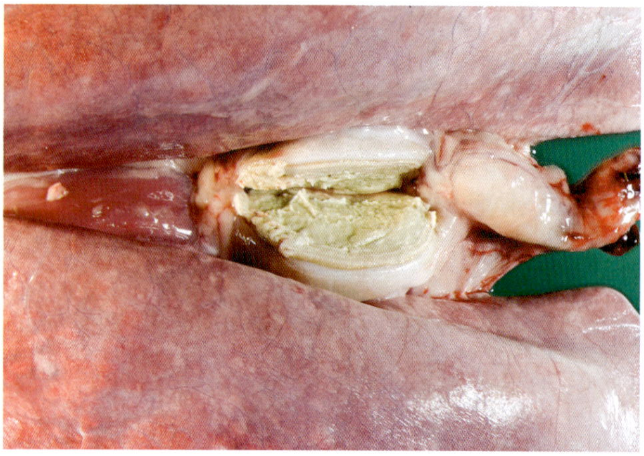

• **Fig. 10.3** The cut surface of a caseous lymphadenitis abscess in the caudal mediastinal lymph node of a sheep. Notice the onion-layer appearance of the abscess. (Courtesy Dr. José Ramos-Vara, Purdue University.)

rule out CL with this finding. Microscopic examination of the purulent material will be more helpful in early infections. Samples should be collected in a sterile manner for culture. Some positive animals will be culture negative because other bacteria present overgrow the *C. pseudotuberculosis* or one simply samples a negative area of the abscess. Likewise, there are numerous tests that can be conducted in asymptomatic stock to determine the CL infection status. Diagnosis of sheep and goats without enlarged external lymph nodes requires serologic testing. Both agglutination tests and hemolysis synergistic inhibition tests may aid in identification. These two tests are not accurate enough for clinicians to base decisions to cull animals that have early nonclinical infections. ELISA is the most frequently used serologic test for CL. It is relatively inexpensive, readily performed, and has good sensitivity. Agar gel immunodiffusion (AGID) can be performed but takes longer to test than ELISA and may be less sensitive. Some ELISA techniques are more accurate in goats than sheep so should be considered as such when used to test for eradication in a flock. PCR for genomic testing is useful when applied to the purulent abscess material; however, it is obviously difficult to sample internal abscesses and blood testing via PCR is not as reliable as sampling purulent material. When trying to eliminate CL from a flock, repeated testing using different methods will need to be done as no single test can identify all cases and stages of the disease.[62]

Treatment. External lymph node abscesses may be removed surgically, but special care needs to be implemented so that the abscess is not opened during surgical removal. Lancing and draining the external abscesses may be done with special care to collect all of the purulent material and flushing solution so as not to contaminate the environment. This collected material should be burned. If lancing and draining the abscess(es) are utilized, a 1-month isolation is recommended to prevent subsequent spread to other susceptible sheep or goats. Treatment and management of the external lymph nodes do not guarantee that the small ruminant is free of CL as internal lymph node infection may also be present. Systemic antibiotics are not considered to be very effective because of the thickness of the lymph node capsule and the intracellular survival (even within activated macrophages) of the bacteria.[63] However, systemic antibiotics with a gram-positive spectrum should be used when treating an external abscess to help prevent spread to other lymph nodes. Injection of formalin into the abscess has been used, with some success. A recent study compared the efficacy of three different treatments for CL.[64] Treatments included (1) opening, draining, flushing (with a diluted iodine solution), and treating with subcutaneous penicillin, (2) closed system lavage (a 16-gauge needle was used to inject saline and withdraw the saline abscess mixture) and intralesional tulathromycin, and (3) closed-system lavage and subcutaneous tulathromycin. All treatments resulted in $> 80\%$ resolution of the treated lesions. Ultimately, the best treatment is to cull the affected animals.[60]

Prevention. The best prevention is to maintain a CL-free flock. Any new stock should be tested for CL and examined for lymph node enlargement prior to entering the flock. Housing should be maintained free of objects that can cause skin injury. Needles, surgical equipment, tattoo pliers, shears, foot trimmers, and dipping vats should be cleansed and disinfected after use. In addition, the control of external parasites is considered important because pruritic stock will rub themselves on items that could produce breaks in the skin.[3] Eradication is possible but difficult in that it requires frequent testing and management of a CL-free and CL-infected group. Vaccines are available and can be helpful especially in herds or flocks that choose to live with the disease in that they can reduce the incidence of abscesses in a flock.[65] Vaccines do not necessarily prevent the disease, but new and better vaccines could lead to a means of prevention or at least control of CL.[66,67]

Goats vaccinated with sheep CL vaccines tend to have more adverse reactions than sheep. Anecdotal reports indicate that goat owners are more satisfied with autogenous CL vaccines. Milk and colostrum transmission is apparently not important, but removal of neonatal lambs and kids from affected dams should lessen the chance of exposure. Likewise, intrauterine transmission has not been reported.

Fungal Diseases

Dermatophytosis (Ringworm, Lumpy Wool, Club Lamb Fungus)

The primary fungal agent of ringworm in sheep and goats is *Trichophyton verrucosum*. However, *Trichophyton mentagrophytes*, *Microsporum canis*, and other less common species have been reported.[2,68] Transmission occurs via direct contact with clinically affected individuals or indirectly via contaminated fomites (fences, water or feed equipment, grooming equipment). The disease tends to be more common in young animals than in adults, likely due to decreased immunity in those young animals not previously exposed to the disease agent. Other potential predisposing factors include immunosuppression, poor nutrition, crowding, high humidity, and other debilitating diseases. The zoophilic dermatophytes exist as spores in the environment. The dermatophytes utilize keratin as a nutrient source, ergo their predilection for skin.[69] Spores typically enter the skin via abrasions. The conidium (the spores) germinates and hyphae appear within the stratum corneum (invasion of living tissue does not occur) and invade the walls of the hair follicles. They then emerge into the follicular canal and grow downward between the hair cuticle and the wall of the follicle. The hyphal tip penetrates into the hair cortex by dissolving the keratin and by mechanical pressure, and multiplication ensues with conidia located outside of the hair shaft.[69] As the hair grows, the fungal elements are carried out of and above the surface of the skin, where hairs may become broken or fall out. Spread occurs centrifugally from the point of invasion, resulting in the classic ring-shaped lesion. Incubation period from exposure to clinical disease is 1 to 6 weeks and is more commonly seen in the fall and winter months.

Lanolin or perhaps full wool tends to protect the sheep skin from ringworm invasion.[49] Show lambs are sheared short and the frequent washing to prepare them for show tends to remove the protective lanolin, allowing the ringworm agents better access to infect the skin (Figure 10.4). Thus, this disease would be unusual in sheep that are not being prepped for show or sale. Club lamb fungus was first reported in 1989. Although typically considered a disease of show lambs due to extensive washing and close shearing, herd outbreaks have occurred in commercial flocks and were associated with recent shearing with possibly contaminated blades.[70,71] The disease is contagious, which is why sheep with evidence of ringworm are not allowed to participate in fair activities. Lesions take ~1 month to become evident. Fungal spores remain viable for years under natural conditions. Those treating or working with the flock or herd should wear protective clothing and gloves as the disease is zoonotic.

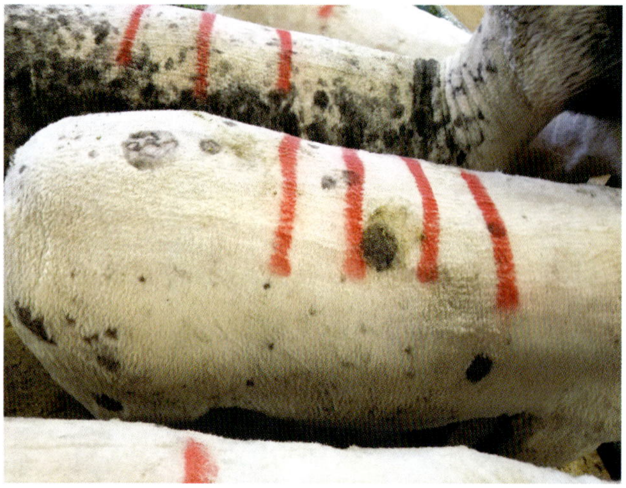

• **Fig. 10.4** Typical presentation of show lamb fungus. Lesions may appear on any haired or wooled body surface. The first sign of club lamb fungus (ringworm) is often a raised area where the wool is clumped and feels stiff. The affected area may be covered by a gray-white scab.

Clinical Signs. In both goats and sheep, lesions affect primarily the ears, head, and neck but any body surface may be affected. Ringworm lesions affecting wooled surfaces were previously considered to be rare, but show lamb fungus is probably as common on the wooled areas as on the more typical locations. Lesions in haired areas consist of circular patches of alopecia, scaling, and crusts, but affected areas may also be uneven and diffuse. Lesions in wooled areas may be covered with matted wool and be inflamed and reddened underneath the matt.[71] Lesions tend to be nonpruritic or only mildly pruritic and are usually not painful. Although lesions typically occur on the face, ears, neck, and shoulder area, lesions may also be dispersed over the body, including the tail head region.[71]

Diagnosis. Although most diagnoses are based on the clinical presentation, this assumption may be faulty as numerous other conditions can be similar. Differentials for sheep and goats should include external parasites, zinc deficiency, dermatophilosis, staphylococcus dermatitis, and immune mediated diseases. Use of the Wood's lamp during clinical examination may help with differential diagnosis. However, Trichophyton species do not fluoresce. Ultimately, fungal culture on Sabouraud's dextrose agar and identification is definitive. Scrapings should occur from the periphery of the lesion as these strictly aerobic fungi die out under the crust in the center of most lesions. The exudation from inflamed epithelial layers, epithelial debris, and fungal hyphae produce the dry crusts that create a more anaerobic environment. Microscopic examination of hairs and keratin from the periphery of an active lesion may reveal ectothrix invasion of hair shafts.[3] A 20% potassium hydroxide solution can be used to prepare wet mounts of arthrospores on the hair shafts for microscopic examination.

Treatment. The first step in dealing with a case of ringworm is the isolation of the affected stock. Care must be taken to eliminate spread of the fungus on hands or other fomites to herd mates. The disease is self-limiting and usually does not adversely affect the health of the affected small ruminant. Healing takes 4 to 16 weeks for spontaneous recovery. Some have reported healing in as short as 2 weeks, but this has not been scientifically validated. Many treatments have been suggested, but few have been studied to determine actual efficacy. Most treatments are extra-label and meat withdrawal times are rarely known. The following treatments should not be considered "the definitive treatment" but are options when clients want their stock treated. Griseofulvin has been suggested for infections that are widespread on the body or chronic. This antifungal agent becomes incorporated into keratin in the skin and hair and treated stock remain resistant for a number of weeks following treatment.[72] Griseofulvin can be expensive and slaughter withdrawal time is not specified. One report indicated that lesions regressed soon after treatment with seven daily doses of 7.5 mg/kg griseofulvin in feed and were almost completely resolved 20 days later. Natamycin has been used with some success but did not cure severe lesions especially those in the wooled areas.[71] Listerine has been suggested for spot treatment (scrubbed into the lesion) with a brush once a day for 7 days. Seven percent iodine mixed with Bag Balm has been applied to lesions once a day for 7 days. 10 to 20% sodium iodide administered IV at 1 g/14 kg at weekly intervals has been reported to be effective.[2] To stop an outbreak, exposed stock should be treated. When treatments are applied as sprays or ointments, treatment should concentrate on the margins of the lesions where the most active growth of the dermatophyte is and should also extend beyond the lesion as dermatophytes may be isolated from normal-appearing skin up to 6 cm.[73] These can be treated with 3% captan or 2 to 5% lime sulfur applied topically daily for 5 days, then weekly for another 3 to 4 weeks. All exposed stock, the environment and fomites should be treated or when practical, properly disposed of. Five percent lime sulfur, 5% sodium hypochlorite, 5% formalin, 3% captan, and 3% cresol have all been suggested for environmental treatment.[2] Chlorhexidine 0.5% is reportedly very effective for show lamb fungus but is inactivated by soap.[70] Exposure to sunlight and treatment with vitamins A and D may hasten healing of lesions.[34,70] However, Scott notes that there is no indication that vitamin and mineral preparations are of any benefit in most cases.[2] Ultraviolet light has proven helpful in treating ringworm; thus, exposure to sunlight may be beneficial.[69] Animals that do not recover within 4 months likely have significant immunosuppressive or predisposing environmental factors that need to be addressed.[2] Alternative and herbal treatments abound, but scientific evidence of successful treatment with herbal remedies is limited.[74]

Prevention. General preventive measures for the herd or flock include good nutrition, proper health care, and a clean, dry, sunny environment. Vaccines are available in some countries. The disease is zoonotic, so wearing protective gloves is strongly advised. The spores may exist for several years, thus once on the farm, always on the farm. Use of antifungal disinfectants on exposed equipment and housing is highly recommended. Various means are used to determine the infection status of show stock at fairs. Nebraska regulations use "inactive if the affected area is not encrusted and hair/wool has begun growth in the area."[75] For both treatment and prevention, the clinician is advised to determine if treatments can be legally used for food animals in a state or country where the animals reside.

Mycetoma

Mycetomas are painless granulomatous infections of the skin, subcutaneous tissues, and bones characterized by sinus formation through which fungal colonies are discharged in the form of grains.[34] Mycetomas may also be formed by bacterial elements or both fungal and bacterial elements.[3] Lesions most often occur on the limbs, are slow growing, and may be initiated by a wound. These lesions cause focal swelling and have an exudate that contains granules composed of microbial organisms coated with host immune elements (e.g., immunoglobulins, fibrin).[76] These granules may be red, yellow, or purple. *Actinomadura madurae* and *Actinomadura pelletierii* have been found in goats with mycetoma, as has *Nocardia brasiliensis*. Although success rates are unknown, treatment strategies include the use of antimicrobial drugs, surgical excision, and limb amputation depending on the severity of the disease. Mycetomas have not been reported in sheep. No reports could be found in white-tailed deer.

Candidiasis

Yeast or Candida dermatitis has been diagnosed in goats.[76,77] *Candida albicans, Candida tropicalis, Candida pseudotropicalis, Candida stellatoidea, Candida parapsilosis, Candida krusei, Candida parakrusei, Candida stellatoidea, Candida guilliermondii*, and other yeasts may be isolated from lesions. If yeast dermatitis is diagnosed, a compromised immune system or malnutrition must be suspected. Chronic moist conditions resulting in maceration of the skin allow the yeast to become established.

Clinical Signs. Clinical signs include alopecia, scales, crusts, a greasy layer to the skin, and lichenification of the skin.

Diagnosis. Diagnosis is made by observation of budding yeasts and pseudohyphae on skin cytology.

Other Fungal Conditions

Several other fungi have been isolated from chronic dermatopathy in goats. *Peyronellaea glomerata* is associated with hyperkeratotic lesions of the ears of goats in the United Kingdom.[76] *Aspergillus* species can cause clinical disease in animals with compromised immune systems. These fungi also may cause granulomatous lesions in the skin. Two cases of *Malassezia* dermatitis in goats have been reported.[78,79] Clinical signs consisted of a seborrheic dermatosis and extensive alopecia over much of the thorax and abdomen with extension to the neck and legs in one case. Pruritus was not evident. Both cases were chronic at presentation (1 month and 5 months) and both had demonstrated weight loss. Lesions of the first case included erythema, hyperpigmentation, mild lichenification, large scales, follicular casts, and a coat that was dull and easily epilated.[78] *Malassezia pachydermatis* was diagnosed by impression smears and culture on Sabouraud's dextrose agar. Treatment, which consisted of weekly baths in a chlorhexidine containing shampoo followed by a 0.2% solution of enilconazole for 4 weeks, resulted in a complete resolution of the infection.[78] The second case had been euthanized because previous treatments (ivermectin and amitraz) were ineffective and the goat's condition was poor.[79] Lesions of this case included diffuse alopecia and thickened skin covered by dense crusts. *Malassezia* species were not recovered from culture media. The diagnosis of *Malassezia slooffiae* was based on visualization of large numbers of yeast and hyphal forms consistent with the genus *Malassezia* and phylogenetic analyses using PCR.[79]

Parasitic Diseases

Parasitic diseases are presented here with respect to their importance in causing lesions in the skin and hair.

Lice (Pediculosis)

Lice infestation tends to be more common in goats than in sheep, at least in the United States. They are commonly found in cervids but rarely cause clinical disease. The sucking louse *(Solenopotes binipilosus)* and two chewing lice (*Tricholipeurus lipeuroides* and *Tricholipeurus parallelus*) are reported as only infecting cervids. There are only a few reports of lice infestation of sheep in the United States.[1,80,81] Most reports of sheep lice come from New Zealand, Australia, and Great Britain.[82] In a telephone questionnaire survey, Australian investigators reported that 21% of sheep flocks had lice infestations.[83] In a postal survey of sheep producers in Great Britain, 10.7% of farmers reported at least one outbreak of infestations by lice in the previous year, but some regions reported up to a 19% prevalence.[84] Lice tend to be a greater problem in the winter when nutrition may be poor and conditions more crowded and long hair or wool provides a more conducive environment for louse reproduction.[1] However, a Minnesota report of experimentally infested sheep, which were housed out of sunlight and rainfall, noted that louse numbers peaked in late spring.[85] Louse activity has been shown to decline significantly in response to higher environmental temperatures. During warm to hot months, only small populations of lice survive in protected areas, such as inside the ears and between the legs.[2] Lice are highly host specific and spend the complete life cycle on the host. However, it is not unusual for some species of lice to infest both sheep and goats. Lice reported in goats include the sucking lice *Linognathus africanus* and *Linognathus stenopsis* and the chewing or biting lice *Bovicola* (formerly *Damalinia*) *limbata*, *Bovicola caprae*, and *Bovicola crassipes*. Lice reported in sheep include the chewing louse *Bovicola ovis* (Figure 10.5) and the sucking lice *Linognathus ovillus* (body louse) and *Linognathus pedalis* (sucking foot louse). The biting lice *B. ovis* and *B. caprae* may be transferred between sheep and goats.[86] Biting or chewing lice feed on epithelial and cutaneous debris, while sucking lice feed on blood and tissue fluid. Although lice can survive off the host for a few weeks, most transmission occurs through direct contact or indirectly through contact with equipment or grooming tools. Louse eggs (nits) are attached to individual hair or wool fibers, hatch within 1 to 2 weeks, and develop into adults in 2 to 4 weeks. The foot louse is usually found in circumscribed areas on the feet or limbs but

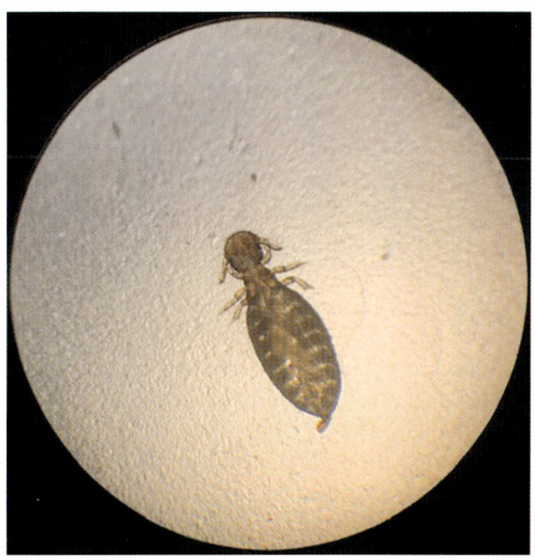

• **Fig. 10.5** A 4× photomicrograph of *Bovicola (Damalinia) ovis* collected from a Katahdin ram that had been showing signs of pruritus for about a month. (Courtesy Dr. Sarah Fadden, Loyal Veterinary Service, Loyal, Wisconsin.)

may be found on abdominal or scrotal areas when large populations develop.[87]

Clinical signs. Clinical signs of lice infestation in goats may present as pruritus, rubbing or scratching, weight loss, decreased production efficiency, and patches of alopecia which give the appearance of a rough, shaggy hair coat. In addition to these general signs seen with most lice infestations, sucking lice may cause anemia, hypoproteinemia, and death. Heavy infestations likely make the animal more susceptible to other diseases. Infestations with sucking lice have been shown to cause immunosuppression, while chewing lice produce significant inflammatory response in goats.[88] In sheep, fleece derangement (rubbed or chewed fleece) was found to be a good early indicator of the presence of lice, and pruritus may be evident well before lice can be readily found by direct inspection.[89] In the aforementioned study, in sheep experimentally infested with lice, fleece derangement was first evident at 5 weeks postinfestation. Lameness may be observed in sheep infested with *L. pedalis.*

Diagnosis. Sucking lice are most common around the poll, nose, eyes, neck, brisket, withers, tail, axillary, and inguinal areas. Biting lice are most common in areas of the neck, withers, and tailhead. *L. pedalis* can typically be found on the short-haired areas, especially the lower leg and foot. Lice are usually visible by the naked eye, but a magnifying glass may help. Collection of the lice and viewing under a microscope is often sufficient to determine whether the lice are sucking or biting. Many cases have been discovered in animals without obvious clinical signs simply by handling the animal and then feeling/seeing lice on oneself.

Treatment. Application of an approved insecticide either as a powder, dust, dip, spray, or pour-on will help control or eliminate most infestations. It is important to treat the entire herd or flock; otherwise, reinfestation will occur. It should be noted that few treatments are approved for goats and special care should be taken to avoid meat and milk residues. Most insecticides are not ovicidal, and thus, treatment needs to be repeated twice at 1- to 2-week intervals. Avermectin injectables at 0.2 mg/kg body weight are useful against sucking lice, but the efficacy against chewing lice is unpredictable. Oral administration of avermectin products is reported to be of limited value. Pour-on ivermectin at a rate of 1 mL/22 lb. body weight applied along the topline in a narrow strip extending from the withers to the tailhead may be effective against lice in goats and cervids. The efficacy of topically applied products for lice treatment of small ruminants requires further study. Lice developing chemical resistance have been reported when annual treatment for lice in sheep was required by law.[90] To obtain greater treatment efficacy, sheep and Angora goats should be shorn prior to externally applied chemicals. Shearing can directly remove > 50% of louse populations.[91] Shearing also allows better contact between the skin and externally applied chemical and allows greater exposure to sunlight. A botanical insecticide, NeemAzal, was found to reduce survival but not eradicate natural infestations of *Damalinia limbata* in Angora goats.[92]

Prevention. Preventing lice infestations via selective breeding to obtain resistance is being conducted and has had some promising results.[93] Louse resistance to backline applications with triflumuron and diflubenzuron has been recently reported.[94] Treatment and isolation of new additions will prevent the disease from entering a herd or flock that has eradicated lice.

Melophagus ovinus (Sheep Ked)

Sheep keds were once relatively common until effective pesticides were developed and utilized. Transmission requires direct contact. Sheep are the only definitive host, but other species may occasionally be infested. Because sheep keds feed on blood, they may transmit other diseases such as bluetongue. These parasites are unique in that the female produces a single egg that hatches within her uterus where the larva then develops for 7 to 12 days. The larva then enters the pupal stage and is attached to the wool, where it will hatch after 2 to 3 weeks. Additional details are available in an extensive review that has been published.[95]

Clinical Signs. The irritation caused by the biting ked results in pruritus, scratching, and rubbing, which cause damage to the wool and skin. Severe infestations can cause weight loss and anemia.

Diagnosis. The sheep ked is a wingless fly and is easily seen with the naked eye. Wool may need to be parted to allow visualization.

Treatment. Most pesticides are effective due to the sucking nature of this parasite. Treatments should be repeated in 14- to 21-day intervals. A 2007 study reported that both pour-on and subcutaneous ivermectin regimens were 100% effective by day 7 against *M. ovinus* in long-haired goats.[96]

Prevention. Shearing removes the majority of the infestation, and when followed by an appropriate pesticide, eradication is possible if the entire flock or herd is treated.

Deer Keds (*Lipoptena* and *Neolipoptena* sp.)

Deer keds or louse flies are fairly common in wild deer. Farmed cervids have few cases due to management practices for internal and external parasites on most farms that kill keds secondary to other pathogens. Visual inspection of the skin will usually reveal the keds and they can be distinguished by having six legs. To speciate the ked requires microscopic examination. Their life cycle is similar to the sheep ked.

Clinical Signs. Usually none, but on heavily infested animals or debilitated animals, they may cause problems.

Diagnosis. The keds are easily seen with the naked eye, but one may have to part the hair to see them.

Treatment. Most topical insecticides will kill the ked. Repeated treatment in 2 to 3 weeks will usually eliminate it from a herd.

Prevention. Isolate and treat new herd members before introducing to main herd. Reinfection may occur from nearby wild cervids.

Mange Mites

Mange is rare in sheep but relatively common in goats.[3,18,35] Mange mites known to infest sheep include *Psoroptes communis* var *ovis, Sarcoptes scabiei ovis, Psorergates ovis, Chorioptes bovis* var *ovis,* and *Demodex ovis.* Mange has been essentially eradicated from sheep in the United States, with the exception of demodectic mange. However, mange exists in bighorn sheep (*Psoroptes* spp.), and where domestic sheep mingle with wild sheep, transmission is possible.[97,98] In goats, clinically important forms of mange include sarcoptic mange, demodectic mange *(Demodex caprae),* psoroptic mange *(Psoroptes cuniculi),* and chorioptic mange. The mange mite of white-tailed deer is *Demodex odocoilei.* Most infections are not evident, but others have small to extensive hair loss, thickened skin, and numerous small pustules.[24]

Diagnosis. Diagnosis is made by demonstration of the mites in skin scrapings. Scrapings are typically acquired by using a scalpel blade and a microscope slide with mineral oil.

Treatment. Treatment for mange is most easily performed after shearing. Various products have been used, with variable success, including coumaphos (0.3% dip), toxaphene (0.5% dip), lime sulfur (2% dip), and phosmet (0.15–0.25% dip). Topical or systemic avermectins may also work.

Psoroptic Mange (*Psoroptes ovis, Psoroptes cuniculi*, Common Sheep Scab)

Psoroptic mange is a reportable disease in the United States.[3,18,35] These mites have elongated heads and are oval in shape, and their first pair of legs are jointed. These mites are transmitted by direct contact, are host specific (no zoonoses), have a 2-week life cycle, and can live off the host for as long as 3 weeks. These mites are highly contagious and the successful transfer of a single ovigerous female to a susceptible sheep is sufficient to establish an infestation.[99] Under optimal conditions, the life cycle from egg to egg production by the adult female takes 11 to 19 days.[100,101] In sheep, clinical disease is most severe in the fall and winter. The saliva of the mite causes an intense inflammatory reaction in the skin, with severe pruritus resulting in self-trauma and alopecia. These lesions of *Psoroptes ovis* are primarily distributed along the trunk. The mites infest heavily wooled areas and cause papules, crusting, and matting of wool. In goats, *Psoroptes cuniculi* usually infests the ears and may cause alopecia, pruritus localized to the ears, and head shaking. Infestation of the ears may be seen in goats as young as 10 days old. These are non-burrowing mites that appear to congregate, feed, and deposit eggs at the interface of affected and nonaffected skin.[102,103] These mites may be observed on the skin surface with a magnifying lens. Local administration of louse medications is curative. Psoroptic mites can be recognized by their round bodies and long-segmented pedicles.

Psoroptes cuniculi typically infests the ears of cervids, causing clinical signs in heavily infected animals. They may become uncoordinated, circle, and appear in a stupor due to secondary bacterial infections of the inner ear. Most deer do not show clinical signs.

Treatments should be applied to all affected and in-contact animals at 5-to 7-day intervals at least twice. Traditionally used dewormers have been effective in treating *Psoroptes*.[104] However, some resistance to macrocyclic lactone has been demonstrated in the United Kingdom.[105]

Raillietia Ear Mites

Raillietia caprae have been isolated from the ears of goats in the United States and other part of the world.[106] One study found *R. caprae* in the ear of 20 of 360 goats at slaughter.[107] *R. caprae* was identified in the ears of 10% of 145 goats from 10 farms in Brazil.[108] The youngest infested was 8 months old and the oldest was 10 years old. Although these mites do not tend to create obvious clinical disease (otitis and neurologic signs are possible), they could be mistaken for *Psoroptes*. *Raillietia* mites tend to be larger than *Psoroptes*, and their longer legs originate from the anterior half of the body.[3]

Sarcoptic Mange

S. scabiei var *ovis* and *S. scabiei* var *caprae* are rare in sheep and goats and are not known to be present in the United States.[3,18,35] Scabies is a reportable disease in the United States and is zoonotic. This mite prefers to infest the skin around the eyes and ears and causes intense pruritus. The mites are round in head and body and have long, nonjointed stalks for the first pair of legs. These mites burrow through the epidermis, and the female lays eggs in these tunnels. The life cycle of *Sarcoptes* ranges from 10 to 17 days. The mites are most commonly transmitted by direct contact but can survive in the environment for variable periods. Excoriations, alopecia, and crusting occur on the face and nonwooled areas but do not spread to the bodies of the affected sheep. Chronic infection causes hyperpigmentation and lichenification of the skin, and affected sheep and goats suffer weight loss and ill thrift because of the discomfort. In goats, sarcoptic mange may affect the entire body, causing alopecia, crusting, pruritus, and subsequent weight loss. Regional lymph nodes may become enlarged because of the severity of skin damage.

Diagnosis requires deep skin scraping of the periphery of active lesions, but mites are difficult to find and diagnosis is often based on clinical signs and response to therapy. Numerous scrapings may be required to find these mites and negative scrapings do not rule out the infestation. Diagnosis may be made on clinical suspicion and response to therapy. An alternative to direct examination is to mix skin scrapings and crusts with sodium nitrate solution, a technique similar to fecal floatation.

Treatment consists of ivermectin anthelmintic administration and dips such as 1% lime sulfur. Dips may be required weekly for 4 to 12 weeks before the condition resolves completely. Spontaneous resolution of sarcoptic mange can occur in goats. An anti-scabies vaccine failed to protect goats in a 2005 study.[109]

Psorergates ovis (Sheep Itch Mite)

The smallest of the sheep mange mites, *Psorergates ovis* has a rounded body with indentations between the attachments of the legs.[3,18,35] This mite has a 4- to 5-week life cycle and lives in the epidermis. Alopecia, crusts, and scales are primarily distributed along the trunk (withers and sides) of the body. Infested sheep demonstrate severe pruritus, including biting at affected regions. These mites may be observed on the skin surface with a magnifying lens. There have been no reports of this mite in the United States since the 1950s.[110]

Chorioptic Mange

The *Chorioptes* mite (*Chorioptes ovis* and *Chorioptes caprae*) has an oval body shape; the first pair of legs are short and unsegmented and have suckers attached to the ends.[3,18,35] *Chorioptes* is host specific (no zoonoses), has a 2- to 3-week life cycle, and can only live off the host for a few days. These mites and their associated lesions are limited to the scrotum and distal rear limbs of sheep and the lower limbs, abdomen, and hindquarters of goats. Lesions include alopecia, erythema, excoriation, crusts, and pruritus. The skin lesions may be combined with and complicated by *Staphylococcus* infections.[1] Infested sheep and goats may be restless, stomp, and chew at their feet because of discomfort. Crusts may be so thick that deep scrapings may be required; conversely, kids tend to have less chronic infestations, increasing the chance of positive scrapings. Scrotal infestation may cause dermatitis and temporary infertility in rams. These mites may be observed on the skin surface with a magnifying lens. Lime sulfur dips are usually curative. Chorioptic mange appears to be the only common mange mite in small ruminants in the United States and is very common in the United Kingdom.[1]

Demodectic Mange

Demodectic mange (*D. ovis*, *D. caprae*, and *D. odocoilei*) affects the face, limbs, and back.[3,18,35] *D. ovis* mites infest hair follicles, causing severe folliculitis often complicated by secondary pyoderma (evidenced by the presence of pustules or abscesses). Disease is characterized by 2- to 12-mm diameter nodules in the skin along the face, neck, shoulders, and trunk, although there appears to be a predilection for the eyelids. These nodules exude a thick exudate. Material expressed from nodules may be examined microscopically for the cigar-shaped mites. Diagnosis may require deep skin scraping and should include follicles bordering active lesions. *D. caprae* infestation may be the most common mange of goats. Fourteen percent of 118 sheep flocks in an Israeli study were positive for demodectic parasites.[111] The Israeli study also found a greater proportion of merino flocks with demodicosis, suggesting a greater susceptibility of this breed to this parasite. Although the exact mode of transmission is not clear, mites are thought to spread among kids and lambs where skin lesions remain unnoticed for many months. Spread among adults is not common; therefore, isolation of affected animals from kids is prudent but not necessary from adult herd members. Severe infestation suggests a compromised immune system. Therefore, clinicians and keepers should pay close attention to the nutrition program and general health of affected goats.

Treatment may include weekly dipping with 0.5% malathion, 0.2% trichlorfon, or 0.5% amitraz. Avermectins, both orally and pour-on application, have been reported to lead to entire healing without any scar formation in two clinically affected goats.[112]

Fly Strike

Although no estimates of the incidence of this condition were found for the United States, fly strike certainly occurs and would be considered common in the United States and has been reported as the most prevalent ectoparasite-mediated disease to affect sheep in the United Kingdom and northern Europe.[84] Screw-worm *(Cochliomyia hominivorax)* has been eradicated from the United States, but continued surveillance for larvae of this fly is prudent. These larvae are 1 to 2 cm long, pink, and tapered. The adult fly is blue-green, with an orange head and three dark longitudinal stripes on the body. Cutaneous myiasis (black blowfly, *Phormia regina*) occurs in sheep in the United States and is most common among breeds that have excessive skin folds such as Merino sheep. In Australia, the sheep blowfly, *Lucilia cuprina*, is the major ectoparasite of sheep, causing severe damage from myiasis and death from secondary infections.[113] However, a variety of fly larvae can infest wounds that have necrotic tissue present. Skin lesions cause staining of wool and alopecia. Larvae, other than *C. hominivorax*, feed on necrotic tissue and wound secretions. Deer may suffer from fly strike at two different stages of life. Young fawns may have fly strike around the tail and anus, especially if afflicted with diarrhea and the dam not keeping them clean, and around the umbilicus (Figure 10.6). Daily observation of fawns (especially mule deer) is very important. The second common event is fly strike to the developing antlers after they have suffered an injury (Figure 10.7). These wounds may become infected and necrotic and draw fly strike. These wounds are very serious, and it is not uncommon for these to lead to septicemia, resulting in the death of the buck.

Clinical Signs. Affected stock may or may not show irritation, but there tends to be a foul odor. Death can result due to secondary infection and toxemia; thus, small ruminants may be sick and depressed. Areas around the tail and perineum that become soiled via diarrhea are especially common locations; however, any wound, such as dehorning sites, castration, tail docking, and shearing nicks, will attract flies.

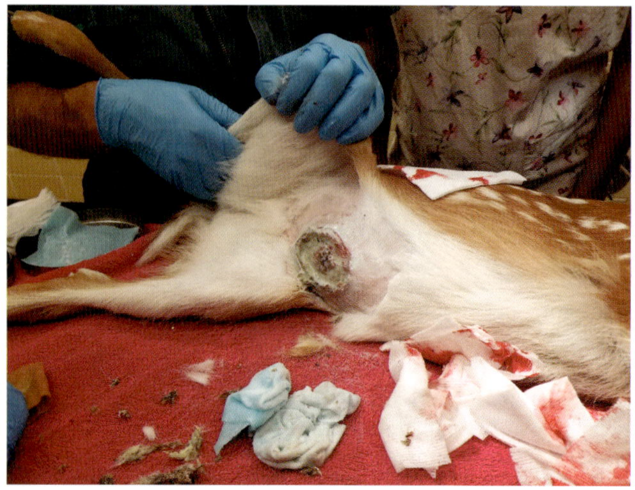

• **Fig. 10.6** Fly strike of the umbilicus in a white-tailed deer fawn.

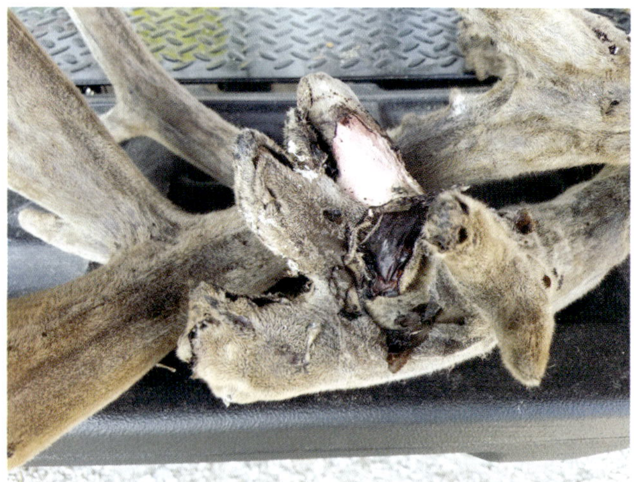

• **Fig. 10.7** Injury to developing antlers of a white-tailed deer. Exudate and a few maggots can be seen along with the injury to the velvet antler.

Diagnosis. Check for maggots in soiled areas.

Treatment. Treatment includes routine spraying with various insecticides. This seems to stimulate the larvae to wiggle out of the sprayed area. It is imperative to identify all of the fly-stricken area; thus, complete clipping of the entire extent of the struck area is necessary. When dealing with heavy fleece, palpation may be necessary to identify hidden areas of fly strike. Cleaning, debriding, and drying the wound will certainly help reduce the attraction for the flies. Bandaging the wound will also help as long as the bandage stays dry. After cleaning the affected area and removing all noticeable maggots, follow up with a systemically administered larvicide (such as ivermectin) that will help kill unseen maggots. Severe cases should also be treated with a broad-spectrum antibiotic.

Prevention. Avoid surgical procedures during fly season, but if procedures must be done, use fly repellants and bandages during the first few days. Fly sprays should be used on and around any wounds. Observe susceptible livestock at least once a day. A preparation of *Bacillus thuringiensis*, a nonpathogenic strain that is commonly isolated from wool, when applied in high concentrations to sheep, protected the sheep from fly strike for up to 6 weeks.[114] In certain parts of the world, routine dipping or spraying with larvicidal compounds is used for prevention and control. Recognize the seasonality of the problem, and treating to reduce the fly population early in the fly season will pay dividends.[115]

Elaeophorosis (Sorehead)

Elaeophora schneideri is a filarial nematode that has been primarily reported in wildlife species in the western United States, including mule deer, white-tailed deer, and bighorn sheep.[116–119] The disease is uncommon in sheep and goats. The filaria cause thrombosis of capillary beds and terminal arteries. Tissue ischemia resulting from vascular injury causes severe lesions that appear similar to those of photosensitization and ulcerative dermatitis. Horse flies (*Hybomitra, Tabanus*) are intermediate hosts that transmit infective larvae from one host to another. Infective larvae migrate and develop to young adults in the leptomeningeal arteries. If thrombosis occurs at this level, circling, opisthotonos, convulsions, and other neurologic signs or sudden death may occur. Alternatively, the young adults may migrate to the common carotid and maxillary arteries and develop into mature adults. These adults produce microfilaria that embolize the capillary beds of the face and may cause ischemia or an allergic reaction. Lesions primarily occur on the face but may develop on other areas of the body. They are focal and consistent with vascular compromise and may require months or years to heal completely. White-tailed deer may commonly have food impactions, tooth loss, and occasional fractures of the jaw.[24] The lesions wax and wane with the appearance of new generations of microfilaria. Elaeophorosis should be included in the differential diagnosis of any unilateral lesions of the head. Skin biopsy may reveal the microfilaria either by histologic examination or by tissue maceration and harvest of larvae. Avermectin drugs (ivermectin 200 μg/kg SC) can kill the microfilaria, but repeated doses may be required. Adult nematodes can be killed by the administration of piperazine salts (50 mg/kg by mouth [PO]) or ivermectin.

Onchocerca Species Infestation

Onchocerca species can parasitize sheep and goats, although there are relatively few reports of the condition. A Finland study reported in 2008 found no evidence of sheep infected with *Onchocerca* species.[120] Adult *Onchocerca* species can live in the connective tissues of sheep and goats, where they induce nodules. Adults produce microfilariae that migrate into the dermis of the ventral abdomen and thorax. Alopecia, erythema, and thickening of the skin develop because of the host's response to dying larvae.

Other nematodes diagnosed in cases of focal dermatitis include *Pelodera strongyloides*, *Strongyloides papillosus*, and *Parelaphostrongylus tenuis*. These nematodes have been associated with dermatitis, but their clinical significance is minimal. Strongyloidiasis is seen on dependent regions of the body; the localized dermatitis is caused by an immune reaction to migrating larvae. *P. tenuis* infestation of the central nervous system may cause focal regions of hyperesthesia. This may lead to self-trauma that the keeper or clinician notes as excoriations or nonhealing ulcers.

Autoimmune Diseases

Pemphigus Foliaceus

Pemphigus foliaceus is a rarely diagnosed autoimmune skin disease of goats, sheep, and cervids characterized by widespread crusty, pruritic lesions.[2,121,122] It has been classified as a type II hypersensitivity reaction. Lesions are often first noted over the face or limbs but may be found on the abdomen, perineum, and scrotum as well. The proposed mechanism is the development of autoantibodies directed against the skin, specifically the glycocalyx of keratinocytes. Loss of intercellular cohesiveness results in blister formation and acantholysis. The dermatopathy developed after a dog bite injury. Lesions were present primarily on the face and ears but were also present on the coronary bands and vulvar area. Lesions continuously dripped serum. The administration of corticosteroids improved healing and decreased serum loss but the condition never resolved.

Diagnosis. A diagnosis of pemphigus foliaceus may be made from skin biopsy specimens obtained from characteristic skin lesions. Numerous biopsies should be taken from suspect animals to improve the accuracy of the diagnosis. The presence of acantholytic keratinocytes within vesicles is a diagnostic feature of pemphigus. Because acantholysis can be seen in other dermatologic conditions, biopsies should be evaluated by a veterinary pathologist with expertise in dermatopathies.

Treatment. Treatment of pemphigus is aimed at diminishing the body's immune response. Prednisolone (1 mg/kg every 24 hours for 7 days) in conjunction with aurothioglucose (1 mg/kg intramuscularly [IM] every 24 hours for 7 days) has been reported effective in controlling symptoms, followed by 1 mg/kg of prednisolone every 48 hours. In another caprine case, remission of dermatitis was obtained with injectable dexamethasone-21-isonicotinate (0.04 mg/kg IM), every 2 months for 1 year.[122] Because no improvement was seen in a sheep with 1 week worth of prednisone at the above dose, a different regimen was tried: an antibiotic and 0.2 mg/kg triamcinolone administered IM once every 7 days with tapering doses for 1 month; this regimen resulted in clinical improvement.[121] Another juvenile Cashmere goat had skin lesions respond to treatment with prednisolone, but the goat was ultimately euthanized because of poor growth and quality of fiber.[123] More recently, a ram was reported to be treated with 2.5 mg/kg of methylprednisolone acetate SC every 4 weeks for 12 injections. The skin lesions resolved, with no adverse effects to the ram from treatment.[124] A 2-month-old Nigerian Dwarf goat diagnosed with pemphigus foliaceus was successfully treated with SC dexamethasone and IM gold sodium thiomalate.[125] The goat was treated for 6 months and was free of clinical signs of pemphigus foliaceus for at least 26 months after discontinuing therapy. Gold sodium thiomalate is not approved for food animal species, and appropriate meat or milk withdrawal times are not known. All of the extended steroid treatments must be critically evaluated in regard to ever-changing regulations in food animals before being used.

Nutritional Diseases

Nutritional deficiencies and excesses are beyond the scope of this chapter and are discussed in other chapters (see Chapter 2). However, changes specific to the skin or hair are briefly discussed in the following paragraphs.

Fescue Toxicity

Fescue toxicosis is caused by ingestion of tall fescue grass (*Lolium arundinaceum*, formerly known as *Festuca arundinacea*) contaminated with an endophyte (*Epichloe coenophiala*, formerly known as *Neotyphodium coenophialum*).[126] During winter months, the toxins may cause a peripheral vasoconstriction leading to a gangrenous necrosis of the distal limbs and tail. Of the 35 to 40 million pasture acres in the United States, approximately 80% is infected. About 8 million acres of fescue grass are not infected with the endophytic fungus and therefore do not contain the ergovaline toxin. Sheep and goats appear to be less sensitive to the toxin than cows are. Feeding noninfested fescue and diluting fescue by planting other species of grasses both help reduce the incidence of this condition. Deer prefer browse and other grasses over fescue when given a choice.

Sheep fed endophyte-infected fescue hay have shown increased rectal temperature, likely related to vasoconstrictive action of the endophyte,[127] while another study found an increase in core body temperature in wethers fed endophyte-infected hay compared to those on endophyte-free hay.[128] There is mostly anecdotal evidence of decreased growth rates and reproductive efficiency in goats fed endophyte-infected fescue.[129]

Copper Deficiency

Copper deficiency or molybdenosis decreases wool quality and color. Wool quality suffers because of decreased crimp and a limp and steely texture. Dark wool loses color intensity until it is gray-white in color. This disease can result from absolute copper deficiency (pasture grass with less than 3 ppm dry matter copper) or excessive molybdenum (pasture grass with more than 10 ppm dry matter molybdenum), sulfur, or iron in the diet. Deer require much more copper in their diet than sheep or goats. It is common to see copper deficiency in deer if a special deer diet is not fed. Diagnosis can be made by assessing copper concentrations in the blood or liver. Copper deficiency is diagnosed if the blood copper concentration is less than 0.7 mg/dL or the liver concentration is less than 80 mg/kg dry weight (see Chapter 2). A report of copper deficiency in goats found alopecia along with other signs in animals presented for respiratory stridor. The affected animals were found to have a laryngeal neuropathy with axonal degeneration of the recurrent laryngeal nerve. The clinically affected animals had a lower serum copper concentration than unaffected herd mates, which had lower serum copper levels than control animals from another herd.[130] Free-choice feeding/offering of a good-quality mineral mixture containing copper in will usually be preventative. In some locales or when excess molybdenum, iron, or other factors that may cause a conditioned copper deficiency exist, organic or chelated sources of copper should be considered

Iodine Deficiency

Iodine deficiency (goiter) of newborn lambs manifests as alopecia, thick scaly skin, weakness, and enlarged thyroid glands.[131] Neonatal death, poor reproductive performance, and abortion may be seen in the flock or herd. Herd outbreaks of goiter, alopecia, poor skeletal development, and increased neonatal lamb deaths may be seen in iodine deficient areas.[132] Familial goiter occurs in Merino sheep, Dutch goats, and Nubian and Angora goats, among others. Iodine deficiency causes kids to be born hairless or with fine hair. The kids may be weak or stillborn and have goiters. Goiter also may be caused by congenital defects or ingestion of goitrogens in the diet. Dietary iodine deficiency is most common in geographic regions with sandy soil and heavy rainfall. Ingestion of large amounts of calcium, cyanogenic glycosides, and cruciferous plants also may induce iodine deficiency. Cruciferous plants are commonly planted for cervids for winter and spring food plots. Diagnosis of iodine deficiency can be made by identifying protein-bound iodine in serum (normal serum protein-bound iodine for adult ewes is 2.4 to 4 μg/dL serum). In herds known to be at risk for iodine deficiency, potassium iodide (250 mg) may be administered at 60 and again at 30 days before lambing. Providing a good-quality iodine-containing trace mineral supplement and removing pregnant animals from pastures containing goitrogenous plants decrease the occurrence of goiter.

Zinc Deficiency

Zinc deficiency is associated with parakeratosis and may cause reduced growth rate, wrinkled skin, swollen hocks, and salivation. Parakeratosis is most pronounced on the face, feet, and scrotum of affected animals. Rams fed a zinc-deficient diet develop abnormal testicles and experience impaired spermatogenesis. In goats, the most prominent clinical signs include rough hair coat; hair loss on the head, limbs, and scrotum; overgrowth of the dental pad; small testicles; and fissures of the feet. Pruritus may or may not be present. The predominant histologic lesions are hyperkeratosis and parakeratosis.[133] Increased calcium and phosphorus intake decreases zinc absorption. Some goats may have a genetic predisposition to depressed zinc absorption. This is magnified in the face of high calcium (and other mineral) intake.[134] Goats with a genetic predisposition may require lifelong zinc supplementation.[135] Diets rich in legumes (high calcium) or "homemade" high-phosphorus grain supplements (corn-soybean, corn-oats-barley) with no added minerals all predispose to zinc deficiency. Deer require significant zinc supplementation, and a "balanced" mineral or complete feed is essential for antler growth and reproduction. A biopsy of the affected area indicating parakeratosis coupled with properly collected serum zinc concentrations of less than 0.8 ppm is diagnostic.[133] Blood drawn for zinc analysis should be collected in a special tube that does not have a butyl rubber stopper. Animals benefit from supplementation of a good-quality trace mineral salt offered free choice. Adding zinc to the feed or administering zinc sulfate (1 g/day PO) is usually effective.[133] If calcium makes up 1.5% of the diet, the zinc sulfate may not be effective and chelated zinc should be administered or added to a premixed salt supplement. Response to zinc supplementation should be rapid (within 14 days) (see Chapter 2), although goats with suspected hereditary malabsorption of zinc required 1 to 3 months for complete resolution.[135] Removing legumes and cereal grains from the diet and feeding grass hay and commercially prepared concentrate feeds (with added zinc) are usually preventative.

Vitamin A Deficiency

Vitamin A deficiency may cause hair loss and night blindness, overgrown hooves, and corneal ulceration in adult goats.[131] Deficiency is rare if animals have access to green forage. If dry, brown forage is fed, inclusion of vitamin A in a supplement (mineral mixture) or use of a commercial injectable product helps prevent deficiency disease. Sheep fed a vitamin A–deficient diet responded to IM injection of 3500 IU/kg of vitamin A palmitate by showing significantly elevated vitamin A levels at 24 hours and for 8 days compared to nontreated controls.[136]

Photosensitization

Photosensitization is segregated into primary and secondary causes based on the pathophysiology of the disease (Table 10.3). *Photosensitization* refers to conditions under which photodynamic chemicals accumulate in the skin and become stimulated by sunlight on exposed and unpigmented areas of the skin.[3,77,131,137] These substances damage the capillary beds and result in skin necrosis and sloughing. *Primary photosensitization* refers to ingested photodynamic substances that do not require alteration in the body to cause disease. Primary photosensitization may occur after ingestion of St. John's wort, which contains hypericin; aphids containing an unknown photodynamic agent; or lush forage with accumulated phylloerythrin. This condition is most common in late summer and early autumn during periods of rapid pasture growth. Ingestion of alfalfa and other plants, including clover, lucerne, vetch, and oats, has been associated with photosensitization. Other plants have Even been reported to cause photosensitization in small ruminants.[138,139] The mechanism of pathology is not well understood. Secondary photosensitization occurs when liver damage results in the accumulation of photodynamic substances such as phylloerythrin in the bloodstream. Liver damage may be caused by the ingestion of plants containing pyrrolizidine alkaloids or carbon tetrachloride, *Pithomyces chartarum*–infected grasses, or blue-green algae *(Anacystis cyanea)*.

Clinical Signs and Diagnosis. Clinical signs of photosensitization include head shaking, restlessness, erythema, and edema of eyelids, muzzle, ears, and tail. Skin lesions characteristically affect exposed, nonpigmented regions of the skin. Yellow serum may seep through the skin within 2 days and pruritus causes self-trauma. The transudate accumulates as a crust and superficial skin sloughing occurs. Secondary bacterial infection is common. Necropsy reveals subcutaneous edema and sloughing tissue. In cases of secondary photosensitization, liver disease may be obvious.

Treatment. Treatment for photosensitization is symptomatic and includes the provision of shade, control of secondary infections, treatment of primary disease if liver damage is present, removal of animals from high-risk forage, allowance of grazing at night only, maintenance of hydration and access to electrolytes, and administration of nonsteroidal antiinflammatory drugs (NSAIDs) and antibiotics in severe cases. Photosensitization can be prevented by good pasture management and provision of adequate shade.

Mycotoxins

Pithomycotoxicosis

Pithomycotoxicosis (facial eczema) occurs in all ages of sheep, cattle, and, to a lesser extent, goats in Australia, New Zealand, South Africa, and some European and South American countries.[140] *P. chartarum* is a fungus that produces the mycotoxin sporidesmin; it is most often found in ryegrass. Sporidesmin is a hepatotoxin that causes hepatogenous photosensitization and phylloerythrin accumulation in the bloodstream. Morbidity is highest in summer and fall, especially when rains follow a period of drought.

Clinical Signs. Clinical signs of pithomycotoxicosis include conjunctivitis, keratitis, restlessness, stomping of the feet, and lethargy. Edema of the eyelids and ears may be noted. Ears may become so swollen that they become pendulous.[141] Erythema and alopecia on the face and around the eyes and ears have also been reported.[141] Exudate accumulates on the skin, which then begins to slough. Sheep may suffer secondary infections and die in 2 weeks to 2 months.

Diagnosis. Sporidesmin is a potent hepatotoxin that causes pericholangitis and the occlusion of bile ducts. Thus, elevated levels of serum gamma glutamyltransferase are suggestive. However, the definitive diagnosis requires the presence of high *Pithomyces* spore counts and confirmation that the *P. chartarum* isolated produces sporidesmin.[140]

Treatment. Feeding zinc sulfate (0.5–2 g/head/day) is protective for sheep grazing infected pastures. Applying thiabendazole (1 kg per acre) to the pasture has been reported to control the fungus.

Stachybotryotoxicosis

Stachybotryotoxicosis (poisoning by fungi of the genus *Stachybotrys*) has been reported in sheep. This fungal mycotoxin causes cutaneous necrosis, ulceration, petechiae, and ulceronecrotic areas, most pronounced in the mucocutaneous junctions. The toxin is a macrocyclic trichothecene that also causes bone marrow suppression, neutropenia, and thrombocytopenia.

Environmental Skin Disease

Intertrigo

Intertrigo occurs in areas of skin-to-skin contact; excessive motion results in moist dermatitis and inflammation because of friction. This most commonly occurs in ruminants between the udder and the inner aspect of the thigh. Treatment includes cleansing the region and applying an astringent ointment with the goal of drying the lesion. The disease is self-limiting in most animals, but pain may cause apparent lameness; moreover, the area may have a foul odor and secondary infection may increase the risk of mastitis.

Callus

A callus is formed on areas of the skin that receive chronic mild to moderate abrasion from objects in the environment. The most common location in small ruminants is the dorsal aspect of the carpi and the sternum. Other locations include the cranial aspect of the stifle and the caudal aspect of the elbow. These lesions are normal unless they have associated exudate, swelling, or pain.

Hematoma

Blunt trauma can result in the formation of a hematoma. Hematomas may develop in exposed highly vascular tissues such as the ears or on the main body. Causes of trauma include injury from horned and antlered animals, fighting injury, attack by dogs or other predators, equipment-related injury, and entanglement with fences or other objects. Spontaneous bleeding under the skin is rare but may occur if ingestion of toxins causes coagulopathy. Ultrasonographic findings may suggest hematoma, but a definitive diagnosis requires needle aspiration of blood following aseptic preparation. Unless the hematoma is enlarging, they are best left to resolve with time.

TABLE 10.3 Causes of Photosensitization in Small Ruminants.

Source	Toxin	Species Affected
Primary photosensitization		
Plants		
St. John's wort	Hypericin	Any ruminant
Buckwheat	Fagopyrin, photofagopyrin	Any ruminant
Bishop's weed	Furocoumarins	Any ruminant
Dutchman's breeches	Furocoumarins	Any ruminant
Wild carrot	Furocoumarins	Any ruminant
Perennial ryegrass	Perloline	Any ruminant
Burr trefoil	Aphids	Any ruminant
Toxins		
Phenothiazine	Phenothiazine alkaloids	Any ruminant
Thiazides		Any ruminant
Methylene blue		Any ruminant
Sulfonamides		Any ruminant
Tetracyclines		Any ruminant
Hepatogenous photosensitization		
Plants		
Rape, kale	Any ruminant	
Kleingrass	Sheep	
Caltrops	Saponins	Sheep
Lantana	Triterpene	Any ruminant
Ragworts, heliotrope	Pyrrolizidine alkaloids	Any ruminant
Mycotoxins		
Pithomyces chartarum (pasture grass, especially ryegrass)	Sporidesmin	Sheep, cattle
Anacystis (blue-green algae)	Alkaloid	Any ruminant
Periconia (Bermuda grass)	Any ruminant	
Phomopsis leptostromiformis (lupin)	Acid-phenolic compounds	Any ruminant
Chemicals		
Copper		Any ruminant
Phosphorus		Any ruminant
Carbon tetrachloride		Any ruminant
Phenanthridium		Any ruminant
Bacterial hepatitis		
Viral hepatitis		
Parasitic hepatitis		
Hepatic neoplasia		

Adapted from Scott DW: *Large animal dermatology,* Philadelphia, 1988, WB Saunders.

Cutaneous Ulceration

Pressure sores (or cutaneous ulcerations) form when bony prominences are in prolonged contact with hard surfaces. They most commonly occur when small ruminants rest in lateral recumbency because of musculoskeletal or neurologic disease. Pressure sores form because of prolonged ischemia and cellular injury (pressure necrosis). They can therefore be prevented or controlled by frequent movement of the animal. Contact with moist surfaces can accelerate this process because hydration of the skin weakens its resistance elasticity.

Foreign Bodies

Foreign bodies can become lodged in the skin by injury or surgery. In a study of skin reaction to suture materials in Borno white goats, researchers found that a prolonged inflammatory phase was associated with nylon and silk but not cotton or stainless steel suture material.[142] Stainless steel and nylon sutures produced a moderate amount of granulation tissue reaction, cotton suture produced a marked granulation response, and silk produced the smallest amount of granulation. Wounds sutured with cotton or stainless steel healed faster than those sutured with nylon or silk.

Subcutaneous Emphysema

Penetrating wounds or full-thickness lacerations that act as one-way valves can result in subcutaneous emphysema. In these cases, air is allowed to enter but not freely exit from the subcutaneous tissues (bellows effect). Subcutaneous emphysema also occurs in sheep and goats with pneumonia, especially after parturition. The weakened lung parenchyma may rupture into the mediastinum if excessive intrathoracic pressure is applied against a closed glottis (as occurs during parturition). The air dissects along tissue planes and exits through the thoracic inlet to the subcutaneous spaces.

Clinical Signs. Subcutaneous emphysema typically is noted along the neck, dorsal to the shoulder; it may dissect along the back. The condition also may occur with clostridial infections. Often affected animals are found dead and subcutaneous emphysema is discovered during necropsy. However, emphysema may be noted on physical examination early in the infectious process. Clostridial disease should be considered in the differential diagnosis if the animal exhibits severe systemic disease in the presence of subcutaneous emphysema. The condition may also occur as a sequela to a transtracheal wash.

Burns

Skin burns are most commonly found on animals that have been trapped in building fires. Pour-on products containing alcohol are flammable but usually do not ignite the hair coat and do not continue to burn after the fluid volume is consumed. Burns may be classified by severity and extent of the body surface area involved. Sequelae of burn injuries include secondary infection, especially with *Pseudomonas*, and hypoproteinemia from protein exudation from the wounds. Severe or extensive burns are more likely to result in fatal infection or protein losses. Smoke inhalation and thermal damage to the lungs also can cause death. The clinician should perform a thorough evaluation of the thorax after the initial injury and follow up later because the onset of clinical disease may be delayed. Burns in neonates are likely to occur as a result of inappropriate heat lamp placement in maternity pens. Lambs, kids, and fawns stand under the lamps for warmth and may burn the dorsum as a result. Pour-on products or irritants such as creosote and strong iodine can cause chemical burns on areas of skin contact.

Clinical Signs. Depending on its severity, a burn may produce only superficial scabbing or it may result in serum exudation and suppuration with deeper skin layer involvement. Because wool is fire-retardant, the most severe burns on sheep exposed to barn or grass fires are likely to be found around the head and limbs, whereas goats are likely to have severe burns over their entire bodies.

Treatment. Evaluation of the patient's overall condition is essential in a fire because smoke inhalation and thermal damage to the respiratory tract may cause death. Treatment is aimed at preventing or controlling secondary infection. Pain management and administration of plasma (if needed to address hypoproteinemia caused by excessive serum exudation from the wounds) are common therapeutic elements.

Sunburn

Sunburn in animals, as in human beings, is caused by skin damage from ultraviolet light. Sunburn is different from photosensitization.[133,134] It is more commonly seen in white-faced sheep (especially on the face and ears), particularly those that have been recently shorn, leucistic and piebald deer, and light-colored goats (especially on the udders, ears, and nose).[133] Fawns that have been bottle raised indoors may suffer severe sunburn, especially on their ears, once they are released outside. Prolonged sun exposure is associated with tumors (e.g., squamous cell carcinoma).

Clinical Signs. Clinical signs of sunburn include erythema, swelling, crusting of skin, head shaking, and pruritus. If the udder is affected, animals will resent milking or being nursed.[143]

Treatment. Treatment includes the application of pigmented teat dips and the application of sunburn lotion on the udder (for dairy goats), the provision of adequate shelter, and gradual light exposure for light-pigmented animals. In cases of secondary bacterial infection, the use of topical or systemic antimicrobial agents is warranted.[133,134]

Frostbite

Prolonged exposure to extremely cold temperatures may result in frostbite. Young stock are most prone to frostbite injury, and the extremities (ears, tail, and feet) are most commonly involved. It is especially a problem in a newborn that is not adequately dried off in cold weather.[144] Death from low body core temperature ensues if treatment is not initiated before vital organs are compromised. Frostbite may occur at a variety of temperatures depending on environmental conditions (sunlight, moisture, wind).[77] Injury is caused by vasoconstriction, subsequent arterial thrombosis, and ischemic necrosis. After sloughing, damaged ears tend to be rounded with alopecic tips.[133] If the surface of the skin is wet, ice crystals can form, accelerating the process. Frostbite injuries occur in four phases.[145,146] Phase 1 (prefreeze) is characterized by arteriolar constriction, venous dilatation, congestion, and serum transudation. Phase 2 (freeze-thaw) begins with extracellular ice crystal formation. Phase 3 (vascular stasis) is denoted by more severe and persistent venous dilatation and arterial spasm, which causes arteriovenous shunting and tissue hypoxia. Phase 4 (ischemia) is denoted by nervous tissue damage caused by prolonged local hypoxia.

Treatment. The therapy for frostbite may result in reperfusion injury. Nevertheless, it should be instituted immediately and continued for at least the first few days after injury. Warming in water of 104° to 106° F is recommended, as is the use of antibiotics and antiinflammatory drugs as needed to control tissue damage. Necrotic tissue should be debrided as needed to facilitate healing and limit secondary bacterial infection.

Prevention. An easily accessible shelter should be provided. For each degree drop in ambient temperature below 0° C, the keeper should offer a 0.5 to 1% increase in feed. Feeding ewes and does in barns keeps them and their lambs, fawns, and kids out of the cold weather and in a warmer condition.

Wool Slip and Wool Break

Goats naturally shed their coats in spring. Sheep, however, continuously grow wool and should not shed it. Shorn sheep being housed for winter can, however, experience complete loss of wool (wool slip).[133,143] The affected skin is smooth and free of ectoparasites and shows no signs of disease. No treatment is required and the wool does grow back.[133,143] Wool slip has been associated in some sheep with copper deficiency (low serum copper and cold stress).[143] Therefore, possible deficiencies in dietary copper should be investigated. Stressors such as parasitism and systemic disease can cause sheep to undergo a cessation in wool growth and can weaken the fiber (wool break). Wool can be lost within days of a systemic stress (anagen defluxion) or within 2 to 3 months after the stress (telogen defluxion). In both cases, the wool does grow back over time. The practical application of this information is in educating the owners of pet sheep that survive a systemic illness—the clinician should warn the neophyte owner of the potential for fiber loss. Anagen defluxion can also occur in goats under stress or due to the stress of disease.

Congenital Pathologies

Several forms of congenital skin disorders are of clinical interest. Because of good identification and culling practices, most are fairly rare.[147]

Hepatogenous Photosensitization

Southdown lambs have an autosomal recessive trait that can result in hepatogenous photosensitization.[147] The defect causes congenital hyperbilirubinemia and subsequent photosensitization. Corriedale lambs have an assumed inherited condition, similar to Dubin-Johnson syndrome in human beings, characterized by a failure to transfer phylloerythrin and conjugated bilirubin. Hepatogenous photosensitization has been reported in a Santa Inesmix sheep, which responded to treatment consisting of avoiding sunlight, fluid therapy, and antiinflammatories.[148]

Epitheliogenesis Imperfecta

Epitheliogenesis imperfecta has been diagnosed in numerous breeds of sheep. It is an autosomal recessive genetic defect in cattle. Epithelial defects in the oral cavity (including the tongue and hard palate) are noted at birth. Hoof horn can easily be separated from the underlying laminae.[149]

Collagen Tissue Dysplasia (Ehlers-Danlos Syndrome)

Collagen tissue dysplasia, or Ehlers-Danlos syndrome, appears to be a hereditary skin disease of Norwegian sheep. Skin wounds develop rapidly after birth because of collagen defects.[147] Affected lambs die soon after birth because of secondary infection. This genetic defect results in the failure of collagen bundles to form in a functional configuration. A similar defect has been reported in crossbred sheep and White Dorper sheep in Brazil.[150,151]

Hypotrichosis Congenita

Hypotrichosis congenita is a viable hypotrichosis—that is, the disease is not immediately fatal to affected neonates. It is hereditary in polled Dorset sheep. Affected lambs have sparse hair fibers, most pronounced on the face and limbs. It has also been reported in a calf and a kid.[152]

Epidermolysis Bullosa

Epidermolysis bullosa is a recessive heritable defect of Weisses Alpenschaf sheep and has been diagnosed in Suffolk and South Dorset Down breeds of sheep as well.[147,153] Affected animals are born without type VII collagen and develop wounds rapidly after epidermal abrasion.[146] Skin biopsy reveals separation of the dermal-epidermal junction in the absence of epidermolysis. The hooves may slough and ulcers of the gingiva, hard palate, tongue, and mouth form rapidly.[153–156] The gene mutation responsible for this disease has been identified in cattle.[157] The application of this gene mapping technology in herds that have occasional cases will allow for genome-based breeding to avoid breeding carrier animals.

Hairy Shaker Disease of Lambs

Border disease, or hairy shaker disease, is a congenital condition caused by a pestivirus that may be transmitted vertically from the ewe to the fetus in utero. The border disease virus is closely related to the bovine viral diarrhea virus (BVDV). Clinical signs of border disease have been found in sheep infected with BVDV-2.[158] Newborn lambs have domed heads, short limbs, and thick trunks. Viral infection of the fetus before day 80 of gestation may interfere with the development of primary hair follicles and result in the formation of "kempy" fibers and long halo fibers in the fleece. Affected lambs appear abnormally hairy and are called *hairy shaker* lambs because tonic-clonic contractions of their skeletal muscles cause them to shake. Diagnosis is confirmed by virus isolation or a necropsy finding of hypomyelinogenesis in the central nervous system. It is unknown exactly how prevalent this disease is in the sheep industry or how much economic impact it has.[159] A persistently infected goat with no clinical signs of disease has been identified as the source of a herd outbreak.[160]

Neoplastic and Related Lesions

Neoplasia is rarely diagnosed in sheep, goats or cervids but a few conditions are described.

Papillomas (Warts, Fibropapillomatosis)

Warts in sheep are caused by species-specific papovaviruses. These DNA viruses cause papillomas on the face, legs, and teats that vary in size but may be as large as 4 cm in diameter and 2 cm in height. These lesions are vascular and bleed when disrupted. Secondary bacterial infection may occur with repeated trauma to the lesion. Teat papillomas may predispose to mastitis in sheep.[161] A cellular immune response eventually clears the lesions, which may

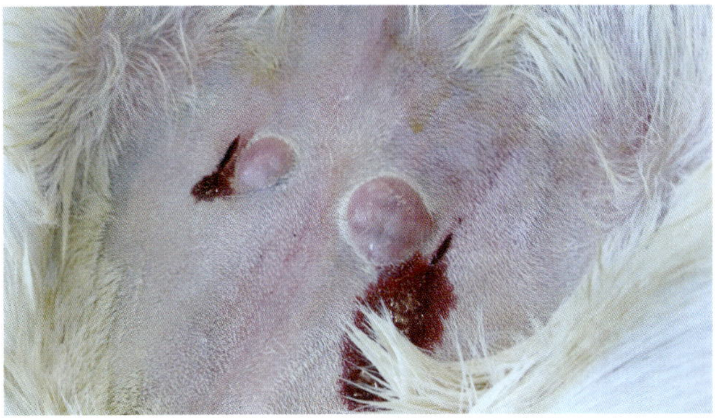

• **Fig. 10.8** Warts on the ventrum of a white-tailed deer at the scope and instrument portal sites after laparoscopic artificial insemination.

require months to regress. Failure of lesions to regress or excessive numbers of lesions suggests that the immune system is not competent. A viral cause has not been confirmed in goats. Papillomas on the udder of Saanen goats have been documented; they tend to persist without undergoing the regression typical of viral papillomas. Warts are fairly common in cervids and are usually self-limiting (Figure 10.8). There are cases, however, where multiple warts in an area may interfere with body functions and put the animal at risk.

Squamous Cell Carcinomas

Squamous cell carcinomas are most commonly diagnosed in Merino sheep and are usually seen in sheep older than 4 years. The peak incidence (12%) was observed in 12-year-old sheep. Tumors occur on the face, ears, and vulva but most commonly involve the ears. Squamous cell carcinoma of the perineum of a Merino ewe and goats has been reported.[162,163] One study determined squamous cell carcinoma to be the third most common skin disease in sheep and goats behind myiasis and contagious ecthyma.[164] An oral squamous cell carcinoma was diagnosed in a 3-year-old sheep presented for weight loss and the presence of an oral mass. Shortly after the diagnosis was confirmed with a biopsy, the animal was euthanized because of deterioration of her condition.[165] The high incidence of this tumor in goats appears to be due to lack of pigmentation at the perineum and the high and short tail of the goats, that exposes the area to intense ultraviolet radiation in the tropics.[162] As the tumor grows, the surface may become ulcerated because of tissue necrosis or self-trauma. Diagnosis is made by histopathologic examination of tissue specimens. Characteristic lesions exhibit acanthosis, pseudoepitheliomatous hyperplasia, and hyperkeratosis. Inflammation associated with ulceration or secondary bacterial infection is not uncommon. Ultraviolet radiation has been implicated in squamous cell carcinoma; photosensitive sheep are at greatest risk. Lesions in the ear, such as from ear tags, are more prone to mutate into squamous cell carcinoma. Treatment is by surgical excision with wide margins, but early culling is recommended. Squamous cell carcinoma in white-tailed deer is very rare and may be seen around the vulva/perineum in older animals (Figure 10.9). Prognosis is poor and culling of the animal is recommended.

Melanoma

Melanoma has an unknown incidence in sheep, goats, and cervids. One survey of the skin of 37,026 sheep and 23,429 goats

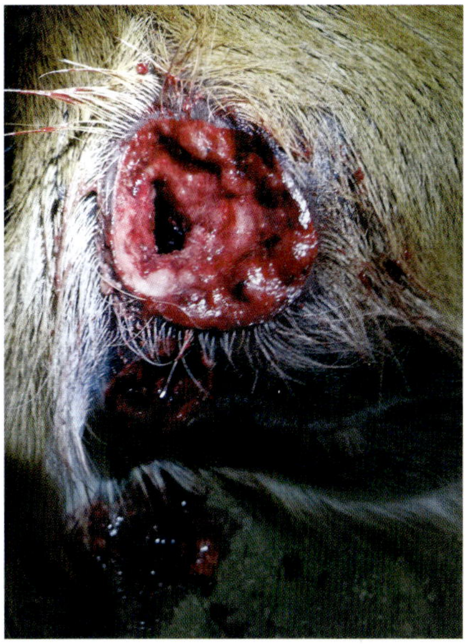

• **Fig. 10.9** Squamous cell carcinoma of the perineal region of a white-tailed deer.

found only two melanomas, both occurring on goats.[166] Another survey indicated an incidence of 0.03% cutaneous melanoma in goats,[167] while yet another reported malignant melanoma second only to squamous cell carcinoma in sheep and goats affected by skin tumors.[168] A case of malignant melanoma, originating at the base of the left horn, was reported in a white 11-year-old Pygora doe.[169] Another case of metastatic malignant melanoma was reported in a 3-year-old sheep without identifying a primary origin lesion.[170]

Hemangioma

Hemangioma has been diagnosed in an ewe with a lesion affecting the distal rear limb. The diagnosis was confirmed by histology after surgical excision. Another case was diagnosed in a lamb with a mass at the umbilicus.[171] Hemangioma has also been reported on the mandibular gingiva of a 5-year-old cross-bred ewe. The lesion in this case was surgically removed with the aid of local anesthesia and histopathologic examination confirmed the diagnosis.[172]

Drug Residue Issues

Preservation of a wholesome product, free of contaminants, is paramount to the small ruminant industry.[173] Nearly all treatments for skin diseases are performed in an extra-label manner because relatively few drugs are approved for use in small ruminants. Veterinarians must work diligently with industry personnel to ensure quality. In the United States, keepers and clinicians should respect the treatment guidelines described in the Animal Medical Drug Use and Clarification Act (AMDUCA) to avoid residue contamination of meat and milk. Small ruminants differ from cattle in both size of drug dosages and drug elimination times. Therefore, whenever possible, drug withdrawal times should be established from research performed specifically on the species being treated if possible.[174]

Removal of Wattles, Scent Glands, and Horns and Other Skin Procedures

Wattles

Wattles are skin appendages that are found in the cervical regions of some goats. The presence of wattles is a dominant genetic trait.[175,176] Although they are usually encountered in the mid-neck, they also may be found on the face or ears.[3] They are composed of connective tissue, nerves, blood vessels, smooth muscles, and a cartilaginous core.[3] Cysts may be found in the bases of some wattles.[3] These cysts may be hereditary and either bilateral or unilateral. If swollen, the cysts will be filled with a clear fluid. Surgical excision has proven to yield better results in treating wattle cysts than lancing or aspiration.[177] Wattles may become injured (e.g., caught in feeders or fences), detract from the appearance of show animals, make clipping and grooming difficult, and may be chewed or nursed by other kids or adults.[3,178] For these reasons, some owners wish to have them removed. Wattles can be easily removed at the time of castration and/or disbudding of very young animals. Slight tension can be placed on the wattle before its base is cut with scissors.[3,178] If excessive bleeding occurs, pressure should be applied. The skin should heal without further therapy.

Disbudding of Goats and Sheep

Some management styles prefer that goats (and occasionally rams) have their horn buds removed during the first 2 weeks of life.[178] However, many meat, fiber, and pet goat owners prefer to keep horned animals. Disbudding is more common among dairy goat producers to reduce fighting-related injuries. Kids can be held or placed in a dehorning box. They can be sedated (xylazine 0.05–0.2 mg/kg), have a ring of tissue around the horn anesthetized (1% lidocaine SC), or be placed under general anesthesia. A dehorning box encloses all of the body except the head. The heat from a commercial electric dehorning iron (for cattle or goats) or an electric cautery unit may be used. Regardless of the method, clipping all hair around the area aids the process. If an electric dehorning iron is used for this purpose, Williams[178] has recommended allowing it to heat and then applying it to a pine board. If the iron makes a slightly depressed black ring on the board, the proper temperature has been achieved.[178] The dehorner should be applied in a rocking manner over the horn buds. The area should be burned until a copper color is attained (Figure 10.10). If the hot iron is correctly applied, the horn "cap" should be easily removed. Williams[178] recommends burning the horn until the central core is removed. Common mistakes with this method are heat-induced meningitis and underheating of the germinal epithelium of the horn, resulting in the regrowth of abnormal horn tissue.[3,178] If the germinal horn tissue is not completely destroyed, the "scur" that regrows can be removed later. The calvarium of a kid is thin and the cornual sinus is small compared with those of calves. Heat-induced malacia of the underlying cerebrum can result in depression, blindness, abscess formation, and death.

Heat-induced meningitis and malacia are rarely reversible. Still, in such cases, immediate treatment with glucocorticosteroids (dexamethasone sodium phosphate 1–2 mg/kg IV), mannitol (0.25–1 mg/kg IV over 5 minutes), and possibly NSAIDs is indicated.

An alternative to cauterization of the horn buds is surgical removal. This can best be accomplished in 2- to 4-day-old kids using a similar method as described for heat removal. Instead of using a dehorning iron or electric cautery, the clinician makes a circumferential incision through the anesthetized skin and removes the horn bud and germinal tissue. To control hemorrhage, the area can be cauterized or firm digital pressure can be applied.

Caustic paste also is used to remove the horns of young kids. Clipping the hair around the horn buds aids in the application of the paste. If caustic paste is used, lanolin or petroleum jelly should be applied around the area, particularly around the eyes. The clinician should take care to prevent the caustic ointment from injuring the kids' eyes or other soft tissues. This method should be relegated to animals kept indoors (out of the rain), kids not nursing their dams, and those not able to rub the caustic ointment onto other kids.

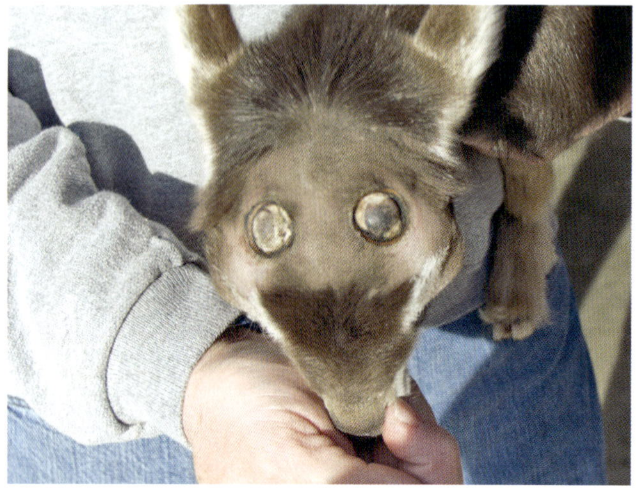

• **Fig. 10.10** The normal disbudding site 5 days after the procedure was done on a 4-day-old Oberhasli cross doe.

Dehorning

In kids older than 2 to 3 weeks of age, those whose previous dehorning has resulted in the growth of an abnormal horn tissue (scur), and adult goats are all candidates for dehorning. It is recommended that general anesthesia is used when dehorning adults and particularly males with large horns. However, sedation (xylazine 0.05–0.2 mg/kg) and local anesthesia of the cornual branches of the lacrimal and supratrochlear nerves may be acceptable. One not familiar to the innervation of the horns in small ruminants (which differs from that of cattle[179]) might consider a ring block around both horns being careful not to exceed the toxic dose of lidocaine. Diluting 2% lidocaine to 1% will help avoid toxic levels of lidocaine. Frequently, sedation and local anesthesia are chosen when the dehorning is done as a field procedure or when economics dictate that the less expensive route is taken.

The owner should be forewarned that this procedure is usually a "bloody mess." The wounds can take 4 to 6 weeks to heal,[180] result in secondary sinusitis, leave holes that never completely heal, or possibly result in brain abscesses (Figure 10.11). The skin around the horns should be clipped and surgically prepared. The clinician makes a circular incision through the skin 2 mm outside of the horn-skin junction. The strip of skin between the two horns should be left intact to improve and shorten healing time. An obstetric wire is then "laid into" the incision. A helper-technician holds the head to prevent excessive motion, and the surgeon stands in front of the

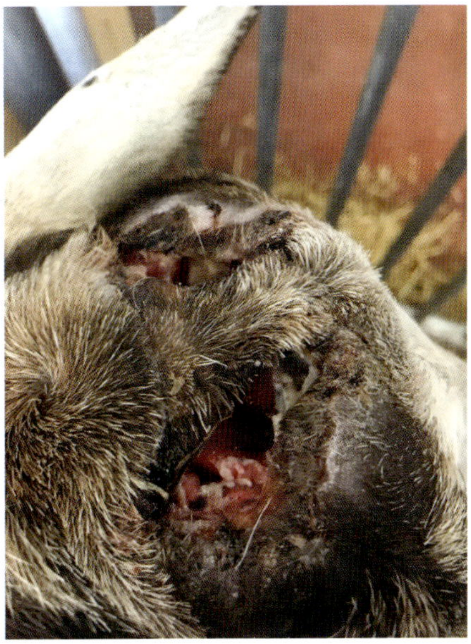

• **Fig. 10.11** The dehorning site of an adult goat approximately 4 weeks after surgery. Notice the open sinus with granulation tissue and some purulent exudate. This animal still requires frequent cleaning and bandaging.

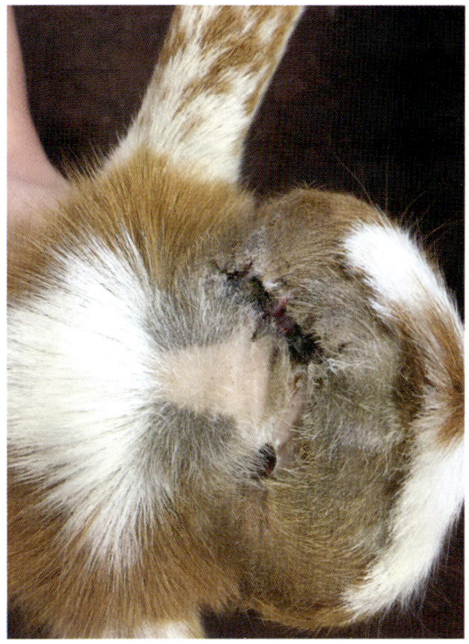

• **Fig. 10.12** The healed cosmetic dehorning site of a pygmy goat 14 days after surgery when sutures were removed. Notice a surgical scar with some scabbing but no communication with sinuses.

animal. The cut should be made in a rostral-ventral direction. Hemorrhage can be controlled by cautery, pressure, or pulling the bleeding vessels with hemostats. If the animal has a small horn base, the surrounding skin can be undermined and stretched over the opening created by the horn removal.[3] Closing the skin over the surgical site allows for a more rapid recovery but is rarely possible in adult males without removing some of the frontal bone, which will described later. An antibiotic ointment (triple antibiotic) can be applied and a gauze pad or other absorbable material can be placed over the site where each horn was removed. The pads can be held in place by tape wrapped around the head or by a piece of orthopedic stockinet with holes cut for the eyes and ears.[3] Animals can be given antibiotics (penicillin 20,000 IU/kg BID), NSAIDs, tetanus prophylaxis (tetanus antitoxin 150–300 IU), or tetanus toxoid. Fly control measures should be instituted. The bandage should be changed and the area examined every 2 to 4 days or as needed.

Some clinicians prefer not to bandage the dehorning site for fear of not being able to appreciate postoperative wound complications. These clinicians recommend instead isolation of the animal and feeding off the ground to avoid contamination of the wound until a scab forms in about 48 hours.[180] Most will bandage these animals.

An alternative to obstetric wire is to use a small Barnes dehorner to cut or nip off the horn tissue. The cut should be made carefully to avoid injuring the thin skull. The area can then be cauterized to control bleeding and destroy all remaining germinal epithelium. This method is not recommended because of the potential for skull damage.

Cosmetic dehorning with primary closure has been described in adult goats.[181] The horns are removed as described above with obstetric wire. After the horns are removed and the surrounding skin is undermined, rongeurs are used to remove small pieces of the frontal bone (taking care not to drop bone fragments into the sinus) until the skin can be closed over the surgical wound. This causes minimal change in the shape of the head, but it allows healing in 10 to 14 days and greatly decreases the aftercare required (Figure 10.12). No bandage is needed. All the animals in the original report healed without complications.[181] Rather than take a lot of frontal bone, the clinician can free more skin for closure by making a release incision in the skin between the horns (Figure 10.13). While this technique leaves a skin wound, it allows closure of the sinus and quicker healing. In some cases, the author (A.N. Baird) has used this technique to partially close the dehorning site when complete closure could not be accomplished without major frontal bone revision. It results in much smaller wounds, which will heal more quickly than larger ones. Complete closure and primary healing are the preferred techniques. The cosmetic dehorning technique is not without the

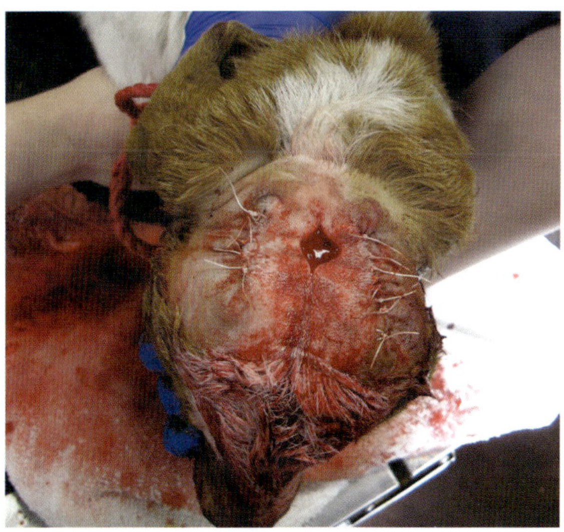

• **Fig. 10.13** An intraoperative photograph of a cosmetic dehorning of a Boer goat. Notice the dehorning sites are completely closed and there is a small gapping release incision between the two surgical incisions, allowing closure of the surgery sites with less tension.

potential for complications, but the complications are usually minor. One study found that 35% of the cases had minor complication such as incisional swelling, nasal discharge, or inappetence, but less than 3% of the cases suffered major complications such as dehiscence or death.[182]

An alternative method to completely removing the horn is to cut the horn off at the tip, mid-horn, or as close to level with the skull as possible, depending on the desire of the owner and the animal's use. This should be done on a sedated or an anesthetized goat. The horn can be cut with obstetric wire or a dehorning saw. The animal should be monitored for sinusitis, and the horn will continue to grow.

Deantlering Cervids

Male cervids have deciduous antlers that can be lethal weapons to others in the group or their human handlers. Although the males are primarily raised for their antlers, they are sometimes removed for safety and other reasons. To prevent antler growth, the male must be castrated prior to pedicle formation, or if pedicle formation has occurred, they must have the pedicle removed at time of castration. Most males have their antlers cut just above the pedicle after going "hard" in the fall as their testosterone rises and they begin to show signs of the rut. During this process, it is important to not cause any damage to the pedicle as it may cause permanent damage to future antler growth. Most antlers can be removed while restrained in a chute, but many deer are anesthetized for the procedure. No local anesthetic is needed with "hard" antler, but removal during the velvet phase of growth should be done with a local anesthetic or under anesthesia. Bleeding is not a problem with hard antler, but sometimes, a tourniquet is applied for velvet antler (Figure 10.14). It is removed after the antler is cut off and minimal bleeding is usually seen. Fly spray may be applied to the affected area to prevent fly strike. Obstetrical wire, dehorning saw, or reciprocating saw are commonly used. Coarse blade saws will work better due to clearance of bony material from cut site.

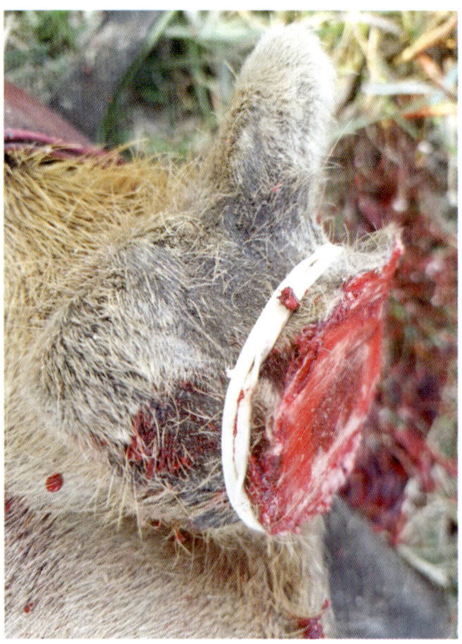

• **Fig. 10.14** A photograph of the amputation of an injured and infected developing antler in a white-tailed deer. Notice the tourniquet to decrease hemorrhage.

Descenting

Because of the smell associated with bucks, some owners request the removal of these animals' sebaceous glands. Removal of these glands may improve the smell, but odor will probably not be completely prevented. In young buck kids, the area behind the horns can be cauterized during dehorning. In the adult, the glands are located in thickened, folded skin caudad-medial to the horn base. The gland opening is a hairless area at the base of a skin fold.[178] Washing the head helps the clinician visualize the scent glands. The buck should be anesthetized or heavily sedated, the hair clipped, and the area surgically prepared. The clinician then makes an incision through the skin 1.5 to 2 cm around the gland opening. The incision should be deepened to the periosteum, the area dissected, and the gland identified and removed.[178] The clinician should attempt to close the skin defect. However, this is most difficult in older males because of the skin hypertrophy in this area. If the skin is not easily sutured, an antibiotic ointment can be applied and the area allowed to granulate.[183]

Acknowledgments

We acknowledge and appreciate the original contributions of Drs. David Anderson and D. Michael Rings (1st edition) and Dr. Jerry R. Roberson (2nd edition), whose work from previous editions of this book has been incorporated into this updated chapter.

References

1. Corke M, Matthews J: Diagnosing and treating skin diseases in goats: an update, *Practice* 40(4):149–156, 2018.
2. Scott DW: *Large animal dermatology*, Philadelphia, 1988, WB Saunders.
3. Smith MC, Sherman DM: Skin. In Smith MC, Sherman DM, editors: *Goat medicine*, ed 2, Ames, IA, 2009, Wiley-Blackwell.
4. Steinhagen O, Bredenhann AEJ: The effect of histological processing on sheep skin samples, *S Afr J Anim Sci* 17:151, 1987.
5. Kromer C, Bierschenk C, Czerny CP, Schön MP1, Buhl T: Orf (ecthyma contagiosum) in a sheep and a shepherd, *Lancet Infect Dis* 18(1):122, 2018.
6. Romero-Mercado CH, McPherson EA, Laing AH, Lawson JB, Scott GR: Virus particles and antigens in experimental orf scabs, *Arch Gesamte Virusforsch* 40:152, 1973.
7. Nettleton PF, Gilray JA, Yirrell DL, Scott GR, Reid HW: Natural transmission of orf virus from clinically normal ewes to orf-naïve sheep, *Vet Rec* 139:364, 1996.
8. de la Concha-Bermejillo A: Orf/contagious ecthyma. In Haskell SRR, editor: *Blackwell's five-minute veterinary consultant*, ed 1, Singapore, 2008, Wiley-Blackwell.
9. Cheng HY, Li WJ, Li XM, et al: Pathogenicity of blood orf virus isolates in the development of dairy goat contagious pustular dermatitis, *Vet Microbiol* 219:178–182, 2018.
10. McElroy MC, Bassett HF: The development of oral lesions in lambs naturally infected with orf virus, *Vet J* 174:663, 2007.
11. Coates JW, Hoff S: Contagious ecthyma: an unusual distribution of lesions in goats, *Can Vet J* 31:209, 1990.
12. Sargison ND, Scott PR, Rhind SM: Unusual outbreak of orf affecting the body of sheep associated with plunge dipping, *Vet Rec* 160:372, 2007.
13. Gumbrell RC, McGregor DA: Outbreak of severe fatal orf in lambs, *Vet Rec* 141:150, 1997.
14. Meynink SE, Jackson PGG, Platt D: Treatment of intraoral orf lesions in lambs using diathermy and cryosurgery, *Vet Rec* 121:594, 1987.

15. Blood DC, Radostits OM, Henderson JA, Arundel JH, Gay CC: *Veterinary medicine*, London, 1983, Bailliere Tindall.
16. de la Concha-Bermejillo A, Ermel RW, Zhang MZ: Contagious ecthyma (ORF) virulence factors and vaccine failure, *Proceedings of the 1999 one hundred and third annual meeting of the United States Animal Health Association,* Pat Campbell & Associates and Carter Printing Company, Richmond, VA San Diego, CA, 1999.
17. Musser JMB, Taylor CA, Guo J, Tizard IR, Walker JW: Development of a contagious ecthyma vaccine for goats, *Am J Vet Res* 69:1366, 2008.
18. Mullowney PC: Skin diseases of sheep, *Vet Clin North Am Large Anim Pract* 6(1):131, 1984.
19. Perez JLT: *Kids Immunity to Contagious Ecthyma (Orf Virus)*, presented at the Goat Diseases and Production, 2nd International Colloquium in Niort, France, June 26–29, 1989 (Abstract, p 24).
20. Renshaw HW, Dodd AG: Serologic and cross-immunity studies with contagious ecthyma and goat pox virus isolates from the western United States, *Arch Virol* 56:201, 1978.
21. USDA-APHIS: *Animal Health Monitoring and surveillance: status of reportable diseases in the United States*, 2008. http://www.aphis.usda.gov/vs/nahss/disease_status.htm#sheep.
22. Venkatesan G, Kumar Teli M, Sankar M, et al: Expression and evaluation of recombinant P32 protein based ELISA for sero-diagnostic potential of capripox in sheep and goats, *Mol Cell Probes* 37:48–54, 2018.
23. Bhanuprakash V, Indrani BK, Hosamani M, Singh RK: The current status of sheep pox disease, *Comp Immunol Microbiol Infect Dis* 29:27, 2006.
24. Davidson WR, Nettles VF: *Field manual of wildlife diseases in the southeastern United States*, ed 2, Southeastern Cooperative Wildlife Disease Study, College of Veterinary Medicine, The University of Georgia, 1997, Athens, GA.
25. Kitching P: Notifiable viral diseases and spongiform encephalopathies of cattle, sheep and goats, *Practice* 19(2):51–63, 1997.
26. Bridges VE, McCluskey BJ, Salman MD, Hurd HS, Dick J: Review of the 1995 vesicular stomatitis outbreak in the western United States, *J Am Vet Med Assoc* 211:556, 1997.
27. Roberts DS: Release and survival of *Dermatophilus dermatonomus* zoospores, *Aust J Agric Res* 14:386, 1963.
28. Martinez D, Prior P: Survival of *Dermatophilus congolensis* in tropical clay soils submitted to different water potentials, *Vet Microbiol* 29:135, 1991.
29. Hauptmanova K, Panev A, Antosova L, et al: Dermatophilosis in sheep, *Veterinarstvi* 64(5):376–380, 2014.
30. Riofrio AC, Lopez JC, Moyano JC, et al: Strawberry footrot in a Blackbelly sheep in the Ecuador Amazonia, *Sustain Agric Res* 5(4):56–57, 2016.
31. Larsen JWA: An outbreak of mycotic dermatitis in goat kids, *Aust Vet J* 64:160, 1987.
32. Yeruham I, Elad D, Perl S: Dermatophilus in goats in the Judean foothills, *Rev Med Vet* 154:785, 2003.
33. Norris BJ, Colditz IG, Dixon TJ: Fleece rot and dermatophilosis in sheep, *Vet Microbiol* 128:217, 2008.
34. Iliyasu D, Munir AS, Auwal U, et al: Consequences of chronic dermatophilosis on semen quality and reproductive performance of Friesian bull in multipurpose farm in Zaria, Nigeria, *Int J Livest Res* 5(6):46–53, 2015.
35. Mullowney PC, Baldwin EW: Skin diseases of goats. In Mullowney PC, editor: *Veterinary clinics North America, large animal dermatology*, Philadelphia, 1984, W. B. Saunders Company.
36. Dalis JS, Kazeem HM: Concurrent infections of a goat with *Dermatophilus congolensis* and *Blastomyces dermatitides*, *J Anim Vet Adv* 6:773, 2007.
37. Munro R: Caprine dermatophilosis in Fiji, *Trop Anim Health Prod* 10:221, 1978.
38. Dixon TJ, Mortimer SI, Norris BJ: 16S rRNA gene microbial analysis of the skin of fleece rot resistant and susceptible sheep, *Aust J Agric Res* 58:739, 2007.
39. Stuart TPA: On green-producing chromogenic micro-organisms in wool, *J Proc R Soc* 28:320, 1894.
40. Seddon HR, McGrath TT: Green coloration in wool, *Aric Gaz* 40:206, 1929.
41. Torell DT, Weir WC, Bradford GE, Spurlock GM: Effects of time of shearing on wool and lamb production, *Calif Agric* 23:16, 1969.
42. El-sukhon SN: Isolation and characterization of *Pseudomonas aeruginosa* from sheep with fleece rot in northern and middle Jordan, *Vet Dermatol* 13:247, 2002.
43. Chin JC, Watts JE: Dermal and serological response against *Pseudomonas aeruginosa* in sheep bred for resistance and susceptibility to fleece-rot, *Aust Vet J* 68:28, 1991.
44. Bonfiglio G, Carciotto V, Russo G: Antibiotic resistance in *Pseudomonas aeruginosa*, an Italian survey, *J Antimicrob Chemother* 41:307, 1998.
45. Gerceker AA, Gürler B: In vitro activities of various antibiotics, alone and in combination with amikacin against *Pseudomonas aeruginosa*, *J Antimicrob Chemother* 36:707, 1995.
46. Costa JLN, Oliveira MMD, Lobato FCF, et al: Outbreak of malignant oedema in sheep caused by *Clostridium sordellii*, predisposed by routine vaccination, *Vet Rec* 160:594, 2007.
47. Cihan H, Yalcin E, Mecitoglu Z, Senturk S: Outbreak of malignant oedema in sheep following vaccination with a multivalent clostridial bacterin-toxoid, *Tierarztl Prax Ausg G Grosstiere Nutztiere* 38(3):165–167, 2010.
48. Morris WE, Uzal FA, Fattorini FR, Terzolo H: Malignant oedema associated with blood-sampling in sheep, *Aust Vet J* 80:280, 2002.
49. Winter A, Clarkson M: Skin and wool. In *A handbook for the sheep clinician*, ed 7, Liverpool University Press, Liverpool, UK, 2012, pp 107–118.
50. Watson WA: The carriage of pathogenic staphylococci by sheep, *Vet Rec* 77:477, 1965.
51. Koutinas AF, Saridomichelakis MN, Argyroudis S, Koutinas CK, Karatzanos P, Giadinis N: Clinical, histopathological and therapeutic considerations in a flock of sheep with facial staphylococcal-associated dermatitis, *Vet Dermatol* 18:211, 2007.
52. Mavrogianni VS, Fthenakis GC: Clinical, bacteriological, cytological and pathological features of teat disorders in ewes, *J Vet Med A Physiol Pathol Clin Med* 54:219, 2007.
53. Schamber G, Alstad AD: Isolation of *Staphylococcus hyicus* from seborrheic dermatitis in a pygmy goat, *J Vet Diag Invest* 1:276, 1989.
54. Wilson DJ, Scott PR, Sargison ND, Bell G, Rhind SM: Effective treatment of severe facial dermatitis in lambs, *Vet Rec* 150:45, 2002.
55. Hardy WT, Price DA: Staphylococcal dermatitis of sheep, *J Am Vet Med Assoc* 119:445, 1951.
56. Stoops SG, Renshaw HW, Thilsted JP: Ovine caseous lymphadenitis: disease prevalence, lesion distribution, and thoracic manifestations in a population of mature culled sheep from western United States, *Am J Vet Res* 45:557, 1984.
57. Seddon HR: A discussion of the method of infection by bacillus of preisz-nocard, *Aust Vet J* 5:49, 1929.
58. Batey RG, Speed CM, Kobes CJ: Prevalence and distribution of caseous lymphadenitis in feral goats, *Aust Vet J* 63:33, 1986.
59. Maddy KT: Caseous lymphadenitis of sheep, *J Am Vet Med Assoc* 122:257, 1953.
60. O'Reilly KM, Green LE, Malone FE, Medley GF: Parameter estimation and simulations of a mathematical model of *Corynebacterium pseudotuberculosis* transmission in sheep, *Prev Vet Med* 83:242, 2008.
61. Faez Firdaus JA, Nur Amirah AL, Chung LT, et al: Changes in the reproductive hormones of non-pregnant does infected intradermally with *Corynebacterium pseudotuberculosis* in chronic form, *Int J Livest Res* 5(7):33–40, 2015.
62. Oreiby AF: Diagnosis of caseous lymphadenitis in sheep and goat, *Small Rumin Res* 123(1):160–166, 2015.
63. Holstad G, Teige J, Larsen HJ: *Corynebacterium pseudotuberculosis* infection in goats VIII. The effect of vaccination against experimental infection, *Acta Vet Scand* 30:275, 1989.
64. Washburn KE, Bissett WT, Fajt VR, et al: Comparison of three treatment regimens for sheep and goats with caseous lymphadenitis, *J Am Vet Med Assoc* 234:1162, 2009.

65. Pugh DG: Caseous lymphadenitis in small ruminants, *Proc North Am Vet Conf* 11:983, 1997
66. Eshra MA, Mahmoud AKA, Elshemey TM, Abdurrahman A, Abbas O: A trial for vaccination of sheep against Caseous lymphadentitis using oil adjuvant bacterin enhanced by Bacillus Calmette-Guerin vaccine, *Alex J Vet Sci* 57(1):140–147, 2018.
67. Silva MTO, Bezerra FSB, de Pinho RB, et al: Association of *Corynebacterium pseudotuberculosis* recombinant proteins rCP09720 or rCP01850 with rPLD as immunogens in caseous lymphadenitis immunoprophylaxis, *Vaccine* 36(1):74–83, 2018.
68. Sharp MW, Lupson GR, Flamank M: *Microsporum canis* infection in sheep, *Vet Rec* 132:388, 1993.
69. Gillespie JH, Timoney JF: *Hagan and bruner's infectious diseases of domestic animals*, London, 1981, Cornell University Press.
70. Hopkins FM, Gill W: Ringworm (Club lamb fungus) in sheep, Agricultural Extension Service, University of Tennessee, http://animalscience.ag.utk.edu/sheep/pdf/Ringworm.pdf.
71. Sargison ND, Thomson JR, Scott PR, Hopkins G: Ringworm caused by *Trichophyton verrucosum*—an emerging problem in sheep flocks, *Vet Rec* 150:755, 2002.
72. Hiddleston WA: The treatment of bovine ringworm, *Vet Rec* 92:123, 1973.
73. Knudsen EA: The areal extent of dermatophyte infection, *Br J Dermatol* 92:413, 1975.
74. Mugnaini L, Nardoni S, Pistelli L, et al: A herbal antifungal formulation of *Thymus serpillum, Origanum vulgare* and *Rosmarinus officinalis* for treating ovine dermatophytosis due to *Trichophyton mentagrophytes, Mycoses* 56(3):333–337, 2013.
75. Grotelueschen DM, Sahara RJ: Club lamb fungus disease. NebGuide, Cooperative Extension, University of Nebraska-Lincoln G92-1075-A, 1992, http://digitalcommons.unl.edu/cgi/viewcontent.cgi?article=1205&context=extensionhist.
76. Scott DW, Smith MC, Manning TO: Caprine dermatology. Part I. Normal skin and bacterial and fungal disorders, *Comp Cont Ed Pract Vet* 6:S190, 1984.
77. Smith MC: Dermatologic diseases of goats, *Vet Clin North Am Large Anim Pract* 5:449, 1983.
78. Pin D: Case report Seborrhoeic dermatitis in a goat due to *Malassezia pachydermatis, Vet Dermatol* 15:53, 2004.
79. Uzal FA, Paulson D, Eigenheer AL, Walker RL: *Malassezia slooffiae*–associated dermatitis in a goat, *Vet Dermatol* 18:348, 2007.
80. Gray GG, Pence DB: Ectoparasites of sympatric Barbary sheep and mule deer in the Texas Panhandle, USA, *J Med Entomol* 16:448, 1979.
81. Boswell E: *MSU researchers run their fingers through wool looking for solutions*, 2007, http://www.montana.edu/cpa/news/nwview.php?article=4553.
82. Cornall K, Wall R: Ectoparasites of goats in the UK, *Vet Parasitol* 207:176-179. 2015.
83. James PJ, Riley MJ: The prevalence of lice on sheep and control practices in South Australia, *Aust Vet J* 82:563, 2004.
84. Bisdorff B, Milnes A, Wall R: Prevalence and regional distribution of scab, lice and blowfly strike in Great Britain, *Vet Rec* 158:749, 2006.
85. James PJ, Moon RD, Brown DR: Seasonal dynamics and variation among sheep in densities of the sheep biting louse, Bovicola ovis, *Int J Parasitol* 28:283, 1998.
86. Hallam GJ: Transmission of *Damalinia ovis* and *Damalinia caprae* between sheep and goats, *Aust Vet J* 62:344, 1985.
87. Livingston CW: Parasitic skin diseases of sheep. In Howard JL, editor: *Current veterinary therapy food animal practice 2*, Philadelphia, 1986, W.B. Saunders.
88. Ajith Y, Dimri U, Singh SK, et al: Lice induced immuno-oxidative wreckage of goats, *Vet Parasitol* 242:24–30, 2017.
89. James PJ, Bartholomaeus FW, Karlsson LJE: Temporal relationship between infestation with lice (*Bovicola ovis* Schrank) and the development of pruritic behaviours and fleece derangement in sheep, *Vet Parasitol* 149:251, 2007.
90. Levot GW: Resistance and control of sheep ectoparasites, *Int J Parasitol* 25:1355, 1995.
91. Heath ACG, Lampkin N Jowett JH: Evaluation of nonconventional treatments for control of the biting louse (*Bovicola ovis*) on sheep, *Med Vet Entomol* 9:407, 1995.
92. Habluetzel A, Carnevali F, Lucantoni L, et al: Impact of the botanical insecticide NeemAzal® on survival and reproduction of the biting louse *Damalinia limbata* on Angora goats, *Vet Parasitol* 144:328, 2007.
93. Pfeffer A, Morris CA, Green RS, et al: Heritability of resistance to infestation with the body louse, *Bovicola ovis*, in Romney sheep bred for differences in resistance or resilience to gastro-intestinal nematode parasites, *Int J Parasitol* 37:1589, 2007.
94. James PJ, Cramp AP, Hook SE: Resistance to insect growth regulator insecticides in populations of sheep lice as assessed by a moulting disruption assay, *Med Vet Entomol* 22:326, 2008.
95. Small RW: A review of *Melophagus ovinus* (*L.*), the sheep ked, *Vet Parasitol* 130:141, 2005.
96. Jafari Shoorijeh S, Noori A, Tamadon A: Comparative efficacy of pour-on and subcutaneous injection of ivermectin on *Melophagus ovinus* (*L.*) in Darab ecotype goats of Southern Iran, *Vet Parasitol* 148:179, 2007.
97. Boyce WM, Weisenberger ME: The rise and fall of psoroptic scabies in bighorn sheep in the San Andres Mountains, New Mexico, *J Wildl Dis* 41:525, 2005.
98. Foreyt WJ: Contact transmission of psoroptic mange from bighorn to stone sheep, *J Wildl Dis* 33:664, 1997.
99. Van den Broek AH, Huntley JF: Sheep scab: the disease, pathogenesis and control, *J Comp Pathol* 128:79, 2003.
100. Downing W: The life history of *Psoroptes communis* var *ovis* with particular reference to latent or suppressed scab. III The clinical aspect of sheep scab, *J Comp Pathol Ther* 49:183, 1936.
101. Sweatman GK: On the life history and validity of the species in *Psoroptes*, a genus of mange mite, *Can J Zool* 36:906, 1958.
102. Kirkwood AC: History, biology and control of sheep scab, *Parasitol Today* 2:302, 1986.
103. Sargison N: Differential diagnosis and treatment of sheep scab, *Practice* 17:3, 1995.
104. Zaman MA, Tauseef-ur-Rehman, Abbas RZ, et al: Therapeutic potential of ivermectin, doramectin and trichlorophan against *Psoroptes ovis* in sheep and cattle of cholistan, *Pak Vet J* 37(2):233–235, 2017.
105. Doherty E, Burgess S, Mitchell S, Wall R: First evidence of resistance to macrocyclic lactones in *Psoroptes ovis* sheep scab mites in the UK, *Vet Rec* 182(4):106, 2018.
106. Friel J, Greiner EC: Ear mites from domestic goats in Florida, *Exp Appl Acarol* 4:345, 1988.
107. Jimena ON, Laura JM, Elena MM, Alonso NH, Teresa QM: Association of *Raillietia caprae* with the presence of Mycoplasmas in the external ear canal of goats, *Prev Vet Med* 92:150, 2009.
108. Faccini JL, Ribeiro VR: *Raillietia caprae* (Acari: Raillietidae) and *Psoroptes ovis* (Acari: Psoroptidae) in the ears of goats in the state of Rio de Janeiro, Southeast Brazil, *Rev Bras Parasitol Vet* 17:59, 2008.
109. Tarigan S, Huntley JF: Failure to protect goats following vaccination with soluble proteins of *Sarcoptes scabiei*: evidence for a role for IgE antibody in protection, *Vet Parasitol* 133:101, 2005.
110. Bell DS, Pounden WD, Edgington BH, Bentley OG: *Psorergates ovis* a cause of itchiness in sheep, *J Am Vet Med Assoc* 120:117, 1952.
111. Yeruham I, Rosen S, Hadani A: Sheep demodicosis (*Demodex ovis* Railliet, 1895) in Israel, *Rev Elev Med Vet Pays Trop* 39:363, 1986.
112. Strabel D, Schweizer G, Gansohr B, Braun U: The use of avermectins in two goats with demodicosis, *Schweiz Arch Tierheilkd* 145:585, 2003.
113. Young AR, Meeusen EN, Bowles VM: Characterization of ES products involved in wound initiation by *Lucilia cuprina* larvae, *Int J Parasitol* 26:245, 1996.
114. Heath ACG, Broadwell AH, Chilcott CN, Wigley PJ, Shoemaker CB: Efficacy of native recombinant Cry1B protein against experimentally induced and naturally acquired ovine myiasis (fly strike) in sheep, *J Econ Entomol* 97:1797, 2004.

115. Wall R: Blowfly strike—approaches to seasonal management in sheep, *Vet Times* 46:32, 16, 18, 2016.
116. Boyce W, Fisher A Provencio H, Rominger E, Thilsted J, Ahlm M: Elaeophorosis in bighorn sheep in New Mexico, *J Wildl Dis* 35:786, 1999.
117. McKown RD, Sterner MC, Oates DW: First observation of *Elaeophora schneideri* Wehr and Dikmans, 1935 (Nematoda: Filariidae) in mule deer from Nebraska, *J Wildl Dis* 43:142, 2007.
118. LeVan IK, Fox KA, Miller MW: High elaeophorosis prevalence among harvested Colorado moose, *J Wildl Dis* 49(3):666–669, 2013.
119. Henningsen JC, Williams AL, Tate CM, et al: Distribution and prevalence of *Elaeophora schneideri* in moose in Wyoming, *Alces* 48:35–44, 2012.
120. Solismaa M, Laaksonen S, Nylund M, Pitkänen E, Airakorpi R, Oksanen A: Filarioid nematodes in cattle, sheep and horses in Finland, *Acta Vet Scand* 50:20, 2008.
121. Brenner DJ, Stokking L, Donovan TA, Lamberski N: Pemphigus foliaceus in a Barbary sheep (*Ammotragus lervia*), *Vet Rec* 165:509, 2009.
122. Pappalardo E, Abramo F, Noli C: Pemphigus foliaceus in a goat, *Vet Dermatol* 13:L331, 2002.
123. Janzen AM, Wiles D, Myers S, Marqués FJ: Pemphigus foliaceus in a juvenile Cashmere goat, and outcome after prednisolone and methylprednisolone therapy, *Can Vet J* 52(12):1345–1349, 2011.
124. Lambacher B, Schoiswohl J, Brunthaler R, Wittek T, Krametter-Frötscher R: Successful treatment of pemphigus foliaceus in a Berrichon du Cher ram with methylprednisolone acetate, *Vet Dermatol* 28(5):499-e117, 2017.
125. Cornish J, Highland M: Successful treatment of juvenile pemphigus foliaceus in a Nigerian Dwarf goat, *J Am Vet Med Assoc* 236:674, 2010.
126. Williamson JA, Aiken G E: Case study: recovery from ergot alkaloid-induced vasoconstriction for steers conditioned to grazing seedhead-suppressed and unsuppressed pastures of toxic endophyte-infected tall fescue, *Prof Anim Sci* 33(6):756–763, 2017.
127. Zanzalari KP, Heitmann RN, McLaren JB, Fribourg HA: Effects of endophyte-infected fescue seed and cimetidine on respiration rates, rectal temperatures and hepatic mixed function oxidase activity as measured by hepatic antipyrine metabolism in sheep, *J Anim Sci* 67:3370–3378, 1989.
128. Aldrich CG, Rhodes MT, Miner JL, Kerley MS, Paterson JA: The effects of endophyte-infected tall fescue consumption and use of a dopamine antagonist on intake, digestibility, body temperature, and blood constituents in sheep, *J Anim Sci* 71:158–163, 1993.
129. Gasparotto SW: *Tall fescue toxicity in goats*, Onion Creek Ranch, Lohn, TX, 2017.
130. Sousa RFA, Almeida VM, Neto JE, et al: Laryngeal neuropathy in adult goats with copper deficiency, *Vet Pathol* 54(4)676–682, 2017.
131. Scott DW, Smith MC, Manning TO: Caprine dermatology. Part II. Viral, nutritional, environmental, and congenitohereditary disorders, *Compend Contin Educ Pract Vet* 6:S473, 1984.
132. Campbell AJD, Croser EL, Milne ME, Hodge PJ, Webb Ware JK: An outbreak of severe iodine-deficiency goitre in a sheep flock in northeast Victoria, *Aust Vet J* 90(6):235–239, 2012.
133. Smith MC: Small Ruminant Dermatology. *Proceedings of the 1998 Symposium on Small Ruminants for the Mixed Animal Practitioner Western Veterinary Conference*, Las Vegas, NV, 1998.
134. Linklater KA, Smith MC: *Color atlas of diseases and disorders of the sheep and goat*, Aylesbury, UK, 1993, Wolfe Publishing.
135. Krametter-Froetscher R, Hauser S, Baumgartner W: Zinc-responsive dermatosis in goats suggestive of hereditary malabsorption: two field cases, *Vet Dermatol* 16:269, 2005.
136. Koutsoumpas AT, Giadinis ND, Lafi SQ, et al: Serum vitamin A and vitamin E concentrations after parenteral vitamin A administration in sheep, *Small Rumin Res* 109(1):28–30, 2013.
137. Kimberling CV: Diseases of the skin. In Kimberling CV, editor: *Jensen and swift's diseases of sheep*, ed 3, Philadelphia, 1988, Lee & Febiger.
138. Santos DS, Silva CCB, Araújo VO, et al: Primary photosensitization caused by ingestion of *Froelichia humboldtiana* by dairy goats, *Toxicon* 125:65–69, 2017.
139. de Araújo VO, Oliveira Neto TS, Simões SVD, da Silva TKF, Riet-Correa F, Lucena RB: Primary photosensitization and contact dermatitis caused by *Malachra fasciata* Jacq. N.V. (Malvaceae) in sheep, *Toxicon* 138:184–187, 2017.
140. Pinto C, Santos VM, Dinis J, et al: Pithomycotoxicosis (facial eczema) in ruminants in the Azores, Portugal, *Vet Rec* 157:805, 2005.
141. Smith BL, Towers NR: Mycotoxicoses of grazing animals in New Zealand, *N Z Vet J* 50:28, 2002.
142. Mohammed A, Rabo JS, Ibrahim AA: Reaction to skin suture materials in Borno white goats, *Small Rumin Res* 16:191, 1995.
143. Mitchell GBB: Non-parasitic skin diseases in sheep. In Boden E, editor: *Sheep and goat practice,* London, 1991, Bailliere Tindall.
144. Smith MC: Caprine dermatologic problems: a review, *J Am Vet Med Assoc* 178(7):724–729, 1981.
145. Gonzalez-Jimenez E, Blaxter KL: The metabolism and thermal regulation of calves in the first month of life, *Br J Nutr* 16:199, 1962.
146. Pelton JA, Callan R, Barrington GM, Parish SM: Frostbite in calves, *Comp Cont Ed Pract Vet* 22:S136, 2000.
147. Basrur PK, Yadav BR: Genetic diseases of sheep and goats, *Vet Clin North Am Food Anim Pract* 6:779, 1990.
148. Vercosa BLA, Vitorino Filho RNL, de Sousa MVC, et al: Clinical aspects and treatment of hepatogenous photosensitization in sheep, *PUBVET* 3:30, unpaginated, 2009.
149. Azimpour S, Gholamhoseini B, Shaghayegh A: First report of congenital epitheliogenesis imperfecta in a lamb from Iran, *Comp Clin Path* 24(2):247–250, 2015.
150. Oliveira MC, Raimundo BPS, Silveira CR, et al: Dermatosparaxis in a sheep: clinical, anatomopathological, and molecular findings, *Acta Sci Vet* 45(Suppl):224, 2017.
151. Andrade DGA, Pavan LF, Amorim RM, et al: Clinical, histopathological and molecular aspects of the dermatosparaxis in White Dorper sheep, *Pesqui Vet Bras* 34(5):443–448, 2014.
152. Rani RU, Kumar AS, Balaji NS: Hypotrichosis congenita in a calf and a kid, *Intas Polivet* 14(2):449–450, 2013.
153. Steffen DJ: Congenital skin abnormalities, *Vet Clin North Am* 9:105, 1993.
154. Benavides J, Suarez-Vega A, Gutierrez J, et al: Generalized severe junctional epidermolysis bullosa with congenital absence of skin in churra lambs, *Vet Dermatol* 26(5):e83, 2015.
155. Medeiros GX, Riet-Correa F: Epidermolysis bullosa in animals: a review, *Vet Dermatol* 26(1):3–e2, 2015.
156. Medeiros GX, Riet-Correa F, Barros SS, et al: Dystrophic epidermolysis bullosa in goats, *J Comp Pathol* 148(4):354–360, 2013.
157. Pausch H, Ammermüller S, Wurmser C, et al: A nonsense mutation in the *COL7A1* gene causes epidermolysis bullosa in Vorderwald cattle, *BMC Genet* 17:149, 2016.
158. Eiras MC, Vina M, Fernandez D, et al: Border disease-like clinical signs in sheep caused by a BVDV-2 type d, *Vet Rec Case Rep* 5(3):e000478, 2017.
159. Crilly JP, Jennings A, Gascoigne E: Border disease: an under-appreciated threat to flock health and productivity? *Livest* 23(2):88–92, 2018.
160. Rosamilia A, Grattarola C, Caruso C, et al: Detection of border disease virus (BDV) genotype 3 in Italian goat herds, *Vet J* 199(3):446–450, 2014.
161. Mavrogianni VS, Cripps PJ, Papaioannou N, Taitzoglou I, Fthenakis GC: Teat disorders predispose ewes to clinical mastitis after challenge with *Mannheimia haemolytica*, *Vet Res* 37:89, 2006.
162. Barbosa JD, Duarte MD, Oliveira CMC, et al: Perineal squamous cell carcinoma in goats in the State of Pará, Brazil, *Pesqui Vet Bras* 29:421, 2009.
163. Bush RD, Toribio J, Windsor PA: The impact of malnutrition and other causes of losses of adult sheep in 12 flocks during drought, *Aust Vet J* 84:254, 2006.

164. Macedo JTSA, Riet-Correa F, Dantas AFM, et al: Diseases of the skin in sheep and goats from the Brazilian semiarid, *Pesqui Vet Bras* 28(12):633–642, 2008.
165. Namjoo AR, Soroori S, Farid M, Nourani H: An unusual squamous cell carcinoma in a sheep: a case report, *Comp Clin Path* 21(6):1383–1386, 2012.
166. Venkatesan RA, Nandy SC, Santappa M: A note on the incidence of melanoma on goat skin, *Ind J Anim Sci* 49:154, 1979.
167. Venkatesan RA, et al: Survey of the incidence of various surface defects in goat and sheep skins in Madras, *Leather Sci* 24:255, 1977.
168. Ahmed AF, Hassanein KM: A Ovine and caprine cutaneous and ocular neoplasms, *Small Rumin Res* 106(2–3):189–200, 2012.
169. Mavangira V, Hughes JM, Middleton JR, Mitchell WJ, Kim DY: Malignant melanoma of the horn base in a Pygora goat, *J Vet Diagn Invest* 20:104, 2008.
170. Oryan A, Ghane M, Ahmadi N, Daneshbod Y: Melanoma of unknown primary origin metastasizing to visceral organs in a sheep, *Braz J Vet Pathol* 11(1):24–27, 2018.
171. Abubakar AA, Sahabi SM, Yakubu AS: Diagnosis and surgical management of umbilical hemangioma in a lamb, *Intas Polivet* 14(1):99–101, 2013.
172. Mohajeri D, Mousavi G, Rezaie A: Gingival hemangioma in a sheep, *Iran J Vet Surg* 3(1):85–89, 2008.
173. Bretzlaff K: Special problems of hair goats, *Vet Clin North Am Food Anim Pract* 6:721, 1990.
174. Fajt VR: Label and extralabel drug use in small ruminants, *Vet Clin North Am Food Anim Pract* 17:2, 2001.
175. Reber I, Keller I, Becker D, Flury C, Welle M, Drögemüller C: Wattles in goats are associated with the *FMN1/GREM1* region on chromosome 10, *Anim Genet* 46(3):316–320, 2015.
176. Aziz A, Das D, Konwar BK: A note on the inheritance pattern of wattles in goats, *Indian Vet J* 78(7):645–646, 2001.
177. Abu-Seida AM: Radiographical examination and treatment of wattle cyst in goats and sheep, *Glob Vet* 12(6):862–864, 2014.
178. Williams CSF: Routine sheep and goat procedures, *Vet Clin North Am Food Anim Pract* 6:737, 1990.
179. Vitums A: Nerve and arterial supply to the horns of the goat with reference to the sites of anesthesia for dehorning, *J Am Vet Med Assoc* 125:284, 1954.
180. Hull BL: Dehorning the adult goat, *Vet Clin North Am Food Anim Pract* 11:183, 1995.
181. Hague BA, Hooper RN: Cosmetic dehorning in goats, *Vet Surg* 26:332, 1997.
182. Hartnack AK, Jordan ME, Roussel AJ: Complications associated with surgical dehorning in goats: a retrospective study of 239 cases, *Vet Surg* 47(2):188–192, 2018.
183. Matthews J: Descenting of male goats, *Goat Vet Soc J* 24:25, 2008.

11

Diseases of the Musculoskeletal System

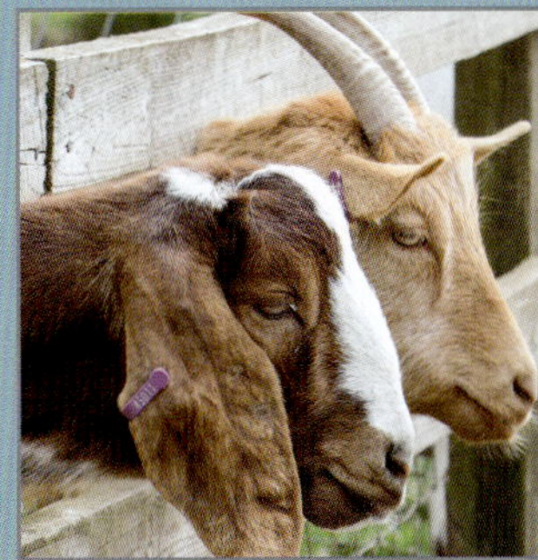

A.N. BAIRD AND CLIFFORD F. SHIPLEY

Examination

Farm-raised sheep, goats, and cervids are naturally herd animals that prefer living and staying in a group. Therefore any examination of these animals on the farm should include initial observation of the entire group if possible. Group observation is probably less important in the evaluation of traumatic musculoskeletal conditions than when several animals are affected by infectious diseases, parasitism, nutritional disorders, and improper management. The practitioner should look for potential hazards around feeders and other areas of the environment when the group has a higher than expected incidence of fractures or injury. Veterinarians should look closely for animals that lie down or walk on their knees when their herd mates are moving around. Animals also should be observed for difficulty in rising; swollen or enlarged joints; lameness; and abnormal stance.

When examining an individual animal, the clinician should perform careful, meticulous palpation and close examination. Some animals may have obvious fractures and wounds. Those with subtle problems require thorough examination. The clinician should first examine the feet for overgrown hooves, abscesses, interdigital lesions, exudate, and any foul smell. The coronary band should be examined for swelling, hyperemia, and proliferative lesions. All limb joints should be evaluated for swelling associated with trauma, septic arthritis, and infectious disease. The clinician should flex and extend the animal's joints through the entire range of motion to detect pain or laxity. In cases of hindlimb lameness, the clinician also should evaluate the patella for laxity, movement, and pain. Any asymmetry associated with swelling or muscle atrophy should be noted. Sciatic or peroneal nerve injury can occur after intramuscular (IM) injections and may produce lameness and muscle atrophy.

Anatomy

Sheep and goats, like cattle, are members of the *Bovidae* family. Deer are members of the *Cervidae* family. They join several other even-toed animals in the order *Artiodactyla.* Animals in this order share three skeletal characteristics: the talus has distal and proximal trochleae; the calcaneus and fibula articulate with each other; and the limb axis divides the fused third and fourth metacarpal-metatarsal bones and the associated digits.[1] Sheep have short, blunt, spinous processes of the cervical vertebra, whereas those of goats are longer and pointed and have sharp edges. Small ruminants have 7 cervical vertebrae, 13 thoracic vertebrae, 6 or 7 lumbar vertebrae, 4 sacral vertebrae, and 16 to 18 caudal vertebrae. The presence of 7 cervical vertebrae is a reliable trait in identification. However, variations are not unusual, such as 12 or 14 thoracic vertebrae or 5 lumbar vertebrae. Occasionally, an unusual transitional vertebra that is difficult to classify is found between the thoracic and lumbar vertebrae.[1] The authors describe a few of the musculoskeletal differences between sheep and goats within this chapter, as well as some of the variations from cattle. However, a thorough description of small ruminant anatomy is beyond the scope of this text.

Congenital Conditions

Myotonia Congenita

Myotonia congenita is a heritable condition of goats in which the animal experiences tetanic muscle contraction when startled. Occasionally, the contraction is severe enough that the goat collapses to the ground. This phenomenon has led to affected animals being referred to as *fainting goats.* This condition is caused by an autosomal dominant trait.[2] Some speculate that the variability in clinical signs and intensity of muscle contractions may be related to the animal being homozygous rather than heterozygous for the trait.[2] The condition closely resembles one form of myotonia congenita in human beings and has therefore been used as a research model for the human disease.[3] The condition is caused by a mutation in the voltage-dependent chloride channel in skeletal muscle, which leads to hyperexcitability of the sarcolemma and delayed relaxation of contracted muscle.[4] Histochemical and ultrastructural abnormalities are present in goats with myotonia congenita.[2,3] A similar condition has been described in a flock of sheep in Spain. The authors reporting this finding recommended identification and culling of rams that sired affected lambs.[5]

Hereditary Chondrodysplasia (Spider Lamb Syndrome)

Spider lamb syndrome is an inherited musculoskeletal condition seen primarily in the Suffolk and Hampshire breeds,[6] while Shropshire and Oxford sheep may also be affected.[7]

Clinical signs may be present at birth or affected lambs may appear normal at birth, only to have the severe skeletal abnormalities develop by 6 weeks of age.[8] This latter group may have longer legs with angular deviations, shallower bodies, and narrower chests than normal lambs,[8] and these animals display the expected radiographic abnormalities associated with this condition at birth. Skeletal abnormalities exhibited by affected lambs vary in severity and type. Chondrodysplasia is evident in the skull, sternum, appendicular skeleton, and vertebrae.

Radiographically, the dorsal silhouette of the skull may be rounded, the occipital condyles may be elongated (occasionally with cartilage erosion), and thickening of the occipital bone between the condyles and the poll may be evident. The sternebrae may be of abnormal size and shape. The sternum is often misaligned, dorsally deviated, and not fused across the midline. The scapula and olecranon usually have more cartilage and less bone distally than normal. Animals with spider lamb syndrome have several islands of ossification near the anconeal process that can be seen on flexed lateral radiographs of the elbow. The distal physis of the radius is flared, and angular limb deformities are common. Generally, the forelimbs are more severely affected than the hindlimbs. Erosion of articular cartilage is common if the lamb survives for a few months. The vertebrae commonly have abnormal and excessive cartilage. Vertebral body abnormalities may contribute to scoliosis or, less commonly, kyphosis.[8] Histologically, the typical osseous lesion is manifested as uneven growth cartilage. The pathologic changes are found by the end of the second trimester of gestation.[8]

Spider lamb syndrome is caused by a mutation in fibroblast growth factor receptor 3 that leads to excessive skeletal growth.[9] Initially considered to follow an autosomal recessive pattern with complete penetrance but variable expression, genetic testing has led to a suggestion of a codominant pattern. Heterozygotes are occasionally affected with spider lamb syndrome but more typically have a phenotype close to normal but with longer bones than animals without the mutation.[9] Carriers were difficult to identify until a DNA test became commercially available. The incidence of spider lamb syndrome has dropped greatly since the test became available.[10]

Arthrogryposis

Arthrogryposis, congenital fixation of multiple joints, has been reported to result from infectious, toxic, and genetic causes. Arthrogryposis and hydranencephaly may result from infection with Akabane virus, Cache Valley virus, Border disease virus, and possibly other organisms such as Schmallenberg virus that affect the developing fetus.[11] Affected animals have severely flexed forelimbs and overextended hindlimbs. A spiral deviation of the spine also is present. Neurologic conditions that may be seen with arthrogryposis and hydranencephaly include cerebellar hypoplasia, hydrocephalus, micromelia, and hydrocephaly.

Maternal ingestion of lupine (*Lupinus* sp.) and hemlock (*Conium maculatum*) has produced arthrogryposis in offspring. The type and severity of disorders vary according to age of gestation, dose, and duration of ingestion. A controlled study feeding *Poincianella pyramidalis* to pregnant does in Brazil resulted in a number of malformations, including arthrogryposis, in kids.[12]

Inherited arthrogryposis has been reported in Suffolk[13] and Corriedale[14] sheep. It appears to follow an autosomal recessive pattern and a site on chromosome 5 has been identified as the likely locus.[15]

Polydactyly

By definition, polydactyly is a congenital anomaly in which extra digits are present. It is seldom seen in small ruminants. The condition is certainly heritable in cattle and probably heritable in pigs, where cleft palate may concurrently be seen. Polydactyly is suggested to be heritable in horses. One report of polydactyly in goats describes an affected female that was sired by a male with polydactyly.[16] Polydactyly usually has only cosmetic consequences for affected animals. However, polydactyly may cause serious gait abnormalities in some animals. The practitioner must thoroughly examine animals with gait abnormalities to determine whether the lameness is because of some other anomaly or clinically significant lesion. Radiographs are necessary to assess the anomaly fully and determine any treatment to be rendered.

Treatment. Treatment involves surgical removal of the extra digits and primary closure of the skin incision. Removal of some of the digits can be done by sharp excision; however, orthopedic instrumentation is sometimes required to disrupt osseous attachment. Appropriate postoperative care should be given after surgical excision.

Patella Luxation

Animals with congenital patella luxation are usually brought to veterinarians shortly after birth because they tend to crouch on the rear legs when attempting to stand. The patella luxation functionally disrupts the quadriceps apparatus, rendering the animal unable to hold the stifle in extension. The primary differential diagnosis that must be ruled out with this presentation is femoral nerve injury, which also causes failure of the quadriceps apparatus because of lack of strength in the quadriceps muscle, producing the same abnormal stance. Femoral nerve injury is more commonly seen in calves after dystocia than it is in small ruminants. A diagnosis of patella luxation is easily made by palpating the patella; a luxated patella easily dislocates either medially or laterally. In severely affected animals, the patella remains luxated and is difficult to reduce into its normal position. This manipulation is more easily accomplished with the stifle held in extension.

Standard radiographic views with the addition of a skyline image demonstrate the position of the patella, the depth of the trochlear groove, and other osseous abnormalities that may be present. The skyline view, which allows the best assessment of the trochlear groove, is taken with the stifle flexed and the x-ray beam directed proximally to distally perpendicular to the tibia. However, the ease of luxation on palpation of the patella is much more important diagnostically than is the location of the patella on a single craniocaudal radiograph. The affected patella is often in a normal position for a given radiograph if it is not purposely luxated by the examiner before the radiograph is taken.

Surgery is usually indicated for young animals with congenital patella luxation. Most young animals respond well to imbrication of the fibrous joint capsule and overlying fascia on the side opposite the direction of patella luxation. However, the veterinarian must fully evaluate the limb before surgery and also assess the joint at surgery. Some severe cases may require trochleoplasty or tibial crest osteotomy and relocation. The reader should refer to small animal surgery texts for detailed descriptions of the more complex stifle surgeries.[17]

Affected animals should be thoroughly examined for other congenital abnormalities. Specifically, severely affected newborns may not be able to stand and suckle. Therefore, failure of passive transfer and associated illness may become more significant to the health of these animals than even the primary patella luxation. Small ruminants may compensate for mild cases of patella luxation (especially if the condition is unilateral) and go undiagnosed until they are seen by veterinarians as adults with lameness caused by luxation or degenerative joint disease caused by intermittent luxation. One report of sheep with common bloodlines developing patellar luxation when as old as 2 years suggests some genetic predisposition to the condition.[18] Adult animals also may exhibit acute lameness as a result of traumatic patella luxation. Surgical treatment of adults tends to be more involved in that orthopedic implants such as screws and wires may be required to secure the patella in the normal position. They may also require wedge trochleoplasty and/or tibial tuberosity transposition in addition to imbrications and fascial release.[18] The prognosis for a return to soundness in adults is not good compared with the prognosis for treated neonates with congenital luxations.[19,20]

Spastic Paresis

Spastic paresis has been described in pygmy goats.[21] Affected goats suffer constant contraction of the gastrocnemius muscles in the hind legs. The contraction produces extension of the tibiotarsal joint and arching of the back. Clinical signs are not significantly different from those described in several breeds of cattle.[22–24] This condition is suspected to be inherited, but the exact mode of transmission is unknown. No lesions have been noted in the spinal cord, tibial or peroneal nerves, or gastrocnemius muscle. The clinical signs appear to be caused by a defect in the myotactic reflex that results in an overstimulation or relative lack of inhibition of the efferent motor neurons.[21] Spastic paresis has been treated in calves by tibial neurectomy. The procedure has reportedly provided some improvement, but complete resolution of signs should not be expected and clinical signs may worsen in time following treatment.[25]

Carpal Contracture

Carpal contracture can occasionally present as a congenital condition in neonates. Many will respond very quickly to treatment with splints and bandages. One should radiograph the limbs to identify any osseous lesion that may contribute to the flexural deformity. Careful palpation of the limb while attempting to straighten it will frequently identify the structures under tension. Tenotomy of the restrictive structure may relieve the flexural deformity. Flexural deformities may develop in older animals following an injury that leads to abnormal weight bearing. This secondary flexural deformity will often involve fibrosis of the joint capsule and seldom respond to tenotomy. Some will not resolve in spite of release incision of the joint capsule and all flexural structures between the skin and joint capsule.

Traumatic Conditions

Predator Attack

Small ruminants are of the stature and disposition to make them susceptible to predators. In the United States, predation accounts for about 28% of sheep and lamb losses and about 25% of goat death loss, primarily (65–75%) due to attacks from coyotes and dogs.[26,27] That amounts to over 122,000 goat deaths. Small ruminants seldom survive attacks by wild carnivores, but there are still over 10,000 goats each year that are injured yet survive predator attacks.[26] Veterinarians are sometimes called to treat survivors of attacks by domestic animals or interrupted attacks by wild animals. These survivors often ultimately die because of either lethal injury to internal organs or physical exhaustion from the chase and the attack. A veterinarian treating animals that survive the initial trauma may face a significant challenge. Although skin wounds are quite obvious after the animal is thoroughly examined and clipped, injuries to deeper structures and serious myopathy are more difficult to assess.

Attacking predators tend to "go for the jugular," which leads to a concentration of wounds in the head and neck area. The associated injury to the great vessels is usually obvious and often fatal. Tracheal puncture can cause respiratory difficulties and subcutaneous emphysema. Subcutaneous emphysema also can result from the undermining skin wounds alone, making diagnosis of tracheal perforation difficult in some cases and adding to the difficulty of detecting a tracheal wound. Perforation of the esophagus is common. Esophageal injury may lead to abscess formation and tissue necrosis as a result of contamination of surrounding tissues by esophageal contents. Abscess formation may physically impinge on the airway and make swallowing difficult. Neurologic damage from the primary injury or damage caused by abscess formation may inhibit normal function of the soft palate.

Tetanus antitoxin should be administered to these animals, as well as broad-spectrum antibiotics (florfenicol 20 mg/kg every 48 hours) to combat wound infection and sepsis. Antibiotics with good efficacy against anaerobic bacteria (penicillin 20,000 IU/kg twice a day [BID]) should be considered in cases in which massive trauma has resulted in some tissue devitalization. All skin wounds must be thoroughly cleaned of organic debris and foreign material. Establishing drainage in undermined skin wounds also is important. Some of these wounds lend themselves to debridement and delayed primary closure, whereas others are best managed by allowing second intention healing. The veterinarian must be conscious of injury to muscle and joints deep beneath these skin wounds. Supportive care in the form of fluids and nonsteroidal antiinflammatory drugs (NSAIDs) (flunixin meglumine 1–2 mg/kg intravenously [IV]) is important in treating any myopathy.

Fractures

The hallmark of long bone fracture in small ruminants is acute non–weight-bearing lameness. A thorough physical examination must be performed to rule out other causes of severe lameness, including septic arthritis, joint luxation, and severe foot rot. The clinician should readily detect instability and crepitance on palpation of the fracture site. The exception is an incomplete or greenstick fracture that manifests itself as a less severe acute lameness that improves with time. The clinician should not overlook the possibility that an incomplete fracture may suffer a catastrophic breakdown and become unstable rather than heal. Because of economic constraints, radiographic examination may be impractical. However, whenever possible, radiographic evaluations before and after repair enhance the success of the procedure.

The most commonly treated fractures occur in the metacarpal and metatarsal bones.[28] These fractures are usually treated successfully with a cast. Fractures of the distal half of the metacarpal and metatarsal bones often respond well to lower limb casts that incorporate the foot and extend proximally to a point just distal to the carpus or tarsus respectively. Proximal or comminuted metacarpal

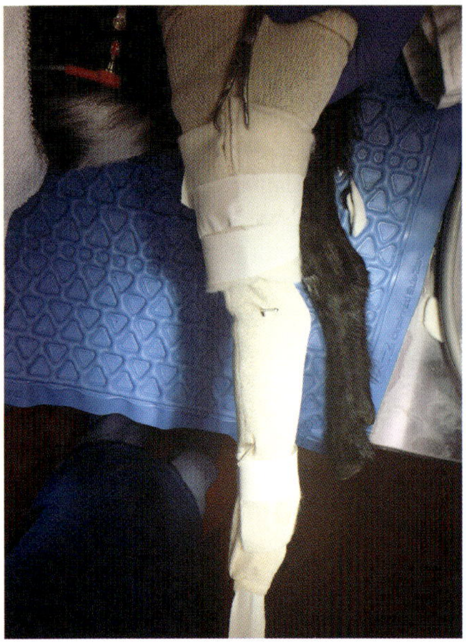

• **Fig. 11.1** A 2-year-old Pygmy goat with a metatarsal III–IV fracture with two transcortical pins placed (one above and one below the fracture) in preparation for application of cast material to construct a transfixation cast.

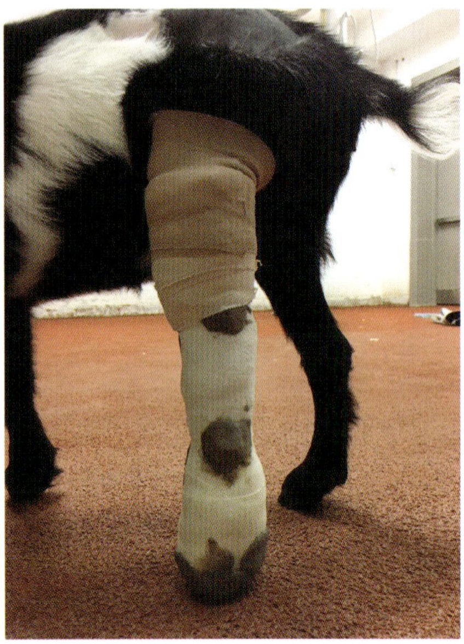

• **Fig. 11.2** The same goat from Figure 11.1 with transfixation casting complete. Notice the acrylic covering the pin ends and the bottom of the cast as well as elastic tape at the top of the cast to seal it.

and metatarsal fractures may require full-limb casting with or without transfixation pins to stabilize the fracture properly and prevent collapse (Figures 11.1 and 11.2).

Many fractures of the carpus or tarsus also respond to treatment with a full-limb cast.[29] However, these injuries are often associated with contamination of the joint, and the incidence of septic arthritis is high. Septic arthritis requires more intensive antibiotic therapy, as well as local treatment through a window in the cast. One complication with using treatment windows in casts is the "window edema" that frequently develops. The cast window should be cut out as one piece. Edema can be minimized by securing this piece in the window with tape between treatments. The management of carpal/tarsal fractures with concomitant septic arthritis is difficult. Ankylosis of the joint often results even if successful fracture healing occurs.[29]

Radius fractures must be evaluated individually to determine the best mode of treatment. Fractures of the distal radius may respond to a full-limb cast. Proximal radius fractures may heal better with the use of an external fixator, a transfixation cast, or possibly a modified Thomas splint. Splints may be very applicable for neonates and need only stay in place for 2 to 4 weeks in most instances.[30] Some radius fractures may be best treated with internal fixation using plates and screws. However, internal fixation is seldom required and often not economically feasible in small ruminants. If a splint is used for a radius fracture, it should extend from the ground or fetlock to the elbow and preferably above it.[30]

Treatment decisions for tibia fractures are very similar to those for radius fractures. Distal fractures heal well with full-limb casting.[31] The fractured tibia responds well to an external fixator or in larger goats (over 60 lb) a transfixation full-limb cast. Fractures of the humerus and femur occur less frequently in small ruminants.[28] Humerus fractures often heal with stall rest alone. However, the distal limb frequently suffers carpal contracture, rendering the animal unsound regardless of fracture healing. Femoral fractures may heal if the limb is taped in a modified Ehmer sling (made of tape placed in figure-of-eights around the limb) that is taped to the abdomen. This method is less costly but is still an effective method in young or lightweight animals.[30] Fractures of the humerus and femur frequently heal better with internal fixation using plates and screws or intramedullary pins. The mode of internal fixation depends on the complexity of the fracture and the experience of the veterinarian. Financial considerations may dictate the use of intramedullary pins rather than plates and screws when possible.

Fractures in other areas such as the scapula and pelvis can be treated much as they are in the dog. Small ruminants are usually good orthopedic patients because of their relatively small size and ability to maneuver well on three limbs. Often, pelvic or scapula fractures heal if the animal is confined for 3 to 6 weeks.[30] The veterinarian can form a plan for treating unusual orthopedic injuries in small ruminants by considering principles of small animal orthopedics and cost-benefit decision-making processes of food animal medicine.

Most lower leg fractures in cervids can be treated as previously mentioned, whereas upper limb fractures generally heal without intervention. The disposition of cervids makes limb care and management sometimes very difficult. Euthanasia should be considered in some cases, but sometimes, the most severe fracture will heal remarkably well on its own. Many will get along on three legs, so amputation may also be a consideration in some cases.

Mandible fractures may occur in small ruminants that have been kicked by a large animal such as a horse or cow and those that have caught the rostral mandible in a fence or some other object. A kick injury may result in any number of fracture configurations; the veterinarian must refer to information on small animal fundamentals to determine whether plates, wires, or pins are the most appropriate surgical stabilizers. Frequently, external fixators can be used to treat mandibular fractures. At this time, the authors prefer using cortical bone screws placed in the mandible via stab incisions, leaving the screw to protrude about 2 to 4 cm out of the skin. Then acrylic is made to fit over the screw heads and act as connecting bars of an external fixator. The screws provide better stability in the mandible than transcortical pins and the acrylic allows more liberty in screw placement than traditional connecting bars would. Rostral fractures may involve mostly teeth and soft tissues but very little bone. They often cause loss of teeth but minimal instability. Therefore, the veterinarian may wish to debride the area, institute antibiotic therapy, and modify the animal's diet (see Chapters 2 and 4). If the mandibular fracture occurs between the incisors and the cheek teeth, it may be stabilized by securing wires from the rostral mandible to the cheek teeth.[32,33] Animals with these types of fractures require nutritional support, either orally or parenterally (see Chapters 2 and 3). Many of these animals can be fed a moistened pelleted diet.

Occasionally, digit or leg amputation is required to treat septic conditions, fractures, or luxations. Amputation can be done with the animal under general anesthesia or with the animal sedated and under local anesthesia (see Chapter 18). For digit amputation, a tourniquet should be applied proximal to the fetlock after the surgical site is prepared in an aseptic manner. A circumferential skin incision is made just proximal to the coronary band. One may then make two incisions perpendicular to the circumferential incision (one dorsal and another palmar or plantar) to create a skin flap that is elevated to allow amputation with Gigli wire. The authors prefer to make one incision over the abaxial aspect of the affected digit perpendicular to the coronary band to create an inverted T incision. The two flaps of the inverted T can be undermined to allow the passage and crossing of the Gigli wire. The amputation should be completed on an angle at the distal aspect of the proximal phalanx, with the clinician removing all of the articular cartilage and synovial membrane of the proximal interphalangeal joint while leaving the interdigital ligaments intact to provide stability to the fetlock. Alternatively, the practitioner may choose to disarticulate the pastern joint rather than cut through distal P1. The corners of the flaps of the inverted T can be trimmed to minimize dead space when the surgical site is closed. The site can be closed completely if the amputation is performed as a treatment for fracture or luxation. However, if infection is present in the form of septic arthritis or osteomyelitis, the clinician should consider the advantages of drainage facilitated by partial closure. With either closure, a bandage should be placed on the foot to aid in hemostasis before the tourniquet is removed. The bandage should be changed as needed until the incision site has healed. The use of broad-spectrum antibiotics (oxytetracycline 10 mg/kg IV or IM BID or 20 mg/kg subcutaneously [SC] every 48 hours) and antiinflammatory drugs should be considered.

If a limb is to be amputated, one should have detailed conversations with the owners to determine the postoperative use, living environment, and management of the animal. Then assess the impact of age and weight on the above considerations. Limbs are usually amputated as high as possible (midhumerus, midfemur) to prevent trauma to the remaining "stump" of the limb. The author (A.N. Baird) has violated this principle, with good results, on the hindlimb of camelids. The amputation done just below the hock allows a partial limb to aid in rising. This does present additional management concerns in that the hock must be protected from trauma by bandages or a protective boot. However, the practitioner should consider this technique when amputating the distal hindlimb in small ruminants. Once the location of the amputation is determined, techniques similar to those used in small animals can be applied to limb removal in sheep, goats, and cervids. One recent review of amputations found that the outcomes for sheep and goats were variable on a case-by-case basis and suggested that owners be advised of the likelihood of complications. Postoperative care and physical therapy should also be planned.[34]

Cast. The previous description of fractures discussed casting as a primary treatment option for fixation of fractures. The clinician should prepare the limb for cast application by removing any organic debris to ensure the leg is clean. Cotton or gauze sponges should be placed in the interdigital space to prevent pinching of the interdigital skin within the cast by the hooves. Orthopedic felt or gauze sponges should be placed over the dewclaws to provide padding; however, holes should be cut to allow the dewclaws to protrude. Without this precaution, pressure from the cast over the dewclaws can cause skin ulcerations and may even result in dewclaw sloughing. The clinician then applies a double layer of stockinette to the limb and places a strip of orthopedic felt around the limb where the most proximal part of the cast will end. The authors prefer to put this proximal felt between two layers of stockinette so the felt is encased in the stockinette when it is rolled down over the felt during application of the cast. However, others place the felt beneath the stockinette. Other padding materials may be used according to preference, but the clinician should remember that the relatively small size of most small ruminants demands that the cast not be overly heavy or bulky. The authors believe no padding beyond the previously mentioned interdigital cotton, orthopedic felt, and stockinette is necessary to prevent skin ulceration under a properly applied cast. If the wool of heavily wooled animals is not clipped, it may act as excellent padding.[30] An exception in which more padding is useful is in very young animals, which are likely to experience significant growth while in the cast and tend to be more prone to cast sores than adults.

Fiberglass casting material has replaced plaster because of its increased strength, lighter weight, and faster drying time. The foot should be included in the cast. The clinician should be careful to apply the cast without wrinkles (which may cause cast sores) and in a timely manner so that all layers bond together as one rather than laminate in several layers. The cast is not as strong if it dries in laminated layers. The solar surface of the cast should be protected from wear in some manner. Methods of protecting this part of the cast include tape alone, a section of tire inner tube and tape, and a walking pad made of hoof acrylic. The particular method chosen is less important than achieving the desired result of preventing exposure of the hoof through a worn cast.

Any animal in a cast must be monitored closely to detect complications as soon as possible. The clinician should consider complications under the cast as the cause of any abnormal clinical signs such as fever, loss of appetite, increased lameness in the cast limb, and swelling proximal to the cast. The cast should be palpated daily to determine its fit and check for any areas of increased heat that may indicate the formation of cast sores. However, some areas of the cast (e.g., over wounds and bony protuberances) are normally warmer than other areas of the cast. Therefore, it is more important to recognize changes in relative warmth in the same area of the cast from day to day than differences in temperature between different areas of the cast. A fiberglass cast applied over stockinette is porous, and exudate from a wound or cast sore will penetrate the cast. If the environment makes fly control difficult, flies may be observed concentrating over these localized areas of the cast before exudate can be seen penetrating the cast. This part of the cast also may have an increased relative temperature before the exudate penetrates it.

Transfixation casts add stability in cases in which cast immobilization alone is not adequate.[28] Transfixation pins help immobilize proximal fractures in ways that casting alone does not. In some cases, comminuted distal fractures collapse unless transfixation pins transfer the weight away from the distal limb to the transfixation pins.[35] Application of a transfixation cast often requires general anesthesia, although transfixation casting of hindlimbs can be done with sedation and spinal anesthesia. Pin diameter and placement depend on animal size, bone diameter, and fracture configuration. The transfixation pins are placed through stab incisions using aseptic technique. Intraoperative radiographs are helpful in the placement of the transfixation pins. However, this technique is usually successful even when pin placement is directed by palpation alone. Antimicrobial ointment ("Zipp" ointment or neomycin-polymyxin B-bacitracin) can be applied to the skin at the pin sites and covered with gauze sponges. The limb is then prepared as previously described for cast application. "Zipp" ointment applied under a cast has an antibacterial effect for as long as 2 weeks. "Zipp" is made from equal parts zinc oxide, iodoform, and mineral oil. The clinician should cut holes into the stockinette to accommodate the pins and cut the pins so that they protrude about 1 to 1.5 cm beyond the anticipated thickness of the cast. The cast material should be applied so that the bone pin ends perforate the cast material or the material placed around the pin. When the cast material has set or become hardened, the pin ends should be covered to prevent injury to the contralateral limb. Hoof acrylic or cotton and tape can be used to cover the pin ends. As the fracture heals, bone resorption occurs around the pins, causing them to loosen. Neither special instrumentation nor general anesthesia is required for pin removal.

External Fixation. External fixators are preferable to simple casts or transfixation casts in some fractures of the radius and tibia. Either traditional fixators or modified fixators using cast material to support the transcortical pins work well in small ruminants. Traditional external fixation techniques described for small animals can be used for sheep and goats.[36] One must be conscious of the hazards associated with treating cervids with external fixators and the exposed hardware. Standard smooth intramedullary pins can be used successfully in this technique, but we prefer positive profile threaded pins for extra stability. A modified fixator designed to treat calf tibia fractures is less technically demanding to apply than a traditional external fixator[37] and allows more flexibility in pin placement. The authors have found this technique to be most useful in tibia fractures but also of value for treatment of other fractures. The procedure is performed on a surgically prepared animal, under general anesthesia (see Chapter 18) and according to aseptic technique. At least two pins must be placed proximal and two pins distal to the fracture site. The pins can be placed through stab incisions from lateral to medial (type II pins) through the skin on each side. One major advantage of this technique is that a single type I pin can be placed from the dorsal aspect. The type I pin passes through one skin surface and both cortices of the bone, but not through the caudal soft tissues and skin (Figures 11.3 and 11.4). A second type I pin is not required because the cast material itself connects and stabilizes the pins. This is a major advantage in fractures (either proximal or distal) in which the fragment size does not allow placement of two type II pins. The pins should be incorporated into a cast as described previously for the transfixation cast and the limb treated with topical ointment. This technique incorporates more padding than that used with a standard cast. Cotton or some other padding should be wrapped around the entire length of the tibia. No stockinette or orthopedic felt is required. Fiberglass cast material should then be placed over the length of the tibia to incorporate the pins, as is done with the transfixation cast. After the cast hardens completely, the caudal quarter to third of the cast can be removed and the padding cut away from the caudal aspect of the limb. This modification allows unencumbered movement of the gastrocnemius. Occasionally, the dorsal distal portion of the cast also must be trimmed to allow flexion of the hock. Some patients initially require a splint or bandage over the fetlock to ensure the animal bears weight on the solar surface of the foot. Most

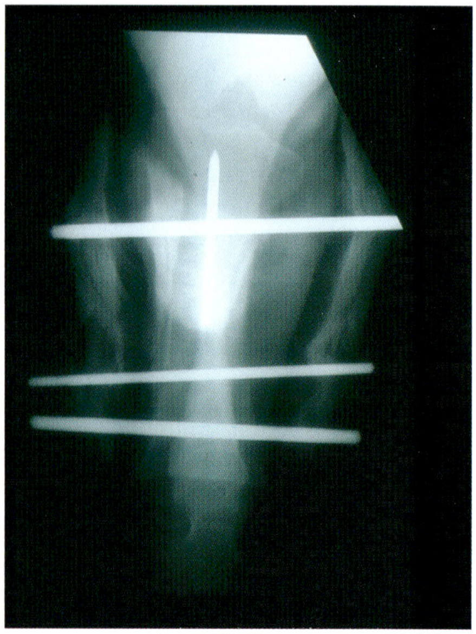

• **Fig. 11.3** A dorsoplantar radiograph of a goat with a modified fixator in place to treat a tibia fracture.

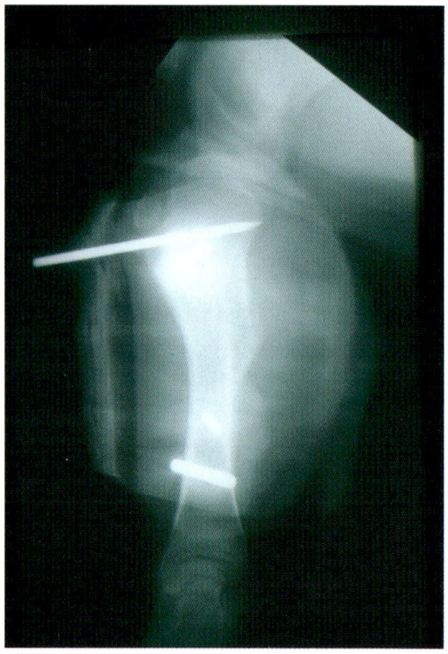

• **Fig. 11.4** A lateral radiograph of the same goat in Figure 11.3. Notice the proximal most pin place from dorsal to plantar to engage but not penetrate the plantar cortex of the tibia.

patients become fully ambulatory in 48 to 72 hours. Treatment of young animals should be tailored to prevent a compensatory tarsal varus of the contralateral limb. This procedure is technically less difficult because the practitioner is allowed more variation in pin placement than if traditional connecting bars are used. The pin ends should be covered as they are in transfixation casting.[37]

Splints. Splints can be useful in treating some musculoskeletal conditions in small ruminants. However, the veterinarian should be selective in using them. Many practitioners are more comfortable using casts and external fixators than applying and monitoring splints. Many of the small ruminants presented to referral centers for malunion or delayed-union healing of fractures have been treated with polyvinyl chloride (PVC) or spoon splints before referral (Figures 11.5 and 11.6). For this reason alone, practitioners should consider using other techniques that achieve more stable fracture fixation. However, splints can be useful in selected cases if the practitioner is skilled at splint management. In emergency situations, a splint can be made of cut PVC pipe or other such material.[33]

A spoon splint, either commercially manufactured or fashioned from cast material, is probably best used to support greenstick fractures of the distal limb. When used in this way, it helps prevent catastrophic breakdown of the fracture. However, a more important role may be in preventing the limb contracture that can occur if the carpus is allowed to remain flexed for a prolonged period in a non–weight-bearing animal. With this technique, a padded bandage is placed on the limb and the splint is conformed to the bandage and secured with adhesive tape.

Another type of splint occasionally used in small ruminants is the traction splint, commonly referred to as the *Schroeder-Thomas splint*. This splint is usually made of aluminum rods and consists of a ring that fits in the axillary or inguinal region of the animal with bars on the dorsal and palmar or plantar aspect of the limb joined distally. The shape of the splint varies, as does the way particular parts of the limb are secured to the splint depending on the specific reason the splint is applied. Traction is applied by securing the foot to the distal splint with adhesive tape or by placing wires through the hoof wall. A soft bandage should be placed on the limb, after which the limb is secured strategically to the splint. Usually, tape is placed over the entire limb and distal splint.[38]

Cases treated with splints or casts without ideal alignment occasionally heal with unacceptable angulation. The animal may have been initially treated with splint or cast and possibly no radiographs for financial reasons, but then the owner feels guilty and pursues osteotomy and fixation to improve the angle of the limb. Fixation after osteotomy can be done with external fixation or a transfixation cast (Figures 11.7 and 11.8).

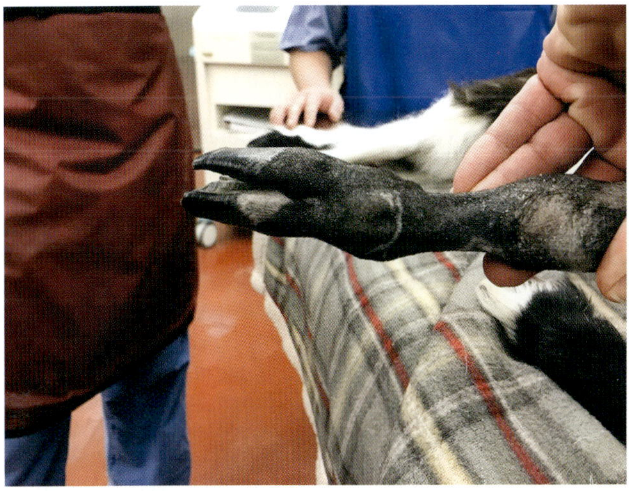

• **Fig. 11.5** A photograph of a yearling pygmy goat with lateral deviation of the right forelimb after a metacarpal III–IV fracture was treated with a bandage and polyvinyl chloride splint.

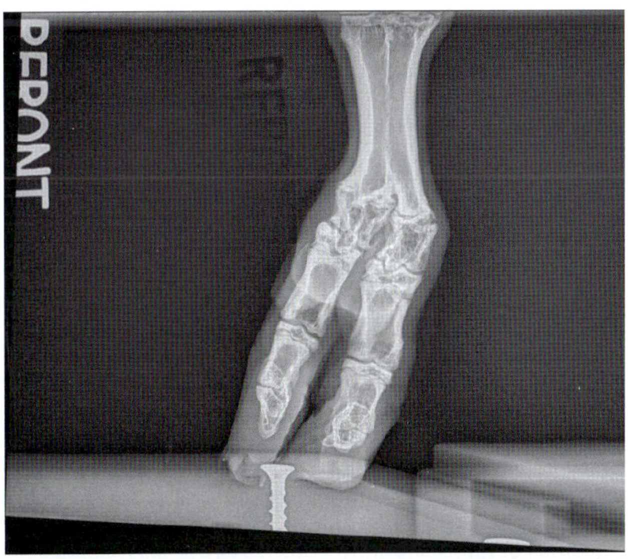

• **Fig. 11.6** A dorsopalmar radiograph of the goat in Figure 11.5. The fracture has healed with a nearly 20-degree lateral deviation due to improper alignment or stability in the polyvinyl chloride splint.

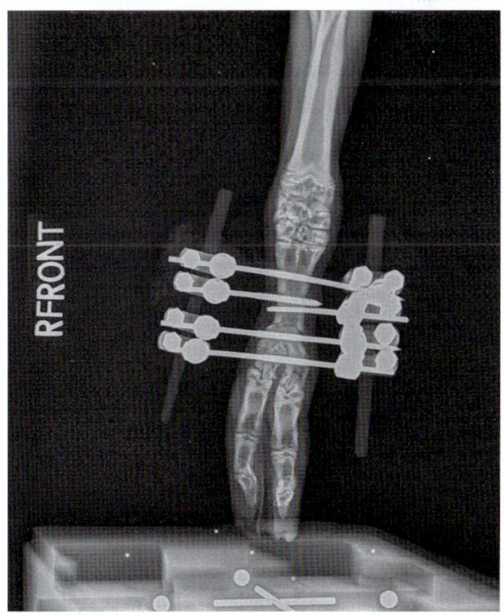

• **Fig. 11.7** A dorsopalmar radiograph of the goat in Figure 11.5 after a dome osteotomy to align the limb and an external fixator to stabilize it. Notice the arced osteotomy seen just above the distal two pins, which allows the surgeon to rotate the bone into proper alignment.

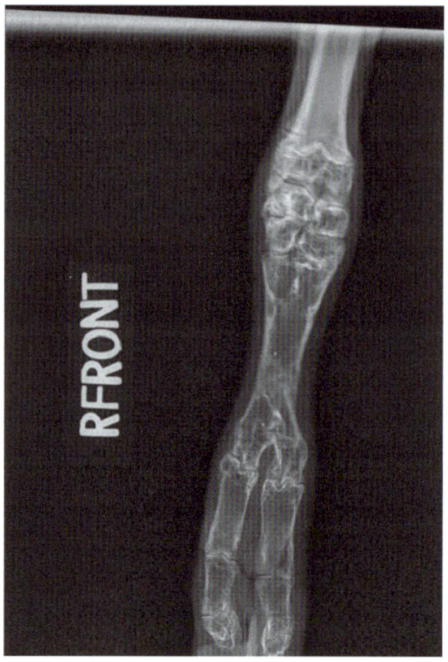

• **Fig. 11.8** A dorsopalmar radiograph of the goat from Figure 11.5 after the osteotomy has healed and the fixator removed. Compare the alignment to Figure 11.6.

Infectious Conditions

Septic Arthritis

Bacterial infections of the joints (septic arthritis) occur most commonly in neonates. However, older animals sporadically suffer from joint infection as a result of a penetrating injury or spread from adjacent infected tissues, as in the case of foot rot. In neonates, septic arthritis is most often a sequela to septicemia and often a consequence of failure of passive transfer.[39] The bacteria isolated from lambs include *Streptococcus, Escherichia coli, Actinomyces pyogenes, Erysipelothrix insidiosa (rhusiopathiae), Pasteurella haemolytica, Corynebacterium pseudotuberculosis,* and *Fusobacterium necrophorum. Staphylococcus aureus* arthritis is associated with tick pyemia, a disease seen in lambs 2 to 6 weeks old in areas infested with *Ixodes ricinus. Streptococcus dysgalactiae* has been reported as a cause of arthritis in dairy goats and was the most common pathogen isolated from arthritic lambs in England and Wales. Other isolates included *E. coli,* coagulase-positive *Staphylococcus, E. rhusiopathiae,* and *A. pyogenes.*[40] Coexisting omphalitis was found in 16% of arthritic lambs.

Erysipelothrix polyarthritis is a nonsuppurative condition usually seen in 2- to 6-month-old lambs, but it also can cause neonatal disease. Outbreaks may affect as many as 40% of the lambs in a flock. Hallmarks of this infection are fever and lameness, with minimal swelling of joints. This nonsuppurative polyarthritis will progress to chronic arthritis if not treated appropriately.[39]

Pathogenesis. Septicemia often contributes to hematogenous seeding of joints with bacteria that localize in the synovial membrane. The resulting synovitis causes the affected animal to exhibit joint pain, heat, swelling, and synovial effusion. Progression of the septic arthritis and associated synovitis causes damage to articular cartilage and subchondral bone. As bacteria proliferate, inflammatory cells produce hydrolytic enzymes that destroy bacteria and normal cartilage, resulting in cartilage erosion. In the chronic stages of infection, animals develop thickening of the synovial tissue, fibrosis of the joint capsule, and signs of degenerative joint disease.

Clinical Signs. The hallmarks of septic arthritis are lameness and warm swelling of the joints. The joints most commonly involved are the carpus, tarsus, and stifle. Any joint may be infected, including the hip, shoulder, or elbow; infection here may be more difficult to diagnose than in the more commonly affected joints. Several joints may be affected, and the practitioner should always perform a thorough examination when one septic joint is discovered to rule out polyarthritis. Lameness may be severe (non–weight-bearing) and animals may remain recumbent. Affected animals are often febrile and anorexic. Other signs of systemic disease such as omphalitis, meningitis, and uveitis may be evident.

Diagnosis. A sterile aspirate of synovial fluid should be obtained and the fluid submitted for culture and cytology. The character of the synovial fluid varies according to the etiology and stage of disease. Synovial fluid from infected joints may be thin and watery (lacking normal viscosity) or thick and cloudy with purulent material. Infected synovial fluid often has characteristic pleocytosis and neutrophilia (more than 30,000–100,000 white blood cells/μL and more than 75% neutrophils), as well as an increased total protein. Not all aspirates from septic joints yield bacteria, but some do. Culture results may improve with the use of enhancement media or synovial membrane biopsy, particularly if the animal has been treated with antimicrobial agents. Radiography may be used to determine the severity of degenerative changes, although bony changes may not be visible for several days after the onset of disease. Radiography may be more important to monitor the progression of septic arthritis during therapy. Ultrasonography also may be useful in evaluating existing soft tissue pathology.

Treatment. The administration of antimicrobial agents and joint lavage are the mainstays of treatment of septic arthritis. Antimicrobials, which may be administered systemically or intra-articularly, should be chosen based on an assessment of specific pathogens (gram-positive bacteria are more likely) and culture results when available.[41] Lavage of the joint with sterile polyionic solution aids in removal of inflammatory products. Light sedation of the animal is usually indicated. The skin over the joint should be clipped and surgically prepared, and the clinician should adhere strictly to aseptic technique. The clinician inserts a needle (16- or 14-gauge) attached to a sterile syringe into the affected joint at the most obviously distended area and aspirates fluid (for culture and cytology). The joint is then distended with an isotonic solution (e.g., saline and lactated Ringer's). A second needle is placed in the joint on the opposite side of the joint. Between 0.5 to 1 L of fluid should be flushed through the joint. The joint should be distended several times during the lavage by occluding the egress needle. The joint should be flushed daily for 2 to 3 days; the need for subsequent flushing should be based on the presence of pain or swelling and cytologic evaluation of joint fluid. Removing inflammatory mediators by lavage can improve clinical signs, although such improvement is often temporary. Some cases have accumulated fibrin within the joint and over the articular cartilage that requires drainage and debridement by arthrotomy or arthroscopy. Lavage of these joints may yield clear fluid after treatment, but any improvement is short-lived. Just after lavage, nonirritating antibiotics should be instilled into the joint. In general, products for IV use are adequate for intraarticular use.

Regional limb perfusion with antibiotics is an adjunctive procedure that may be beneficial in some cases.[41,42] This technique entails instilling small volumes of antimicrobial agents in targeted locations to achieve high concentrations in infected areas. Regional perfusion can be accomplished with intramedullary administration of antimicrobial agents but is more easily and commonly performed by IV injection distal to a tourniquet. Sheep and goats generally should be sedated before this procedure and cervids will likely need to be anesthetized. The skin over the peripheral vein is aseptically prepared. The clinician inserts a needle (20- or 21-gauge) into the vein in a proximal direction and infuses the antibiotic of choice (potassium or sodium penicillin [1 million IU] or ampicillin [1 g]). For repeated administration in chronic conditions, a catheter (22-gauge) can be placed in the vein and the leg wrapped to help maintain catheter patency.[42] The prognosis for septic arthritis is guarded and chronic lameness is a sequela in many cases.

Prevention. Ensuring adequate passive transfer in neonates helps prevent septicemia and septic arthritis resulting from hematogenous spread of bacteria to joints. Maintaining a clean environment for parturition and providing appropriate umbilical care also help prevent neonatal septicemia.

Chlamydial Polyarthritis

Chlamydial polyarthritis is a common contagious disease of feedlot lambs in the United States. The disease is suspected to occur in goats as well.[43] The causative agent was formerly considered to be a strain (immunotype 2) of *Chlamydia psittaci* but has been reclassified as *Chlamydophila pecorum.*[44,45] Economic losses associated with chlamydial arthritis result from weight loss and treatment costs. Disease occurs in 1- to 8-month-old lambs, with 3- to 5-month-old lambs most commonly affected.[46] In feedlots, outbreaks often occur a few weeks after lambs are introduced.[46] Morbidity can be as high as 80%, with less than 1% mortality.[45]

Pathogenesis. *C. pecorum* is present in nasal and ocular secretions, feces, and urine of infected animals.[46] As many as half the lambs on some farms shed *C. pecorum* in feces without signs of clinical disease.[44] One abattoir study found *C. pecorum* in over 6% of synovial tissue samples from abnormal joints.[47]

Clinical Signs. Affected lambs have fever (up to 108° F) and are reluctant to move, often appearing "tucked up" or becoming recumbent. Lameness is apparent in one or more limbs, and affected joints are typically enlarged.[43,46] Chlamydial conjunctivitis may occur concurrently.[46,48,49] The course of the disease is about 10 to 14 days without treatment. Most lambs recover, but some remain lame.[43] Significant necropsy findings include fibrinous exudate in joints and edema of surrounding tissue. The articular cartilage is minimally affected.[43,49]

Diagnosis. Joint fluid may contain fibrin but is not purulent. Elementary inclusion bodies may be seen on Giemsa-stained smears of synovial fluid. Isolation of *Chlamydia* requires special media and is not routinely performed. The use of DNA-based tests should aid and improve the understanding of the epidemiology of different chlamydial infections.[50] Currently, complement fixation and specific polymerase chain reaction (PCR) may aid the practitioner in diagnosis when suspected from clinical signs.[51]

Differential diagnoses for chlamydial polyarthritis include white muscle disease and nutritional osteodystrophy. These diseases lack fever and synovial effusion, however, and laboratory testing should help differentiate these conditions.

Treatment and Prevention. Oxytetracycline (20 mg/kg SC or IM every 48–72 hours), erythromycin (3–5 mg/kg IM three times a day [TID] or BID), and tylosin (20 mg/kg IM BID) may be useful.[45] Treatment early in the course of disease speeds recovery.[43,49] During an outbreak, lame and febrile lambs should be isolated from healthy lambs to minimize the spread of infection.

A vaccine is available for chlamydial abortion, but researchers have not determined whether it provides protection against *C. pecorum* arthritis.

Mycoplasmal Polyarthritis

Mycoplasmal arthritis is a highly fatal disease of goats marked by polyarthritis, septicemia, and mastitis. This disease is usually caused by *Mycoplasma mycoides* subspecies *mycoides* large-colony (*Mmm*LC), currently classified as a serovar of *M. mycoides* subspecies *capri.*[52] Other mycoplasmas (*Mycoplasma agalactiae, Mycoplasma capricolum,* and *Mycoplasma putrefaciens*) cause similar syndromes.[53] This is distinct from the small-colony or bovine biotype of *Mmm* that causes contagious bovine pleuropneumonia, a disease eradicated from the United States in 1892. Sheep may be experimentally infected, and natural infection in sheep is suspected to occur.[54]

Mycoplasmal arthritis occurs as an epizootic condition in many countries throughout the world. In the United States, most outbreaks are in large goat dairies. Morbidity and mortality rates as high as 90% have been reported in kids.[55] *M. putrefaciens* was responsible for the loss of 700 goats in one California dairy.[56]

Mmm is usually introduced to a farm by an asymptomatic shedder. The bacteria are shed in the colostrum and milk of infected does, and ingestion is thought to be the primary source of infection of kids.[54–56] In one outbreak, about half of the does shed *Mmm* in milk. Some animals were intermittent asymptomatic shedders, but most ultimately developed clinical mastitis.[57] Horizontal transmission was documented among kids housed together and is likely to occur among adults, especially in the milking parlor.[57,58] Illness often follows stresses such as castration, dehorning, concurrent disease, bad weather, and overcrowding.[56,57,59]

Pathogenesis. Infection leads to mycoplasmosis and involvement of numerous body systems, with fibrinous polyarthritis, pneumonia, peritonitis, mastitis, conjunctivitis, and pericarditis being among the more common presentations. If animals recover, the organism may be shed in ocular and nasal secretions and in milk.[60]

Clinical Signs. Kids of 3 to 8 weeks old are most susceptible, but animals of any age may be affected. Clinical signs include fever, warm swellings of numerous joints, mastitis, lameness, conjunctivitis, weight loss, and pneumonia. Three syndromes have been described in kids. A peracute form results in death in 12 to 24 hours, with fever being the only sign. A second group of kids showed signs of brain disease (opisthotonos) and died in 24 to 72 hours. The third syndrome was characterized by fever, warm swollen joints, lameness, recumbency, and pneumonia. Many in this group died within a few days, but some lame kids recovered over a few weeks.[55] Adult females may develop acute or peracute mastitis, the latter causing death in 1 to 3 days. Does that recover may have udder fibrosis and may shed *Mmm* intermittently. Arthritis is a less common finding in adults compared with kids. Mastitis and severe lameness without fever were observed in an *M. putrefaciens* outbreak.[56]

Diagnosis. Laboratory work usually shows leukocytosis, neutrophilia, and hyperfibrinogenemia. Peracute cases may exhibit neutropenia with a left shift. Synovial fluid has an elevated cell count with neutrophilia and fibrin clots. *Mycoplasma* can be cultured using special media.

Postmortem findings include suppurative polyarthritis, osteomyelitis, fibrinous pleuritis, pneumonia, peritonitis, meningoencephalitis, and pericarditis.[55,57,59] The joints most commonly affected are the carpus, stifle, tarsus, hip, and elbow. Joint fluid is purulent and contains fibrin, and the joint capsules are thickened, with erosions of articular cartilage. *Mmm* can be cultured from synovial fluid and from many internal sites.[57]

Treatment. Antibiotic treatment does not eliminate infection in most cases. Some animals appear to improve only to relapse later. Tylosin is the antibiotic that has been most commonly recommended (10–50 mg/kg TID), but its efficacy is uncertain.[60] Antimicrobial susceptibility may vary with strain, but an in vitro study suggests that tylosin, erythromycin, oxytetracycline, or enrofloxacin may be effective.[61] This would currently be an extra-label use of enrofloxacin, which is prohibited in food-producing animals by some jurisdictions, so the practitioner should become familiar with regulations before using.

Prevention. Effective preventive measures for kids include the feeding of heat-treated colostrum and pasteurized goat milk. Disease in adults can be controlled by identifying carriers by milk culture and either culling carriers or isolating infected animals and milking them after uninfected animals. Cultures of individual does and the bulk tank should be performed periodically to identify newly infected animals or intermittent shedders, and colostrum should be cultured at the time of freshening. No vaccine is currently commercially available.

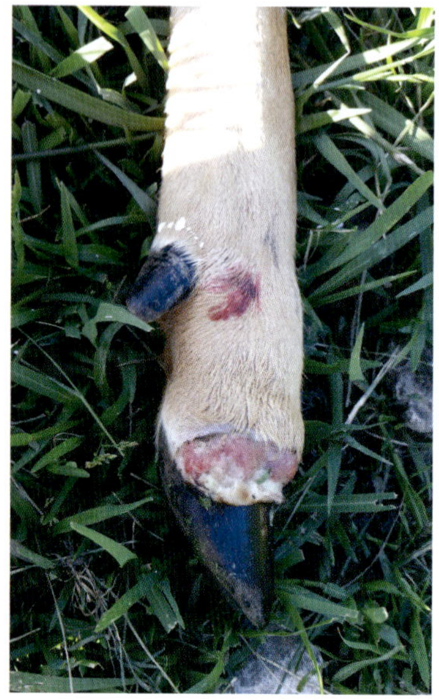

• **Fig. 11.10** The white-tailed deer from Figure 11.10 immediately after claw amputation before partial closure and bandaging.

Osteomyelitis

Bone infections usually result from hematogenous spread of organisms or from direct inoculation associated with trauma to soft tissues covering the bone. The soft tissue damage may be from either an acute injury (trauma or surgical incision) or decubital ulcers in a recumbent animal. Occasionally, the ulcers develop during normal recumbency when animals are housed on hard, rough surfaces and are not sequelae of debilitation. The infectious agents include *Corynebacterium*, *A. pyogenes*, *Rhodococcus equi*,[62] and *E. coli*. Cervids are especially prone to *Fusobacterium* infections (Figures 11.9 and 11.10). Cervids could be treated with long-acting systemic or regional antibiotics if the condition was discovered before irreversible damage was done by the infection.

Clinical Signs. Lameness, pain on palpation, and focal swelling are common clinical signs of osteomyelitis. Severe lameness may result in recumbency. Infection of vertebrae may produce signs of spinal cord dysfunction.[45]

Diagnosis. Radiographic changes usually cannot be seen before the infection has persisted for 10 to 14 days. When radiographic changes are present, they consist of a combination of lysis and proliferation. Avascular fragments of dead bone and sequestra also may be seen. If the osteomyelitis is related to a surgical infection, the incision usually dehisces and the surrounding skin shows signs of inflammation or even vascular compromise. The site may be aspirated for culture. Laboratory tests may reveal leukocytosis, leukopenia, or hyperfibrinogenemia.

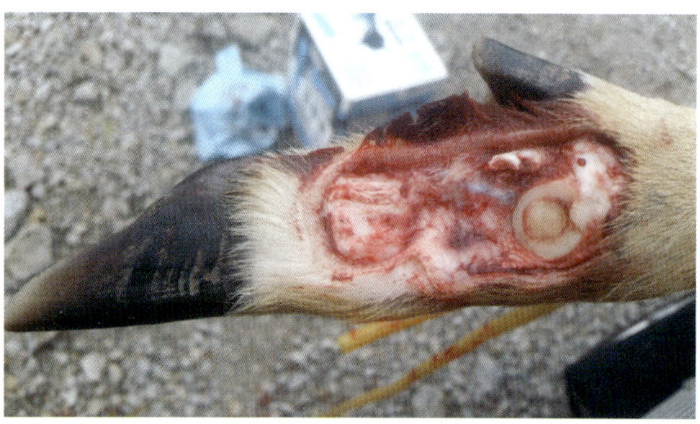

• **Fig. 11.9** A white-tailed deer with osteomyelitis of the digit.

Trauma without bone infection must be considered as a differential diagnosis for this condition. These cases exhibit soft tissue inflammation but no osseous radiographic changes. The radiographic changes of lysis and proliferation also may resemble the changes seen in response to neoplasia. Osteomyelitis may predispose the animal to pathologic fracture if bone lysis becomes severe enough. The distinction must be made between a pathologic fracture related to neoplasia and a fracture that is infected or becoming a proliferative nonunion.

Treatment and Prevention. The prognosis is guarded. Antimicrobial therapy alone is rarely successful because of its poor penetration of infected bone. Surgical debridement of infected tissue is an important component of therapy. Antibiotics, particularly those used based on culture and sensitivity patterns, should be continued for several weeks after surgical debridement. Regional perfusion of antibiotics may be useful in treating osteomyelitis. Amputation is the only possible way to rid the animal of infection in some cases. The possibility of control of infection varies with the cause of the infection. Environmental control is probably the most important mechanism to prevent trauma to the animal. Adherence to aseptic technique when performing any surgery on or near osseous structures decreases surgical infection.

Small Ruminant Lentivirus

Small ruminant lentivirus (SRLV) is in the Lentivirus genus and the retrovirus family. These viruses cause chronic disease in small ruminants. Caprine arthritis encephalitis virus (CAEV) of goats and visna maedi virus (VMV) of sheep, which is also referred to as ovine progressive pneumonia (OPP) in the United States, were originally believed to be similar organisms in the retrovirus family. They have been determined to be the same virus by epidemiologic and phylogenetic analysis.[63] The virus causes chronic lifelong infection and slowly progressive, yet different, clinical disease in sheep and goats. Persistent lifelong infection with SRLV may be related to a selection for antigenic variants, thus creating a reservoir of latent virus.[64,65] However, there has been a report of a lameness outbreak from arthritis in sheep caused by an adaptation of the CAEV to affect sheep so there is evidence of similar disease across species.[66] The main source of infection is through the dam's milk, but aerosol spread from infected animals to noninfected ones also occurs, making housing important.[67] In milking herds, any infected animals should be milked after the noninfected ones to prevent potential spread of the virus by milking procedures.

An evaluation of acute phase proteins (APP) in SRLV-positive animals showed an increase in serum amyloid A (SAA) in the leukocytes of infected goats, but no other APP showed changed expression, which may mean that the SRLV can modify the animal's immune response to the virus, which in turn facilitates the chronic infection. The SAA was lower in milk of infected animals, which could support a different immune response to the virus in the udder.[63] Macrophages play a key role in immune response against viral infections in general, but the SRLV specifically attacks macrophages for replication, likely causing the inability of the immune system to fight off this infection, again contributing to the lifelong infections of SRLV.[65] PCR has confirmed clinical cases of OPP with gross and histopathologic signs.[68] While PCR is a good test for SRLV, the low viral load early in the disease may lead to false-negatives. It is best to combine enzyme-linked immune-specific assay (ELISA) and PCR in repeated testing when trying to eradicate SRLV from a flock.[65] Repeated testing is also important because of the slow progression of the infection.[65]

There is genomic evidence of some animals having natural resistance to SRLV while others may be more sensitive. Genetic marker-assisted selection of breeding animals may help in control or even eradication of SRLV in a flock.[65,69]

Control or eradication of SRLV from a flock is dependent on how aggressive owners wish to be. At a minimum, neonates must be removed from dams and raised on bovine milk, and positive animals must be removed from the flock.[63] A more aggressive (and successful) approach is described in an OPP-positive sheep dairy flock. All the animals were tested and the seropositive animals (66% of the flock) were segregated from the negative animals. Testing was repeated every 6 to 12 months. New positive animals were moved out of the negative group. Replacement females came only from the negative group. The positive sheep were slowly culled so herd size, and thus, milk production was not drastically cut. The seropositive rate in the segregated part of the flock dropped from 66% to 0.2% in 2 years. The last of the positive group was culled 6 years from the start of the testing and eradication process. The flock was back at the original number in 8 years.[66] Discussions specific to caprine arthritis encephalitis (CAE) and OPP will follow.

Caprine Arthritis Encephalitis

CAE is a chronic multisystemic disease of goats caused by a retrovirus (SRLV). Infection with CAEV is widespread and chronic polyarthritis is the most common clinical manifestation.[70] Some subtypes of these viruses occur in both sheep and goats, and there is evidence of transmission of SRLV between the species.[71] There is some evidence of experiment transmission in red and roe deer, but none reported in white-tailed deer at this time.

The seroprevalence of CAEV in goats in the United States, Canada, and Europe ranges from 38 to 81%.[70,72,73] Seroprevalence in England, Australia, and developing countries is usually less than 10%.[74] Clinical arthritis is estimated to occur in less than 25% of seropositive animals, but it may be more prevalent in some herds.[70,73] The prevalence of other clinical syndromes is not known. Infection occurs by transmission of fluids that contain infected macrophages from an infected animal to an uninfected animal. The most efficient manner of transmission is from dam to kid by ingesting colostrum or milk from infected does.[75] The presence of antiviral antibodies in colostrum is not protective. Feeding nonpasteurized milk increases the risk of infection.[72,73] Horizontal transmission of CAEV is also important.[75–77] When uninfected goats are housed with infected goats for long periods, a significant number seroconvert.[75] Uninfected does readily seroconvert when milked with infected does, presumably as a result of transfer of the virus during the milking process.[75] Venereal transmission is possible, especially if one of the animals is clinically affected.[78,79]

Transmission from doe to kid before or during parturition has been documented.[76] No evidence supports transmission by an insect vector. Iatrogenic transmission (by dehorning equipment or needles) also is possible. The likelihood of transmission from a contaminated environment is very low.[77,78]

Pathogenesis. CAEV infects monocytes and macrophages and induces a persistent (lifelong) infection despite host antibody production. "Restricted replication" allows the virus to remain latent in the host's monocytes and undetected by the immune system. The virus localizes in the macrophages of the synovium, lung, central nervous system, and mammary gland. Initially, the virus proliferates rapidly and induces a vigorous immune response that limits but does not eliminate the virus. Virus-infected macrophages may be more prone to activation and thereby induce proliferation of lymphocytes and macrophages. Lymphocyte proliferation is a hallmark pathologic lesion seen in CAEV infection. The important target tissues of CAEV include the joints, mammary glands, lungs, and brain. At these target sites, CAEV induces chronic inflammation by invoking the host's immune responses. The virus is capable of making antigenic variants to help it evade the host immune response. CAEV can often be isolated from the synovial fluid and milk of infected animals.[70,75] Disease results from inflammation elicited by the reaction of the immune system to the virus. Infected macrophages express viral proteins near major histocompatibility complex antigens, which are recognized by T lymphocytes and stimulate cytokine production. Goats usually seroconvert in 2 to 8 weeks but can have a long clinical latency (years).

Clinical Signs. CAEV can cause chronic disease in several body systems; however, most infected animals remain asymptomatic. Four clinical syndromes have been described for CAEV-infected goats: arthritis, leukoencephalomyelitis, interstitial pneumonia, and mastitis.

Chronic progressive arthritis is seen in goats older than 6 months and is usually characterized by swelling of one or both carpal joints. Arthritis of the hock, stifle, hip, and atlantooccipital joints occurs but is not usually detected clinically. In the initial stages, joint swelling may wax and wane, and lameness is minimal. Some animals experience a sudden onset of lameness. The time course is variable, with some animals deteriorating over a few years and others remaining stable for several years.[70] As the disease progresses, animals become lame or recumbent and debilitated. Effusion of the atlantooccipital and supraspinous bursae may be detected. Radiographs of joints show soft tissue swelling initially, and calcification of periarticular structures occurs in more advanced cases. The synovial fluid has a decreased protein concentration and an increased cell count comprised of 90% mononuclear cells, primarily lymphocytes.[70] Postmortem examination usually reveals pathology in numerous joints in addition to the carpus. The joint capsule is thickened, often with periarticular mineralization, but articular cartilage is usually intact. Histopathology shows chronic proliferative synovitis with infiltration by lymphocytes, macrophages, and plasma cells.

Diagnosis. No abnormalities are typically seen on hematology or blood chemistry except for mild anemia in some cases.[70] Routine diagnosis is based on serologic testing, although sensitivity and specificity are not well defined due to lack of a "gold standard" for infection. The agar gel immunodiffusion (AGID) test is widely used because of its low cost and rapid results. It has good specificity and fair sensitivity. The ELISA test is another test suitable for screening, which is more sensitive than the AGID.[80] PCR assays can detect viral proteins in blood, milk, and tissue; however, the low viral load and heterogeneity of virus limit its usefulness in clinical investigations.[80] The combined use of ELISA and PCR with repeated testing is the best way to detect positive animals.[65] Virus isolation takes 3 to 4 weeks and sensitivity is poor.

A positive antibody test signifies infection, although animals may remain asymptomatic for years. The time to seroconversion varies and may not occur for months after infection. Therefore, false-negatives may occur early in the disease process. Intermittent negative AGID tests have been reported in seropositive animals.[81]

Treatment. No specific treatment exists or is likely to be developed. Affected animals are a source of infection to others, and their symptoms worsen over time. Most symptomatic animals are ultimately culled or euthanized because of lameness, recumbency, weight loss, or poor production. Supportive care for affected goats consists of nutritional management and the provision of high-quality, easily digestible, readily accessible feed. Goats with the arthritic form of the disease require frequent proper foot trimming, administration of NSAIDs, good pasture management, and soft and thick bedding to prevent trauma to the limbs. Treatment as described for degenerative joint disease may be of benefit.

Prevention. Attempts to induce immunity to CAEV with formalin-inactivated virus in adjuvants have not been successful.[82] Vaccines employing genetically modified viruses or recombinant plasmids have shown some promise in conferring protection but are still under investigation.[83]

A program of periodic testing and culling of all positive animals can help control the virus in a herd.[84] The more aggressive testing, segregation of positive and negative animals, and selective breeding are better ways to eradicate SRLV.[66] This method is not often chosen because of the large number of animals likely to be culled from herds with high infection rates.

The following management protocol should reduce the prevalence of CAEV in a herd by eliminating the transmission of CAEV in colostrum and milk. Kids should be removed from the dam at birth to prevent nursing. They should be removed immediately because licking of the kid by the doe may allow transmission of CAEV, via saliva or respiratory droplets.[77,78] Kids should be isolated from older animals and given colostrum that has been heat treated at 56° C (133° F) for 1 hour. At this temperature, the virus is inactivated but the immunoglobulins remain intact.[78] Kids then are kept isolated and raised on pasteurized (74° C [165° F] for 15 seconds) goat or cow milk or milk replacer. At least every 6 months, keepers should test kids for CAEV and cull animals that test positive. Kids fed pasteurized milk are less likely to seroconvert than kids fed unpasteurized milk. However, cases presumed to result from horizontal transmission may continue to occur.[72,73] Contact transmission of CAEV infection has been demonstrated in goats of all ages, although the exact nature of the contact required for transmission is unknown. Transmission during breeding or gestation (transplacental) is unlikely. In a dairy herd, CAEV-infected does should be milked last. New additions should be quarantined and tested within 60 days of arrival. If sheep are housed with goats, they should be tested for OPP and a similar protocol followed due to the possibility of cross-species infection.

Chemical disinfection of equipment between use with seropositive and seronegative animals should include the use of phenolic and quaternary ammonium compounds. Complete eradication of CAEV infection in a herd may be impossible without the culling of seropositive goats. Nevertheless, iatrogenic transmission by needles or instruments can be avoided through the use of aseptic technique. Segregation of seropositive and seronegative does by a solid wall or 2-m alley is advisable.[78]

Ovine Progressive Pneumonia

OPP is a chronic disease of sheep caused by SRLV. Predilection sites for this virus include the lung, udder, and, less commonly, joints. OPP is the term used to describe this condition in the United States, which in much of the world is called visna maedi virus. The arthritis caused by OPPV in sheep closely resembles that caused by CAEV in goats. Cross-infection with CAEV in sheep and OPPV in goats is uncommon but has been documented.[71] Lentiviruses induce persistent infections (lifelong) and replicate by integrating DNA into the host genome. One study in the western United States found 47% of sheep flocks had OPP-positive sheep. And in those infected flocks, the individual sheep prevalence varied from 4 to 96% of a flock.[85] At this time, it is thought that these viruses do not affect cervids.

Clinical Signs. The majority of sheep infected with OPPV are asymptomatic.[86] Clinically apparent illness, which usually occurs years after infection, may involve one or more body systems. The lungs and udder are the sites most commonly affected, but chronic arthritis also occurs in association with OPPV infection.[87–89] In some sheep, lameness is the chief clinical sign, although other body systems (typically lung or udder) may be concurrently affected.[87,88]

Because of OPP's long incubation period, clinical signs are observed in adults. Slowly progressive joint swelling, lameness, and weight loss despite good appetite are the typical musculoskeletal manifestations of OPPV infection. The carpi are the joints most commonly affected; the tarsi are affected less frequently.[86,88,89] Examination of the affected joints reveals firm soft tissue swelling.[87,88] Radiography may reveal mineralization of soft tissue and osseous proliferation of adjacent bones.[87] Sheep usually die within 1 year of developing clinical signs.[89] Postmortem examination reveals severe degenerative changes of the joints, with fibrosis of the joint capsule, proliferation of synovial membranes, and erosion of the articular cartilage. Histology reveals nonsuppurative lymphoid infiltration.[89] OPPV can frequently be isolated from the synovial fluid of affected joints.[88] The joint pathology is very similar to that reported in goats with CAEV infection.[88] Differential diagnoses include mycoplasmosis, chlamydial arthritis, and laminitis.

Diagnosis. Serologic tests are useful in diagnosing OPPV infection. The PCR and ELISA tests are widely used for OPP diagnosis because they are quick, inexpensive, very specific, and fairly sensitive. A diagnosis of OPP infection also may be made by virus isolation or identification of viral nucleic acid, but these methods are costly and rarely useful in clinical case management.

Because OPPV infection is lifelong, the presence of antibodies confirms infection, except in the instance of passive transfer of antibodies to a neonate from a positive dam.[90]

The majority of infected animals are asymptomatic, so the clinician should rule out other differential diagnoses before concluding that clinical signs are caused by OPP. Obviously, a negative test helps rule out infection. Reasons for false-negative results include early infection (seroconversion may not take place for months after infection) and seroreversion, which is seen rarely in advanced stages of the disease.

Treatment. No specific treatment is available for OPPV. Palliative treatment with antiinflammatory drugs could be considered in certain cases; however, affected animals are a source of infection to others.

Prevention. A surveillance and segregation program as outlined above for SRLV should reduce the prevalence of OPP in flocks.

Lyme Disease

Lyme disease is a multisystemic infection caused by a spirochete, *Borrelia burgdorferi. Ixodes* species ticks transmit the organism from rodents such as the white-footed mouse *(Peromyscus leucopus)*, the primary reservoir species in the eastern United States, to larger mammals, including deer, humans, cattle, horses, sheep, and goats. A small study in the southeastern United States found that ticks collected from hunter-harvested white-tailed deer were PCR positive for Ehrlichia and Anaplasma but none were found to carry Borrelia.[91]

Clinical Signs. Common clinical signs in human beings and dogs include arthritis, skin rash, neuritis, meningitis, and cardiac disease. Arthritis, abortion, poor milk production, and laminitis have been linked with *B. burgdorferi* infection in cattle.[92] Few cases of Lyme disease have been reported in sheep or goats. It is thought to be a nonpathogen for deer. Sheep reportedly infected with *B. burgdorferi* showed clinical signs of lameness, anorexia, and weight loss.[93] Borreliosis has also been suggested as a cause of arthritis in lambs even when *B. burgdorferi* could not be isolated.[94] A seroprevalence study using sheep from nine farms in Scotland revealed that 40% of 1-year-old ewes were seropositive although no clinical disease was reported. The tick *I. ricinus* was present on these farms.[95] Similar seroprevalence studies have shown that 26% of over 2700 sheep and goats in China were seropositive,[94] while testing over 500 small ruminants in Tunisia found seropositive rates of 30% in goats and 6% in sheep. Those animals in humid areas of the country had higher infection rates.[93] Experimental infection of lambs produced no signs of disease.[96]

Diagnosis. Ideally, diagnosis depends on the identification of *B. burgdorferi* by culture, PCR, or other techniques, but the organism is difficult to culture and other techniques are not widely available.[93,97] Serology is often used to confirm a diagnosis, but the high seropositive rate in the absence of clinical disease is a confounding factor. Frequently, in endemic regions, a clinical diagnosis is made based on clinical signs, elimination of other causes of lameness, and response to treatment.

Treatment. An optimal treatment for Lyme disease in ruminants has not been determined. A typical treatment regimen is a prolonged (2- to 4-week) course of oxytetracycline, ceftiofur, or penicillin. Prevention of the disease currently relies on eliminating the tick with insecticides. A vaccine has been developed for use in dogs, but none is available for large animals.

Clostridial Myonecrosis (Blackleg)

Clostridial myonecrosis is a highly fatal infection of muscle caused by the anaerobic spore-forming bacterium *Clostridium chauvoei*. Other clostridial species (chiefly *Clostridium septicum* and *Clostridium novyi*) have been isolated from cattle with blackleg, either alone or with *C. chauvoei*. The disease is most common in cattle, but sheep also may be affected. It has also been reported in cervids and goats appear less susceptible than sheep.[98]

Clostridial myonecrosis is not contagious but often occurs in outbreaks in small ruminants because the predisposing conditions affect many animals simultaneously. Infection is usually associated with wounds from castration, dehorning, tail docking, shearing, dystocia, or injections.[45] Animals of any age, including neonates, may be affected.[99] The mortality rate is close to 100%. *C. chauvoei* is ubiquitous and persistent in the soil and is frequently identified in the gastrointestinal tract. Soil subject to flooding and high rainfall have been linked to outbreaks of disease in cattle.[100]

Pathogenesis. In cattle, most cases of blackleg arise when endogenous clostridial spores that have lodged in tissues after absorption through the gastrointestinal tract begin to proliferate and produce toxins. These cases do not usually have an associated break in the skin, although the animal may have a history of blunt trauma that might create a hypoxic environment conducive to clostridial growth in the muscle. In contrast, clostridial myositis in sheep most often develops after contamination of a wound by spores from the environment. The vegetative organisms liberate exotoxins that induce severe necrotizing myositis, followed by systemic toxemia and death. Clostridial cardiac myositis has been reported in lambs.[45]

Clinical Signs. Clostridial myonecrosis progresses very rapidly and animals are often found moribund or dead. Systemic signs observed early in the disease include fever, anorexia, and depression. Local signs depend on the site of infection. If a wound is infected, severe swelling and a malodorous discharge are often evident.[99] Blackleg is almost always fatal.

Diagnosis. Diagnosis is made based on culture of a clostridial pathogen from wounds or necrotic muscle as well as necropsy findings. Samples for anaerobic culture should be taken quickly because the normal proliferation of clostridial organisms in tissue after death can confound results. A Gram stain of material from diseased muscle may show large gram-positive rods. On gross examination, affected muscle is darker than normal and has a rancid smell. Lesions tend to be deeper and have less associated gas than lesions typically found in cattle.[99] When external wounds are involved, edema is evident. Histology shows myonecrosis, edema, and neutrophilic inflammation; clostridial organisms can usually be visualized. Identification of *C. chauvoei* is aided by fluorescent antibody tests and PCR because culture of this organism may be difficult. Differential diagnoses include lightning strike and peracute infections such as anthrax and other clostridial diseases.

Treatment. The rapid death of most patients precludes treatment. However, if animals are detected by their early signs, high doses of penicillin (44,000 IU/kg IV every 4–6 hours) are indicated until the animal's condition stabilizes. Surgical incision of the skin and fascia over the affected area is thought to be beneficial. Supportive measures include IV fluids and NSAIDs.

Prevention. Vaccination against *C. chauvoei*, *C. novyi*, and *C. septicum* is recommended to reduce losses at parturition and shearing time. Dams should receive two doses, the second being administered 1 month before parturition. Annual boosters are necessary to protect dams and neonates. Some of the literature also recommends vaccinating older lambs before shearing. The efficacy of vaccination programs is unknown. Carcasses should be buried deeply or burned to reduce contamination of soil.[99]

Sarcocystosis

Sarcocystis species parasites are coccidia that cycle between a carnivorous host and an herbivorous intermediate host. In ruminants, infection is often subclinical, but abortion, failure to thrive, and neuromuscular disease have been reported.[101] The development of clinical disease depends on the species of *Sarcocystis* as well as the dose ingested. *Sarcocystis tenella* is considered the most pathogenic species for sheep, and *Sarcocystis capracanis* is most pathogenic in goats.[101] The sarcocysts from some species (*Sarcocystis gigantea* and *Sarcocystis medusiformis*) are large enough to be seen macroscopically and result in carcass condemnation.

The prevalence of infection in small ruminants is high, but clinical disease is uncommon. A postmortem survey of range goats in Texas revealed microscopic *Sarcocystis* species in 60% of the animals, with the tongue being the most commonly affected site.[102] The presence of working dogs that are fed raw meat is associated with sarcocystosis in a herd. Administration of monensin may predispose to the development of clinical disease.[103]

Pathogenesis. The definitive host, a carnivore, becomes infected by eating tissue from an intermediate host that contains sarcocysts. The parasite develops into a sporocyst that is passed in the feces of the definitive host. The intermediate herbivore host is infected by consuming contaminated feed or water. After ingestion, sporozoites penetrate the mucosa of the small intestine and lodge in the endothelial cells of the blood vessels. This causes damage to the vasculature, resulting in hemorrhage and anemia. The parasites ultimately enter muscle and nerve cells, where they develop into sarcocysts.

Clinical Signs. Common clinical signs in sheep include muscular weakness, ataxia, and flaccid paralysis. Poor growth and anemia also have been reported. Neonates are most susceptible. *Sarcocystis* infection also has been associated with esophageal dysfunction in sheep.[101] Experimental infection of two sheep with coyote-origin *Sarcocystis* produced fever, anorexia, and anemia; one sheep exhibited abnormal behavior. Myositis was found in many sites.[102–105] There is a report of *Sarcocystis tenella* being diagnosed in a stillborn lamb with microscopic lesions in the central nervous system and placenta.[106]

Goats experimentally infected with *S. capracanis* showed a range of clinical signs. Goats receiving the smallest dose remained clinically normal, but goats receiving higher doses developed fever, depression, and weakness, and many died acutely in the first weeks after infection. Microscopically, stages of the parasite were detected in the endothelial cells of arteries in many organs. Myocardial necrosis was observed in many goats. Multifocal necrosis, gliosis, and vasculitis of the central nervous system were noted, and sarcocysts were found in the brain and spinal cord.[104,107]

Diagnosis. Laboratory findings reported in cattle include a regenerative anemia, and elevations of the muscle enzymes creatine phosphokinase, aspartate aminotransferase (AST), and lactate dehydrogenase. Similar results are expected in small ruminants. Demonstration of a rise in antibody titer after acute illness aids in diagnosis. Development of PCR tests should improve the ability to diagnose infections with pathogenic species of *Sarcocystis*.[108] Histology of skeletal or cardiac muscle reveals the presence of sarcocysts. There may be edema in multiple organs and atrophy of fat.[105] Differential diagnoses include the numerous other causes of fever, anemia, and poor growth.

Treatment and Prevention. No approved treatment exists for sarcocystosis. The use of amprolium (100 mg/kg/day) or salinomycin has been reported.[102] Carnivores should be kept away from small ruminants and exposure to uncooked meat or carcasses should be minimized to help control this disease. However, removing carnivorous guard dogs may increase losses to predators. No vaccine is currently available (see Chapter 6).

Foot and Mouth Disease

Foot and mouth disease (FMD) is a highly contagious viral disease of ruminants and swine characterized by fever and vesicles of the mouth, feet, and teats. Cattle and pigs are most severely affected, but sheep, goats, and cervids are susceptible.[109] FMD often produces a mild clinical syndrome in sheep and goats, and therefore, these species may be inapparent sources of the virus during outbreaks.[110,111] In the 2001 FMD outbreak in the United Kingdom, movement of apparently normal virus-excreting sheep contributed to widespread dissemination of the disease.[112] FMD has significant economic impact resulting from loss of production and limitations on movement of animals from affected areas. FMD is endemic in Asia, Africa, South America, and parts of Europe. North America, Central America, and Australia are currently free of FMD.[113] FMD usually occurs as an outbreak that spreads rapidly. All hoof stock except for horses are susceptible. Morbidity is high (close to 100%), although mortality is low. Most deaths are seen in young animals as a result of myocardial necrosis.[110,111]

FMD is readily spread by direct contact with affected animals; aerosolization of the virus is another important source of infection. Ruptured vesicles, respiratory secretions, saliva, milk, urine, and semen are sources of the virus. FMD also may be spread to new premises by human beings, animal products, fomites, and even wind currents.[113] Most animals stop shedding the virus within a few days of vesicle rupture, but cases of long-term (weeks to years) carriers have been reported.[110,111] The virus may persist in the environment for months, and it is not destroyed by common disinfectants. Wild hoof stock is susceptible to FMD and in some cases may act as reservoirs for the virus.

Pathogenesis. The FMD virus, an aphthovirus (family *Picornaviridae*), consists of seven serotypes (O, A, C, Asia 1, SAT 1, 2, and 3) and more than 60 subtypes that vary in virulence and species specificity.[45] FMD virus gains access to the animal through the mucosal epithelium, viremia ensues, and the virus localizes to epithelial sites throughout the body. Lesions are most evident in the oral mucosa and feet. Necrotizing myocarditis has been reported to affect primarily young animals. Immunity conferred by infection is fairly short-lived (a few years), and cross-protection against other strains is poor.[45]

Clinical Signs. In cattle, infection with FMD virus produces fever, vesicles, erosions, and ulcers of the oral mucosa, teats, coronary band, and interdigital area. The lesions seem to be very painful, and the resulting clinical signs include anorexia, depression, salivation, agalactia, and lameness. Weight loss, mastitis, and secondary bacterial infections are common sequelae.[45] Most animals recover within 2 to 3 weeks.

Sheep and goats usually show milder clinical signs than cattle; however, severe outbreaks have been reported in sheep. Deer have lesions similar to cattle, sheep and goats. Oral lesions are usually mild and transient, and foot lesions and lameness are the predominant symptoms noted.[110,111] If the oral lesions are not detected, FMD may resemble infectious foot rot. In the 2001 UK outbreak, lameness and fever were the most evident signs in sheep. Vesicles in the interdigital area, heel, and coronary band required careful inspection to detect, and shallow oral erosions were found in some cases, primarily involving the dental pad, tongue, hard palate, and lips.[114]

Lesions detected on postmortem examination include vesicles, erosions, and ulcers of the mouth and feet. The udder, pharynx, trachea, esophagus, forestomachs, and intestines also may be affected. The myocardia of neonates often have pale streaks caused by necrosis, an appearance known as *tiger heart.*[45]

Diagnosis. Rapid confirmation of FMD is essential because of the far-reaching consequences of this disease. The clinical signs of FMD resemble those of other vesicular diseases such as bluetongue, vesicular stomatitis (which rarely causes disease in small ruminants), and poxvirus infection, as well as infectious foot rot. If FMD is suspected, a state veterinarian should be contacted immediately. Development of rapid diagnostic tests will greatly aid diagnosis and management of FMD outbreaks.

Treatment. FMD has no specific treatment. Antiinflammatory agents and topical dressings may be used to alleviate discomfort.

Control. FMD-free regions maintain their status by restricting the entry of live animals and animal products from endemic areas. Outbreaks in nonendemic areas are generally controlled by quarantine and eradication of affected animals and those with which they have had contact. In endemic regions, vaccination is employed to control FMD. Ideally, the vaccine should contain local strains of virus. The immunity provided by killed vaccine is short-lived (6–8 months) and is protective against only a few strains of virus. Cattle are usually the focus of a vaccination program, but vaccination of sheep and goats in endemic regions is recommended.[110,111]

Degenerative Joint Disease

Degenerative joint disease is a complex physiologic process that can destroy articular cartilage and cripple animals. Lameness is the most common clinical sign seen in animals with degenerative joint disease. This lameness results from normal destructive processes in the joint overriding the balancing repair processes normally present. This lack of balance in the joint leads to inflammation that produces heat, swelling, and pain. Degenerative joint disease in small ruminants is most often a sequela to infectious arthritis. However, trauma such as direct injury to a joint also can result in degenerative joint disease. Pet goats and sheep (particularly geriatric animals) tend to develop degenerative joint disease, and the condition can be exacerbated by CAE infection in goats.[107] Other joints may be affected as well because of abnormal stresses resulting from aberrant gait or weight-bearing patterns used by the animal to compensate for the injured joint. Unfortunately, small ruminants function well with mild lameness, and therefore, degenerative disease is often quite advanced before an affected animal is brought to the attention of a veterinarian. If a clinician can examine an animal early in the process of degenerative joint disease, he or she may be able to address the etiology directly or at least change management procedures in order to slow the progression of the disease. Some affected animals refuse to walk or have a stiff gait; many often have overgrown feet.

Treatment

Several dietary supplements and chondroprotective agents are available to veterinary practitioners today. No scientific studies support the efficacy of these agents in small ruminants, but anecdotal reports suggest some may be beneficial.[107] Injections of a polysulfated glycosaminoglycan (Adequan) (125 mg/week for 4 weeks) have been suggested. Issues of expense and management regarding long-term treatment of individual animals must be addressed by the owner before instituting therapy with chondroprotective agents. Administration of NSAIDs (aspirin 100 mg/kg BID), provision of proper care, maintenance of good body condition scores (2–3) in animals, and avoidance of obesity are all valuable parts of the therapeutic plan.[107] Some animals severely lame due to degenerative joint disease will experience increased comfort when the painful joint fuses over time (ankylosis) or has a surgical arthrodesis performed.

Metabolic and Nutritional Conditions

Nutritional Muscular Dystrophy

Nutritional muscular dystrophy (NMD), also known as *white muscle disease,* is a disease of all large animals caused by a deficiency of selenium and/or vitamin E. The disease affects skeletal and cardiac muscle and is most common in young, rapidly growing animals. Selenium and vitamin E deficiencies also produce syndromes of ill thrift and reproductive losses.[45]

NMD occurs in selenium-deficient areas throughout the world. It is a significant disease in North America, the United Kingdom, Europe, Australia, and New Zealand. In the United States, the northeast, southeast, and northwest regions are deficient in selenium; the central region has sufficient selenium in its soil.[115] Even within a region, the selenium content of soil and forage may vary depending on pH, season, and type of plants grown. For example, alkaline soils encourage selenium uptake by plants, whereas plants grown in areas of high rainfall and acidic soils are usually low or marginal in selenium content.[116] In most instances, the selenium content of pasture is lowest in the spring. Nitrogen and, to a certain degree, phosphorus fertilization and irrigation may decrease selenium uptake by plants. Faster-growing plants have lower selenium content; this condition is exacerbated when plants are grown on soils already marginal in selenium. Hay grown in drier areas tends to have a higher selenium concentration. Hay analysis is crucial in determining dietary selenium intake.

Selenium is absorbed, as are other minerals, in the small intestine. Therefore, high concentrations of other minerals (e.g., calcium, sulfur, and copper) may decrease its absorption. Also, certain feed contaminants (e.g., nitrate, unsaturated fats, and sulfates) may further suppress selenium uptake and availability.[117] Forage with less than 0.1 ppm of selenium on a dry matter basis is deficient.

Vitamin E helps prevent peroxidation of cell membrane lipids, aiding in the maintenance of membrane integrity. It also is somewhat protective against selenium deficiency. Of the forms of vitamin E, the D-isomer of alpha-tocopherol has the greatest biologic activity. It also is absorbed in the upper small intestine.[118] Because bile acids are needed for proper absorption, derangements in small intestine function can decrease the absorption of vitamin E, even if dietary concentrations are adequate. Vitamin E–deficient small ruminants probably absorb 50 to 75% of dietary tocopherol, whereas animals receiving adequate vitamin E absorb only

20 to 30%. Vitamin E activity is good in green pasture and good hay. Legumes often have less available vitamin E than grass does.[116] Vitamin E can be destroyed by oxidative destruction, particularly if large amounts of unsaturated fats and certain minerals (e.g., copper, iron) are added to the same supplement or mineral mixture. Long-term storage of feedstuffs decreases vitamin E activity by as much as 50% per month.[116]

Deficiencies occur when animals are fed poor-quality hay or straw and lack access to pasture. Diets high in polyunsaturated fatty acids contribute to the development of NMD by increasing the requirement for vitamin E. Vitamin E requirements also are increased if vitamin C and/or carotenoids are deficient or if dietary nitrate intake is increased. However, adequate vitamin C and beta-carotene in the diet help lower vitamin E requirements. Adequate dietary selenium is almost completely protective against vitamin E deficiency.[119]

Limited vitamin E transport occurs across the placenta, but colostrum has a large quantity of vitamin E. Therefore, neonates deprived of colostrum need supplemental vitamin E.

NMD occurs most commonly in neonates whose mothers were fed a selenium-deficient diet. Most cases occur in animals less than 6 months old, and NMD has been reported in neonates. Kids are believed to be more susceptible than lambs, possibly because they have a higher requirement for selenium. Further, sudden muscular activity in deficient animals unaccustomed to exercise often triggers episodes of NMD.[45]

Hydrogen peroxide and other free radicals are toxic byproducts of cell metabolism that have the ability to cause oxidative damage to biologic membranes. Selenium is a cofactor in several enzyme systems in the body, but much of the pathology associated with selenium deficiency is caused by an impairment of the enzyme glutathione peroxidase (GPx). GPx protects cell membranes against destruction by these endogenous peroxides by converting them to relatively benign hydroxy fatty acids. The lipid-soluble vitamin E molecule acts as a free radical scavenger within the cell membrane. High concentrations of dietary fat can overwhelm the vitamin E protection system.[119] Selenium and vitamin E act as antioxidants by separate mechanisms; diets that are deficient in selenium or vitamin E permit oxidative damage, which leads to muscle degeneration. The deficiency of these two nutrients results in a buildup of free radicals and increases in subsequent damage. Muscles with high metabolic activity are most susceptible (e.g., heart, diaphragm). This syndrome and other selenium-responsive diseases are most commonly encountered in young growing lambs, particularly those 2 to 4 months of age.[116,120] Selenium deficiency also may impair the body's immune system. In cattle and possibly in small ruminants, deficient selenium intake can result in reduced neutrophilic response, a higher incidence of mastitis and metritis, and poor overall body condition. Because of their compromised immune systems, many of these lambs are more susceptible to other contagious diseases. Sheep consuming selenium-deficient diets produce low wool yields and may have an increased incidence of periodontal disease. Adults consuming a deficient diet may have these signs, whereas growing neonates exhibit NMD.

Clinical Signs. Two syndromes of NMD are classically described: an acute to peracute cardiac form and the more common subacute skeletal muscle form. Animals with involvement of cardiac muscle show acute signs that include recumbency, respiratory distress, and death. Respiratory signs include tachypnea and frothy nasal discharge resulting from pulmonary edema. Tachycardia is common, sometimes accompanied by a heart murmur. Animals are often alert and their struggles to arise may be interpreted as seizures. A history of collapse after exercise is typical. Differential diagnoses include toxicities, fulminant infectious diseases, pneumonia, and neurologic disease such as polioencephalomalacia or tetanus.

Animals with skeletal muscle degeneration have a different appearance. These animals have a stiff gait and tremble while standing. Many prefer to remain in sternal recumbency. The muscles may feel firm. Signs described in this form of the disease include hunched appearance, stiff gait, and overall poor production.[116] Neonates continue to weaken and eventually become unable to nurse.[120] Many young have aspiration pneumonia resulting from dysfunction of the glottis. Some adult animals continue to eat, but others are dysphagic because of involvement of the tongue. Skeletal and cardiac muscle disease may occur concurrently. Careful assessment of flock/herd history and a through physical examination are required to determine the underlying cause of the pneumonia. Other diseases that may appear similar include enzootic ataxia, polyarthritis, and nutritional osteodystrophy. Vitamin E–associated NMD is most commonly encountered in lambs and yearling ewe lambs.[116]

Diagnosis. Elevated creatine kinase (CK) is a good indicator of subclinical NMD.[116] Marked elevations in CK (10–50 ×) can occur in NMD. CK has a short half-life (2–4 hours), so elevations indicate recent or ongoing muscle damage. CK levels return to normal as the animal recovers. AST also is elevated with muscle injury; however, it is not specific to muscle disease—hepatic disease also may cause elevations in AST. AST has a longer half-life than CK does, and concentrations are elevated for several days after an episode of NMD. Elevations in CK and AST are not specific for NMD, and these enzymes may be elevated in any recumbent animal. However, CK and AST generally occur in much higher serum concentrations in the presence of primary muscle disease such as NMD.

Selenium deficiency can be confirmed by measuring selenium levels in whole blood or tissues. In cases of flock/herd problems, 10% of the animals or 7 to 10 animals should have blood collected for selenium analysis.[116] Erythrocyte GPx concentrations are highly correlated with selenium concentration, and the activity of this enzyme is a useful diagnostic test. However, GPx samples must be handled with care, and many diagnostic laboratories do not offer the test. Testing for serum selenium levels may be of value for assays if the diet has been maintained for weeks to months. It is of questionable value in assessing individuals, particularly those that have experienced any dietary changes. Obviously, most sick animals have undergone a diet change, and many have anorexia. Evaluating whole-blood selenium is the easiest and most reliable test. Selenium concentration in whole blood reflects the selenium level of the diet over the life of a red blood cell.[121] More than 95% of blood selenium is located inside the red blood cell and was placed there when the cell was manufactured. Vitamin E status can be assessed by measuring serum tocopherol. Some specialized laboratories offer a vitamin E assay. This chapter does not provide guidelines for adequate or deficient concentrations because of the variance in techniques and assays among laboratories. Instead, the clinician should inquire about normal values from the laboratory where samples are assayed.

At necropsy, affected muscles are friable and contain pale streaks that correspond with regions of degeneration and mineralization. The distribution is bilaterally symmetric. Similar changes are seen in the myocardium if animals have cardiac involvement. Histology of muscle shows hyaline degeneration, necrosis, and mineralization.

Chronic infections (caused by depressed immune function) and aspiration pneumonia (resulting from compromised glottis-closing ability) also may be encountered.[45,115,116]

Treatment. One injection of a vitamin E and/or selenium preparation should result in improvement within a few days. The treatment can be repeated in 24 hours. Following the label doses of some commercial products will provide adequate selenium but very little vitamin E, and supplementation may be required. If other animals show clinical signs, they also should be treated. The clinician should avoid exposing the animals to stress or exertion during treatment. Most animals respond to treatment; however, those with cardiac involvement have a poor recovery rate.

Prevention. NMD can be prevented by supplementing the diet of susceptible animals with selenium and vitamin E. Supplementation of pregnant animals helps reduce disease in newborns because selenium is transferred across the placenta and also is present in colostrum and milk. Clinicians and keepers should pay careful attention to the proper dosage of selenium to prevent toxicosis in the animals and should adhere to withdrawal periods to limit concentrations in tissues at slaughter. Pasture, hay, and any grain supplements should be assayed to determine the amount of selenium to be added to a supplemental pellet, grain, or mineral mixture.

Selenium and vitamin E supplementation can take many forms. The dietary concentration of selenium should be more than 0.1 to 0.3 mg/kg.[45,120] Feed supplementation is commonly recommended. In some circumstances, higher levels of selenium are necessary to prevent NMD in lambs. Dietary supplementation appears to be the least expensive, most efficient method of ensuring selenium adequacy. Current regulations in the United States limit selenium supplementation for sheep to 0.7 mg/head/day or 90 ppm in the mineral mixture for free-choice feeding.[116] Although the use of free-choice mineral supplementation is an excellent mode of selenium supplementation, ensuring a complete diet or providing a dietary supplement of 0.2 ppm selenium ensures more consistent mineral intake.[120] Fresh legumes and grasses are good sources of vitamin E.[122] Silage, oil seeds, cereal grains, and dry hays tend to be poor sources of vitamin E.[118] Therefore, diets high in grain content should be supplemented with vitamin E.

Alternatively, selenium and vitamin E can be incorporated in mineral mixes that are fed free choice to pregnant and lactating dams. If feedstuffs contain oxidizing agents (e.g., copper, iron), fats, or a high content of disulfide bonds (onions), vitamin E potency may be reduced, with resultant deficiency.[116] Whenever these dietary factors are encountered, supplemental vitamin E is indicated. Diets high in corn also may be associated with vitamin E deficiency because a lowered rumen pH reduces vitamin E activity. This condition can be clinically significant in the young growing neonate.

If it is not practical to supplement the diet, monthly injections of a commercial vitamin E–selenium selenite compound may be useful, although they may need to be repeated more often in lambs.[45] Injecting the dam 30 days before birth can help prevent NMD.[116,120] Injecting lambs with selenium–vitamin E preparations at tail docking (1 mg selenium) and again at weaning (2 mg selenium) may be protective on some farms. In addition to injected supplements, another source of vitamin E should be provided because the amount in commercially available injectable compounds is too low to prevent disease in deficient animals. Access to pasture or quality forage should provide adequate levels of vitamin E.

Other options for selenium supplementation are practiced in some regions. A slow-release formulation of selenite can be given by SC injection. A dose of 1 mg/kg selenium given to ewes 3 weeks before lambing protects lambs for as long as 12 weeks after birth. An intraruminal selenium pellet also is available for sheep. Top-dressing of pasture with sodium selenite at a dose of 10 g selenium/hectare is practiced in some countries. This method is safe and prevents NMD for at least 12 months.[45] When neonates are bottle-fed, the keeper should ensure an intake of adequate vitamin E in the milk replacer (see Chapter 2).

Rickets and Osteomalacia

Rickets is a disease of young animals caused by a failure of proper cartilage mineralization. Vitamin D deficiency is the most common cause, but rickets may occur as a result of deficiencies in phosphorus and calcium as well. In older animals, the same deficiencies result in abnormal mineralization of osteoid, a condition known as *osteomalacia.* An inherited form of rickets has been reported in Corriedale sheep in New Zealand.[123] There have also been reported cases of nutritional congenital rickets in lambs in New Zealand when ewes were on phosphorus-deficient grazing during gestation.[124]

Rickets occur mostly in rapidly growing animals that have low vitamin D levels because of limited sun exposure. Animals housed indoors, those fed green (uncured) forage, and those living at high latitudes in winter are most prone. Animals that consume a diet low in calcium or phosphorus occasionally develop rickets. Ingestion of some poisonous plants, particularly those containing oxalates (which bind calcium in the intestine); chronic lead or fluoride aluminum toxicity; and chronic parasitism can all produce or add to the pathogenesis of rickets.[119]

Pathogenesis. The primary problem is failure of mineralization of cartilage and osteoid, which leads to persistence of cartilage and irregular osteoid deposition.[117] Irregular osteochondral junctions and widened physes result. The metaphyses at the costochondral junctions are noticeably affected. In the long bones, the persistent soft tissue in the physis is deformed by weight bearing. In the diaphysis, osteoid is not properly mineralized.[125] Long-haired or woolly animals raised in latitudes closer to the earth's poles, those raised indoors, and those fed milk replacers with inadequate vitamin D concentrations may be particularly deficient in vitamin D and predisposed to NMD. Twin lambs may be more susceptible to disease in the neonatal period.[126]

Clinical Signs. Affected animals are usually less than 1 year old and have a stiff gait, shifting legs, lameness, and recumbency. Joints and bones of the distal aspects of the limbs may be enlarged, and enlargements of the ribs at the costochondral junctions (rachitic rosary) are frequently seen. Limbs are frequently deformed and may be bowed. Teeth may be mottled and their eruption delayed. Animals may be thin because of failure to graze adequate forage.[121] Differential diagnoses include NMD and infectious arthritis.

Diagnosis. Blood chemistry shows elevations in alkaline phosphatase greater than those seen in normally growing animals. Blood levels of calcium and phosphorus may be low. Serum vitamin D is low but usually within normal ranges. Radiographic changes include widened growth plates, bowing of long bones, and thinned cortices.[125] Radiographic examination of adult animals with osteomalacia will reveal porous bone.

Postmortem examination reveals thickening of growth plates and epiphyseal enlargement of long bones. Rib fractures are often apparent. Normal bone contains an ash–to–organic matter ratio of 3:2, whereas the ratio in rachitic bone is 1:2 to 1:3.

Careful investigation of feed content; access to sunlight; and vitamin D, calcium, and phosphorus levels aid in determining the underlying cause of rickets.

Treatment. Vitamin D_3 injections (10,000–30,000 IU/kg) may be beneficial if dietary supplementation of calcium and phosphorus occurs concurrently.[126] Recovered animals frequently maintain a short stature with limb deformities.

Prevention. Rickets and osteomalacia can be managed by providing access to sunlight and properly cured forage. Dietary calcium and phosphorus levels should be adjusted if they are low, and a calcium-to-phosphorus ratio of 1:1 to 2:1 should be maintained. Any potentially toxic substances or plants should be removed from the diet.

Osteodystrophia Fibrosa

Osteodystrophia fibrosa is a metabolic disease of goats and sheep in which bone mineral is resorbed as a result of prolonged hypersecretion of parathyroid hormone (PTH). In a brief search, no cases could be found in cervids, but it is likely to occur. High phosphorus or low calcium levels in the diet frequently contribute to osteodystrophia fibrosa.[127] Clinically, this disease is similar to rickets.

Osteodystrophia fibrosa is most commonly seen in animals consuming a high-phosphorus diet. Diets with a high proportion of bran or other cereal grains are often associated with this disease. Cereal grains have an inappropriate calcium-to-phosphorus ratio, and much of the phosphorus in cereal grains is in the form of phytic acid. High phytic acid content can further depress calcium absorption from the intestine. The dietary calcium-to-phosphorus ratio should be maintained at 1:1 to 2:1. Many cereal grains or byproduct feeds (bran) have a ratio of 1:6 or greater.

Pathogenesis. Primary hyperparathyroidism caused by hyperplasia or neoplasia of the parathyroid gland is extremely rare. Most cases of hyperparathyroidism are sequelae of nutritional or metabolic conditions that produce hypocalcemia. Diets with low levels of calcium, high levels of phosphorus, or deficient amounts of vitamin D may result in hyperparathyroidism; frequently, more than one factor is present. PTH stimulates vitamin D production, which in turn induces resorption of bone in the animal to maintain calcium homeostasis. Renal failure also may result in hyperparathyroidism, but this manifestation is uncommon in sheep and goats. All the bones of the body are affected, but the bones of the face and mandible are most obviously abnormal.

Clinical Signs. Bilateral enlargement of the mandible is typically the most obvious sign. The mandible feels soft and the animal may not be able to open its mouth properly. Lameness and stiffness are often observed as a result of pathologic fractures. Animals are often thin because of decreased food intake.

Diagnosis. Radiographs show enlargement of the mandible, decreased bone density, and rotation of the cheek teeth with the occlusal surfaces pointed lingually. Fractures of other bones may be apparent.[128] Laboratory results may show low calcium or high phosphorus levels, but these tests often fall within the normal range. Postmortem examination shows the mandible to be quite soft and malleable. Histology of the mandible shows a lack of mineralization of bone and replacement of bone by an extensive fibrous matrix.

Caseous lymphadenitis (CL) commonly causes enlargement of the mandibular region as a result of abscess formation in the submandibular and retropharyngeal lymph nodes. Palpation and radiographs should aid in distinguishing between CL and osteodystrophia fibrosa.

Treatment. Animals may recover if placed on a diet with a calcium-to-phosphorus ratio of 1:1 or 2:1. The enlarged mandible may not improve.[129] Formulation of a ration that ensures a calcium-to-phosphorus ratio of 1:1 or greater should prevent nutritional hyperparathyroidism and osteodystrophia fibrosa.

Epiphysitis

Epiphysitis is a condition of rapidly growing animals in which improper ossification of the physes occurs. The etiology is complex, with both genetic and dietary factors believed to play roles. It is seen in young rams being fed to maximize growth and is associated with pregnancy in about 1% of yearling dairy does.[98]

Clinical Signs. Clinical signs reported in a pregnant yearling Nubian doe included insidious onset of lameness progressing to recumbency. Enlargement of the carpi, tarsi, and fetlock joints was observed, as was angular limb deformity. Radiographs revealed delayed maturation of cartilage and overgrowth of new bone. The animal's gait improved shortly after parturition, but a degree of limb deformity resulting from premature closure of a portion of the physes remained. The cause was attributed to trauma to the physes as a result of advanced pregnancy.[46] After noting epiphysitis in animals, the keeper should examine the diet to assess the adequacy of copper and maintain a proper calcium-to-phosphorus ratio of 4:1 to 6:1. Adequate calcium, phosphorus, protein, and energy should all be maintained. Proper foot trimming, the provision of pain relief (NSAIDs), and the removal of animals from hard surfaces may all be of benefit.[130]

Osteochondrosis

Osteochondrosis is a disease of abnormal endochondral ossification. It is common in pigs and chickens and occurs in most domestic animals, but reports are rare in small ruminants. Osteochondrosis was observed in a Suffolk flock,[131] and it should be considered on the differential diagnosis list when animals that have been fed diets high in grain to produce rapid weight gain develop lameness or joint swelling. Radiographs of affected animals reveal osteochondrosis lesions as seen in other domestic animals.

Toxic Conditions

Selenium Toxicity

Selenium toxicity may result from grazing pastures with high selenium content or from exogenous administration of selenium by injection or feed supplementation. Acute poisoning may result in death, but chronic overdose leads to hoof malformation and lameness. The toxic dose for sheep has been reported to be 2.2 mg/kg orally as a single dose or chronic ingestion of 0.25 mg/kg body weight.[45] Sheep are considered more susceptible to selenium toxicosis than cattle. Little information is available about the natural occurrence of selenium toxicosis in goats, but the administration of high doses of selenium can result in death.[132]

Soils in specific regions of North America, Ireland, Australia, and South Africa have high selenium content because of the composition of the underlying rock.[45] Soils in areas of low annual rainfall often have an alkaline pH and are more likely to have high selenium levels. Plants extract selenium from the soil, and certain plants are concentrators of selenium. These plants are not highly palatable, but animals that graze in these areas may develop signs of toxicity if more palatable forage is lacking. Documented cases of naturally occurring selenium toxicity are uncommon.[115]

Selenium poisoning also occurs when incorrect doses of selenium are administered to flocks/herds in an attempt to prevent NMD.[133] Organic selenium compounds (i.e., those found in plants) are considered more toxic than inorganic compounds such as selenite and selenium dioxide. This reported difference does not always correlate with clinical disease.[45]

Pathogenesis. Selenium concentrates in the kidney, liver, and keratinized tissue and has a dystrophic effect on skeletal muscle. Toxic concentrations of selenium may displace sulfur in some of the amino acids (methionine, cystine), preventing them from forming disulfide bonds and thereby weakening keratin formation. Hoof material has high concentrations of methionine and cystine. The mechanism of toxicity has not been determined, but selenium also may interfere with the function of certain enzymes. A high-protein diet is protective against selenium toxicosis in sheep.[45]

Clinical Signs. Acute poisoning may result in dyspnea, tachycardia, fever, depression, and death. White or blood-tinged froth is often observed at the nostrils and mouth.[133] Signs of chronic toxicity include poor hair coat, alopecia, ill thrift, abnormal appetite, respiratory failure, and lameness. Hoof lesions are apparent in all feet and include edema of the coronary bands and deformity or separation of hooves. Neonates may have hoof abnormalities apparent at birth.

Diagnosis. Diagnosis is based on identifying toxic levels of selenium in the animal. Selenium levels in blood, urine, and hair are all elevated. Anemia and low hemoglobin levels are characteristic of chronic selenium poisoning. Necropsy findings in chronic selenium poisoning show myopathy of skeletal and cardiac muscle and hoof and hair coat abnormalities as described previously. Lesions in many other organs also have been described.

Treatment. No specific treatment is effective. If possible, the source of excess selenium should be removed.

Prevention. Selenium supplementation should be carefully monitored to ensure safe dosage. In regions with seleniferous soils, supplemental forage can be provided to reduce consumption of selenium-containing plants and increase dietary protein. Rich sources of sulfur-containing amino acids (soybean meal) in the diet are partially protective. Alternate grazing of areas with plants that do not accumulate toxic concentrations of selenium is another option. The addition of 0.01% arsanilic acid or 20 ppm copper to the ration also may be preventive, but these substances are potentially toxic.

Ergot Toxicosis

Ergot toxicity results from ingestion of alkaloid compounds produced by the fungus *Claviceps purpurea.* This fungus infects cereals and grasses, most commonly rye, wheat, and oats. The seeds of the plants turn dark as they are filled with the fungal sclerotia, and this grossly visible structure is referred to as an "ergot." *C. purpurea* is the fungal species most frequently linked with ergotism, but *Acremonium coenophialum* may cause a similar syndrome.[45]

The pathology occurs in animals grazing ergot-infested pasture or eating grain or hay made from such plants. It is fairly common in cattle, but reports in sheep and goats are rare. It has been seen in wapiti, but deer are very selective grazers and tend to avoid fescue unless there is nothing else to graze. In one report of goats and sheep co-grazing a fescue pasture, only goat kids were affected.[134] The condition usually occurs after a warm wet season, conditions that favor growth of the fungus.

Pathogenesis. Ergots contain alkaloid compounds and other pharmacologically active compounds known as *ergotoxins.* The effects of this group of toxins, which includes ergotamine, ergotoxine, and ergometrine, include constriction of arterioles and endothelial damage leading to gangrene of the extremities.

Clinical Signs. Clinical signs of ergotism include swelling, coolness, and hair loss, followed by drying and discoloration of the skin of the distal limbs, tail, and ears. A distinct demarcation between normal and gangrenous skin is observed and affected tissue may slough. Lameness is evident, and animals may remain recumbent. Clinical signs reported in goats include lameness, most often in the hindlimbs, with separation of the hoof in the most severe cases.[135] Ulceration of the oral, ruminal, and intestinal mucosa has been reported in sheep.[45]

Diagnosis. Feed samples should be analyzed for ergot or similar compounds. Differential diagnoses include thrombosis secondary to sepsis and trauma.

Treatment. No specific treatment exists for ergot toxicity. Animals should be removed from the source of toxin.

Prevention. Feed should contain less than 0.1% infected seedheads.[45] Pastures with severe ergot infestations should not be used for grazing or hay.

Fluorosis (Fluorine Poisoning)

Chronic fluorine poisoning (fluorosis) occurs after the ingestion of toxic amounts of fluorine compounds by feed or water. The severity of disease depends on the fluorine compound ingested. Sodium fluoride is more toxic than rock phosphate; calcium fluoride or sodium fluorosilicate are much less toxic. Deer are usually exposed to fluorine from contaminated sites and show clinical signs more severe than cattle.[136] Sheep and goats are reported to be less susceptible than cattle.[135]

Fluorine occurs naturally in rocks, usually in association with phosphate. Soils derived from these rocks and water that percolates through these rock formations may contain high levels of fluorine. Other sources of fluorine include industrial contamination (as far as 14 km downwind), deep water wells, volcanic ash, and phosphatic supplements given to combat hypophosphatemia.[45]

Pathogenesis. The mechanism of fluorine toxicity has not been determined. Excess fluorine is deposited in bones and teeth. Bony lesions may develop at any time in the animal, but dental lesions occur only if fluorine levels are high during the formation of the teeth. Urinary excretion of fluorine, accompanied by calcium and phosphorus, leads to mobilization of calcium and phosphorus and results in osteomalacia and osteoporosis. Many other sites, including the bone marrow, undergo degenerative changes.[45]

Clinical Signs. Acute fluorine toxicity is marked by gastrointestinal signs, tetany, and death. Chronic ingestion leads to decreased feed consumption and unthriftiness. Dental lesions, which consist of surface pitting and increased wear caused by improper enamel formation, are the first to appear, although they may not be noticed. With time, rapid wear and tooth breakage occurs, leading to impaired mastication.[137,138]

Signs of osteofluorosis include ill thrift, stiffness, and lameness that is most prominent in the hindlimbs. Pathologic fractures, often of the third phalanx (P3), may occur in several animals in the group. The affected bones are painful to palpation and may be enlarged.[45]

Differential diagnoses include other causes of lameness on a herd or flock basis, including hypophosphatemia, vitamin D deficiency, selenium toxicity, and selenium deficiency.

Diagnosis. Serum fluorine levels are often elevated in toxicosis (the normal level for cattle is 0.2 mg/dL), but normal levels do not rule out toxicity because of the storage of fluorine in bone. Urinary fluorine is often elevated (16–68 mg/kg is normal for cattle). Serum alkaline phosphatase levels are usually elevated.[45,137]

Radiographic abnormalities include increased bone density, enlarged bones, narrowing of the marrow cavity, and spontaneous fractures that heal poorly.

Postmortem examination reveals chalky, brittle bones with diaphyseal exostoses. Histology shows abnormal calcification of bone. Hypoplasia of enamel is observed in animals with dental disease. Degenerative changes of many tissues, including bone marrow, are observed. The fluorine content of bones can be measured to confirm the diagnosis. The mandible and metacarpal and metatarsal bones are considered the most reliable sources of bone for fluorine assay.[44]

Treatment. Keepers should remove animals from the source of fluorine. Cases of acute toxicity can be treated with aluminum salts (to neutralize hydrofluoric acid in the stomach) and IV calcium salts to control tetany. Dental and bone lesions do not usually improve. Animals should be fed good-quality hay. The addition of calcium carbonate or aluminum sulfate to the diet at 1% of the dry matter intake may be beneficial in decreasing bone fluoride content.

Prevention. Phosphate feed supplements for cattle should not contain more than 0.2 to 0.3% fluorine. A phosphorus-to-fluoride ratio greater than 100:1 should be maintained. Rock phosphate can be a source of fluorine, and deep-water wells should be assayed for fluorine levels before use. Careful management of grassland and water in high-fluorine areas may reduce losses caused by fluorine toxicosis.[139] Some guidelines recommend feeding aluminum salts to bind fluorine and reduce accumulation in tissue, but these compounds are unpalatable.[45]

Plant Toxicity

Australian sheep eating lupine stubble infested with the fungus *Phomopsis (Diaporthe toxica)* developed a myopathy of skeletal muscle marked by stiff gait and recumbency.[140] Ingestion of *Cassia roemeriana* (twin-leaf senna) is believed to cause a similar syndrome in cattle and sheep in Texas, New Mexico, and Mexico.[141,142]

Neoplasia

Neoplasia of the musculoskeletal system is extremely rare in sheep, goats, and cervids. A study of 673 ovine neoplasms submitted to a veterinary laboratory in South Africa revealed that 21 of them were of connective tissue origin. Types of tumors included chondroma, chondrosarcoma, fibroma, fibrosarcoma, osteoma, rhabdomyosarcoma, leiomyoma, and fibrolipoma.[143] Most other reports of small ruminant neoplasia are single case reports rather than large studies as described.

A 9-year-old pygmy goat was diagnosed with a spindle cell tumor of the rumen with metastasis to the liver and adhesions throughout the abdomen including spleen, liver, diaphragm, and body wall.[144] Squamous cell carcinoma of the prepuce has been described in a Boer buck with chronic posthitis.[145] Also, adenocarcinoma and leiomyosarcoma of the uterus have been reported in a mixed-breed doe.[146] Osteosarcoma and pathologic fracture developed in a 9-year-old Toggenburg goat 4 years after a comminuted humeral fracture had been repaired with an intramedullary pin. The animal also was reported to have pulmonary nodules, but these were not examined histologically.[147] Osteoma of the frontal bone and compromise of the nasal cavity were reported in a sheep.[148] Mandibular osteoma was diagnosed in a 10-year-old Toggenburg cross, and osteochondrosarcoma of the rib and sternum of a goat also has been described.[147,149]

A diagnosis of neoplasia is based ultimately on histopathology. Bony enlargement, lameness, and radiographic evidence of lysis or proliferation may suggest a diagnosis of neoplasia, especially in an older animal. Successful treatment of connective tissue tumors has not been reported.

Tail Docking (Sheep)

Tail removal or "docking" is usually performed during the first 2 weeks of life.[150,151] Some lambs sold in niche markets do not have their tails docked, and in some breeds (e.g., Karakul), the tail should be left long because the fat at the base of the tail is considered a prized commodity. Still, in most environments in which lambs are kept, long tails can become soiled with loose stool or diarrhea (as a result of high-grain diets, lush pasture, or internal parasites), leading to fly strike or infestation of the wool with maggots. Furthermore, long tails in females appear to depress normal reproductive performance. For these and other reasons, tails are usually removed. If the lamb is less than 24 hours old, the stress associated with tail removal may decrease absorption of colostral antibodies and result in the diseases associated with failure or partial failure of passive transfer. Therefore, lambs should be 2 to 3 days to 2 weeks old at docking. One of the authors (DGP) prefers to dock tails at 3 days on alert, healthy animals that are being cared for by their dams. The docking can take place after the lambs and their dams are moved to a single-family unit (jug) or holding area. Placing the new lamb and dam together helps prevent the ewe from wandering off or abandoning the lamb after the procedure. Anesthesia is seldom required, with the obvious exception of adult or pet animals (on owner's request). If anesthesia is required, either a sedative or a caudal epidural and ring block will suffice.[150] Some studies suggest that a tail ring block of a local anesthetic can reduce the stress associated with tail removal.[152] Still, Hooper[150] has suggested, and the authors of this chapter agree, that the neonatal lamb responds as much, or possibly more, to the injection of a local anesthetic as to the surgical removal of the tail without anesthesia. The pain associated with lidocaine injection can be partially alleviated by adding sodium bicarbonate (1–10) to the lidocaine. There is evidence that sheep undergoing tail docking benefit from analgesics such as meloxicam and local anesthetics.[153–155]

The tail should be left long enough to cover the anus and may be extended to the dorsal aspect of the vulva on females.[151] The wool-less distal attachment of the paired caudal skinfolds on the ventral tail surface provides a good landmark for the site of tail removal. Many owners of show or club lambs prefer to remove the tail as close to the body as possible. However, docking too close to the sacrum may result in an increased incidence of rectal and possibly vaginal prolapse.[150] The short docking has also been found to correlate with the presence of septic arthritis and carcass loss in an abattoir review of over 63,000 lambs.[156]

The tail can be crushed, cut, cauterized, or removed with a combination of these methods.[151] Equipment used for tail removal includes an emasculator, an emasculatome, a hot chisel, a knife, or elastrator bands. Tails should be cleaned of dirt and feces. The lamb should be manually restrained as the clinician determines the exact spot of tail removal; the tail should not be excessively stretched. Leaving some skin proximal to the point of removal provides redundant skin to cover the spinal stump.[150] Use of a cautery unit (e.g., hot chisel, suture heated wedge, electric wedge, and electric cautery) minimizes hemorrhage. If hemorrhage does occur, the ventral blood vessels can be clamped and sutured if needed. If cautery units are used and the wool is burned, some ewes may reject the lambs.[150] Removing wool over the docking site before the procedure and gently washing or cleansing the tail after removal can minimize ewe rejection. Ewe rejection caused by cautery docking is rare, and this method of docking is very acceptable. Cautery equipment should be used cautiously because of the possibility of burning the vulva, anus, or perineal skin. Regardless of the method, in the absence of complications, the tail stump will heal within 2 weeks. Tetanus toxoid or antitoxin should be routinely administered on farms where tetanus is a problem; it also can be provided for all docked animals.

If an elastrator or rubber band is used, the tail sloughs because of ischemic necrosis. This procedure is controversial, and elastrator band use should always be accompanied by tetanus prophylaxis.

The tail of an adult sheep can be removed as it would be in other animals. The animal can be placed under general anesthesia or sedated, restrained, and given an epidural or ring block with local anesthetic. The surgical area is clipped and aseptically prepared, and the site for tail excision is determined. The clinician then makes a wedge-shaped skin incision distal to the intervertebral space where the tail is to be removed. This leaves enough skin to suture over the stump.[150] The clinician cuts the tail between the vertebrae, removes the tail, and closes the skin. If excessive hemorrhage occurs, the vessels can be cauterized or sutured with absorbable material. Animals can be placed on a broad-spectrum antibiotic and given tetanus prophylaxis.

General Hoof Care

Most lameness in small ruminants is associated with pathology of the foot. Surveys have found that the incidence of foot disorders varies from approximately 10 to 19%.[157,158] Overgrown hooves are one of the most common foot disorders. Many foot disorders can be attributed to environmental, nutritional, and anatomic factors, but some can be prevented by proper trimming and management. With increased nutritional intake, and particularly with enhanced protein intake, hooves tend to grow more rapidly.

The hooves of small ruminants have fewer problems in a dry environment. The incidence of hoof disorders is higher in seasons of more precipitation and when housing is allowed to become humid, wet, or muddy. Fewer problems are seen when the animals can move about on hard, dry surfaces. Most sheep and goats require hoof trimming because of lack of adequate exercise on a hard, dry surface to wear down hoof material naturally; because of chronic laminitis; or because of fast hoof growth resulting from intensive feeding practices designed to increase production. Deer rarely require foot trimming, but hoof overgrowth may occur on soft wet soils or as sequelae to hemorrhagic disease (Figure 11.11). Some herds/flocks may require foot trimming every 6 weeks to 2 months to minimize the incidence of foot disorders. Hooves can usually be trimmed adequately with shears, although a hoof knife also may be useful.[157]

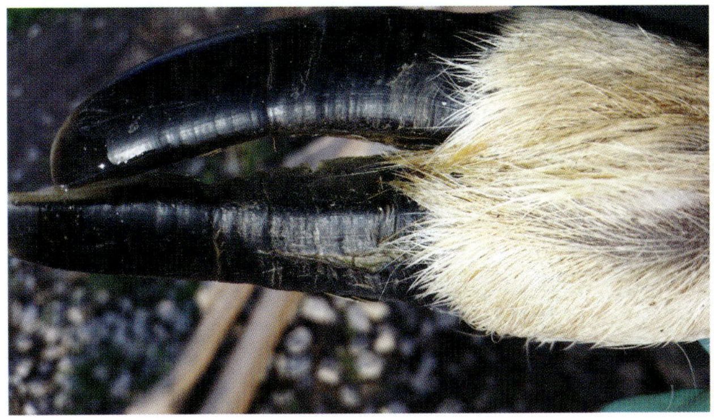

• **Fig. 11.11** A white-tailed deer with overgrown toes and a crack in the proximal dorsal aspect of one toe.

During trimming, some goats will stand, others need to be "set up" on their rumps, and others will stand in a stanchion. Some individuals prefer to trim the feet of sheep with them restrained in a tilt chute. The authors of this chapter prefer to trim the feet of sheep with them sitting on their rumps; foot trimming in goats is easier if the animals stand and the operator stands to the side. If an animal is allowed to stand, it should be tied. This allows the animal to be secured between the operator and a wall during foot trimming.[157] Regardless of the method, complete restraint is crucial to proper hoof care. Almost all deer (except possibly reindeer) will require deep sedation or anesthesia to trim feet safely for both the animal and the handler.

The clinician or keeper should shape the foot to match the angle of the coronary band while trimming the toe wall and sole. Dirt that has become packed into the toe should be removed so the operator can determine the amount of toe horn to be removed. After trimming, the hoof wall and the coronary band should be almost parallel. Trimming of the lateral wall corrects many hoof problems. After trimming the toe and lateral wall, the clinician or keeper should cut the inner wall shorter than the outer wall. The rubbery heel should be cut if it is excessively long or overgrown. The outer hoof wall should be slightly longer than any other hoof structure because it is a weight-bearing surface. If the hoof is improperly trimmed, the animal may walk on the toe or side of the foot or on the heel with the toe pointing up. A common cause of foot problems is an inward-turning outer wall that produces areas that accumulate debris and become infected. The inner wall may occasionally overgrow toward the interdigital cleft and predispose the animal to interdigital disease. The foot will be better balanced if the operator removes the toe curl by trimming the solar surface of the hoof and keeping it level rather than dubbing or shortening the toe. In groups kept on soft pastures or paddocks, placing feeders on rough surfaces helps decrease the amount of trimming needed. Building or stacking rough material (cement or concrete blocks) for goats to play on also may help minimize the need for frequent trimming.

Feeding affects hoof condition and growth. Animals being overfed energy and protein and living on soft ground may be more prone to some abnormalities. As a general rule, a well-balanced feeding program with a free choice mineral salt supplement consisting of calcium, phosphorus, and trace minerals is all that is required. However, some feeding programs may enhance hoof growth and health and are useful in special circumstances.

In other ruminants (cattle), diets that change normal rumen function by increasing the fermentation rate negatively affect the hoof health.[159] The ingestion of high-energy feeds, coupled with inadequate fiber intake, can result in suboptimal hoof health. In rations in which concentrates and roughage are fed separately, the concentrated portion of the diet should be divided into two or more equal feedings each day. This not only promotes overall health but also may help reduce the microflora changes that alter normal rumen fermentation and predispose animals to founder. Forage should always make up more than 30 to 50% of the dry matter content of the ration. Lush, young forage rarely provides enough effective fiber to optimize rumen fermentation. The feeding of buffers, particularly in high-concentrate diets, may help the rumen resist digestive upsets and thereby prevent subsequent hoof disease. Abnormal rapid hoof growth can occur when abnormal rumen fermentation is induced by the ingestion of lush, well-fertilized pastures.[159]

Hoof health also can be affected by certain vitamins and minerals. The addition of 20 mg of biotin improves short-term healing of hoof and claw lesions and decreases hoof disease in cattle.[159] Furthermore, diets that acidify the rumen decrease the microbial synthesis of biotin. One of the authors (DGP) prefers to include biotin (3–4 mg/day) in sheep and goat rations for animals with a history of hoof disease. Other vitamins that play major roles in hoof health include vitamins A and E and the vitamin A precursor beta-carotene. Adequate dietary vitamin A and beta-carotene are needed for normal cell replication, epithelial repair, and immune function. Vitamin E maintains cellular integrity and normal immune function. Diets should be fortified with both of these nutrients if hoof problems occur and in cases in which production practices predispose to hoof disease.

Calcium is the largest mineral component of hooves and is required for normal hoof growth. Dietary calcium concentrations should range between 0.6 and 0.8% of the diet, with the calcium-to-phosphorus ratio being maintained between 1:1 and 2:1. Of the trace minerals that appear to affect hoof growth, zinc, copper, and, to a lesser extent, molybdenum and manganese are most crucial.[159] Zinc is required for normal immunity, horn tissue production, vitamin A metabolism, epithelial repair, and hoof hardness. Studies in range, dairy, and feedlot cattle have all shown improved hoof health and decreased lameness when zinc is added to the diet, particularly in a chelated form (zinc methionine).[159] The use of such minerals also may be of value in improving overall hoof health. In sheep, the administration of oral zinc sulfate (0.5 g daily) to prevent foot rot has shown mixed results.[160–162] In cases of high legume intake (high calcium), zinc in the chelated form (zinc methionine) may be beneficial. Copper is needed for keratin synthesis and normal immune function and as a cofactor for many enzyme systems in the body. Copper deficiency in the body may be primary (inadequate copper in the diet) or conditioned by other dietary factors (excessive dietary molybdenum, sulfur, or iron). The dietary copper-to-molybdenum ratio should be maintained between 4:1 and 6:1 to maintain adequate copper availability (see Chapter 2).

Excessive nitrogen fertilization and liming of soils may depress copper and selenium uptake by plants. Heavily fertilized forage and roughage harvested after a drought may be sources of nitrates, which are reduced to nitrites by anaerobic microbial metabolism in the rumen. Nitrites can have a direct effect on hoof growth, resulting in abnormal horn tissue in cattle and possibly other ruminants.[159]

The key to maintaining healthy hoof tissue with respect to nutrition lies in minimizing rumen acidosis and fortifying the diet with certain nutrients (e.g., biotin, calcium, zinc).

Diseases of the Foot

Infectious Foot Rot

Infectious foot rot is a severe, contagious disease of sheep, and to a lesser extent goats, that leads to significant economic losses as a result of weight loss, low fleece weight, labor and treatment costs, decreased milk production,[163] and premature culling. It does not appear to be a significant disease of deer, but *Fusobacterium* by itself leads to severe foot disease in deer. Many factors contribute to the disease, but the primary agent is the anaerobic bacterium *Dichelobacter nodosus (Bacteroides nodosus)*. Previous infection by *F. necrophorum* contributes to the development of foot rot. The presence of both organisms in a large percentage of symptomatic foot rot sheep gives reason for added consideration in managing an outbreak as well as quarantine of herd additions.[164] *Corynebacterium (Actinomyces) pyogenes* infection may increase the susceptibility of the hoof to the other two bacteria. One study suggested that a number of spirochetes may also be associated with both sheep foot rot and digital dermatitis in cattle.[165] The spirochete is most likely a secondary invader in foot rot where it is the primary organism causing lameness in cattle, sheep goats, and some cervids (see Hairy Heel Wart, later in this chapter).

Many strains of *D. nodosus* have been identified, and some have classified the different strains as benign or virulent. Virulent strains have a greater keratolytic ability, which is associated with the production of a heat-stable protease.[157,158,166–168] A study of 735 *D. nodosus* isolates from 247 farms in Western Australia found 181 molecular types by pulsed-field gel electrophoresis. Three common clonal groups made up most of the isolates and were also found in cases from other parts of Australia. The molecular type was stable over several years on some farms, while it changed within flocks and even within feet on other farms.[169] Recent research supports that *D. nodosus* is present in high numbers days to weeks prior to clinical signs of foot rot. This is associated with the less severe or benign foot rot. *F. necrophorum* numbers increase after the initial infection as a secondary infection. This secondary infection is then associated with the more virulent or severe foot rot.[170]

Foot rot occurs worldwide wherever periods of warmth and prolonged wetness occur. In many regions, the spring and fall are the times when transmission is most likely. If conditions are favorable, a significant portion of the flock can be affected. All ages are susceptible, but the severity of disease generally increases with age. Merino sheep are most susceptible to disease, and some breeds (Gulf Coast native) are more resistant. Some individuals do not become infected or have less severe signs, and a genetic basis for resistance is suspected.[167,168] Some believe that excessive hoof growth and, anecdotally, hoof color (white) may predispose to the condition.[160] Recent theories suggest that the excessive hoof growth is a result of foot rot, not a predisposition. The hooves tend to be worn naturally after resolution of clinical signs regardless of trimming.[171]

The source of *D. nodosus* is the feet of infected animals, which transfer the organism to the soil where it contacts the feet of other sheep.[167] The organism was thought to survive only a few days to a few weeks in the environment but can persist for years in carrier sheep and goats. Studies suggest that the organism survives more than 30 days under all conditions and soil types. It survived even longer in cool soils and clay.[172] New infections usually are preceded by the introduction of new animals or exposure to ground that has recently been occupied by an infected flock. Management practices that allow the concentration of animals in small areas, irrigated pastures, long grass (which may abrade the interdigital skin), and wet or rainy conditions all predispose to infection.[160,167]

Pathogenesis. Wet conditions leading to maceration of tissue encourage infection with *F. necrophorum* (and occasionally *A. pyogenes*), which is thought to be necessary for infection by *D. nodosus* to occur in cattle.[160] When sheep or goats with interdigital dermatitis are exposed to *D. nodosus*, the soft horn becomes under-run but no further pathology occurs. This condition is known as benign (or nonprogressive) foot rot. If sheep develop a secondary infection with *F. necrophorum*, they develop a much more severe disease known as virulent foot rot.[170]

Clinical Signs. Foot rot usually affects both claws in more than one foot. Benign foot rot is characterized by inflammation and necrosis of the interdigital tissue. The soft horn is pale and pitted and may be separated from the skin, but this separation does not involve the hard horn. With benign foot rot, often, only one or a few animals in a flock are affected. Virulent foot rot, in contrast, is marked by severe lameness in numerous animals in the flock, with under-running of the hard horn beginning near the heel on the axial surface. In severe cases, the entire horn may separate from the underlying tissue. Affected areas produce a malodorous exudate. Animals may carry the affected leg, graze on their knees, or remain recumbent. Some animals develop fever, anorexia, and weight loss. Secondary bacterial infection and fly strike may complicate foot rot infection.

Foot rot in goats is generally less severe than in sheep, although significant lameness may develop. Interdigital dermatitis is a more prominent sign, and under-running of the horn is a less prominent sign compared with sheep infected with the same virulent strain of *D. nodosus*.[166,173]

Diagnosis. The diagnosis of virulent foot rot is usually based on the clinical presentation of interdigital dermatitis and lameness in numerous flock members (virulent foot rot). A Gram stain of the interdigital exudate may show the large, curved, gram-negative, barbell-shaped rods characteristic of *D. nodosus*; however, they may not always be isolated because of their special growth requirements.[174] Serologic tests may aid in identifying carrier animals. Antibody levels are elevated for a short time only and are not always accurate. Vaccination may confound the interpretation of the antibody tests. Foot rot is the most common cause of lameness in sheep. However, other differential diagnoses include foot abscess, laminitis, bluetongue, and FMD.

Treatment. The mainstay of therapy for years has been proper hoof trimming. While trimming in the face of disease has fallen out of favor with some because it can increase short-term lameness and delay healing by up to 6 days,[171] others have historically believed that appropriate trimming can produce very high cure rates without other forms of therapy.[160] Applying antibacterial agents to the foot after trimming it further improves cure rates and may be more critical than trimming. Topical treatments include antibiotics (tetracycline) and antiseptics (copper sulfate, zinc sulfate, cetrimide, or 4 to 5% formalin). If only a few animals are affected, these agents may be applied with a spray applicator or brush; bandaging ensures contact of the medication with affected tissue.[167] Chitosan, which is a by-product of the seafood industry, has been shown to have an antibacterial effect on both *D. nodosus* and *F. necrophorum* in vitro, but it was not effective in treating the clinical disease in field trials.[175] Time will tell if future studies with higher doses will show effectiveness.

The use of foot baths is a more practical method to treat numerous animals. Typically, affected animals should be separated from unaffected animals. Both groups of animals are passed through a foot bath and then kept in a dry place for a few hours before being placed on separate clean pastures. If this procedure is repeated several times, the majority of the animals will be cured, and the rest should be culled. A prolonged soaking time (1 hour) may be more effective than brief passes through foot baths, even when they are performed every 10 days.[176] Copper sulfate (5%), zinc sulfate (10%), and formalin (5%) have been used in foot baths and seem to have similar efficacy. Zinc sulfate is preferred because it is less hazardous and causes less discomfort than formalin, does not stain the wool, and has a reduced risk of toxicity compared with copper sulfate.[177]

An anionic surfactant, sodium lauryl sulfate, appears to enhance penetration of the zinc sulfate solution.[167,176] Dry foot baths (85% powdered limestone, 15% zinc sulfate) also may be beneficial. The clinician should remember that sheep are capable of jumping long distances and goats can walk on the thin edge of a small plank. Therefore, foot baths should have solid sides and be at least 2.5 to 3 m long. Regardless of the type of foot bath used, trimming the feet before the therapy greatly enhances its effectiveness.

Several systemic antibiotics have been shown to be effective in the treatment of foot rot. Penicillin (20,000–30,000 IU/kg IM BID), long-acting oxytetracycline (20 mg/kg SC every 72 hours), erythromycin (3–5 mg/kg IM BID), lincomycin, spectinomycin, and florfenicol (20 mg/kg IM every 48 hours) have been used successfully, especially when conditions are dry. These treatments are not approved in all countries.[178,179]

Sheep with foot rot had a quicker resolution of clinical signs when supplemented with selenium than control sheep treated with saline. The clinically normal sheep at the beginning of the study had higher whole blood selenium levels than the sheep with clinical signs.[180]

A randomized study of treatment of sheep with foot rot looking at time to resolution of foot lesions and lameness showed no difference with use of NSAIDs, while parental antibiotics shortened recovery time and foot trimming soon after diagnosis prolonged the time to resolution of lesions and lameness. Therefore, it was suggested that use of parental antibiotics and not trimming feet in animals with clinical disease would shorten the time to resolution of clinical signs in sheep with foot rot.[181] Foot rot in sheep can be controlled to a degree by antibiotic use. Routine trimming of diseased and normal feet may exacerbate the clinical disease either through environmental contamination or an increased susceptibility to disease in recently trimmed feet.[181,182]

Vaccination has been shown to shorten the course of disease in flocks. However, a significant number of injection reactions have been reported.[167] While the decision to vaccinate during an outbreak must be carefully considered, the use of present serogroup-specific monovalent or bivalent vaccines is recommended.[183] There are 10 serogroups to the fimbriated *D. nodosus* organism. Vaccines using fimbrial proteins can be very effective, but cultures are required to determine the specific serogroup responsible for a given outbreak. Multivalent vaccines are not effective because there is no cross-protection and even competitive immunity between the different serogroups.[184]

Prevention. Eradication of virulent foot rot is possible but often difficult, especially in areas that are wet most of the year.[166,167]

• BOX 11-1 Foot Rot Prevention Program[a]

- Separate infected animals, and when trimming feet, disinfect trimming equipment between animals.
- Move all animals through a 15% zinc sulfate foot bath. Where possible, have them stand in the foot bath for 30 minutes. Foot baths should be repeated two to four times at weekly intervals.
- Put both affected and nonaffected sheep in a previously unused (clean) pasture or paddock.
- Cull all severely affected animals and those not responding to treatment.
- Vaccinate with specific serogroup (monovalent or bivalent) vaccines based on farm isolates 8 to 12 weeks before the season when large numbers of foot rot cases are anticipated (disease tends to occur at the same time each year).
- Selectively breed for animals that appear less susceptible.

[a]*Some or all of these procedures can be employed. The main ingredient in any protocol for foot rot prevention is vigilance.*

Box 11.1 describes a foot rot prevention program. Treating affected animals, culling chronic cases, and isolating new animals are the mainstays of an eradication program. New animals should be segregated through a wet season before they are placed with a foot-rot–free flock. Obviously, any animal showing signs of foot rot during quarantine should be culled.

In flocks with endemic foot rot, vaccination may be useful in reducing the number and severity of foot rot cases, but foot bathing and culling should be continued to complement a good vaccination program targeted at the specific serogroups isolated from diseased animals on the farm. Several types of vaccines are available. Two doses given at least 6 weeks apart, followed by boosters a few weeks before the wet season may improve effectiveness.[160] Knowledge of seasonal infection patterns and vaccination before the predicted increase in clinical cases improves vaccination effectiveness.[160] Genetic selection for resistance to foot rot should be a primary adjunct to disease control.

There have been a lot of exciting developments in the area of foot rot vaccination in recent years that have led to better immune response and, thus, better protection from disease. Administration of melatonin with foot rot vaccination produced better immune response to the vaccine[185,186] reportedly due to a positive effect on platelet function.[187,188] Melatonin also enhanced the immune response in animals previously vaccinated for foot rot when given after vaccination.[185]

Commercial foot rot vaccines that contain as many as nine fimbrial serogroups of *D. nodosus* will stimulate short-lived and low antibody responses because of antigenic competition. Vaccines with one or two serogroups will provide better responses for longer time periods. Giving two different bivalent vaccines 3 months apart will produce better immunity without the serogroups interfering with each other. This would work better to eradicate foot rot on farms that are affected by several different strains of *D. nodosus*.[187,188]

One study reported the eradication of foot rot from two farms in Australia by using farm-specific monovalent whole cell vaccine in the entire flock for 1 year and culling the few animals that did not respond.[183] An autogenous *D. nodosus* serogroup B vaccine administered to an entire flock for two consecutive years eradicated virulent foot rot from the farm (that had seen cases for 10 years) with no other foot rot treatments given.[189] Novel strains within the serogroups of *D. nodosus* have been identified. These strains being associated with disease could be important when attempting to use specifically targeted vaccinations to eradicate foot rot on a given farm.[188–190]

Laminitis

Laminitis (inflammation of the dermal and epidermal laminae) is fairly common in sheep and goats but relatively uncommon in white-tailed and mule deer. The history often includes consumption of a highly concentrated or lush forage diet. Laminitis also may be associated with systemic illness such as pneumonia, mastitis, and metritis; it can occur after parturition.[98]

Clinical Signs. Clinical signs of laminitis include lameness and warm feet. Animals move with a stiff gait and prefer recumbency. In chronic cases, foot deformity, marked by "turning up" of the toes, occurs. Laminitis is often accompanied by signs of primary gastrointestinal illness such as bloat, diarrhea, and toxemia. Differential diagnoses include foot rot, CAE, and nutritional conditions that produce lameness, stiff gait, and recumbency.

Treatment and Prevention. The mainstay of treatment is NSAIDs such as flunixin meglumine (1 mg/kg SID) and aspirin (100 mg/kg PO BID), as well as treatment of the primary disorder. If the inciting cause can be corrected, many animals recover.[46] The risk of laminitis can be reduced by *slowly* increasing the amount of grain being fed. Preventing accidental exposure to large amounts of concentrate, ensuring adequate forage intake, and adding rumen buffers to the diet all help decrease the incidence of laminitis.

Hairy Heel Wart

Cases of unusually severe lameness in sheep have been described in the United Kingdom in which the animals are infected with *Treponema* sp. enzymatically and biochemically very similar, if not identical, to the spirochetes responsible for dermal dermatitis (hairy heel warts) in cattle.[191–193] Affected animals usually have only one digit involved, but the severe undermining of the hoof wall causes pain that leaves the animal unable to bear weight. The condition is called contagious ovine digital dermatitis (CODD).[192–194] The same *Treponema* sp. has crossed species to cause similar clinical disease in goats (called caprine digital dermatitis [CDD]).[193,195,196] Elk have also been diagnosed with this spirochete-related lameness in North America (Washington state) after sharing wet pasture with cattle.[193,197] This condition may become severe enough that amputation is the treatment of choice. However, systemic antibiotics, topical therapy with tetracycline, and foot baths an should be attempted before resorting to amputation. Tetracycline can be placed in a foot bath, injected, or painted onto the lesion. While *Treponema* is considered the primary agent in these conditions, there is also evidence that some cases are complicated by the presence of anaerobic bacteria as secondary infections.[195]

Maintaining a closed herd may also help control the disease.[192,198] Other management techniques that will help minimize transmission of the *Treponema* is to avoid aggressive hoof trimming as hoof bleeding when trimmed is associated with a higher incidence of CODD.[171] Foot trimming equipment such as hoof knives and even gloves worn when working with feet have been shown to harbor *Treponema* with the potential to transmit it from animal to animal. Iodine disinfection of the equipment lowers the contamination rate but does not eliminate all organisms.[196,199]

Vaccines are being developed using genomic analysis of the organism to attack proteins of the outer layer of the spirochete, which, if successful, could help eliminate CODD (and CDD) from flocks.[192] Selection of replacement animals from parents never affected by lameness also appears to help control the spirochete-related lameness.[171]

Interdigital Fibromas

Interdigital fibromas occasionally occur in small ruminants but are much more common in cattle. This hyperplasia of the interdigital skin may not cause lameness until the lesion is quite large or infected. Some reports speculate that predisposing factors include obesity, foot rot, and abnormal hoof conformation.[178] Complete surgical excision under general anesthesia or sedation and local anesthesia is the treatment of choice, although cryotherapy, cautery, and topical caustic agents also have been employed. After surgery, the foot is bandaged. Healing may be enhanced by securing the toes with wire to prevent spreading and movement of the interdigital skin. Recurrence of interdigital fibromas is not uncommon.[178]

Acknowledgments

The authors acknowledge the work of Dr. Laura K. Reilly on this chapter in the previous editions of this text.

References

1. Getty R, Sisson S: *Sisson and grossman's the anatomy of domestic animals*, ed 5, Philadelphia, 1975, WB Saunders.
2. Bryant SH, Lipicky RJ, Herzog WH: Variability of myotonia signs in myotonic goats, *Am J Vet Res* 29(12):2371, 1968.
3. McKerrell RE: Myotonia in man and animals: confusing comparisons, *Equine Vet J* 19:266, 1987.
4. Beck CL, Fahlke C, George AL: Molecular basis for decreased muscle chloride conductance in the myotonic goat, *Proc Natl Acad Sci U S A* 93:11248–11252, 1996.
5. Monteagudo LV, Ferrer LM, Tejedor MT, et al: Myotonia congenital in lambs, XXXVIII Congreso Nacional y XIV Internacional de la Sociedad Espanola de Ovinotecnia y Caprinotecnia (SEOC), Malaga, Espana, 18–20 de Septiembre de 2013, 575–583, 2013.
6. Rook JS, Trapp AL, Krehbiel J, et al: Diagnosis of hereditary chondrodysplasia (spider lamb syndrome) in sheep, *J Am Vet Med Assoc* 193(6):713, 1988.
7. Kaczor U, Kucharski M, Martyniuk E, et al: Polymorphism analysis of FGFR3 gene in Suffolk sheep. Annales Universitatis Mariae Curie-Sklodowska, *Sectio EE Zootechnica* 33(1):11–15, 2015.
8. Oberbauer AM, East N, Pool R, et al: Developmental progression of the spider lamb syndrome, *Small Rumin Res* 18:179, 1995.
9. Beever JE, Smit MA, Meyers SN, et al: A single-base change in the tyrosine kinase II domain of ovine FGFR3 causes hereditary chondrodysplasia in sheep, *Anim Genet* 37:66–71, 2006.
10. Jolly RD, Blair HT, Johnstone AC: Genetic disorders of sheep in New Zealand: a review and perspective, *N Z Vet J* 52:52–64, 2004.
11. Lievaart-Peterson K, Luttikholt S, Peperkamp K, Van den Brom R, Vellema P: Schmallenberg disease in sheep or goats: past, present and future, *Vet Microbiol* 181(1–2):147–153, 2015.
12. Santos Dos Reis SD, de Oliveira RS, Correia Marcelino SA, et al: Congenital malformations and other reproductive losses in goats due to poisoning by *Poincianella pyramidalis* (Tul.) L.P. Queiroz (=*Caesalpinia pyramidalis* Tul.), *Toxicon* 118:91–94, 2016.
13. Doherty ML, Kelly EP, Healy AM: Congenital arthrogryposis: an inherited limb deformity in pedigree Suffolk lambs, *Vet Rec* 146:748–753, 2000.
14. Whittington RJ, Glastonbury JR, Plant JW, Barry MR: Congenital hydranencephaly and arthrogryposis of Corriedale sheep, *Aust Vet J* 65:124–127, 1988.
15. Murphy AM, MacHugh DE, Park SD, et al: Linkage mapping of the locus for inherited ovine arthrogryposis (IOA) to sheep chromosome 5, *Mamm Genome* 18:43–52, 2007.
16. Al-Ani FK, Hailat NQ, Fathalla MA: Polydactyly in Shami breed goats in Jordan, *Small Rumin Res* 26:177, 1997.
17. Hulse DA, Shires PK: *Textbook of small animal surgery*, Philadelphia, 1985, WB Saunders.
18. Shettko DL, Trostle SS: Diagnosis and surgical repair of patellar luxations in a flock of sheep, *J Am Vet Med Assoc* 216(4):564, 2000.
19. Baron RJ: Laterally luxating patella in a goat, *J Am Vet Med Assoc* 191(11):1471, 1987.
20. Gahlot TK, Rathor SS, Chouhan DS, et al: Correction of patella luxation in goats, *Mod Vet Pract*, 64:418, 1983.
21. Baker J, Ciszewski D, Lowrie C: Spastic paresis in pygmy goats, *J Vet Int Med* 3(2):113, 1989.
22. Leipold HW, Huston K, Guffy MM, Noordsy JL: Spastic paresis in beef shorthorn cattle, *J Am Vet Med Assoc* 151(5):598, 1967.
23. Thomason KJ, Beeman KB: Spastic paresis in Gelbvieh calves: an examination of two cases, *Vet Med* 82(5):548, 1987.
24. Harper PAW: Spastic paresis in Brahman crossbred cattle, *Aust Vet J* 70(12):456, 1993.
25. de Vlamynck C, Pille F, Vlaminck L: Long term outcome of conservative management or surgical treatment of bovine spastic paresis: 79 cases, *Vet Surg* 45(2):187–193, 2016.
26. *Goat and kid predator and nonpredator death loss in the United States, 2015*, Fort Collins, CO and USDA, 2015 USDA-APHIS-VS-CEAH.
27. *Sheep and lamb predator and nonpredator death loss in the United States, 2015*, Fort Collins, CO, 2015 USDA-APHIS-VS-CEAH-NAHMS.
28. Kaneps AJ: Orthopedic conditions of small ruminants, *Vet Clin North Am Food Anim Pract* 12(1):211, 1996.
29. Nyack B, Padmore CL, White M: External fixation of carpal and metacarpal fractures in a goat, *Bov Pract* 3(3):23, 1982.
30. Smith MC: Practice Tips for Small Ruminant Veterinarians. *Proceedings of the 1998 Symposium on Small Ruminants for the Mixed Animal Practitioner Western Veterinary Conference*, Las Vegas, NV, 1998.
31. Mbiuki SM, Byagagaire SD: Full limb casting: a treatment for tibial fractures in calves and goats, *Vet Med* 79(2):243, 1984.
32. Monin T: Tension band repair of equine mandibular fractures, *J Equine Med Surg* 1(10):325, 1977.
33. DeBowes RM: *Equine fracture repair*, Philadelphia, 1996, WB Saunders.
34. Gamsjaeger L, Chigerwe M: Indications for and outcomes of limb amputation in goats and sheep, *J Am Vet Med Assoc* 252(7):860–863, 2018.
35. Nunamaker DM, Richardson DW, Butterweck DM, et al: A new skeletal fixation device that allows immediate full weight bearing application in the horse, *Vet Surg* 15(5):345, 1986.
36. Egger EL, Greenwood KM: *Textbook of small animal surgery*, Philadelphia, 1985, WB Saunders.
37. St-Jean G, Clem MF, DeBowes RM: Transfixation pinning and casting of tibial fractures in calves: five cases (1985–1989), *J Am Vet Med Assoc* 198:139, 1991.
38. Arnoczky SP, Blass CE, McCoy L: External coaptation and bandaging. In Slatter DH, editor: *Textbook of small animal surgery*, Philadelphia, 1985, WB Saunders.
39. Watkins GH: Arthritis. In Aitken ID, editor: *Diseases of sheep*, Ames, Iowa, 2007, Blackwell Publishing.
40. Watkins GH, Sharp MW: Bacteria isolated from arthritis and omphalitic lesions in lambs in England and Wales, *Vet J* 156:235, 1998.
41. Trent AM, Plumb D: Treatment of infectious arthritis and osteomyelitis, *Vet Clin North Am Food Anim Pract* 7:747, 1991.

42. Navarre CB, Zhang L, Sunkara G, Duran SH, Kompella UB: Ceftiofur distribution in plasma and joint fluid following regional limb injection in cattle, *J Vet Pharmacol Ther* 22:13, 1999.
43. Adams DS: Infectious causes of lameness proximal to the foot, *Vet Clin North Am Food Anim Pract* 5:499, 1983.
44. Everett KDE: Chlamydia and chlamydiales: more than meets the eye, *Vet Microbiol* 75:109, 2000.
45. Radostits OM, Gay C, Hinchcliff K, Constable Peter: *Veterinary medicine*, ed 10, Philadelphia, 2007, WB Saunders.
46. Bulgin MS: Diagnosis of lameness in sheep, *Compend Contin Ed Pract Vet* 8:F122, 1986.
47. Lloyd J, Yang R, Kessell A, et al: Detection of *Chlamydia pecorum* in joints trimmed from ovine carcasses with arthritis at an abattoir in southern Australia, *Small Rumin Res* 150:80–86, 2017.
48. Stephenson EH, Storz J, Hopkins JB: Properties and frequency of isolation of *Chlamydia* from eyes of lambs with conjunctivitis and polyarthritis, *Am J Vet Res* 35:177, 1974.
49. Cutlip RC, Smith PC, Page LA: Chlamydial polyarthritis of lambs: a review, *J Am Vet Med Assoc* 161:1213, 1972.
50. Sachse K, Vretou E, Livingstone M, Borel N, Pospischil A, Longbottom D: Recent developments in the laboratory diagnosis of chlamydial infections, *Vet Microbiol* 135:2–21, 2009.
51. Walker E, Moore C, Shearer P, et al: Clinical, diagnostic and pathologic features of presumptive cases of *Chlamydia pecorum*–associated arthritis in Australian sheep flocks, *BMC Vet Res* 12:193, 2016.
52. Manso-Silvan L, et al: Mycoplasma leachii sp. nov. as a new species designation for *Mycoplasma* sp. bovine group 7 of Leach, and reclassification of *Mycoplasma mycoides* subsp. *mycoides* LC as a serovar of *Mycoplasma mycoides* subsp, *Capri, Int J Syst Evol Microbiol* 59:1353–1358, 2009.
53. DaMassa AJ, Wakenell PS, Brooks DL: Mycoplasmas of goats and sheep, *J Vet Diagn Invest* 4:101, 1992.
54. Rosendal S: Experimental infection of goats, sheep, and calves with the large colony type of *Mycoplasma mycoides* subsp. *Mycoides, Vet Pathol* 18:71, 1981.
55. DaMassa AJ, Brooks DL, Adler HE: Caprine mycoplasmosis: widespread infection in goats with *Mycoplasma mycoides* subsp *mycoides* (large colony type), *Am J Vet Res* 44:322, 1983.
56. DaMassa AJ, Brooks DL, Holmberg CA, Moe AI: Caprine mycoplasmosis: an outbreak of mastitis and arthritis requiring the destruction of 700 goats, *Vet Rec* 120:409, 1987.
57. East NE, DaMassa AJ, Logan LL, Brooks DL, McGowan B: Milkborne outbreak of *Mycoplasma mycoides* subspecies *mycoides* infection in a commercial goat dairy, *J Am Vet Med Assoc* 182:1338, 1983.
58. DaMassa AJ, Brooks DL, Holmberg CA: Induction of mycoplasmosis in goat kids by oral inoculation with *Mycoplasma mycoides* subsp *mycoides, Am J Vet Res* 47:2084, 1986.
59. Rosendal S: *Mycoplasma mycoides* subspecies *mycoides* as a cause of polyarthritis in goats, *J Am Vet Med Assoc* 175:378, 1979.
60. East NE: *Mycoplasma mycoides* polyarthritis in goats. In Smith BP, editor: *Large animal medicine,* ed 2, St Louis, 1996, Mosby.
61. Al-Momani, Nicholas RA, Janakat S, Abu-Basha E, Ayling RD: The *in vitro* effect of six antimicrobials against *Mycoplasma putrefaciens, Mycoplasma mycoides* subsp. *mycoides* LC and *Mycoplasma capricolum* subsp. *capricolum* isolated from sheep and goats in Jordan, *Trop Anim Health Prod* 38:1–7, 2006.
62. Davis WP, Steficek BA, Watson GL, et al: Disseminated *Rhodococcus equi* infection in two goats, *Vet Pathol* 36:336–339, 1999.
63. Reczynska D, Zalewska M, Czopowicz M, Kaba J, Zwierzchowski L, Bagnicka E: Small ruminant lentivirus infection influences expression of acute phase proteins and cathelicidin genes in milk somatic cells and peripheral blood leukocytes of dairy goats, *Vet Res* 49:113, 2018.
64. Anarson H, Palsson A, Gudnadottir M, Andresdottir V: Maedi-visna virus persistence: Antigenic variation and latency, *Comp Immunol Microbiol Infect Dis* 55:6–12, 2017.
65. de Pablo-Maiso L, Doménech A, Echeverría I, et al: Prospects in innate immune responses as potential control strategies against non-primate lentiviruses, *Viruses* 10(8):435, 2018.
66. Pérez M, Muñoz JA, Biescas E, et al: Successful Visna/maedi control in a highly infected ovine dairy flock using serologic segregation and management strategies, *Prev Vet Med* 112(3–4):423–427, 2013.
67. Bojar W, Junkuszew A, Dudko P, et al: Risk factors associated with small-ruminant lentiviruses in sheepfold buildings, *Ann Agric Environ Med* 25(3):383–387, 2018.
68. Singh R, Kumar P, Singh R, et al: Pathology and polymerase chain reaction detection of ovine progressive pneumonia (maedi) cases in slaughtered sheep in India, *Vet World* 10(11):1401–1406, 2017.
69. White SN, Knowles DP: Expanding possibilities for intervention against small ruminant lentiviruses through genetic marker-assisted selective breeding, *Viruses* 5(6):1466–1499, 2013.
70. Crawford TB, Adams DS: Caprine arthritis-encephalitis: clinical features and presence of antibody in selected goat populations, *J Am Vet Med Assoc* 178:713, 1981.
71. Shah C, Huder JB, Böni J, et al: Direct evidence for natural transmission of small ruminant lentiviruses of subtype A4 from goats to sheep and vice versa, *J Virol* 78:7518–7522, 2004.
72. Rowe JD, East NE, Franti CE, Thurmond MC, Pedersen NC, Theilen GH: Risk factors associated with the incidence of seroconversion to caprine arthritis-encephalitis virus in goats on California dairies, *Am J Vet Res* 53:2396, 1992.
73. East NE, Rowe JD, Madewell BR, Floyd K: Serologic prevalence of caprine arthritis-encephalitis virus in California goat dairies, *J Am Vet Med Assoc* 190:182, 1987.
74. Adams DS, Oliver RE, Ameghino E, et al: Global survey of serological evidence of caprine arthritis-encephalitis virus infection, *Vet Rec* 115:493, 1984.
75. Adams DS, Klevjer-Anderson P, Carlson JL, McGuire TC, Gorham JR: Transmission and control of caprine arthritis-encephalitis virus, *Am J Vet Res* 44:1670, 1983.
76. East NE, Rowe JD, Dahlberg JE, Theilen GH, Pederson NC: Modes of transmission of caprine arthritis-encephalitis virus infection, *Small Rumin Res* 10:251, 1993.
77. Blacklaws BA, Berriatua E, Torsteinsdottir S, et al: Transmission of small ruminant lentiviruses, *Vet Microbiol* 101:199–208, 2004.
78. Rowe JD, East NE: Risk factors for transmission and methods for control of caprine arthritis-encephalitis virus infection, *Vet Clin North Am Food Anim Pract* 13:35, 1997.
79. Chang CC, Yang WS: Detection of caprine arthritis-encephalitis virus (CAEV) in semen of bucks, *J Taiwan Livest Res* 49(2):121–129, 2016.
80. Peterhans E, Greenland T, Badiola J, et al: Routes of transmission and consequences of small ruminant lentiviruses (SRLVs) infection and eradication schemes, *Vet Res* 35:257–274, 2004.
81. Hanson J, Hydbring E, Olsson K: A long term study of goats naturally infected with caprine arthritis-encephalitis virus, *Acta Vet Scand* 37:31, 1996.
82. McGuire TC, Adams DS, Johnson GC, Klevjer-Anderson P, Barbee DD, Gorham JR: Acute arthritis in caprine arthritis-encephalitis virus challenge exposure of vaccinated or persistently infected goats, *Am J Vet Res* 47:537, 1986.
83. Reina R, Berriatua E, Luján L, et al: Prevention strategies against small ruminant lentiviruses: an update, *Vet J* 182:31–37, 2009.
84. Tavelta A, Bettini A, Ceol M, et al: Achievements of an eradication programme against caprine arthritis encephalitis virus in South Tyrol, Italy, *Vet Rec* 182(2):51, 2018.
85. Gerstner S, Adamovicz JJ, Duncan JV, et al: Prevalence of and risk factors associated with ovine progressive pneumonia in Wyoming sheep flocks, *J Am Vet Med Assoc* 247(8):932–937, 2015.
86. de la Concha-Bermejillo A: Maedi-visna and ovine progressive pneumonia, *Vet Clin North Am Food Anim Pract* 13:13, 1997.
87. Oliver RE, Gorham JR, Parish SF, Hadlow WJ, Narayan O: Ovine progressive pneumonia: pathologic and virologic studies on the naturally occurring disease, *Am J Vet Res* 42:1554, 1981.

88. Cutlip RC, Lehmkuhl HD, Wood RL, Brogden KA: Arthritis associated with ovine progressive pneumonia, *Am J Vet Res* 46:65, 1985.
89. Cutlip RC, Lehmkuhl HD, Schmerr MJ, Brogden KA: Ovine progressive pneumonia (maedi-visna) in sheep, *Vet Microbiol* 17:237, 1988.
90. Knowles DP: Laboratory diagnostic tests for retrovirus infections of small ruminants, *Vet Clin North Am Food Anim Pract* 13(1):1–11, 1997.
91. Mays SE, Hendricks BM, Paulsen DJ, Houston AE, Trout Fryxell RT: Prevalence of five tick-borne bacterial genera in adult ixodes scapularis removed from white-tailed deer in western Tennessee, *Parasit Vectors* 7:473, 2014.
92. Parker JL, White KK: Lyme borreliosis in cattle and horses: a review of the literature, *Cornell Vet* 82:253, 1992.
93. Ben Said M, Belkahia H, Alberti A, et al: First molecular evidence of *Borrelia burgdorferi* sensu lato in goats, sheep, cattle and camels in Tunisia, *Ann Agric Environ Med* 23(3):442–447, 2016.
94. Fridriksdóttir V, Overnes G, Stuen S: Suspected Lyme borreliosis in sheep, *Vet Rec* 130:323, 1992.
95. Mitchell GBB, Smith IW: Lyme disease in Scotland: results of a serological study in sheep, *Vet Rec* 133:66, 1993.
96. Stuen S, Fridriksdóttir V: Experimental inoculation of sheep with *Borrelia burgdorferi*, *Vet Rec* 129:315, 1991.
97. Yang J, Liu Z, Li Y, et al: Comprehensive surveillance of the antibody response to *Borrelia burgdorferi* s.l. in small ruminants in China, *Ann Agric Environ Med* 22(2):208–211, 2015.
98. Guss SB: *Management and diseases of dairy goats*, Scottsdale, AZ, 1977, Dairy Goat Journal Publishing.
99. Glastonbury JR, Searson JE, Links IJ, Tuckett LM: Clostridial myocarditis in lambs, *Aust Vet J* 65:208, 1988.
100. Useh NM, Ibrahim ND, Nok AJ, Esievo KA: Relationship between outbreaks of blackleg in cattle and annual rainfall in Zaria, Nigeria, *Vet Rec* 158:100–101, 2006.
101. Dubey JP, Livingston CW: *Sarcocystis capracanis* and *Toxoplasma gondii* infections in range goats from Texas, *Am J Vet Res* 47:523, 1986.
102. Jeffrey M, Low JC, Uggla A: A myopathy of sheep associated with *Sarcocystis* infection and monensin administration, *Vet Rec* 124:422, 1989.
103. Dubey JP, Fayer R, Seesee FM: *Sarcocystis* in feces of coyotes from Montana: prevalence and experimental transmission to sheep and cattle, *J Am Vet Med Assoc* 173:1167, 1978.
104. Dubey JP, Weisbrode SE, Speer CA, Sharma SP: Sarcocystosis in goats: clinical signs and pathologic and hematologic findings, *J Am Vet Med Assoc* 178:683, 1981.
105. Dubey JP, Lindsay DS: Neosporosis, toxoplasmosis, and sarcocystosis in ruminants, *Vet Clin North Am Food Anim Pract* 22(3): 645–671, 2006.
106. Agerholm JS, Dubey JP: Sarcocystosis in a stillborn lamb, *Reprod domest Anim* 49:6, e60–e63, 2014.
107. Smith ME: Exotic disease of small ruminants. Geriatric medicine for small ruminants. *Proceedings of the 1998 Symposium on Small Ruminants for the Mixed Animal Practitioner Western Veterinary Conference,* Las Vegas, NV, 1998.
108. Heckeroth AR, Tenter AM: Development and validation of species-specific nested PCRs for diagnosis of acute sarcocystosis in sheep, *Int J Parasitol* 29:1331–1349, 1999.
109. Jaisree S, Hemaltha S, Mahaprabhu R, et al: Outbreak of foot and mouth disease in an organized sheep and goat farm, *Indian Vet J* 93(11):31–33, 2016.
110. Sharma SK: Foot and mouth disease in sheep and goats, *Vet Res J* 4(1):1–21, 1981.
111. Barnett PV, Cox SJ: The role of small ruminants in the epidemiology and transmission of foot and mouth disease, *Vet J* 158:6, 1999.
112. Mansley LM, Dunlop PJ, Whiteside SM, Smith RG: Early dissemination of foot-and-mouth disease virus through sheep marketing in 2001, *Vet Rec* 153:43–50, 2003.
113. Scott GR: Foot-and-mouth disease. In Sewell MMH, Brocklesby DW, editors: *Handbook on animal diseases in the tropics,* ed 4, Philadelphia, 1990, Bailliere Tindall.
114. Kitching RP, Hughes GJ: Clinical variation in foot-and-mouth disease: sheep and goats, *Rev Sci Tech* 21:505–512, 2002.
115. Edmondson AJ, Norman BB, Suther D: Survey of state veterinarians and state veterinary diagnostic laboratories for selenium deficiency and toxicosis in animals, *J Am Vet Med Assoc* 202:865, 1993.
116. Maas J, Valberg SJ: Nutritional myodegeneration. In Smith BP, editor: *Large animal internal medicine,* St Louis, 2009, Mosby.
117. Maxie MG: *Jubb*, kennedy and palmer's *pathology of domestic animals,* ed 5, Orlando, FLA, 2007, Saunders.
118. Bulgin MS: Diagnosing nutritional difficulties. *Proceedings of the 1998 Symposium on Small Ruminants for the Mixed Animal Practitioner Western Veterinary Conference,* Las Vegas, NV, 1998.
119. Smart ME, Cymbaulk: Trace minerals. In Naylor JM, Ralston SL, editors: *Large animal clinical nutrition,* St Louis, 1991, Mosby.
120. Naylor JM: Vitamins. In Naylor JM, Ralston SL, editors: *Large animal clinical nutrition,* St Louis, 1991, Mosby.
121. Ogilvie TH: Musculoskeletal disorders. In Ogilvie TH, editor: *Large animal internal medicine,* Baltimore, 1998, Williams & Wilkins.
122. Bretzlaff K, Haenlein G, Huston E: Common nutritional problems feeding the sick goat. In Naylor JM, Ralston SL, editors: *Large animal clinical nutrition,* St Louis, 1991, Mosby.
123. Thompson KF, Dittmer KE, Blair HT, Fairley RA, Sim DF: An outbreak of rickets in Corriedale sheep: evidence for a genetic aetiology, *N Z Vet J* 55:137–142, 2007.
124. Dittmer KE, Morley RE, Smith RL: Skeletal deformities associated with nutritional congenital rickets in newborn lambs, *N Z Vet J* 65(1):51–55, 2017.
125. Goff J: Calcium, magnesium and phosphorus. In Smith BP, editor: *Large animal internal medicine,* ed 4, St Louis, 2007, Mosby.
126. Van Saun RJ: Vitamin D–responsive rickets in neonatal lambs, *Can Vet J* 45:841–844, 2004.
127. Bonniwell MA, Smith BS, Spence JA, Wright H, Ferguson DA: Rickets associated with vitamin D deficiency in young sheep, *Vet Rec* 122:386, 1988.
128. Sasidharan M, Varughese G: Osteodystrophia fibrosa in goat—a case report, *J Indian Vet Assoc, Kerala* 9(3):53–54, 2011.
129. Andrews AH, Ingram PL, Longstaffe JA: Osteodystrophia fibrosa in young goats, *Vet Rec* 112:404, 1983.
130. Pawar VN, Dighe DG, Velhankar RD, et al: Osteodystrophia fibrosa in a kid—a case report, *Indian J Vet Med* 30(2):138–139, 2010.
131. Anderson KL, Adams WM: Epiphysitis and recumbency in a yearling prepartum goat, *J Am Vet Med Assoc* 183:226, 1983.
132. Scott CA, Gibbs HA, Thompson H: Osteochondrosis as a cause of lameness in purebred Suffolk lambs, *Vet Rec* 139:165–167, 1996.
133. Ahmed KE, Adam SE, Idrill OF, Wahbi AA: Experimental selenium poisoning in Nubian goats, *Vet Hum Toxicol* 32:249, 1990.
134. Smith BI, Donovan GA, Rae DO: Selenium toxicosis in a flock of Katahdin hair sheep, *Can Vet J* 40:192–194, 1999.
135. Hibbs CM, Wolf N: Ergot toxicosis in young goats, *Mod Vet Pract* 63:126, 1982.
136. Choubisa SL: Some observations on endemic fluorosis in domestic animals in southern Rajasthan (India), *Vet Res Commun* 23:457, 1999.
137. Haigh JC, Hudson RJ: *Farming wapiti and red deer*, Mosby, 1993.
138. Botha CJ, Naudé TW, Minnaar PP, Van Amstel SR, Janse van Rensburg SD: Two outbreaks of fluorosis in cattle and sheep, *J S Afr Vet Assoc* 64:165, 1993.
139. Schultheiss WA, Van Niekerk JC: Suspected chronic fluorosis in a sheep flock, *J S Afr Vet Assoc* 65:84, 1994.
140. Wang JD, Hong JP, Li JX: Studies on alleviation of industrial fluorosis in Baotou goats, *Fluoride* 28:131, 1995.

141. Allen JG, Steele P, Masters HG, Lambe WJ: A lupinosis-associated myopathy in sheep and the effectiveness of treatments to prevent it, *Aust Vet J* 69:75, 1992.
142. Rowe LD, Corrier DE, Reagor JC, Jones LP: Experimentally induced *Cassia roemeriana* poisoning in cattle and goats, *Am J Vet Res* 48:992, 1987.
143. Bastianello SS: A survey on neoplasia in domestic species over a 40-year period from 1935 to 1974 in the republic of South Africa. II. Tumours occurring in sheep, *Onderstepoort J Vet Res* 49:205, 1982.
144. Pesato ME, Boyle AG, Fecteau ME, Hamberg A1, Smith BI: Gastrointestinal spindle cell tumor of the rumen with metastasis to the liver in a goat, *J Vet Diagn Invest* 30(3):451–454, 2018.
145. Grimmer ED, Canisso IF, Hsiao SH, et al: Squamous cell carcinoma and papilloma virus in the prepuce of a Boer buck, *Clin Theriogenology* 9(4):595–599, 2017.
146. Dockweiler JC, Cossic B, McDonough SP, et al: Tumor collision of uterine adenocarcinoma and leiomyosarcoma in a goat, *J Vet Diagn Invest* 29(5):696–699, 2017.
147. Steinberg H, George C: Fracture-associated osteogenic sarcoma and a mandibular osteoma in two goats, *J Comp Pathol* 100:453, 1989.
148. Pèrez V, Rúa P, Benavides J, Ferreras MC, García Marín JF: Osteoma in the skull of a sheep, *J Comp Pathol* 130:319–322, 2004.
149. Cotchin E: Tumors of farm animals, *Vet Rec* 40:816, 1960.
150. Hooper RN: General surgery techniques—part I. *Proceedings of the 1998 Symposium on Small Ruminants for the Mixed Animal Practitioner Western Veterinary Conference,* Las Vegas, NV, 1998.
151. Johnson JH, Lowe JE, Fessler JF et al: The musculoskeletal system. In Oehme FW, Prier JE, editors: *Textbook of large animal surgery,* Baltimore, 1976, Williams & Wilkins.
152. Kent JE, Molong V, Graham MJ: Comparison of methods for the reduction of acute pain produced by rubber ring castrating or tail docking of week-old lambs, *Vet J* 155:39, 1998.
153. Small AH, Marini D, Floch M le, et al: A pen study evaluation of buccal meloxicam and topical anaesthetic at improving welfare of lambs undergoing surgical mulesing and hot knife taildocking, *Res Vet Sci* 118:270–277, 2018.
154. Small AH, Marini D, Dyall T, et al: A randomised field study evaluating the effectiveness of buccal meloxicam and topical local anaesthetic formulations administered singly or in combination at improving welfare of female Merino lambs undergoing surgical mulesing and hot knife tail docking, *Res Vet Sci* 118:305–311, 2018.
155. Marini D, Colditz IG, Hinch G, et al: Self-administration by consumption of flunixin in feed alleviates the pain and inflammation associated with castration and tail docking of lambs, *Appl Anim Behav Sci* 188:26–33, 2017.
156. Lloyd J, Kessell A, Barchia I, Schröder J, Rutley D: Docked tail length is a risk factor for bacterial arthritis in lambs, *Small Rumin Res* 144:17–22, 2016.
157. Cottom DS, Pinsent PJ: Lameness in the goat, *Goat Vet Soc J* 9(1):14, 1988.
158. Chakrabarti A: Incidence of foot disorders in goats in Tripura, *Indian Vet J* 74:342, 1997.
159. Greenough PR, Schugel LM, Johnson AB: *Illustrated handbook on cattle lameness*, Eden Prairie, MN, 1996, ZinPro.
160. Morgan K: Footrot. In Boden E, editor: *Sheep and goat practice,* London, 1991, Bailliere Tindale.
161. Cross RF, Parker CF: Oral administration of zinc sulfate for control of ovine footrot, *J Am Vet Med Assoc* 178(7):704, 1981.
162. Cross RF, Parker CF: Zinc sulfate foot bath for control of ovine foot rot, *J Am Vet Med Assoc* 178(7):706, 1981.
163. Christodoulopoulos G: Foot lameness in dairy goats, *Res Vet Sci* 86(2):281, 2009.
164. Bennett G, Hickford J, Sedcole R, Zhou H: *Dichelobacter nodosus,* Fusobactrium necrophorum and the epidemiology of footrot, *Anaerobe* 15(4):173, 2009.
165. Dhawi A, Hart CA, Demirkan I, Davies IH, Carter SD: Bovine digital dermatitis and severe virulent ovine foot rot: a common spirochaetal pathogenesis, *Vet J* 169(2):232, 2005.
166. Egerton JR: Footrot of cattle, goats, and deer. In Egerton JR, Yong WK, Riffkin GG, editors: *Footrot and foot abscess of ruminants,* Boca Raton, FL, 1989, CRC Press.
167. Stewart DJ: Footrot in sheep. In Egerton JR, Yong WK, Riffkin GG, editors: *Footrot and foot abscess of ruminants,* Boca Raton, FL, 1989, CRC Press.
168. Kimberling CV, Ellis RP: Advances in the control of foot rot in sheep, *Vet Clin North Am Food Anim Pract* 6:671, 1990.
169. Buller NB, Ashley P, Palmer M, Pitman D, Richards RB, Hampson DJ: Understanding the molecular epidemiology of the footrot pathogen *Dichelobacter nodosus* to support control and eradication programs, *J Clin Microbiol* 48(3):877, 2010.
170. Witcomb LA, Green LE, Kaler J, et al: A longitudinal study of the role of *Dichelobacter nodosus* and *Fusobacterium necrophorum* load in initiation and severity of footrot in sheep, *Prev Vet Med* 115: 48–55, 2014.
171. Green L: A Multidisciplinary Approach Changing the Paradigm of Footrot in Sheep. 18th International Symposium and 10th Conference on Lameness in Ruminants 53–58, 2015.
172. Muzafar M, Green LE, Calvo-Bado LA, et al: Survival of the ovine footrot pathogen *Dichelobacter nodosus* in different soils, *Anaerobe* 38:81–87, 2016.
173. Ghimire SC, Egerton JR, Dhyngyel OP: Transmission of virulent footrot between sheep and goats, *Aust Vet J* 77:450, 1999.
174. Rings DM: Ovine contagious foot rot. In Howard JL, Smith RA, editors: *Current veterinary therapy 4, food animal practice,* Philadelphia, 1999, WB Saunders.
175. Bekhit AEA, Mros S, Ali MA, McConnell M: Brief communication: chitosan is a highly effective *in vitro* antibacterial agent against the strains of bacteria causing footrot, but is not effective in treating stage-four footrot on farm, *Proc N Z Soc Anim Prod* 75:172–174, 2015.
176. Bulgin MS, Lincoln SD, Lane VM, Matlock M: Comparison of treatment methods for the control of contagious ovine foot rot, *J Am Vet Med Assoc* 189:194, 1986.
177. Ortolani El, Antonelli AC, de Souza Sarkis JE: Acute sheep poisoning from a copper sulfate footbath, *Vet Hum Toxicol* 46(6):315, 2004.
178. Radostits OM, Blood DC, Gay CC, et al: *Veterinary medicine,* ed 9, Philadelphia, 2000, WB Saunders.
179. Vandyke S, Wallace L, Sterle SW, et al: Treatment of ovine foot rot: use of florfenicol versus oxytetracycline for treatment of ovine foot rot, *Sheep and Goat Res J* 15:54, 1999.
180. Hall JA, Bailey DP, Thonstad KN, Van Saun RJ: Effect of parental selenium administration to sheep on prevalence and recovery from footrot, *J Vet Intern Med* 23(2):352, 2009.
181. Kaler J, Daniles SL, Wright JL, Green LE: Randomized clinical trial of long-acting oxytetracycline, foot trimming, and flunixine meglumine on time to recovery in sheep with footrot, *J Vet Intern Med* 24(2):420, 2010.
182. Green LE, Wassink GJ, Grogono-Thomas R, Moore LJ, Medley GF: Looking after the individual to reduce disease in the flock: a binomial mixed effects model investigating the impact of individual sheep management of footrot and interdigital dermatitis in a prospective longitudinal study on one farm, *Prev Vet Med* 78(2):172, 2007.
183. Dhungyel OP, Lehmann DR, Whittington RJ: Pilot trials in Australia on eradication of footrot by flock specific vaccination, *Vet Microbiol* 132(3–4):364, 2008.
184. McPherson AS, Dhungyel OP, Whittington RJ: Detection and serogrouping of *Dichelobacter nodosus* infection by use of direct PCR from lesion swabs to support outbreak-specific vaccination for virulent footrot in sheep, *J Clin Microbiol* 56(4):1–12, 2018.
185. Ramos A, Laguna I, de Lucia ML, Martin-palomini P, Regodon S, Miguez MP: Evolution of oxidative/nitrosative stress biomarkers during an open-field vaccination procedure in sheep: effect of melatonin, *Vet Immunol Immunopathol* 133(1):16, 2010.

186. Regodon S, del Prado Miquez M, Jardin I, et al: Melatonin, as an adjuvant-like agent, enhances platelet responsiveness, *J Pineal Res* 46(3):275, 2009.
187. Regodon S, Ramos A, Morgado S, Tarazona R, Martin-palomino P, Rosado JA, Miquez Mdel P: Melatonin enhances the immune response to vaccination against A1 and C strains of *Dichelobacter nodosus, Vaccine* 27(10):1566, 2009.
188. Dhungyel OP, Whittington RJ: Modulation of inter-vaccination interval to avoid antigenic competition in multivalent footrot (*Dichelobacter nodosus*) vaccines in sheep, *Vaccine* 28(2):470, 2009.
189. Gurung RB, Dhungyel OP, Tshering P, Egerton JR: The use of an autogenous *Dichelobacter nodosus* vaccine to eliminate clinical signs of virulent footrot in a sheep flock in Bhutan, *Vet J* 172(2):356, 2006.
190. Zhou H, Lottner S, Ganter M, Hickford JG: Identification of two new *Dichelobacter nodosus* strains in Germany, *Vet J* 184(1):115, 2010.
191. Naylor RD, Martin PK, Jones JR: Isolation of a spirochete from a case of severe virulent ovine footrot, *Vet Rec* 25:690, 1998.
192. Staton GJ, Ainsworth S, Blowey RW, Evans NJ, Carter SD: Developing a Vaccine for Digital Dermatitis of Cattle and Sheep: A Reverse Vaccinology Approach, Proceedings of the Cattle Lameness Conference, Sixways, Worchester 65–66, 2014.
193. Clegg SR, Sullivan LE, Bell J, Blowey RW et al: The Expanding Host Range of Digital Dermatitis Treponemes, Proceedings of the Cattle Lameness Conference, Sixways, Worchester 55–56, 2014.
194. Sindhu K, Somashekhar H, Ashok W, et al: The incidence of foot ailments in few districts of central and north Karnataka with emphasis on management of lameness in large ruminants, *Pharma Innov J* 7(7):28–34, 2018
195. Sullivan LE, Evans NJ, Clegg SR, et al: Digital dermatitis treponemes associated with a severe foot disease in dairy goats, *Vet Rec* 176(11):283, 2015.
196. Carter S: Digital Dermatitis—How is it spread and can we stop it? Proceedings of the Cattle Lameness Conference, Sixways, Worchester 43–48, 2014
197. Han S, Mansfield KG, Bradway DS, et al: Treponeme-associated hoof disease of free-ranging elk (*Cervus elaphus*) in southwestern Washington state, USA, *Vet Pathol* 1–15, 2018. (online publication).
198. O'Connell NE: Practical solutions to digital dermatitis problems, Proceedings of the Cattle Lameness Conference, Sixways, Worchester 49–53, 2014.
199. Sullivan LE, Blowey RW, Carter SD, et al: A High Association of Digital Dermatitis Treponemes on Cattle and Sheep Hoof Trimming Equipment, Proceedings of the Cattle Lameness Conference, Sixways, Worchester 59–60, 2014.

12 Diseases of the Urinary System

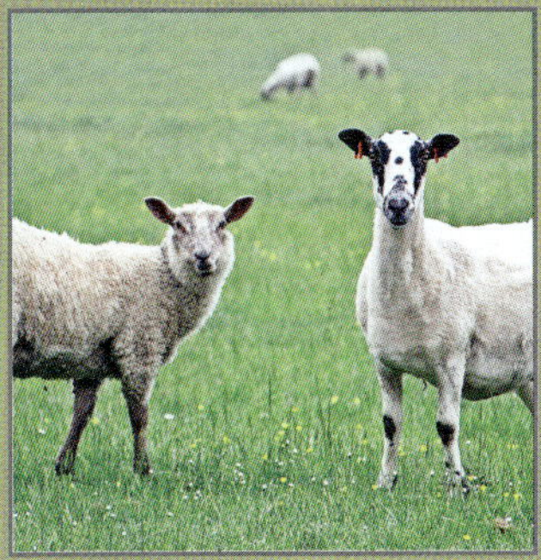

MEREDYTH JONES, MATT MIESNER, AND MISTY A. EDMONDSON

Initial Evaluation of the Urinary Tract

History

A thorough health and husbandry history is very useful in the management of all cases presented for veterinary care. The most common urinary tract diseases of sheep and goats are related to management, and information about previous management assists with the diagnosis and recommendations for management modifications that can benefit the entire herd or flock.

For animals with signs referable to the urinary tract, owners should be questioned regarding dietary history, duration and progression of clinical signs, treatments administered, response to therapy, and the quality of the last observed urination. For females, pregnancy status, parturition history, and history of dystocia may provide diagnostic direction. For males, age at castration should be determined. It is also important to remember that animals with urinary tract disease will often present with an owner complaint of gastrointestinal (GI) or reproductive tract disease (e.g., straining and abdominal distension), making early identification of these signs at the time of initial consultation imperative to initiate appropriate care.

Physical Examination

Due to the common nature of urinary tract disease, particularly in male small ruminants, any ill animal should receive a urinary tract evaluation. This evaluation should begin with a thorough, systematic physical examination, with the presence of signs of systemic illness, including mental depression, dehydration, fever, abdominal distension and rumen hypomotility, noted and used to localize urinary tract disease. During the examination, the animal should be observed for urination behaviors, with classification of these as normal micturition, dysuria, pollakiuria, or polyuria as well as observation for urine scalding.

Palpation of the abdomen of small ruminants is generally easy to perform after determination of abdominal contour. Palpation of the urinary bladder, ballottement, and succussion can provide characterization of the abdominal contents. In males, the urethra can be indirectly observed as it exits the pelvis and traces the body wall to the external urethral orifice. Pulsations and generalized or focal swellings along this length are suggestive of obstruction, urethral rupture, hematoma, or abscess formation. The vulvar and preputial hairs should be examined for the presence of grit, blood, purulent matter, or urine, consistent with recent urination.

The penis should be exteriorized and the prepuce and free portion of the penis examined. This can be accomplished in unsedated animals by placing them either on their rump or in lateral recumbency with the upper hindlimb pulled forward (see Chapters 1 and 8). Distressed animals may require local anesthesia or sedation. Sedation may be achieved by use of acepromazine (0.05–0.1 mg/kg, intravenously [IV] or intramuscularly [IM]) or (diazepam 0.1 mg/kg, slow IV), while a lumbosacral epidural of 2% lidocaine (1 mL/7 kg) may be used instead of sedation to relieve discomfort and aid in exteriorization of the penis. The use of xylazine should be avoided in animals with potential obstruction due to its diuretic effects,[1,2] increasing the risk of urinary tract rupture.

Ancillary Diagnostic Testing

Complete Blood Count and Serum Biochemistry

The results of a complete blood count (CBC) and serum chemistry can provide assistance in the diagnosis, prognosis, management, and monitoring of diseases involving the urinary tract. Blood analyses in animals with urinary tract disease, however, may be within reference ranges, depending on disease severity and duration. For this reason, this section will focus on interpretation of abnormalities once they are identified (see Appendix 2).

Abnormalities noted on the CBC may include anemia of chronic inflammation or renal failure, stress, or inflammatory leukogram and hyperfibrinogenemia. Anemia of chronic inflammation is a nonregenerative anemia characterized by normocytic, normochromic red blood cells and the anemia is typically mild to moderate in severity.[3] The mechanisms of this anemia include increased concentrations of inflammatory mediators that reduce red blood cell lifespan and impair bone marrow function. Anemia of chronic renal failure (CRF) is also normocytic and normochromic, but the anemia may become more severe than anemia of chronic inflammation. The mechanism for this anemia is decreased renal production of erythropoietin in the kidneys.[3] The long red blood cell lifespan in ruminants (125–160 days)[4] precludes the development of anemia in acute renal failure (ARF).

Inflammatory diseases are common in sheep and goats and the leukogram may reflect inflammatory processes primarily affecting the upper urinary tract. Most ruminants have a neutrophil-to-lymphocyte (N:L) ratio of 1:2, while adult goats typically have a ratio of 1:1. The N:L ratio is a more important consideration than is the actual numbers of each. Sheep and goats have a small circulating pool of neutrophils that results in neutropenia 24 to 8 hours after the onset of severe inflammation, reducing the N:L ratio. The presence of immature neutrophils (bands) is termed a left-shift and indicates severe inflammation. This is a common finding in the acute phase of severe inflammation but is associated with a poor prognosis if the left-shift persists. Increases in the N:L ratio with the presence of bands indicates an inflammatory leukogram. A reversal of the N:L ratio to greater than 2:1, without the presence of bands, is indicative of a stress leukogram. The stress leukogram occurs as a result of corticosteroid administration or endogenous steroid release, generally from noninflammatory diseases. Fibrinogen is a positive acute phase protein, increasing over a period of 2 days after initiation of inflammation in ruminants.[5,6]

The serum biochemistry includes renal enzymes as well as electrolytes, which may be altered by renal disease. Blood (serum) urea nitrogen (BUN) is interpreted as a measure of glomerular filtration rate (GFR), indicating the perfusion and function of the kidneys. BUN is influenced by the protein level of the diet and the ability of the rumen to recycle urea. Creatinine is produced and eliminated in constant amounts in the body and is not influenced by superfluous factors, making it superior for evaluation of renal disease in ruminants. Azotemia, or elevations in BUN or creatinine, may be of pre-renal, renal, or post-renal causes. Pre-renal azotemia is caused by decreased GFR due to volume depletion and dehydration. Renal azotemia occurs when greater than 75% of functional nephrons are lost and indicates renal failure. Animals with pre-renal or renal azotemia may both show clinical dehydration, so differentiation is based upon urine specific gravity (USG). The production of adequately concentrated urine (see "Urinalysis" section in this chapter) indicates that enough functional nephrons exist to concentrate urine and the azotemia is classified as pre-renal. The production of dilute urine would indicate renal failure, but other causes of urine dilution should be considered, including fluid therapy, diuretic or corticosteroid therapy, and hyponatremia or hypokalemia. Further clarification of a renal azotemia involves the determination of fractional excretion (FE) of electrolytes, namely sodium. FE is a sensitive indicator of renal function, reflecting the percentage of an electrolyte that is filtered through the glomerulus and lost in urine. The procedure involves concurrent collection of serum and urine and analysis of each for creatinine and sodium. The following formula is then used to calculate the FE[7]:

$$FE_{Na+} = ([Na+]_{urine}/[Na+]_{serum})/([Creatinine]_{urine}/[Creatinine]_{serum}) \times 100$$

Normal sheep have an FE of sodium of $< 1\%$,[7] while an FE of sodium $> 1\%$ indicates primary renal tubular disease or sodium toxicity. Post-renal azotemia is most commonly caused by urinary tract obstruction, which is identified by findings in the history, physical examination, and imaging studies. With prolonged urinary tract obstruction, renal damage may occur, worsening the azotemia.

Hyponatremia and hypochloremia may be present with renal disease due to renal losses and decreased dietary intake. Hyperkalemia, as is seen in monogastrics with renal failure, is not consistently seen in ruminants with urinary obstruction or renal disease. This is due to aldosterone release in response to hypovolemia, which preserves sodium.[8] This allows potassium to replace sodium as the major cation in the saliva, resulting in sequestration in the GI tract. Animals with metabolic acidosis may also show hyperkalemia as potassium is shifted extracellularly. Phosphorus is primarily excreted by ruminants into the saliva, not the kidney, as in other species.[9] In lambs, only 3% of total phosphorus excretion occurs through the kidney.[9] Therefore, conditions that cause a reduced GFR do not necessarily result in increased serum phosphorus. When phosphorus is elevated, however, it should be considered significant. Mild hypocalcemia may also be noted, particularly in hyperphosphatemic animals as a result of complexing of these two ions. Hypermagnesemia is also associated with decreased GFR. The acid-base status of animals with urinary tract disease is variable and can be partially evaluated by total carbon dioxide (TCO_2) on serum chemistry, with a high TCO_2 indicating metabolic alkalosis, the opposite being true for metabolic acidosis (see Appendix 2).

Urinalysis

Urinalysis should be performed in any animal with suspected urinary tract disease or any other systemic disease for which the disease or treatment may impact urinary health. Free-catch urine may be obtained spontaneously during physical examination or animals may be encouraged to urinate by occlusion of the nostrils (sheep), placement in a new clean stall, exposure to a new animal, or by allowing the animal to lie down for a time and then getting them up. Animals which do not voluntarily provide a urine sample and have a patent urinary tract may be catheterized or have cystocentesis performed. All male artiodactyls also possess a urethral diverticulum or recess, at the level of the ischial arch, which communicates with the urethra and contains the ducts of the bulbourethral glands.[10] This structure readily accepts a urinary catheter, preventing retrograde catheterization of the urinary bladder. Catheterization of males is possible through the use of J-curved human cardiac catheters.[11] In ewes and does, a suburethral diverticulum is present below the external urethral orifice, which must be bypassed to allow retrograde catheterization of the urinary bladder.

Urine should be grossly examined for color and clarity, be placed on a commercial dipstick for biochemical testing, and placed on a handheld refractometer for specific gravity determination and be centrifuged at 450G for 3 to 5 minutes for subsequent examination of the sediment and supernatant.[12]

USG is useful for determination of the origin of azotemia and should be determined with a refractometer rather than urine dipsticks, which have an upper limit of 1.025 to 1.030.[11] Urine concentrating ability is lost prior to the occurrence of azotemia so that the production of dilute urine in azotemic animals suggests loss of renal function, with USG > 1.025 considered adequately concentrated in ruminants. USG should be interpreted carefully and not based upon a single sample, as one of the authors (MJ) has observed clinically normal goats without added dietary salts to have USG ranging from as low as 1.003.

Biochemical tests commonly available on urine dipsticks include urine pH, protein, glucose, ketones, occult blood, bilirubin, urobilinogen, nitrites, and USG. Urine pH is best determined on a pH meter,[13] but urine dipstick measurement can provide a useful indication. In ruminants, the pH is normally alkaline, with urine pH generally 7.5 to 8.5.[14] Ruminants commonly experience a paradoxic aciduria in the presence of metabolic alkalosis as a result of abomasal or proximal intestinal obstructions,[15] but this can occur with significant metabolic and acid/base derangements, which occur with severe urinary tract disease. This occurs via a variety of physiologic mechanisms related to volume, sodium, chloride, and potassium depletion.[15]

Urine normally contains very low quantities of protein, and urine dipstick analysis normally reveals negative to trace amounts. However, the normal alkaline urine of sheep and goats influences the protein reaction, leading to falsely elevated protein readings[14] of 1+ or 2+. To definitively determine if elevated protein levels exist, the sulfosalicylic acid turbidity test or colorimetric assays should be performed. If proteinuria is determined to be present, post-renal contributions should be considered when urine was obtained free-catch. These include cystitis, urethritis, and other exudative processes of the distal urinary tract. Proximal causes of proteinuria include pre-renal (e.g., which include hemoglobin from intravascular hemolysis and myoglobin) and post-renal (e.g., inflammatory or degenerative glomerular or tubular damage) causes.[14] Glomerular protein losses tend to be of greater magnitude and result in significant reductions in blood protein levels. Proteinuria may be present in neonatal lambs and kids until about 2 days of age as a result of renal permeability to colostral proteins.[16]

Normally, the urine glucose reaction should be negative. The renal threshold for glucose in ruminants is considered to be 100 to 140 mg/dL,[17] although one study reported a renal glucose threshold in goats to be as low as 81 mg/dL.[18] Blood glucose levels above this threshold range will result in glucosuria, with common causes including *Clostridium perfringens* type D enterotoxemia,[19] corticosteroid, xylazine,[1] or dextrose administration. Less common causes include stress and renal tubular disease.[14]

Urine ketone concentrations are useful for detecting excessive fat metabolism, as are seen with negative energy balance syndromes, including pregnancy toxemia and starvation (see Chapters 2 and 8). Urine ketone concentration is the single most useful test for diagnosis of pregnancy toxemia in ewes and does. There are three ketone bodies produced by the body, with urine ketone strips detecting acetoacetate and acetone, but not β hydroxybutyrate, the primary ketone produced.[14] False-negative or underestimated ketone concentrations may therefore occur due to the volatility of ketone bodies if sample testing is delayed or if β hydroxybutyrate is not a large portion of the ketone bodies produced in an individual animal.

A positive test for urine occult blood can indicate the presence of hemoglobin, myoglobin, or whole blood in the urine sample. Differentiating these can be performed in a stepwise fashion, particularly if the urine is visibly pigmented. Red or brown color cannot be relied upon to indicate the presence of hemoglobin or myoglobin, respectively (Figure 12.1). First, the urine sample should be centrifuged and the sediment examined. If the supernatant loses pigmentation and the sediment is composed of primarily red blood cells, hematuria is present and indicates hemorrhage or an inflammatory condition. If the supernatant remains red or brown and no sediment is produced or does not contain intact red blood cells, hemoglobinuria or myoglobinuria exists. At this time, a blood sample should be drawn and centrifuged in a microhematocrit tube and observed for evidence of hemolysis, including pink plasma and anemia. If no evidence of hemolysis exists, myoglobinuria is the most likely diagnosis and may be confirmed by clinical examination, history, and elevations of muscle enzymes on a serum chemistry panel. Myoglobin is a much smaller molecule than is hemoglobin and passes more readily into the urine. It will be present in the urine without being visible in the plasma. Hemoglobin, however, accumulates in the blood and then, upon exceeding the renal threshold, will be filtered into the urine. Hemoglobin, if visible in the urine, will therefore be visible in the plasma. Differential diagnoses for hematuria, hemoglobinuria, and myoglobinuria may be found in Table 12.1. Diseases which cause purely extravascular or spleen-mediated hemolysis

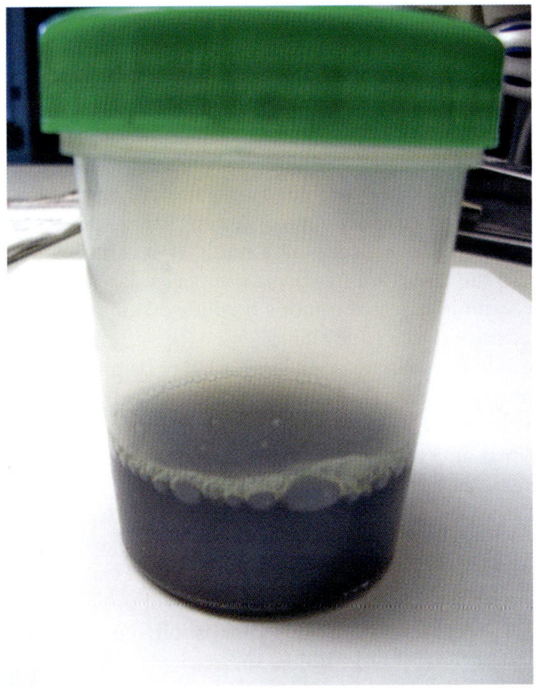

• **Fig. 12.1** Appearance of the urine from a sheep with copper toxicity. This brown-colored urine actually contains large amounts of hemoglobin, not myoglobin, as the color may suggest.

TABLE 12.1 Differential Diagnoses for Red/Brown Pigmented Urine.

Hematuria (Whole Blood)
Cystitis
Pyelonephritis
Contamination from reproductive tract
Bracken fern toxicity
Nonobstructive urolithiasis
Trauma
Disseminated Intravascular Coagulation
Hemoglobinuria
Copper toxicity
Water intoxication/isoerythrolysis (most common in goats)
Leptospirosis
Bacillary hemoglobinuria *(Clostridium haemolyticum)*
Plant toxicity: *Brassica*, onion
Phosphorus deficiency
Myoglobinuria
Severe myodegeneration/myositis
Prolonged recumbency

(e.g., anaplasmosis) will not result in hemoglobinuria, which is produced only when intravascular hemolysis exists. Hypophosphatemic hemoglobinuria has been rarely reported in sheep and goats with feeding histories, including *Brassica* species.[20,21] Neonatal isoerythrolysis has been reported in lambs and kids fed cow colostrum,[22] but hemoglobinuria does not appear to be a common clinical finding. Cold water isoerythrolysis has been reported in a variety of species rapidly consuming large amounts of cold water. The condition occurs as a result of fragility of red blood cells from the reduction in plasma osmolality. The red blood cells of goats exhibit increased osmotic fragility, making this species the most sensitive to the condition.[23]

Bilirubinuria (conjugated bilirubin) may be present as a result of hemolytic disease, hepatic insufficiency, and biliary obstruction. It should be noted that urobilinogen, nitrites, and USG, as determined on a dipstick, are not considered diagnostic in veterinary medicine.[12,14]

Urinary gamma glutamyltransferase (GGT), available through reference laboratories, has been shown to be of diagnostic value of nephropathies in sheep and goats due to its presence in proximal tubular cells, where serum concentrations will not be affected.[24,25] Urine GGT concentrations in normal adult sheep have been reported to be 5 to 33 U/L (mean, 13.9 U/L)[7] and 6.8 to 24.6 U/L (mean, 15.7 U/L).[26] Urinary GGT levels have been shown to increase a mean of 4.5 days after experimental aminoglycoside-induced nephrotoxicosis in sheep.[27]

Urine sediment examination is performed to determine the presence of cells, bacteria, casts, crystals, or other debris. Cells, typically erythrocytes, leukocytes, and epithelial cells, may originate from any level of the urinary tract. Red and white blood cells degenerate quickly in urine and can be accurately identified only in fresh samples. Large amounts of erythrocytes indicate the presence of hematuria as a cause of red urine or a positive fecal occult blood test, and differential diagnoses are listed in Table 12.1. The presence of large numbers of leukocytes, particularly neutrophils, indicates the presence of inflammatory exudates, which most commonly originate from the renal pelvis or urinary bladder. If bacteria are noted on urinalysis, it is important to determine if they are contaminants or the cause of urinary tract inflammation. The presence of white blood cells, in addition to bacteria, suggests legitimate bacterial presence. A cystocentesis sample, along with bacterial culture, should be obtained to further clarify this. When accompanied by dysuria or stranguria, this exudate likely originates from the lower urinary tract, while signs of systemic illness would indicate an origin in the upper urinary tract. Differential diagnoses for pyuria include contamination of the prepuce or female reproductive tract, pyelonephritis, cystitis, urolithiasis, and neoplasia. Epithelial cells are normally present in low numbers in the urine and, if present in large numbers, generally indicate contamination at collection but should be confirmed to be nonneoplastic.[14]

Urinary casts are forms of proteins and/or cells that originate in the kidney. Hyaline casts are protein-only casts and indicate glomerular protein leakage, and the formation of these casts is increased with highly concentrated or acidic urine. Cellular casts may be made up of red or white blood cells or epithelial cells and indicate hemorrhage, infection, or tubular sloughing, respectively, all of renal origin. Granular casts and waxy casts are casts that were cellular but have been degraded. Casts may be broken down in alkaline urine and should only be interpreted from freshly obtained urine.[14]

Crystalluria is important in small ruminant urinalysis, due to the commonality of urolithiasis in small ruminants. The most common urolith components include struvite (magnesium ammonium phosphate), apatite (calcium phosphate), calcium carbonate, and silicate. Crystals may be present in clinically normal animals due to the alkaline urine of ruminants and dietary contributors and should be interpreted in light of other risk factors for urolithiasis to determine case management. Alternatively, in the authors' experience, the urine of obstructed animals obtained from cystocentesis or cystotomy is often free of crystals.

Ultrasound Examination

Transabdominal ultrasound is more frequently utilized than transrectal examination for urinary tract evaluation in small ruminants. The kidneys and urinary bladder are readily evaluated, as well as surrounding soft tissue structures, swellings, and the peritoneal cavity. The ureters and urethra may be impossible to identify in normal sheep or goats.[28,29] For transabdominal evaluation, a 3.5- or 5-mHz curvilinear or linear probe is typically used, with the left kidney situated in the dorsal region of the right paralumbar fossa and the right kidney visualized dorsally in the 11th and 12th intercostal spaces.[30] In sheep, goats and cervids, the kidney is smooth, lacking the lobulation seen in cattle[28,29] (see Figures 12.2 and 12.3). Reference ranges for the ultrasonographic evaluation of the urinary tracts of sheep have been published.[28,29] In ewes weighing between 41 and 89 kg, the mean length, width, and depth of the left kidney was 8.2 cm, 4.4 cm, and 4.0 cm, respectively.[29] Rams of the same size range had mean left kidney measurements of 8.4 cm in length, 4.7 cm in width, and 4.4 cm in depth, similar to measurements seen in the right kidney.[28]

Abnormalities frequently noted on renal ultrasound include hydronephrosis, pyelonephritis, cysts, neoplasms, and perirenal fluid accumulation. Hydronephrosis is evidenced by a dilated collection system filled with anechoic fluid. Pyelonephritis is marked by renal enlargement with dilated renal sinus, containing echogenic debris in varying amounts.[31] The ureters may also be dilated.[31] Cysts and neoplastic masses may also be noted as hypoechoic fluid-filled or solid masses on the surface of the kidney or within the renal parenchyma. Perirenal fluid accumulation may be inflammatory in origin but is more commonly seen secondary to urinary tract rupture, where the fluid will be anechoic.

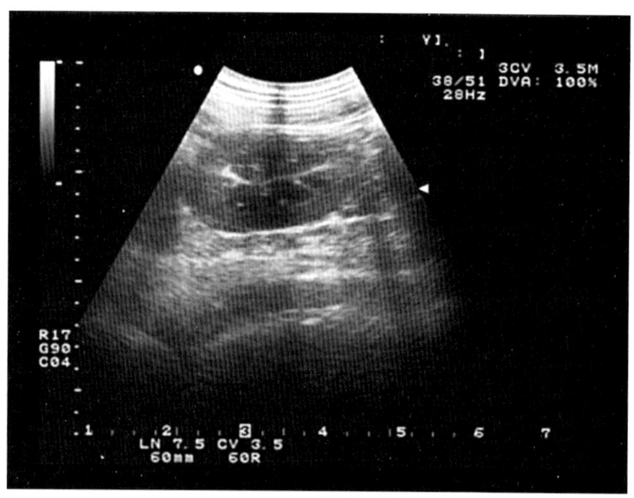

• Fig. 12.2 Transabdominal ultrasound of the right kidney of a healthy ram. This image is taken in the dorsal aspect of the right paralumbar fossa using a 3.5-mHz curvilinear probe.

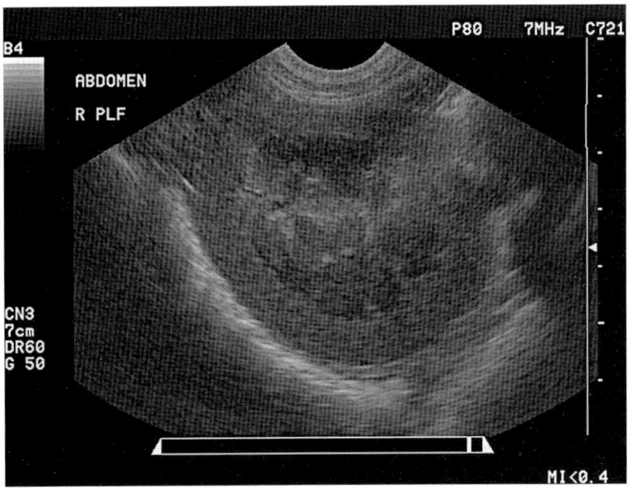

• **Fig. 12.3** Ultrasound of the right kidney obtained from the right paralumbar fossa of a 3-year-old LaMancha cross doe demonstrating the characteristic echogenic renal pelvis and the nearly anechoic appearance of the medulla compared to the echogenic renal cortex. The corticomedullary junction is easily distinguished. This ultrasound was obtained with a 7-MHz microconvex transducer. Dorsal is to the left of the image. (Courtesy Dr. Karine Pader, Purdue University.)

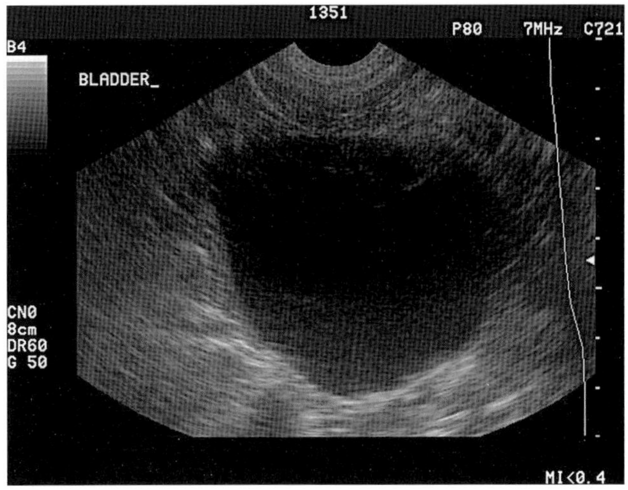

• **Fig. 12.4** Ultrasound of the bladder obtained from a 2-year-old crossbred ram. The bladder appears as an oval shaped, anechoic, fluid-filled structure with echogenic margins that represent the bladder walls. Echogenic material is normally seen at the ventral aspect of the bladder and represents mucus and sedimentation within the bladder. This ultrasound was obtained from the inguinal region with a 7-MHz microconvex transducer and the ram in dorsal recumbency. (Courtesy Dr. Karine Pader, Purdue University.)

The urinary bladder is visualized in the right inguinal region or may be examined transrectally. Urinary bladder diameter, wall thickness, mural changes, and intraluminal contents may be evaluated. In female sheep, the diameter of the urinary bladder ranged from 0.3 to 6.9 cm in 96.8% of sheep, with a mean diameter of 3.6 ± 1.6 cm.[29] In rams, urinary bladder diameter ranges between 1.8 and 13.2 cm, with a mean of 7.5 ± 2.8 cm. In goats with obstructive urolithiasis, the urinary bladder was distended to 4 to 15 cm (mean, 7 cm) and 8 to 12 cm (mean, 9.5 cm) in small and large breed goats, respectively,[32] so there is overlap between bladder diameter in goats with patent and nonpatent urinary tracts. Wall thickness varies based upon bladder fullness, with the wall thickness normally decreasing as bladder volume increases.[29] Therefore, a thick wall in a distended bladder may indicate inflammation or other mural infiltration. The wall of the urinary bladder should also be examined for the presence of nodules or other abnormalities along the interior or exterior of the urinary bladder. Normal urine within the urinary bladder is anechoic, but it is common to note some minor, echogenic debris within the bladder lumen (Figure 12.4). With hematuria, pyuria, or urinary calculosis, the ventrum of the urinary bladder may contain hyperechoic material. During transabdominal ultrasound, with the probe in contact with the abdominal wall, the operator may shake the probe and abdominal wall vigorously to determine and demonstrate the presence of cellular debris, blood clots, or uroliths within the urinary bladder, differentiating this from masses associated with the bladder wall.

Transabdominal ultrasound is also useful for determining the presence of excess free abdominal fluid. Visual determination of the character of the fluid on ultrasound is the first step in identification and classification of the fluid type. Anechoic fluid signifies a transudate or modified transudate, as would be seen with urine leakage, whereas fluid with echoic (cells or protein) debris is consistent with inflammatory or exudative processes. For thorough characterization of fluid, abdominocentesis should be performed as described later in this chapter (see also Chapter 5).

Cystocentesis

Needle aspiration of urine directly from the urinary bladder avoids potential contamination of urine by the lower urinary tract, providing superior samples for laboratory evaluation, including bacterial culture, and may also be used in the treatment of obstructive urolithiasis where the urinary bladder is intact.[33]

With the animal restrained in left lateral recumbency, the urinary bladder should be identified low in the right flank by deep abdominal palpation or transabdominal ultrasonography. The skin surface is clipped and aseptically prepared and an 18-gauge, 2- to 3.5-inch (5–9 cm) needle with syringe attached is inserted perpendicularly through the skin and abdominal wall and quickly thrust into the bladder lumen. The needle is steadied, at least 10 mL of urine is aspirated, and the needle is quickly withdrawn. Quick, sharp insertion and removal of the needle from the bladder ensure that only a small circular perforation of the urinary bladder wall is made, which will be quickly sealed. Larger, slit-shaped perforations, particularly those made into a distended urinary bladder wall with poor wall integrity, may result in uroperitoneum or sepsis, although this appears to be rare.[33]

Abdominocentesis

Abdominocentesis is useful for determining the character and elucidating the etiology of excess free peritoneal fluid. The most common use of peritoneal fluid analysis in sheep and goats is the diagnosis of uroperitoneum; however, inflammatory exudates and other fluid types may point to other disease conditions.

Abdominocentesis can be performed with ultrasound guidance upon identification of fluid pockets, or the abdomen can be blindly sampled at four sites to increase likelihood of obtaining fluid. The cranial two sites are just caudal to the xiphoid and 1 to 2 inches (2.5–5 cm) to the right or left of midline. The caudal sites are just cranial to the mammary gland or scrotum, also 1 to 2 inches (2.5–5 cm) lateral to the midline. The selected sampling site should be aseptically prepared and a 20- to 18-gauge, 1- to 1.5-inch (2.5–4 cm) needle inserted perpendicular through the skin and into the peritoneal cavity. Alternatively, the skin may be anesthetized with a small volume of 2% lidocaine and a stab incision made through the skin and a teat cannula inserted into the peritoneal cavity for collection. The latter method reduces the likelihood of puncture of abdominal viscera but typically increases blood contamination of the sample.

Fluid obtained should be examined for total protein (TP) level, cytologic count, and differential and creatinine level, if uroperitoneum is suspected. Normal peritoneal fluid from ruminants should be clear and colorless to straw colored. Normal values for TP, total nucleated cell count (TNCC), and differential vary widely in cattle.[34–36] The authors typically consider peritoneal fluid to be within normal limits if it is not present in large amounts, has a TP < 3.0 g/dL and a TNCC < 5000 cells/μL. For abnormal exudates, it is preferable to classify them based upon the pathophysiology behind their creation, rather than simply based upon protein and cell counts.[37]

Protein-poor transudates result from excess diffusion of water or lymph from the vascular space as a result of abnormalities of hydraulic or oncotic pressure. They typically have a TP < 2.0 g/dL and a TNCC < 1500 cells/μL. Causes include protein losing enteropathy or nephropathy, lymphatic obstruction, and portal hypertension. Protein-rich transudates result from inflammatory processes, which increase vascular permeability so that plasma exits the vasculature, often along with leukocytes. These generally have a TP > 2 g/dL and a TNCC > 5000 cells/μL and are caused by bacteria, some viruses, protozoa, parasites, neoplasms, foreign bodies, or uroperitoneum. Hemorrhagic effusions must be differentiated into iatrogenic (occurring at the time of abdominocentesis) and pathologic causes, based on several criteria.[37] These effusions have a TP > 2.0 g/dL and a TNCC > 2000 cells/μL and may be caused by trauma, bleeding disorders, and neoplastic diseases. Effusions caused by a rupture of a hollow organ or other tissue include those resulting from urinary tract rupture, biliary leakage, and GI rupture. In early phases of the disease, uroperitoneum will have the character of urine (very low TP and TNCC) but, with time and irritation to the peritoneum, will take on the characteristics of an exudate with increased TP and TNCC, which may be diluted by high volumes of urine leakage. Early uroperitoneum will usually have a TP < 2.0 g/dL and a TNCC < 1500 cells/μL but with chronicity will have a variable TP and TNCC > 1500 cells/μL.[37,38] Figure 12.5 shows the cytology of peritoneal fluid obtained from an animal with uroperitoneum of a few days' duration. Additional, but less common, effusions include lymphorrhage from lymphatic leakage and multiple-process effusions where multiple pathophysiologic processes alter the character of the peritoneal fluid.[37]

The most common biochemical test performed on peritoneal fluid samples from ruminants is a creatinine concentration. This can definitively diagnose the presence of urine in the abdomen, with creatinine levels greater than two times the serum creatinine indicating that uroperitoneum exists.[39]

Radiography

Survey Radiography. Small ruminants are well suited in size and disposition for table-top radiography, although sedation may be required to achieve full extension of the hindlimbs. Related to urinary tract disease, survey radiography may be utilized to evaluate the peritoneum, body wall, kidneys, ureters, urinary bladder, and the urethra when there is adequate contrast with surrounding tissues. The loss of serosal detail and inability to visualize abdominal organs may be due to decreased intraabdominal fat and abdominal effusions, including blood and urine. Abdominal effusions may be localized or generalized, with generalized effusion typically visible as bilateral ventral abdominal distension. Such effusions may be confirmed by ultrasonography and abdominocentesis. The retroperitoneal space surrounding the kidneys is also evaluated, with fluid and free gas being common abnormalities. These changes are consisted with renal abscessation, body wall trauma, and foreign body presence.

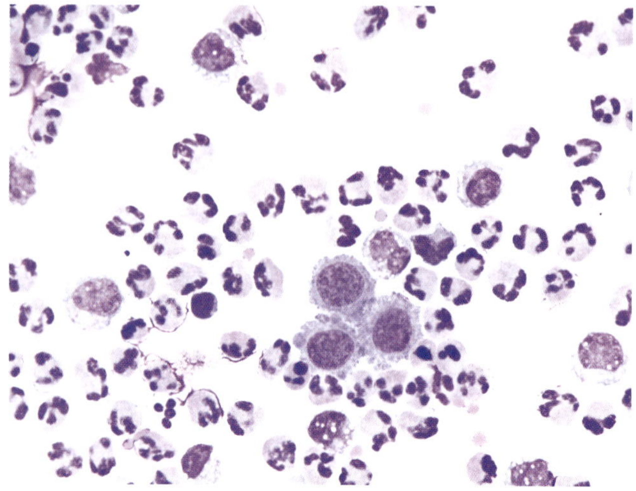

• **Fig. 12.5** Cytologic evaluation of a peritoneal fluid sample from an animal with bilateral ventral abdominal distension. The fluid had a total nucleated cell count of 3.2 K/μL and a total protein of 1.4 g/dL. The blood creatinine was 17.5 mg/dL, while the peritoneal fluid contained 55.7 mg/dL, confirming uroperitoneum. The high number of neutrophils, in the absence of bacteria, is seen with the chemical peritonitis of uroperitoneum.

The number, size, shape, and density of the kidneys are evaluated. Unilateral and bilateral renal agenesis has been reported in lambs.[40,41] In goats, normal kidneys have been found to be 2 to 2.5 times the length of the second lumbar vertebra.[42] Enlarged kidneys may be seen with hydronephrosis, amyloidosis, glomerulonephritis, cysts, or compensatory hypertrophy of a functional kidney. These conditions may also result in kidneys of normal size early in the disease process. Small kidneys typically result from end-stage, chronic renal diseases. Air or mineral opacities may be present in the kidneys, suggestive of abscesses or trauma (air) and uroliths (mineral). The ureters are best visualized with contrast radiography, but air or mineral opacities may be present within the lumen.

The urinary bladder is readily visualized on survey radiographs and most easily evaluated in the lateral view. If the urinary bladder is not visible, potential causes include an empty bladder, decreased intraabdominal fat, and superimposition by other abdominal viscera. The position of the bladder should be evaluated, with ventral displacement occurring from pregnancy, hernias, or urachal remnants. The size of the urinary bladder varies greatly with filling, but an abnormally large urinary bladder suggests obstruction or neurologic deficits, while an abnormally small bladder over time suggests congenital urinary bladder bypass, including ectopic ureter, fistulas, or cystitis and neoplasia inducing frequent bladder emptying. Gas and mineral opacities may also be present in the urinary bladder, with gas introduced via catheterization or infection. If cystic calculi are suspected, horizontal beam radiography can be useful to visualize sediment in the ventral bladder.

The urethra of rams, bucks, and castrated males is an important structure to be evaluated in imaging studies. Survey radiographs are most useful to evaluate the tissues surrounding the urethra and opacities within the urethra. In one study,[32] cystic or urethral calculi were visible in 8 of 10 obstructed goats. The visible stones seen in these studies were calcium carbonate or struvite in composition, while apatite and silicate stones were not seen radiographically.[32] In other studies,[11,43] survey radiographs were of limited usefulness for diagnosing uroliths. Negative survey radiographs should not be interpreted to rule out urolithiasis. Evaluation of the pelvic bones is also important due to fracture impacts on urethral and bladder patency. The urethra is best studied by contrast radiography or endoscopy. Endoscopy is not frequently used in small ruminant urethral studies due to the requirements for diameter and length of the endoscopy unit.

Contrast Radiography. An excretory urogram provides an anatomic and qualitative functional view of the kidneys. The procedure involves the injection of an ionic contrast media intravenously, with sequential radiographs taken up to 40 minutes postinjection. Patients undergoing excretory urography should be adequately hydrated, as opacification of the kidneys is dependent upon glomerular filtration. In normal goats, the kidneys are best visualized if radiographs are taken immediately postinjection.[42] Delayed or reduced opacification indicates dehydration or inadequate glomerular filtration. When evaluating ureteral patency, it should be noted that normal peristalsis can appear as a stricture or narrowing of the lumen. Ureteral patency can be altered by uroliths, blood clots, inflammatory exudates, trauma, or stricture. Excretory urography, in some patients, may not provide visualization of the urinary bladder and urethra.[43]

Contrast cystography and urethrography may be performed in normograde or retrograde fashion and with negative (air) or positive (organic iodide) contrast media. Barium should never be used for urinary imaging. Indications for such procedures include dysuria, pollakiuria, and chronic hematuria. Cystourethrography is best performed in a normograde fashion via a cystotomy tube.[43] For retrograde studies, catheterization may be performed completely only in the female ruminant but may be partially completed in male ruminants. Occlusion of the distal urethral orifice after partial catheter passage allows for the instillation of contrast media in a retrograde fashion. Alternatively, a precurved cardiac catheter may be utilized to bypass the urethral diverticulum.[11] For retrograde studies, a ballooned catheter is used and passed into the urinary bladder in females or a nonballooned catheter is passed a few inches into males and contrast material instilled. The presence of intraluminal contrast material allows for assessment of degree of patency and wall thickness of the urinary bladder and urethra. Mural masses may be visualized and may be caused by cellular or fibrous infiltration. Filling defects of the urinary bladder may be caused by polyps, air, calculi, blood clots, or inflammatory exudates, and urachal diverticula may be seen.[44] Filling defects of the urethra may be caused by air bubbles, calculi, which may be radiopaque or radiolucent, blood clots, neoplasms, inflammation, scar tissue, and extramural compression. Extravasation of contrast material results from traumatic lacerations, fistulas (urethrorectal and urethrovaginal), and diverticula. Fistula between the urethra and corpus spongiosum has been diagnosed by contrast radiography in a goat-sheep after surgery for obstructive urolithiasis.[44]

Renal Biopsy

Renal biopsy is not commonly performed but may provide antemortem diagnosis of metabolic, neoplastic, and toxic diseases of the kidney. In cases where renal abscess is suspected, it is preferable that renal biopsy be performed by fine needle aspiration to reduce the risk of localized or generalized peritonitis. Renal biopsy should be performed in a well-restrained or sedated animal under ultrasound guidance. The skin overlying the last two to three ribs and paralumbar region is aseptically prepared, the skin and body wall are anesthetized with 2% lidocaine, and a stab incision is performed. The ultrasound probe may be placed in a sterile glove filled with ultrasound gel to maintain asepsis and to locate the target kidney. A 14-gauge biopsy instrument is directed into the kidney parenchyma and a sample obtained. Depending on the testing required, obtained tissue should be divided, with both fresh and fixed tissue submitted to a reference laboratory. Potential complications of renal biopsy include hematuria, hematoma, hemoabdomen, and peritonitis. In a retrospective study in 25 cattle, ultrasound-guided percutaneous renal biopsy resulted in six animals having a small subcapsular hematoma (< 2 cm) after the procedure, but no gross or occult hematuria.[45] Another study using serial laparoscopic biopsies in cattle resulted in microscopic hematuria for 1 to 5 days.[46]

DISEASES OF THE KIDNEYS

Clinically, kidney disease is not commonly encountered as a primary problem in small ruminants; however, incidental kidney pathology can often be identified at necropsy.[47] Kidney disease is described based on duration (acute versus chronic) and the character of renal damage leading to dysfunction (glomerular, tubular, and vascular). The clinician's challenge is to recognize situations resulting from primary renal disease and/or risks leading to secondary or induced renal damage. Clinical tendencies of kidney disease are anuria, oliguria, dysuria, abdominal pain, and abnormal urinary constituents. Clinical signs in small ruminants are often synchronized with the multisystem disease processes that lead to renal damage. Therefore, recognition of risk factors, preemptive case management practices, ancillary diagnostics, and postmortem diagnosis are important in overall disease management and prevention.

The general causes of kidney disease are:

- Infectious (bacterial, viral, and parasitic)
- Toxic (chemical, heavy metals, medications, and plant origin)
- Obstruction and trauma (nephroliths, direct)
- Secondary hydronephrosis from ureteral, cystic, and urethral calculi
- Vascular (infarcts, hyperdynamics of sepsis, and toxemia)
- Chronic inflammation (glomerulonephritis, amyloidosis)
- Congenital

Renal Failure

Renal failure occurs when diminished renal function results in persistent metabolic abnormalities such as azotemia as well as the inability to concentrate urine. Renal failure that develops rapidly, within a few hours or days, illustrates ARF and is usually due to intrinsic (vascular, toxic) causes from systemically absorbed toxins, body origin toxins (myoglobin, hemoglobin, and urea), administered therapeutics, or dynamic changes in renal blood flow during sepsis, shock, or toxemia. The kidneys receive a large

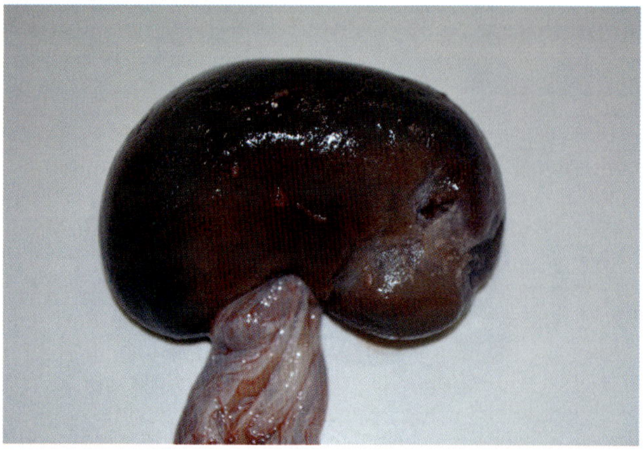

• **Fig. 12.6** This photo was taken of an infarcted kidney, from a mature, farm-raised white-tailed deer doe, who was found dead. *Pasteurella multocida* was cultured out of multiple tissues. Histopathologic examination of the kidney showed a focally extensive region of the cortex expanded by many lymphocytes, plasma cells, and some macrophages. The interstitium was filled with fibrous connective tissue. (Courtesy Dr. Kelley Steury, Auburn, Alabama.)

proportion of circulating blood volume, resulting in high rates of toxin exposure, as well as increased vulnerability to ischemia and reperfusion injury with diseases causing hyperdynamic changes in nutrient blood flow. Toxin exposure is amplified as renal tubules resorb filtered toxins in conjunction with the normal function of urine concentration. Damage to this sensitive portion of the nephron may result in acute tubular necrosis, resulting in loss of urine concentrating ability, protein, glucose, and electrolytes. Consequently, the kidneys provide a good postmortem diagnostic sample for toxins, and urinalysis can provide objective information about the nature of disease (Figure 12.6). The clinician can assume that a degree of damage is occurring during shock, septicemia, dehydration, or toxemia and should take preemptive steps in the preservation and protection of renal function during case management. Changes in blood flow or oxygen delivery to the kidney cause renal insufficiency, potentially leading to ARF or CRF. Dehydration, heat stress, severe rumen bloat, sepsis, and anemia result in physiologic and metabolic changes leading to kidney dysfunction due to decreased cardiac output and renal vasoconstriction and dilation. Exertional (capture) myopathy in cervids may result in ARF[48,49] (see Chapter 20).

Treatment of ARF should include removing any offending toxin or source, promoting diuresis through IV fluid administration and diuretic medications, correcting acid-base and electrolyte derangements, and close monitoring of positive or adverse responses to treatment. Intravenous fluids of choice are 0.9% saline or 0.45% saline + dextrose. Additional IV potassium can be substituted if indicated after initial therapy, being cautious to remain below the generally recommended toxicity rate of 0.5 mEq/kg/h. Diuresis should continue until the patient is producing sufficient volumes of urine. Monitor serum potassium levels and provide parenteral support when using furosemide (1 mg/kg every 2 to 3 hours, to effect). Alternatively, mannitol (1 g/kg bolus) can be used to provide osmotic diuresis. Additional supportive therapy may include secure broad-spectrum antimicrobials against susceptible infectious agents, plasma to treat hypoproteinemia, antiinflammatories, and nutritional support through parenteral nutrition or rumen transfaunation. Urinalysis and FE of electrolytes can be measured in conjunction with serum monitoring parameters during intensively managed cases (see "Ancillary Diagnostic Tests" section in this chapter).

Vasopressors and inotropes can be instituted as adjunct therapy but need to be administered as carefully calibrated constant rate infusions have wide and debated ranges of therapeutic efficacy, and scientific data for use in small ruminants are largely extrapolated from other species, including humans. Much of the human literature, however, is based on information gained from sheep models of disease. Treatment of persistent oliguria or anuria has been addressed by the author using intravenous dopamine (2–5 μg/kg/min), dobutamine (5–10 μg/kg/min), and combination norepinephrine (0.4 μg/kg/min) + dobutamine (5 μg/kg/min), based on information gathered from other sources.[50] It should be noted that the use of dopamine alone in cases of ARF may not be as beneficial as once thought and more potential adverse effects have been discovered.[51,52]

Progressive loss of renal function over a period of months or years describes CRF. In contrast to ARF, where nephron repair and compensatory hypertrophy can occur spontaneously and with treatment, chronic disease results in progressive, permanent, and irreparable damage and fibrosis to the nephron. CRF is may be due to secondary glomerulonephritis or tubulointerstitial disease resulting from immune complex deposition secondary to a distant chronic inflammatory process (abscess and pneumonia). Clinical signs may be nonexistent or limited to failure to thrive. Polyuria/polydipsia is not a frequent historical complaint but may be detected during hospitalization. Antemortem diagnosis is supported by serum markers of azotemia, urine dilution, urinalysis (proteinuria, pyuria), renal biopsy, and ultrasound characteristics of the kidney. Unique characteristics of serum urea nitrogen and creatinine metabolism in ruminants should reviewed for accurate interpretation (see Ancillary Diagnostic Tests section in this chapter). Ultrasound may reveal small, irregular, echodense kidney parenchyma with loss of detail at the cortico-medullary junction, evidence of fluid accumulation (pyelonephritis and hydronephrosis), or echodense foci within the renal calices possibly representing nephroliths. Nonregenerative anemia, hyperkalemia, and other electrolyte abnormalities may be detected on bloodwork. General causes of CRF may be from lasting effects and insufficient compensation of a previous acute episode, pyelonephritis, amyloidosis, congenital, or idiopathic causes. Treatment is supportive to palliative.

Acute Renal Diseases

Infectious Diseases

***C. perfringens* type D.** Disease syndromes caused by *C. perfringens* type D are referred to as enterotoxemia, overeating disease, and pulpy kidney disease. The U.S. Department of Agriculture (USDA)–National Animal Health Monitoring System (NAHMS) Sheep 2001 survey revealed that 38.8% of sheep flocks had suspected or confirmed cases of enterotoxemia, with 30.9% confirmed by veterinary or laboratory examination, in the previous 3 years.[53] Enterotoxemia is most commonly seen in young, growing animals consuming diets high in rapidly fermentable carbohydrates. High milk or starch content allows for excess colonization of the jejunum with *C. perfringens* type D, which produces alpha and epsilon toxins,[54] of which epsilon is the most significant in disease. Epsilon toxin is activated in the intestine and is systemically absorbed, resulting in increased capillary permeability from a loss of endothelial integrity[54,55] and an influx of protein and fluid occurs in the organs and body cavities. Sheep more often experience the systemic form of the disease, characterized by edema throughout the body, including the brain, lungs, and kidneys, often resulting in acute death, while goats develop hemorrhagic enterocolitis.[56,57] The systemic form most often seen in sheep commonly results in acute death, but live animals may exhibit seizures, blindness, recumbency, dyspnea,[58] and other signs consistent with fluid accumulation in and around organs.

At necropsy, visceral edema, serosal hemorrhage, and cavitary effusions may be present, but death from *C. perfringens* type D may also result in no gross lesions. The cortices of the kidney may be softened and have subcapsular petechiae.[58] Epsilon toxin promotes liver glycolysis, resulting in hyperglycemia and glucosuria, making dipstick evaluation of bladder urine a useful test in lambs and kids presented for acute death. After experimental infection in sheep, ileum has been found to be the best sample for isolation of epsilon toxin by enzyme-linked immunosorbent assay (ELISA).[59] Histopathology of the brain reveals microangiopathy with protein surrounding the arteries and veins, which is pathognomonic for *C. perfringens* type D infection,[58,60] but no lesions may be seen in the kidneys.[60] Negative testing for *C. perfringens* type D through any of these means does not necessarily preclude it as the cause of disease.[58,60]

Prevention of *C. perfringens* type D is of utmost importance and should include management using vaccination and gradual dietary adaptation. Bacterin-toxoid as well as antitoxins are commercially available. Antitoxins are most useful in outbreak situations, as they provide rapid passive immunity, but preemptive use of bacterin-toxoids for prolonged, active immunity is preferred for protection against systemic disease. It is recommended that ewes be vaccinated using a *C. perfringens* type D toxoid-containing vaccine 3 to 4 weeks prepartum, which provides passive protection in lambs up to 12 weeks of age.[61] No benefit has been seen in vaccination of lambs prior to 6 weeks of age,[61] so a potential recommendation is to vaccinate lambs at 6 to 10 weeks of age with a booster vaccination given a month later. Although the vaccine is readily available, inexpensive, and effective, currently only 48.4% of flocks in the United States vaccinate breeding or replacement ewes and 66.9% vaccinate nursing lambs and 44.8% vaccinate feeder lambs postweaning, demonstrating a need for producer education based on available research.[61]

Leptospirosis. Sheep and goats may become infected by a number of serovars of *Leptospira interrogans*, resulting in several clinical syndromes, bacterial clearance, or a subclinical carrier state.[62] The kidneys are damaged via hemolysis and interstitial nephritis.

Infected urine is the primary source of infection, with animals obtaining the bacteria from contaminated water or the urine of herdmates, wildlife, rodents, or other domestic animals.[63] In one study of experimental infection of sheep with *L. interrogans* serovar Pomona, clinical disease occurred 34 days after experimental infection.[64] Because the bacteria can penetrate intact mucous membranes and is considered to be the most widespread zoonosis in the world,[65] it should be respected as an occupational hazard for veterinarians, staff, and livestock producers. Leptospiral seropositivity occurs in cervids,[66–68] but the clinical importance or their role in transmission is not well defined.

Animals presented with leptospirosis may show general malaise, fever, icterus, anemia, azotemia, and hemoglobinuria.[69] Hemolytic changes to blood analysis occur 4 to 8 days postinfection.[69] Total white blood cell counts are often elevated with a neutrophilia.[70] A positive result for hemoglobin may occur 3 to 8 days postinfection.[69] Urine sediment exam may show cellular or proteinaceous tubular casts. The herd or flock history may reveal reproductive manifestations as well, including infertility, abortions, and stillbirths. On necropsy, the carcass is icteric[69] and the kidneys are dark red and swollen, with pale foci in the cortices and the liver is often yellow or copper colored.[71] Histopathology reveals a diffuse acute or chronic interstitial nephritis,[70,72] and organisms may be observed. There is often loss of the brush border and necrotic epithelial cells found within the tubules.[64]

Diagnosis is based upon increasing serological titers in the acute and convalescent periods, using the microscopic agglutination test,[73] complement fixation (CF), or ELISA. CF antibodies are short lived (13–18 weeks), while Microscopic Agglutination Test (MAT) antibodies can be detected for longer periods after infection.[69] For urine samples, polymerase chain reaction (PCR), darkfield microscopy, or culture may be used. PCR is preferred as darkfield microscopy has shown false-negative results in infected animals[69] and culture of urine is generally unrewarding due to difficulties in growth in artificial media and intermittent shedding.[74] Histopathology and immunofluorescent antibody[75] may identify organisms in renal tissue. One study has determined that, in herd or flock situations, using MAT for herd-level screening, followed by urine PCR, is suitable for identification of carrier animals.[74]

Several serovars are reported in small ruminants, including *L. interrogans* serovar Pomona, Hardjo, Grippotyphosa, Icterohemorhagiae, Canicola, and Bratislava.[73–78] *L. interrogans* serovar Pomona appears to be the most commonly associated with interstitial nephritis and hepatic centrilobular necrosis.[64,72] It has also been shown to cause severe hemolytic anemia in lambs.[67,72] In one case in lambs, the kidneys were negative for leptospiral organisms, but a rising titer to the Pomona serovar was observed.[70] Ewes administered the hemolysin of *L. interrogans* serovar Pomona experienced a reduction in hemoglobin levels to 57% of the normal range within 48 hours and had lesions similar to animals infected with the whole organism.[71] At necropsy, there was placental separation and autolysis of caruncles and cotyledons in some pregnant ewes.[71] Pigs are the natural reservoir host of *L. interrogans* serovar Pomona.

L. interrogans serovar Hardjo is host adapted to cattle[72] and sheep.[74,76] It has also been reported in a sheep found acutely dead[78] with organisms found in the renal tubular epithelium and tubular lumen. Flockmates of this animal were seropositive against serovar Hardjo, with small numbers seropositive against other serovars.[78] One study comparing the hemolytic properties of three serovars of leptospires found serovar Hardjo to be more hemolytic than serovar Pomona.[76] Sheep with renal infections of serovar Hardjo may not harbor the bacterium in their reproductive tracts,[79,80] while sheep experimentally infected with serovar Hardjo-bovis show renal localization and harbor the bacteria up to 242 days postinfection.[80] Treatment of leptospirosis consists of intravenous crystalloid fluid therapy combined with blood transfusion in clinically anemic animals. Because of the difficulty in culturing the organism, antimicrobial therapy is based upon anticipated spectrum of coverage. In cattle shedding leptospires in the urine, the following antibiotic regimens were shown to clear urinary shedding of organisms: oxytetracycline (20 mg/kg IM, once), tilmicosin (10 mg/kg subcutaneously [SC], once), dihydrostreptomycin-penicillin G (25 mg/kg IM, once), or ceftiofur sodium (2.2 or 5 mg/kg IM every 24 hours for 5 days or 20 mg/kg IM every 24 hours for 3 days). It should be noted that tilmicosin is toxic to goats and should be used only in sheep.[81,82]

Vaccination for control of leptospirosis may be useful in reducing urinary shedding but should not be relied upon for protection from disease. Bovine-labeled vaccines are commonly used and suffer from questionable efficacy and duration of immunity even in label species.[83–85] In designing management plans for leptospirosis, consideration should be given to biosecurity for new additions, control of access to wild and domestic animals, and the accessibility of potentially contaminated water sources.

Adenovirus. Many serotypes of adenovirus infect sheep worldwide with varied tissue tropism and unpredictable pathogenicity. Exposure and seroconversion are common, and it was identified in the interstitial vasculature of lamb kidneys during routine postmortem examination.[86,87] The virus can be isolated from nasal secretions and feces of healthy sheep as well as those with respiratory or GI disease. Many infections go unnoticed; however, the virus was the cause of acute mortality in an outbreak involving several young lambs in the United States.[88] Histopathology revealed a highly cellular, mainly cortical interstitial nephritis, with intranuclear inclusion bodies, in all three lambs where the virus was identified. Evidence of systemic disease was also apparent with hepatic necrosis. Experimental infection with some strains has resulted in similar pathologic findings.[89]

General supportive therapy could be beneficial; however, clinical observations indicate rapid progression of disease once recognized. Recognition and preventive management practices should be carried out if problems develop. Specific vaccines are not available.

Lamb Nephrosis. A yet to be determined cause for acute necrotic nephrosis in young (~1-month-old) lambs has been described as a condition seen during the early grazing season, particularly in the United Kingdom and surrounding regions.[90–93] Occasional sporadic occurrences are documented in various governmental disease surveillance reports to date. Associated causes for nephrosis such as coccidia and other GI parasites, *Salmonella*, pestivirus, and plant, chemical, and gentamicin toxicities should be ruled out before diagnosing idiopathic nephrosis. Nephrosis and associated staphylococcal skin scald syndrome has also been reported in two approximately 5-month-old Merino lambs.[94]

A progressive, terminal illness develops over a few days. Lethargy, weakness, and ataxia progress to recumbency and death. Diarrhea and dehydration are also common. Serum chemistry and urinalysis are consistent with a nephrotic syndrome with azotemia, hypoalbuminemia, and proteinuria and inactive urine sediment. Gross necropsy findings reveal large, soft, pale kidneys. Microscopic examination reveals renal tubular degeneration and necrosis focusing on the proximal convoluted tubules and renal cortices. Hyaline to fibrin-like casts may be seen in the distal tubules and collecting ducts with dilation of the distal convoluted tubules. Focal glomerular lesions may also be observed.[91]

Supportive fluid and electrolyte therapies are indicated. Institute preventive measures aimed at concurrent disease processes.

Toxic Diseases

Toxic insult to the kidney occurs with a wide variety of substances (bacterial endotoxins, plants, metals, and body metabolites) and array of severities. Toxic nephropathy generally occurs due to vascular (ischemia and reperfusion) dynamics and direct tubular injury. Glomerular damage may also occur. Endogenous toxicity from hemolytic disease and myopathies may lead to delivery of large of amounts of hemoglobin and/or myoglobin causing renal vasoconstriction and tubular obstruction from protein coagulation.

Plants. Nephrotoxic plants are common sources of acute kidney disease, and a summary table is provided in Table 10.2. Tannins (oak), soluble and insoluble oxalate-containing plants

TABLE 12.2 Summary of Some Commonly Implicated Nephrotoxic Plants Including Family, Genus, Species, and Common Names Generated to Serve as a Guide to Finding More Specific Information.

Plant Family	Common Names and Species	Toxic Principle (Renal)	Comments
Chenopodiaceae	Lamb's quarters (*Chenopodium* spp.) Halogeton *(H. glomerulatus)* Greasewood *(Sarcobatus vermiculatus)* Russian thistle (*Salsola* spp.) Mexican fireweed *(Kochia scoparia)* Smother weed *(Bassia hyssopifolia)*	Soluble sodium and potassium oxalates. Plants are often weeds found in disturbed alkaline or acidic soils such as seen with overgrazed pastures, along roadsides or railways, dry watersheds or lakes, floodplains, etc. Plants are generally not considered palatable and toxic consumption dose is variable, partially due to rumen adaptation during gradual introduction but also due to variable oxalate concentration between plants. Green and dried forms of the plants are considered toxic. Often cause mixture of systemic clinical signs.	*Chenopodium* spp. may cause GI signs due to irritation from terpenes found in the plant oils. *Kochia* may also cause photosensitivity, toxic hepatitis, and polioencephalomalacia. Commonly accumulate nitrates.
Polygonaceae	Rhubarb *(Rheum rhaponticum)* Beets/sugarbeets *(Beta vulgaris)* Dock Orchard sorrel, Indian tobacco (*Rumex* spp.)		*Beta* and *Rumex* spp. are nitrate accumulators
Oxalidaceae	Wood sorrel Oxalis, Lady's sorrel (*Oxalis* spp.)		Potassium oxalates, very acidic
Amaranthaceae	Pigweed (*Amaranthus* spp.)		May see perirenal edema and nephrosis at necropsy. Nitrate accumulators.
Solanaceae	Jessamine/jasmine *(Cestrum diurnum)* Nightshades *(Solanum malacoxylon)*	Vitamin D–containing plants.	Cause generalized soft tissue mineralization including glomerular and interstitial fibrosis. Often concomitant GI and/or nervous clinical signs due to toxic alkaloids
Fagaceae	Oak (*Quercus* spp.)	Tannins (tannic acids) and pyrogallol from rumen conversion. Direct GI, liver, and kidney toxins. Pyrogallol can cause methemoglobinemia in sheep.	All oak species considered toxic. Prolonged consumption of immature leaf stages (spring) or acorns (fall).

GI, Gastrointestinal.

(many), vitamin D plants *(Cestrum, Solanum)*, and sudan/sorghum are potential sources of nephrotoxins in grazing and fed animals.[95,96] Seasonal variations in toxicity are observed as seen with *Quercus* spp. (oak), and ruminants may undergo rumen adaptation to safely graze toxic plants such as those containing oxalates. Herbicides such as paraquat, a defoliant, if grazed soon after application, may result in acute renal tubular necrosis in addition to respiratory symptoms. Pet sheep and goats or those escaping pastures to explore may become exposed to ornamental plants with toxic principles (lilies, ivy, and oleander).[97,98] Many of the nephrotoxic plants, particularly those causing oxalate toxicity, are also nitrate accumulators. Plant origin nephrotoxins often also exhibit mixed effects on cardiac, GI, respiratory, and hepatic systems. Specific mechanisms of action may not yet be determined in some direct nephrotoxic plants such as *Isotropis* spp.[99] and the kidneys are susceptible to secondary damage from toxins primarily affecting other organ systems.

In general, browsing animals are considered relatively resistant to the effects of toxic plants.

Clinical manifestation and pathologic lesions are most often consistent with acute tubular necrosis in those plants with affinity for inducing nephrotoxicity. Clinical signs are usually acute-onset lethargy, depression, oliguria, and neurologic signs often expected. Anticipated clinicopathologic findings are hyponatremia, hypochloremia, hypocalcemia, hyperkalemia, metabolic alkalosis, azotemia, hyposthenuria, enzymuria, glucosuria, dark tubular casts, and changes in the FE of electrolytes. Gross necropsy observations usually reveal swollen, pale to dark, edematous kidneys and peri-renal edema. Histopathologic lesions are generally focused on tubular damage characterized by necrotic epithelial tubular desquamation, hyaline casts forming with distal tubular obstruction, intact basement membranes, and relatively unaffected glomeruli. Oxalate toxicity may cause urolith and nephrolith formation and polarizing calcium oxalate crystals may be see in the tubular lumen.[95] Gross and microscopic pathologic changes reveal generalized calcification of tissues that accompany nephrotoxicity involving vitamin D containing plants.

Acute toxicity is often treatable as tubular regeneration is possible. The animals should be removed from the offending toxin. Rumenotomy and evacuation can be considered if history indicates exposure is less than 12 to 24 hours' duration (see Chapter 5). Fluid and electrolyte replacement therapy and correction of acid-base are indicated (see Chapter 3). Fluids should contain sodium chloride with added potassium and calcium. Saturated calcium hydroxide solution orally may bind unabsorbed soluble oxalates.

A key management strategy is to prevent or minimize exposure by recognizing plants with potential to cause disease as well as seasonal variations. This allows for better grazing management and implementation of measures to avoid exposure. Animals that are hungry or starved will more likely consume dangerous plants when given the opportunity. Ruminants can safely graze many oxalate-contaminated pastures if given time to adapt and not grazing during rapid growth phases of the plants. Feeding dicalcium phosphate, salt, and supplemental hay can minimize toxicity.

Ethylene Glycol. Another oxalogenic nephrotoxin of potential risk to small ruminants is ethylene glycol (EG). EG is a compound found in automotive antifreeze coolants, brake, transmission fluid, and windshield cleaning fluids, as well as a component of many industrial solvents and detergents, all of which are commonly found in farm environments. EG converts to nephrotoxic metabolites, mainly glycolic acid, by the liver, which then cause renal damage. Calcium oxalate crystals also form and are deposited in renal tubules causing further kidney damage.[100] Toxicity is commonly encountered in dogs and cats, but poisoning is rarely reported in farm animals. An early report in a calf was followed by experimental reproduction in cattle.[101] Lethal doses are 5 to 10 mL/kg in mature cattle and 2 mL/kg in preruminating calves.[101,102] The rumen provides some resistance to toxicity through normal oxalate metabolic degradation by microbes but also serves as a reservoir prolonging absorption EG. Contaminated feedstuffs and byproducts may serve as a source of EG; thus, feed analysis may be indicated with compatible clinical and diagnostic findings.[103,104] A clinical case of EG intoxication has been reported in a pygmy goat with similar clinical signs and progression as reported in other species.[105]

Central neurologic signs (ataxia, depression, and loss of menace), hypersalivation, tachypnea, GI atony, and rumen bloat are typically described as presenting clinical complaints. Clinical signs are a result of initial degradation of EG to glyoxylic acid by dehydrogenases resulting in central nervous system (CNS) depression and acidosis. A more commonly occurring differential diagnosis would be polioencephalomalacia. Hemolytic anemia, hemoglobinuria, and ocular signs may occur less commonly. Progressive depression and recumbency follow with oliguric/anuric renal failure, leading to death in 2 to 10 days, depending on exposure rate. Recovery is possible as described in calves (4–5 months old) with experimental toxicity dosed at 7.5 mL/kg for 2 consecutive days.[102] Azotemia, metabolic acidosis, hypocalcemia, and hyperphosphatemia are expected serum chemistry findings. Urinalysis reflects tubular disease with proteinuria and oxalate crystalluria.

Necropsy findings are consistent with oxalate toxicosis and histopathology revealing birefringent crystals seen in the renal tubules. Frothy rumen contents may be present and may have a sweet smell if intoxication was due to antifreeze consumption. Differentiate EG poisoning from plant oxalate poisoning through tissue testing. Chemical analysis for EG and glycolic acid should be performed on rumen contents, urine, renal tissue, and ocular fluid.

Aggressive fluid therapy with isotonic sodium chloride and bicarbonate should be instituted early; additional calcium and potassium can be added later. Ethanol 20% IV saturates alcohol dehydrogenase enzymes preventing glycosylation of EG, thus allowing excretion of unaltered nontoxic EG. Bolus doses of 20% ethanol (5 mL/kg) at 6- to 8-hour intervals for 24 to 36 hours as well as doses of 50 mL/hour have been recommended. In ruminants, EG lingers in the rumen for days, allowing for prolonged absorption. 4-Methylpyrazole, an alcohol dehydrogenase inhibitor, is a reported antidote for EG toxicity that works well in dogs but not cats, and information does not exist about use in ruminants.[106] Oral cathartics or activated charcoal are indicated to help prevent absorption of EG. Supplemental thiamine may also help reduce the toxic effects of glycolic acid.[96] Rumenotomy and rumen evacuation could be attempted, but patient stability should be closely assessed (see Chapter 5).

Heavy Metals. Metals (zinc, lead, mercury, cadmium, copper, and arsenic) are potential sources of nephrotoxicity arising from environmental as well as feed sources.[107] Copper toxicosis is the most clinically recognized toxicity in small ruminants. Other metals only occasionally cause or have the potential to cause secondary kidney disease; however, the kidneys provide a diagnostic tissue source for evaluating exposure. Cadmium, an environmental contaminant that can cause acute endothelial renal tubular disease, has been reproduced experimentally only in sheep, although exposure and accumulation of the toxin in ruminants have been documented.[108] Lead poisoning is more commonly recognized as a neurologic disease arising from consumption of batteries, lead-based paints, oil, and contaminated water, but lesions indicating chronic kidney degeneration may be discovered at necropsy. Mercury toxicosis is very unlikely to be a cause of toxicity in sheep or goats and has never been reported. Zinc and arsenic are primarily GI toxins but affect cells with high metabolic rates, including the kidneys.

Copper Toxicity. Acute copper toxicity results from ingestion of high copper feeds, copper salts, pesticides, poultry litter, and other high-copper substances. Acute copper poisoning can occur at copper intakes of 20–50 mg/kg in sheep,[109] while goats are tolerant of copper. Chronic copper toxicity occurs when high levels of copper are ingested over time but at doses below the acutely toxic level. Sheep are the most susceptible species to chronic copper toxicity because their liver cells have a high affinity for copper and they excrete copper into the bile at a very low rate, leading to a build-up of liver copper concentration over time. The USDA-NAHMS Sheep 2001 survey reported that 2.9% of flocks incurred at least one case of copper toxicity in the preceding 3 years.[53] One of the most common causes of toxicity in sheep is the accidental feeding of feedstuffs intended for other livestock. Molybdenum reduces the accumulation of copper in the liver. The ratio of copper to molybdenum in the feed is therefore an important factor determining the risk of copper poisoning. Chronic copper toxicity typically involves the ingestion of feeds that have a high copper-to-molybdenum ratio. Any feed that tests to have copper levels >20 ppm copper is potentially toxic to sheep, while a copper-to-molybdenum ratio of >10:1 approaches toxicity for sheep.[109] It is important to note that the feeding of monensin to sheep increased hepatic copper and copper retention in the liver compared with animals that consumed a diet not supplemented with monensin.[110] Serum copper levels have been shown to be higher in steers fed monensin or lasalocid.[111]

Copper is a strong oxidizing agent. It binds to proteins in the liver cells and is stored in lysosomes within hepatocytes.[112] If the copper remains stored in lysosomes, it does not cause tissue damage. Copper can, however, be spontaneously released or released at times of stress, including shearing, weather extremes, or transport. Chronic copper poisoning is often described as a stress-related disease. When copper enters the blood, it partitions into red cells, elevating red cell copper levels 15 to 20 times, while plasma copper levels only increase two to three times. It causes oxidative injury to hemoglobin, inducing Heinz body formation and converting it to methemoglobin, which cannot bind O_2 or CO_2. The sulfhydryl groups of the red blood cell membrane also undergo oxidative change,[113] resulting in significant hemolysis and anemia. Finally, this massive release of hemoglobin can result in hemoglobinuric nephrosis and renal failure.

Many animals affected by copper toxicity are simply found dead. Necropsy findings will include icterus and "gun metal blue" kidneys. In the live animal, icterus, red or brown urine, anorexia, pallor, weakness, and recumbency are common signs. Brown blood or pink serum may be noted on blood collection and processing; anemia and, in some cases, evidence of red blood cell regeneration will be present on blood work. Elevations in creatinine are expected in animals with renal involvement. Hepatocellular injury and bile duct occlusion occur as the copper release and the enzymes AST and GGT levels may be used to predict animals at risk of copper toxicity and risk of death and have been shown to rise above normal at least 9 weeks before clinical signs in some animals.[114]

Animals presenting alive ill exhibit anorexia, weakness, icterus, and hemoglobinuria.[115] Once these clinical signs are recognized, the current feed for the flock should be withdrawn pending testing for both copper and molybdenum. Because copper may be stored in the liver for up to 18 months, it is common to find that the current feed is not the source. On necropsy, fresh samples of liver and kidney should be submitted to a diagnostic laboratory for copper levels. Serum copper levels are unreliable in live animals due to the primary storage in liver. If serum copper levels are elevated (>2.0 ppm), this is diagnostic. If the levels are below this level, copper toxicity cannot be excluded because the elevation in serum copper concentration is often transient. Liver copper levels should also be interpreted with caution because the release of copper from the liver during the disease process can significantly reduce liver copper concentrations.

Treatment is complicated by economic restrictions and antidote availability. *Methylene blue* (4–10 mg/kg slow IV; given to effect) is important in controlling the acute methemoglobinemia. Doses up to 15 mg/kg have been shown to be safe in sheep.[116] Response is typically rapid with a noticeable effect expected within 15 minutes. The low end of the dose range may be repeated if additional doses are required. Methylene blue is a potential carcinogen, and because of the lack of residue studies that account for bound methylene blue in tissues, a slaughter withholding of 180 days has been recommended by the U.S. Food and Drug Administration (FDA) in any species.[117] Free methylene blue is not readily retained in the body and is almost completely eliminated by 14 days, this being the current recommendation for withholding in cattle published by the Food Animal Residue Avoidance Database (FARAD),[117] but all withdrawals should be confirmed to be current by direct contact with FARAD. *Sodium thiosulfate* (1000 mg per animal) is administered orally once daily for 3 weeks. This usually comes in an injectable form, which is administered orally. This drug is considered by FARAD to not be a concern for slaughter, but it is recommended to impose a slaughter withdrawal of 24 hours.[117] *D-penicillamine* (26 mg/kg orally twice daily for 6 days) is a heavy metal chelator and increases copper excretion via urine. The recommended slaughter withdrawal is 21 days.[114] *Ammonium tetrathiomolybdate* (1.7 mg/kg IV every other day for three treatments) decreases the absorption of copper and increases removal from liver.[118] A 10-day slaughter withdrawal is recommended, along with a 5-day milk withholding.[117] *Vitamin C* (500 mg subcutaneously) may also be useful in treating copper toxicity as ascorbic acid counters red blood cell oxidative damage, as may zinc and vitamin E supplementation.[119,120] Supportive treatments, including blood transfusions and aggressive intravenous fluid therapy, should be considered as indicated by clinical and economic parameters. When addressing individual ill animals, it is also important to consider flock management. It is recommended that sodium thiosulfate, at the above listed dosage, be administered to all at-risk animals daily for 3 weeks to facilitate copper removal from the liver.

There is considerable overlap of adequate and toxic copper levels in the serum of sheep and goats, making serum an inadequate sample for definitive diagnosis.[109] Liver copper levels in goats above 180 ppm wet weight and above 100 ppm wet weight in sheep are considered high, with levels >250 in sheep and >230 in goats considered toxic.[109] Liver and kidney levels of copper should be accompanied by histopathology in order to document organ damage and failure due to heavy metal toxicosis.

Antibiotic Toxicity. Some antibiotics have the potential to cause acute kidney disease, particularly when used in dehydrated animals or during episodes of altered renal perfusion such as shock. Due to concerns about violative residues with aminoglycoside usage in farm animals, aminoglycoside (gentamicin, neomycin) usage has greatly diminished. Gentamicin concentrations are cumulative in the renal tubules and may cause cell death through mitochondrial oxidation or other mechanisms.[95,121] In addition to cardiac affects, tetracyclines can cause nephrotoxicity when given at high doses or in dehydrated cattle, although similar occasions have not been documented in small ruminants.[122,123] Sulfonamides have the potential of causing renal disease due to deposition of precipitates in the renal tubules, resulting in decreased blood flow and urine concentration.

Judicious use of antibiotics, patient status recognition, risk factors, and prompt detection of adverse effects should eliminate severe consequences regarding antibiotic toxicity.[121] Clinical signs of toxicity are consistent with tubular nephrosis, and crystalluria may be seen with sulfonamide toxicity. Discontinuing potentially nephrotoxic substances, providing intravenous fluids, and diuresis can reverse toxic insult and result in recovery.

Chronic Renal Diseases

Systemic Disease

Acute and chronic respiratory, GI, and dermal diseases are common and have the potential to lead to direct renal pathology and dysfunction through seeding infection and abscess formation within the kidney or embolic showering. Often, lesions seen in the kidneys secondary to a primary disease are subclinical. Sheep and goats are susceptible to infection with *Corynebacterium pseudotuberculosis*, leading to chronic systemic abscess formation including the kidney. *Staphylococcus* spp., *Streptococcus* spp., *Salmonella*, *Escherichia coli*, *Chlamydia*, *Klebsiella* spp., as well as other environmental contaminants can cause embolic disease, renal infarcts, and abscesses. Conidiobolomycosis, a fungal disease seen in tropical regions, primarily affects the upper airway/ethmoids but can also disseminate to the kidney.[124] Chronic intravenous catheterization is a risk factor for renal infarction and kidney dysfunction. Evaluation of indwelling catheter effects on kidneys in sheep revealed immune-mediated glomerulonephritis; however, clinical disease was not apparent.[125] Renal lipomatosis was reported as more of an incidental finding in a 5-month-old lamb with severe coccidiosis as the primary problem.[126]

Pyelonephritis. Urinary tract infections (UTIs) may cause chronic kidney disease in small ruminants but is a less commonly reported condition than in cattle. As with other species, infection of the kidney results most commonly from ascending infection of pathogenic bacteria. Bacterial infections may arise from normal inhabitants of the genitourinary epithelium, GI tract, or the environment. Infection may ascend from the urinary bladder to cause unilateral or bilateral disease of the ureters and kidneys. Pyelonephritis of the left kidney is more common, thought to be due to a shorter ureteral distance from the bladder, although bilateral disease may be present. Ascending infection originating from the lower urinary tract is more likely in females due to the shorter urethra and is often reported with a history of decreased frequency of urination and with post-parturient diseases. Dehydration, spinal disease, and anatomical anomalies may result in lower volumes of urine produced and decreased urine flow. Down animals that are unable to rise often urinate infrequently, if at all without assistance, and are in closer prolonged proximity to environmental contaminants. Other origins for ascending infection may be from an infected urachus in neonates, indwelling transabdominal cystostomy tubes and cystic-cutaneous marsupialization for urethral obstruction, or introduced through urethral catheterization and obstetric manipulation. Hematogenous spread is possible and inflammatory urinary diseases or trauma may increase the likelihood of establishing infection. Inflammation within the urinary tract from trauma or urinary calculi increases the risk of an established UTI, although *E. coli* and *Corynebacterium renale* can establish primary infections in normal mucosa.

The most commonly isolated organisms from pyelonephritis cases are *E. coli* and *C. renale*. *E. coli* is more commonly considered an environmental or opportunistic pathogen, whereas *C. renale* is commonly considered the agent of "infectious" epithelium. Poor on-farm environmental hygiene increases the frequency of clinical disease. *C. renale* disseminates into the environment from infected animals and may survive there for 2 months.[127] Other *Corynebacterium* species, coliforms, and *Arcanobacterium pyogenes* are also capable of causing disease. Some recognized pathogens have been isolated from the male genital tract, *Corynebacterium* spp. in bulls and *Eubacterium suis* (formerly *Corynebacterium*) in boars, which makes venereal transmission possible.[128,129] Since *C. renale* and *E. coli* can be recognized as normal flora in healthy animals, bacterial fimbriae attachments, urine pH, and other factors enhance the chances of establishing clinical infection in individuals. *Mycobacterium avium* subsp. *paratuberculosis* has been associated with pyelonephritis in a free-ranging red deer in Portugal.[130]

Ill thrift, fever, and vague colic signs may accompany a diagnosis of pyelonephritis. There may also be a history of straining to urinate or pus in the urine. Ancillary diagnostics should include urinalysis for evidence of hematuria, leukouria, bacteriuria, and proteinuria. Isosthenuria with an alkaline pH is expected. It is important to observe the complete urination period as debris may have settled to the ventral bladder and only be voided terminally in the urination process. Transabdominal palpation should be performed in an attempt to determine pain elicited on palpation of the kidneys. Percutaneous ultrasound may be diagnostic.[131]

Promoting diuresis is an important adjunctive therapy in flushing the urinary tract. Intravenous fluids may be used initially or in severe cases. Encouraging water intake or administering oral fluids should be done at a minimum. Providing salt and feeding ammonium chloride (maximum 200 mg/kg per day) will encourage water consumption. Ammonium chloride has the added benefit of urine acidification, which may prevent adhesion of some organisms.

Antibiotic selection should be based on culture and sensitivity; however, penicillin is the most common initial treatment of choice. Overwhelming infection may result in a lack of therapeutic response despite bacterial susceptibility. Long-term antibiotic administration should extend several weeks. Limited studies have suggested relapse rates in cattle of nearly 10% and overall mortality or culling rates of one-third of clinical cases.[132]

Confirming bilateral disease can be important for prognosis, and extent of renal function is more difficult to determine in ruminants. Measuring USG, azotemia response to fluid therapy, and physical exam findings should be combined to determine response to therapy. Nephrectomy may be an option in select cases, and both kidneys can be carefully evaluated with palpation and ultrasound during the exploratory.[133]

Amyloidosis. Amyloidosis is a systemic disease associated with deposition of insoluble extracellular hyaline protein throughout bodily organs. Insoluble β-pleated sheets of amyloid fibrils develop from partial degradation of circulating precursor proteins and deposit in multiple tissues. Many forms of amyloid can develop and cause disease in all species. The proteinaceous complex can develop as a result of chronic inflammatory disease, generally termed reactive amyloid (AA), be immunologically derived (AL) from lymphoid origin neoplasia, namely myeloma, and genetic development is recognized in some species/breeds. Cases of amyloidosis in small ruminants due to myeloma or genetic susceptibility, disregarding scrapie, were not located in the veterinary literature. Only one case of systemic AL amyloidosis in a cow can be located in the literature.[134] Chronic suppurative, inflammatory, and neoplastic conditions, which are commonly regarded as risk factors for development of reactive amyloidosis, often occur in small ruminants; however, clinical cases of amyloidosis are infrequently reported.[135,136] Subclinical amyloidosis may be an incidental finding in ruminant species.[137] Amyloidosis can be induced experimentally, is more common in hyperimmunized animals for product development or research, and usually presents a more systemic process.[138]

Amyloidosis is a systemic disease that commonly affects kidney function as chronic noninflammatory glomerular disease with a history of chronic weight loss, decreasing apatite to anorexia. Clinical presentation is usually that of nephrotic syndrome and hypoalbuminemia characterized by edema, ascites, pleural and pericardial effusion, dyspnea, exercise intolerance, and possibly diarrhea. A recent case report described severe chemosis as the presenting complaint in a goat.[139] Multiorgan dysfunction, including hepatic, hematopoietic, and GI, with associated clinical signs are expected in addition to renal signs.

Clinical pathology exposes hyperkalemia, hyperphosphatemia, and elevated BUN with normal serum creatinine levels.[140] Normal to decreased serum TP may be found with hypoalbuminemia, hyperglobulinemia and a decreased albumin-to-globulin ratio. Proteinuria is a consistent urinalysis finding with an elevated urine protein-to-creatinine ratio. Urine concentration is inconsistent as well as variable sedimentation characteristics of epithelial cells and cellular casts. However, unless secondary infection is present, the cellular sediment is not active. Enzymuria and elevated serum amyloid markers may also support diagnosis. Ultrasonography may reveal renal enlargement and peri-renal edema with hyperechogenic parenchyma. Renal biopsy can be performed as an additional antemortem test with variable results.

Necropsy findings are somewhat dependent upon the severity of amyloidosis and include normal size to grossly enlarged kidneys, diffusely pale, or pale miliary foci on the surface and throughout the parenchyma.[141] Microscopic changes with amyloid deposition reveals extracellular hematoxylin and eosin (H&E)–positive tissue staining mostly affecting the glomerulus. Congo red staining confirms the presence of amyloid.

Treatment is supportive and symptomatic including diagnosis and treatment of potential inciting causes. Prognosis is generally regarded as poor to grave. Steroids and nonsteroidal antiinflammatory drugs can be administered, and several sources indicate use of dimethyl sulfoxide (DMSO) may be efficacious for dissolving amyloid protein. Only medical-grade DMSO is allowable for use in food production animals, and FARAD should be consulted for withdrawal times.

Glomerulonephritis. Glomerular inflammation and pathology occur in both mature and young animals for various reasons. As opposed to amyloidosis, the glomerular damage is inflammatory with deposition of immune-mediated components of antigen, immunoglobulin, and complement and can occur spontaneously in sheep and goats.[142] In older animals, the inciting cause is usually due to a distant chronic inflammatory process, often pneumonia or abscesses. Immune complex deposition affects the glomerular capillary basement membranes, causing thickening and overgrowth leading to both clinical and subclinical renal disease. Proliferative glomerulonephritis is a common incidental finding and often has no clinical significance in sheep and goats. Sheep suffering from pregnancy toxemia may develop toxic and vascular damage to the glomeruli, resulting in edema and epithelial and endothelial cell destruction.

A well-described spontaneous glomerulonephritis occurs in purebred and crossbred Finnish Landrace lambs called spontaneous mesangiocapillary glomerulonephritis (MCGN).[143] Literature and research regarding this condition are lacking within the last few decades. MCGN has a genetic predisposition of C3 complement deficiency with a recessive mode of inheritance, affecting lambs under 4 months of age.[144] Initially presumed to be isolated to Scotland, several cases were diagnosed in northern Alberta in the mid-1980s.[145] This form of glomerulonephritis is considered terminal, with lambs developing clinical signs of lethargy, abdominal pain, and renal failure within weeks after parturition.

With the exception of MCGN, glomerulonephritis is not rapidly progressive in sheep and goats. A relatively non-specific clinical appearance of failure to thrive is noted and may be confused with more common conditions such as metabolic disease or GI parasitism. Historical evidence of disease (i.e., pregnancy toxemia, abscesses, and pneumonia), in addition to concurrent clinical signs of active infection or inflammation, should be considered. Depending on the degree of glomerular disease leading to hypoproteinemia, pleural and peritoneal effusion may develop. The hallmark of glomerular disease is proteinuria. Renal biopsy can be definitive. Gross and microscopic examination at necropsy reveals pale, contracted kidneys with glomerular fibrosis, interstitial thickening, tubular fibrosis, and capillary occlusion.

Treatment of the inciting cause should be implemented, if apparent. Immunosuppressive and chronic steroidal therapy may suppress glomerular inflammation, but long-term prognosis is poor.

Mesangiocapillary Glomerulonephritis. MCGN is an immune-mediated renal disease characterized by immunoglobulin deposition in the glomerular capillary walls and a third component of complement deficiency in affected lambs.[146] This congenital,[147] heritable condition is best described as recessive, although the mode of inheritance is complex[144] and colostral intake has not been shown to play a primary role in disease development.[148] Affected lambs have been mostly described in Finnish Landrace lambs less than 4 months of age, but it has been documented in crossbred lambs from "low risk" Finnish Landrace ewes and Dorset rams.[149] Clinical signs include isolation, anorexia, conjunctival edema, cerebral neurologic signs, and acute death.[145] The kidneys are grossly enlarged and animals become uremic[145] and hypoalbuminemic.

Diagnosis is based on histopathology of the kidney, which demonstrates crescent lesions of neutrophilic infiltration, fibrosis, and glomerular hypertrophy.[146] Ultrastructural studies have shown this condition to be similar to human MCGN type I.[149] Edema, immunoglobulin G deposition, and cellular infiltration have also been seen in the choroid plexus of affected lambs.[150] Treatment is generally not attempted in affected lambs, but alternate day prednisone therapy has been shown to ameliorate the disease in children.[151]

Renal Abscesses. Abscessation of the kidneys typically occurs from hematogenous spread, and abscesses are often revealed in other organs of the body. Worldwide, the most common cause of abscesses in sheep and goats is *C. pseudotuberculosis*, the cause of caseous lymphadenitis. Abscesses may be superficial, in the subcutaneous tissues and superficial lymph nodes, or visceral, primarily affecting the lungs, mediastinal lymph nodes, and other organs, including the kidneys.[152]

Corynebacterium spp. shares a family with *Rhodococcus*, *Mycobacterium*, and *Nocardia* spp. and are associated with chronic, pyogranulomatous inflammation, and infection should be considered lifelong, as viable bacteria may be cultured from older abscesses for several years after infection.[125] Sheep tend to have more frequent and more severe visceral manifestations of caseous lymphadenitis than do goats.[152] The purulent material contained in the abscess contains large numbers of the bacteria and is extremely contagious, with transmission generally occurring from respiratory, integumentary, oral, and other routes. The bacteria invade local lymph nodes and disseminate, producing thickly encapsulated pyogranulomas throughout the lymphatic system and visceral organs.

Other bacteria have been reported to cause abscesses in sheep and goats and serve as differential diagnoses for caseous lymphadenitis. *Mycobacterium bovis* has been demonstrated in an infected sheep flock with abscesses throughout the body, including the kidneys.[153] An avirulent strain of *Rhodococcus equi* has caused disseminated abscesses in goats, but renal involvement did not specifically exist in these cases.[154] *Staphylococcus* spp., *Streptococcus* spp., *Salmonella* spp., and *Chlamydia* spp. have also been associated with renal abscesses in lambs.[155]

Burkholderia (Pseudomonas) pseudomallei has been cultured from abscesses in a Boer doe in South Africa, involving the mammary gland and the cortex of one kidney.[156] This bacterium inhabits soil and water in endemic areas, occurring in Asia, Africa, Australia, and Central and South America.

Diagnosis of renal abscesses is most readily made on ultrasonographic examination of the kidneys and retroperitoneal space, where fluid pockets or gas accumulation may be encountered. Fine needle aspiration of suspected abscesses is recommended over needle biopsy to minimize peritoneal contamination. Culture of abscesses provides etiologic diagnosis, along with antimicrobial sensitivities. In the case of *C. pseudotuberculosis*, cultured bacteria frequently demonstrate sensitivity to several antimicrobials in vitro; however, in vivo performance is poor, likely due to the thick encapsulation of the abscesses and intracellular activity of the organism.[152] A course of rifampin and oxytetracycline has been shown to result in clinical resolution of caseous lymphadenitis abscesses in sheep, but it was not determined if animals remained infected.[157] Serologic tests for hemagglutination inhibition as well as ELISA and other serologic tests are available, as is PCR.[152]

Surgical removal of abscesses in their entirety has been performed. If renal involvement is unilateral, nephrectomy may be performed, relying on compensatory changes in the remaining kidney,[158] although it is likely that other visceral manifestations exist. Animals affected with caseous lymphadenitis should be considered lifelong, systemic carriers, serving as a potential source of infection to other animals and humans, which often makes culling the most appropriate management decision.

Miscellaneous Causes of Renal Disease

Parasites Affecting the Kidneys

Protozoa, cestodes, trematodes, and nematodes have been shown to infect or have effects on the kidneys of sheep and goats. Disseminated disease with *Toxoplasma gondii* has been documented in a 2-year-old goat, in which the kidneys showed white streaks in the cortex and a necrotizing glomerulonephritis.[159] *Toxoplasma* bradyzoites were present in the kidney, and other systemic involvement included cystitis, respiratory, and GI lesions.[159] A 4-year-old pregnant goat exhibited encephalitis and abortion and was found to have hepatic and renal presence of organisms consistent with *Toxoplasma* spp.[160] *Encephalitozoon (Nosema) cuniculi* has been shown to infect sheep[161] and goats.[162] Renal tubular cells contain the organism and cause a chronic interstitial nephritis.[161,162] Congenital sarcocystosis has been documented in a stillborn goat, with *Sarcocyst* organisms present in the kidneys.[163] Of particular concern with many protozoan parasites is their zoonotic potential. Control of protozoal parasites should include the limitation of contact of flocks and herds with cats and rabbits.

Infertile cysts and cysticerci of the cestodes *Echinococcus granulosis* and *Taenia hydatigena* have been found in the kidneys of sheep,[164] with mesangial and membranoproliferative glomerulonephritis, a common change noted with hydatidosis in sheep.[165] An acute nephrosis believed to be caused by *Nematodirus battus* has been shown at affect lambs primarily less than 1 month of age, but the exact etiology of this condition is unknown.[166] *Fasciola hepatica* also causes anemia and hemosiderin deposition in the proximal renal tubules in lambs.[167] Control of these systemic manifestations of parasites includes the control of carnivores, stocking density, regular monitoring for parasitism, and appropriate application of parasiticides with owner education regarding food safety issues.

Cloisonnè Kidney

This condition was previously termed caprine cloisonnè kidney, as it was originally described exclusively in male white Angora goats in Texas[168,169] but has since been reported in sheep[170,171] as well. Grossly, the kidneys are of normal size but appear brown, with this discoloration extending throughout the renal cortex.[168] Histopathologically, the lesion includes a thickened, brown-pigmented proximal tubular basement membrane.[169] This pigment has been characterized as containing a glycolytic group, inorganic material, amino acids,[172] and ferritin[173] with repeated intravascular hemolysis proposed as an etiology.[173] Initially, the condition was believed to have a restricted geographic presence[168] but has been described in North America and Eurasia.[169–172] The condition is generally subclinical, frequently demonstrated on postmortem surveys[168,170–172] or survey renal biopsies[169,173] but may have clinical significance in some animals.[170] Management and treatment principles for this condition have not been proposed.

Congenital Anomalies of the Kidneys and Ureters

Several congenital anomalies are reported to involve the kidneys and ureters, with most of the reports involving lambs. Reported anomalies include unilateral and bilateral renal agenesis, cystic and polycystic kidneys, hydronephrosis, lobulated kidney, and renal dysgenesis in fetal and neonatal lambs, with congenital polycystic kidney disease also reported in a stillborn white-tailed deer fawn.[174–180] Polycystic renal disease in lambs is believed to be an autosomal recessive trait.[174] Renal agenesis has been reported in young goats where the kidneys were pale and slightly small, with cysts, fibrosis, cellular infiltrates, and oxalate crystals were present in the renal tubules of one goat.[181] In one case of cystic renal dysplasia of lambs, 30% of one ram's offspring were affected, and the condition was associated with abortions and stillbirths.[178] Polycystic renal disease has been reported in a female adult European roe deer with features similar to an autosomal dominant form in humans.[182] Ectopic ureter has been reported in a goat examined for a ventricular septal defect.[183] Animals diagnosed with a congenital anomaly frequently have concurrent anomalies,[175,177,183] which are important considerations in case management.

Neoplasia of the Kidneys

Multicentric lymphosarcoma has been reported to involve the kidney of sheep experimentally infected with the bovine leukemia virus (BLV).[184] With this experiment, sheep developed tumors at a much higher rate (34.7%)[184] than is reported in cattle. Goats appear to be more resistant to the development of lymphosarcoma as a consequence of BLV infection, but renal involvement has been noted. Nephroblastoma has been reported in an aborted lamb.[185] Embryonal nephroma with pulmonary metastases has been reported in an emaciated 1.5-year-old female elk.[186]

DISEASES OF THE URINARY BLADDER

Cystitis

Inflammation of the urinary bladder is a common condition, primarily affecting females because of ascending infection. This commonly occurs postpartum as a result of contamination from the genital tract or iatrogenic from fetal manipulation. Cystitis may also result from the presence of uroliths, as an ascending infection from an infected urachus in neonates and from bladder atony resulting from neurological disorders. Animals experiencing prolonged recumbency may not urinate frequently, predisposing them to the development of UTIs. The most common etiologic organisms are *C. renale*, *E. coli*, *Staphylococcus* spp., and *Streptococcus* spp. Animals with cystitis are often pollakiuric and stranguric[187] and may have blood clots or purulent debris on the vulvar or preputial hairs.

Urinalysis will reveal hematuria or pyuria, with red blood cells, neutrophils, and, in some cases, bacteria, visible in microscopic sediment. Ultrasound examination of the urinary bladder may reveal a thickened wall, hyperechoic urine, and blood clots or purulent debris on the bladder floor. Horizontal-beam radiography is useful for demonstrating sediment in the bladder, and survey and contrast radiography can be utilized to demonstrate bladder wall thickening.[188] Endoscopy is useful for visualizing the interior of the urinary bladder to rule out differential diagnoses, including urolithiasis and enzootic hematuria.[187] Urine obtained as a midstream, free-catch sample or via cystocentesis may be submitted for bacterial culture and sensitivity. Cystocentesis provides the preferred samples for culture, as contamination is minimized. The presence or absence of renal involvement in animals with UTIs should be determined. Animals with renal involvement or pyelonephritis will often be systemically ill, febrile, and azotemic and will require more aggressive treatment.

Consideration should be given to the administration of antimicrobials, antiinflammatory drugs,[187] promotion of diuresis, and urinary acidification in the management of animals with UTIs. In selecting an antimicrobial, the agent should be broad-spectrum, based on culture and sensitivity, and be excreted through urine. The beta-lactam antibiotics, ceftiofur and penicillin, are most commonly utilized. Sulfonamide and tetracycline products may also be used. For lower UTIs, a treatment duration of 7 to 10 days is generally recommended, followed by repeat urinalysis to determine the ongoing need for treatment. Antiinflammatory medications may be used in the first 2 to 3 days of therapy to provide relief of discomfort but should be used with caution if renal involvement is suspected. When selecting an antimicrobial and antiinflammatory protocol for individual patients in the United States, the Minor Use Minor Species approved drug lists and the FARAD should be consulted for drug approval and appropriate withdrawals.[189,190] Encouraging the frequent voiding of urine may be achieved with fluid therapy and salt consumption for frequent bacterial removal from the bladder. An indwelling urinary catheter provides a consistent outlet for urine and the opportunity for bladder lavage. Catheters must be placed and maintained in a hygienic manner to avoid further contamination of the urinary tract. Urine acidification is particularly useful for infections with *C. renale*, as it possesses pili that adhere to uroepithelium in an alkaline environment.

Urinary Incontinence

Urinary incontinence arises primarily from neurologic disorders and is of clinical concern due to urine scalding and risk of UTI from urine retention or inadequate urethral sphincter activity. On examination of affected animals, the urinary bladder should be classified as upper motor neuron (UMN) or lower motor neuron (LMN). Those affected with UMN lesions (spinal segment L4-S2) exhibit a distended bladder that is difficult to manually express. The urinary bladder affected by a LMN lesion (spinal segment S2-caudal) will also be distended but will be easily expressed and animals may dribble urine. These animals also exhibit ataxia and decreased tail tone and perineal reflexes.

Causes of urinary incontinence include trauma to lumbosacral spinal cord segments, detrusor atony secondary to urinary tract obstruction, and a variety of diseases affecting the spinal cord. Urinary incontinence has been reported as a clinical sign in a case series of enzootic ataxia in goat kids.[191] Enzootic ataxia is a disease of animals in the first few months of life characterized by low tissue copper levels and Wallerian degeneration and dysmyelinogenesis of the cervical and thoracic spinal cord segments.[192] Urinary incontinence has been reported in a heifer affected with CNS migration of *Parelaphostrongylus tenuis*,[193] which also occurs in goats.[194] West Nile Virus has been reported to cause encephalomyelitis in an ewe whose clinical signs included a distended urinary bladder and urinary incontinence.[195] Urinary incontinence is well recognized as a result of axonal degeneration and demyelination in horses consuming *Sorghum* species but was not recognized in lambs affected by CNS lesions after grazing *Sorghum* pastures.[196] Lesions in lambs differed from those in horses in distribution and severity, as axonal degeneration and demyelination were not significantly present in lambs. One study in lambs evaluated tail docking and its effects on health, using urine staining as one parameter.[197] There was no significant difference in urine staining between docked and undocked lambs, but tail docking is believed to be a risk factor for urinary incontinence in dogs.[198] Urinary incontinence may also result from primary urinary tract disease, including cystitis, ectopic ureter, and hypospadias, which have been reported in goats and sheep and may result in urinary incontinence.[199–201]

Treatment of urinary incontinence has not been specifically described in small ruminants and should focus on management of the primary disease, adequate nursing care, and prevention of potential sequelae, including hydronephrosis and UTI. Urinary catheterization may be performed in females and cystocentesis in males to provide relief of the bladder distension and urine outflow until neurologic recovery occurs. Animals with detrusor atony may be treated with cholinergic drugs such as bethanechol (0.04–0.08 mg/kg SC, TID) to stimulate detrusor activity but should not be used in animals with urethral obstruction or increased urethral tone.

Congenital Anomalies of the Urinary Bladder

A heritable, congenital hypoplasia or aplasia of the urinary bladder has been reported in Sufolk lambs along with renal dysplasia which was fatal within the first 5 days of life.[202] Patent urachus has been reported in lambs,[200,201] with other concurrent anomalies, including atresia ani and vaginalis. These cases occurred in the absence of omphalitis,[203] the most common cause of patent urachus in ruminant neonates.

Neoplasia of the Urinary Bladder

Leiomyoma, a smooth muscle tumor, has been reported to occur with hepatocellular carcinoma and phaeochromocytoma in a 12-year-old male goat.[204] Multicentric lymphosarcoma involving the kidneys, ureter, and urinary bladder wall has been reported in sheep experimentally infected with BLV.[205] Renal and cardiac metastases of a goat with Jaagsiekte disease or pulmonary adenomatosis have been reported.[206] Multiple neoplasias such as hemangiosarcoma, hemangioma, and transitional cell carcinoma along with chronic cystitis have been reported in a captive fallow deer and are believed to have resulted from Bracken fern ingestion.[207]

DISEASES OF THE URETHRA

The anatomy of the distal urinary tract of male ruminants differs significantly from that of males of other species. The penis is sigmoid in arrangement,[208] with two major bends occurring between the urinary bladder and the distal glans penis. The glans penis of the small ruminant also has a vermiform appendage, or urethral process, which is an extension of the urethra 2 to 4 cm beyond the distal end of the penis.[208] It has a narrowed diameter compared to the more proximal portions of the urethra.

Obstructive Urolithiasis

Obstructive urolithiasis is the single most common urinary tract disease of small ruminants, with significant economic significance. The USDA-NAHMS study in 2001 reported that 20% of surveyed sheep operations had at least one case of urinary calculi in the previous 3 years.[209] Urolithiasis has been reported in a 6-month-old white-tailed deer and an adult elk.[210,211] Males are most commonly obstructed, but uroliths may form in females, as well.

Uroliths are solid crystalline formations in the urine, which are composed of organic matrix and organic and inorganic crystalloids that precipitate in supersaturated urine.[212] Factors affecting urine supersaturation include the rate of renal excretion of crystalloids, negative water balance, urine pH, and the presence or absence of crystallization inhibitors.[212] Metaplasia of uroepithelium, as a result of vitamin A deficiency, may contribute cells and protein for nuclear formation.[213] Suture, tissue debris, blood clots, or bacteria may also serve as nuclear components initiating urolith formation.[212] Infection, however, is considered to be a minor factor in urolith formation in ruminants.

Urolithiasis is a multifactorial disease with diet, urine pH, and body water balance playing significant roles. Struvite (magnesium ammonium phosphate) and apatite (calcium phosphate) may be commonly seen in animals fed high-grain diets, while animals consuming legumes are predisposed to calcium carbonate uroliths. Silicate stones may be observed in animals grazing siliceous plants and soils in the western United States and Canada. Calcium oxalate stones may be associated with oxalate-containing plants. A significant factor in availability of urolith components and their binding ability is urine pH.[214] Struvite, apatite, and calcium carbonate uroliths are known to precipitate in alkaline urine.[212,214] Struvite crystallization occurs only at a pH range of 7.2 to 8.4, while apatite stones develop at a urine pH of 6.5 to 7.5.[215] Calcium carbonate stones also tend to form in alkaline urine, while pH may have little or no effect on silicate or calcium oxalate uroliths. Total body water balance plays an important role in calculogenesis by its effects on urine volume and concentration. This may be seen in winter and during times of other systemic illness when animals consume decreased volumes of water, thus reducing urine output.

Uroliths may obstruct urine flow anywhere from the renal pelvis to the distal urethra, although the most common sites of obstruction are at the distal sigmoid flexure or the vermiform appendage in sheep and goats (Figure 12.7A, B). Obstruction at these sites may result in either rupture of the urethra or of the urinary bladder.

Although hematuria may be noted, urolithiasis without obstruction rarely results in clinical disease. Animals presenting with clinical disease related to urolithiasis are often obstructed and signs are dependent upon the degree of obstruction, location of the obstruction, and the duration of disease. Uroliths may not completely obstruct urine flow yet manifest as an incomplete or even intermittent obstruction. Initial incomplete obstruction often becomes complete obstruction with time due to inflammation of damaged urethral mucosa.

Clinical signs of urinary obstruction may range from nonspecific inappetence and lethargy to overt colic. Restlessness, persistent straining, repetitive posturing to urinate, and vocalization

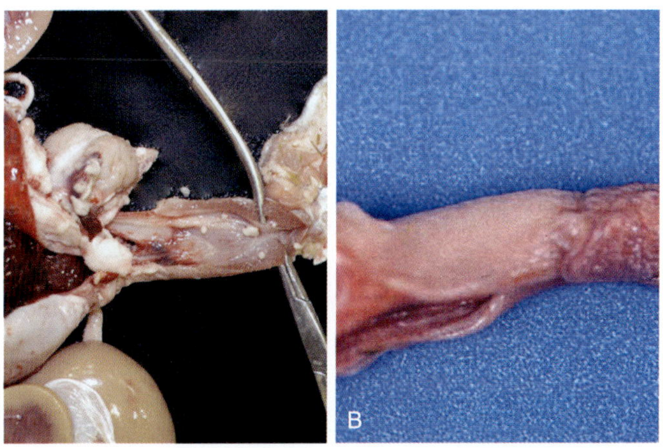

• **Fig. 12.7 A.** The pelvic urethra from an 8-month-old male goat with urinary calculi. **B.** The urethral process of this buck was occluded by a urinary calculi. This was a postmortem finding. (Courtesy of Dr John Roberts, University of Florida, College of Veterinary Medicine.)

are common. Swelling around the prepuce or bilateral ventral abdominal distension may be noted with rupture of the urethra or urinary bladder, respectively.

Clinical pathology findings are related to the duration of obstruction and sequela, such as uroabdomen and hydronephrosis. In a retrospective study of goats with urolithiasis, the most common abnormalities were azotemia and hypophosphatemia.[216] Animals may also have slight decreases in sodium and chloride with elevations in potassium and a metabolic alkalosis.[216] Unlike monogastric species, the azotemia is often mild or may not be present early in the disease as ruminants have the ability to more effectively manage uremia. In addition, ruminants often maintain adequate phosphorus and potassium homeostasis through salivary secretions,[217,218] without experiencing the large increases of these analytes as seen in obstructed monogastric animals.

The principles of management for obstructive urolithiasis include establishing a patent route of urine excretion, providing analgesia, correcting fluid deficits and electrolyte derangements, decreasing inflammation, and preventing infection. The presence of the urethral diverticulum prevents passage of a urinary catheter retrograde from the urethral orifice to the urinary bladder.[208] Retrograde catheterization or retropulsion of uroliths is not recommended as further trauma or puncture of the urethra is possible. Attempts at retropulsion of uroliths may result in over distention of the urinary bladder as the stone is diverted into the diverticulum, allowing fluid to pass into the bladder, followed by the urolith falling back into the urethra. Occasionally, removal of the vermiform appendage (Figure 12.8) in male sheep and/or goats establishes a patent urethra; however, inflammation in the proximal urethra from passage of the uroliths may still prevent normal urination. Uroliths tend to occur in multitudes in the urinary bladder and most animals initially relieved by amputation of the vermiform appendage will often reobstruct with subsequent stone passage. Relief of urinary obstruction often requires surgical intervention.

The systemic health of the patient is an important consideration when selecting drugs to facilitate treatment. Acepromazine (0.05–0.1 mg/kg IV or IM) has been utilized in the medical management of urolithiasis.[218–220] Unproven arguments for utilization of acepromazine have been to relax urethral tone through α-antagonistic effects on smooth muscle and relaxation of the retractor penis muscle. Acepromazine may also suppress the anxiety associated with the inability to urinate. Caution should be taken when using phenothiazine tranquilizers in patients, which may already be hypotensive and hypothermic. Diazepam (0.1 mg/kg, slow IV) may also be used for urethral relaxation and as an anxiolytic. Xylazine (0.05–0.1 mg/kg, IV or IM) or other α-2 agonists may be used in attempt to restrain the patient for examination of the penis and have excellent analgesic properties in ruminants. Caution should be exercised when utilizing xylazine prior to relief of the obstruction, as it promotes dieresis[221] as well as enhances hypotension. Lumbosacral epidurals using 2% lidocaine (1 mL/7 kg) may be utilized in the place of sedation to relieve discomfort and aid in exteriorization of the penis.

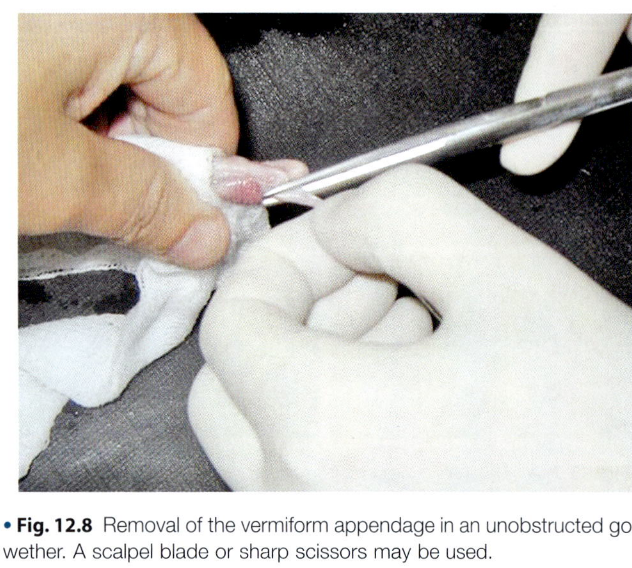

• **Fig. 12.8** Removal of the vermiform appendage in an unobstructed goat wether. A scalpel blade or sharp scissors may be used.

Fluid therapy should be instituted as indicated by the clinical examination. After relief of the obstruction, diuresis is important to replace dehydration, reduce azotemia, and flush the urinary tract. Normal (0.9%) NaCl is a good choice for intravenous fluid therapy, although additional electrolyte and acid-base abnormalities should be considered. If the animal has been obstructed for longer than 36 to 48 hours or has a ruptured bladder, potassium is likely to be elevated and electrolyte panels are very helpful in guiding the correction of electrolyte and acid-base abnormalities. Potassium levels may be used as a marker for determining the degree of intervention and high levels exert inhibitory effects on the heart causing bradycardia. If the potassium levels are high, dextrose may be added to make a 2.5% to 5% solution (50–100 mL of 50% solution per liter of fluid) or insulin may be utilized to move potassium intracellularly, protecting the heart. The addition of 20 mL of 23% calcium borogluconate per liter of fluids can improve cardiac contractility, and atropine 0.04 mg/kg can be used in bradycardic patients. Sodium bicarbonate can be used to correct acidosis and decrease hyperkalemia but should not be mixed with calcium-containing fluids. Nonsteroidal antiinflammatory drugs should be administered to decrease inflammation and aid in the prevention of urethral stricture formation but should be used with caution until adequate renal perfusion is attained. Broad-spectrum antibiotic therapy should be instituted to prevent or treat infection resulting from devitalized or inflamed urinary tissues or cavitational accumulation of urine. Beta-lactam antimicrobials (penicillins and cephalosporins) may be chosen, as they have good spectrum of activity and are excreted in the urine.

There are many methods for relieving urethral obstruction due to urolithiasis. Methods with practical application include vermiform appendage amputation, urethrotomy, urethrostomy, cystotomy, tube cystostomy, and urinary bladder marsupialization. Other methods including prepubic urethrostomy, extrapelvic and urethropreputial anastomosis, buccal mucosal urethral grafting, and laser lithotripsy are described much less commonly.[222–225] Relieving the obstruction by retrograde urinary catheterization is highly unlikely to be achieved in ruminants and pigs due to the urethral diverticulum present at the ischial arch of the penis.[226] Although traditional straight polypropylene catheters often fail, the use of angiographic catheters has been investigated as a more successful option in retrograde catheterization.[227] On the occasions when an obstruction is cleared by retrograde catheterization, the relief is temporary and some surgical treatment will be required to resolve the condition. In addition, dynamic and physiologic healing characteristics of the ruminant urethra result in a strong likelihood for luminal stricture formation as a result of trauma from calculi, attempted catheterization or surgery (i.e., urethrostomy).

Surgeries such as urethrotomy and perineal urethrostomy are considered palliative or salvage treatments, as the surgical site will likely stricture within months resulting in reobstruction.[228] It should, however, be considered as the treatment of choice for long-term survival when the urethra has ruptured and there is significant damage to the distal portion of the penis and surrounding tissues due to urine accumulation. A modified perineal urethrostomy technique involving extensive release of penile connective tissue proximally has shown promise in reducing postoperative stricture formation.[229] Perineal urethrostomy is not a viable option for maintaining intact breeding males. Tube cystostomy is a viable option for curative (long-term) relief of urethral obstruction as well as maintaining functional breeding males. Short- and long-term prognoses, complication rates and reobstruction rates for each procedure have been recently reviewed.[230]

Vermiform Appendage Amputation

One of the first procedures to attempt relief of urethral obstruction is to visualize the vermiform (urethral process) for evidence of lodged calculi. This is a narrow appendage at the terminal urethra that is prone to calculi obstruction (Figure 12.7B). The patient is restrained in a sitting position (Figure 12.9), while the penis is extended and visualized. Visualization of the penis may not be possible without general anesthesia in very young males as diffuse preputial-penile attachments are still present before the effects of testosterone and maturity allow release. Sponge forceps may be used to extend the penis when the obstructed male is under general anesthesia, which will allow the clinician to then carefully free the distal portion of the penis from the prepuce. Amputation of the vermiform is done with either a pair of Mayo scissors or a scalpel blade. Amputation is usually performed even if calculi are not visualized. Hemorrhage is expected but not profuse and may continue for some time (hours) due to the effects of urine on coagulation.

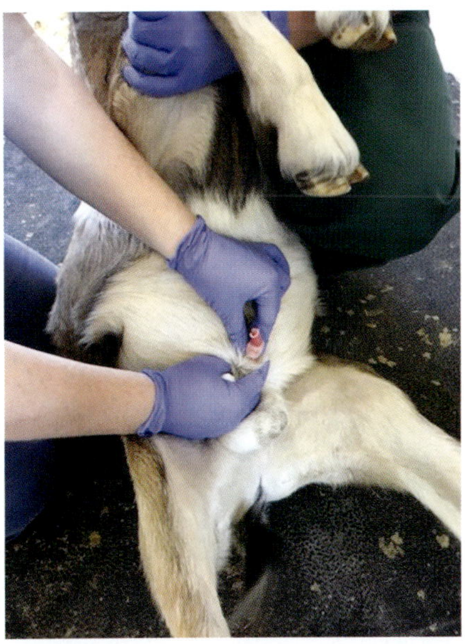

• **Fig. 12.9** A buck being "set up" to facilitate exteriorization of the penis for examination of the vermiform appendage and glans. This method of restraint may be used for both sheep and goats.

Urethrotomy, Urethrostomy, and Penile Transection and Transposition (With or Without Penile Amputation)

Urethrotomy and urolith removal can be attempted when stones are located by palpation, radiographs, or ultrasound. The distal sigmoid flexure is another common site where uroliths may lodge. A urethral incision may be made directly over the stone or in healthy urethra adjacent to it, followed by urolith removal. Suturing the urethra is recommended by most, but allowing second intention healing of the urethrotomy site is also acceptable and much less technically challenging. Stricture formation is a high-risk complication for urethral surgery in small ruminants regardless of the specific technique employed.

Urethrostomy can be performed in different ways to allow for a prolonged or permanent stoma for urinary diversion. The most commonly performed method is perineal urethrostomy. A combination of local and epidural anesthesia is provided, and an incision is made on midline in the perineum somewhere between the ischial arch and dorsal to the sigmoid flexure, which is just dorsal to the scrotum. The author prefers to incise the skin and subcutaneous tissue as distal as possible since the dissected penis will be more mobile for urethrostomy with less tension. The distal urethrostomy also provides extra tissue proximally for surgical reconstruction should stricture develop. Alternatively, the approach can be at the level of the ischial arch that may have the benefit of urinary bladder catheterization as the urethral diverticulum can be bypassed. Once the penis is dissected free from the subcutaneous tissue, the urethra can be incised longitudinally and a stoma sutured to the skin.

Alternatively, the penis can be transected and dorsal segment repositioned. Amputation of the penis provides a simple approach to relieving urethral obstructions. However, this procedure may not be cosmetically appealing and strictures often occur within months after surgery. The surgery can be accomplished under either general or epidural anesthesia. Many clinicians prefer to perform this surgery after administering epidural anesthesia on an animal in sternal recumbency with the hindlimbs off the end of the table. A midline incision is made in the perineum dorsal to the sigmoid flexure at the point where the perineum turns ventrocranially. Careful, sharp dissection is performed to expose the penis. The distal sigmoid flexure is identified and pulled to the incision site. If there has been significant urine damage to the preputial tissues due to urine leakage, the entire distal penis can often be extracted from the wound with moderate pressure. The penis is avulsed from its preputial attachment. A point on the penis 4 to 7 cm distal to the dorsal edge of the skin incision is chosen for the amputation site. The dorsal penile vessels are ligated dorsal to this point and the retractor penis muscles are ligated and transected as far proximally as possible. The distal part of the penis is very difficult to remove (and not recommended) if the surrounding tissues are normal. If the distal penis in not removed, the dorsal penile vessels should be reflected off the penis and left intact. The penis is transected as far distal as the perineal skin incision will allow. A wedge-shaped piece of tunica albuginea and the underlying cavernous tissue of the corpus cavernosum penis (CCP) are removed to allow for better closure of the CCP and thus minimize hemorrhage when an intact male is sexually stimulated. The transected CCP is closed with a simple continuous or continuous mattress pattern using 2-0 absorbable suture in the tunica albuginea surrounding the CCP. The urethra and tunica albuginea of the corpus spongiosum penis (CSP) are split longitudinally for 2 to 3 cm in order to spatulate the new urethral opening. The urethral mucosa is sutured to the tunica albuginea down each side and at the transected end of the penis with a continuous pattern using 3-0 absorbable material. This suture line seals the CSP and lessens hemorrhage during urination. A suture can be placed into the tunica albuginea at the mucosal closure near the transected end of the penis, around the dorsal aspect of the penis (opposite the urethra), and into the tunica albuginea again near the mucosa of the opposite side. The suture is then tied on the dorsal aspect of the penis. This suture creates a bigger opening of the spatulated urethra. The penile stump is secured to the skin with a mattress suture. A "bite" is taken through the skin where the penile stump will exit the incision. The next bite is into the tunica albuginea of the CCP and then the skin on the opposite side. The second half of the mattress suture is placed through the skin as normally done ventral to the first bite. This suture will secure the penis in place as well as direct the transected end of the penis out of the skin incision. The remainder of the skin incision is closed in a routine fashion of the clinician's choosing. Castration at the same time as the penile amputation is prudent.[231]

Tube Cystostomy

Surgical success when dealing with urinary obstruction largely depends on duration of disease and correction of fluid and electrolyte derangements prior to or during surgery. Not using hypotensive drugs and quickly replacing fluid volume is probably of primary importance. The electrolyte abnormalities to correct are hypochloremia, hyponatremia, and hyperkalemia. The severity of these electrolyte changes varies with duration and if the bladder has ruptured.

Potassium levels can be variable in ruminants, even with ruptured bladder. A ruptured bladder may quickly lead to hyperkalemia and acidosis in many species, but ruminants manage pH and electrolyte derangements better through salivary metabolism. Small ruminants (especially sheep), however, seem to be affected more often with the hyperkalemic acidosis syndrome as seen in small animals and foals. This is most likely due to the duration of obstruction prior to recognition. Several anesthetic and preanesthetic protocols can be used to combat these life- threatening changes.

Tube cystostomy can be successfully performed in field situations with percutaneous introduction of the catheter. A method for percutaneous tube cystostomy and vesicular irrigation has been described.[232] Risks with this procedure include bowel perforation and increased risk of peritonitis.[233] A disadvantage of this technique is that it does not allow normograde urethral flushing or removing stones via cystotomy. Therefore, the tube will likely need to be left in the bladder longer before resolution of the condition. Guafenesin (5%) with 1 mg/mL of ketamine added is adequate for intubation and could also be used to maintain a surgical plane of anesthesia.[234] For surgical induction or intubation, the dose of the "double drip" mixture is about 0.75 to 1 mL per pound of body weight. The onset of anesthesia is slow and the drug should be dosed slowly and to effect. In patients to be intubated, the use of a stylet to guide the endotracheal tube through the larynx and the use of a long laryngeal blade facilitate the procedure.

General anesthesia is not essential for successfully performing a tube cystostomy; however, it provides the surgeon more time to flush the bladder and attempt normograde catheterization for hydropulsion of stones from the urethra. Induction with "double drip" (guafenesin and ketamine) and tracheal intubation with maintenance on a small animal anesthesia machine is easily performed in small ruminants. An alternative to general anesthesia would be lidocaine epidural and local anesthesia with xylazine/ketamine sedation. Care should be taken when using lidocaine in goats (toxic dose 5–10 mg/kg). Xylazine should also be used with caution due to its hypotensive and diuretic effects. Metabolic and electrolyte imbalances should be considered (hyponatremia, hypochloremia, and possibly hyperkalemia) and either measured or empirically treated. Hyperkalemic animals can have significant adverse cardiovascular effects with xylazine, and it also sensitizes the heart to catecholamine induced tachyarrhythmias (see Chapter 18).

Laparotomy procedures are performed with the patient in dorsal recumbency. The abdomen should be clipped and prepped for abdominal surgery. A paramedian approach should be used to avoid the penis. The incision should be approximately 15 cm long (anterior to posterior), with the posterior extent of the incision ending just anterior to the teat. Care should be taken to avoid the caudal superficial epigastric vessels.

The tip of the distended bladder is easily exteriorized through the body wall incision and packed off with moistened towels. Two stay sutures are placed in the bladder wall to maintain the bladder at the incision once it is decompressed. A sharp stab incision is made with a scalpel blade between the stay sutures, taking care to avoid abdominal contamination with urine and calculi. Suction is very helpful in limiting contamination, if available. The bladder incision is enlarged to adequately allow intraluminal palpation of the trigone of the bladder for stones. The bladder should be lavaged with saline to remove any stones, blood clots, and debris. One may find a small spoon or scoop useful in removing stones (Figure 12.10). Normograde passage of a polypropylene urinary catheter can be attempted to flush stones from the urethra. It may be difficult to pass the catheter in many cases, but unsuccessful attempts do not predict eventual failure to relieve urethral calculi. One technique that aids in placing a catheter in a normograde fashion is to put a finger in the trigone area and push the catheter under the finger into the urethra. A syringe casing can also be used to fill the trigone. This technique more easily directs the catheter into the urethra, whereas it may curl in the trigone otherwise. Prolonged attempts at normograde catheterization should be avoided to prevent excessive trauma to the urethral mucosa.

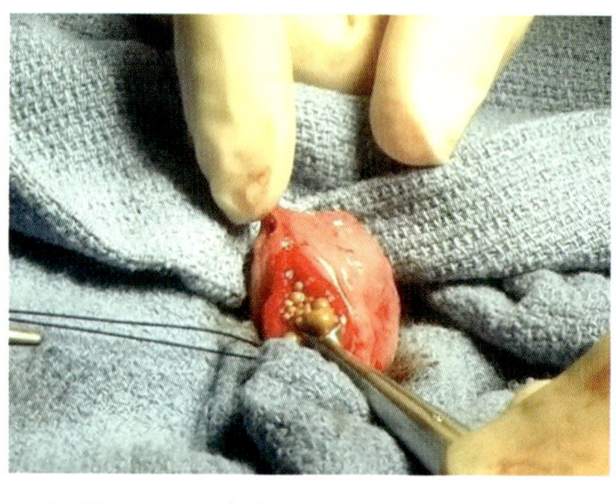

• **Fig. 12.10** Uroliths removed via cystotomy from a 2-year-old castrated Pygmy goat with obstructive urolithiasis. Calcium carbonate stones tend to be smooth and yellow-white to golden and resemble BB's. Struvite crystals tend to be "sand like" in appearance. (Courtesy Dr. AN Baird, Purdue University.)

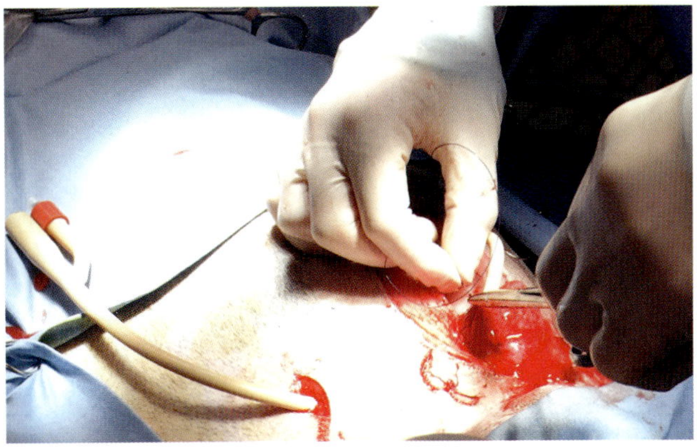

• **Fig. 12.11** An intraoperative photograph showing a distended, inflamed bladder due to an urethral obstruction in a 50-lb Pygmy wether. The Foley catheter has been placed through the abdominal wall, pleated through part of the omentum, then secured into the decompressed yet still inflamed bladder with a purse-string suture. (Courtesy Dr. AN Baird, Purdue University.)

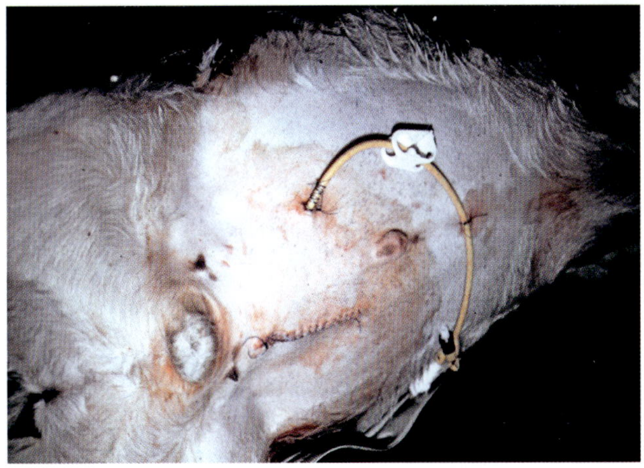

• **Fig. 12.12** An immediate postoperative photograph of the Pygmy wether, showing the left paramedian abdominal incision closed with a continuous suture pattern and the Foley catheter exiting the body wall in the right paramedian area. (Courtesy Dr. AN Baird, Purdue University.)

The tube cystostomy involves placing a Foley catheter through the abdominal wall and into the bladder to allow urine flow to bypass the urethra while the obstruction resolves, and the urethral mucosa heals. The size of the tube should be large enough to allow passage of small blood clots without becoming obstructed. A stab incision is made in a caudal paramedian location contralateral to the laparotomy incision. The tip of the catheter is then passed through the abdominal wall. It is easiest to pass a hemostat from interior (peritoneum) to exterior (skin) and pull the catheter through. The Foley is then pleated through the omentum several times before being inserted into the bladder via a stab incision about 2 cm lateral to the cystotomy incision (Figure 12.11). The bulb is then filled with approximately 10 mL of saline. Some surgeons will then place a purse-string suture around the insertion of the catheter into the bladder. The cystotomy incision is then closed with a one- or two-layer, inverting pattern. Finally, the laparotomy incision is closed in routine fashion. The portion of the Foley catheter exiting the abdomen should be anchored to the skin using a "finger trap" suture, where it exits the body wall and as needed cranially with interrupted sutures to prevent the tube from dragging the ground (Figure 12.12). An Elizabethan-type collar can be placed on the patient to prevent chewing or dislodging the Foley. The Foley catheter should be clamped off 3 to 4 days after surgery to assess urethral patency. Obstruct the catheter and monitor for urination or patient discomfort indicating persistent obstruction. If the animal becomes uncomfortable, the clamp is removed to allow urine drainage through the Foley. This process is repeated until the patient is able to urinate comfortably with the Foley occluded for 48 hours, at which time the Foley is removed. The Foley is removed by simply cutting any retention sutures, deflating the bulb, and pulling the catheter out of the bladder and through the skin. The surgeon should be cognizant that the clamp occluding urine flow through the Foley also prevents saline flow from the bulb so unclamp the catheter before attempting to decompress the bulb. Regardless of when the animal urinates normally, the Foley is left in place at least 7 days to allow formation of a fibrous tract around the catheter from the bladder to the body wall. This prevents urine from diffusely filling the abdomen while the catheter site in the bladder heals closed. Urine leakage from the insertion site may be noted but will soon close. The clinician should expect approximately 14 days before the patient is able to urinate, including some instances where urethral calculi were present after surgery. However, tube retention may be necessary for a longer time. Success rate for long-term cure (greater than 1 year) is about 70% in one retrospective study.[230]

Walpole's solution can also be used to dissolve stones in cases treated by tube cystostomy. It is infused into the bladder through the Foley catheter and the catheter is occluded to retain the solution in the bladder. This is frequently done twice a day with the catheter remaining occluded for up to 30 minutes as long as the animal is comfortable. One could be more aggressive with the pH testing as described above.

Potential complications from urethral obstruction are hydronephrosis, cystitis, pyelonephritis, atonic bladder from overdistention, urethral stricture due to trauma from the calculi, failure to pass the obstruction, and erectile dysfunction in breeding males due to damage to the CCP.[233,235] The potential complications should be discussed with the client prior to treatment.

Urinary Bladder Marsupialization

Urinary bladder marsupialization provides direct drainage of urine from the bladder. A paramedian approach is made similar to tube cystostomy. When anticipating an empty or contracted bladder, make the approach more caudal than for a tube cystostomy. The bladder is localized, and the apex is sutured to the body wall and skin at a 3 to 5 cm paramedian incision site contralateral to the laparotomy incision. The seromuscular layer of the bladder is secured to the external rectus sheath then the bladder is opened, and the mucosa is sutured to the skin. Interrupted or short continuous segments of absorbable suture are used to create this stoma for permanent drainage of urine (Figure 12.13). Problems may arise with localized or ascending UTIs, urine scald, and obstruction of the stoma due to bladder mucosal proliferation and prolapse.

Nonsurgical Therapy

The use of Walpole's solution (sodium acetate and glacial acetic acid) has been published as an alternative therapy for obstructed

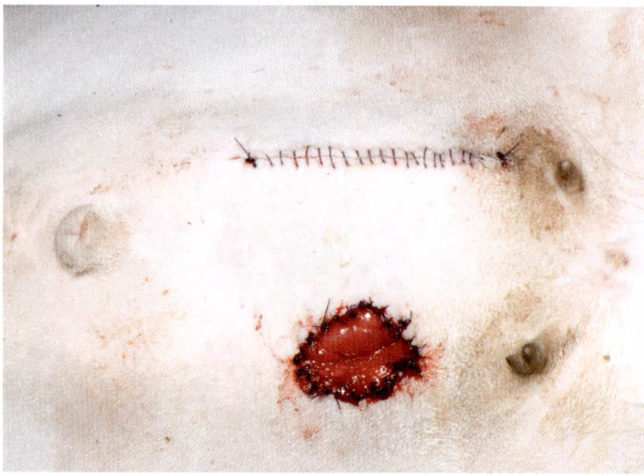

• **Fig. 12.13** An immediate postoperative photograph of a 2-year-old castrated Pygmy goat with obstructive urolithiasis. A bladder marsupialization has been performed with the goat under general anesthesia in dorsal recumbency. For orientation, the preputial orifice is the left and the rudimentary teats are to the right. The skin at the left paramedian laparotomy site has been closed with a simple continuous suture pattern. The bladder mucosa has been sutured to the skin edge to the right of midline in a simple interrupted pattern. (Courtesy Dr. AN Baird, Purdue University.)

cases with an intact urinary bladder in which surgery is not elected.[235] The procedure involves sedation of the animal and performance of an ultrasound-guided cystocentesis to withdraw urine. Then, 50 mL of Walpole's solution is infused into the bladder. The solution is allowed to remain in the bladder for 2 minutes, followed by withdrawal of urine and pH testing. This procedure is repeated until the urine pH is 4 to 5, making sure that sufficient urine remains in the bladder to maintain the cystocentesis needle in place. Reportedly, 80% of obstructions are resolved in the short-term using this method, but about 30% of those animals reobstructed after discharge.[236]

Once the obstruction is relieved, dietary and management modifications should be instituted to prevent reoccurrence in the individual animal and in the herd. Risk factors addressed in preventative strategies include high phosphorus relative to calcium, high magnesium, and low fiber content of rations, as well as low urine output and alkaline urine. Additional factors, including selective grazing and castration timing, may be addressed.

Medical Management and Prevention. An elevated level of phosphorus in the diet with a calcium-to-phosphorus ratio of less than 2:1 increases the excretion of phosphorus in the urine and provides an ion to bind to organic matrix.[237] Increasing the level of calcium in the diet markedly decreases the incidence of urolithiasis, probably due to competition with phosphorus for intestinal absorption and matrix binding.[237] Phosphorus should not comprise greater than 0.6% of the total ration,[214] and it is recommended that a 2.5:1 or 2:1 calcium-to-phosphorus ratio be achieved by the use of calcium salts, if necessary.[235] Calcium oversupplementation should be avoided as increased calcium excretion in the urine may contribute to calcium-containing uroliths. High phosphorus levels are present in grains, particularly sorghum, wheat, corn, milo, and oats. A reduction in phosphorus excretion into the urine is also desirable. Excessive dietary levels of phosphorus may saturate the salivary pathway of excretion,[218] causing the excess to be excreted in the urine. Urine phosphorus excretion is greater in animals fed pelleted rations as compared to meal-type rations[237] due to a decrease in saliva production, the pathway for excess phosphorus excretion. Increases in the roughage component of diets are important from this standpoint as they increase the amount of saliva that must be produced for proper mastication. Particularly in the case of struvite stones, but also with apatite stones, an increase in magnesium excretion into the urine is contributory to crystallization. It is recommended that magnesium not exceed 0.6% of the total ration of ruminants.[214]

Increasing water intake and urine volume is an important preventive measure for urolithiasis. The provision of adequate palatable water at desirable temperatures according to the ambient environment is desirable.[214] Ruminants demonstrate a reduction in water intake for grain feeding over roughage feeding. Additionally, the feeding of intermittent meals may cause shunting of body water into the rumen due to increased osmotic pull from generated volatile fatty acids, resulting in a decrease in urine output. This has led to the recommendation that ruminants be fed ad libitum to maintain urine output.[214]

Increasing forage versus grain in the diet of animals at-risk for urolithiasis has many benefits. Grain results in increased magnesium, phosphorus, and peptides in the urine and forage consumption encourages saliva production for phosphorus excretion, potentially reduces magnesium uptake, reduces overall grain consumption, and increases water intake. Legumes and their hays should be avoided, as they have high levels of calcium and are associated with calcium carbonate urolithiasis.

The role of urine pH in urolithiasis is well documented; urine pH goals of 5.5 to 6.5 are recommended, based on the solubilities of the common stone compositions. Due to an ability to alter acid-base balance and body water balance, salts have been widely used and recommended for the prevention of urolithiasis. Anionic salts containing primarily chlorides have been popular and used extensively, as they reduce urine pH, increase urine output, and ultimately prevent urolithiasis. Sodium chloride (1–4%), calcium chloride (1–2%), and ammonium chloride (0.5–2%) have been traditionally added to as percentages of rations to increase water intake and produce acidic urine, with inconsistent results. The traditional addition of these salts as a simple percentage of the diet without consideration for the components of the total ration commonly leads to inconsistent and unsuccessful maintenance of a low urinary pH. Dietary cation anion difference (DCAD) is a concept based upon the strong ion difference theory and the effects on the body of dietary concentrations of the major physiologic cations and anions, represented by the formula $[Na + K] - [Cl + S] = \text{mEq/kg}$ of feed. With increased anions in the diet, the feed has a more negative DCAD, which produces a metabolic acidosis and aciduria in the animal. Few controlled studies for target DCAD levels currently exist, but a DCAD of 0 mEq/kg appears to achieve urine pH of intact and castrated goats of less than 6.5.[238,239] To accurately assess the efficacy of salts in the diet, whether DCAD balanced or not, owners should be encouraged to periodically assess urine pH at home 5 to 7 hours after feeding.

Castration is significantly associated with the development of obstructive urolithiasis,[215] and early castration is thought to reduce the positive influence of testosterone on urethral diameter as well as diminish normal preputial to penile attachments that are present in the neonate. Delaying castration in pet animals may serve to increase urethral diameter as well as increase the ability to examine the penis. A 2.5× increase in cross-sectional urethral diameter at the level of the distal sigmoid flexure was noted when castration of lambs was delayed from 2 weeks to 3 months of age.[240] When castration was delayed to 5 months, a 3.5 times increase in urethral diameter was seen.[240] Other considerations should be made regarding prophylactic removal of the vermiform appendage in young animals and limiting the grazing of males on silicaceous pastures (see Chapter 2).

Ulcerative Posthitis/Vulvovaginitis

Ulcerative posthitis, also known as enzootic balanoposthitis, pizzle rot, and sheath rot, is an infectious disease of the external genitalia of male small ruminants with lesions also occurring in females. The primary etiologic agent is *C. renale,* a normal inhabitant of the skin and external genitalia of small ruminants. Parapoxviruses, *Corynebacterium pilosum*, *Corynebacterium cystitidis*,[241] *Acholeplasma oculi*,[241] Caprine herpesvirus-I,[241,242] orf (parapoxvirus),[243] *Mycoplasma* ovine/caprine serogroup 11,[244] *Mycoplasma mycoides* ssp. *mycoides*,[245] *Ureaplasma* spp.[246,247] *Mycoplasma capricolum* ssp. *Capricolum*,[247] have all been demonstrated to cause ulcerative or granular posthitis or vulvovaginitis in sheep and goats.

Risk factors for infection include high-protein diets, legume diets, thick fiber, and wet conditions, and several of these organisms are transmitted venereally. *C. renale* proliferates on genital mucosa in the presence of urea, which increases in concentration in the urine of animals fed high protein, legume pasture, and nonprotein-nitrogen (NPN) diets.[248] It then acts to hydrolyze urea to ammonia, resulting in necrosis of the surrounding tissue. There is increased incidence in Merino and Angora animals due to dense fiber coats.[249] Symptomatic or asymptomatic carriers may spread large numbers of the bacteria venereally.

The clinical signs associated with ulcerative posthitis in rams, bucks, and wethers include moist ulcers and thin, brown, malodorous scabs at the mucocutaneous junction of the prepuce.[250] The infection may become internalized, with diffuse swelling of the prepuce, and the presence of necrotic tissue and exudate. Eventually, fibrinous or fibrous adhesions may form between the penis and prepuce and stenosis of the preputial orifice may occur. In some cases, the preputial orifice may be reduced to a pinhole-sized stoma.[249] The lesions are quite painful and lead to dysuria, vocalization during urination, and a stilted gait, and chronic weight loss may occur. In does and ewes, ulcerative lesions of the perineum and vulva occur with vulvar swelling. Dysuria may result in cases where infection and inflammation involve the urethral orifice and longstanding cases may result in fibrosis and contracture of the vulva. Lesions of herpesvirus include hyperemia of the penis, ulcerative lesions of prepuce, discrete punctate areas of epithelial desquamation of prepuce and petechiae and ecchymoses.[241] Other clinical syndromes are known to occur from the agents of posthitis/vulvovaginitis, including abortions with caprine herpesvirus-1 keratoconjunctivitis with *A. oculi*[241] and inflammation of the entire female reproductive tract, polyarthritis, pneumonia, and mastitis with *Mycoplasma* spp.[244,246] Outbreaks may occur with up to 95% incidence when nutritional factors contribute.[241]

Diagnosis of this condition is usually based on lesion characteristics of preputial or vulvar hyperemia, scabs, nodules, and proliferative masses[243,244] and dietary information. Histopathology, bacterial culture, and PCR can provide a definitive diagnosis, which assists with planning control and prevention programs. Serology may show high titers to caprine herpesvirus-1, which is antigenically related to bovine herpesvirus (IBR).[249] Serum chemistry may reveal an increased BUN, creatinine, and potassium if urinary outflow is obstructed. Mild lesions may resolve spontaneously.[241]

Medical treatment involves reducing the protein or NPN levels in diet to less than 16%, which may alone effect a cure with no further treatment in mild cases. Shearing fiber away from the external genitalia to allow airflow and irrigation of the sheath and application of nonirritating antiseptic/antibiotic solutions is useful. Iodine solutions should be avoided due to their encouragement of adhesions and production of granulation tissue. Systemic use of penicillin or oxytetracycline should be initiated in internalized cases and continued until lesions are dry and inflammation is reduced. Surgical management may involve lesion debridement or, as a salvage procedure, 2- to 4-cm incisions may be made through the ventral skin into the prepuce to allow drainage and lavage. In order to retain animals for breeding, preputial resection to allow urine flow and prevent adhesions may be attempted. After treatment, patients should be monitored closely to ensure patency of the urinary tract. Three months after a large outbreak, 33% of animals had residual posthitis and scarring may develop after lesion resolution.[241]

Control and prevention of ulcerative posthitis should involve isolation of affected individuals and a reduction in dietary protein to less than 16%. Supplementation with grass hay may limit intake of high-protein feeds and legume pastures. Shearing animals at times of high protein intake, the inclusion of the urinary acidifier ammonium chloride, or chlortetracycline added to the feed may reduce disease incidence. Shearing of the entire ventrum has been shown to reduce lesion incidence, while shearing only 3" around the preputial orifice was minimally effective.[251] The fiber of affected animals should be burned, and the bacterium is environmentally resistant in exudate. The lesion material from wethers was able to induce lesions on other wethers, ewes, and steers.[250] Venereal transfer readily occurs from rams to ewes, and flies may play a role in mechanical transmission.

The prognosis for recovery depends largely on the severity of signs when treatment is initiated. Without a reduction in dietary protein, it is unlikely that any treatment or preventative regime will be successful. If the disease is recognized prior to fibrosis, there may be a good prognosis for a full recovery with appropriate medical and dietary management. Potential sequelae in males include loss of breeding soundness due to adhesion of penis to prepuce, scarring of the preputial orifice, urethritis, and urethral obstruction. In females, there may be urine scalding and loss of breeding soundness due to impaired vulvar conformation. Fibrosis of the vulva may be severe enough to cause dystocia.

Congenital Anomalies of the Urethra

Hypospadias appears to be the most common congenital anomaly of the urethra reported in lambs,[251–253] and the urethral exposure may range from a small opening ventrally on the glans up to exposure along the full length of the urethra.[253] Lambs with hypospadias frequently have concurrent anomalies, including cleft scrotum and atresia ani.[252]

A condition of ventral urethral dilatation has been reported in an intersex goat where the urethra was not associated with the rudimentary penis.[254] Congenital narrowing of the urethral process with subsequent formation of a urethral diverticulum has been documented and repaired surgically in a goat kid.[255] Congenital urethral diverticulum and surgical correction has been reported in male kids.[256,257]

References

1. DeRossi R, Juniqueira AL, Beretta MP: Analgesic and systemic effects of ketamine, xylazine, and lidocaine after subarachnoid administration in goats, *Am J Vet Res* 64(1):51–56, 2003.
2. Thurmon JC, Nelson DR, Hartsfield SM, Rumore CA: Effects of xylazine hydrochloride on urine in cattle, *Aust Vet J* 54:178–180, 1978.
3. Waner T, Harrus S: Anemia of inflammatory disease. In Feldman BF, Zinkl JG, Jain NC, editors: *Schalm's veterinary hematology*, ed 5, Philadelphia, 2000, Lippincott Williams and Wilkins, pp 205–209.
4. Kramer JW: Normal hematology of cattle, sheep, and goats. In Feldman BF, Zinkl JG, Jain NC, editors: *Schalm's veterinary hematology*, ed 5, Philadelphia, 2000, Lippincott Williams and Wilkins, pp 1075–1084.
5. Braun U, Stehle C, Ehrensperger F: Clinical findings and treatment of listeriosis in 67 sheep and goats, *Vet Rec* 150:38–42, 2002.
6. de la Concha-Bermejillo A, Guo J, Zhang Z, Waldron D: Severe persistent orf in young goats, *J Vet Diagn Invest* 15:423–431, 2003.
7. Garry F, Chew DJ, Rings DM, Tarr MJ, Hoffsis GF: Renal excretion of creatinine, electrolytes, protein, and enzymes in healthy sheep, *Am J Vet Res* 51(3):414–419, 1990.
8. Mitchell AR, Moss P: Responses to reduced water intake, including dehydration natriuresis, in sheep excretion sodium predominately in urine or in feces, *Exp Physiol* 80:265–274, 1995.
9. Ammerman CB, Forbes RM, Garrigus US, Newmann AL, Norton HW, Hatfield EE: Ruminant utilization of inorganic phosphates, *J Anim Sci* 16:796–810, 1957.
10. Garrett PD: Urethral recess in male goats, sheep, cattle, and swine, *J Am Vet Med Assoc* 191(6):689–691, 1987.
11. Reppert EJ, Streeter RN, Simpson KM, Taylor JD: Retrograde catheterization of the urinary bladder in healthy male goats by use of angiographic catheters, *Am J Vet Res* 77(11):1295–1299, 2016.
12. Osborne CA, Stevens JB: Urinalysis: *A clinical guide to compassionate patient care*, Shawnee Mission, Kansas, 1999, Bayer Corporation.
13. Nappert G, Naylor JM: A comparison of pH determination methods in food animal practice, *Can Vet J* 42(5):364–367, 2001.
14. Stockham SL, Scott MA: Urinary system. In Stockham SL, Scott MA, editors: *Fundamentals of veterinary clinical pathology*, ed 2, Ames, 2008, Blackwell, pp 277–336.
15. Lunn DP, McGuirk SM, Smith DF, MacWilliams PS: Renal net acid and electrolyte excretion in an experimental model of hypochloremic metabolic alkalosis in sheep, *Am J Vet Res* 51(11):1723–1731, 1990.
16. McDougall EI: Proteinuria of newborn suckling ruminants, *Biochem J* 94:101–105, 1965.
17. Carlson GP: Clinical chemistry tests. In Smith BP, editor: *Large animal internal medicine*, ed 3, St. Louis, 2002, Mosby, pp 389–412.
18. Cutler JT: Studies of the carbohydrate metabolism of the goat, *J Biol Chem* 106:653–666, 1934.
19. Uzal FA, Kelly WR: Experimental *Clostridium perfringens* type D enterotoxemia in goats, *Vet Pathol* 35:132–140, 1998.
20. Setty DRL, Narayana K: A case of non-febrile haemoglobinuria in a she goat, *Indian Vet J* 52:149, 1975.
21. Stamp JT, Stewart J: Haemolytic anaemia with jaundice in sheep, *J Comp Path* 63:48–52, 1953.
22. Winter A, Clarkson M: Anaemia in lambs and kids caused by feeding cow colostrum, *In Pract* 14(6):283–286, 1992.
23. Perk K, Frie YF, Herz A: Osmotic fragility of red blood cells in young and mature domestic and laboratory animals, *Am J Vet Res* 25: 1241–1248, 1964.
24. Fernandez A, Mensua C, Biescas E, Lujan L: Clinicopathological features in ovine AA amyloidosis, *Res Vet Sci* 75:203–208, 2003.
25. Price RG: Urinary enzymes, nephrotoxicity and renal disease, *Toxicology* 23(2–3):99–134, 1982.
26. Garry F, Chew DJ, Rings DM, Tarr MJ, Hoffsis GF: Renal excretion of creatinine, electrolytes, protein, and enzymes in healthy sheep, *Am J Vet Res* 51(3):414–419, 1990.
27. Garry F, Chew DJ, Hoffsis GF: Enzymuria as an index of renal damage in sheep with induced aminoglycoside nephrotoxicosis, *Am J Vet Res* 51(3):428–432, 1990.
28. Braun U, Schefer U, Fohn J: Urinary tract ultrasonography in normal rams and in rams with obstructive urolithiasis, *Can Vet J* 33(10):654–659, 1992.
29. Braun U, Schefer U, Gerber D: Ultrasonography of the urinary tract of female sheep, *Am J Vet Res* 53(10):1734–1739, 1992.
30. Hallowell GD: Abdominal ultrasound. In *Proceedings of the 26th Annual American College of Veterinary Internal Medicine Forum*, San Antonio Texas, 2008.
31. Floeck M: Sonographic application in the diagnosis of pyelonephritis in cattle, *Vet Radiol Ultrasound* 48(1):74–77, 2007.
32. Halland SK, House JK, George LW: Urethroscopy and laser lithotripsy for the diagnosis and treatment of obstructive urolithiasis in goats and pot-bellied pigs, *J Am Vet Med Assoc* 12:1831–1834, 2002.
33. Janke JJ, Osterstock JB, Washburn KE, Bissett WT, Roussel AJ, Hooper RN: Use of Walpole's solution for treatment of goats with urolithiasis: 25 cases (2001–2006), *J Am Vet Med Assoc* 234(2):249–252, 2009.
34. Kopcha M, Schulze AE: Peritoneal fluid. II. Abdominocentesis in cattle and interpretation of noneoplastic samples, *Comp Cont Ed Pract Vet* 13(4):703–710, 1991.
35. Anderson DE, Cornwell D, Anderson LS, St-Jean G, Desrochers A: Comparative analyses of peritoneal fluid from calves and adult cattle, *Am J Vet Res* 56(8):973–976, 1995.
36. Wilson AD, Hirsch VM, Osborne AD: Abdominocentesis in cattle: technique and criteria for diagnosis of peritonitis, *Can Vet J* 26(2):74–80, 1985.
37. Stockham SL, Scott MA: Cavity effusions. In Stockham SL, Scott MA, editors: *Fundamentals of veterinary clinical pathology*, ed 2, Ames, 2008, Blackwell, pp 831–868.
38. Wilson DG, MacWilliams PS: An evaluation of the clinical pathologic findings in experimentally induced urinary bladder rupture in pre-ruminant calves, *Can J Vet Res* 62(2):140–143, 1998.
39. Sockett DC, Knight AP, Fettman MJ, Kiehl AR, Smith JA, Arnold SM: Metabolic changes due to experimentally induced rupture of the bovine urinary bladder, *Cornell Vet* 76(2):198–212, 1986.
40. Dennis SM: Urogenital defects in sheep, *Vet Rec* 105(5):344–347, 1979.
41. Hartley WJ, Kater JC: Perinatal disease conditions of sheep in New Zealand, *N Z Vet J* 12(2):49–57, 1964.
42. Cegarra IJ, Lewis RE: Excretory urography in the goat (*Capra hircus*), *Am J Vet Res* 38(8):1129–1132, 1977.
43. Palmer JL, Dykes NL, Love K, Fubini SL: Contrast radiography of the lower urinary tract in the management of obstructive urolithiasis in small ruminants and swine, *Vet Radiol Ultrasound* 39(3):175–180, 1998.
44. Cruz-Arámbulo Rde J, Tan L, Callan RJ, Van Metre DC, Park RD: What is your diagnosis? Communication between the urethra and the corpus spongiosum, urethral stricture, mild cystitis, and presence of a urachal diverticulum, *J Am Vet Med Assoc* 222(9):1211–1212, 2003.
45. Mohamed T, Oikawa S: Efficacy and safety of ultrasound-guided percutaneous biopsy of the right kidney in cattle, *J Vet Med Sci* 70(2):175–179, 2008.
46. Naoi M, Kokue E, Takahashi Y, Kido Y: Laparoscopic-assisted serial biopsy of the bovine kidney, *Am J Vet Res* 46(3):699–702, 1985.
47. Sankarappa EV, Rao PR: Renal lesions in sheep and goats in Andhra Pradesh, *Indian Vet J* 59:705–708, 1982.
48. Wallace RS, Bush M, Montali RJ: Deaths from exertional myopathy at the National Zoological Park from 1975 to 1985, *Wildl Dis Assoc* 23(3):454–462, 1987.
49. Nuvoli S, Burrai GP, Secci F, et al. Capture myopathy in a Corsican red deer *Cervus elaphus corsicanus* (Ungulata: Cervidae), *Italian J Zoo* 81(3):457–462, 2014.
50. Corley KT: Inotropes and vasopressors in adults and foals, *Vet Clin N Am Equine Prac* 20(1):77–106, 2004.
51. Trim CM, Moore JN, Clark ES: Renal effects of dopamine infusion in conscious horses, *Equine Vet J Suppl* (7):124–128, 1989.

52. Kellum JA, Decker JM: Use of dopamine in acute renal failure: a meta-analysis, *Crit Care Med* 29(8):1526–1531, 2001.
53. National Animal Health Monitoring Service: *Sheep 2001 Part II: reference of sheep health in the United States 2001*, USDA; 2003.
54. Niilo L: *Clostridium perfringens* in animal disease: a review of current knowledge, *Can Vet J* 21(5):141–148, 1980.
55. Gardner DE: Pathology of *Clostridium perfringens* type D enterotoxemia. II. Structural and ultrastructural alterations in the tissues of lambs and mice, *J Comp Pathol* 83:509–524, 1973.
56. Fernandez Miyakawa ME, Uzal FA: The early effects of *Clostridium perfringens* type D epsilon toxin in ligated intestinal loops of goats and sheep, *Vet Res Commun* 27(3):231–241, 2003.
57. Blackwell TE, Butler DG, Prescott JF, Wilcock BP: Differences in signs and lesions in sheep and goats with enterotoxemia induced by intraduodenal infusion of *Clostridium perfringens* type D, *Am J Vet Res* 52(7):1147–1152, 1991.
58. Uzal FA, Kelly WR, Morris WE, Bermudez J, Baisón M: The pathology of peracute experimental *Clostridium perfringens* type D enterotoxemia in sheep, *J Vet Diagn Invest* 16:403–411, 2004.
59. Layana JE, Miyakawa MEF, Uzal FA: Evaluation of different fluids for detection of *Clostridium perfringens* type D epsilon toxin in sheep with experimental enterotoxemia, *Anaerobe* 12(4):204–206, 2006.
60. Uzal FA, Songer JG: Diagnosis of *Clostridium perfringens* intestinal infections in sheep and goats, *J Vet Diagn Invest* 20:253–265, 2008.
61. de la Rosa C, Hogue De, Thonney ML: Vaccination schedules to raise antibody concentrations against epsilon-toxin of *Clostridium perfringens* in ewes and their triplet lambs, *J Anim Sci* 75: 2328–2334, 1997.
62. Ellis GR, Partington DL, Hindmarsh M, Barton MD: Seroprevalence to *Leptospira interrogans* serovar Hardjo in Merino stud rams in South Australia, *Aust Vet J* 71(7):203–206, 1994.
63. Heath SE, Johnson R: Leptospirosis, *J Am Vet Med Assoc.* 205(11): 1518–1523, 1994.
64. Marshall RB: Ultrastructural changes in renal tubules of sheep following experimental infection with *Leptospira interrogans* serotype Pomona, *J Med Microbiol* 7(4):505–508, 1974.
65. Adler B, de la Peña MA: Leptospira and leptospirosis, *Vet Microbiol* 140(3–4):287–296, 2010.
66. Aguirre AA, Hansen DE, Starkey EE, McLean RG: Serologic survey of wild cervids for potential disease agents in selected national parks in the United States, *Prev Vet Med* 21(4):313–322, 1995.
67. Bender LC, Hall PB: *Leptospira interrogans* exposure in free-ranging elk in Washington, *J Wildl Dis* 32(1):121–124, 1996.
68. Pedersen K, Anderson TD, Maison RM, et al: *Leptospira* antibodies detected in wildlife in the USA and the US Virgin Islands, *J Wildl Dis* 54(3):450–459, 2018.
69. Hodges RT: Some observations on experimental Leptospira serotype Pomona infection in sheep, *N Z Vet J* 22(8):151–154, 1974.
70. Smith BP, Armstrong JM: Fatal hemolytic anemia attributed to leptospirosis in lambs, *J Am Vet Med Assoc* 167(8):739–741, 1975.
71. Sleight SD, Langham RF: The effects of Leptospira Pomona hemolysin on pregnant ewes, cows, and sows, *J Infect Dis* 111(1):63–77, 1962.
72. Vermunt JJ, West DM, Cooke MM, Alley MR, Collins-Emerson J: Observations on three outbreaks of *Leptospira interrogans* serovar Pomona infection in lambs, *N Z Vet J* 42:133–136, 1994.
73. Harrington R: Leptospiral antibodies in serum from cattle, swine, horses, deer, sheep and goats: 1973–1974, *Am J Vet Res* 36(9):1367–1370, 1975.
74. Lilenbaum W, Varges R, Ristow R, et al: Identification of Leptospira spp. carriers among seroreactive goats and sheep by polymerase chain reaction, *Res Vet Sci* 87:16–19, 2009.
75. Kingscote B: Leptospirosis in sheep in western Canada, *Can Vet J* 26:164–168, 1985.
76. Prusty PK, Srivastava SK: Haemolytic properties of different Leptospira strains, *Ind J Anim Sci* 61(2):129–134, 1991.
77. Hathaway SC, Marshall RB: Experimental infection of sheep with *Leptospira interrogans*: serovars Hardjo and Balcanica, *N Z Vet J* 27(9):197, 1979.
78. Mitchell G, Leonard J: Leptospira interrogans serovar Hardjo infection in a sheep, *Aust Vet J* 62(10):346–347, 1985.
79. Cerri D, Nuvoloni R, Ebani V, et al: *Leptospira interrogans* serovar Hardjo in the kidneys and genital tracts of naturally infected sheep, *New Microbiol* 19:175–178, 1996.
80. Farina R, Cerri D, Renzoni G, et al: *Leptospira interrogans* in the genital tract of sheep. Research on ewes and rams experimentally infected with serovar Hardjo (hardjobovis), *New Microbiol* 19: 235–242, 1996.
81. Webb AI, Baynes RE, Craigmill AL, Riviere JE, Haskell SR: Drugs approved for small ruminants, *J Am Vet Med Assoc* 224(4):520–523, 2004.
82. Anonymous: Adverse reaction to tilmicosin use in goats, *Large Anim Vet Rep* 7:95, 1996.
83. Bolin CA, Thiermann AB, Handsaker AL, Foley JW: Effect of vaccination with a pentavalent leptospiral vaccine on *Leptospira interrogans* serovar Hardjo type hardjo-bovis infection of pregnant cattle, *Am J Vet Res* 50:161–165, 1989.
84. Bolin CA, Zuerner RL, Trueba G: Effect of vaccination with a pentavalent leptospiral vaccine containing *Leptospira interrogans* serovar Hardjo type hardjo-bovis on type hardjo-bovis infection in cattle, *Am J Vet Res* 50:2004–2008, 1989.
85. Bolin CA, Cassells JA, Zuerner RL, Trueba G: Effect of vaccination with a monovalent *Leptospira interrogans* serovar Hardjo type hardjo-bovis vaccine on type hardjo-bovis infection in cattle, *Am J Vet Res* 52:1639–1643, 1991.
86. Lehmkuhl HD, Cutlip RC, Brogden KA: Seroepidemiologic survey for adenovirus infection in lambs, *Am J Vet Res* 54:1277–1279, 1993.
87. Finnie JW, Swift JG: Adenovirus infection in ovine kidney and liver, *Aust Vet J* 68:184, 1991.
88. DeBey BM, Lehmkuhl HD, Chard-Bergstrom C, Hobbs LA: Ovine adenovirus serotype 7–associated mortality in lambs in the United States, *Vet Pathol* 38:644–648, 2001.
89. Belák S, Vetési F, Pálfi V, Papp L: Isolation of a pathogenic strain of ovine adenovirus type 5 and a comparison of its pathogenicity with that of another strain of the same serotype, *J Comp Pathol* 90(2):169–176, 1980.
90. Angus KW, Hodgson JC, Hosie BD, et al: Acute nephropathy in young lambs, *Vet Rec* 124:9–14, 1989.
91. Angus KW, Hodgson JC: Recognition and management of nephrosis in lambs, *In Pract* 12(1):3–5, 1990.
92. Angus KW: Nephropathy in young lambs, *Vet Rec* 126:525–528, 1990.
93. Benson JA, Williams BM: Acute renal failure in lambs, *Br Vet J* 130:475–481, 1974.
94. Yeruham I, Perl S, Elad D, Avidar Y: A generalized staphylococcal scalded skin-like disease in lambs, *Zentralbl Veterinarmed B* 46: 635–640, 1999.
95. Plumlee KH: Clinical Veterinary Toxicology. In Plumlee KH, editor: St. Louis, 2004, Mosby.
96. Radostits OM, Gay CC, Blood DC, Hinchcliff KW: Diseases of the kidney. In Radostits OM, Gay CC, Hinchcliff KW, editors: *Veterinary medicine: a textbook of the diseases of cattle, sheep, pigs, goats and horses*, Philadelphia, 2000, Saunders.
97. Barbosa RR, Fontenele-Neto JD, Soto-Blanco B: Toxicity in goats caused by oleander (*Nerium oleander*), *Res Vet Sci* 85:279–281, 2008.
98. Wisløff H, Flåøyen A, Ottesen N, Hovig T: *Narthecium ossifragum* (L.) huds. causes kidney damage in goats: morphologic and functional effects, *Vet Pathol* 40:317–327, 2003.
99. Cooper TB, Huxtable CR, Vogel P: The nephrotoxicity of *Isotropis forrestii* in sheep, *Aust Vet J* 63(6):178–182, 1986.
100. McMartin K: Are calcium oxalate crystals involved in the mechanism of acute renal failure in ethylene glycol poisoning? *Clin Toxicol (Phila)* 47(9):859–869, 2009.
101. Crowell WA, Whitlock RH, Stout RC, Tyler DE: Ethylene glycol toxicosis in cattle, *Cornell Vet* 69:272–279, 1979.

102. Singh DP, Kumar M, Varshney KC: Pathological changes in experimental ethylene glycol intoxication in cow calves: clinico-haematological and biochemical changes, *Ind J Anim Sci* 64: 1361–1363, 1994.
103. Barigye R, Mostrom M, Dyer NW, Newell TK, Lardy GP: Ethylene glycol toxicosis in adult beef cattle fed contaminated feeds, *Can Vet J* 49(10):1018–1020, 2008.
104. Church AS, Witting MD: Laboratory testing in ethanol, methanol, ethylene glycol, and isopropanol toxicities, *J Emerg Med* 15(5): 687–692, 1997.
105. Boermans HJ, Ruegg PL, Leach M: Ethylene glycol toxicosis in a pygmy goat, *J Am Vet Med Assoc* 193(6):694–696, 1988.
106. Dial SM, Thrall MA, Hamar DW: Comparison of ethanol and 4-methylpyrazole as treatments for ethylene glycol intoxication in cats, *Am J Vet Res* 55(12):1771–1782, 1994.
107. Ammerman CB, Miller SM, Fick KR, Hansard SL: Contaminating elements in mineral supplements and their potential toxicity: a review, *J Anim Sci* 44(3):485–508, 1977.
108. Stoev SD, Grozeva N, Simeonov R, et al: Experimental cadmium poisoning in sheep, *Exper Tox Path* 55(4):309–314, 2003.
109. Puls R: *Mineral levels of animal health*, ed 2, Clearbrook BC, 1994, Sherpa International.
110. van Ryssen JB: Effect of monensin and its metabolites in broiler litter on sheep consuming the broiler litter, *J S Afr Vet Assoc* 62(3):94–99, 1991.
111. Starnes SR, Spears JW, Froetschel MA, Croom WJ Jr: Influence of monensin and lasalocid on mineral metabolism and ruminal urease activity in steers, *J Nutr* 114(3):518–525, 1984.
112. Nederbragt H, van den Ingh TSGAM, Wensvoort P: Pathobiology of copper toxicity, *Vet Quart* 6(4):179–185, 1984.
113. Hochstein P, Kumar KS, Forman SJ: Mechanisms of copper toxicity in red cells, *Prog Clin Biol Res* 21:669–686, 1978.
114. Lewis NJ, Fallah-Rad AH, Connor ML: Copper toxicity in confinement-housed ram lambs, *Can Vet J* 38:496–498, 1997.
115. Roubies N, Giadinis ND, Polizopoulou Z, Argiroudis S: A retrospective study of chronic copper poisoning in 79 sheep flocks in Greece (1987–2007), *J Vet Pharmacol Ther* 31(2):181–183, 2008.
116. Burrows GE: Methylene blue: effects and disposition in sheep, *J Vet Pharmacol Ther* 7(3):225–231, 1984.
117. Haskell SR, Payne M, Webb A, Riviere J, Craigmill AL: Antidotes in food animal practice, *J Am Vet Med Assoc* 226(6):884–887, 2005.
118. Humphries WR, Mills CF, Greig A, Roberts L, Inglis D, Halliday GJ: Use of ammonium tetrathiomolybdate in the treatment of copper poisoning in sheep, *Vet Rec* 119:596–598, 1986.
119. Gaetke LM, Chow CK: Copper toxicity, oxidative stress, and antioxidant nutrients, *Toxicology* 189:147–163, 2003.
120. Schilsky ML, Blank RR, Czaja MJ, et al: Hepatocellular copper toxicity and its attenuation by zinc, *J Clin Invest* 84:1562–1568, 1989.
121. Garry F, Chew DJ, Hoffsis GF: Urinary indices of renal function in sheep with induced aminoglycoside nephrotoxicosis, *Am J Vet Res* 51(3):420–427, 1990.
122. Lairmore MD, Alexander AF, Powers BE, Milisen WB, McChesney AE, Spraker TS: Oxytetracycline-associated nephrotoxicosis in feedlot calves, *J Am Vet Med Assoc* 185(7):793–795, 1984.
123. Vaala WE, Ehnen SJ, Divers TJ: Acute renal failure associated with administration of excessive amounts of tetracycline in a cow, *J Am Vet Med Assoc* 191(12):1601–1603, 1987.
124. Silva SM, Castro RS, Costa FA, et al: Conidiobolomycosis in sheep in Brazil, *Vet Pathol* 44:314–319, 2007.
125. Rao VP, Poutahidis T, Marini RP, Holcombe H, Rogers AB, Fox JG: Renal infarction and immune-mediated glomerulonephritis in sheep (*Ovis aries*) chronically implanted with indwelling catheters, *J Am Assoc Lab Anim Sci* 45(4):14–19, 2006.
126. Wobeser G, Haas S: Renal lipomatosis in a lamb, *Can Vet J* 45:863–864, 2004.
127. Hayashi A, Yanagawa R, Kida H: Survival of *Corynebacterium renale*, *Corynebacterium pilosum* and *Corynebacterium cystitidis* in soil, *Vet Microbiol* 10(4):381–386, 1985.
128. Pijoan C, Lastra A, Leman A: Isolation of *Corynebacterium suis* from the prepuce of boars, *J Am Vet Med Assoc* 183(4):428–429, 1983.
129. Tubbs RC: Cystitis, pyelonephritis, and miscellaneous diseases of swine. In Howard JL, Smith RA, editors: *Current veterinary therapy: food animal practice*, ed 4, Philadelphia, 1999, WB Saunders, pp 631–632.
130. Matos AC, Figueira L, Martins MH, et al: Detection of *Mycobacterium avium* subsp. *paratuberculosis* in kidney samples of red deer (*Cervus elaphus*) in Portugal: evaluation of different methods, *J Vet Med Sci* 79(3):692–698, 2017.
131. Floeck M: Sonographic application in the diagnosis of pyelonephritis in cattle, *Vet Rad Ultrasound* 48(1):74–77, 2007.
132. Markusfeld O, Nahari N, Kessner D, Adler H: Observations on bovine pyelonephritis, *Br Vet J* 145(6):573–579, 1989.
133. Miesner MD, Anderson DE: Unilateral nephrectomy of cattle, *Vet Clin North Am Food Anim Pract* 24(3):497–500, 2008.
134. Taniyama H, Yamamoto S, Sako T, Hirayama K, Higuchi H, Nagahata H: Systemic kappaAL amyloidosis associated with bovine leukocyte adhesion deficiency, *Vet Pathol* 37:98–100, 2000.
135. Rings DM, Garry FB: Amyloidosis associated with paratuberculosis in a sheep, *Comp Cont Ed Food Animal* 10:381–385, 1988.
136. Tham VL, Bunn CM: Amyloidosis in an angora goat, *Aus Vet J* 69:40–41, 1992.
137. Woolf A, Kradel DC: Mortality in captive bighorn sheep—clinical, hematological, and pathological observations, *J Wildlife Dis* 9:12–17, 1973.
138. Biescas E, Jirón W, Climent S, et al: AA amyloidosis induced in sheep principally affects the gastrointestinal tract, *J Comp Pathol* 140:238–246, 2009.
139. Stummer P, Fuchs-Baumgartinger A, Franz S, Nell B: Severe chemosis caused by nephrotic syndrome in a goat: a case report, *Vet J* 175:141–143, 2008.
140. Fernández A, Ménsua C, Biescas E, Luján L: Clinicopathological features in ovine AA amyloidosis, *Res Vet Sci* 75:203–208, 2003.
141. Ménsua C, Carrasco L, Bautista MJ, et al: Pathology of AA amyloidosis in domestic sheep and goats, *Vet Pathol* 40:71–80, 2003.
142. Lerner RA, Dixon FJ, Lee S: Spontaneous glomerulonephritis in sheep. II. Studies on natural history, occurrence in other species, and pathogenesis, *Am J Pathol* 53(4):501–512, 1968.
143. Angus KW, Sykes AR, Gardiner AC, Morgan KT, Thomson D: Mesangiocapillary glomerulonephritis in lambs. I. Clinical and biochemical findings in a Finnish Landrace flock, *J Comp Pathol* 84:309–317, 1974.
144. Young GB, Sales DI, Waddington D, Angus KW, Gardiner AC: Genetic aspects of mesangiocapillary glomerulonephritis in Finnish sheep, *Br Vet J* 137(4):368–373, 1981.
145. Frelier PF, Pritchard J, Armstrong DL, Nagge WT, Lewis RM: Spontaneous mesangiocapillary glomerulonephritis in Finn cross lambs from Alberta, *Can J Comp Med* 48:215–218, 1984.
146. Frelier PF, Armstrong DL, Pritchard J: Ovine mesangiocapillary glomerulonephritis type I and crescent formation, *Vet Pathol* 27(1):26–34, 1990.
147. Angus KW, Gardiner AC, Mitchell B, Thomson D: Mesangiocapillary glomerulonephritis in lambs: the ultrastructure and immunopathology of diffuse glomerulonephritis in newly born Finnish Landrace lambs, *J Pathol* 131(1):65–74, 1980.
148. Angus KW, Gardner AC, Mitchell B, Aitchison GU, Thomson D: The role of colostrum in glomerulonephritis of Finnish Landrace lambs: effect of cross-fostering newly born Finnish Landrace and Cheviot lambs, *Res Vet Sci* 19(2):222–224, 1975.
149. Angus KW, Gardiner AC: Mesangiocapillary glomerulonephritis in Dorset-Finnish landrace cross lambs, *Vet Rec* 105(20):471, 1979.
150. Morgan KT, Gardiner AC, Angus KW: A choroid plexus lesion in lambs with mesangiocapillary glomerulonephritis, *J Comp Path* 87(1):15–25, 1977.
151. Tarshish P, Bernstein J, Tobin JN, et al: Treatment of mesangiocapillary glomerulonephritis with alternate-day prednisone—a report

of The International Study of Kidney Disease in Children, *Ped Neph* 6(2):123–130, 1992.
152. Baird GJ, Fontaine MC: *Corynebacterium pseudotuberculosis* and its role in ovine caseous lymphadenitis, *J Comp Pathol* 137:179–210, 2007.
153. Cordes DO, Bullians JA, Lake DE, Carter ME: Observations on tuberculosis caused by Mycobacterium bovis in sheep, *N Z Vet J* 29:60–62, 1981.
154. Davis WP, Steficek BA, Watson GL, et al: Disseminated *Rhodococcus equi* infection in two goats, *Vet Pathol* 36:336–339, 1999.
155. Angus KW, Hodgson JC: Renal ultrastructure in lamb nephrosis, *J Comp Pathol* 103(3):241–245, 1990.
156. Van der Lugt JJ, Henton MM: Melioidosis in a goat, *J S Afr Vet Assoc* 66(2):71–73, 1995.
157. Senturk S, Temizel M: Clinical efficacy of rifamycin SV combined with oxytetracycline in the treatment of caseous lymphadenitis in sheep, *Vet Rec* 159:216–217, 2006.
158. Ziada G, Youseif H, Khalil M: Compensatory changes in the function of the remaining kidney immediately after unilateral nephrectomy in sheep, *Tohoku J Exp Med* 219(2):165–168, 2009.
159. Mehdi NA, Kazacos KR, Carlton WW: Fatal disseminated toxoplasmosis in a goat, *J Am Vet Med Assoc* 183(1):115–117, 1983.
160. Hartley WJ, Seaman JT: Suspected toxoplasma infection in an adult goat, *Vet Pathol* 19(2):210–212, 1982.
161. Pang VF, Shadduck JA: Susceptibility of cats, sheep, and swine to a rabbit isolate of *Encephalitozoon cuniculi*, *Am J Vet Res* 46(5):1071–1077, 1985.
162. Khanna RS, Iyer PK: A case of Nosema cuniculi infection in a goat, *Indian J Med Res* 59(7):993–995, 1971.
163. Mackie JT, Dubey JP: Congenital sarcocystosis in a Saanen goat, *J Parasitol* 82(2):350–351, 1996.
164. Oryan A, Moghaddar N, Gaur SN: Metacestodes of sheep with special reference to their epidemiological status, pathogenesis and economic implications in Fars Province, Iran, *Vet Parasitol* 51 (3–4):231–240, 1994.
165. Lizardo-Daudt HM, Albano Edelweiss MI: Ultrastructural alterations in glomerulonephropathy associated with hydatidosis in sheep, *Bol Chil Parasitol* 53(3–4):52–57, 1998.
166. Angus KW: Nephropathy in young lambs, *Vet Rec* 126:525–528, 1990.
167. Pullan NB, Sewell MM, Hammond JA: Studies on the pathogenicity of massive infections of *Fasciola hepatica* L. in lambs, *Br Vet J* 126(10):543–558, 1970.
168. Light FW Jr: Pigmented thickening of the basement membranes of the renal tubules of the goat ("cloisonné kidney"), *Lab Invest* 8:228–238, 1960.
169. Altman NH, Grossman IW, Jernigan NB: Caprine cloisonné renal lesion. Clinicopathological observations, *Cornell Vet* 60(1):83–90, 1970.
170. Oryan A, Razavi M, Maleki M: Observations on cloisonné kidney in sheep, *N Z Vet J* 41:210, 1993.
171. Hatipoglu F, Erer H: Lesions of cloisonné kidney in sheep: report on four cases, *Revue Med Vet* 152(4):313–315, 2001.
172. Thompson SW, Bogdon TR, Yost DH: Some histochemical studies of "cloisonné kidney" in the male Angora goat, *Am J Vet Res* 22:757–763, 1961.
173. Grossman IW, Altman NH: Caprine cloisonne renal lesion. Ultrastructure of the thickened proximal convoluted tubular basement membrane, *Arch Pathol* 88(6):609–612, 1969.
174. Johnstone AC, Davidson BI, Roe AR, Eccles MR, Jolly RD: Congenital polycystic kidney disease in lambs, *N Z Vet J* 53(5): 307–314, 2005.
175. Krotec K, Meyer BS, Freeman W, Hamir AN: Congenital cystic disease of the liver, pancreas, and kidney in a nubian goat (*Capra hircus*), *Vet Pathol* 33:708–710, 1996.
176. Newman SJ, Leichner T, Crisman M, Ramos J: Congenital cystic disease of the liver and kidney in a pygmy goat, *J Vet Diagn Invest* 12:374–378, 2000.
177. Dennis SM: Urogenital defects in sheep, *Vet Rec* 105(15):344–347, 1979.
178. Jones TO, Clegg FG, Morgan G, Wijeratne WV: A vertically transmitted cystic renal dysplasia of lambs, *Vet Rec* 127(17):421–424, 1990.
179. O'Toole D, Jeffrey M, Jones T, Morgan G, Green R: Pathology of renal dysplasia and bladder aplasia-hypoplasia in a flock of sheep, *J Vet Diagn Invest* 5:591–602, 1993.
180. Palmer MV, Carpenter JG: Congenital polycystic kidney in a white-tailed deer (*Odocoileus virginianus*), *J Vet Diagn Invest* 16(5):475–477, 2004.
181. Gomez-Villamandos JC, Carmona JM, Castellano J, et al: Possible renal dysplasia in two related, juvenile goats, *Small Rum Res* 13:311–314, 1994.
182. Blutke A, März K, Matenaers C, Oswald K, Hermanns W, Wanke R: Polycystic kidney disease in a European roe deer (*Capreolus capreolus*), *J Zoo Wildl Med* 44(2):487–490, 2013.
183. Scarratt WK, Lombard CW, Buergelt CD: Ventricular septal defects in two goats, *Cornell Vet* 74(2):136–145, 1984.
184. Olson C, Baumgartener LE: Pathology of lymphosarcoma in sheep induced with bovine leukemia virus, *Cancer Res* 36:2365–2373, 1976.
185. Raperto F, Damiano S: Nephroblastoma in an ovine foetus, *Zentralbl Veterinarmed A* 28:504–507, 1981.
186. Snyder SP, Davies RB, Spraker TR, et al: Embryonal nephroma in a wapiti, *J Wildl Dis* 15:303–306, 1979.
187. Halland SK, House JK, George LW: Urethroscopy and laser lithotripsy for the diagnosis and treatment of obstructive urolithiasis in goats and pot-bellied pigs, *J Am Vet Med Assoc* 220(12):1831–1834, 2002.
188. Cruz-Arámbulo Rde J, Tan L, Callan RJ, Van Metre DC, Park RD: What is your diagnosis? Communication between the urethra and the corpus spongiosum, urethral stricture, mild cystitis, and presence of a urachal diverticulum, *J Am Vet Med Assoc* 222(9): 1211–1212, 2003.
189. Food Animal Residue Avoidance Database. Available at: http://www.farad.org/.
190. The Minor Use Animal Drug Program. Available at: http://www.nrsp-7.org/mumsrx/.
191. Wouda W, Borst GH, Gruys E: Delayed swayback in goat kids, a study of 23 cases, *Vet Q* 8(1):45–56, 1986.
192. O'Sullivan BM: Enzootic ataxia in goat kids, *Aust Vet J* 53(9): 455–456, 1977.
193. Duncan RB, Patton S: Naturally occurring cerebral parelaphostrongylosis in a heifer, *J Vet Diagn Invest* 10:287–291, 1998.
194. Kopcha M, Marteniuk JV, Sills R, Steficek B, Schillhorn van Veen TW: Cerebrospinal nematodiasis in a goat herd, *J Am Vet Med Assoc* 194:1439–1442, 1989.
195. Tyler JW, Turnquist SE, David AT, Kleiboeker SB, Middleton JR: West Nile virus encephalomyelitis in a sheep, *J Vet Intern Med* 17:242–244, 2003.
196. Bradley GA, Metcalf HC, Reggiardo C, et al: Neuroaxonal degeneration in sheep grazing Sorghum pastures, *J Vet Diagn Invest* 7:229–236, 1995.
197. French NP, Wall R, Morgan KL: Lamb tail docking: a controlled field study of the effects of tail amputation on health and productivity, *Vet Rec* 134(18):463–467, 1994.
198. Holt PE, Thrusfield MV: Association in bitches between breed, size, neutering and docking, and acquired urinary incontinence due to incompetence of the urethral sphincter mechanism, *Vet Rec* 133:177–180, 1993.
199. Scarratt WK, Lombard CW, Buergelt CD: Ventricular septal defects in two goats, *Cornell Vet* 74(2):136–145, 1984.
200. Dennis SM: Hypospadias in Merino lambs, *Vet Rec* 105(5):94–96, 1979.
201. Hartley WJ, Kater JC: Perinatal disease conditions of sheep in New Zealand, *N Z Vet J* 12(3):49–57, 1964.
202. O'Toole D, Jeffrey M, Jones T, Morgan G, Green R: Pathology of renal dysplasia and bladder aplasia-hypoplasia in a flock of sheep, *J Vet Diagn Invest* 5:591–602, 1993.

203. Dennis SM: Patent urachus in a neonatal lamb, *Cornell Vet* 59(4):581–584, 1969.
204. Lairmore MD, Knight AP, DeMartini JC: Three primary neoplasms in a goat: hepatocellular carcinoma, phaeochromocytoma and leiomyoma, *J Comp Pathol* 97:267–271, 1987.
205. Olson C, Baumgartener LE: Pathology of lymphosarcoma in sheep induced with bovine leukemia virus, *Cancer Res* 36:2365–2373, 1976.
206. Al-Dubaib MA: Renal and cardiac metastases of Jaagsiekte-like tumour in a goat, *Small Rum Res* 58(1):75–58, 2005.
207. Scala C, Ortiz K, Catinaud J, Lemberger K: Hematuria and urinary bladder lesions compatible with Bracken fern *(Pteridium aquilinum)* intoxication in captive fallow deer *(Dama dama)*, *J Zoo Wildl Med* 45(2):380–385, 2014.
208. Dyce KM, Sack WO, Wensing CJG: The pelvis and reproductive organs of male ruminants. In *Textbook of veterinary anatomy*, ed 3, Philadelphia, 2002, Saunders, pp 713–722.
209. National Animal Health Monitoring Service: *Sheep 2001 Part II: reference of sheep health in the United States 2001*, USDA, 2003.
210. Hattel AL, Shaw DP, Love BC, Wagner DC, Drake TR, Brooks JW: A retrospective study of mortality in Pennsylvania captive white-tailed deer (*Odocoileus virginianus*): 2000–2003, *J Vet Diagn Invest* 16:515–521, 2004.
211. Larsen RS, Cebra CK, Wild MA: Diagnosis and treatment of obstructive urolithiasis in a captive Rocky Mountain wapiti (*Cervus elaphus* nelsoni), *J Zoo Wildl Med* 31(2):236–239, 2000.
212. Osborne CA, Polzin DJ, Abdullahi SU, Leininger JR, Clinton CW, Griffith DP: Struvite urolithiasis in animals and man: formation, detection, and dissolution, *Adv Vet Sci Comp Med* 29:1–101, 1985.
213. Packett LV, Coburn SP. Urine proteins in nutritionally induced ovine urolithiasis. *Am J Vet Res* 26(10):112–129, 1965.
214. Hay L: Prevention and treatment of urolithiasis in sheep, *Vet Record Suppl: In Practice* 12:87–91, 1990.
215. Elliot JS, Quaide WL, Sharp RF, Lewis L: Mineralogical studies of urine: The relationship of apatite, brushite and struvite to urinary pH, *J Urol* 80(4):269–271, 1958.
216. George JW, Hird DW, George LW: Serum biochemical abnormalities in goats with uroliths: 107 cases (1992–2003), *J Am Vet Med Assoc* 230(1):101–106, 2007.
217. Michell AR, Moss P: Responses to reduced water intake, including dehydration natriuresis, in sheep excreting sodium predominantly in urine or in faeces, *Exp Physiol* 80:265–274, 1995.
218. Ammerman CB, Forbes RM, Garrigus US, et al: Ruminant utilization of inorganic phosphates, *J Anim Sci* 16:796–810, 1957.
219. Oehme FW, Tillmann H: Diagnosis and treatment of ruminant urolithiasis, *J Am Vet med Assoc* 147:1331–1339, 1965.
220. Van Metre DC, House JK, Smith BP, et al: Obstructive urolithiasis: medical treatment and urethral surgery, *Compend Cont Edu* 18:317–328, 1996.
221. DeRossi R, Junqueira AL, Beretta MP: Analgesic and systemic effects of ketamine, xylazine, and lidocaine after subarachnoid administration in goats, *Am J Vet Res* 64(1):51–56, 2003.
222. Mann FA, Cowart RP, McClure RC, Constantinescu GM: Permanent urinary diversion in two Vietnamese pot-bellied pigs by extrapelvic urethral or urethropreputial anastomosis, *J Am Vet Med Assoc* 205(8):1157–1160, 1994.
223. Stone WC, Bjorling DE, Trostle SS, Hanson PD, Markel MD: Prepubic urethrostomy for relief of urethral obstruction in a sheep and a goat, *J Am Vet Med Assoc* 210(7):939–941, 1997.
224. Gill MS, Sod GA: Buccal mucosal graft urethroplasty for reversal of a perineal urethrostomy in a goat wether, *Vet Surg* 33:382–385, 2004.
225. Deleted in review.
226. Garrett PD: Urethral recess in male goats, sheep, cattle, and swine, *J Am Vet Med Assoc* 191(6):689–691, 1987.
227. Reppert EJ, Streeter RN, Simpson KM, Taylor JD: Retrograde catheterization of the urinary bladder in healthy male goats by use of angiographic catheters, *Am J Vet Res* 77(11):1295–1299, 2016.
228. Haven ML, Bowman KF, Engelbert TA, Blikslager AT: Surgical management of urolithiasis in small ruminants, *Cornell Vet* 83(1):47–55, 1993.
229. Tobias KM, van Amstel SR: Modified proximal perineal urethrostomy technique for treatment of urethral stricture in goats, *Vet Surg* 42(4):455–462, 2013.
230. Ewoldt JM, Jones ML, Miesner MD: Surgery of obstructive urolithiasis in ruminants, *Vet Clin North Am Food Anim Pract* 24(3):455–465, 2008.
231. May KA, Moll HD, Wallace LM, Pleasant RS, Howard RD: Urinary bladder marsupialization for treatment of obstructive urolithiasis in male goats, *Vet Surg* 2:583–588, 1998.
232. Streeter RN, Washburn KE, McCauley CT: Percutaneous tube cystostomy and vesicular irrigation for treatment of obstructive urolithiasis in a goat, *J Am Vet Med Assoc* 221(4):546–549, 2002.
233. Fortier LA, Gregg AJ, Erb HN, Fubini SL: Caprine obstructive urolithiasis: requirement for 2nd surgical intervention and mortality after percutaneous tube cystostomy, surgical tube cystostomy, or urinary bladder marsupialization, *Vet Surg* 33:661–667, 2004.
234. Abrahamsen EJ: Ruminant field anesthesia. In Anderson DE, Rings DM, editors: *Current vet therapy 5, food animal practice*, St. Louis MO, 2009, Saunders Elsevier, p 558.
235. Todhunter P, Baird AN, Wolfe DF: Erection failure as a sequela to obstructive urolithiasis in a male goat, *J Am Vet Med Assoc* 209(3):650–652, 1996.
236. Janke JJ, Osterstock JB, Washburn KE, Bissett WT, Roussel AJ, Hooper RN: Use of Walpole's solution for treatment of goats with urolithiasis: 25 cases (2001–2006), *J Am Vet Med Assoc* 234(2):249–252, 2009.
237. Hoar DW, Emerick RJ, Embry LB: Potassium, phosphorus and calcium interrelationships influencing feedlot performance and phosphatic urolithiasis in lambs, *J Anim Sci* 30(4):597–600, 1970.
238. Stratton-Phelps M, House JK: Effect of a commercial anion dietary supplement on acid-base balance, urine volume, and urinary ion excretion in male goats fed oat or grass hay diets, *Am J Vet Res* 65(10):1391–1397, 2004.
239. Jones ML, Streeter RN, Goad CL: Use of dietary cation anion difference for control of urolithiasis risk factors in goats, *Am J Vet Res* 70(1):149–155, 2009.
240. Bani Ismail ZA, Al-Zghoul MF, Al-Majali A, et al: Effects of castration on penile and urethral development in Awassi lambs, *Bulg J Vet Med* 10(1):29–34, 2007.
241. Tarigan S, Webb RF, Kirkland D: Caprine herpesvirus from balanoposthitis, *Aust Vet J* 64(10):321, 1987.
242. de la Concha-Bermejillo A, Guo J, Zhang Z, Waldron D: Severe persistent orf in young goats, *J Vet Diagn Invest* 15:423–431, 2003.
243. Kumar D, Gupta PP, Rana JS, Banga HS: Granular vulvovaginitis (GVV) in sheep experimentally induced with Mycoplasma ovine/caprine serogroup 11, *Acta Vet Brno* 61:241–249, 1992.
244. Bergonier D, Berthelot X, Poumarat F: Contagious agalactia of small ruminants: current knowledge concerning epidemiology, diagnosis and control, *Rev Sci Tech* 16(3):848–873, 1997.
245. DaMassa AJ, Wakenell PS, Brooks DL: Mycoplasmas of goats and sheep, *J Vet Diagn Invest* 4:101–113, 1992.
246. Doig PA, Ruhnke HL: Isolation of *Ureaplasma* from sheep with granular vulvitis, *Vet Rec* 100:179–180, 1977.
247. McMillian KR, Southcott WH: Aetiological factors in ovine posthitis, *Aust Vet J* 49:405–408, 1973.
248. Shelton M, Livingston CW Jr: Posthitis in Angora wethers, *J Am Vet Med Assoc* 167(2):154–155, 1975.
249. Whetstone CA, Evermann JF: Characterization of bovine herpesviruses isolated from six sheep and four goats by restriction endonuclease analysis and radioimmunoprecipitation, *Am J Vet Res* 49(6):781–785, 1988.

250. Southcott WH: Epidemiology and control of ovine posthitis and vulvitis, *Aust Vet J* 41:225–234, 1965.
251. Dennis SM: Hypospadias in Merino lambs, *Vet Rec* 105(5):94–96, 1979.
252. Hartley WJ, Kater JC: Perinatal disease conditions of sheep in New Zealand, *N Z Vet J* 12(3):49–57, 1964.
253. Dennis SM: Urogenital defects in sheep, *Vet Rec* 105(15):344–347, 1979.
254. Karras S, Modransky P, Welker B: Surgical correction of urethral dilatation in an intersex goat, *J Am Vet Med Assoc* 201(10):1584–1586, 1992.
255. Temizoylu MD: Penile urethral diverticulum in a kid, *Ankara Univ Vet Fak Derg* 52:185–187, 2005.
256. Nair NR, Tiwari SK: Congenital urethral anomaly in a kid and its surgical reconstruction, *Indian Vet J* 66:762–763, 1989.
257. Gahlot TK, Ranka AK, Chouhan DS, et al: Congenital urethral diverticulum in a male goat *(Capra hircus)*—surgical management, *Indian Vet Surg* 3(2):95–97, 1982.

13 Diseases of the Neurologic System

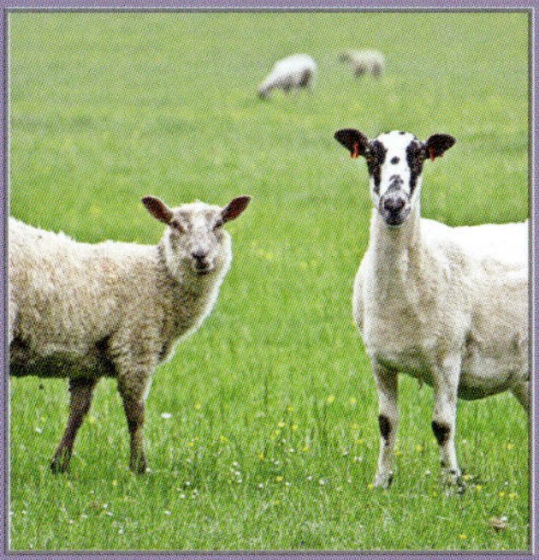

THOMAS PASSLER AND PAUL H. WALZ

Examination of the Neurologic System

The central nervous system (CNS) is a complex organ, and clinical signs of neurologic disease depend on the location of the disease process within the nervous system. Diseases of diverse etiologic origins can produce similar or identical neurologic signs in small ruminants (sheep, goats, and cervids). In addition, accurate diagnosis can be challenging because many systemic diseases can manifest with clinical signs referable to the nervous system. Specific examples are hypocalcemia, hypoglycemia, pregnancy toxemia, grain overload, hepatoencephalopathy, and severe endotoxemia. Thus, the objectives in the management of sheep, goats, or cervids with a clinical problem that could be related to the nervous system are (1) to verify that the underlying disorder is truly of neurologic origin and (2) to localize the lesion to a certain segment or segments of the nervous system (neuroanatomic localization). Of note, clinical signs associated with nervous system disease usually reflect the location of the pathologic process within the nervous system, rather than the specific cause of disease. However, determining the cause of the pathologic changes and the extent of the lesion is important for prognosis and for estimating costs associated with treatment. Finally, obtaining an accurate diagnosis is important because some neurologic diseases carry herd health implications or are zoonotic, so preventive measures are important for limiting or avoiding disease in at-risk populations.

Complete Neurologic Examination

Assessment of Chief Complaint. Obtaining information on signalment and history and performing a thorough physical examination including assessment of the nervous system constitute the complete neurologic examination. Information on signalment is important because disease susceptibility can be linked to age, species, breed, and sex. For example, Suffolk sheep older than 2 years of age are more likely to be affected by scrapie than younger animals or animals of different breeds. The signalment often is ascertained by simple observation, but specific details such as production status and exact age are more accurately determined through client interview. Some diseases capable of causing neurologic signs are species specific, especially those diseases with an infectious or genetic basis. In general, young animals with neurologic problems are more likely to have congenital, inherited, or infectious disorders, whereas older animals are more likely to be affected by neoplastic and degenerative diseases. Knowledge of common neurologic diseases, in either individual animals or groups, related to gender or a particular breed or age can greatly assist the clinician in developing a list of entities to consider in the differential diagnosis. Many sheep and goats are production animals, so the expenses associated with evaluation and treatment must be weighed against the prognosis for future productivity. Although captive cervids can vary in economic value, the expense and stress of capture and treatment must be considered. Great care and forethought should be employed when capturing cervids with neurologic disease, as sedatives and anesthetics can result in exacerbation of neurologic signs and mortality. Because small ruminants reside in social groups, the interests of the population also must be considered.

The clinical history is an important step in the diagnosis of neurologic disease. Information related to onset, duration, and progression of the chief complaint can assist with an etiologic diagnosis *(What is the cause?)* after the anatomic diagnosis *(Where is the lesion?)* has been made. In collecting historical information, it is important to determine the nature of the first clinical signs but also to define the relationship between the severity of clinical signs with respect to time (as on a sign-time graph). Some neurologic diseases occur acutely, with all clinical signs apparent within hours. Traumatic, toxic, infectious, and metabolic diseases can manifest with this pattern, whereas degenerative, neoplastic, or some viral disorders may develop more slowly, requiring days to weeks before the full complement of clinical signs becomes apparent. In addition to specific information related to the chief complaint, information on diet, housing, gestational status, and vaccination and deworming regimens should be part of the information gathered from the client. In interviewing clients for historical information, ambiguous or leading questions should be carefully avoided, because the information thus obtained may be inaccurate.

A thorough physical examination should be performed in conjunction with every neurologic examination. The nervous system is integrated within many other body systems, and diseases of the cardiovascular, respiratory, musculoskeletal, and endocrine and metabolic systems can manifest with clinical signs similar to those observed with nervous system disease. Before being subjected to the stress of handling or capture, the animal should be observed in its normal surroundings to assess behavior, mental status, gait, tremors, and head, neck, and limb postures. Cervids are best visualized in their natural environment using a spotting scope or binoculars.

Mentation. Evaluation of mentation can assist the clinician in differentiating intracranial from extracranial disease processes. As described previously, some systemic diseases will result in depression without nervous system pathology. During the period of initial observation, the animal's mental status and behavior can be assessed, but this must be done when the animal is not stimulated. For animals to be alert and oriented, the cerebral cortex and the ascending reticular activating system must be functioning properly. The ascending reticular activating system makes up the major portion of the brain stem parenchyma and is responsible for arousal and sleep-wake transitions in animals. Consequently, disorders involving the ascending reticular activating system can cause somnolence. The ascending reticular activating system is composed of several neuronal circuits connecting the brain stem to the cortex. External stimuli, such as light, touch, sound, smell, and temperature, help to maintain consciousness. An animal should appear as sensitive to its environment as its herdmates. If removed from its usual environment, the normal animal will be alert and cautious of new situations and aware of the examiner. The animal should follow the examiner's movement with its head, eyes, and ears. All animals should avoid painful stimuli. Abnormal mentation in ruminants can be placed into one of the following categories: (1) excitement, mania, or hyperesthesia; (2) seizures; (3) depression; (4) aimless circling, stupor, and coma; (5) abnormal vocalization; and (6) blindness.[1] Stupor is characterized as a condition of unresponsiveness to environmental stimulation such as light and sound, with retention of response to painful stimuli. By contrast, a comatose animal is nonresponsive to either environmental or painful stimulation.

Behavioral changes may be difficult to assess if the animal's environment has been changed. Alterations in behavior include aggression, vocalization, compulsive activities such as circling or walking or gazing, yawning, head pressing, and increased or abnormal sexual activity. The neuroanatomic localization of behavioral disorders may be difficult because the components of the limbic system—hypothalamus, hippocampus, amygdala, and portions of the cerebral cortex—all are associated with complex behavior.

Gait and Posture. To properly assess gait and posture, the small ruminant should be allowed to move freely within an enclosed area. A pet or tame animal can be walked at a slow pace by the client using a halter. Observations on forelimb gait are made as the animal is walked toward the examiner, and observations on hindlimb gait should be made as the animal is walked away from the examiner. *Gait* is defined as a regularly repeating series of leg movements during walking or running. Goats and sheep walk by first flexing the hindlimb on one side and then the forelimb on the same side. This process is then repeated for the opposite side. Animals integrate multiple neural processes in order to walk. The cerebrum initiates voluntary locomotion and adjusts movements according to learned functions. The cerebellum contributes to the coordination of movement. The vestibular system maintains balance and helps anticipate alterations in the animal's center of gravity so that it can compensate appropriately. Spinal cord reflexes are responsible for maintaining the limbs in extension, supporting the animal's weight, and initiating stepping motion. The organization of stepping motion is performed at the brain stem in the reticular formation.

Diseases of the nervous system, muscles, bones, joints, and associated connective tissues can affect gait. When associated with conditions originating in the nervous system, gait abnormalities can result from lesions within the cerebellum, brain stem, spinal cord, or peripheral nerves. *Ataxia* is a term used to describe an abnormal gait characterized by incoordination, but without spasticity, weakness, or involuntary movements. Ataxia can be classified by the quality of signs observed and the pathway involved; the three types are vestibular ataxia, cerebellar ataxia, and proprioceptive ataxia. In general, vestibular ataxia is associated with a head tilt, while cerebellar ataxia is characterized by hypermetria and no proprioceptive deficits. Proprioceptive ataxia also is referred to as spinal ataxia because it is associated with spinal cord lesions and is characterized by abnormal proprioception, weakness, and lack of head tilt, circling, or other intracranial signs.

Posture typically is evaluated with the animal at rest in a comfortable position and unrestrained. Head, neck, trunk, and limb posture should be assessed and abnormalities identified. Head tilt, rotation of the neck and thoracic, and wide-based stance are examples of abnormal head, neck, trunk, and limb posture, respectively. A "base-wide" stance can be caused by lesions within the vestibular system, cerebellum, or spinal cord. The inverse posture, or "base-narrow" stance, can result from muscle weakness due to peripheral nerve disease, abnormalities of neuromuscular junctions, or disorders of the skeletal muscles. *Spasticity* is a condition of increased tone of skeletal muscles producing abnormal limb posture. Abnormal distribution of weight to one side should be noted, because this finding can indicate either weakness of ipsilateral extensor muscles from a peripheral nerve disorder or increased tone of contralateral extensor muscles, which would indicate an upper motor neuron (UMN) lesion.[2]

Assessment of Cranial Nerves. Twelve pairs of cranial nerves (CNs), labeled I to XII, are described as follows: CN I, the olfactory nerve; CN II, the optic nerve; CN III, the oculomotor nerve; CN IV, the trochlear nerve; CN V, the trigeminal nerve; CN VI, the abducent (or abducens) nerve; CN VII, the facial nerve; CN VIII, the vestibulocochlear nerve; CN XI, the glossopharyngeal nerve; CN X, the vagal nerve; CN XI, the spinal accessory nerve; and CN XII, the hypoglossal nerve. Clinical evaluation of CN I (olfactory nerve) and CN XI (spinal accessory nerve) cannot be reliably performed in ruminants. Because the intact sense of smell is important for nutritional intake, CN I is assumed to be intact in sheep, goats, and cervids that are eating. CN XI (spinal accessory nerve) has axonal inputs from cervical spinal nerves and innervates specific muscles of the neck. Damage to CN XI is rare because the nerve is protected throughout much of its course by the muscles it innervates, and injury to the spinal canal or base of the skull is accompanied by neurologic deficits that can mask clinical signs of CN XI damage.

Abnormalities in the function of CNs result from localized lesions involving neuronal cell bodies within the brain or the specific nerves themselves. With the exception of CN I and CN II, which are located within the cerebral cortex, all CNs arise from the brain stem. Knowledge of the location of CN nuclei assists the clinician in neuroanatomic localization of lesions. The presence of neurologic deficits involving CNs III to XII in small ruminants that are severely depressed or somnolent would indicate that the responsible lesion is most likely to be within the brain stem.

CN II (Optic Nerve): Menace Response Vision is the function of CN II. The nerve transmits sensory information from electrochemical receptors in the retina to the visual cortex in the occipital lobe of the cerebrum. The visual pathway (Figure 13.1) is an afferent pathway and consists of an extraparenchymal portion (retinas, optic nerves, and optic chiasm) and an intraparenchymal portion (optic tracts, lateral geniculate nucleus in the thalamus, optic radiations, and visual cortices). In ruminants, 90% of optic

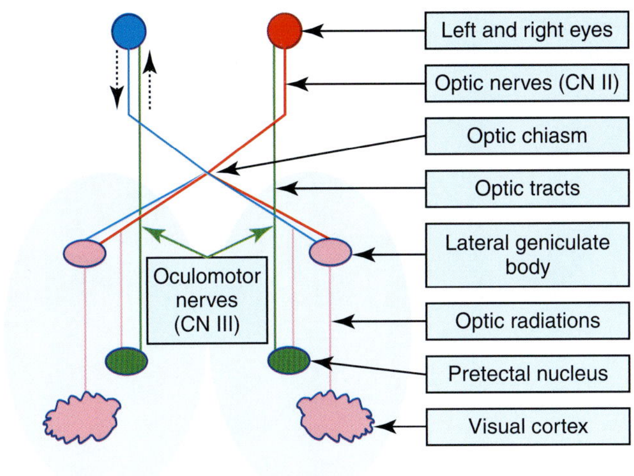

• **Fig. 13.1** Schematic of the simplified pathways of vision and pupillary light reflex (see text for details). *CN*, Cranial nerve.

nerve fibers cross at the chiasm to enter the contralateral optic tract; this arrangement has important implications in evaluating lesions of the visual pathways. During assessment of the chief complaint, the client may report that the animal appears blind, but an important consideration is that depressed or somnolent animals or animals with loss of balance due to cerebellar or vestibular disease can stumble and appear blind.

The clinical assessments of visual ability include the menace response test and the obstacle test. Eliciting the menace response, which also is referred to as the blink response or eye preservation response, is the easiest method for evaluation of vision impairment; however, the obstacle test, if performed accurately, is superior for assessing vision in ruminants. For this test, objects are placed in the path of the animal, and then its ability to negotiate around the objects is assessed. Degrees of blindness can occur with ocular disease, and the simplest obstacle test is to determine if the blind animal moves toward the lighted opening when placed in a dark environment.

The menace response evaluates the entire visual pathway, CN VII, and the cerebellum. This test assesses a response, rather than a reflex, because the response involves the cerebrum and thus is a learned response. The presence of a response or its magnitude parallels the maturity of the cerebellum—thus, a reduced response is expected in kids, lambs, and fawns less than a week of age. A diminished or absent menace response also can be observed in animals that are severely depressed or have cerebellar disease or CN VII lesions. The normal response is characterized by an eyelid blink, ocular retraction, and head aversion as the examiner rapidly moves a finger toward the eye from a rostral direction. It is important to limit air movement toward the eye and not to touch the eye or adnexa, because such maneuvers may result in a response in animals with intact facial sensation (CN V). Alternatively, the examiner can drop an object into the animal's visual field from above, which should elicit the menace response from the animal. This method is considered imprecise, with a stimulus that is too slow, for adequate evaluation of this reflex in ruminants. When a visual deficit is observed during the menace response or obstacle test, pupillary light reflexes are tested to assist in localizing the lesion and in characterizing the blindness as central or peripheral.

CN III (Oculomotor Nerve): Pupillary Light Reflex The oculomotor nerve contains parasympathetic fibers responsible for constriction of the pupils and motor fibers, which influence movement of the eye. The sympathetic nervous system is responsible for pupil dilation, so as a result of such stimulation, stressed and frightened animals can have dilated pupils. The pupillary light reflex assesses CN II and CN III. The afferent pathway for pupillary constriction during light stimulation follows a similar pathway as the afferent pathway for vision (optic nerve, optic chiasm, and optic tract); however, before reaching the synapse in the lateral geniculate nucleus in the thalamus, nerve fibers associated with the pupillary light reflex diverge from those of the optic tract and synapse on the pretectal nucleus, which sends a majority of its neurons to the contralateral oculomotor nucleus (see Figure 13.1), which forms the basis for the direct pupillary light reflex. The pretectal nucleus also sends some of its neurons to the ipsilateral nucleus of CN III; this neuroanatomic arrangement forms the basis for the indirect or consensual pupillary light reflex. Before performing the pupillary light reflex test, the examiner should assess the pupils for size at rest and symmetry and check the eyes for the presence of primary ocular disease. The normal small ruminant often has large pupillary diameters owing to sympathetic stimulation from fear. Ideally, animals are moved to a dimly lit location so that external light does not influence the examination. Pupils that are very small are considered miotic, and dilated pupils are mydriatic. Occasionally, inequality in pupil size may be observed, but if the size difference is not extremely pronounced, this may be a normal finding for the animal. Severe asymmetry is termed *anisocoria*. To assess for irregularity in pupil size, the clinician can move the animal from a dark to a bright area. Although a sympathetic lesion will prevent the affected pupil from dilating in the dark, lesions of CN III (parasympathetic nerve) will prevent the pupil from constricting in bright light. To assess the pupillary light reflex, a strong light source should be used to overcome sympathetic pupil dilation. The light beam is directed into one eye in a nasotemporal direction toward the temporal region of the retina. The direct response should be constriction of the examined pupil, and the opposite eye also should constrict as a result of the consensual pupillary reflex, although this is difficult to assess by a single examiner. If the intraparenchymal visual pathways are affected by a neurologic disorder (central or cortical blindness), the menace response is absent on the side contralateral to the lesion, but the pupillary light reflexes are intact. With involvement of the extraparenchymal visual pathway (retina, optic nerve, and optic chiasm), blindness on the side of the lesion is characteristic, and the pupillary light reflexes are abnormal.

CNs III (Oculomotor Nerve), IV (Trochlear Nerve), and VI (Abducent Nerve): Movement of Eye CNs III, IV, and VI are responsible for conjugate eye movements through innervations of the somatic extraocular muscles, and these nerves are examined as a functional unit. CN III provides a majority of innervations for eye movements because it is responsible for the function of the dorsal, ventral, and medial rectus muscles; the ventral oblique muscle; and the levator palpebrae muscle. The trochlear nerve (CN IV) is responsible for innervation to the dorsal oblique muscle of the eye; the abducent nerve (CN VI) is responsible for innervations to the lateral rectus and retractor bulbi muscles of the eye.

The clinician should first examine the eye position in relationship to the head at rest and note if strabismus (abnormal position of the eyeball) exists. Strabismus can be the result of damage to the nerves or the muscles they innervate. Further evaluation of the motor function of CNs III, IV, and VI can be performed by moving the animal's head. Ruminants should drop the eyes as the head is lifted. When the nose is elevated, the eyes tend to maintain a horizontal axis, and ventral strabismus becomes apparent. Slow, lateral (horizontal) motion of the head should cause the animal's eye to try to remain focused straight ahead, with the result that the eye moves slowly in the opposite direction of head movement. However, as the head continues to turn, vestibular influences will then move the eye quickly in the same direction. This movement pattern is referred to as *physiologic nystagmus*, or normal inducible vestibular nystagmus, and indicates normal function of extraocular muscles, the vestibular system, and CNs III, IV, and VI and their connections in the medial longitudinal fasciculus. Clinical assessment for lesions affecting CNs III, IV, and VI can be performed by moving the animal's head and observing the ocular position. Cerebellar and vestibular diseases also produce nystagmus, but the strabismus changes whenever the head and neck are moved. With paralysis of CN III, IV, or VI, the strabismus should be present with all positions of the head. Lesions involving CN III can result in ipsilateral ventrolateral strabismus and mydriasis, usually without vision loss in either eye. In addition, CN III is responsible for innervation of the levator palpebrae muscle, but ptosis (eyelid droop) occurring as a result of CN III lesions is not commonly observed in sheep, goats, or cervids because the frontalis muscle can lift the upper eyelid. Lesions in CN IV can result in ipsilateral, contralateral, or bilateral dorsomedial strabismus. Bilateral dorsomedial strabismus occurs in several diffuse encephalopathies such as polioencephalomalacia (PEM) and listeriosis, but whether this abnormality is the result of a true bilateral lesion involving the CN VI nucleus is unclear.[2] Lesions involving CN VI result in ipsilateral medial strabismus with a more forward positioning of the eye. In addition, failure to retract the globe may be noted during assessment of the palpebral reflex. This is not entirely specific to CN VI, because eyeball retraction also may require function of all extraocular muscles, including those innervated by CN III and CN IV.

CN V (Trigeminal Nerve): Corneal and Palpebral Reflexes The large CN V contains motor nerve fibers that innervate the muscles of mastication and acquires sensory information from most parts of the head. The nerve is divided into three branches: ophthalmic, maxillary, and mandibular. All three branches have sensory nerves, but only the mandibular branch contains motor nerve fibers. The mandibular nerve innervates the masseter, temporal, rostral digastric, pterygoid, and mylohyoid muscles. The masticatory muscles should be palpated for symmetry and atrophy. Bilateral loss of motor function of the mandibular nerve is rare but would result in muscle atrophy of the temporal and masseter muscles, a flaccid and lowered jaw, inability to chew, and excessive drooling, which can result in bicarbonate loss. The animal's tongue may protrude from the mouth as a result of fatigue, but the tongue can be withdrawn to appropriate stimulation. Unilateral lesions can cause asymmetric muscle atrophy and a slightly lowered position of the jaw. This may not result in dysphagia, but abnormal wear of teeth and dental problems may be evident.

Function of the sensory branches is tested by corneal and palpebral reflexes (Figures 13.2 and 13.3) and assessing sensation across multiple areas of the face. In the palpebral and corneal reflexes, CN V is the afferent (sensory) portion, whereas CN VII is the efferent (motor) portion of the reflex. The corneal reflex is performed by slowly advancing a finger or cotton swab toward the animal's eye and placing it directly on the cornea. The palpebral reflex is performed by touching a finger on periocular skin without the animal visualizing the finger. The corneal reflex and touching the medial canthus of the eye for the palpebral reflex assess the ophthalmic branch of CN V, which innervates the eye and surrounding skin and is responsible for the maintenance of corneal epithelium. The maxillary branch of CN V can be assessed by touching the lateral canthus of the eye during elicitation of the palpebral reflex. The normal reflex response with intact CN V, CN VI, and CN VII is closure of the lid, retraction of the eye, and aversion of the head, respectively. The mandibular branch of CN V can be assessed by touching the ear base and observing for closure of the lid. A deficient palpebral reflex with a normal menace response suggests a lesion in the trigeminal nerve or ganglion. Loss of CN V innervation to the corneal epithelium can result in neurotropic or exposure keratitis, because the affected animal cannot sense corneal dryness or the presence of ocular foreign bodies.

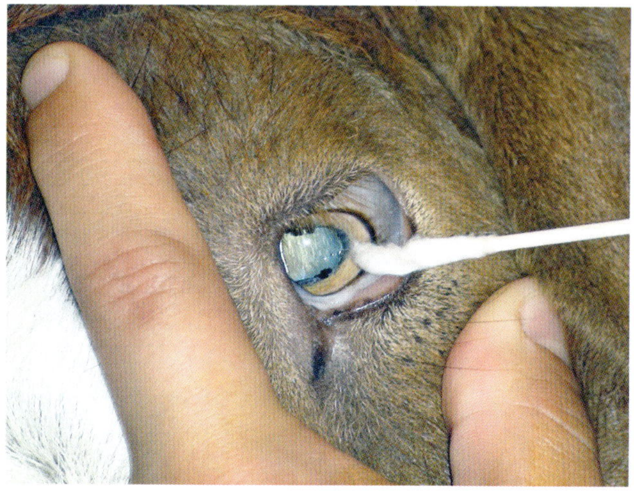

• **Fig. 13.2** The corneal reflex is assessed by gently placing a finger or the loosened fibers of a cotton tip applicator directly on the cornea.

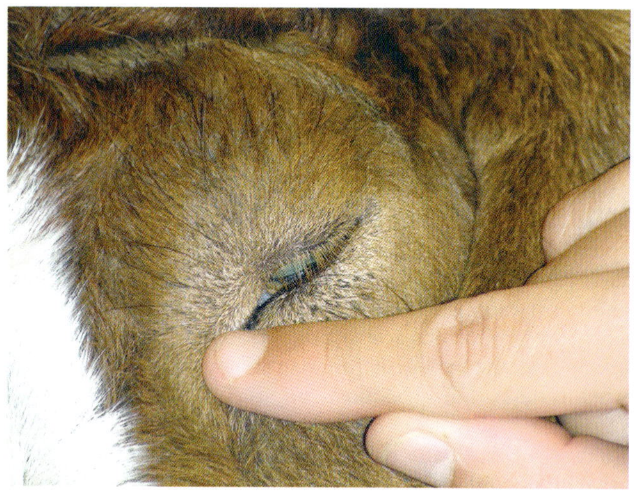

• **Fig. 13.3** The palpebral reflex is tested by touching the periorbital skin with the examiner's finger while keeping the animal from seeing the approaching finger.

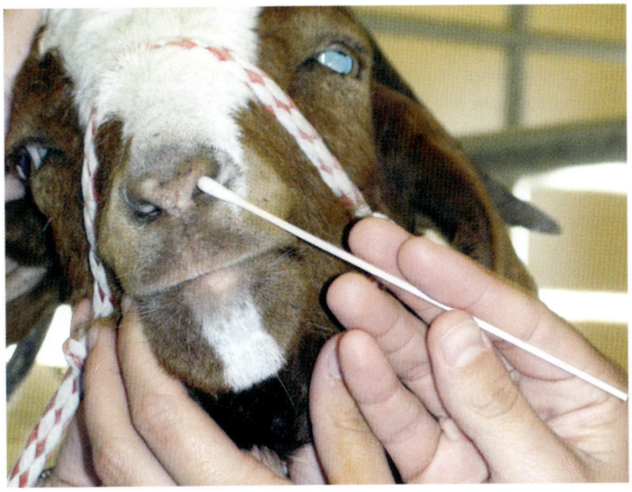

• **Fig. 13.4** Assessment of the conscious recognition of a noxious stimulus by way of the maxillary branch of cranial nerve V to the contralateral parietal cortex. The animal demonstrates the appropriate response of blinking and attempting to withdraw the head from the stimulus.

Damage to any branch of the trigeminal nerve results in sensory losses to the areas it innervates. Deficits in CN V function manifests as the ipsilateral loss of sensation over the face and affected animals do not reflexively blink or twitch the face. This is a subcortical reflex and does not require conscious input. The consciously mediated, coordinated movement of the head away from the noxious stimuli is assessed by stimulating the nasal septum. The examiner applies stimulation using a finger or cotton swab to the inner (medial) surface of the nasal septum (Figure 13.4). The response in a normal animal is blinking and facial twitching; the head is pulled away in response to a painful stimulus. This response requires conscious recognition of the noxious stimulus by way of CN V maxillary nerve to the contralateral parietal cortex. This determination is important because an animal with a CN V maxillary branch abnormality will have neither sensation nor conscious recognition of pain, whereas small ruminants with a contralateral cerebral cortical lesion have normal sensation but no conscious recognition of the painful stimulus.

CN VII (Facial Nerve): Facial Expression, Other Brain Stem Function The facial nerve (CN VII) is predominantly a motor nerve, providing innervations to muscles responsible for facial expression, but CN VII also contains parasympathetic nerve fibers that provide innervations to the lacrimal gland and mandibular and submandibular salivary glands. The CN VII neurons supplying innervations to the muscles of facial expression are located within the brain stem. Assessment of CN VII motor function is performed through the menace response test and eliciting the corneal and palpebral reflexes as discussed previously. It is important to evaluate the symmetry and posture of the eyelids, ears, and lips; abnormal findings can provide initial evidence of CN VII dysfunction. Goats and sheep of breeds with erect ears should hold them upright, whereas those with pendulous ears should be able to move the base of the ear canal to follow external stimuli. In small ruminants with compromised CN VII motor function, eyelid droop (ptosis), lack of ear movement, ear droop, and deviation of the nasal philtrum can be observed. CN VII is most easily assessed by the menace response and palpebral reflex. Simultaneous loss of the menace response and the palpebral reflex, characterized by a failure to blink rapidly and completely, suggests a lesion in CN VII innervations to the orbicularis oculi muscle.[3] The animal's vision is intact when lesions are limited to CN VII. CN VII dysfunction results in protrusion of the tongue on the affected side of the mouth, and the animal may drool. Feedstuff often is found packed into the cheek pouch on the affected side. Damage to CN VII can be localized according to the clinical signs.

Lesions in the brain stem can result in a number of discrete or diffuse clinical signs in affected animals. Listeriosis in sheep and goats can cause discrete lesions throughout the brain stem, which may result in abnormal function of the ipsilateral facial muscles. An additional manifestation of CN VII dysfunction is the presence of neurotropic (exposure) keratitis and corneal ulceration, because affected animals cannot blink to distribute the tear film. Because of close proximity of CN VIII and CN VII nuclei in the brain stem, as well as the proximity of the CNs in the periphery, vestibular signs often accompany those of facial nerve palsy.

CN VIII (Vestibulocochlear Nerve): Head Tilt and Other Reflections of Vestibular Function CN VIII has two main divisions: vestibular and cochlear. The vestibular division is responsible for maintaining the position of the head and other structures relative to gravity; the cochlear division functions in hearing.[4] The objective assessment of hearing loss in large animals is difficult and requires the use of electrodiagnostic testing (brain stem auditory evoked response). Animals that have bilateral hearing losses may be easier to assess because they do not respond to loud environmental noises.

The vestibular part of CN VIII supplies the major input to the vestibular system and is evaluated by observing the animal's head and body position. Clinical signs of vestibular dysfunction of CN VIII include a head tilt, abnormal nystagmus, ataxia, staggering, and positional strabismus. With vestibular dysfunction, many of these signs are observed at presentation without being elicited. The presence of a head tilt is best assessed with the examiner looking face on at the animal's head. A head tilt is an abnormal posture when sustained and can be visualized as ventral deviation of one ear compared with the opposite, or as deviation of an imaginary line drawn across the eyes from the normal horizontal plane. The head tilt is continuously directed toward the side of the lesion whenever CN VIII or the vestibulocochlear nucleus is affected. Animals that are recumbent with vestibular disease tend to lie on the side of the lesion.

CNs IX (Glossopharyngeal Nerve) and X (Vagus Nerve): Laryngeal and Pharyngeal Function The glossopharyngeal nerve, or CN IX, carries motor and sensory fibers to and from the rostral pharynx, palate, larynx, and tongue. The glossopharyngeal nerve also contains a parasympathetic component that innervates the parotid and zygomatic salivary glands. The vagus nerve, or CN X, provides motor innervation to the pharynx, larynx, palate, and striated muscles of the esophagus by the recurrent laryngeal nerve. The parasympathetic branch of CN X arises from the vagal nucleus in the medulla and innervates the abdominal and thoracic viscera, with the exception of the pelvic viscera. Damage to CN IX and CN X results in clinical signs related to laryngeal and pharyngeal function. Affected animals have difficulty swallowing and may drool from an inability to swallow saliva. Choke also may be observed. The gag reflex can be used to assess normal function. In normal animals, placing a tongue depressor in the back of the mouth elicits the gag reflex, in which the caudal portion of the tongue pushes the tongue depressor forward. The clinician should always wear gloves when examining a small ruminant with suspected CN IX or X disease, because oropharyngeal paralysis is common in rabid animals. Inspiratory stertor may be heard as a result of unilateral or bilateral paresis of the pharynx and larynx. Animals with pharyngeal paralysis can regurgitate food through the nose. In small ruminants, disease of CNs IX and X is rare.

CN XII (Hypoglossal Nerve): Tongue Function The hypoglossal nerve, or CN XII, is the motor pathway to the muscles of the tongue, allowing its protrusion and retraction. Animals with damage to CN XII often have a history of difficulty apprehending and masticating food. The tongue should be examined for atrophy and tone. Normal animals attempt to retract the tongue with strength when it is pulled by the examiner. A palatable substance or loose salt can be placed on the animal's lips, and with normal CN XII function, the animal will lick the substance off the area. Unilateral damage to CN XII causes deviation or protrusion of the tongue toward the affected side, because the tongue is pushed by the intact muscles on that side.

Postural Reactions. Postural reactions complement the evaluation of gait. Postural reactions are easily examined in sheep and goats but difficult to evaluate in cervids. Postural reactions include hopping, wheelbarrowing, hemi-standing, hemi-walking, placing, and proprioception. Testing for the *hopping* postural reaction is performed by lifting three limbs off the ground while walking the animal forward. Each of the front limbs should be evaluated for the hopping postural reaction; a normal animal will lift and place the limb as it would with normal locomotion. *Wheelbarrowing* is similar, but only the two hindlimbs are lifted off the ground as the animal is walked forward. *Hemi-standing* and *hemi-walking* are similar postural reactions that are assessed by lifting the ipsilateral front limbs and hindlimbs while the animal is observed at rest and during locomotion, respectively. *Placing* is assessed by lifting the goat or sheep and advancing it to the edge of a table; normal animals lift the front legs to place them on the table. *Proprioception* reflects the animal's ability to consciously recognize an abnormal limb posture. To test for the proprioception reaction, the standing animal's distal limb is flexed at the fetlock joint, resulting in weight-bearing at the dorsum of the digit. A normal proprioceptive reaction quickly results in correction of the abnormal weight bearing.

Spinal Reflexes. Five spinal reflexes should be evaluated in sheep and goats with suspected neurologic disease: the extensor reflex of the front limb, the panniculus reflex, the patellar reflex, the perineal reflex, and the withdrawal reflexes of the forelimbs and hindlimbs. The spinal reflexes are best examined with the animal in lateral recumbency, with the side to be evaluated in the upper position. Spinal reflexes involve a local reflex arc that includes a stretch or touch receptor, an afferent peripheral nerve that relays information to the spinal cord gray matter, spinal cord interneurons that can stimulate or inhibit other neurons, an efferent motor neuron that exits the spinal cord, and a muscle. Spinal reflexes do not require conscious or voluntary input for normal function.

Assessment of spinal reflexes tests the integrity of the lower motor neuron (LMN) but also can provide some information on influences of the UMNs on the LMN (Table 13.1). The UMNs are a group of neurons that do not physically exit the nervous system and provide stimulatory or inhibitory influences to the LMN. The LMNs are composed of the peripheral nerves and the effector organs (primarily skeletal muscles). Several responses can be observed when spinal reflexes are tested. A normal response can be observed, which indicates normal sensory and motor components of the reflex arc. An exaggerated response often is observed with UMN pathway abnormalities. A diminished or absent response indicates LMN disease in either its sensory or motor components. In addition to diminished responses, animals with LMN disease exhibit muscle atrophy, hyporeflexia or areflexia, hypotonia or atonia, and paresis.

Testing the extensor reflex of the front limb assesses the radial nerve. The radial nerve is responsible for weight bearing of the front limb and innervates the triceps muscle group. With the animal in lateral recumbency, the extensor reflex is assessed by placing a hand under the foot of the animal and pushing the limb gently toward the animal until extensor tone is noted. The normal reflex is for the animal to "push back" with its leg. Animals with LMN disease display decreased or absent resistance, and those with UMN disease may exhibit increased tone of the triceps muscle.

Testing the patellar reflex evaluates motor and sensory components of the femoral nerve. The femoral nerve innervates the quadriceps muscles, which are responsible for extension of the stifle and weight-bearing in the hindlimb. The patellar reflex is a

TABLE 13.1 Summary of Lower and Upper Motor Neuron Signs.

Parameter	Lower Motor Neuron Segmental Signs	Upper Motor Neuron Long Tract Signs
Motor function	Paralysis—loss of muscle power, flaccidity	Paresis to paralysis—loss of voluntary movements
Reflexes	Hyporeflexia to areflexia	Normal to hyperreflexia (especially myotatic reflexes)
Muscle atrophy	Early and severe: neurologic; contracture after several weeks	Late and mild: disuse
Muscle tone	Decreased	Normal to increased
Electromyographic changes	Abnormal potentials (fibrillation, positive sharp waves) after 5 to 7 days	No changes
Associated sensory signs	Anesthesia of innervated area, paresthesia or hyperesthesia of adjacent areas	Decreased proprioception; decreased perception of superficial and deep pain

From Oliver JE Jr, Lorenz MD: *Handbook of Veterinary Neurologic Diagnosis,* Philadelphia, 1983, WB Saunders.

tendinous reflex and is elicited by lightly tapping the patellar tendon with a reflex hammer while observing an extension of the stifle. Patellar reflex testing is a subjective assessment, and clinicians should be as consistent as possible in technique. To begin, the limb should be in relaxed flexion with the patellar tendon just barely tightened. The tendon is palpated, and then, while the examiner's fingers are kept on the tendon, the limb is flexed until the tendon feels tight. To raise tension in the tendon, the clinician can place a hand under the foot while extending the digits. The tapping on the tendon is done with a pendulum motion. The reflex cannot be elicited if the limb is tense, but by tapping the tendon rhythmically, the animal relaxes over time. The strength of the patellar reflex is proportional to the force applied to the tendon. The plexor (hammer) used for examination of large dogs is adequate for testing the reflex of small ruminants. The patellar reflex, combined with the proprioceptive reaction, is used to determine the integrity of the LMN. With LMN lesions, deficits exist in conscious proprioception and patellar reflexes, whereas deficits of conscious proprioception in animals with intact patellar reflexes indicate lesions in the UMN.

Withdrawal reflexes also are referred to as flexion reflexes, and testing is performed by applying a noxious stimulus to the medial or lateral digits of the front limbs and hindlimbs. A hemostat often is used to apply the stimulus. In the front limb, the withdrawal reflex evaluates the axillary, median, and ulnar nerves. In the hindlimb, the reflex evaluates the sciatic nerve on the lateral part of the limb and the femoral nerve on the medial part of the limb. A normal response is the flexion of the limb fully away from the stimulus.

Testing the perineal reflex is performed by pinching the skin around the anus. The perineal reflex tests the afferent pudendal nerve, whereas the efferent nerve fibers are part of the caudal nerves. The normal response is anal sphincter contraction and downward contraction of the tail. During the reflex test, the tail should not be manipulated because this may cause contraction of the anus.

The panniculus reflex or cutaneous trunci reflex also relies on a reflex arc. This test is performed by applying stimuli to both sides of the body, starting caudally at the wing of the ileum to the cranial thoracic area (at the T2 level). The stimulus usually is applied with the tip of a ballpoint pen or a hemostat. The sensory fibers from the skin enter the dorsal root of the spinal cord and then ascend to the C8 and T1 segments, where the efferent limb of the reflex is the motor neurons of the lateral thoracic nerve. A normal reflex is flinching of the skin. If twitching of the skin occurs at the level of the wing of the ileum, then the afferent limb is intact in its entirety. However, a transection of the spinal cord caudal to T1 may result in a decreased or absent cutaneous response in the area caudal to the transection.

Pain. Whereas spinal reflexes test the LMN, assessments of conscious proprioception, voluntary motor functions, superficial pain sensation, and deep pain sensation are used to test UMNs. With compromise to the spinal cord, conscious proprioception is the first deficit observed, followed in order by voluntary motor function, superficial pain sensation, and deep pain sensation. Superficial pain sensation can be assessed by applying a noxious stimulus over a dermatome or cutaneous zone, which is an area of skin on the animal's body surface that is innervated by a single nerve. A two-step pinch technique is recommended to test superficial pain sensation. First, a small area of skin is lightly tented using a hemostat. After a slight pause, a second, sharp skin pinch is applied. Intact superficial pain sensation is present if a reflex withdrawal occurs, and the UMN is intact if the animal demonstrates conscious recognition of the pain through an aversion response, vocalization, or both. Deep pain sensation is determined by placing a large hemostat or needle-holders across the digit just above the coronary band and progressively pinching to stimulate the periosteum. As with the superficial pain sensation, a positive response is conscious recognition of the stimulus, as evidenced by aversion, vocalization, or both. The assessment of deep pain sensation is important for prognosis for the recumbent small ruminant with neurologic disease because deep pain is the last function to be lost with a severe spinal cord lesion.

Localization of Neurologic Lesions

During the complete neurologic examination, abnormalities of nervous system function should be identified, characterized, and recorded. Some abnormalities in nervous system function can be readily ascribed to specific segments of the nervous system, whereas for others, the origin of dysfunction is more difficult to identify. Determining the neuroanatomic location of lesions or abnormalities within the nervous system is important with respect to management and prognosis for the sheep or goat with neurologic disease. For small ruminants with suspected neurologic disease, clinical signs or specific pathologic processes should be ascribed to four functional areas of neuroanatomy: (1) the cerebrum, (2) the cerebellum, (3) the brain stem and CNs, and (4) the spinal cord and peripheral nerves (Table 13.2). If the location of a lesion is not readily apparent after the complete neurologic examination, repeating all or specific portions of the neurologic examination can reveal subtle abnormalities missed earlier.

Cerebral Disease. Nervous system disorders involving the cerebrum can be variable in severity and frequently are characterized by alterations in mental acuity, behavioral changes, seizures, and blindness. Diffuse or symmetric cerebral disease often does not affect the gait on flat surfaces, but gait can appear abnormal on ascending or descending slopes. Likewise, postural and proprioceptive reflexes are normal with diffuse cerebral disorders unless the affected animal is moved across slopes. In most animals with diffuse cerebral disease, spinal reflexes are normal. Of note, metabolic abnormalities are considered the most common cause of symmetric cerebral disease in ruminants.[1] Dehydration and acid-base and electrolyte abnormalities often result in depression in small ruminants.

With unilateral lesions located within the cerebrum, a majority of clinical signs will be observed contralateral to the lesion, with the exception of circling and head turn, which usually are in the direction of the lesion. Specific examples of clinical signs associated with asymmetric cerebral disease are contralateral hemiparesis, circling with the head turned toward the side of the lesion, contralateral facial sensation deficits, and presence of a contralateral menace deficit with normal palpebral reflexes and normal pupillary light reflexes.

Cerebellar Disease. The cerebellum functions by providing input data to motor areas of the cerebral cortex and brain stem; thus, clinical signs of cerebellar dysfunction reflect failure of smooth, coordinated movements of the head, body, and limbs. Clinical cerebellar disease with lack of coordinating input results in ataxia, truncal sway, dysmetria, intention tremors, pupillary abnormalities, and vestibular signs. Small ruminants with clinical cerebellar disease are characterized by normal mentation and abnormal gait; however, depression and stupor can be observed in

TABLE 13.2 Association of Neurologic Signs With Functional Deficits of Clinically Relevant Neuroanatomic Locations.

Neurologic Sign/ Disorder	Cerebral Diseases	Cerebellar Diseases	Diseases of Brain Stem and Cranial Nerves	Diseases of Spinal Cord and Peripheral Nerves
Mentation	Abnormal	Normal	Abnormal or normal	Normal
Gait	Normal	Abnormal	Abnormal or normal	Abnormal
Posture	Normal	Abnormal	Abnormal or normal	Abnormal
Spinal reflexes	Normal	Abnormal or normal	Abnormal or normal	Abnormal or normal
Disorders discussed within chapter	• Bacterial meningitis • *Clostridium* enterotoxemia • Lentiviral encephalitis • Louping-ill • Polioencephalomalacia • Thiamine deficiency • Sulfur toxicosis • Lead toxicosis • Sodium toxicosis • Pseudorabies • Rabies • Transmissible Spongiform Encephalopathy (TSE) • Urea toxicity • West Nile virus encephalitis	• Grass staggers	• Listeriosis • Otitis	• Botulism • Cerebrospinal nematodiasis • Enzootic ataxia • Organophosphate toxicity • Spastic paresis • Spinal cord trauma • Tetanus • Tick paralysis

Modified from Constable PD: Clinical examination of the ruminant nervous system, *Vet Clin North Am Food Anim Pract* 20:185, 2004.

kids, lambs, and fawns with congenital cerebellar disease as a result of failure to nurse with subsequent dehydration and hypoglycemia (metabolic disease). In small ruminants with cerebellar ataxia, strength is preserved in the front and hindlimbs, and proprioceptive deficits are not observed. Strength of the limbs is assessed by applying pressure on the withers and the pelvis. Although diffuse cerebellar disease, which is more common in large domestic animals/livestock, causes ataxia of all four limbs, unilateral cerebellar lesions result in ipsilateral ataxia of front and rear limbs.

Brain Stem and CN Diseases. Small ruminants with brain stem lesions may have normal or abnormal mentation. Because the ascending reticular activating system in the rostral brain stem frequently is affected by diseases of the brain stem, profound depression and stupor are common. CN deficits in a small ruminant with abnormal mentation characterized as depression and stupor suggest that the lesion is localized to the brain stem. During the complete neurologic examination, the evaluation of CN function should receive much attention. Clinical signs associated with brain stem disease include CN deficits (as described previously), ipsilateral hemiparesis, coma, and stupor (with abnormalities of the ascending reticular activating system). In addition, respiratory and cardiovascular abnormalities may be noted because the respiratory center is located in the caudal brain stem.

Spinal Cord and Peripheral Nerve Diseases. Clinical signs of spinal cord disease depend on the location of the disease within the spinal cord. In examining a small ruminant with suspected spinal cord or peripheral nerve disease, differentiating LMN disease from UMN disease is useful. As described previously, the UMNs are a group of neurons that do not physically exit the nervous system and provide stimulatory or inhibitory influences to the LMNs. The LMNs are composed of the peripheral nerves and the effector organs (primarily skeletal muscles). Clinical signs of UMN disease include proprioceptive deficits, weakness, and paralysis, but exaggerated reflexes and increased extensor tone also are observed. Lesions of the LMN result in clinical signs consisting of paresis or paralysis combined with absent or diminished spinal reflexes.

Peripheral nerve injuries are uncommon in small ruminants but result in clinical signs referable to LMN disease, including paresis, paralysis, diminished or absent spinal reflexes, and muscle atrophy. The radial nerve and brachial plexus can be traumatized in the forelimb. In the hindlimb, the sciatic, peroneal, femoral, or obturator nerve can become damaged.

Radial nerve paralysis can result from fractures of ribs or the humerus or from avulsion of the brachial plexus, and the severity of clinical signs often is dependent on the location of traumatic injury. Damage to the radial nerve causes a lack of innervations to the triceps muscle group and the inability to extend the elbow joint. The more distal the injury on the limb, the less the animal's gait is affected. Trauma to the distal radial nerve results in paralysis of the extensor muscles of the carpus and digits and knuckling of the lower limb. A loss of sensory innervation to the dorsum of the leg below the elbow also may be evident. The animals may have scuffed or abnormally shaped hooves, as well as abrasions on the front of the fetlocks.

The *femoral nerve* provides innervations to the quadriceps muscle group. Animals with femoral nerve paralysis drag or carry the affected rear limb while hopping on the unaffected leg. Injury to this nerve can occur as a result of extreme extension of the hindlimb or as a result of injection sites that have become infected. Sensation of medial skin surfaces often is preserved through the saphenous branch of the femoral nerve, because this branch separates from the rest of the femoral nerve proximally at the level of the iliopsoas muscle.

Obturator nerve paralysis occurs as a result of extreme abduction of the rear limb or as a lambing or kidding injury. When the nerve is damaged, the animal is unable to adduct its rear limb. Unilateral involvement of the obturator nerve is associated with gait abnormalities less frequently than is bilateral involvement. Radiographs of the pelvis are warranted to rule out pelvic fracture.

Sciatic (ischiadic) nerve paralysis can occur after pelvic or lumbosacral fractures. The nerve arises from spinal cord segments L6 to S2 and travels in the vertebral canal before its fibers exit. The sciatic nerve innervates the muscles that extend the hip and flex the stifle before dividing into the peroneal and tibial branches. The *tibial nerve* provides motor innervations to the gastrocnemius muscle, whereas the peroneal provides motor innervations to the extensors of the digits. The tibial and peroneal nerves also collect sensory input from the distal portion of the hindlimb. Whereas lumbosacral fractures usually cause bilateral hindlimb paresis or paralysis, damage to the proximal sciatic nerve, which can be a consequence of acetabular and femoral fractures, results in dysfunction of flexor muscles only. The extensor muscles of the stifle remain functional, allowing the animal to bear weight but not flex the stifle. The animal exhibits a dropped hock, and the limb will be knuckled over. On testing, the animal's flexor response is greatly inhibited, and with pinching of the medial claw, the animal flexes its hip without flexing the rest of the limb. This differential response occurs because the medial side of the limb still has intact sensory innervation through the saphenous branch of the femoral nerve. Many of these injuries resolve over time, but a poor prognosis is associated with the complete loss of deep pain.

The *peroneal nerve* supplies the muscles that flex the hock and extend the digits and provides cutaneous sensory innervation to the dorsal aspect of the foot and cranial surface of the hock and tibia. Improperly administered injections may injure this nerve, resulting in knuckling onto the dorsum of the fetlock and overextension of the hock. Animals appear to be able to compensate fairly well with this type of injury by extenuated flexing of the hip and extension of the stifle at walk. The flexor response is depressed when the dorsum of the fetlock is stimulated; however, if the sole of the hoof is stimulated, the animal flexes its leg but keeps the hock fixed.

Ancillary Tests

As noted previously, the objectives of the neurologic examination are to verify that the small ruminant has disease of nervous system origin and to determine the anatomic location of the lesion within the nervous system. Once the neuroanatomic location has been identified, additional diagnostic testing can be performed to identify a specific causative disorder or contributing factor. A precise etiologic diagnosis is important because individual sheep, goats, and cervids typically are members of a herd or a flock, and elucidation of the etiology allows implementation of preventive strategies aimed at reducing the potential for disease in other at-risk animals. A number of diagnostic tests are available for the neurologic workup of a small ruminant, but owing to cost and availability of testing equipment, only a few tests can be routinely used in practice settings for the diagnosis of neurologic diseases in sheep and goats. Complete blood count (CBC) and serum biochemistry profile, cerebrospinal fluid (CSF) analysis, and routine imaging studies such as survey radiographs can be used during the diagnostic evaluation of sheep and goats with suspected nervous system disease.[5,6] For captive and wild cervids, postmortem evaluation is often most cost-effective approach for diagnosing the cause of neurologic dysfunction rather than attempting ancillary tests in support of a diagnosis.

CBC and Serum Biochemistry Panel. Because metabolic disorders are the most frequent cause of symmetric cerebral dysfunction, the CBC and serum biochemistry panel should be performed to evaluate for the presence of hypocalcemia, hypoglycemia, acid-base disorders, electrolyte abnormalities, and inflammatory conditions. Anomalies observed during routine blood workup may be primary or secondary to the nervous system disorder[6] (see Appendix 2).

CSF Analysis. CSF is located within the subarachnoid space; therefore, diseases involving the CNS can lead to alterations in the normal composition of the CSF. The CSF can be collected from the atlantooccipital space but is more easily obtained at the lumbosacral site. General anesthesia or heavy sedation is required for atlantooccipital CSF collection, and anesthesia for neurologically impaired animals often is contraindicated. Positioning and restraint are critically important for successful collection of CSF (Figure 13.5A). Sampling can be performed in the standing small ruminant provided that restraint is sufficient to prevent lateral motion, or the animal can be sedated. If recumbent, most animals can be manually restrained in sternal recumbency, but mild sedation may be necessary. Ideally, the animal is positioned such that the hips are flexed and the pelvic limbs extended alongside the abdomen, with the pelvis kept straight and level. The skin over the lumbosacral space should be clipped and aseptically prepared. A palpable indentation should be felt at the lumbosacral space, and this site should be infiltrated with 2% lidocaine (0.5 mL administered subcutaneously) (see Figure 13.5B). A final scrub should be applied, and the clinician should don sterile gloves.

For lambs, kids, and fawns weighing less than 30 kg, a 20- or 21-gauge, 1-inch needle can be used; an 18- or 20 gauge, 1.5-inch needle can be used for adult sheep and goats. A disposable needle or a stylet-type spinal needle can be used. The needle should be inserted on midline halfway between the last palpable lumbar dorsal spinous process and the first palpable sacral dorsal spinous process. The needle should be placed perpendicular to the spine from the lateral view and straight up and down as viewed from the back of the animal. If bone is encountered, the needle should be redirected either cranially or caudally. The needle is advanced until a slight "pop" is felt as the needle passes through both the interarcuate ligament and the subarachnoid membrane. The animal may move or jump slightly when the needle punctures the dura mater, or the tail and anus may reflexively contract. The clinician can periodically remove the stylet to check for the presence of CSF in the hub of the needle. Approximately 1 mL of fluid/5 kg of body weight can be safely removed, but only 1 to 2 mL is necessary for cytologic evaluation. Gently and slowly aspirating CSF or allowing it to flow freely from the needle prevents excessive movement and blood contamination (see Figure 13.5C). The CSF samples should be placed in ethylenediamine tetraacetic acid (EDTA) for cytologic analysis and in a serum separator tube for culture. For biochemical analysis, CSF should be placed in a serum separator or lithium heparin tubes. Cytologic evaluation of CSF should be performed rapidly, ideally within 60 minutes of collection. If this is not possible, the CSF can be mixed with an equal volume of 40% ethanol to preserve the cells.

Once collected, CSF can be evaluated for gross appearance, cytology, protein concentration, biochemical composition, and

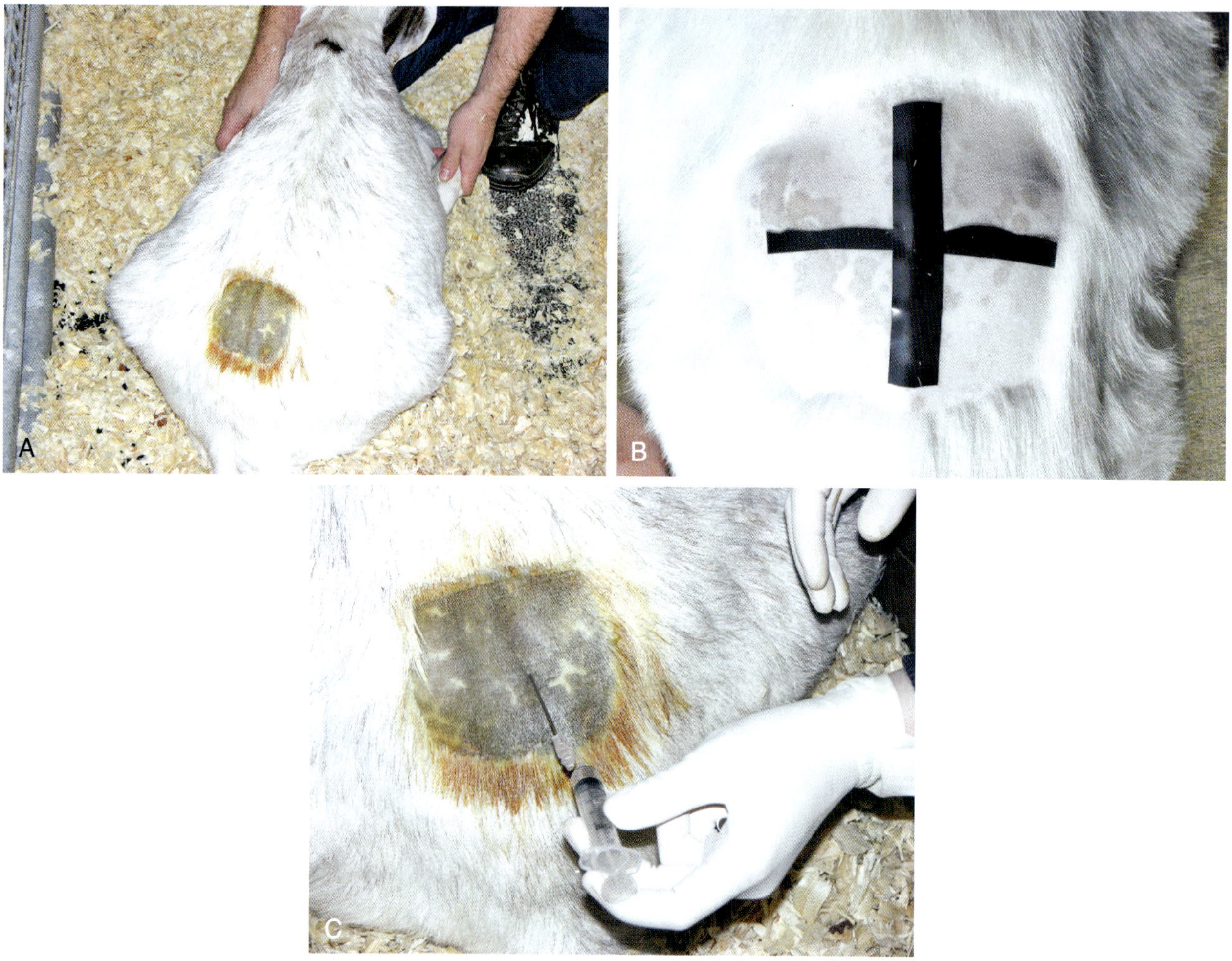

• **Fig. 13.5** Collection of cerebrospinal fluid. **A.** Correct positioning of an animal for collection of cerebrospinal fluid from the lumbosacral space. The animal is placed in sternal recumbency, and both pelvic limbs are pulled cranially to arch the spinal column. **B.** The lumbosacral space is identified at the intersection of a line connecting the caudal aspects of the tuber coxae with the vertebral midline (between L6 and S1). **C.** Cerebrospinal fluid is collected by free catch or aspiration using a 5- to 10-mL syringe and immediately placed into tubes for analysis.

presence of bacteria. Normal CSF is clear and colorless. Red discoloration indicates the presence of blood in the CSF, and the hemorrhage may be iatrogenic (Figure 13.6A) or from previous hemorrhage within the CSF. In general, blood from a previous hemorrhage is evenly mixed with the CSF and often does not clot, as opposed to iatrogenic hemorrhage during collection, in which the red discoloration may lessen as additional fluid is collected and the CSF will clot. Xanthochromia is orange or yellow discoloration of the CSF, and this finding can be observed for up to 10 days after the occurrence of bleeding within the CSF. Turbid CSF usually indicates a high white blood cell count, as can occur with bacterial meningitis. The total nucleated cell and differential counts should be performed to assist with an etiologic diagnosis. Normal CSF contains less than 10 nucleated cells/μL, with a majority of cells being mononuclear. Bacterial infections of the nervous system usually are characterized by a neutrophilic pleocytosis (see Figure 13.6B), with the exception of listeriosis in small ruminants in which mononuclear pleocytosis (see Figure 13.6C) is usually present. Mononuclear pleocytosis can also be observed with viral encephalitides and PEM. Cerebrospinal nematodiasis (CSN), secondary to aberrant migration of nematode parasites, often results in marked elevations of eosinophils, which may be the predominant CSF leukocyte in affected animals (see Figure 13.6D). Normal protein concentrations in CSF are considerably lower than in blood. CSF protein concentration of healthy sheep is less than 40 mg of protein/dL and that of healthy goats less than 15 mg of protein/dL. CSF glucose content generally is low compared with that in the peripheral blood. Glucose concentrations normally are 80% of the value in peripheral blood, and decreased concentrations are detected in animals with bacterial meningoencephalitis as a consequence of bacterial glucose consumption.

Medical Imaging. After a lesion has been localized within the CNS, plain survey films may be helpful to identify luxations of the vertebral column, osteomyelitis, or fractures of the pelvis. Survey radiographs of the skull can be used to diagnose fractures or assess involvement of the tympanic bulla in cases of otitis. Radiographic techniques used in medium to large dogs are applicable to most small ruminants. For UMN disease of the forebrain, brain stem, or cerebellum, several diagnostic imaging

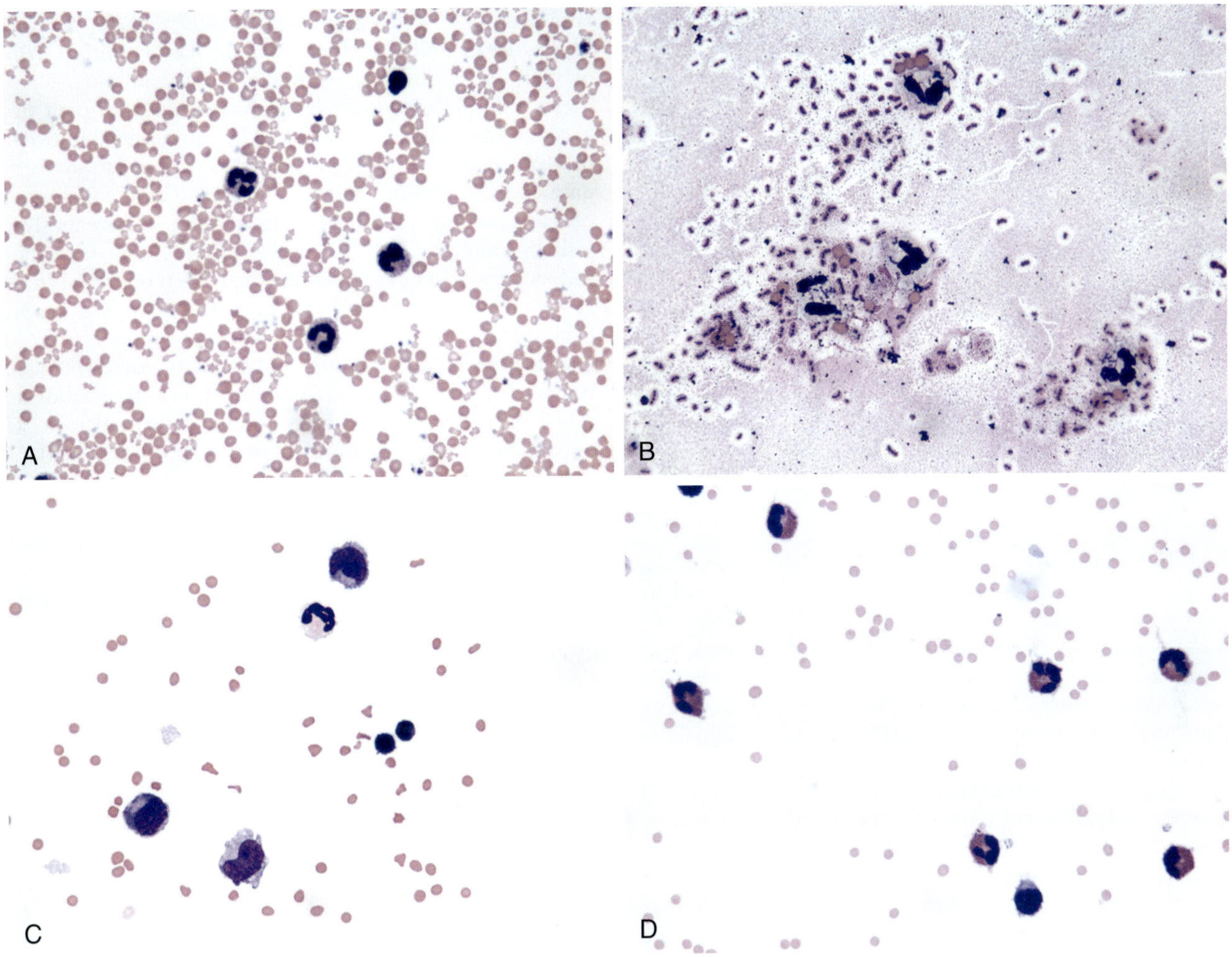

• **Fig. 13.6** **A.** Iatrogenic blood contamination during collection of a cerebrospinal fluid (CSF) sample. This can be differentiated from histopathologic evidence of disease by the presence of red and white blood cells in ratios similar to those in blood samples and the presence of thrombocytes. Similar findings are detected in cases of traumatic injury occurring within 30 minutes of CSF collection. **B–D.** CSF cytology for different neurologic diseases. **B.** Findings in a goat with streptococcal meningitis. A majority of nucleated cells are neutrophils that show degenerative changes. The identification of many small cocci in pairs or short chains suggests streptococcal meningitis. **C.** Findings in a goat with listeriosis include a mixed-cell mononuclear pleocytosis, with a predominance of mononuclear cells, small lymphocytes, and presence of neutrophils. **D.** Findings in a goat with cerebrospinal nematodiasis include predominance of eosinophils, which is seen in cases of aberrant spinal migration by *Parelaphostrongylus tenuis.* (Courtesy Dr. Elizabeth Spangler, Auburn, Alabama.)

procedures can be performed. The structural integrity of the UMN anatomy can be evaluated by the use of computed tomography (CT) and magnetic resonance imaging (MRI). Myelography can be used to identify compressive or expansive lesions in the spinal cord. Electromyography also can be used to determine whether specific neurons are responsible for neuromuscular disease by assessing the electrical activity of the muscle after a neuron is stimulated. Electroencephalography can be used to assess the electrical activity in various parts of the brain. It is used primarily in cases of presumed neurologic disease manifested by seizures, narcolepsy, and encephalopathy.

Cerebral Diseases

Bacterial Meningitis and Encephalitis

Etiology and Pathophysiology. Meningitis is defined as inflammation of one or more of the three layers (dura mater, arachnoid, and pia mater) covering the CNS, and involvement of adjacent structures (CNS or spinal cord) is common. Meningitis and meningoencephalitis can be caused by many etiologies, but principally result from extension of local processes or hematogenous spread of bacteria.[7] Infections extending into the meninges and nervous tissues may be caused by surgical procedures such as dehorning and tail docking, thermal osteonecrosis after cauterization at dehorning, sinusitis, otitis interna, and skull fractures. In male adult white-tailed deer, infections by *Trueperella (Arcanobacterium) pyogenes* and other bacteria can cause intracranial abscessation and suppurative meningoencephalitis (Figure 13.7 and Chapter 20, Figure 20.19), and while the pathophysiology is poorly understood, development of the infection may be associated with antler development.[8,9]

Hematogenous spread of bacteria in cases of pneumonia, omphalophlebitis, mastitis, endocarditis, and other septic processes may also cause meningoencephalitis and is especially

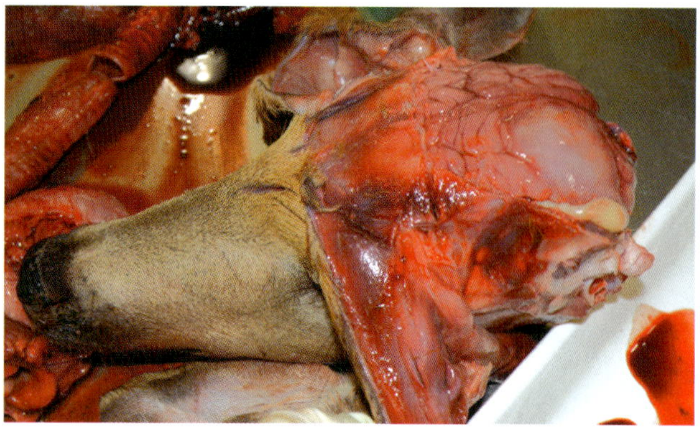

• **Fig. 13.7** Brain abscess in a 4-and-a-half-year-old male white-tailed deer. *Trueperella pyogenes* and *Escherichia coli* were cultured from the contents of this abscess. (Courtesy Dr. Kelley Steury, Auburn, Alabama.)

common in neonates with failure of passive transfer. Depending on the etiology, various bacterial pathogens may be involved in the disease. In neonatal meningoencephalitis, *Escherichia coli*, *Pasteurella multocida*, *Streptococcus* spp., *Staphylococcus* spp., and *T. (Arcanobacterium) pyogenes* are commonly isolated. Infection with *Mycoplasma mycoides* (ssp. *mycoides* large colony (LC) type or ssp. capri) may cause meningoencephalitis in juvenile and adults goats, which is typically, but not always, associated with other systemic signs such as polyarthritis, pneumonia, and mastitis.[10] *Pseudomonas aeruginosa* can cause septicemia and meningitis in goats secondary to mastitis.[11] In the CSF, host immune defense mechanisms provide limited protection as antibody and complement concentrations in CSF are low.[7,11] Bacterial and inflammatory insults lead to congestion and infarction of arachnoidal or subependymal veins, decreased CSF absorption and hypertension, and necrosis of nerve cells.[7,11]

Clinical Signs. Affected animals are often severely lethargic and depressed or may be hyperexcitable. In cases associated with neonatal septicemia, diarrhea and dysthermia are common. Hyperesthesia, a stiff, extended neck, and signs of pain upon manipulation of head and neck are observed. Passive manipulation of the neck may result in sudden tonic extension and rigidity of the limbs.[11] Loss of CN functions may be observed as nystagmus, strabismus, and facial palsy.[7,11] With progression of the disease, decreases of sensory function, propulsive walking, seizures, and coma develop.

Diagnosis. Meningitis should be suspected based on clinical signs, especially in neonates with signs of failure of passive transfer and sepsis. To differentiate the disease from metabolic abnormalities, serum electrolytes and glucose should be evaluated. Confirmation of meningitis is based on CSF analysis or postmortem examination. Marked increases in protein concentration, total leukocyte count, and proportion of neutrophils in CSF samples are characteristic of bacterial meningitis. The CSF glucose concentration is below that of serum, reflecting bacterial consumption of glucose in the CSF.[7] Xanthochromia and free or intracellular bacteria can also be present. Bacteriological culture and susceptibility testing should be attempted if therapy is intended.

Treatment. Case fatality rates in farm animals with bacterial meningitis are high, which can be attributed, in part, to late recognition of the disease. Therapy is based on aggressive and prolonged administration of antibiotics, supplemented with antiinflammatory drugs and anticonvulsive therapy as needed. The choice of antibiotic should be guided by an initial Gram stain of CSF, or culture and antimicrobial susceptibility, but initial therapy should broadly cover gram positive and gram negative bacteria. Antibiotic therapy should be administered intravenously to attain maximum peak blood and CSF concentrations.[11] Recommended antibiotic choices for treatment of meningitis include: ceftiofur sodium (5–10 mg/kg q24h–q8h, intravenously [IV]), sodium ampicillin (10–20 mg/kg q8h IV), and trimethoprim-sulfonamide (5 mg/kg based on the trimethoprim q12h to q8h IV), which can be administered in combination (e.g., ampicillin-ceftiofur or ampicillin-trimethoprim-sulfonamide).[12] The use of antiinflammatory therapy for treatment of bacterial meningitis has not been evaluated in farm animals, but steroidal or nonsteroidal antiinflammatory drugs should be considered. Seizures should be controlled using diazepam (0.01–0.2 mg/kg every 30 minutes).[7] In neonates with failure of passive transfer, plasma should be administered (15–30 ml/kg IV).

Prevention. Timely administration of adequate colostrum is the most important method of preventing bacterial meningitis in neonates. Proper sanitation should be provided during surgical procedures, and dehorning of goats should be performed with great care for hygiene, analgesia, and limited thermal cauterization. Early therapy of predisposing conditions may prevent their extension to the nervous system.

Clostridium perfringens

Etiology and Pathophysiology. *C. perfringens* types C and D (and less commonly type E) are important pathogens of sheep and goats, and clinical disease has been sporadically reported in farmed deer, often associated with overconsumption of energy-dense diets.[13] *C. perfringens* manifests mainly as enteric disease and peracute death, with associated pathologic changes such as edema and petechiation in the nervous system. The organisms are ubiquitous in the environment and feces of farm animals. *C. perfringens* type C produces α and β toxins, which are not degraded in young animals (< 10 days of age) due to low intestinal concentrations of proteolytic enzymes. β Toxin forms ion-conductive channels in membranes of excitable cells, leading to irreversible depolarization and neurologic disease.[14] Disease associated with *C. perfringens* type D is usually seen in young small ruminants consuming overly plentiful diets, allowing clostridial overgrowth and production of α and ϵ toxins in the small intestine; however, neonatal lambs in unvaccinated flocks may also be affected.[15] Activation of ϵ toxin from its precursor occurs by enteric proteases. Subsequently, the toxin causes disruption of tight junctions of vascular endothelial cells and vasogenic edema in different organs, including the brain, lungs, and kidneys.[16]

Clinical Signs. The duration of the disease is limited to a few hours, and clinical signs preceding death may not be observed. Abdominal discomfort and signs of colic, such as teeth-grinding and vocalization, may be noticed. Hemorrhagic diarrhea may be present in some cases and is regularly observed in goats with type D enterotoxemia.[17] Neurologic signs include depression, tetany, opisthotonus, convulsions, and coma.[17,18] In type D enterotoxemia, focal encephalomalacia may develop, which is characterized by aimless wandering, blindness, and walking into inanimate objects.[17]

Diagnosis. The short duration of clinical disease precludes most antemortem diagnostics. Identification of large numbers of clostridia in fecal smears is suggestive but certainly not definitive.

Following postmortem examination, the histologic presence of enteritis with numerous clostridia in the upper small intestine and, in cases of type D enterotoxemia, edematous tissues supports the diagnosis. Toxin assays may be performed using polymerase chain reaction (PCR), enzyme-linked immunosorbent assay (ELISA), or mouse inoculation assays.

Treatment. Affected animals usually die prior to systemic antibiotics possessing a Gram positive spectrum and fluid therapy can provide a therapeutic benefit. The administration of C and D antitoxin is likely more beneficial to prevent disease in at-risk herd-mates than in the treatment of moribund animals.[18]

Prevention. Routine vaccination of sheep and goats against *C. perfringens* C and D is critical and should be performed in captive deer.[13] Annual to biannual boosters are recommended for all breeding stock. Administration of C and D antitoxin shortly after birth should provide protection to lambs and kids of unvaccinated dams for approximately 2 weeks.[18] Sudden feed changes and overconsumption of high-energy diets (grain, lush pasture, or milk) should be avoided.[13]

Lentiviral Encephalitis: Caprine Arthritis-Encephalitis and Maedi-Visna

Etiology and Pathophysiology. Lentiviral leukoencephalomyelitis is caused by caprine arthritis encephalitis virus (CAEV) in goats and either maedi-visna virus (MVV) or, less commonly, ovine progressive pneumonia virus (OPPV) in sheep. In North America, OPPV is usually associated with respiratory disease; however, neurologic disease in sheep has also been described.[19] Small ruminant lentiviruses (SLRVs) belong in the genus *Lentivirus*, family *Retroviridae*, and have a worldwide distribution, although prevalence varies widely among herds.[20] While different in certain clinical aspects, SLRVs share many virological, epidemiological, and pathophysiological features. The nomenclature may indicate SLRVs to be species specific, but natural infection of sheep with CAEV and goats with MVV is possible, and crossing of species barriers is not uncommon.[21] The SRLVs are enveloped RNA viruses that, upon infection of host cells, transcribe their genome into a double-stranded DNA, which is inserted into the host's genome, resulting in lifelong infection.[20] Monocytes and macrophages are the primary cells infected by SRLVs, and invasion of target organs is believed to be in macrophages.[21,22] Transmission of SRLVs is primarily by vertical transmission from dam to offspring through viral shedding in colostrum and milk. Less frequently, horizontal transmission from respiratory, urogenital, or gastrointestinal secretion and excretions can cause infections in all age groups. In utero infections are possible, but their relative importance is unclear.[20,22] Inflammatory changes associated with SRLV infection may occur in the CNS, lungs, udder, joints, lymph nodes, and blood vessels and result in progressive dysfunction of the affected organ(s).

Clinical Signs. Clinical signs associated with SLRV infection are slowly progressive and initially nonspecific. Neurologic disease (leukoencephalomyelitis) is relatively rare in comparison to respiratory disease in adult sheep and arthritis in adult goats.[20] In sheep, clinical signs usually occur in animals older than 1 to 3 years of age but are possible at a younger age.[20,23] Initial signs include weight loss, hindlimb weakness, and an abnormal stance that progress to ascending paresis and paralysis. Death occurs several months after initial signs are noticed and may be preceded by neurologic signs of the head such as lip twitching, nystagmus, and blindness.

Affected goats are usually 1 to 5 months of age; however, adult goats may be affected.[22] The clinical course of neurologic disease is more rapid in goats than in sheep. Because the virus can induce a demyelinating leukoencephalomyelitis, clinical signs include a short, choppy gait and unilateral or bilateral posterior paresis and ataxia. Some kids may appear to be straining to urinate as part of the clinical picture. Initially, the mentation appears to be unaffected, and animals eat, drink, or nurse normally. Progression of the disease leads to tetraparesis, and head tilt, circling, torticollis, opisthotonos and blindness may develop.

Diagnosis. Neurologic disorders associated with SRLV infection are relatively rare, and other conditions should be considered in the workup. The presence of interstitial pneumonia may suggest SRLV infection, but clinical sigs of respiratory disease are often absent. On CSF analysis, increased protein concentrations and mononuclear pleocytosis may be present. Identification of SRLV antibodies is performed by AGID or ELISA techniques. The presence of antibodies in serum implies infection but not disease causation. PCR techniques may be used to detect SLRV infections before antibodies are produced.[24] Postmortem diagnosis is based on identification of a nonsuppurative, demyelinating encephalomyelitis and lymphocytic infiltration of the CNS.

Treatment. Effective therapies to slow or halt the disease do not exist and affected animals should be euthanized.

Prevention. Successful vaccination strategies, suitable for field conditions, are not available.[25] One option for eradication of SRLVs from a herd is a test-and-cull program, which may not be feasible in herds with high prevalence rates. Control measures should be chosen according to herd prevalence of infection.[25] In herds with mixed populations of sheep and goats, cross-specific transmission is possible and both CAEV and MVV/OPPV must be controlled. Control and eradication are based on identification of seropositive animals and segregation of infected from uninfected animals, removal of infected animals, and continued serologic testing. Prevention of perinatal transmission is achieved by separation of lambs and kids from their dam immediately after birth and by cleaning uterine and placental fluids off of newborns.[20] Because consumption of colostrum and milk from infected dams is an important method of transmission, these products should be harvested only from uninfected dams. Alternatively, bovine colostrum-sourced colostrum replacers or pasteurized colostrum can be used. Heating of colostrum to 56° C for 60 minutes decreases the load of infectious virus and decreases immunoglobulin concentrations only minimally.[26] Use of milk replacers or pasteurized milk is recommended in kid and lamb raising protocols. Iatrogenic transmission by needles, tattooing equipment, and other surgical instruments must be prevented by use of disposable instruments or sterilization.[20]

Louping-Ill (Ovine Encephalomyelitis)

Etiology and Pathophysiology. Louping-ill is a tick borne viral encephalomyelitis of sheep that also affects red grouse *(Lagopus lagopus scotica)* and occasionally other species, including goats, deer, and people. The disease is caused by louping ill virus (LIV), a member of the tick-borne encephalitis group, in the genus *Flavivirus*, in the family *Flaviviridae.* LIV is closely related to other tick-borne flaviviruses that cause similar disease but demonstrate antigenic and geographical variations, including Turkish sheep encephalitis virus, Spanish sheep encephalitis virus, and Greek goat encephalitis virus.[27] Louping-ill occurs in moorland pastures in upland United Kingdom, Ireland, and Norway, where the tick vector *Ixodes ricinus* is supported by a ground layer microclimate of high humidity. *I. ricinus* is a three-host tick that becomes infected with LIV by feeding on viremic hosts, which occurs mainly in the spring, but also in the early fall, when lambs have lost colostral immunity.[20,28] Following infection of the tick, LIV survives in salivary glands, and infection of a new susceptible host occurs when the tick feeds during its next life cycle in the following season. Although mainly maintained by the sheep-tick cycle, LIV is also amplified by red grouse and hare, in which high levels of viremia sustain transmission. After ticks transmit the pathogen to sheep, replication of LIV occurs in lymphatic tissues, followed by viremia and invasion of the CNS after 6 to 20 days. Viral replication in the CNS results in nonsuppurative inflammation, neuronal degeneration, and associated clinical signs.[29]

Clinical Signs. Sheep that have acquired protective antibody levels through previous infection, vaccination, or by ingestion of colostrum are protected from infection, and clinical signs are most common in lambs older than 3 months of age and yearlings.[20,28] Pyrexia, anorexia, constipation, and depression are observed during the initial stages of infection. Progression of the disease leads to generalized muscle tremors and rigidity, hyperesthesia, ataxia, hypermetria, and a stiff, bounding gait. Severely affected animals develop cerebral disease and display head pressing, recumbency, convulsion, coma, and death.[20]

Diagnosis. When neurologic signs develop, viremia has ceased and virus isolation from blood is unsuccessful. High levels of specific antibodies develop in the CSF of affected animals. CSF should be handled with caution due to the zoonotic potential of LIV.[22,30] Detection of hemagglutinating immunoglobulin M antibodies that occur early in the disease may be used diagnostically.[30] No gross lesions are observed on postmortem examination. Histologic lesions include perivascular cuffing of mononuclear cells and neutrophils in the meninges, brain, and spinal cord. Neural degeneration is most evident in cerebellar Purkinje cells. Virus isolation, immunohistochemistry (IHC), or PCR procedures are used to demonstrate LIV in tissues.[20]

Treatment. No specific therapy is available, and affected animals should receive supportive care.

Prevention. LIV may infect humans, and veterinarians, shepherds, and abattoir workers are at increased risk.[31] Infection of susceptible sheep may be prevented by vaccination and acaricide treatments.[32]

Polioencephalomalacia

The histopathological changes in the cerebral gray matter referred to as PEM can result from diverse etiologies. All causes of PEM involve a disruption of the cerebral energy metabolism, resulting in intracellular sodium and water accumulation. These pathophysiological changes cause edema, swelling, and subsequent pressure necrosis of cerebral neurons, which have a limited capacity to expand within the bony calvarium.[33] In small ruminants, PEM is most commonly caused by thiamine deficiency but may also result from sulfur toxicosis, sodium toxicosis and water deprivation, or lead toxicosis. Regardless of etiology, clinical signs are similar in most cases of PEM, and further diagnostics may be warranted before initiating specific therapies.

Thiamine Deficiency

Etiology and Pathophysiology. Ruminants rely on thiamine (vitamin B_1) production by ruminal microorganisms for adequate amounts of this vitamin, and sufficient quantities are produced by the healthy rumen microflora. Thiamine phosphate serves as a cofactor for transketolase, the rate-limiting enzyme of the glycolytic pathway (pentose phosphate pathway) that provides most ATP to the brain. In thiamine deficiency, reduced availability of ATP results in dysfunction of neuronal Na1K1ATPases causing intracellular sodium and water accumulation and, subsequently, PEM. In sheep, ruminal thiamine synthesis is estimated to be approximately 1.5 to 3 mg/day,[34] which implies that little excess to daily requirements (e.g., 2.9 mg for a 75-kg pregnant ewe) exists.[35] Thiamine requirements are altered by certain physiological and environmental conditions, such as pregnancy, lactation, and availability of pasture.[35] As is true for all water-soluble vitamins, long-term storage of thiamine is impossible and any disruption of the ruminal fauna can quickly lead to a state of deficiency. Subclinical thiamine deficiency may result from increased thiaminase production when dietary changes are made without prior adaptation.[36]

PEM as a result of thiamine deficiency is most commonly associated with ruminal acidosis.[37] Under acidic conditions, a decrease in thiamine-producing bacteria is exacerbated by increasing numbers of bacteria that produce thiaminases. The activity of bacterial thiaminase type II is enhanced in acidic conditions such as rumen acidosis. This etiology of PEM most frequently occurs in lambs and kids on low-roughage, high-concentrate diets such as in feedlots or in preparation for shows but may affect ruminants of any age. In cases of PEM in captive and free-ranging deer, access to supplemental feed high in carbohydrates was also reported.[38] In pre-ruminants, the feeding of low-quality milk replacers with insufficient thiamin content may also cause PEM. Plant-derived thiaminases, produced by bracken fern *(Pteridium aquilinum)*, horsetail *(Equisetum arvense)*, Nardoo fern *(Marsilea drummondii)*, and prostrate pigweed *(Amaranthus blitoides)*, have been implied in experimental and natural cases of thiamine deficiency–associated PEM.[39–42] Administration of thiamine analogs, such as the commonly used anticoccidial drug amprolium, may cause PEM by competitive inhibition.[43]

Clinical Signs. Typical clinical signs of PEM are bilaterally symmetric, develop rapidly, and may progress. The occurrence of clinical signs may be peracute, and a rapid development of severe clinical signs warrants a poor prognosis.[33] Affected animals are often found wandering aimlessly but become recumbent and display central blindness (absent menace response and intact PLR), opisthotonus, muscle tremors, extensor rigidity, periodic tonic-clonic convulsions, and nystagmus (Figure 13.8). Affected animals may walk along their confinement's enclosure and into inanimate objects (head-pressing). Behavioral changes, such as a lack of flight response, depression, stupor, coma, or hyperexcitability, and excessive chewing may observed. Dorsomedial strabismus, although difficult to assess in the presence of opisthotonus, was suggested to be typical of PEM caused by thiamine deficiency. An ophthalmoscopic examination may reveal papilledema resulting from increased intracranial pressure. Normal rumen function may be present initially, but inappetence and underlying ruminal acidosis result in rumen atony and diarrhea. In addition to neurological disease, thiamine deficiency and the presence of thiaminases in feces have been associated with poor growth and development in lambs.[44]

Diagnosis. Clinical signs of symmetric cerebral disease, signalment, and history are the basis for a presumptive diagnosis of PEM and initial therapy. A rapid response to thiamine therapy suggests the correct diagnosis. CBC and serum chemistry findings

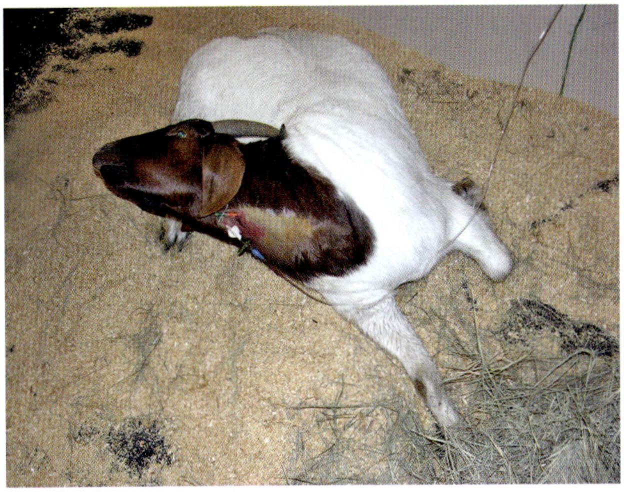

• **Fig. 13.8** A goat with thiamine-responsive polioencephalomalacia, displaying opisthotonos, incoordination, recumbency, and central blindness.

are usually unrewarding but may serve to rule out other conditions. CSF analysis may reflect mild increases in protein concentrations and mononuclear cell count, and increases in CSF pressure are present. Specific diagnostic tests include measurements of blood thiamine concentrations, erythrocyte transketolase activity, and ruminal or fecal thiaminase concentrations, but these tests are not widely available. Erythrocyte transketolase activity is determined using the thiamine diphosphate (TPP) effect that measures the increase in transketolase activity when TPP is added to the sample in excess. A TPP effect above 70 to 80% is detected in animals affected by PEM.[45] Sheep affected by acute ruminal acidosis had a mean TTP effect of 109 ± 28% as compared to 22.2 ± 3.7% in normal sheep.[37]

On postmortem examination, evidence of diffuse cerebral edema is present. Cerebral gyri are flattened and widened and may be yellowish discolored. The cerebellum may be dislocated caudally into the foramen magnum. Using ultraviolet illumination, lesions may autofluoresce, indicating necrosis and engulfment of necrotic tissues by lipophages.[45] Histologically, bilateral cortical laminar necrosis, edema, and presence of phagocytic cells are detected.

Treatment. Therapy is based on immediate thiamine replacement, and initial intravenous administration at a dose of 10 mg/kg is recommended.[33] Because adverse reactions, including sudden death, may occur with intravenous administration of thiamine, the injection should be given slowly. Thiamine hydrochloride therapy should be continued for several days at a dose of 10 mg/kg administered every 3 to 6 hours by subcutaneous or intramuscular route. Improvement is often noticed in 6 to 24 hours, and the frequency of thiamine administrations can be slowly reduced. In severely affected animals, treatment of cerebral edema using mannitol (20%, 1–2 g/kg IV), followed by dexamethasone 3 hours later (1 mg/kg IV), has been recommended.[46] Oral administration of thiamine hydrochloride (1 g) has been recommended when deficiencies are caused by thiaminases, or in herd outbreak situations, in which other animals are likely affected. Oral thiamine administrations may also be beneficial in cases of acute ruminal acidosis.[37]

Prevention. Adequate provision of good-quality roughage (1.5 kg/100 kg), allowing slow adaptation to dietary changes, prevention of ruminal acidosis, and avoidance of phytothiaminases are cornerstones to preventing thiamine deficiency. Diets for animals at risk for thiamine deficiency may be supplemented with oral thiamine. Although protective levels of oral thiamine are not well established, rates of 3 to 30 mg of thiamine per kilogram of feed have been recommended.[45]

Sulfur Toxicosis

Pathophysiology. High dietary intake of sulfur or sulfates has been associated with PEM in ruminants without thiamine deficiency. Potential sources for sulfur include elemental sulfur, feed intake limiters such as gypsum (calcium sulfate), urinary acidifiers such as ammonium sulfate, cruciferous crops, *Kochia scoparia* (burningbush, "poor man's alfalfa"), and molasses.[33] Coproducts of ethanol production, such as distillers grain with solubles, are an important source of sulfur toxicosis for beef cattle[47] and may cause PEM in small ruminants if fed in sufficient amounts. High levels of sulfates have also been found in some water sources, such as new wells. Seasonal occurrence of sulfur toxicosis is possible in the summer months, when concentrations of sulfates in water sources may be elevated, coinciding with increased water intakes during high ambient temperatures. Although not completely understood, the pathophysiology of sulfur-induced PEM is likely associated with sulfides produced from ingested sulfur compounds in the rumen. Sulfides are normally incorporated into bacterial de novo synthesis of amino acids, eructated as hydrogen sulfide (H_2S), or absorbed across the rumen wall. Sulfides are detoxified by hepatic oxidation, but may reach the brain when large amounts are intestinally absorbed and overwhelm hepatic capacities. Alternatively, sulfides may circumvent hepatic detoxification when inhaled as eructated H_2S. Sulfides are thought to inhibit the cellular electron transport chain, reducing neuronal ATP availability, resulting in PEM.[48]

Clinical Signs. Clinical signs of bilaterally symmetric cerebral disease are principally those described under thiamine deficiency. A larger percentage of animals at risk may develop clinical PEM due to sulfur toxicosis, compared to thiamine deficiency–induced PEM.[49,50] In sheep with PEM due to sulfur toxicosis, clinical signs included depression, central blindness, and head pressing, but not hyperesthesia, nystagmus, or opisthotonus.[50] Sulfur toxicosis may also be suspected if evidence of acidosis or scouring is absent.[49] The ruminal contents of affected animals may smell of rotten eggs (H_2S).[49]

Diagnosis. Sulfur toxicosis may be suspected in cases of PEM that do not respond rapidly to thiamine therapy.[49,50] In suspected cases, all sources of feed and water should be tested for sulfur content. Reported cases of PEM have occurred with sulfur contents of 0.43% of a diet fed ad libitum.[50] Dietary sulfur contents of greater than 4000 ppm and water sulfur contents of greater than 1000 ppm are suggestive of sulfur toxicosis.[33] Assessment of H_2S in the ruminal gas cap may be useful to detect sulfur toxicosis. Although ruminal H_2S concentrations above 1000 ppm are considered diagnostic, ruminal H_2S concentrations may decline rapidly due to anorexia in affected animals. Comparing the ruminal H_2S concentrations of affected animals with those of unaffected herd mates may be more informative. On postmortem examination, cerebrocortical necrosis similar to thiamine deficiency–induced PEM is detected. In cases of sulfur toxicosis, the distribution of lesions may be different, with lesions distributed multifocally rather than the laminar pattern seen in PEM due to thiamine deficiency. Severe involvement of the rostral neuroaxis, thalamus, and midbrain without lesions in cerebellum and hippocampus may be observed in animals affected by sulfur toxicosis.[51]

Treatment. Specific therapies do not exist and treatment as described for thiamine deficiency is recommended.

Prevention. Prevention relies on avoidance of feed and water sources with high sulfur contents as determined by testing. Other measures to reduce the incidence of PEM include allowing free access to a good-quality trace mineral salt, closely monitoring animals fed diets containing calcium sulfate, and providing free-choice access to good-quality forage. Oral thiamine supplementation may prevent clinical signs of PEM in animals fed a diet high in dietary sulfur.[47]

Lead Toxicosis

Etiology and Pathophysiology. Lead poisoning is among the most frequent intoxications of ruminants, although the acute form of the disease is more common in cattle than in small ruminants.[52,53] In recent years, various new sources for lead have been eliminated in many countries, but reports of environmental contamination continue to be of concern.[53] Concomitant pollution with other heavy metals may occur in areas or situations in which lead contamination is detected.[53] Sources for lead include lead arsenical insecticides and herbicides, lead-acid batteries, lead-containing paints, gasoline, crankcase oil, shotgun pellets, and discharges from smelting plants.[33,53]

The pathophysiology of lead poisoning is affected by various factors. The route and chronicity of exposure influence the type and severity of clinical signs. Young animals are more susceptible to lead toxicosis due to higher rates of intestinal lead absorption.[54] Metallic or sulfide lead compounds are intestinally absorbed less efficiently than are lead acetate, phosphate, carbonate, and hydroxide salts; however, chronic toxicities may result from entrapment of metallic lead in the reticulum. Once absorbed, most lead is irreversibly bound to erythrocyte proteins. When aged erythrocytes are removed from the blood stream, lead is again released and deposited in bone and, in smaller quantities, in kidneys and liver. Lead adversely affects many biological processes and enzyme systems. Lead damages capillary endothelial cells and interferes with mitochondrial functions and neuronal ATPases, resulting in dysfunction of cerebral energy metabolism and subsequently to neurologic disease. Gastrointestinal damage results from caustic actions of the ingested lead salts. Interference with enzymes of heme synthesis, such as δ-aminolevulinic acid dehydratase and ferrochelatase, as well as other red cell proteins results in a shortened erythrocyte lifespan, anemia, and increases in blood δ-aminolevulinic acid and porphyrin concentrations. Lead readily crosses the placental barrier and accumulates in fetal tissues, especially bones.

Clinical Signs. In cases of acute toxicosis, clinical signs of neurologic disease and gastrointestinal irritation predominate. Affected animals show bilaterally symmetric cerebral disease with weakness, ataxia, either dullness or excitability, cortical blindness, muscle tremors, and skin twitching. Clinical signs of intestinal irritation include abdominal pain, anorexia, and scant feces, followed by foul-smelling diarrhea. Subacute and chronic exposures, such as those caused by industrial pollutants, may result in emaciation, anorexia, weakness, and anemia.[53] In chronically exposed sheep, infertility and abortions have been reported.[55] Environmental contamination was demonstrated to cause increased testicular lead concentrations and reduce sperm quality in exposed deer.[56,57] Young lambs grazing lead-contaminated pastures may develop stiffness, lameness, and hindlimb paralysis as the result of osteoporosis and weakness of vertebral bones that results in spinal compression. Posterior paresis in lambs with high tissue levels of lead, but without evidence of osteoporosis, has also been described.[58]

Diagnosis. In animals with clinical signs of PEM, the presence of fetid diarrhea and abdominal pain suggests lead toxicosis. Measurement of lead concentrations in whole blood samples is the standard method of diagnosis, and levels up to 0.3 ppm are considered the maximum normal concentration.[59] Because blood lead concentrations may vary significantly by laboratory and test assay, the interpretation of test results as well as the choice of blood tubes for sample collection should be discussed with the laboratory. Blood lead concentrations do not reflect the length of exposure or tissue concentrations. In some chronic cases, blood lead concentrations may be normal. In these cases, submission of blood and urine samples after initiation of therapy with calcium disodium EDTA has been recommended.[59] The activity of erythrocyte δ-aminolevulinic acid dehydratase was demonstrated to be a sensitive indicator of lead poisoning in sheep.[60] In chronically exposed animals, a normocytic, normochromic anemia may be present. Basophilic stippling and other pathologic changes of red cells may be detected, but they are neither specific nor sensitive diagnostic tools.[60] For postmortem diagnostics, liver, kidney, fetuses, and feed samples should be submitted either fresh or fixed in formalin.

Treatment. Calcium disodium EDTA is used for chelation therapy and removes lead from osseous, but not soft, tissues. Slow intravenous administration of EDTA for 3 to 5 days (70–75 mg/kg IV, once daily) followed by 2 days without treatment and then 3 to 5 days of additional administrations once daily has been recommended. An alternative treatment regimen uses 110 mg/kg of EDTA twice daily for 2 days, followed by 2 days without treatment, after which 2 more days of twice daily treatment are administered.[59] At the time of this edition, no commercially available products containing Ca-EDTA are available. While the use of compounded products is allowed with restrictions, their use in food animals requires that no violative residues occur. Administration of adjunctive thiamine therapy (20 mg/kg or 500 mg/sheep and goats and, where applicable, cervids, once daily SC) enhances the success of chelation therapy and reduces lead deposition in soft tissues.[61,62] Oral administration of magnesium sulfate enhances fecal lead excretion by formation of insoluble salts. Further treatments may include supportive fluid therapy, nutritional care (oral or total parenteral nutrition), and the control of seizures (0.5–2 mg/kg IV of diazepam or midazolam).

Sodium Toxicosis and Water Deprivation (Salt Poisoning)

Etiology and Pathophysiology. Sodium toxicosis may result either from ingestion of excessive amounts of sodium chloride in feed or water or from normal sodium chloride intake during restricted access to water. Susceptibility to sodium toxicosis varies between species and age groups, but it is plausible that all ruminants can be affected, especially when access to free-choice water is limited. High saline concentrations are found in certain water sources (e.g., artesian wells), oral electrolyte solutions, or when salt is used to limit feed intake. Animals without prior access to salt may consume excessive amounts when salt becomes available. Limited access to water may be a factor in bottle-fed neonates and transported animals or may become an issue when water sources malfunction or freeze. Regardless of etiology, the resulting hypernatremia causes fluid shifts from extracellular spaces and increases in CSF sodium concentrations. As a protective response to prevent neuronal water loss, increased concentrations of electrolytes and idiogenic osmoles are maintained within the CNS. If hypernatremic animals are allowed unrestricted access to water, or are rapidly rehydrated, the serum sodium concentration decreases and cerebral edema and PEM result as fluids follow the osmotic gradient into the CNS.

Clinical Signs. High dietary salt concentrations may result in reduced feed intake, depression, and gastroenteritis. The neurologic disorder is characterized by the classic clinical signs of PEM, which include ataxia, central blindness, behavioral changes, nystagmus, opisthotonus, coma, and death. Brown-discolored serum and urine may result from accompanying intravascular hemolysis.[33]

Diagnosis. Historical overexposure to salt and/or water deprivation and the presence of hemolysis may be suggestive of salt poisoning. Hypernatremia may be present but may be masked by water intake prior to serum chemistry analysis. Sodium concentrations in CSF in excess of those in serum are diagnostic for salt poisoning.

Treatment. The type and route of administration of fluid therapy depend on the number of animals affected and severity of clinical signs. Oral and intravenous fluids should be isotonic or hypertonic to prevent the development of cerebral edema. Affected animals and herd-mates that are still able to drink should be provided with restricted access to water four to six times a day until free-choice water can be offered after 3 to 4 days. For initial therapy, water should be made isotonic by the addition of 9 g of sodium chloride per liter. More severely depressed animals should be given fluids by oral or intravenous route. Intravenous fluids should be isotonic or hypertonic, and a slow correction of the serum sodium concentration is desirable, especially in chronically affected animals. Although higher rates of correction may be tolerated, a reduction of the serum sodium concentration by 1 mEq/L/hour has been recommended.[63] Cerebral edema may be treated by administration of intravenous mannitol (20%, 1–2 g/kg IV) and, possibly, dexamethasone.

Prevention. The provision of free-choice water of high quality to animals of all ages and the proper preparation of milk replacers and electrolyte solutions are important in preventing salt poisoning.

Pseudorabies (Aujeszky's Disease, Mad Itch)

Etiology and Pathophysiology. Pseudorabies, also called Aujeszky's disease and "mad itch," is caused by Suid alphaherpesvirus 1 (SuHV-1), an alphaherpesvirus of swine. Other domestic and free-ranging species, including small ruminants, may develop clinical disease but are considered dead-end hosts.[20] In young piglets, high morbidity and mortality rates occur and are associated with neurological disease. Case fatality rates decrease with age, and older pigs serve as the reservoir for SuHV-1. Few reports of pseudorabies encephalomyelitis in small ruminants exist, but infection may occur by bite of an infected pig, exposure of open wounds or mucous membranes, iatrogenically, and by airborne route. The virus is neurotropic and spreads centripetally from peripheral neurons to the CNS, resulting in progressive encephalomyelitis. The incubation period and duration of clinical signs are short, and death occurs within 2 to 7 days.[20]

Clinical Signs. In infected ruminants, paresthesia and intense local pruritus at the site of inoculation are common.[20,64] Pyrexia and self-mutilation result in abrasions, swelling, and alopecia. Other clinical signs include fever, ataxia, circling, and depression; however, excitement and aggression can also be observed. Death is preceded by recumbency, convulsions, vocalization, and other signs of severe cerebral disease.[64]

Diagnosis. Pseudorabies should be suspected in ruminants that had contact with pigs and show clinical signs of severe pruritus and cerebral disease. At postmortem examination, superficial trauma is noted, and signs of meningoencephalitis, including histological evidence of nonsuppurative inflammation, are present. Affected ruminants die before the development of serum antibodies; thus, serology is not useful. Diagnostic confirmation is made by identification of SuHV-1 by virus isolation, IHC, or PCR.

Treatment. Effective therapeutic measures are not available, and affected animals should be euthanized. Pseudorabies is a reportable disease and regulatory authorities should be alerted when suspicious clinical signs are noticed.

Prevention. SuHV-1 has been eradicated from domestic swine in many developed countries; however, the virus remains endemic in some populations of Eurasian wild boar and feral pigs. Contact of ruminants with infected pig populations should be avoided. Contaminated barns and paddocks can be sanitized with quaternary ammonium or phenol-containing compounds.[65]

Rabies

Etiology and Pathophysiology. Infections with rabies lyssavirus (rabies virus) result in a fatal nonsuppurative encephalomyelitis in all mammals. With the exception of a few countries, the disease has a worldwide distribution. In 2015, 5508 cases were detected in animals and three cases in humans in the United States.[66] In the same year, seven sheep and goats and one deer were confirmed to be positive for rabies virus.[66] Rabies is relatively rare in U.S. deer, but cases have been reported in free-ranging and captive deer, which accounted for 0.07% of all reported rabies cases between 1990 and 2009.[67,68] Rabies lyssavirus belongs to the genus *Lyssavirus* in the family *Rhabdoviridae.* Several viral strains exist that are adapted to a particular host-species. In ruminants, the disease is associated with spillover infections from infected wildlife populations, which include the skunk (south-central to north-central United States and California), raccoon (southeastern United States and East Coast), fox (southern United States and Alaska), and mongoose (Puerto Rico).[66] Bat-associated rabies variants exist, which, while a public health concern, appear to be of limited importance for small ruminants.[69] Maintenance of the virus within wildlife is influenced by migration, expansion, and density of populations. Natural barriers, such as mountain ranges and rivers, contain the disease geographically.[20,70] Principally, transmission of rabies virus occurs by bite of an infected animal that contains the virus in its saliva. After infection, the virus replicates in muscle cells and subsequently spreads toward the CNS by centripetal axoplasmic flow. The virus replicates in the CNS gray matter and, via parasympathetic nerves, invades several tissues, including salivary glands.[71] Shedding of rabies virus may occur before clinical signs are noticeable. The length of the incubation period may be from 2 weeks to several months and depends on the proximity of the bite wound to the CNS.

Clinical Signs. Rabies should be a differential diagnosis in any animal with neurologic disease as clinical signs can be quite variable. Although the disease usually affects individual animals, a rabid animal may infect and cause clinical signs in multiple herd- or flock-mates.[67,72] Early clinical signs may include depression, ataxia, and anorexia. Proprioceptive deficits, hyperesthesia, muscle twitching, and ascending paralysis develop as the disease progresses. Pharyngeal paralysis results in inability to swallow, stertorous breath, and accumulation of frothy saliva around the oral cavity. Behavioral abnormalities, such as aggression toward handlers and inanimate objects and sexual hyperactivity, may be intermittent. The disease is rapidly progressive and affected animals become recumbent within 3 to 5 days, followed by coma and death by 10 days of onset of clinical illness.[73]

Diagnosis. Whenever rabies is suspected, efforts must be focused on preventing the exposure of personnel handling the animal, and diagnostic samples must be appropriately labeled before submission. Antemortem diagnostics aid in ruling out other diseases but are not available for rabies testing. Collection of CSF should be avoided because of its zoonotic potential. The diagnosis of rabies is based on examination of brain sections by histopathology and fluorescent antibody test (FAT) on fresh tissues. When fresh tissues are unavailable, an immunoperoxidase test can be used on formalin-fixed samples. Tissues should be submitted cooled, but not frozen. The entire brain or head of suspect cases should be submitted intact. Methods of euthanasia that traumatize brain tissue (i.e., captive bolt or gunshot) should be avoided. Classically, diagnosis has been based on histopathological detection of Negri bodies within the hippocampus, medulla oblongata, and cerebellum, but false-negative and false-positive findings are not uncommon. The FAT is a highly accurate test and detects viral antigen in the thalamus, pons, and medulla, among other regions.

Treatment. Rabies is consistently fatal and effective treatments are not available.

Prevention. In endemic areas, vaccination of sheep and goats with a killed vaccine may be appropriate, and vaccines labeled for sheep are available. While the efficacy of rabies vaccination and duration of immunity in deer are limited, vaccination may be considered for valuable animals or those in frequent contact with potential host species.[67,74,75] Postexposure prophylaxis depends on the animal's vaccination history and the value of the animal and should be discussed with regulatory authorities. After cleaning and disinfecting all bite wounds, vaccinated animals should be revaccinated immediately and observed for 45 days in quarantine. Unvaccinated animals may be culled immediately or vaccinated and observed for at least 90 days to 6 months with further booster vaccinations during quarantine.[20]

Transmissible Spongiform Encephalopathy

Transmissible spongiform encephalopathies (TSEs) are a group of slowly progressive neurodegenerative diseases of humans and animals. While other factors may be involved in the pathophysiology, TSEs are caused by prions (proteinaceous infectious particle), which are transmissible, self-replicating proteins that induce misfolding of host proteins. Misfolded proteins are not removed from the body and accumulate in host tissues. Over time, accumulation of prion proteins in nervous tissues results in cell death and the typical spongy appearance of affected tissues. There are many similarities between the TSE affecting small ruminants, such as length of incubation time, uniform fatality in affected animals, alimentary route of infection, and presence of abnormal prion protein in lymphatic tissues allowing antemortem testing. While infection of sheep, goats, and European red deer with bovine spongiform encephalopathy (BSE) by the alimentary route is possible,[76,77] the principle TSEs of sheep and goats and cervids are scrapie and chronic wasting disease (CWD), respectively. For information on appropriate collection of samples for scrapie and CWD testing, please see Chapter 20.

Scrapie

Etiology and Pathophysiology. Scrapie is the earliest known member of the TSEs and is characterized as a uniformly fatal, progressive neurodegenerative disease of sheep and, less frequently, goats. The disease is classified as "classical scrapie" or "atypical scrapie" according to immunobiochemical differences and variations in the localization of neuropathological lesions. Both classical and atypical forms of scrapie have been reported in sheep and goats.[78] In addition, BSE can occur naturally in goats.[79,80] Scrapie is endemic in most countries but appears to have been eliminated from Australia and New Zealand by extensive slaughter campaigns. Prevalence rates of 0.1 to 0.3% have been reported, but accurate estimates are difficult to obtain. Bias from testing sensitivity, underreporting of fallen animals, and differences among tested populations (e.g., fallen, culled, or adult slaughtered sheep) exists.[81–84] Since the institution of a mandatory surveillance program in the European Union (EU) in 2002, larger numbers of classical and atypical scrapie have been discovered, of which many were in a preclinical stage. From 2002 to 2008, scrapie was detected in 15,034 sheep and 3292 goats in the EU.[78] While prions are the most widely accepted cause of scrapie, other hypothesized agents including bacteria and small virions might be involved in the pathophysiology of TSEs and the production of the characteristic abnormal protein found in affected animals.[85,86]

Scrapie-associated prion protein (PrP^{Sc}) is highly resistant to many methods of disinfection and can be recovered from fresh-frozen or formaldehyde-fixed tissues.[87] Common to all TSEs is the misfolding and accumulation of PrP^{Sc}, an abnormal isoform of a host-encoded glycoprotein that is found in high concentrations in lymphoreticular and nervous tissues. Accumulation of PrP^{Sc} in nervous tissues is associated with the development of clinical signs. Transmission of the agent is not fully understood; however, infected animals contaminate pastures by shedding from the placenta and fetal fluids and possibly by other routes.[88] Shedding of the pathogen occurs during the extended incubation period, and transmission occurs likely only by the horizontal route. Susceptible sheep and goats ingest the pathogen, and young sheep appear most susceptible to infection.[89] Susceptibility and length of incubation time are strongly associated with polymorphisms of the prion protein gene. In sheep, polymorphisms at codons 136, 154, and 171 (A136V/T, R154H/L, and Q171R/H/K) are linked to susceptibility or resistance to classical scrapie. While various polymorphisms exist, the ARR/ARR genotype is most resistant to scrapie and therefore recommended for breeding. The greatest risk for classical scrapie is found in sheep with genotypes VRQ/VRQ, VRQ/ARQ, VRQ/ARH, and VRQ/AHQ.[90] Less complex than in other breeds, the increased susceptibly of Suffolk sheep is associated with homozygosity for glutamine (Q) at codon 171. Genotype ARR/ARR does not protect from atypical scrapie, in which polymorphisms of codons 141 and 154 are of importance for disease susceptibility.[90] In goats, susceptibility to scrapie is also associated with PrP gene polymorphisms; however, these are not completely understood. Codons 142, 154, 211, and 222 appear to be influential for classical scrapie in goats, while codon 154 was related to atypical caprine scrapie.[78,91] After ingestion, the agent crosses the intestinal mucosa and invades gut-associated lymphoid tissues, where it replicates and disseminates to other lymphoid organs, before invasion of the nervous system. The agent reaches the CNS by way of the enteric nervous system, following the sympathetic and parasympathetic nerve fibers.[88] Initial infection of the brain is localized in the diencephalon and medulla oblongata, with subsequent replication in other areas of the brain. A noninflammatory, vacuolar degeneration (spongiform) of the gray matter with the presence of PrP^{Sc} in scrapie-associated fibrils follows and results in clinical signs.

Clinical Signs. Scrapie is a progressive and protracted neurological and dermatological disease characterized by intense wasting, pruritus, behavioral changes, and gait abnormalities. The clinical course may last from 2 to 12 months, but in sheep is commonly around 6 months and in goats is 2 to 24 weeks.[92] Affected animals are usually between 2 and 5 years of age but may be older. Initial clinical signs are subtle and noticed intermittently. Behavioral changes such as aggression toward people and objects, fixed gaze, charging dogs or gates, and failure to respond to herding are noticed. Affected animals begin rubbing and biting especially on tail head, rump, thighs, and dorsum, and ataxia, and weight loss becomes apparent. As clinical signs worsen, pruritus becomes more persistent and leads to wool loss and self-inflicted trauma, which may manifest as aural hematomas, facial swelling, and secondary bacterial infections (Figure 13.9). Application of pressure to affected areas may provoke a "scratch reflex," during which the animal nibbles on the distal extremities, smacks and licks its lips, or performs rhythmic head movements. Gait abnormalities begin as hindlimb ataxia and are progressive (Figure 13.10). Poor postural reactions, exaggerated gaits, hypermetria, "bunny-hopping," and falling can be observed. Affected animals separate from the flock or herd and become severely anorectic, which may predispose to pregnancy toxemia. Other clinical signs may include nystagmus, inability to swallow, dysphonia, blindness, and vomiting. Severely affected animals are emaciated and weak and become recumbent with convulsions and hyperextension of the limbs.[87,92]

Diagnosis. Scrapie is a reportable disease, and early contact with regulatory authorities limits the potential for misdiagnosis and errors in the enforcement of control and eradication strategies. Clinical signs of scrapie are variable and nonspecific and may

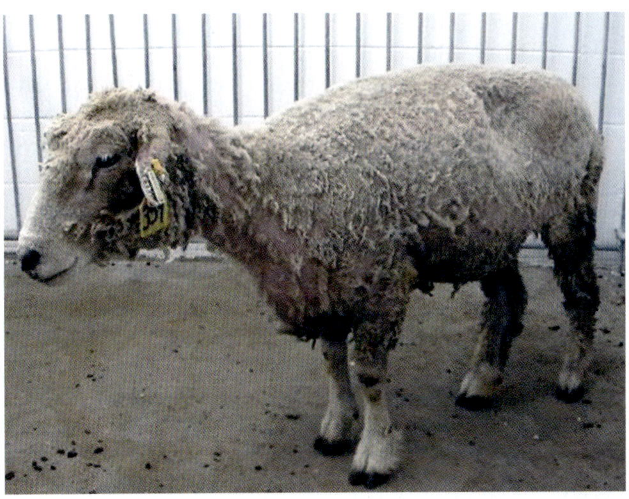

• **Fig. 13.9** Patchy wool loss in a Southdown sheep with clinical scrapie. (Courtesy Dr. Michelle L. Crocheck, Ames, Iowa.)

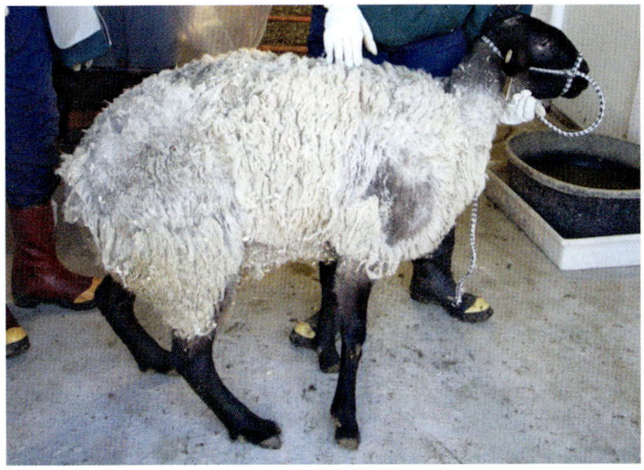

• **Fig. 13.10** Hunched posture and wool loss in a Suffolk sheep with clinical scrapie. (Courtesy Dr. Michelle L. Crocheck, Ames, Iowa.)

go unnoticed in early cases. Antemortem diagnostics for scrapie rely on the detection of PrP^{Sc} in lymphoid tissues; therefore, successful detection depends on the stage of the disease, the genotype of the affected animal, and the collection of sufficient lymphatic tissue.[93] IHC is used on biopsies from tonsils, pharyngeal lymph nodes, or lymphoid follicles in the rectal mucosa or third eyelid.[94] Detection of PrP plaques in lymphoid tissues enables the identification of preclinical animals, before involvement of the nervous system. Tonsillary biopsies are better samples for analysis but are difficult to collect. Third eyelid biopsies are easier to obtain but may not contain sufficient amounts of lymphoid tissue, especially in early cases, when PrP^{Sc} is less evenly distributed.[94] For collection of third eyelid biopsies, animals are sedated and topical analgesia is applied. Visualization of the lymphoid tissue may be enhanced by adding histamine to the topical analgesic. Following eversion of the third eyelid, lymphoid biopsies are excised using a pair of scissors.[87] Rectal biopsies are relatively easy to collect and can have similar sensitivity rates as tonsil samples if at least 10 lymphoid follicles are obtained.[95]

Postmortem diagnostics are based on histological identification of degenerative changes in the CNS gray matter. Submitted samples must be of good quality. Distribution of lesions varies by the genotype of infected animal and infecting scrapie agent.[94] In classical scrapie, typical PrP^{Sc} distribution is observed in the medulla oblongata and the peripheral lymphoreticular system, but in atypical scrapie, PrP^{Sc} accumulates preferentially in cerebellar cortex. Identification of PrP^{Sc} is performed by IHC, western blot, ELISA, or conformation-dependent immunoassay[94] (see Chapter 20).

Treatment. An effective treatment is not available. Early diagnosis and removal of affected animals are important for preventing disease transmission and should be performed in collaboration with regulatory authorities.

Prevention. Scrapie prevention is based on removal of affected and high-risk animals from herds, biosecurity, and selective breeding for resistant animals. When affected small ruminants are identified, regulatory authorities may require removal and testing of the entire flock or affected and high-risk animals (sheep born in the same year as affected, offspring of affected sheep, lambs born in the year affected ewe gave birth).[87] In the United States, the Voluntary Scrapie Flock Certification Program identifies and monitors enrolled flocks and, if scrapie is not detected, assigns the certified status. These herds avoid trade restrictions that are otherwise impeding the U.S. sheep industry. National breeding efforts to perpetuate resistant genotypes and increased testing strategies are utilized in scrapie eradication efforts in countries of the EU. In the United Kingdom, where widespread testing of breeding sheep has been performed since 2001, genotypic selection has effectively altered the national PrP genotype, while having little influence on performance traits or increased inbreeding.[96] While genetic selection for resistance is utilized for the prevention of classical scrapie in sheep, breeding for resistance against atypical scrapie and scrapie resistance in goats still proves challenging.

Chronic Wasting Disease

Etiology and Pathophysiology. CWD is a prion disease of captive and free-ranging cervids that was first described in captive mule deer in Colorado in 1967 and later classified as a TSE.[97] In addition to mule deer, CWD can affect other North American cervids, including elk (wapiti), white-tailed deer, and, less commonly, moose.[98,99] Since the first description of CWD, the disease has expanded rapidly and has been detected in captive and/or free-ranging deer in 23 U.S. states and two Canadian provinces.[100] The disease also occurred in Canadian elk imported to South Korea and was detected, more recently, in free-ranging reindeer in Norway.[101,102] The prevalence of CWD in affected free-ranging populations is dependent upon species, geographic location, age, and sex. While the prevalence in free-ranging populations is generally lower than in captive cervid populations, rates exceeding 10% can be observed in endemic areas.[103] In contrast to the relatively stable dispersion of the disease in free-ranging cervids, captive herds can experience epidemics, during which the incidence of disease may approach 90%.[104,105]

Transmission of CWD is mainly by horizontal spread of infectious prions, either directly by contact with infected animals or indirectly by exposure to contaminated environmental sites while foraging. Infected deer shed prions in saliva, urine, velvet, and feces, and shedding of sufficient amounts to cause transmission can occur from preclinical and clinical deer.[104] In addition to excretions from infected deer, decomposing carcasses also serve as a source of environmental contamination and infection.[106] Similar to scrapie prions, CWD prions are very stable in the environment and can persist for years. Prions can bind to soil, which, depending on soil type, enhances environmental persistence and infectivity and may influence the CWD epidemiology.[107,108]

Infection is the result of ingestion or inhalation of the infectious prion, which crosses the mucosal barriers and invades oropharyngeal lymphatic tissues. Following several weeks, prions invade systemic lymphoid tissues and reach high concentrations, prior to neuroinvasion.[109] Ascending fibers of the autonomic nervous system allow prion invasion of the CNS, with widespread distribution at the onset of clinical signs.[104]

As with scrapie, susceptibility to CWD and length of incubation time are associated with genetic variation in the prion protein gene, and polymorphisms associated with reduced susceptibility have been identified in white-tailed deer, mule deer, and elk.[110] CWD was demonstrated to cause a population decline in some deer populations, and there exist a selection pressure toward the CWD-resistant genotype.[111,112]

Clinical Signs. The incubation time of CWD varies based on genetic susceptibility but is generally at least 1 to 2 years.[113,114] Clinically, CWD is characterized by progressive weight loss and behavioral changes. Behavioral changes and subtle locomotive changes are among the first clinical signs.[104] Affected animals have difficulty swallowing, ptyalism, polydipsia, and polyphagia. Abnormal gastrointestinal function including esophageal dilatation and abnormal rumen content may be associated with aspiration pneumonia. Additional clinical signs include proprioceptive deficits, ataxia, head tremors, altered posture, low head carriage, and increased time spent recumbent. Affected captive deer may survive for several weeks to months.[97] CWD increases the likelihood of free-ranging animals dying from predation or vehicular trauma, shortening the clinical course of disease.[115,116]

Diagnosis. As described for scrapie, there exist methods for antemortem and postmortem diagnosis of CWD. However, while sensitive assays that may allow routine antemortem testing of captive and wild cervids have been developed in the last 20 years, currently approved CWD tests use tissues (medial retropharyngeal lymph nodes or brainstem [obex]) from dead deer. On necropsy of CWD-affected deer, pathognomonic CNS lesion can be detected, including microcavitation of the neuropil, intracytoplasmic vacuolization, astrocytic hypertrophy and hyperplasia, and neuronal degeneration. Within these lesions, amyloid plaques can be visualized by Congo red or Bodian silver staining.[117] Confirmation of the presence of abnormal prion protein can be performed by use of immunoassays including Western blot, IHC, and enzyme immunoassay. For testing by IHC, tissues should be submitted in 10% buffered formalin. More recently, an ELISA assay (Bio-Rad ELISA BioRad, Hercules, CA, USA) has been approved for CWD detection, for which either chilled or frozen tissues should be submitted. The retropharyngeal lymph node and dorsal motor nucleus of the vagus in the obex are tissues in which abnormal protein is found relatively early in the disease progression and are therefore considered the gold standard for postmortem diagnosis[117] (see Chapter 20, Figures 20.20, 20.21, and 20.22).

While immunoassays are very accurate for postmortem diagnosis of CWD in clinically affected animals, they may lack sufficient sensitivity for reliable detection of abnormal prions for antemortem diagnosis in clinically normal animals and are insufficient for other sample types such as bodily fluids and soil. To achieve greater test sensitivity, in vitro amplification of low levels of abnormal prion in a sample can be performed using assays such as protein misfolding cyclic amplification or real-time quaking-induced conversion assay. The use of these in vitro conversion assays may allow accurate antemortem detection of CWD-infected animals using easily obtainable samples; however, proper sample collection and handling remains crucial.[117]

Treatment. There currently exists no effective treatment for CWD.

Prevention. In captive deer, prevention of CWD is centered around surveillance for infected animals and biosecurity. In the United States, a Voluntary National CWD Herd Certification Program was instituted in 2012 and directs enrolled herd owners to identify and maintain records of individual animals, control deer movement with adequate fencing, test all animals over 12 months of age that die or are killed for CWD, and limit new herd additions to animals obtained from certified herds. Herds that are free from CWD for 5 years are certified as low risk for CWD and are allowed interstate transport of deer. Some U.S. states are not participating in this federal program but may have similar or stricter requirements for CWD control.

CWD control in free-ranging animals is based upon surveillance, preventing unauthorized introduction of deer through interstate transport, preventing aggregation of deer at supplemental feeding and baiting sites, and reduction of population densities by increased hunting. Selective and nonselective removal and control strategies have been evaluated, and while some successful control strategies were identified, they may not be generally applicable to all environments.[118]

Urea (Ammonia) Toxicity

Etiology and Pathophysiology. Sheep, goats, or cervids fed urea as a source of nonprotein nitrogen, or those accidentally exposed to large quantities as a result of fertilizer spills, mixing errors, or contamination of water sources, may develop toxicity.[119,120] The toxic dose (minimal lethal dose) in ruminants is approximately 500 mg/kg.[121] In the rumen, urea is catabolized to ammonia and assimilated into microbial proteins, provided that adequate carbohydrates are available. If this process is overwhelmed, ammonia is absorbed from the rumen and detoxified by the liver. Absorption of ammonia exceeding the liver capacity results in clinical signs. Risk factors for the development of toxicity include lack of adaption, high rumen pH (associated with poor-quality forages), concurrent feeding of soybean meal (high in urease), and the lack of readily fermentable carbohydrates in the diet.[122]

Clinical Signs. Affected animals may display signs of severe abdominal pain, become bloated, regurgitate, and froth at the mouth. Muscle tremors, hyperesthesia, incoordination, weakness, ataxia, violent struggling, convulsions, and recumbency may be observed.[123] Severely affected animals die from cardiac or respiratory failure.

Diagnosis. History of exposure and clinical signs may suggest urea toxicity. On serum chemistry analysis, markedly increased glucose and potassium concentrations, elevated aspartate aminotransferase (AST) and alanine aminotransferase (ALT) activities, and decreased sodium concentrations may be present.[123,124] The ruminal pH is markedly increased (~7.5–8), and ammonia concentrations are elevated in rumen, blood, and ocular samples.

Treatment. Infusion of cold water and 5% acetic acid (vinegar, 0.5–1 L) into the rumen reduces the degradation of urea to ammonia and decreases its absorption. This treatment may need to be repeated. In valuable animals, intravenous fluid therapy and a rumenotomy to remove rumen contents should be considered.

Prevention. Rations containing urea should be slowly introduced and never contain more than 3% of the chemical. The adaptation to urea feeding is lost rapidly (1–3 days), and animals must be reintroduced to such rations when urea feeding is interrupted.

West Nile Virus Encephalitis

Etiology and Pathophysiology. West Nile virus (WNV) is a flavivirus in the family *Flaviviridae* with wide geographic distribution. After its first introduction in 1999, the virus has become endemic in the United States. Although different studies have demonstrated antibodies in sheep and goats, disease caused by WNV appears to be rare in small ruminants.[125,126] WNV has caused sporadic cases of fatal meningoencephalomyelitis in sheep.[127,128] Similarly, there is serologic evidence of infection of deer in Europe and North America, but reports of clinical disease are rare.[129] Maintenance of WNV relies on an endemic cycle that involves mosquitoes (mainly *Culex* spp.) and various species of birds. When a susceptible bird is bitten by an infected mosquito during the vector season (July to October), an amplifying viremia develops that allows transmission of WNV to another mosquito. Large warm-blooded animals appear to be dead-end hosts that do not develop viremia sufficient to transmit the virus to uninfected mosquitoes.

Clinical Signs. The disease typically affects only individual animals within a herd.[128] The duration from initial clinical signs to death has been reported to be as short as 8 hours to over 1 week.[128,130] Initial clinical signs include fever, depression, ataxia, and teeth grinding. Muscle fasciculations, ataxia, and spasms are typical signs of WNV infection in horses and have been described in sheep and deer. Affected animals become recumbent and may convulse preceding death.[131,132]

Diagnosis. Low viral titers often make attempts of detecting WNV in blood samples unrewarding. Hyperfibrinogenemia and increased muscle enzymes due to muscle fasciculation and recumbency may be present on blood samples. On CSF analysis, increased protein concentrations and mononuclear pleocytosis can be observed. Definitive diagnosis is based upon comparison of acute and convalescent antibody titers or postmortem examination. Nonsuppurative encephalitis with lymphocytic, plasmacytic perivascular inflammation may be suggestive histopathologically. The virus can be detected in nervous tissue by virus isolation, PCR, or IHC.

Treatment. Reports of effective therapy in small ruminants do not exist and treatment is supportive. In addition to fluids, nutritional support, provision of deep bedding, and antiinflammatory therapy have been recommended.[20] However, studies evaluating the efficacy of steroidal or nonsteroidal antiinflammatory drugs or oral vitamin E supplementation for its antioxidant properties have not been published.

Prevention. Currently, an approved WNV vaccine for use in ruminants does not exist, but several vaccines are approved for use in horses. Seroconversion and apparent safety were demonstrated in reindeer vaccinated with a killed equine vaccine,[133] but routine vaccination of small ruminants and deer against WNV appears to be unnecessary. Prevention of mosquito bites by application of repellants, housing animals indoors at dusk and dawn, and use of fans to limit indoor invasion and feeding of mosquitoes has been recommended.[20]

Cerebellar Diseases

Grass Staggers

Grass staggers refers to any plant-associated tremor syndrome caused by the ingestion of endophytic or intrinsic toxins of grasses. Since these toxins confer protection from parasites and overgrazing (plant-defensive compounds), infested grasses often have a selective advantage over noninfested grasses.[134] Although toxic principles vary among grasses, the clinical characteristics of grass-associated tremor syndromes are similar.

Etiology and Pathophysiology

Annual Rye Grass *(Lolium rigidum)* Toxicity is caused by corynetoxin produced by *Clavibacter toxicus*, which infects seed galls of annual rye grass infested with the nematode *Anguina agrostis*. The disease has been reported in Oregon, but principally is a problem in Australia and South Africa.[134,135] Although clinically similar to perennial rye grass staggers, toxicosis associated with annual rye grass causes severe brain pathology and may be lethal.[134]

Bermuda Grass *(Cynodon dactylon)* The toxic principle of offending Bermuda grass pastures has been uncertain but proposed to be intrinsic alkaloids or mycotoxins.[136] Production of tremorgenic indole-diterpenoid mycotoxins by *Claviceps cynodontis* similar to those of *Claviceps paspali* was detected on ergotized Bermuda grass samples and reported to cause clinical signs.[137]

Canary Grass (Phalaris spp.) Tryptamine alkaloids present in certain species of canary grass inhibit the breakdown of serotonin by monoamine oxidase, increasing the responses to excitatory stimuli in specific brain and spinal cord nuclei.[138] Canary grass intoxication manifests in the cardiovascular and nervous systems, with an acute form of the disease affecting the cardiovascular system, while nervous system disease occurs with prolonged exposure to the toxin.[139] Only weaned animals are affected in an outbreak, and morbidity rates of up to 80% and mortality rates of 20% have been described.[140]

Dallis Grass (Paspalum spp.) Infestation of grasses of the genus *Paspalum*, including Dallis grass, water couch grass, and Argentine bahia grass, with the ergot fungus *C. paspali* results in production of tremorgenic mycotoxins (paspalitrems). The fungus infects seed heads, and large amounts of toxin are found in the reddish-brown to black sclerotia.[139]

Perennial Rye Grass (Lolium perenne) Infestation with *Acremonium loliae* and production of tremorgenic mycotoxins (lolitrems) mainly occur during ambient temperatures over 23° C (73.4° F) in closely grazed pastures, and the concentration of toxin varies seasonally.[139] Fungal growth is greatest in basal leaf sheaths, and lolitrem B levels of 1800 to 2000 ppb are considered the threshold of disease.[141] In addition to sheep and goats, the disease has been reported in farmed elk (wapiti), red deer, and fallow deer in Australia and New Zealand, with wapiti appearing to be more susceptible than red deer.[142,143]

Clinical Signs. Findings are similar for any of the tremorgenic grass staggers, regardless of the grass species involved. Multiple animals in an affected herd often show clinical signs including muscle tremors, stiffness, and ataxia. Affected animals exhibit a spastic, hypermetric gait and are prone to falling. Excitement or external stimuli exacerbate clinical signs and can produce intention tremors of the head.[136] In addition to ataxia and tremors, ingestion of phalaris grass could result in signs of cardiovascular disease including arrhythmia, dyspnea, cyanosis, and sudden death.

Diagnosis. Antemortem diagnosis is based on identification of the typical clinical signs in animals on contaminated pastures and detection of the toxin in plant or seed head. In cases of canary grass staggers, severe pathological lesions can be observed in lungs, heart, kidneys, and CNS.

Treatment. Animals should be quietly removed from offending pastures and provided alternate feed sources. Although severely affected animals may have to be euthanized, spontaneous recovery from grass staggers is possible but may take several months.

Prevention. Grasses in which the toxic principle resides in the seed head (annual rye grass, Bermuda grass, and Dallis grass) can be mowed before seed head development. Mowing and raking seed heads or intermittent grazing has also been recommended.[139] Pastures may have to be burned or sprayed, tilled, and reseeded.[139] Toxins produced by claviceps fungi in Bermuda and Dallis grass survive drying and remain toxic for years.

Diseases of Brain Stem and CNs

Listeriosis

Etiology and Pathophysiology. Infections with *Listeria monocytogenes* are common in sheep, goats, and deer worldwide, but the disease is most often encountered in temperate climates. In addition to focal encephalitis, which is the most common form in ruminants, *L. monocytogenes* may cause septicemia, abortions, mastitis, and ophthalmitis, which usually present as separate disease entities.[144,145] The gram-positive, facultatively intracellular bacteria are ubiquitous in the environment of domestic and free-ranging animals and can be shed by healthy carrier animals.[146] *L. monocytogenes* is shed in feces, milk, tears, nasal secretions, and uterine fluid of sick and apparently healthy ruminants. Shedding in milk is of concern because the organism is an important food-borne zoonotic pathogen. *L. monocytogenes* survives for months to years in soil, feces, and contaminated feed and is able to grow at broad ranges of pH and temperatures, including refrigeration temperatures.[147] Classically, listeriosis is associated with feeding of improperly fermented silage with pH > 5.5, but sources of infection also include other spoiled forages, such as the bottom of round bales and rotten vegetation (e.g., grass clippings). Goats consuming woody browse can also be at increased risk for the disease.[148] Although listeriosis can occur during any time of the year, greater morbidity rates are observed during the winter months,[149] coinciding with silage feeding and crowded winter housing. In a listeriosis outbreak in fallow deer that occurred during the winter and early spring, suspected risk factors included poor beech-mast crop, increased stocking density, and sudden weather changes.[150]

Following ingestion, *L. monocytogenes* crosses mucosal surfaces, resulting in bacteremia, septicemia, and infection of placenta and fetus. Although the bacteria may breach the blood-brain barrier within infected leukocytes or by direct invasion of endothelial cells, invasion of the CNS in ruminants is thought to be most commonly by centripetal migration within axons of CNs.[151] In small ruminants, axonal migration within the trigeminal nerve has been demonstrated, and other CNs may serve as ports of entry.[151,152] Abrasions in the oral cavity associated with hard feedstuffs and the replacement of teeth appear to allow entrance of the bacteria into CN rootlets, but invasion through intestinal and conjunctival mucosae may also be possible.[144,151] Once in the CNS, *L. monocytogenes* induces the formation of microabscesses, focal neuronal necrosis, and neuronophagia. Clinical signs depend on the location of lesions. Commonly, the brainstem and roots of CNs are affected. Lesions may also extend into more rostral regions of the brain, including the cerebellum, midbrain, and thalamus.[151]

Clinical Signs. Listeriosis commonly causes unilateral loss of function of multiple CNs. Affected animals are anorectic and depressed, which may result from metabolic abnormalities, meningitis, and involvement of rostral brain regions. Listeriosis is an acute disease that, in the absence of therapy, rapidly progresses. Fever is observed only in the early stages of the disease, and affected animals are often dehydrated and have decreased rumen motility. The impaired function of CNs results in facial hypalgesia, dropped jaw, and dysphagia (CN V); drooped lips and ears, nasal deviation, and ptosis with secondary exposure keratitis (CN VII); head tilt, circling, and nystagmus (CN VIII) (Figure 13.11); pharyngeal paresis, dysphagia, and upper respiratory stertors (CN IX and X); and unilateral tongue paresis and dysphagia (CN XII). Involvement of other areas of the nervous system may cause further clinical signs, and spinal cord deficits may result in limb paresis or paralysis.[153] The case fatality rate in untreated animals approaches 100%. Recumbency, torticollis, and opisthotonus are observed in moribund animals.[144,154]

Diagnosis. Listeriosis is one the most common CNS diseases of ruminants and should be suspected when clinical signs of

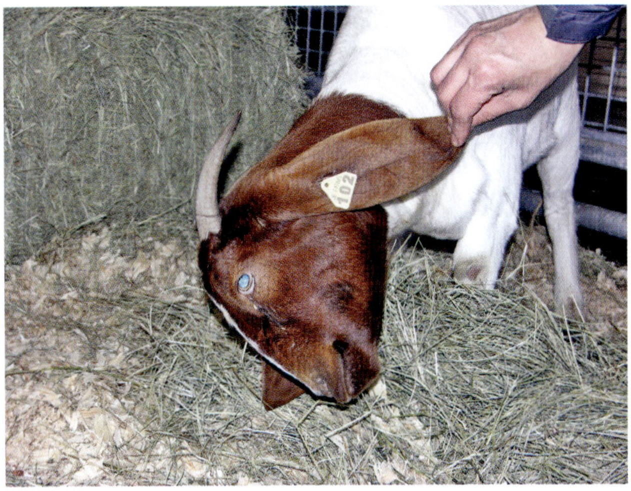

• **Fig. 13.11** Severe head tilt in a goat with listeriosis. Other clinical signs in this animal included circling, nystagmus, ataxia, and inability to blink.

unilateral brainstem disease are present. Clinical signs are not pathognomic for listeriosis, and specific antemortem tests are not available. Clinical pathology reflects metabolic derangements associated with dehydration (azotemia, increased hematocrit, and increased total protein concentration) and metabolic acidosis, which results from loss of salivary bicarbonate in dysphagic animals.[155] Identification of elevated protein concentrations and mononuclear pleocytosis in CSF is useful in diagnosing listeriosis. Mononuclear cells often predominate in the CSF of affected animals, but neutrophils (see Figure 13.6C) are also elevated. *L. monocytogenes* is rarely identified in CSF, and microbiological culture or PCR techniques on CSF samples are unrewarding.[156] On gross postmortem examination, severe pathologic lesions are usually absent, but CNS microabscessation and neuronal necrosis are characteristic histopathological findings. In tissues, the bacteria may be identified using fluorescent antibody or IHC techniques.[157]

Treatment. Treatment of listeriosis includes antibiotic, antiinflammatory, and supportive therapy. Therapy must be initiated early in the disease course, as the treatment of severely ill and recumbent animals is rarely successful.[155] Commonly used antibiotics include oxytetracycline (5–10 mg/kg slow IV twice a day), penicillin (22,000–44,000 IU/kg IM as procaine penicillin twice a day or IV as potassium penicillin two to four times a day), and florfenicol (20 mg/kg IM every 48 hours). Antibiotic choices should not include cephalosporins to which *Listeria* are intrinsically resistant, or aminoglycosides, which are discouraged for use in food animals and appear not to increase the likelihood of successful therapy.[158] Nonsteroidal antiinflammatory drugs (flunixin meglumine 1.1–2.2 mg/kg IV SID to BID) and fluid therapy to correct dehydration and acid-base abnormalities are recommended. In cases of conjunctivitis or keratitis, broad-spectrum ophthalmic antibiotics (tetracycline) and ophthalmic atropine may be indicated. Supportive care involves provision of good bedding and maintaining animals in sternal recumbency. Enteral force-feeding of alfalfa or beet-pulp slurries, moist feeds, green browse, improvement of ruminal microflora by transfaunation, and administration of vitamin B complex might provide additional benefit. Recumbent animals should be turned often, supported in sternal recumbency, and given adequate supportive care. Animals that are treated before becoming recumbent have a fair to good prognosis if appropriate antibiotic and supportive therapy are provided. Therapy appears to be less effective in sheep than in goats.

Prevention. Proper storage and handling of feedstuffs to prevent growth of *L. monocytogenes* are important in preventing exposures. Removal of improperly fermented silages and rotten forages decreases exposure to the organism. As many healthy ruminants, including wildlife, shed *L. monocytogenes*, fecal contamination of feed sources should be prevented. Adequate animal hygiene, prevention of overcrowding, and providing access to pasture decrease the risk of listeriosis.[149]

Otitis Media and Interna

Etiology and Pathophysiology. Infections of the ear are common in ruminants, and involvement of the middle and/or inner ear may be associated with clinical signs of vestibular disease and loss of facial nerve function. Invasion of the middle ear by pathogens can occur by three routes: (1) invasion of pathogens through the auditory tube, which extends from the nasopharynx to the middle ear; (2) extension of an infection from the external ear canal through the tympanic membrane; and (3) hematogenous spread secondary to bacteremia. Hematogenous spread is believed to be least common because bacteremia is uncommon in cases of otitis media.[144] Otitis media/interna most commonly occurs by invasion of respiratory bacterial pathogens through the auditory tube, and young animals, such as feedlot lambs, are at an increased risk.[159,160] Inflammation and accumulation of exudate caused by infection of the middle ear result in clinical signs of facial nerve dysfunction. Otitis media may remain localized or extend through the tympanic membrane into the external ear canal. Extension of otitis media into the inner ear is also possible, resulting in otitis interna and clinical signs of vestibular disease.

Various bacteria have been isolated from sheep and goats affected by otitis. While reports of bacterial isolation from cervine otitis cases are sparse, bacterial pathogens associated with respiratory disease in deer are likely to be causative. Mixed bacterial populations are often present in otitis cases, and the composition of bacterial populations depends on the route of infection. In small ruminants, reported bacteria include *Mannheimia haemolytica*, *P. multocida*, *P. aeruginosa*, *Neisseria catarrhalis*, coagulase-positive, hemolytic and mixed hemolytic *Staphylococcus* spp., hemolytic *Streptococci* spp., and coliforms.[159–161] Several species of *Mycoplasma*, some of which are pathogenic, have been recovered from the external ear canal of goats; however, their importance in otitis media/interna is uncertain.[162–164] A role of ear mites in the transmission of *Mycoplasma* spp. has been suggested, and the presence of *Mycoplasma* in ear-swap samples was associated with the presence of ear mites.[165,166] Ear mites occur in all ages and both sexes of animals, but breeds with dependent ears and younger animals may be at increased risk.[167,168] In goats, the ear mites species *Psoroptes cuniculi* and *Raillieta caprae* are commonly detected, but infestations are usually subclinical.[167,169] Signs of otitis externa, including an increased amount of cerumen, drainage of purulent material, and head-shaking are present in a small percentage of infested animals.[167,168] Similarly, otitis externa and, less commonly, otitis media caused by *P. cunniculi* can occur in mule deer and white-tailed deer, and rates of infestation appear to be greater in captive deer.[170–172] Infestation of sheep with *Psoroptes ovis*, which is endemic in many herds, results in clinical sheep scab that is characterized by exuberant yellowish scab on the ears and body, intense pruritus, wool loss, and secondary lesions.[173]

Clinical Signs. Otitis externa may be subclinical. Clinical signs, when present, include excessive head shaking, ear twitching, and scratching. Excessive production of cerumen and formation of casts at the base of the ear are common findings. In addition, scabs and infected crusty lesions may be noted. In more severe cases, aural hematomas and abscesses resulting in thickening and distortion of the pinnae (cauliflower ears) might be present.[174] Animals affected by uncomplicated otitis media are usually alert and appetent, which can assist in ruling out listeriosis.[144] Visible discharge from the external ear canal may be present in some cases. Loss of facial nerve function results in ear droop, the most common clinical sign in affected animals.[144] Ptosis, lip droop, exposure keratitis on the side of the lesion, and deviation of lips and nostrils to the opposite side might also be observed. Vestibulocochlear nerve dysfunction may follow extension of the infection into the inner ear and is characterized by head tilt, incoordination, falling to the affected side, and occasionally nystagmus. Circling is observed to the same side as the head tilt and the tightness of circles may aid in differentiation from central vestibular disease, in which the diameter of circles is smaller.[1]

Diagnosis. In addition to the physical and neurologic examinations, an otoscopic examination of the ear canal for presence of foreign bodies, severity of inflammation, and integrity of the tympanic membrane should be performed. Visualization of the tympanic membrane is often complicated, and endoscopy is a useful adjunct when evaluating the external ear canal. The presence of ear mites may support a diagnosis of otitis media, but this finding may be incidental. Mites may be localized deep in the ear canal at the tympanic membrane, which complicates their recovery by swabbing or irrigation. Bacterial culture of exudate from the external ear should include testing for *Mycoplasma* spp. and antimicrobial sensitivity testing. Ancillary diagnostic tests such as CBC, serum chemistry, and CSF analysis typically are not helpful for diagnosing otitis media/interna, except when meningitis or secondary systemic illness is present. Radiographically, thickening and loss of definition of the temporal bulla and sclerosis of the petrous temporal bone may be visualized. Injection of contrast media into the ear canal may improve visualization of the ear canal and aid in assessment of the integrity of the tympanic membrane.[144,175]

Treatment. In cases of otitis externa, therapy is based on the removal of the inciting cause and treatment of inflammation and secondary infections. Solutions used to flush and cleanse the ear must be chosen based on the integrity of the tympanic membrane, and mild solutions should be chosen when the tympanic membrane is suspected to be ruptured. Warm physiologic saline is the safest solution to use, but microbicidal solutions can be appropriate (Table 13.3). Irrigation, cleansing, and subsequent drying of the ear canal should be repeated before topical treatments are administered. Ear mite infestations can be successfully treated using parental administration of ivermectin (0.2 mg/kg once or twice) or topical solutions containing rotenone or fenthion.[176] *P. cunniculi* was successfully controlled in captive white-tailed deer by feeding of ivermectin-treated corn (200 μg/kg).[177] In cases of otitis media, extended systemic antibiotic and antiinflammatory therapy may be successful, but chronic cases might not respond. Surgical lateral ear resection facilitates access to the horizontal ear canal in animals that do not respond to medical therapy and in which adequate drainage cannot be achieved.

Prevention. Prevention is based on decreasing metabolic and environmental stress in animals at high risk and on early and appropriate treatment of respiratory disease. Parental administrations of macrocyclic lactone anthelmintics repeated at 2- to 3-week intervals are useful in controlling ear mite infestations.[144,176]

Diseases of Spinal Cord and Peripheral Nerves

Botulism

Etiology and Pathophysiology. Botulism is caused by any of the seven antigenically distinct toxins (A–G) produced by the gram positive, spore-forming, anaerobic bacteria *Clostridium botulinum*. The distribution of these toxin types varies geographically. Small ruminants are most commonly affected by types C and D. Toxin production occurs in warm, moist, anaerobic environments such as spoiled forages (forage botulism) and animal carcasses (carrion-associated botulism). Contamination of feedstuff with carrion, feeding of poultry litter, presence of dead rodents around feeding sites, and factors that promote pica (e.g., hypophosphatemic animals chewing on bones) increase the risk for toxin ingestion.[18,178–180] In ruminants, botulism is almost always associated with ingestion of preformed toxin, although wound contamination or toxico-infectious botulism (proliferation of *C. botulinum* in the intestinal tract) are also possible.[18] Because the degradation of ingested toxin by the ruminal microflora provides a degree of protection, young animals are at a greater risk than adults. Following intestinal absorption, the toxin

TABLE 13.3 Bactericidal Solutions for Flushing the External Auditory Meatus.

Solution	Concentration	Toxicity	Susceptible Organisms	Resistant Bacteria
Chlorhexidine	2%, 0.05%	Ototoxic	Gram negative and gram positive bacteria; fungi	*Pseudomonas*
Povidone-iodine	0.1 to 1%; smaller concentrations are more effective	Ototoxic	Gram negative and gram positive bacteria; fungi	Gram negative bacteria
Acetic acid	1:1, 1:2, or 1:3 dilution of a 5% solution	Ototoxic	*Pseudomonas, Staphylococcus, Streptococcus, Escherichia coli,* and *Proteus*	Very few bacteria are resistant at 5% concentration, but it is irritating to mucosa

is distributed to cholinergic nerve terminals by the bloodstream. Similar to tetanus neurotoxin, botulinum toxin attaches to nerve cell walls by binding to gangliosides and is translocated into the cell. The toxic effects and flaccid paralysis are caused by inhibition of synaptic acetylcholine release at the motor endplate and parasympathetic nerve endings.

Clinical Signs. After a variable incubation period, generalized muscular weakness, reluctance to move, and a stumbling gait develop. Initial weakness and ataxia are more prominent in the rear limbs.[18] As the disease progresses, animals become recumbent with flaccid paralysis. Weakness of the neck musculature results in low head carriage and head bobbing. Protrusion of the tongue, dysphagia, and drooling may be observed. Rumen hypomotility, rumen tympany, regurgitation, and bladder distention can occur. Death results from respiratory paralysis and can occur without premonitory signs.

Diagnosis. Specific hematologic, serum chemistry, or postmortem findings are lacking, and the diagnosis often relies on clinical signs. Definitive diagnosis is based on identification of toxin in feed, gastrointestinal contents, or liver samples. Botulinum toxin can be identified using the mouse bioassay or ELISA techniques, but detection may not be successful in all affected animals.[45]

Treatment. Extended nursing care is the mainstay of therapy, with the goal of supporting the animal until toxin has degraded and new nerve synapses have formed. Such care includes fluid and nutritional support and, in severe cases, prolonged mechanical ventilation. Repeated bladder catheterizations and relief of rumen tympany may also be necessary. Drugs that deplete acetylcholine from the neuromuscular junction, such as neostigmine, or that enhance muscular weakness, such as penicillin or oxytetracycline, should be avoided.[181] When feasible, polyvalent antisera may be beneficial if administered early in the disease.

Prevention. Adequate feed hygiene and removal of contaminated feeds are important factors in prevention. Other measures include proper fermentation of silage, rodent control, and the removal of carcasses. Nutritional deficiencies that lead to pica should be corrected. Vaccination is practiced in endemic areas of the world; however, vaccines are only available in the United States for horses (type B toxoid) and mink (type C bacterin-toxoid).[18]

Cerebrospinal Nematodiasis (Meningeal Worm)

Etiology and Pathophysiology. CSN results from aberrant migration of nematode larvae within the spinal cord. In North America, *Parelaphostrongylus tenuis* is endemic in white-tailed deer, and CSN has been reported in various ruminant species including sheep, goats, elk, moose, mule deer, caribou, reindeer, fallow deer, sika deer, red deer, black-tailed deer, bison, and cattle when collocated with white-tailed deer. In white-tailed deer, adult parasites reside in the subarachnoid space, where they produce eggs that are removed from the CNS via venous sinuses. First-stage larvae hatch and enter the lungs and trachea, are coughed up and swallowed, and passed in the feces. Larvae enter snails or slugs, their intermediate hosts, in which they develop into the infectious third stage and are protected from environmental conditions. Deer accidentally ingest the intermediate host when feeding. Larvae are released in the gastrointestinal tract and migrate to the dorsal horn of the spinal cord, where they mature to adulthood and enter the subarachnoid space, completing the life cycle.[182] In dead-end hosts, such as sheep, goats, and other deer species, the life cycle is not completed, and larvae migrate aberrantly in the spinal cord, inciting inflammation. Although uncommon, aberrant larval migration may extend further rostrally, causing brain involvement and more severe disease.[183,184] CSN may also be associated with infection of small ruminants and deer with nematodes in the genus *Elaphostrongylus* in Europe and New Zealand[185–188] and the filarial nematode *Setaria digitata* in Asia.[189–191]

Clinical Signs. Infection with *P. tenuis* occurs most commonly from late summer to winter.[192] Clinical signs depend on the number of infecting larvae and their migration pattern. Unilateral to bilateral hindlimb paresis and ataxia are most common. Affected animals refuse to rise and display neurologic deficits typical of UMN disease. Neurologic deficits often progress, and generalized ataxia and recumbency can develop. Affected animals are typically bright and alert and maintain a good appetite unless larvae have migrated into the brain. Brain involvement is uncommon but may result in depression, blindness, and death.

Diagnosis. Definitive diagnosis can be made only by identification of migrating larvae in the spinal cord during postmortem examination. Histopathologic changes include demyelination, axonal degeneration, malacia, and presence of larval sections and leukocytes. Antemortem diagnosis is based on clinical signs and CSF analysis. In a majority of affected animals, eosinophilic pleocytosis with 7 to 97% eosinophils may be detected, but monocytes might predominate in some cases.[183,192] Other CSF findings include increased concentrations of proteins, erythrocytes, and leukocytes (see Figure 13.6D). Serum chemistry and CBC findings are usually normal, but increases in muscle enzyme concentrations may be present.

Treatment. Although spontaneous recovery has been reported, CSN is usually a progressive disorder. Many treated animals retain residual neurologic deficits, and full recovery is slow. Treatment protocols for CSN include administration of anthelmintics, antiinflammatory drugs, and supportive care. Fenbendazole (15–50 mg/kg PO SID for 5 days) may be administered alone or in combination with macrocyclic lactone anthelmintics and appear to provide good clinical efficacy. Disagreement exists as to the effectiveness of ivermectin (200–400 μg/kg SC once or twice), as this anthelmintic does not cross the intact blood-brain barrier, but as the integrity of the blood-brain barrier is disrupted in CSN, administration of ivermectin should be efficacious. Moxidectin, a milbemycin with enhanced lipid solubility and potential to cross the blood-brain barrier, might be an alternative to ivermectin. Nonsteroidal antiinflammatory drugs (flunixin meglumine 1.1 mg/kg IV for 3–5 days) or glucocorticoids in nonpregnant animals aid in the suppression of inflammation that is believed to be central to the pathophysiology of CSN. Vitamin E given as an antioxidant, physical therapy, and supportive care may promote recovery and improve outcome.

Prevention. Removal of susceptible animals from moist, low-lying areas that support the intermediate hosts of *P. tenuis* or fencing off these areas could potentially decrease exposure. The use of molluscicides is regulated and may be impractical in larger production systems. Geese and ducks have been used to reduce snail populations. Reduction of contact with white-tailed deer, which shed *P. tenuis* larvae in the feces, is difficult. Preventive deworming programs using injections of avermectins every 4 to 6 weeks are commonly used in at-risk New World camelids and disrupt larval migration from the abomasum to the spinal cord. Although apparently effective, these programs may be too costly for some operations, require repeated handling, and are likely to promote anthelmintic resistance of other nematode parasites.

Enzootic Ataxia (Swayback)

Etiology and Pathophysiology. In sheep, goats, and cervids, primary or secondary copper deficiency can cause neurologic disease. Clinical signs in sheep and goats occur in perinatal and nursing lambs and kids. Two types of the disease are recognized: a congenital form and a delayed form.[193] The congenital form affects neonates born to dams on diets with very low copper content. The delayed form is characterized by slower progression and later onset of clinical signs. In contrast to sheep and goats, enzootic ataxia in deer occurs in young adult and adult animals and has been reported in captive and semicaptive red deer, fallow deer, and sika deer.[194–197]

Copper is a cofactor for many biological processes. Deficiencies cause abnormal mitochondrial function and cytochrome-c oxidase activity in the cerebral white matter and spinal cord, which result in oxidative degeneration and demyelination.[193] Secondary copper deficiencies may develop when the copper metabolism is disturbed by excess molybdenum, iron, cadmium, or sulfate.

Clinical Signs. Neonatal sheep and goats with congenital swayback may be stillborn or are weak and unable to stand and nurse. Affected animals show spastic tetraparalysis and die in the first week of life.

Delayed enzootic ataxia affects lambs and kids at 2 to 4 months of age. The disease begins as pelvic limb ataxia and is less severe than the congenital form. With progression of the disease, ataxia and paresis involve all limbs, resulting in recumbency and death in most affected animals. In deer, clinical signs of rear limb ataxia and incoordination progress over several weeks. Affected animals may be observed to be dog-sitting, eventually becoming recumbent and losing body condition, all the while having normal mentation and appetite.[196] In affected herds, abnormal hair coat and lameness caused by abnormal bone development may be observed in younger deer.[198]

Diagnosis. Measurements of copper concentrations in diet, serum or plasma, and liver biopsy samples are useful to confirm a clinical suspicion. Neonatal values may differ from those of adults, complicating the evaluation. A plasma copper concentration of 4.5 to 9 μmol/L (approximately 0.29–0.57 ppm) has been proposed as a marginal concentration in sheep.[199] Serum or plasma concentrations below 0.4 ppm are considered to be indicative of copper deficiency. Hepatic copper concentrations below 35 ppm (dry matter basis) are considered deficient. Liver samples are preferred to blood samples; however, at least 100 mg of tissues are required for analysis, necessitating a biopsy instrument with at least 3- to 5-mm internal diameter.[200]

Treatment. Affected animals may be supplemented with copper either orally or parenterally. Many of the CNS changes appear to be irreversible, and supplementation of copper may have little effect.

Prevention. Prevention is based on dietary supplementation in deficient areas and maintaining proper ratios of copper to interacting minerals. Increasing the dietary copper to 5 to 15 ppm and maintaining a copper-to-molybdenum ratio of 6:1 in pregnant females are usually protective. Copper sulfate (35 mg per head twice a week) has been advocated to prevent swayback in lambs.[200] Sheep have increased susceptibility to copper toxicity, so supplementation of copper in the diet should be monitored.

Organophosphate Polyneuropathy

Etiology and Pathophysiology. Organophosphate toxicity can result from exposure to insecticides for crop use or overdosing of medicinal insecticides and anthelmintics containing organophosphate or carbamate chemicals. These chemicals bind with and inhibit acetylcholinesterase, resulting in accumulation of acetylcholine in tissues.[136] In addition to typical clinical signs of acute toxicosis (acronym SLUD: *s*alivation, *l*acrimation, *u*rination, and *d*efecation), delayed neurotoxicity may occur. Axonal degeneration and secondary demyelination result from phosphorylation of the enzyme esterase.[122,201] Some sheep appear to have a familial predisposition.[202]

Clinical Signs. Clinical signs occur 8 to 90 days after exposure. Posterior incoordination, weakness, and loss of proprioceptive ability are signs of neuropathy. Animals become recumbent and lose tail, rectal, and bladder function. Additional signs include anorexia, depression, ruminal stasis, and diarrhea.[122]

Diagnosis. History of exposure and clinical signs may suggest the disease. On postmortem examination, histological evidence of degeneration in peripheral nerves and spinal cord are evident.

Treatment. In contrast to cases of acute intoxications, treatments are unavailable for delayed neurotoxicity. In young animals, peripheral nerve lesions may improve upon removal of the offending chemical. Acute cases may be treated with high doses of atropine (0.2–0.4 mg/kg IV) or pralidoxime (2-pyridine aldoxime methyl chloride, 20 mg/kg).

Prevention. Use of organophosphates in accordance with label instructions aids in the prevention of intoxication and neurologic disease.

Spastic Paresis

Etiology and Pathophysiology. Spastic paresis is a sporadic disease of goats and has been reported in different breeds, including Pygmies and Saanens.[203,204] The condition is characterized by progressive and intermittent or continuous contraction of the gastrocnemius muscles of one or both hindlimbs. Spastic paresis appears to be inherited, although the mode of inheritance and pathophysiology are currently poorly understood and other etiologic mechanisms are under discussion.[205] The exaggerated tone of the gastrocnemius muscle is believed to be consequence of overstimulation of myotatic reflexes in the muscle spindle of the affected muscles.[206]

Clinical Signs. Spastic paresis affects goats between 1 and 3 years of age and results in progressive clinical signs. Contraction of the gastrocnemius muscles results in extension of the tibiotarsal joint, weight shifting to the front limbs, and apparent lameness. The pelvic limbs may barely touch the ground or may be extended behind the animal. Clinical signs are abolished or reduced when the animal lies down.

Diagnosis. Diagnosis is based on typical clinical signs and severe contracture of the gastrocnemius muscle. Other diseases, such as CAE, may cause similar clinical signs and must be ruled out. Epidural injection of diluted procaine solution briefly abolishes clinical signs of spastic paresis and helps confirm the clinical diagnosis of spastic paresis.[203,206]

Treatment. Different surgical techniques including tenectomy and partial tibial neurectomy have been utilized in cattle and may be successful in goats. Alternatively, medical treatment with lithium (Li) (0.2 mEq/kg) and/or tryptophan potentiated by manganese and especially copper (20–50 mg/kg per day of tryptophan) may be effective in early cases.[205]

Spinal Trauma, Abscesses, and Tumors

Etiology and Pathophysiology. Various clinical entities may be associated with impaired function of the spinal cord, either by external compression or damage as a result of injuries. Space-occupying lesions may be neoplastic, infectious, or inflammatory. Neoplastic tissue compressing the spinal cord might originate in the CNS (e.g., meningioma) or other organs or might be systemic (e.g., lymphosarcoma).[207,208] Abscesses of the spinal cord usually result from vertebral osteomyelitis following hematogenous infection as a sequela of bacteremia.[209] Septicemia in neonates, rumenitis secondary to acidosis, pneumonia, and sepsis developing at injection sites are common causes of bacteremia. Fractures of the spinal cord may be traumatic or pathological and may result from nutritional imbalances of calcium and phosphorous. Traumatic injuries to the spinal are commonly inflicted by other animals (predators, horses, and donkeys), a result of motor vehicle accidents, or result from high-velocity impacts with inanimate objects (e.g., collision with fence during handling of fractious animals). Identifying the cause of an injury can be challenging.

Clinical Signs. Clinical signs depend on the location of the lesion in relation to spinal nerve roots and the degree of damage. In addition to paresis or paralysis of the extremities, animals can display signs of pain associated with movement of the spinal column. The head and neck may be held in extension, and a stiff gait may be noted. Spinal abscesses that extend through the dura mater cause clinical signs of septic meningitis.[209]

Diagnosis. In addition to clinical signs and palpation of the vertebral column, radiographs are useful in obtaining a diagnosis of demineralization, spinal cord abscessation, osteomyelitis, or fractures. Osteomyelitis is characterized by a random pattern of hyperlucency and increased bone density in the affected vertebrae.[209] If indications of bone demineralization are present, calcium and phosphorus contents of feed and serum parathyroid hormone concentrations should be evaluated.[193] Myelography and advanced imaging techniques (CT and MRI) may be required to visualize lesions from soft tissue compression and internal concussions.[193] While CBC and serum chemistry may not reflect diagnostic alterations, analysis of CSF may be useful. In cases of trauma, xanthochromia and elevations in total protein and mononuclear cells can be observed. Although localized abscesses that do not infiltrate the meninges may change the CSF composition only marginally, protein elevations and neutrophilic pleocytosis have been reported.[210] Cytologic examination of CSF may also suggest the presence of neoplasia.

Treatment. Therapy is based on the etiology and involves administration of antibiotics and antiinflammatory drugs and surgical stabilization or decompression. Antimicrobial drugs must be given for several weeks to treat vertebral osteomyelitis, but prognosis for cure is guarded. Regimens for antiinflammatory therapy have not been formally evaluated, and medications should be selected according to the etiology.

Tetanus

Etiology and Pathophysiology. Tetanus is caused by toxins of the gram positive, anaerobic, spore-forming bacteria *Clostridium tetani*. The organism is ubiquitous in soil and in the intestinal tract of herbivores. Under aerobic conditions, *C. tetani* produces tenacious spores that have a drumstick-like appearance and can remain viable in soil for years. Contamination of and entrance into tissues are usually the consequence of penetrating wounds or surgical procedures (tail docking, castration [especially band castration], velvet harvest, or shearing). Sometimes, the point of entry cannot be found because the wound itself may be minor or has healed. The organism also can be introduced into the reproductive tract during parturition. The disease appears to be less common in cervids than in sheep and goats. Although usually a sporadic disease, outbreaks of tetanus have been associated with contaminated vaccines and injectable dewormers, or following ear-tagging of unvaccinated sheep.[211,212] Tetanus occurs when suitable anaerobic conditions develop within tissues, allowing spores to enter the vegetative state and begin production and release of toxins.[18] The necrotizing toxin tetanolysin enhances anaerobic conditions and proliferation of the bacteria. The tetanus neurotoxin (tetanospasmin) affects the nervous system and is responsible for clinical signs. After receptor-specific binding of tetanospasmin to cell-wall gangliosides on target motor neurons at the site of infection, the neurotoxin is translocated into the neuronal cytoplasm. Following retrograde axonal flow, tetanospasmin crosses into inhibitory interneurons of the spinal cord and blocks their function. Additionally, effects on the brainstem and midbrain may occur with further axonal or circulatory transport. Disruption of the synaptic membrane transport protein synaptobrevin prevents release of glycine and gamma-aminobutyric acid, blocking the inhibitory effect of affected interneurons.[213]

Clinical Signs. The incubation period varies with the time of development of an anaerobic tissue environment, and a wound may not be visible by the time clinical signs are present. Early clinical signs include changes in gait, including stiffness or apparent lameness. The disease is progressive, and generalized stiffness with involvement of head, neck, extremities, and tail (pump-handle tail) ensues (Figure 13.12). The animal may be in a "saw-horse" stance or recumbent. Trismus (lockjaw), erect ears, retraction of lips (sardonic grin), and third-eyelid prolapse are observed during examination of the animal's head. Tetanus affecting laryngeal and pharyngeal muscles decreases the ability to swallow, and drooling of saliva, regurgitation, bloat, and aspiration pneumonia may develop. External stimuli such as loud noises can result in accentuated symptoms and tetanic convulsions.[18] In animals that recover, clinical signs may last for weeks as toxin binding is irreversible. Death from respiratory paralysis is common.

Diagnosis. Clinical signs are typical of tetanus and suggest the diagnosis. A definitive diagnosis is based on identification of *C. tetani* in infected wounds. Blood work reflects dehydration

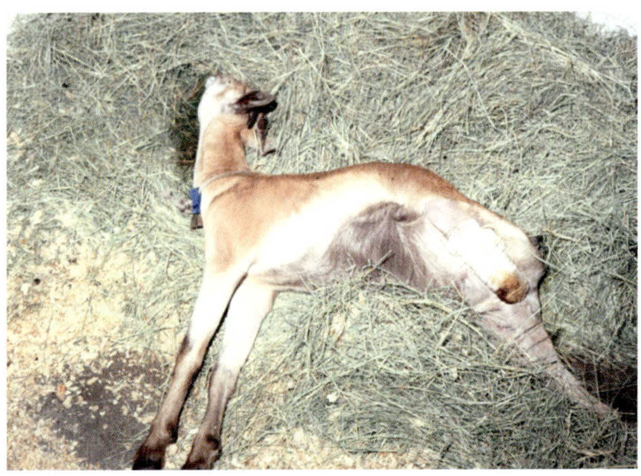

• **Fig. 13.12** Severe clinical signs of tetanus, including recumbency and generalized stiffness of the head, neck, and extremities, in a goat that sustained traumatic injury to the hindlimb.

(azotemia), loss of salivary bicarbonate (acidosis), stress (hyperglycemia and stress leukogram), and increased concentrations of muscle enzymes.

Treatment. Animals affected by tetanus should be handled in a calm and quiet fashion. Treatment is aimed at eliminating the infection, neutralizing unbound toxins, relieving muscle spasms, and provision of nursing care. Identification and debridement of the infected wound removes the anaerobic and necrotic tissues and exposes the bacteria to oxygen. Penicillins are the antibiotic of choice and are given at high doses and frequency (22,000–44,000 IU/kg IM SQ as procaine penicillin or IV as potassium penicillin two to four times a day). The administration of tetanus antitoxin (1500–15,000 IU SQ for 3–5 days) neutralizes only unbound toxin and may not be effective in advanced cases. Sedation and muscle relaxation can be achieved using acepromazine (0.05–0.1 mg/kg IM BID), diazepam (0.5 mg/kg IV), or xylazine (0.02–0.05 mg/kg IV) until signs have improved. Soft, deep bedding and a quiet, dark environment are important supportive measures. Ruminal tympany and anorexia may be alleviated by a rumenotomy to allow escape of free gas as well as enteral feeding.

Prevention. Immunization against tetanus is efficacious and cost effective. Vaccines containing tetanus toxoid often include other clostridial toxoids such as *C. perfringens* C and D (CD/T). Vaccination of captive deer may be appropriate in some herds when risk factors (such as surgical procedures or harvest of velvet) are anticipated; however, efficacy of vaccination and duration of immunity appear to be unknown. Lambs and kids benefit from improved colostral immunity when dams are vaccinated with tetanus toxoid during pregnancy.[214] Lambs and kids should be vaccinated at 2 to 3 months of age, followed by a booster vaccination 3 weeks later, and then revaccinated annually. Adequate hygiene should be maintained during predisposing surgical procedures, and nonvaccinated animals should receive tetanus antitoxin (150–200 IU) prior to surgery, which provides protection for 2 to 3 weeks.

Tick Paralysis

Etiology and Pathophysiology. Tick paralysis is a rapidly progressing, ascending LMN paralysis of many species, including sheep, goats, and possibly deer. In North America, the disease mainly occurs west of the Rocky Mountains, despite broader distribution of the causative ticks, *Dermacentor* spp.[182] Globally, various tick species have been reported to cause tick paralysis.[215] The disease occurs during greatest tick activity—from April to June in North America.[182] Following attachment to the host by a female tick, a salivary neurotoxin is secreted, which impairs acetylcholine release at the motor endplate and causes neuromuscular blockade.[216,217]

Clinical Signs. Clinical signs are observed approximately 1 week after ticks begin feeding on infested animals.[218] Initially, pelvic limb weakness and ataxia may be present, but flaccid quadriplegia rapidly develops.[182,218] Affected animals show typical LMN deficits, are recumbent, and have diminished spinal and withdrawal reflexes. Menace response and corneal and palpebral reflexes may be absent.[218]

Diagnosis. The rapid development of flaccid paralysis and the presence of feeding ticks help to differentiate the disease from CSN and botulism.

Treatment. Removal of all ticks is curative, and clinical signs resolve within 24 hours. Animals must be examined carefully and possibly shorn to detect all ticks. Application of acaricides may be beneficial but should not replace manual removal of ticks.[182]

Prevention. In high-risk areas, use of acaricides, such as pyrethrins or avermectins, aids in the prevention of the disease.

Congenital and Perinatal Neurologic Diseases

A great degree of differentiation, complexity, and long duration of development render the CNS prone to congenital disorders. The type and severity of congenital defect depend on the gestational age and, therefore, stage of fetal brain development, at exposure to a teratogen or pathogen. Developmental dysfunctions may result from hereditable, environmental, or infectious disorders, and a combination of lesions within and outside of the CNS may be detected in affected animals. Elucidating the cause of a congenital defect helps to prevent exposure of other susceptible animals to a pathogen or environmental stressor and excludes carriers of inheritable conditions from breeding programs. Affected fetuses should be evaluated thoroughly and submitted for postmortem examination. In neonates displaying neurologic deficits, the presence of common neonatal disorders such as hypoglycemia, meningitis, hypoxia, and hypothermia should be ruled out when congenital disorders are suspected.[219] Before the discussion of specific etiologies, common congenital disorders affecting the cerebrum (hydrocephalus and hydranencephaly) and cerebellum (hypoplasia and abiotrophy) are briefly described under separate headings, although they may be encountered in combination. Various factors, including maternal hyperthermia, plant toxins (e.g., false hellebore *[Veratrum californicum]* or hemlock *[Conium maculatum]*), and medications (e.g., certain benzimidazoles), may have teratogenic effects that injure the developing fetal CNS.[219,220]

Hydrocephalus and Hydranencephaly

Accumulation of excessive fluid in the ventricular system of the cranium can be the consequence of infectious, inherited, environmental, nutritional, and neoplastic conditions.[219] The disorder can be classified as either normotensive (hydranencephaly) or hypertensive hydrocephalus, depending on the underlying pathophysiology. Both conditions may develop as congenital defects in ruminants, with hydranencephaly occurring more commonly.[221] In hydranencephaly, fetal cerebral tissues fail to develop or undergo necrosis as a result of viral infection or cerebrovascular insults. The cerebral hemispheres and basal ganglia are nearly completely replaced by CSF, surrounded by a thin layer of cerebrum. Affected fetuses do not develop cranial enlargement because of the normotensive character of hydranencephaly. Hypertensive hydrocephalus is caused by stenosis of the ventricular system that prevents absorption of CSF and increased intracranial pressures. Developmental anatomical malformations or alterations as result of inflammation may cause stenosis and hypertension. The resulting compression causes ischemia and necrosis of cerebral hemispheres and enlargement and deformation of the calvarium.

Cerebellar Hypoplasia and Abiotrophy

Two distinct pathogeneses may cause cerebellar dysfunction and associated clinical signs in neonates and young animals. Cerebellar hypoplasia refers to an arrested development of fetal cerebellar tissue, commonly caused by viral infection of the fetus. The severity of cerebellar dysfunction depends on the gestational age and duration of the developmental arrest and may range from aplasia to hypoplasia.[219] In contrast, cerebellar abiotrophy occurs in postnatal animals and describes the premature degeneration of formed cerebellar tissues and especially Purkinje cells.[219] Affected animals may appear healthy at birth but develop clinical signs in the first months of life.

Infectious Causes of Congenial and Perinatal Neurologic Disease

Akabane Virus. Akabane virus, an orthobunyavirus in the family *Bunyaviridae*, causes clinical disease in cattle and small ruminants in Africa, Japan, Israel, Korea, and Australia. Transmission of the virus is by arthropod vectors, including midges (*Culicoides* spp.) and mosquitos (*Aedes* and *Culex*). In Australia, *Culicoides brevitarsis* is considered the major vector, and occurrence of disease is closely linked to vector distribution.[222] Disease in postnatal animals is rare, and infection in nonpregnant animals produces protective immunity. Infection of pregnant, susceptible animals without sufficient immunity (e.g., vector/virus spread to novel locations) results in viremia.[222] Transplacental invasion of the developing fetus results in a persistent infection of fetal membranes with subsequent spread to fetal tissues.[223] Sheep fetuses infected at a gestational age of 30 to 36 days are susceptible to damage of nervous tissues, because the CNS develops rapidly at this time and fetuses are not yet immunocompetent. Viral activity is greatest in the CNS and skeletal muscles, resulting in nonsuppurative encephalomyelitis and polymyositis. Necrosis of subventricular zones of the developing cerebrum prevents migration of neuroblasts and results in accumulation of CSF (hydranencephaly). Arthrogryposis appears to be a consequence of polymyositis and the neurotropic failure of muscle development, which results in joint contracture.

Bluetongue Virus and Epizootic Hemorrhagic Disease Virus. Infections with bluetongue virus (BTV) and epizootic hemorrhagic disease virus (EHDV), orbiviruses in the family *Reoviridae*, cause vascular injury and systemic disease in a variety of domesticated and free-ranging ruminants. In North America, BTV infections have been reported in cattle, sheep, goats, alpacas, white-tailed deer, mule deer, pronghorn, bighorn sheep, and American bison.[224] In white-tailed deer, BTV infection is indistinguishable from infection with EHDV based on clinical signs or postmortem examination.[224] White-tailed deer are the principal host for EHDV in North America, but the virus can also infect domestic cattle, elk, mule deer, pronghorn, bighorn sheep, and mountain goats.[224] At least 24 serotypes of BTV exist worldwide, with infections occurring in all continents except Antarctica.[225] Similarly, seven serotypes of EHDV are recognized worldwide,[226] of which serotypes 1, 2, and 6 are detected in North America. Transmission of BTV and EHDV between mammalian hosts occurs by biting insects of the genus *Culicoides*, which serve as the vector and are able to introduce the viruses into new geographic areas when climatic conditions are permissive. Under field conditions, transplacental infection and congenital defects are not caused by all orbiviruses and have only been associated with attenuated live BTV vaccine strains and BTV serotype 8.[227,228] However, under experimental conditions, other BTV and EHDV serotypes are capable of teratogenisis,[229,230] and orbiviruses should be considered as etiologic agents in cases of fetal encephalopathies. Various factors determine the virulence of an infecting viral isolate, including nutritional and immune statuses, environmental stresses, or breed (e.g., more severe disease in European fine-wool sheep).[225] Infections at the time of development of the fetal CNS may result in congenital defects. Neuronal and glial precursor cells that reside at subepidermal regions before migrating into the developing cerebrum are susceptible to BTV infection and undergo necrotizing cytolysis.[225] Fetal lambs infected between days 55 and 60 develop hydranencephaly and retinal dysplasia (blindness), while infections at days 70 to 80 result in porencephaly and cerebral cysts without ocular defects. Other congenital lesions in affected fetuses include brachygnathia and arthrogryposis. After day 100 of gestation, fetuses may develop meningoencephalitis without destructive lesions.[231]

Cache Valley Virus. Cache Valley virus (CVV) is a member of viral family *Bunyaviridae* that is endemic in North America, and subtypes of CVV have been detected in Central and South America.[232,233] Transmission of CVV is by arthropods, especially mosquitoes, in which the virus replicates and persists. White-tailed deer are believed to be an amplification and reservoir host for CVV.[234] Infection of ruminants with CVV is common and widespread in North America, as evidenced by high seroprevalence rates.[235] The presence of antibodies in mammalian hosts is correlated with the distribution of mosquito vectors, and infections are most common in late summer and fall. Seropositive animals and their fetuses are protected from clinical disease, but fetuses of seronegative sheep are commonly affected by congenital abnormalities.[233] Seronegative status is common in animals that live either in areas previously unaffected by infected mosquitoes or in areas in which vector populations have been diminished by repeated years of drought and winter frosts.[233] In warm and wet years when mosquitoes thrive, infection of seronegative ewes may result in transplacental infection of fetuses. While infections between 27 and 35 days of gestation result in fetal mortality, fetuses infected between 36 and 45 days of gestation may develop hydranencephaly, skeletal muscle abnormalities, arthrogryposis, hydrocephalus, microcephalus, porencephaly, cerebellar hypoplasia, and deformities of the spinal cord. Older fetuses are protected from congenital abnormalities and may seroconvert.[236,237]

Pestiviral Infections. Border disease virus and bovine viral diarrhea virus are members of the genus *Pestivirus*, family *Flaviviridae*, and both infect sheep and goats, and several species of cervids.[238–240] Pestiviral infections in nonpregnant, postnatal animals are often mild, but infection of susceptible pregnant small ruminants may result in substantial clinical disease. In addition to pregnancy loss by fetal resorption or abortion, transplacental infection of the developing fetus may result in the birth of stillborn fetuses, congenital anomalies, or birth of persistently infected offspring. Persistent infections occur when fetuses are infected before development of immunocompetence and have been reported in sheep and goats as well as captive and free-ranging deer, including white-tailed deer, mule deer, Lesser Malayan mouse deer, and pudú[241,242] In congenitally infected fetuses, CNS malformations may include cerebellar hypoplasia, hydranencephaly, hydrocephalus, microencephaly, and ocular lesions, such as bilateral microphthalmia and cataracts. Affected neonates may be bright and alert but have typical cerebellar deficits (intention tremors, ataxia, limb tremors, and inability to stand) that worsen when attempting to nurse. In addition, fleece or hair coat changes and brachygnathia may be apparent.

Schmallenberg Virus. Schmallenberg virus (SBV) is a member of viral family *Bunyaviridae* and emerged in Northwestern Europe in 2011. Since the first description in Germany, SBV has spread widely within and beyond Europe.[243] Transmission of SBV occurs by different midges of the genus *Culicoides*. Originally recognized as a disease of cattle, infection with SBV has been documented in various domestic and free-ranging ruminant species, either by virus identification or seroconversion.[243] In nonpregnant adult ruminants infected with SBV, clinical signs are typically absent or mild and can include fever, reduced milk production, reduced fertility, and diarrhea.[244,245] Among small ruminants, goats appear to be less susceptible to SBV infection than sheep.[246] Infection of pregnant ruminants may result in fetal infection, and the outcome of infection depends on gestational age.[247] In polytocous species, normal and abnormal fetuses may be born to the same dam, and the extent of fetal malformation varies among affected animals. Congenital defects in affected fetuses include arthrogryposis, torticollis, scoliosis, and other skeletal malformations. CNS malformations include porencephaly, hydranencephaly, cerebellar dysplasia, and dysplasia of the brainstem and spinal cord.[247,248] Fetuses surviving SBV infection may be weak, may have neurologic disease, or may appear normal at birth.

Heritable Diseases and Plants Associated With Neurologic Disorders

Table 13.4 summarizes the features of heritable diseases of sheep and goats that have significant neurologic manifestation. Plants associated with neurologic disease are listed in Table 13.5.

TABLE 13.4 Congenital and Perinatal Neurologic Diseases of Sheep and Goats With Heritable Etiology.

Condition	Breeds	Inheritance	Clinical Findings	Additional Information	Reference(s)
Cerebellar abiotrophy	*Sheep*: Charollais, Merino, Wiltshire	Suspected autosomal recessive	Cerebellar dysfunction in lambs beginning at 1 to 4 months of age, tremors, equilibrium disturbances	Severe loss of cerebellar Purkinje cells, proliferation of Bergmann glial cells	16–18
Cerebellar cortical atrophy (daft lamb disease 1)	*Sheep*: Corriedale, Drysdale, Welsh Mountain	Suspected autosomal recessive	Weak lambs, inability to stand, wide-based stance	Severe loss of cerebellar Purkinje cells, cell loss, and gliosis of the granular layer	17, 19
Star-gazing lambs (daft lamb disease 2)	*Sheep*: Border Leicester, Coopworth	Suspected autosomal recessive	Clinically similar to cerebellar cortical atrophy: newborn lambs with dorsal arching of the neck	No loss of Purkinje cells or reactive changes, histopathologic changes in neck muscles and nerves	20, 21
Dandy-Walker syndrome	*Sheep*: Suffolk	Probably autosomal recessive	Usually stillborn with enlarged domed skull; dystocia common	Hydrocephalus, agenesis or hypoplasia of cerebellar vermis	22
GM_1 gangliosidosis (lysosomal beta-D-galactosidase deficiency)	*Sheep*: "Coopworth Romney," Suffolk, Suffolk crosses	Autosomal recessive	Normal at birth; at 4–6 months: rapidly progressive ataxia, recumbency, blindness	Evidence of intraneuronal lipid storage, deficiency of β-galactosidase in leukocytes	23
Holoprosencephaly	*Sheep*: Border Leicester	Autosomal recessive	Facial abnormalities, inability to stand, depression, blindness	Lack of longitudinal cerebral fissure, fusion of cerebral hemispheres, and single lateral ventricle	24
Mucopolysaccharidosis IIID (lysosomal *N*-acetylglucosamine 6-sulfatase deficiency)	*Goats*: Nubian	Autosomal recessive	Neurologic deficiencies at birth, clinical sign of cerebral disease	Accumulation of lysosomal heparan sulfate glycosaminoglycan in central nervous system and other organs, leading to cytoplasmic vacuolation	25, 26
Neuraxonal dystrophy	*Sheep*: Coopworth, Merino, Perendale, Romney, South Suffolk	Likely autosomal recessive	Onset of sign varies by breed, progressive ataxia, recumbency, cerebellar signs	Spheroidal swellings of axons in spinal cord and peripheral nerves	17, 27
Neuronal ceroidlipofuscinosis	*Sheep*: Rambouillet, South Hampshire	Autosomal recessive	Progressive signs from 7–10 months of age, blindness, circling, proprioceptive deficits, reduced cognition	Accumulation of lysosomal ceroidlipofuscin in neurons of the brain, spinal cord, eye, and dorsal root ganglia	28, 29
Spina bifida	*Sheep*: Icelandic sheep	Autosomal recessive	Paralysis of hindlimbs, arthrogryposis, tail defect hairless slit in lumbar area	Failure of closure of dorsal arches of lumbar and sacral vertebrae	30, 31

TABLE 13.4 **Congenital and Perinatal Neurologic Diseases of Sheep and Goats With Heritable Etiology.—Cont'd**

Condition	Breeds	Inheritance	Clinical Findings	Additional Information	Reference(s)
Spongiform leukoencephalopathy	*Sheep*: Romney	Suspected hereditary	Posterior paralysis in 2- to 3-month-old lambs developing to flaccid paralysis	*Diagnosis*: histopathologic evidence of spongy vacuolation of brain and spinal cord	32
Thalamic cerebellar neuropathy	*Sheep*: Merino	Suspected hereditary	Onset at 2 years or older, clinical signs of cerebellar and spinal cord dysfunction, ataxia, tremors, hypermetria	Swelling and degeneration of neurons in cerebellum, thalamus, and spinal cord	33
β-Mannosidosis (lysosomal β-mannosidase deficiency)	*Goats*: Nubian	Autosomal recessive	Recumbency and inability to stand in neonates, carpal contraction, hindlimb extension, excessive gingival tissue, thickened skin, intention tremors, deafness, nystagmus, domed head	Vacuolation and demyelinization of neurons, increases in urine mannose and *N*-acetylglucosamine, reduced β-mannosidase in plasma in homozygotes and heterozygotes	1, 34

TABLE 13.5 **Plants Associated With Neurologic Diseases.[a]**

Disease Category	Plant	Clinical Signs and Symptoms
Paralysis	*Astragalus, Oxytropis*—locoweed	Emaciation, proprioceptive deficits, staggering, paralysis
	Delphinium—larkspur	Rapid onset, "nervous" behavior, muscle twitching, paralysis, death
Seizures or central nervous system stimulation	*Apocynum*—Indian hemp	Convulsions, weakness, coma
	Asclepias—milkweed	Convulsions, coma, death
	Cicuta—water hemlock	Rapid onset, extremely toxic, convulsions, muscle spasms, grinding teeth, coma, death
	Conium—poison hemlock	Trembling, incoordination, respiratory paralysis
	Corydalis—fitweed	Rapid onset, ataxia, seizures, twitching facial muscles, chewing movements
	Delphinium—larkspur	Excitability, staggering, vomiting, convulsions
	Lupinus—lupines	Nervousness, convulsions, coma
Central nervous system stimulation and depression or mixed central nervous effects	*Aesculus*—buckeye, horse chestnut	Vomiting, ataxia, trembling, convulsions, hyperesthesia excitement, or depression
	Datura—jimson weed	Ataxia, tremors, hallucinations, mydriasis, tachycardia, tachypnea
	Eupatorium—white snakeroot	Trembling in the muzzle and legs after exercise, weakness, difficulty breathing
	Haplopappus—rayless goldenrod	Depression, stiff gait, trembling, weakness, recumbency, coma, death
	Kalmia, Rhododendron—mountain laurel, rhododendron, azaleas	Convulsions, vomiting, weakness, paralysis, death
	Leucothoe—fetterbush	Incoordination, vomiting, weakness, spasm, coma, death
	Lupinus—lupines	Nervousness, depression, twitching, convulsions, death
	Ricinus—castor bean	Diarrhea, dullness, weakness, trembling, incoordination
	Solanaceae—ground cherry, nightshade, horsenettle, soda apple	Depression, mydriasis, bradycardia, incoordination
	Veratrum—false hellebore	Vomiting, arrhythmias, weakness, convulsions, coma
	Zigadenus—death camas	Weakness, staggering, convulsions, coma, excess salivation

Continued

TABLE 13.5 Plants Associated With Neurologic Diseases.—Cont'd

Disease Category	Plant	Clinical Signs and Symptoms
Depression or weakness	Halogeton	Rapid and shallow breathing, coma
	Helenium—sneezeweed, bitterweed	Depression, weakness, chronic vomiting
	Hymenoxys—rubberweed	Depression, weakness, bloat, green nasal discharge
	Oxytenia—copperweed	Depression, weakness, coma
	Sarcobatus—greasewood	Dullness, nasal discharge, drooling, weakness
	Tetradymia—horsebrush	Depression, weakness, swelling around head, peeling skin

[a]Cyanogenetic plants such as *Triglochin* (arrowgrass) and *Prunus* (wild cherry), as well as plants that contain nitrates, may cause signs that mimic neurologic deficits. Treatment of animals that have ingested any of these toxic plants should include oral charcoal (0.5 kg PO) and diazepam (0.25–0.5 mg/kg) to control seizures, maintenance of hydration status, and nutritional support.

References

1. Constable PD: Clinical examination of the ruminant nervous system, *Vet Clin North Am Food Anim Pract* 20(2):185–214, 2004.
2. Mayhew IG: Neurologic evaluation. In Mayhew IG, editor: *Large animal neurology,* Ames, IA, 2009, Blackwell Publishing.
3. Bagley RS: *Fundamentals of veterinary clinical neurology,* Ames, IA, 2005, Blackwell Publishing Professional.
4. Parent J: Clinical examination. In Anderson DE, Rings DM, editors: *Current veterinary therapy: food animal practice,* St. Louis, MO, 2009, Saunders Elsevier, pp 274–278.
5. Francoz D: Ancillary tests. In Anderson DE, Rings DM, editors: *Current veterinary therapy: food animal practice,* St. Louis, MO, 2009, Saunders Elsevier, pp 279–283.
6. Scott PR: Diagnostic techniques and clinicopathologic findings in ruminant neurologic disease, *Vet Clin North Am Food Anim Pract* 20(2):215–230, v, 2004.
7. Fecteau G, George LW: Bacterial meningitis and encephalitis in ruminants, *Vet Clin North Am Food Anim Pract* 20(2):363–377, vii, 2004.
8. Cohen BS, Belser EH, Killmaster CH, et al: Epizootiology of cranial abscess disease in white-tailed deer (*Odocoileus virginianus*) of Georgia, USA, *J Wildl Dis* 51(3):609–618, 2015.
9. Davidson WR, Nettles VF, Hayes LE, Howerth EW, Couvillion CE: Epidemiologic features of an intracranial abscessation/suppurative meningoencephalitis complex in white-tailed deer, *J Wildl Dis* 26(4):460–467, 1990.
10. Schumacher VL, Hinckley L, Liao X, Tulman E, Geary SJ, Smyth JA: Meningitis caused by *Mycoplasma mycoides* subspecies capri in a goat, *J Vet Diagn Invest* 23(3):565–569, 2011.
11. Bowen RA: Meningitis (suppurative meningitis). In Smith BP, editor: *Large animal internal medicine: diseases of horses, cattle, sheep, and goats,* ed 3, St. Louis, MO, 2002, Mosby Inc., pp 896–900.
12. Fecteau G, Smith BP, George LW: Septicemia and meningitis in the newborn calf, *Vet Clin North Am Food Anim Pract* 25(1):195–208, vii–viii, 2009.
13. Scala C, Duffard N, Beauchamp G, Boullier S, Locatelli Y: Antibody response to epsilon toxin of *Clostridium perfringens* in captive red deer (*Cervus elaphus*) over a 13-month period, *J Zoo Wildl Med* 47(1):38–44, 2016.
14. Shatursky O, Bayles R, Rogers M, Jost BH, Songer JG, Tweten RK: *Clostridium perfringens* beta-toxin forms potential-dependent, cation-selective channels in lipid bilayers, *Infect Immun* 68(10): 5546–5551, 2000.
15. Scholes SF, Welchman Dde B, Hutchinson JP, Edwards GT, Mitchell ES: *Clostridium perfringens* type D enterotoxaemia in neonatal lambs, *Vet Rec* 160(23):811–812, 2007.
16. Watson PJ, Scholes SF: *Clostridium perfringens* type D epsilon intoxication in one-day-old calves, *Vet Rec* 164(26):816–817, 2009.
17. Songer JG: Clostridial enteric diseases of domestic animals, *Clin Microbiol Rev* 9(2):216–234, 1996.
18. Rings DM: Clostridial disease associated with neurologic signs: tetanus, botulism, and enterotoxemia, *Vet Clin North Am Food Anim Pract* 20(2):379–391, vii–viii, 2004.
19. Biescas E, Preziuso S, Bulgin M, DeMartini JC: Ovine lentivirus-associated leucomyelitis in naturally infected North American sheep, *J Comp Pathol* 132(2–3):107–116, 2005.
20. Callan RJ, Van Metre DC: Viral diseases of the ruminant nervous system, *Vet Clin North Am Food Anim Pract* 20(2):327–362, vii, 2004.
21. Highland MA: Small ruminant lentiviruses: strain variation, viral tropism, and host genetics influence pathogenesis, *Vet Pathol* 54(3):353–354, 2017.
22. Radostits OM, Gay CC, Hinchcliff KW, Constable PD: 22. Diseases associated with viruses and chlamydia–II. In Radostits OM, Gay CC, Hinchcliff KW, Constable PD, editors: *Veterinary medicine. A textbook of the diseases of cattle, horses, sheep, pigs and goats,* ed 10, St. Louis, MO, 2007, Saunders Elsevier, pp 1307–1438.
23. Benavides J, Garcia-Pariente C, Ferreras MC, Fuertes M, Garcia-Marin JF, Perez V: Diagnosis of clinical cases of the nervous form of Maedi-Visna in 4- and 6-month-old lambs, *Vet J* 174(3):655–658, 2007.
24. de Andres D, Klein D, Watt NJ, et al: Diagnostic tests for small ruminant lentiviruses, *Vet Microbiol* 107(1–2):49–62, 2005.
25. Reina R, Berriatua E, Lujan L, et al: Prevention strategies against small ruminant lentiviruses: an update, *Vet J* 182(1):31–37, 2009.
26. Trujillo AJ, Castro N, Quevedo JM, Arguello A, Capote J, Guamis B: Effect of heat and high-pressure treatments on microbiological quality and immunoglobulin G stability of caprine colostrum, *J Dairy Sci* 90(2):833–839, 2007.
27. Grard G, Moureau G, Charrel RN, et al: Genetic characterization of tick-borne flaviviruses: new insights into evolution, pathogenetic determinants and taxonomy, *Virology* 361(1):80–92, 2007.
28. Laurenson MK, Norman R, Reid HW, Pow I, Newborn D, Hudson PJ: The role of lambs in louping-ill virus amplification, *Parasitology* 120(Pt 2):97–104, 2000.
29. Doherty PP, Smith W, Reid HW: Louping-ill encephalomyelitis in the sheep. V. Histopathogenesis of the fatal disease, *J Comp Pathol* 82(3):337–344, 1972.
30. Reid HW, Doherty PC: Experimental louping-ill in sheep and lambs. I. Viraemia and the antibody response, *J Comp Pathol* 81(2):291–298, 1971.
31. Davidson MM, Williams H, Macleod JA: Louping ill in man: a forgotten disease, *J Infect* 23(3):241–249, 1991.

32. Laurenson MK, McKendrick IJ, Reid HW, Challenor R, Mathewson GK: Prevalence, spatial distribution and the effect of control measures on louping-ill virus in the Forest of Bowland, Lancashire, *Epidemiol Infect* 135(6):963–973, 2007.
33. Cebra CK, Cebra ML: Altered mentation caused by polioencephalomalacia, hypernatremia, and lead poisoning, *Vet Clin North Am Food Anim Pract* 20(2):287–302, vi–vii, 2004.
34. Breves G, Hoeller H, Harmeyer J, Martens H: Thiamin balance in the gastrointestinal tract of sheep, *J Anim Sci* 51(5):1177–1181, 1980.
35. Rammell CG, Hill JH: A review of thiamine deficiency and its diagnosis, especially in ruminants, *N Z Vet J* 34(12):202–204, 1986.
36. Ramos JJ, Marca C, Ferrer LM, Loste A, Cebrian LM: Faecal thiaminase, plasma lactate and pyruvate concentrations and erythrocyte transketolase activity changes in apparently normal replacement ewes after the initiation to the pasture, *Res Vet Sci* 80(1):11–16, 2006.
37. Karapinar T, Dabak M, Kizil O, Balikci E: Severe thiamine deficiency in sheep with acute ruminal lactic acidosis, *J Vet Intern Med* 22(3):662–665, 2008.
38. Smits JE, Wobeser G: Polioencephalomalacia in a captive fallow deer, *Can Vet J* 31(4):300–301, 1990.
39. Ramos JJ, Ferrer LM, Garcia L, Fernandez A, Loste A: Polioencephalomalacia in adult sheep grazing pastures with prostrate pigweed, *Can Vet J* 46(1):59–61, 2005.
40. Pritchard D, Eggleston GW, Macadam JF: Nardoo fern and polioencephalomalacia, *Aust Vet J* 54(4):204–205, 1978.
41. Bakker HJ, Dickson J, Steele P, Nottle MC: Experimental induction of ovine polioencephalomalacia, *Vet Rec* 107(20):464–466, 1980.
42. Meyer P: Thiaminase activities and thiamine content of *Pteridium aquilinum, Equisetum ramosissimum, Malva parviflora, Pennisetum clandestinum* and *Medicago sativa, Onderstepoort J Vet Res* 56(2): 145–146, 1989.
43. Spicer EM, Horton BJ: Biochemistry of natural and amprolium-induced polioencephalomalacia in sheep, *Aust Vet J* 57(5):230–235, 1981.
44. Thomas KW, Griffiths FR: Natural establishment of thiaminase activity in the alimentary tract of newborn lambs and effects on thiamine status and growth rates, *Aust Vet J* 64(7):207–210, 1987.
45. Radostits OM, Gay CC, Hinchcliff KW, Constable PD: 36. Specific diseases of uncertain etiology. In Radostits OM, Gay CC, Hinchcliff KW, Constable PD, editors: *Veterinary medicine. A textbook of the diseases of cattle, horses, sheep, pigs and goats,* ed 10, 2007, St. Louis, MO, Saunders Elsevier, pp 1981–2044.
46. Radostits OM, Gay CC, Hinchcliff KW, Constable PD: 12. Diseases of the nervous system. In Radostits OM, Gay CC, Hinchcliff KW, Constable PD, editors: *Veterinary medicine. A textbook of the diseases of cattle, horses, sheep, pigs and goats,* St. Louis, MO, 2007, Saunders Elsevier, pp 575–620.
47. Drewnoski ME, Pogge DJ, Hansen SL: High-sulfur in beef cattle diets: a review, *J Anim Sci* 92(9):3763–3780, 2014.
48. Dorman DC, Moulin FJ, McManus BE, Mahle KC, James RA, Struve MF: Cytochrome oxidase inhibition induced by acute hydrogen sulfide inhalation: correlation with tissue sulfide concentrations in the rat brain, liver, lung, and nasal epithelium, *Toxicol Sci* 65(1): 18–25, 2002.
49. Bulgin MS, Lincoln SD, Mather G: Elemental sulfur toxicosis in a flock of sheep, *J Am Vet Med Assoc* 208(7):1063–1065, 1996.
50. Low JC, Scott PR, Howie F, Lewis M, FitzSimons J, Spence JA: Sulphur-induced polioencephalomalacia in lambs, *Vet Rec* 138(14): 327–329, 1996.
51. Jeffrey M, Duff JP, Higgins RJ, et al: Polioencephalomalacia associated with the ingestion of ammonium sulphate by sheep and cattle, *Vet Rec* 134(14):343–348, 1994.
52. Hoff B, Boermans HJ, Baird JD: Retrospective study of toxic metal analyses requested at a veterinary diagnostic toxicology laboratory in Ontario (1990–1995), *Can Vet J* 39(1):39–43, 1998.
53. Liu ZP: Lead poisoning combined with cadmium in sheep and horses in the vicinity of non-ferrous metal smelters, *Sci Total Environ* 309(1–3):117–126, 2003.
54. Ammerman CB, Miller SM, Fick KR, Hansard SL II: Contaminating elements in mineral supplements and their potential toxicity: a review, *J Anim Sci* 44(3):485–508, 1977.
55. Sharma RM, Buck WB: Effects of chronic lead exposure on pregnant sheep and their progeny, *Veterinary Toxicology* 18(4):186–188, 1976.
56. Castellanos P, del Olmo E, Fernandez-Santos MR, Rodriguez-Estival J, Garde JJ, Mateo R: Increased chromatin fragmentation and reduced acrosome integrity in spermatozoa of red deer from lead polluted sites, *Sci Total Environ* 505:32–38, 2015.
57. Reglero MM, Taggart MA, Castellanos P, Mateo R: Reduced sperm quality in relation to oxidative stress in red deer from a lead mining area, *Environ Pollut* 157(8–9):2209–2215, 2009.
58. Radostits OM, Gay CC, Hinchcliff KW, Constable PD: 32. Diseases associated with inorganic and farm chemicals. In Radostits OM, Gay CC, Hinchcliff KW, Constable PD, editors: *Veterinary medicine. A textbook of the diseases of cattle, horses, sheep, pigs and goats,* ed 10, St. Louis, MO, 2007, Saunders Elsevier, pp 1798–1850.
59. Loneragan GH, Gould DH: Lead poisoning. In Smith BP, editor: *Large animal internal medicine: diseases of horses, cattle, sheep, and goats,* ed 3, St. Louis, MO, 2002, Mosby Inc., pp 932–936.
60. Rolton CE, Horton BJ, Pass DA: Evaluation of tests for the diagnosis of lead exposure in sheep, *Aust Vet J* 54(8):393–397, 1978.
61. Bratton GR, Zmudzki J, Kincaid N, Joyce J: Thiamin as treatment of lead poisoning in ruminants, *Mod Vet Pract* 62(6):441–446, 1981.
62. Maiti SK, Swarup D, Chandra SV: Therapeutic potential of thiamine hydrochloride in experimental chronic lead intoxication in goats, *Res Vet Sci* 48(3):377–378, 1990.
63. Moritz ML, Ayus JC: Preventing neurological complications from dysnatremias in children, *Pediatr Nephrol* 20(12):1687–1700, 2005.
64. Schlipf JW: Pseudorabies (mad itch; Aujeszky's disease). In Smith BP, editor: *Large animal internal medicine: diseases of horses, cattle, sheep, and goats,* St. Louis, MO, 2002, Mosby, pp 887–888.
65. Brown Jr TT: Laboratory evaluation of selected disinfectants as virucidal agents against porcine parvovirus, pseudorabies virus, and transmissible gastroenteritis virus, *Am J Vet Res* 42(6):1033–1036, 1981.
66. Birhane MG, Cleaton JM, Monroe BP, et al: Rabies surveillance in the United States during 2015, *J Am Vet Med Assoc* 250(10): 1117–1130, 2017.
67. Petersen BW, Tack DM, Longenberger A, et al: Rabies in captive deer, Pennsylvania, USA, 2007–2010, *Emerg Infect Dis* 18(1):138–141, 2012.
68. Tack DM, Blanton JD, Holman RC, Longenberger AH, Petersen BW, Rupprecht CE: Evaluation of knowledge, attitudes, and practices of deer owners following identification of a cluster of captive deer with rabies in Pennsylvania in July 2010, *J Am Vet Med Assoc* 242(9):1279–1285, 2013.
69. Tjornehoj K, Fooks AR, Agerholm JS, Ronsholt L: Natural and experimental infection of sheep with European bat lyssavirus type-1 of Danish bat origin, *J Comp Pathol* 134(2–3):190–201, 2006.
70. Brookes SM, Klopfleisch R, Muller T, et al: Susceptibility of sheep to European bat lyssavirus type-1 and -2 infection: a clinical pathogenesis study, *Vet Microbiol* 125(3–4):210–223, 2007.
71. Jackson AC: Update on rabies, *Curr Opin Neurol* 15(3):327–331, 2002.
72. Zhu Y, Zhang G, Shao M, Lei Y, Jiang Y, Tu C: An outbreak of sheep rabies in Shanxi province, China, *Epidemiol Infect* 139(10): 1453–1456, 2011.
73. Bowen RA: Rabies. In Smith BP, editor: *Large animal internal medicine: diseases of horses, cattle, sheep, and goats,* St. Louis, MO, 2002, Mosby, pp 892–895.
74. Prosperi S, Poglayen G, Irsara A: Rabies vaccination trial in wild ruminants, *Vet Res Commun* 4(4):283–285, 1981.

75. Sihvonen L, Kulonen K, Soveri T, Nieminen M: Rabies antibody titres in vaccinated reindeer, *Acta Vet Scand* 34(2):199–202, 1993.
76. Dagleish MP, Martin S, Steele P, et al: Susceptibility of European red deer (*Cervus elaphus elaphus*) to alimentary challenge with bovine spongiform encephalopathy, *PLoS One* 10(1):e0116094, 2015.
77. Foster JD, Hope J, Fraser H: Transmission of bovine spongiform encephalopathy to sheep and goats, *Vet Rec* 133(14):339–341, 1993.
78. Vaccari G, Panagiotidis CH, Acin C, et al: State-of-the-art review of goat TSE in the European Union, with special emphasis on PRNP genetics and epidemiology, *Vet Res* 40(5):48, 2009.
79. Eloit M, Adjou K, Coulpier M, et al: BSE agent signatures in a goat, *Vet Rec* 156(16):523–524, 2005.
80. Jeffrey M, Martin S, Gonzalez L, et al: Immunohistochemical features of PrP(d) accumulation in natural and experimental goat transmissible spongiform encephalopathies, *J Comp Pathol* 134(2–3): 171–181, 2006.
81. Morignat E, Cazeau G, Biacabe AG, et al: Estimates of the prevalence of transmissible spongiform encephalopathies in sheep and goats in France in 2002, *Vet Rec* 158(20):683–687, 2006.
82. Gubbins S, McIntyre KM: Prevalence of sheep infected with classical scrapie in Great Britain, 1993–2007, *Epidemiol Infect* 137(6): 787–791, 2009.
83. Gubbins S: Prevalence of sheep infected with classical scrapie in Great Britain: integrating multiple sources of surveillance data for 2002, *J R Soc Interface* 5(28):1343–1351, 2008.
84. APHIS Veterinary Services: Scrapie, 2004. Accessed September 2, 2009.
85. Bastian FO, Sanders DE, Forbes WA, et al: *Spiroplasma* spp. from transmissible spongiform encephalopathy brains or ticks induce spongiform encephalopathy in ruminants, *J Med Microbiol* 56(Pt 9): 1235–1242, 2007.
86. Manuelidis L, Yu ZX, Barquero N, Mullins B: Cells infected with scrapie and Creutzfeldt-Jakob disease agents produce intracellular 25-nm virus-like particles, *Proc Natl Acad Sci U S A* 104(6): 1965–1970, 2007.
87. Tyler JW, Middleton JR: Transmissible spongiform encephalopathies in ruminants, *Vet Clin North Am Food Anim Pract* 20(2):303–326, vii, 2004.
88. van Keulen LJ, Bossers A, van Zijderveld F: TSE pathogenesis in cattle and sheep, *Vet Res* 39(4):24, 2008.
89. Hamir AN, Kunkle RA, Greenlee JJ, Richt JA: Experimental oral transmission of United States origin scrapie to neonatal sheep, *J Vet Diagn Invest* 21(1):64–68, 2009.
90. Goldmann W: PrP genetics in ruminant transmissible spongiform encephalopathies, *Vet Res* 39(4):30, 2008.
91. Colussi S, Vaccari G, Maurella C, et al: Histidine at codon 154 of the prion protein gene is a risk factor for Nor98 scrapie in goats, *J Gen Virol* 89(Pt 12):3173–3176, 2008.
92. Radostits OM, Gay CC, Hinchcliff KW, Constable PD: 23. Diseases associated with prions. In Radostits OM, Gay CC, Hinchcliff KW, Constable PD, editors: *Veterinary medicine. A textbook of the diseases of cattle, horses, sheep, pigs and goats,* ed 10, St. Louis, MO, 2007, Saunders Elsevier, pp 1439–1454.
93. Greenlee JJ, Greenlee MHW: The transmissible spongiform encephalopathies of livestock, *Ilar J* 56(1):7–25, 2015.
94. Gavier-Widen D, Stack MJ, Baron T, Balachandran A, Simmons M: Diagnosis of transmissible spongiform encephalopathies in animals: a review, *J Vet Diagn Invest* 17(6):509–527, 2005.
95. Gonzalez L, Dagleish MP, Martin S, et al: Diagnosis of preclinical scrapie in live sheep by the immunohistochemical examination of rectal biopsies, *Vet Rec* 162(13):397–403, 2008.
96. Dawson M, Moore RC, Bishop SC: Progress and limits of PrP gene selection policy, *Vet Res* 39(4):25, 2008.
97. Williams ES, Young S: Chronic wasting disease of captive mule deer: a spongiform encephalopathy, *J Wildl Dis* 16(1):89–98, 1980.
98. Baeten LA, Powers BE, Jewell JE, Spraker TR, Miller MW: A natural case of chronic wasting disease in a free-ranging moose (*Alces alces shirasi*), *J Wildl Dis* 43(2):309–314, 2007.
99. Miller MW, Williams ES: Chronic wasting disease of cervids, *Curr Top Microbiol Immunol* 284:193–214, 2004.
100. Anonymous: Map—chronic wasting disease in North America, 2018. Available at: http://cwd-info.org/map-chronic-wasting-disease-in-north-america/. Accessed Mar 21, 2018.
101. Benestad SL, Mitchell G, Simmons M, Ytrehus B, Vikoren T: First case of chronic wasting disease in Europe in a Norwegian free-ranging reindeer, *Vet Res* 47(1):88, 2016.
102. Kim TY, Shon HJ, Joo YS, Mun UK, Kang KS, Lee YS: Additional cases of chronic wasting disease in imported deer in Korea, *J Vet Med Sci* 67(8):753–759, 2005.
103. Miller MW, Conner MM: Epidemiology of chronic wasting disease in free-ranging mule deer: spatial, temporal, and demographic influences on observed prevalence patterns, *J Wildl Dis* 41(2):275–290, 2005.
104. Haley NJ, Hoover EA: Chronic wasting disease of cervids: current knowledge and future perspectives, *Annu Rev Anim Biosci* 3: 305–325, 2015.
105. Miller MW, Williams ES: Prion disease: horizontal prion transmission in mule deer, *Nature* 425(6953):35–36, 2003.
106. Miller MW, Williams ES, Hobbs NT, Wolfe LL: Environmental sources of prion transmission in mule deer, *Emerg Infect Dis* 10(6):1003–1006, 2004.
107. Saunders SE, Bartelt-Hunt SL, Bartz JC: Occurrence, transmission, and zoonotic potential of chronic wasting disease, *Emerg Infect Dis* 18(3):369–376, 2012.
108. Wyckoff AC, Kane S, Lockwood K, et al: Clay components in soil dictate environmental stability and bioavailability of cervid prions in mice, *Front Microbiol* 7:1885, 2016.
109. Hoover CE, Davenport KA, Henderson DM, et al: Pathways of prion spread during early chronic wasting disease in deer, *J Virol* 91:10, 2017.
110. Robinson SJ, Samuel MD, O'Rourke KI, Johnson CJ: The role of genetics in chronic wasting disease of North American cervids, *Prion* 6(2):153–162, 2012.
111. Edmunds DR, Kauffman MJ, Schumaker BA, et al: Chronic wasting disease drives population decline of white-tailed deer, *PLoS One* 11(8):e0161127, 2016.
112. Robinson SJ, Samuel MD, Johnson CJ, Adams M, McKenzie DI: Emerging prion disease drives host selection in a wildlife population, *Ecol Appl* 22(3):1050–1059, 2012.
113. Johnson CJ, Herbst A, Duque-Velasquez C, et al: Prion protein polymorphisms affect chronic wasting disease progression, *PLoS One* 6(3):e17450, 2011.
114. O'Rourke KI, Spraker TR, Zhuang D, Greenlee JJ, Gidlewski TE, Hamir AN: Elk with a long incubation prion disease phenotype have a unique PrPd profile, *Neuroreport* 18(18):1935–1938, 2007.
115. Krumm CE, Conner MM, Miller MW: Relative vulnerability of chronic wasting disease infected mule deer to vehicle collisions, *J Wildl Dis* 41(3):503–511, 2005.
116. Miller MW, Swanson HM, Wolfe LL, et al: Lions and prions and deer demise, *PLoS One* 3(12):e4019, 2008.
117. Haley NJ, Richt JA: Evolution of diagnostic tests for chronic wasting disease, a naturally occurring prion disease of cervids, *Pathogens* 6(3):E35, 2017.
118. Uehlinger FD, Johnston AC, Bollinger TK, Waldner CL: Systematic review of management strategies to control chronic wasting disease in wild deer populations in North America, *BMC Vet Res* 12(1):173, 2016.
119. Ortolani EL, Mori CS, Rodrigues Filho JA: Ammonia toxicity from urea in a Brazilian dairy goat flock, *Vet Hum Toxicol* 42(2): 87–89, 2000.
120. Campagnolo ER, Kasten S, Banerjee M: Accidental ammonia exposure to county fair show livestock due to contaminated drinking water, *Vet Hum Toxicol* 44(5):282–285, 2002.
121. Ertell KG: *A review of toxicity and use and handling considerations for guanidine, guanidine hydrochloride, and urea.* Pacific Northwest National Laboratory (PNNL), Richland, WA, 2006.

122. Radostits OM, Gay CC, Hinchcliff KW, Constable PD: 32. Diseases associated with farm chemicals. In Radostits OM, Gay CC, Hinchcliff KW, Constable PD, editors: *Veterinary medicine. A textbook of the diseases of cattle, horses, sheep, pigs and goats,* ed 10, St. Louis, MO, 2007, Saunders Elsevier, pp 1798–1850.
123. Edjtehadi M, Szabuniewicz M, Emmanuel B: Acute urea toxicity in sheep, *Can J Comp Med* 42(1):63–68, 1978.
124. Roy A, Tiwari SP, Kumari K, Gendley MK, Gupta R: Subchronic toxicity study of urea molasses mineral block in kids, *Vet Res Commun* 33(2):183–190, 2009.
125. Filipe AR, de Andrade HR: Arboviruses in the Iberian Peninsula, *Acta Virol* 34(6):582–591, 1990.
126. Ozkul A, Yildirim Y, Pinar D, Akcali A, Yilmaz V, Colak D: Serological evidence of West Nile virus (WNV) in mammalian species in Turkey, *Epidemiol Infect* 134(4):826–829, 2006.
127. Kecskemeti S, Bajmocy E, Bacsadi A, Kiss I, Bakonyi T: Encephalitis due to West Nile virus in a sheep, *Vet Rec* 161(16):568–569, 2007.
128. Yaeger M, Yoon KJ, Schwartz K, Berkland L: West Nile virus meningoencephalitis in a Suri alpaca and Suffolk ewe, *J Vet Diagn Invest* 16(1):64–66, 2004.
129. Root JJ: West Nile virus associations in wild mammals: a synthesis, *Arch Virol* 158(4):735–752, 2013.
130. Tyler JW, Turnquist SE, David AT, Kleiboeker SB, Middleton JR: West Nile virus encephalomyelitis in a sheep, *J Vet Intern Med* 17(2):242–244, 2003.
131. Palmer MV, Stoffregen WC, Rogers DG, et al: West Nile virus infection in reindeer (*Rangifer tarandus*), *J Vet Diagn Invest* 16(3):219–222, 2004.
132. Miller DL, Radi ZA, Baldwin C, Ingram D: Fatal West Nile virus infection in a white-tailed deer (*Odocoileus virginianus*), *J Wildl Dis* 41(1):246–249, 2005.
133. Palmer MV, Waters WR, Pedersen DD, Stoffregen WC: Induction of neutralizing antibodies in reindeer *(Rangifer tarandus)* after administration of a killed West Nile virus vaccine, *J Wildl Dis* 40(4):759–762, 2004.
134. Cheeke PR: Endogenous toxins and mycotoxins in forage grasses and their effects on livestock, *J Anim Sci* 73(3):909–918, 1995.
135. Galloway JH: Grass seed nematode poisoning in livestock, *J Am Vet Med Assoc* 139:1212–1214, 1961.
136. Scarratt WK: Cerebellar disease and disease characterized by dysmetria or tremors, *Vet Clin North Am Food Anim Pract* 20(2): 275–286, vi, 2004.
137. Uhlig S, Botha CJ, Vralstad T, Rolen E, Miles CO: Indole-diterpenes and ergot alkaloids in *Cynodon dactylon* (Bermuda grass) infected with *Claviceps cynodontis* from an outbreak of tremors in cattle, *J Agric Food Chem* 57(23):11112–11119, 2009.
138. Bourke CA, Carrigan MJ, Dixon RJ: The pathogenesis of the nervous syndrome of *Phalaris aquatica* toxicity in sheep, *Aust Vet J* 67(10):356–358, 1990.
139. George LW: Grass staggers. In Smith BP, editor: *Large animal internal medicine: diseases of horses, cattle, sheep, and goats,* St. Louis, MO, 2002, Mosby, pp 966–970.
140. Simpson BH, Jolly RD, Thomas SH: *Phalaris arundinacea* as a cause of deaths and incoordination in sheep, *N Z Vet J* 17(12): 240–244, 1969.
141. Tor-Agbidye J, Blythe LL, Craig AM: Correlation of endophyte toxins (ergovaline and lolitrem B) with clinical disease: fescue foot and perennial ryegrass staggers, *Vet Hum Toxicol* 43(3):140–146, 2001.
142. Brooks HV, Cahill JJ: The susceptibility of Canadian wapiti to ryegrass staggers, *New Zeal Vet J* 33(8):126–126, 1985.
143. Mitchell PJ, McCaughan CJ: Perennial ryegrass staggers in fallow deer (*Dama dama*), *Aust Vet J* 69(10):258–259, 1992.
144. Morin DE: Brainstem and cranial nerve abnormalities: listeriosis, otitis media/interna, and pituitary abscess syndrome, *Vet Clin North Am Food Anim Pract* 20(2):243–273, vi, 2004.
145. Walker JK, Morgan JH: Ovine ophthalmitis associated with *Listeria monocytogenes*, *Vet Rec* 132(25):636, 1993.
146. Weindl L, Frank E, Ullrich U, et al: *Listeria monocytogenes* in different specimens from healthy red deer and wild boars, *Foodborne Pathog Dis* 13(7):391–397, 2016.
147. Sanders BD, Wiedmann M: Ecology of *Listeria* species and *Listeria monocytogenes* in the natural environment. In Ryser ET, Marth EH, editors: *Listeria, listeriosis, and food safety,* ed 3, Boca Raton, FL, 2007, CRC Press, pp 21–54.
148. Johnson GC, Maddox CW, Fales WH, et al: Epidemiologic evaluation of encephalitic listeriosis in goats, *J Am Vet Med Assoc* 208(10):1695–1699, 1996.
149. Nightingale KK, Fortes ED, Ho AJ, Schukken YH, Grohn YT, Wiedmann M: Evaluation of farm management practices as risk factors for clinical listeriosis and fecal shedding of *Listeria monocytogenes* in ruminants, *J Am Vet Med Assoc* 227(11):1808–1814, 2005.
150. Eriksen L, Larsen HE, Christiansen T, Jensen MM, Eriksen E: An outbreak of meningo-encephalitis in fallow deer caused by *Listeria monocytogenes*, *Vet Rec* 122(12):274–276, 1988.
151. Oevermann A, Di Palma S, Doherr MG, Abril C, Zurbriggen A, Vandevelde M: Neuropathogenesis of naturally occurring encephalitis caused by *Listeria monocytogenes* in ruminants, *Brain Pathol* 20(2):378–390, 2010.
152. Otter A, Blakemore WF: Observation on the presence of *Listeria monocytogenes* in axons, *Acta Microbiol Hung* 36(2–3):125–131, 1989.
153. Seaman JT, Carter GI, Carrigan MJ, Cockram FA: An outbreak of listerial myelitis in sheep, *Aust Vet J* 67(4):142–143, 1990.
154. Vazquez-Boland JA, Dominguez L, Blanco M, et al: Epidemiologic investigation of a silage-associated epizootic of ovine listeric encephalitis, using a new Listeria-selective enumeration medium and phage typing, *Am J Vet Res* 53(3):368–371, 1992.
155. Braun U, Stehle C, Ehrensperger F: Clinical findings and treatment of listeriosis in 67 sheep and goats, *Vet Rec* 150(2):38–42, 2002.
156. Peters M, Pohlenz J, Jaton K, Ninet B, Bille J: Studies of the detection of Listeria monocytogenes by culture and PCR in cerebrospinal fluid samples from ruminants with listeric encephalitis, *Zentralbl Veterinarmed B* 42(2):84–88, 1995.
157. Loeb E: Encephalitic listeriosis in ruminants: immunohistochemistry as a diagnostic tool, *J Vet Med A Physiol Pathol Clin Med* 51(9–10):453–455, 2004.
158. Krawczyk-Balska A, Markiewicz Z: The intrinsic cephalosporin resistome of *Listeria monocytogenes* in the context of stress response, gene regulation, pathogenesis and therapeutics, *J Appl Microbiol* 120(2):251–265, 2016.
159. Macleod NS, Wiener G, Barlow RM: Factors involved in middle ear infection (otitis media) in lambs, *Vet Rec* 91(15):360–361, 1972.
160. Jensen R, Pierson RE, Weibel JL, Tucker JO, Swift BL: Middle ear infection in feedlot lambs, *J Am Vet Med Assoc* 181(8):805–807, 1982.
161. Davies IH, Done SH: Necrotic dermatitis and otitis media associated with *Pseudomonas aeruginosa* in sheep following dipping, *Vet Rec* 132(18):460–461, 1993.
162. Tardy F, Mercier P, Solsona M, Saras E, Poumarat F: *Mycoplasma mycoides* subsp. *mycoides* biotype large colony isolates from healthy and diseased goats: prevalence and typing, *Vet Microbiol* 121(3–4): 268–277, 2007.
163. Gil MC, Hermoso De Mendoza M, Rey J, Alonso JM, Poveda JB, Hermoso De Mendoza J: Isolation of mycoplasmas from the external ear canal of goats affected with contagious agalactia, *Vet J* 158(2):152–154, 1999.
164. DaMassa AJ: The ear canal as a culture site for demonstration of mycoplasmas in clinically normal goats, *Aust Vet J* 67(7):267–269, 1990.
165. Jimena ON, Laura JM, Elena MM, Alonso NH, Teresa QM: Association of *Raillietia caprae* with the presence of Mycoplasmas in the external ear canal of goats, *Prev Vet Med* 92(1–2):150–153, 2009.

166. Cottew GS, Yeats FR: Mycoplasmas and mites in the ears of clinically normal goats, *Aust Vet J* 59(3):77–81, 1982.
167. Friel J, Greiner EC: Ear mites from domestic goats in Florida, *Exp Appl Acarol* 4(4):345–351, 1988.
168. Faccini JL, Ribeiro VR: *Raillietia caprae* (Acari: Raillietidae) and *Psoroptes ovis* (Acari: Psoroptidae) in the ears of goats in the state of Rio de Janeiro, Southeast Brazil, *Rev Bras Parasitol Vet* 17(1):59–61, 2008.
169. Williams JF, Williams CS: Psoroptic ear mites in dairy goats, *J Am Vet Med Assoc* 173(12):1582–1583, 1978.
170. Roberts IH, Meleney WP, Pillmore RE: Ear-scab mites, *Psoroptes cuniculi* (Acarina: Psoroptidae), in captive mule deer, *J Parasitol* 56(5):1039–1040, 1970.
171. Rollor EA III, Nettles VF, Davidson WR, Gerrish RR: Otitis media caused by Psoroptes cuniculi in white-tailed deer, *J Am Vet Med Assoc* 173(9):1242–1243, 1978.
172. Schmitt SM, Cooley TM: Psoroptes cuniculi in captive white-tailed deer in Michigan, *J Wildl Dis* 18(3):349–351, 1982.
173. van den Broek AH, Huntley JF: Sheep scab: the disease, pathogenesis and control, *J Comp Pathol* 128(2–3):79–91, 2003.
174. Morgan KL: Parasitic otitis in sheep associated with psoroptes infestation: a clinical and epidemiological study, *Vet Rec* 130(24):530–532, 1992.
175. Koenig JB, Watrous BJ, Kaneps AJ, Adams JG, Parker JE: Otitis media in a llama, *J Am Vet Med Assoc* 218(10):1619–1623, 1582, 2001.
176. George LW: Diseases presenting principally with brainstem and cranial nerve dysfunction. In Smith BP, editor: *Large animal internal medicine: diseases of horses, cattle, sheep, and goats,* St. Louis, MO, 2002, Mosby, pp 946–956.
177. Garris GI, Prullage JB, Prullage JL, Wright FC, Miller JA: Control of Psoroptes cuniculi in captive white-tailed deer with ivermectin-treated corn, *J Wildl Dis* 27(2):254–257, 1991.
178. Chamberlain P, Thomas RJ: An outbreak of botulism in a deer herd in Queensland, *Aust Vet J* 72(11):427–428, 1995.
179. Otter A, Livesey C, Hogg R, Sharpe R, Gray D: Risk of botulism in cattle and sheep arising from contact with broiler litter, *Vet Rec* 159(6):186–187, 2006.
180. van der Lugt JJ, Henton MM, Steyn BG: Type C botulism in sheep associated with the feeding of poultry litter, *J S Afr Vet Assoc* 67(1):3–4, 1996.
181. Radostits OM, Gay CC, Hinchcliff KW, Constable PD: 17. Diseases associated with bacteria—II. In Radostits OM, Gay CC, Hinchcliff KW, Constable PD, editors: *Veterinary medicine. A textbook of the diseases of cattle, horses, sheep, pigs and goats,* ed 10, St. Louis, MO, 2007, Saunders Elsevier, pp 821–846.
182. Nagy DW: *Parelaphostrongylus tenuis* and other parasitic diseases of the ruminant nervous system, *Vet Clin North Am Food Anim Pract* 20(2):393–1412, viii, 2004.
183. Mayhew IG, deLahunta A, Georgi JR, Aspros DG: Naturally occurring cerebrospinal parelaphostronglylosis, *Cornell Vet* 66(1):56–72, 1976.
184. Alden C, Woodson F, Mohan R, Miller S: Cerebrospinal nematodiasis in sheep, *J Am Vet Med Assoc* 166(8):784–786, 1975.
185. Gajadhar AA, Tessaro SV: Susceptibility of mule deer (*Odocoileus hemionus*) and two species of North American molluscs to *Elaphostrongylus cervi* (Nematoda: Metastrongyloidea), *J Parasitol* 81(4):593–596, 1995.
186. Handeland K: Cerebrospinal nematodiasis in a moose in Norway, *J Wildl Dis* 38(4):817–821, 2002.
187. Handeland K, Slettbakk T: Epidemiological aspects of cerebrospinal elaphostrongylosis in small ruminants in northern Norway, *Zentralbl Veterinarmed B* 42(2):110–117, 1995.
188. Pusterla N, Caplazi P, Hertzberg H, Ehrensperger F, Braun U: *Elaphostrongylus cervi* infection in a Swiss goat, *Vet Rec* 148(12):382–383, 2001.
189. El-Azazy OM, Ahmed YF: Patent infection with *Setaria digitata* in goats in Saudi Arabia, *Vet Parasitol* 82(2):161–166, 1999.
190. Shirasaka S, Suzuki M, Endou G, Adachi Y, Taira N: Efficacy of ivermectin against Setaria microfilariae in calves and cerebrospinal setariosis in sheep and goats, *J Vet Med Sci* 56(6):1213–1214, 1994.
191. Bush DL: Lumbar paralysis of ovine species in Japan reportedly caused by *Setaria digitata, J Am Vet Med Assoc* 118(891):388–394, 1951.
192. Kopcha M, Marteniuk JV, Sills R, Steficek B, Schillhorn van Veen TW: Cerebrospinal nematodiasis in a goat herd, *J Am Vet Med Assoc* 194(10):1439–1442, 1989.
193. Divers TJ: Acquired spinal cord and peripheral nerve disease, *Vet Clin North Am Food Anim Pract* 20(2):231–242, v–vi, 2004.
194. Geisel O, Betzl E, Dahme E, Schmahl W, Hermanns W: [Enzootic spinal ataxia in fallow and wild red deer in Upper Bavaria], *Tierarztl Prax Ausg G Grosstiere Nutztiere* 25(6):598–604, 1997.
195. Millar M, Barlow A, Gunning R, Cosser J: Enzootic ataxia in farmed red deer, *Vet Rec* 152(13):408, 2003.
196. Wilson PR, Orr MB, Key EL: Enzootic ataxia in Red deer, *N Z Vet J* 27(11):252–254, 1979.
197. Yoshikawa H, Seo H, Oyamada T, et al: Histopathology of enzootic ataxia in Sika deer (*Cervus nippon* Temminck), *J Vet Med Sci* 58(9):849–854, 1996.
198. Audige L, Wilson PR, Morris RS, Davidson GW: Osteochondrosis, skeletal abnormalities and enzootic ataxia associated with copper deficiency in a farmed red deer (*Cervus elaphus*) herd, *N Z Vet J* 43(2):70–76, 1995.
199. Laven R, Smith S: Copper deficiency in sheep: an assessment of relationship between concentrations of copper in serum and plasma, *N Z Vet J* 56(6):334–338, 2008.
200. Maas J, Smith BP: Copper deficiency in ruminants. In Smith BP, editor: *Large animal internal medicine,* ed 5, St. Louis, MO, 2015, Elsevier Mosby, pp 837–840.
201. Lotti M, Moretto A: Organophosphate-induced delayed polyneuropathy, *Toxicol Rev* 24(1):37–49, 2005.
202. Williams JE, Dade AW, Benne R: Posterior paralysis associated with anthelmintic treatment of sheep, *J Am Vet Med Assoc* 169(12):1307–1309, 1976.
203. Baker J, Ciszewski D, Lowrie C, Mullaney T: Spastic paresis in pygmy goats, *J Vet Int Med* 3(2):113, 1989.
204. Kral E, Hlousek A: Spasticka pareza panevnich koncetin u kozla, *Veterinarstvi* 23:425–426, 1973.
205. Ledoux JM: Bovine spastic paresis: etiological hypotheses, *Med Hypotheses* 57(5):573–579, 2001.
206. De Ley G, De Moor A: Bovine spastic paralysis—results of selective gamma-efferent suppression with dilute procaine, *Vet Sci Commun* 3(4):289–298, 1980.
207. Gygi M, Kathmann I, Konar M, Rottenberg S, Meylan M: [Paraparesis in a dwarf goat: clarification by means of magnetic resonance imaging], *Schweiz Arch Tierheilkd* 146(11):523–528, 2004.
208. Watt NJ, Scott PR: Cervical spine meningioma causing acute-onset quadriplegia in an aged sheep, *Vet Rec* 136(21):543–544, 1995.
209. George LW: Spinal abscesses, spinal tumors. In Smith BP, editor: *Large animal internal medicine: diseases of horses, cattle, sheep, and goats,* St. Louis, MO, 2002, Mosby, pp 982–984.
210. Scott PR, Penny CD, Murray LD: A field study of eight ovine vertebral body abscess cases, *N Z Vet J* 39(3):105–107, 1991.
211. Driemeier D, Schild AL, Fernandes JC, et al: Outbreaks of tetanus in beef cattle and sheep in Brazil associated with disophenol injection, *J Vet Med A Physiol Pathol Clin Med* 54(6):333–335, 2007.
212. Aslani MR, Bazargani TT, Ashkar AA, Movasaghi AR, Raoofi A, Atiabi N: Outbreak of tetanus in lambs, *Vet Rec* 142(19):518–519, 1998.
213. Cook TM, Protheroe RT, Handel JM: Tetanus: a review of the literature, *Br J Anaesth* 87(3):477–487, 2001.
214. Reynolds GE, Griffin JFT: Humoral immunity in the ewe 3. The influence of adjuvants and immunisation regimes on Immune reactivity in the breeding ewe and her progeny, *Vet Immunol Immunopathol* 25(2):167–175, 1990.

215. Radostits OM, Gay CC, Hinchcliff KW, Constable PD: 28. Diseases associated with arthropod parasites. In Radostits OM, Gay CC, Hinchcliff KW, Constable PD, eds. *Veterinary medicine. A textbook of the diseases of cattle, horses, sheep, pigs and goats,* ed 10, St. Louis, MO, 2007, Saunders Elsevier, pp 1585–1612.
216. Shelton GD: Disorders of neuromuscular transmission, *Semin Vet Med Surg (Small Anim)* 4(2):126–132, 1989.
217. Krishnan AV, Lin CS, Reddel SW, McGrath R, Kiernan MC: Conduction block and impaired axonal function in tick paralysis, *Muscle Nerve* 40(3):358–362, 2009.
218. Schofield LN, Saunders JR: An incidental case of tick paralysis in a Holstein calf exposed to *Dermacentor andersoni*, *Can Vet J* 33(3): 190–191, 1992.
219. Washburn KE, Streeter RN: Congenital defects of the ruminant nervous system, *Vet Clin North Am Food Anim Pract* 20(2):413–434, viii, 2004.
220. Graham JM Jr, Edwards MJ, Edwards MJ: Teratogen update: gestational effects of maternal hyperthermia due to febrile illnesses and resultant patterns of defects in humans, *Teratology* 58(5): 209–221, 1998.
221. Mayhew IG: Disorders of behavior and personality (including diffuse CNS disorders). In Mayhew IG, editor: *Large animal neurology: A handbook for veterinary clinicians,* ed 1, Philadelphia, PA, 1989, Lea & Febiger, pp 73–112.
222. Murray MD: Akabane epizootics in New South Wales: evidence for long-distance dispersal of the biting midge *Culicoides brevitarsis*, *Aust Vet J* 64(10):305–308, 1987.
223. Parsonson IM, McPhee DA, Della-Porta AJ, McClure S, McCullagh P: Transmission of Akabane virus from the ewe to the early fetus (32 to 53 days), *J Comp Pathol* 99(2):215–227, 1988.
224. Ruder MG, Lysyk TJ, Stallknecht DE, et al: Transmission and epidemiology of bluetongue and epizootic hemorrhagic disease in North America: current perspectives, research gaps, and future directions, *Vector Borne Zoonotic Dis* 15(6):348–363, 2015.
225. Maclachlan NJ, Drew CP, Darpel KE, Worwa G: The pathology and pathogenesis of bluetongue, *J Comp Pathol* 141(1):1–16, 2009.
226. Anthony SJ, Maan S, Maan N, et al: Genetic and phylogenetic analysis of the outer-coat proteins VP2 and VP5 of epizootic haemorrhagic disease virus (EHDV): comparison of genetic and serological data to characterise the EHDV serogroup, *Virus Res* 145(2):200–210, 2009.
227. Worwa G, Hilbe M, Ehrensperger F, et al: Experimental transplacental infection of sheep with bluetongue virus serotype 8, *Vet Rec* 164(16):499–500, 2009.
228. Flanagan M, Johnson SJ: The effects of vaccination of Merino ewes with an attenuated Australian bluetongue virus serotype 23 at different stages of gestation, *Aust Vet J* 72(12):455–457, 1995.
229. Maclachlan NJ, Osburn BI: Teratogenic bluetongue and related orbivirus infections in pregnant ruminant livestock: timing and pathogen genetics are critical, *Curr Opin Virol* 27:31–35, 2017.
230. van der Sluijs MT, Schroer-Joosten DP, Fid-Fourkour A, et al: Transplacental transmission of Bluetongue virus serotype 1 and serotype 8 in sheep: virological and pathological findings, *PLoS One* 8(12):e81429, 2013.
231. Machen MR, Waldridge BM, Cebra C, et al: Diseases of the neurologic system. In Pugh DG, editor: *Sheep and goat medicine,* ed 1, Philadelphia, PA, 2002, Saunders, pp 277–316.
232. Calisher CH, Sabattini MS, Monath TP, Wolff KL: Cross-neutralization tests among Cache Valley virus isolates revealing the existence of multiple subtypes, *Am J Trop Med Hyg* 39(2):202–205, 1988.
233. de la Concha-Bermejillo A: Cache Valley virus is a cause of fetal malformation and pregnancy loss in sheep, *Small Rumin Res* 49(1):1–9, 2003.
234. Blackmore CG, Grimstad PR: Cache Valley and Potosi viruses (Bunyaviridae) in white-tailed deer (*Odocoileus virginianus*): experimental infections and antibody prevalence in natural populations, *Am J Trop Med Hyg* 59(5):704–709, 1998.
235. Uehlinger FD, Wilkins W, Godson DL, Drebot MA: Seroprevalence of Cache Valley virus and related viruses in sheep and other livestock from Saskatchewan, Canada, *Can Vet J* 59(4):413–418, 2018.
236. Chung SI, Livingston CW Jr, Edwards JF, Gauer BB, Collisson EW: Congenital malformations in sheep resulting from in utero inoculation of Cache Valley virus, *Am J Vet Res* 51(10):1645–1648, 1990.
237. Edwards JF, Livingston CW, Chung SI, Collisson EC: Ovine arthrogryposis and central nervous system malformations associated with in utero Cache Valley virus infection: spontaneous disease, *Vet Pathol* 26(1):33–39, 1989.
238. Nettleton PF, Gilray JA, Russo P, Dlissi E: Border disease of sheep and goats, *Vet Res* 29(3–4):327–340, 1998.
239. Passler T, Riddell KP, Edmondson MA, et al: Experimental infection of pregnant goats with bovine viral diarrhea virus (BVDV) 1 or 2, *Vet Res* 45:38, 2014.
240. Passler T, Walz PH: Bovine viral diarrhea virus infections in heterologous species, *Anim Health Res Rev* 11(2):191–205, 2010.
241. Nelson DD, Duprau JL, Wolff PL, Evermann JF: Persistent bovine viral diarrhea virus infection in domestic and wild small ruminants and camelids including the mountain goat (*Oreamnos americanus*), *Front Microbiol* 6:1415, 2015.
242. Salgado R, Hidalgo-Hermoso E, Pizarro-Lucero J: Detection of persistent pestivirus infection in pudu (*Pudu puda*) in a captive population of artiodactyls in Chile, *BMC Vet Res* 14(1):37, 2018.
243. Anonymous: OIE technical factsheet: Schmallenberg virus, 2017. Available at: http://www.oie.int/fileadmin/Home/eng/Our_scientific_expertise/docs/pdf/A_Schmallenberg_virus.pdf. Accessed May 23, 2018.
244. Lechner I, Wuthrich M, Meylan M, van den Borne BHP, Schupbach-Regula G: Association of clinical signs after acute Schmallenberg virus infection with milk production and fertility in Swiss dairy cows, *Prev Vet Med* 146:121–129, 2017.
245. Lievaart-Peterson K, Luttikholt S, Peperkamp K, Van den Brom R, Vellema P: Schmallenberg disease in sheep or goats: past, present and future, *Vet Microbiol* 181(1–2):147–153, 2015.
246. Valas S, Baudry C, Ehrhardt N, et al: Serosurvey of Schmallenberg virus infection in the highest goat-specialized region of France, *Transbound Emerg Dis* 62(5):e85–e88, 2015.
247. Laloy E, Breard E, Trapp S, et al: Fetopathic effects of experimental Schmallenberg virus infection in pregnant goats, *Vet Microbiol* 211:141–149, 2017.
248. Peperkamp NH, Luttikholt SJ, Dijkman R, et al: Ovine and bovine congenital abnormalities associated with intrauterine infection with Schmallenberg virus, *Vet Pathol* 52(6):1057–1066, 2015.

14

Diseases of the Eye

RICHARD J. MCMULLEN JR. AND THOMAS PASSLER

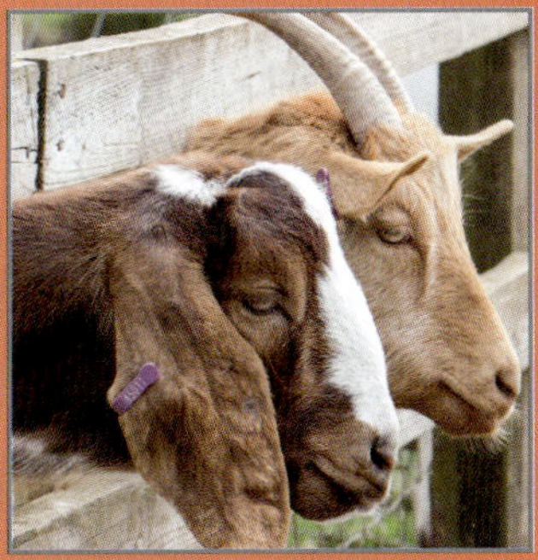

Ocular and Adnexal Anatomy

It is important to have a general and functional understanding of the anatomy of the eye and surrounding tissues. Without this knowledge, it can be very difficult to determine if a lesion or an abnormality is actually present. Although individual differences are present among each of the species covered in this section, deer, goats, and sheep are all arrhythmic ruminants and are equally active diurnally and nocturnally. Thus, the ocular, orbital, and adnexal anatomy is relatively similar.[1,2]

Adnexa

Orbit. Sheep, goats, and deer have an enclosed orbit, typical of most grazing animals. The bony fossa of the orbit in each of these species is comprised of the lacrimal, zygomatic, frontal, sphenoid, and palatine bones. Additionally, the maxillary bone forms part of the orbit in sheep. The size, shape, and position of the orbit are closely associated with visual activity and feeding behavior.[1,2] In general, prey species such as small ruminants have eyes that are located more laterally on the skull, resulting in enhanced monocular vision with an increased panoramic line of vision, allowing these species to scan their surroundings for predators.[1,2] Nerves and blood vessels enter into the orbital region via the rostral alar, ethmoidal, lacrimal, orbital, ovale, optic, rotundum, and supraorbital foramina or fissures. The pterygopalatine region has nerves and vessels associated with the orbit as well, including the caudal palatine, maxillary, and sphenopalatine foramina.[1] Glands of the infraorbital sinus, or preorbital glands, are present in sheep and cervids and are better developed in rams and bucks than in ewes or does, respectively. These are specialized cutaneous glands that produce pheromones; their secretions exit from the infraorbital sinus in a depression just rostral to the eye (Figure 14.1A, B).[3–7]

Orbital Fascia and Fat. The globe is surrounded by three fascial layers. The periorbita is the most external layer and is attached near the optic foramen and the apex of the muscle cone at the exit of the optic nerve from the orbit.[1,2,8] The superficial muscular fascia lies within the periorbita and encloses the lacrimal gland and the levator palpebrae superioris muscle. The deep muscular fascia is more fibrous than the other two fascial layers and originates at the upper and lower eyelid and from the limbus. It sheaths the extraocular muscles and optic nerve.[1,2,8] The orbital fat occupies the spaces between the extraocular muscles and fills the orbital dead space providing a cushion that protects the globe and extraocular muscles.[1,2,8]

Extraocular Muscles. The extraocular muscles suspend the globe within the orbit and are responsible for ocular motility.[1] There are four rectus muscles (dorsal, ventral, medial, and lateral recti) that move the globe in their respective directions. The recti originate from the orbital apex at the annulus of Zinn and insert posteriorly to the limbus at variable distances depending upon the species and muscle in question.[1] The dorsal oblique muscle originates from the medial orbital apex, passes anteriorly on the dorsomedial wall of the orbit, and is then deflected around the trochlea, a cartilaginous pulley attached to the anterior aspect of the medial wall of the orbit, to insert on the dorsolateral aspect of the globe beneath the tendon of the dorsal rectus muscle.[8,9] The dorsal oblique muscle rotates the dorsal aspect of the globe both medially and ventrally. The ventral oblique muscle originates from a depression in the ventromedial wall of the orbit, specifically the anterolateral margin of the palatine bone. It passes laterally beneath the globe, crossing the ventral rectus tendon before inserting on the ventrolateral aspect of the globe.[1,2,8] The ventral oblique muscle moves the globe medially and dorsally. The retractor bulbi muscle, which forms an almost complete cone around the optic nerve, originates from the orbital apex and inserts just posteriorly to the equator beneath the recti muscles.[1,2,8] The retractor bulbi muscle retracts the globe towards the apex of the globe for additional protection and allows the nictitating membrane (third eyelid) to move across the surface of the cornea.[1,2,8] The oculomotor nerve (cranial nerve [CN] III) innervates the dorsal, ventral, and medial recti muscles. The dorsal oblique muscle is innervated by the trochlear nerve (CN IV), and the lateral rectus and retractor bulbi muscles are innervated by the abducens nerve (CN VI).[1,2,8]

Eyelids and Conjunctiva. The superior and inferior palpebrae (eyelids) are two musculofibrous folds of thin skin continuous with the facial skin. The superior eyelid is more mobile than the inferior eyelid. The opening formed by the free edges of the eyelids is the palpebral fissure.[1,2,8,9] Histologically, the eyelids have four tissue layers: the skin, the orbicularis oculi muscle, the tarsus and stromal layer, and the palpebral conjunctiva. The palpebral skin is thin and elastic and is covered by a dense coat of short hairs with small tubular and sebaceous glands. The superior palpebrae have a row of cilia, and vibrissae are present a short distance from the superior and inferior palpebral margins in small ruminants. The arrectores ciliorum are bundles of smooth muscle fibers that extend from the eyelash follicles toward the tarsus and are present in ruminants, but not in carnivores.[1,2] The superior palpebral skin receives sensory innervation by the ophthalmic branch of the

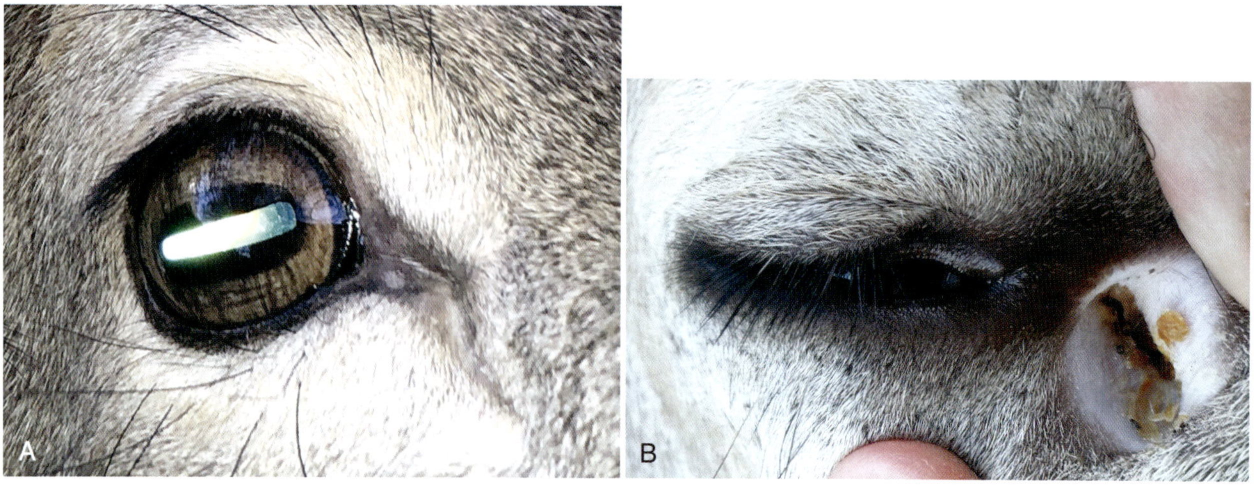

• **Fig. 14.1** **A.** Closed preorbital gland in a young male fallow deer. **B.** Manually dilated preorbital gland in a young white-tailed deer. (Courtesy Dr. Kelley Steury, Alabama Veterinary Diagnostic Laboratory, Auburn, AL.)

trigeminal nerve (CN V), and the inferior palpebral skin is innervated by the maxillary branch of the trigeminal nerve. The orbicularis oculi muscle encircles the entire palpebral fissure and functions to close the palpebral fissure. It receives motor innervation by the palpebral branch of the facial nerve (CN VII). The superior eyelid is elevated by the levator palpebrae superioris muscle, which receives motor innervation from the oculomotor nerve. The levator palpebrae superioris originates at the orbital apex and extends along the dorsal half of the mid-stroma. The sympathetically innervated Müller's muscle complements the function of the levator palpebrae superioris. Other muscles associated with eyelid function include the corrugator supercilii muscle, which assists in elevating the superior eyelid, and the retractor anguli oculi muscle, which lengthens the lateral palpebral fissure. Both of these muscles are innervated by the facial nerve. The tarsus is a poorly developed narrow layer of dense collagenous connective tissue that separates the eyelid muscles from the palpebral conjunctiva. The tarsus is continuous with the septum orbitale in both the superior and inferior palpebrae. The septum orbitale is attached to the periosteum of the bony orbital rim.[1,2] Near the margin of both eyelids are the tarsal gland openings. The tarsal glands are sebaceous glands that produce the lipid component of the preocular tear film. These glands open onto the edge of both eyelids through small openings arranged longitudinally. The tarsal glands are parasympathetically innervated by the oculomotor nerve.[1] The palpebral conjunctiva is the mucous membrane that lines the inner aspect of the eyelids. It consists of stratified columnar epithelium that becomes more stratified and squamous as it nears the eyelid margin. The stratified columnar epithelia have numerous goblet cells that contribute to the mucus layer of the preocular tear film. The palpebral conjunctiva continues onto the globe as the bulbar conjunctiva where it meets and is continuous with the corneal epithelium. The palpebral and bulbar conjunctivae meet at the fornix, and this region is lined with stratified cuboidal epithelium. The potential space created by the conjunctivae is the cul-de-sac. The palpebral, bulbar, and nictitans conjunctivae are named based on their anatomic locations, but they are continuous. The vascular supply to the conjunctiva is from the anterior ciliary arteries (branches of the external ophthalmic artery).[1,2] Ventromedially, the lacrimal caruncle is seen as a small mucosal elevation that may or may not be pigmented and contain hair follicles.

The nictitating membrane (third eyelid, nictitans) is located ventromedially between the lacrimal caruncle and the globe. It is completely lined by conjunctiva and contains a T-shaped cartilaginous plate with a gland (gland of the nictitating membrane or nictitans) at its base. The horizontal part of the T lies at the free edge of the fold. The gland of the nictitating membrane surrounds the stem of the cartilage. The anterior and posterior aspects of the nictitating membrane are lined with nonkeratinized stratified squamous epithelium. The nictitating membrane moves passively over the eye in a dorsolateral direction when the globe is retracted by contraction of the retractor oculi muscle and displacement of the orbital fat.[1,2]

Lacrimal and Nasolacrimal Systems

The lacrimal system consists of the lacrimal gland, the gland of the third eyelid, the accessory glands of Krause and Wolfring, the glands of Zeis, the tarsal glands, and the nasolacrimal duct system.[1,2,8,9] The lacrimal gland lies in the dorsolateral wall of the orbit between the dorsolateral wall of the orbit and the globe. Histologically, the lacrimal gland of the sheep and goat is a compound tubuloalveolar mixed gland.[10,11] The lacrimal gland receives its blood supply from the lacrimal artery. The lacrimal nerve sends sensory innervation to the gland, and the secretory portion of the gland is sympathetically innervated by postganglionic fibers from the cranial cervical ganglion. Two large and four to five small excretory ducts originate from the central surface of the lacrimal gland in small ruminants.[8,10] The lacrimal fluid drains into the dorsal fornix of the conjunctival sac and mixes with the secretions of the accessory glands.[8] The glands of Zeis and the tarsal glands produce the outer lipid layer of the preocular tear film. The lacrimal gland, the gland of the third eyelid, and the accessory glands of Krause and Wolfring produce the middle aqueous component of the preocular tear film. The inner mucin layer is produced by the conjunctival goblet cells.[1,2] The three layers of the preocular tear film are continuously spread across the eye's surface by the eyelids and nictitating membrane during blinking. Unlike cattle, sheep and goats have high lysozyme (an antibacterial enzyme) tear film concentrations.[12,13] Excess preocular tear film pools in the lacrimal lake at the ventromedial angle of the eye. Mechanical pumping action draws the tear fluid into the superior and inferior puncta lacrimale (lacrimal puncta). The puncta are located on the palpebral conjunctiva, just inside the edge of the eyelid and medial to the last tarsal gland.[1,2] Smooth muscle in the puncta contract during blinking to remove pooled tear fluid. The superior and inferior lacrimal puncta continue as the superior and inferior canaliculi. The canaliculi coalesce at the nasolacrimal sac located in the lacrimal fossa of the lacrimal bone.[1,2] The lacrimal sac empties into the nasolacrimal duct, which initially continues rostrally through the osseous lacrimal canal and the osseous lacrimal groove of the maxilla. It then parallels the mucous membrane of the middle meatus and opens on the nasal mucous membrane at the junction of pigmented and nonpigmented skin.[11]

The Harderian gland (glandula palpebrae tertiae profundus) and the nictitans gland (glandula palpebrae tertiae superficialis) have traditionally been considered to be two distinct individual glands. Although the ducts for both glands open on the bulbar conjunctival surface of the nictitating membrane, there are distinct anatomical, histological, and histochemical characteristics that vary among the species possessing both glands.[14] Rehorek et al. (2007) suggest that the two glandular structures known as the Harderian and nictitans glands both originate from a single inception point and, following differentiation at a later time point, separate into two distinct lobes in both the Chinese muntjac *(Muntiacus reevesi)* and fallow deer *(Dama dama)*.[14]

Vascular Supply of the Eye

In domestic mammals, the majority of the ocular and adnexal vascular supply is from the external ophthalmic artery, a branch of the maxillary artery. The arteries supplying the globe originate from the external ophthalmic and the malar artery, a smaller branch of the maxillary artery. The nasal and lateral long posterior ciliary arteries (LPCAs) branch off of the external ophthalmic arteries. The lateral and nasal LPCAs branch to the choroid and ciliary processes; in the periphery, each LPCA divides again into dorsal and ventral branches that form the major arterial circle of the iris. The LPCAs give off the short posterior ciliary arteries (SPCAs). The SPCAs penetrate the globe adjacent to the optic nerve to supply the inner layers of the retina and then ramify into the choroidal vasculature. The SPCAs also branch to the perilimbal region and the anterior ciliary body. The smaller internal ophthalmic artery supplies the optic nerve and anastomoses with the external ophthalmic artery or one of its branches.[1] The external ophthalmic artery then gives off two muscular branches: the ventral and the dorsal branches. These branches supply the extraorbital muscles, the gland of the nictitating membrane, the lacrimal gland, and the levator palpebrae superiors.[1]

Globe

The small ruminant globe (bulbus oculi) is nearly spherical in shape. Little published data exist on the globe dimensions of small ruminants. Anterior to posterior (axial) globe length increases with age in Saanen goats, with the average values being: 18.66 mm (45 days), 22.29 mm (180 days), and 24.37 mm (549 days) in this particular breed.[15] In Barbary sheep, or aoudad *(Ammotragus lervia)*, the average axial globe length was determined to be 28.43 mm in a group of 18 animals.[16] These results are similar to previously reported values from the early 20th century (28.85 mm).[1,17] The globe is composed of three tunics (distinct layers): the fibrous, vascular, and nervous tunics. The external fibrous tunic is composed of dense collagenous connective tissue that resists the eye's internal pressure and gives the globe its round shape. The fibrous tunic is composed of the cornea and sclera, which coalesce at the corneoscleral junction or limbus. This transition is obvious, as the disorganized collagen fibers of the sclera transition into the highly organized (i.e., transparent) fibers of the cornea (Figure 14.2).[18] The middle vascular tunic is comprised of the uvea, which includes the iris, ciliary body, and choroid. The inner nervous tunic includes the retina and optic nerve. The three tunics surround the aqueous humor, lens, and vitreous humor.[1,2]

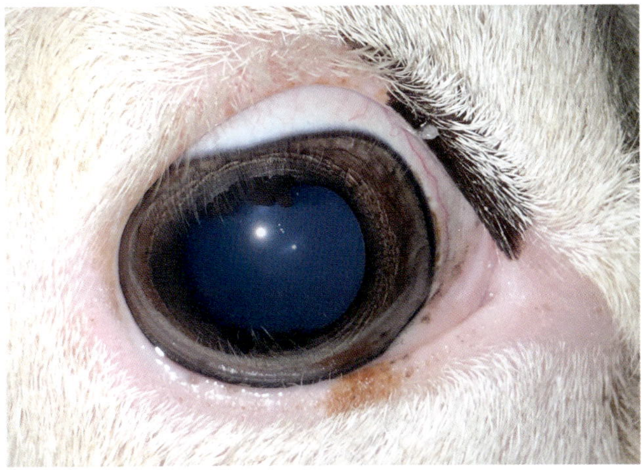

• **Fig. 14.2** Image of the right eye of a young female sheep. The white sclera (dorsal) and clear (transparent) cornea comprise the outer fibrous tunic of the globe.

Fibrous Tunic

Cornea. The cornea is the transparent, avascular, and colorless anterior 20% of the fibrous tunic. It is composed of dense collagenous connective tissue arranged in a regular lamellar pattern. This lamellar pattern, combined with the physiologic pump of the posterior epithelium, maintains the cornea's transparency and deturgescence. The nonkeratinized anterior surface epithelium and the small diameter of the collagen fibrils also contribute to the cornea's transparency.[18,19]

The cornea is the most powerful refractive surface of the eye. In small ruminants, the shape of the cornea is elliptical, with its horizontal diameter greater than its vertical diameter. In sheep, the average width of the cornea is 22.4 mm and the average height is 15.4 mm.[1,19] The sheep cornea is thickest at its center (0.8–2.0 mm) and thinnest at its edge (0.3–0.5 mm).[1] A recent study evaluating the central corneal thickness via optical coherence tomography has shown the average corneal thickness to be 616.9 ± 7.1 μm in goats and 741 ± 9.9 μm in sheep.[20] Not only can the overall corneal thickness be evaluated using this imaging modality, but the various individual corneal layers (epithelium, stroma, Descemet's membrane, and endothelium) can be readily identified and observed under significant magnification (Figure 14.3A, B).[20] Corneal innervation is achieved by the long ciliary nerves, which originate from the ophthalmic branch of the trigeminal nerve.[1]

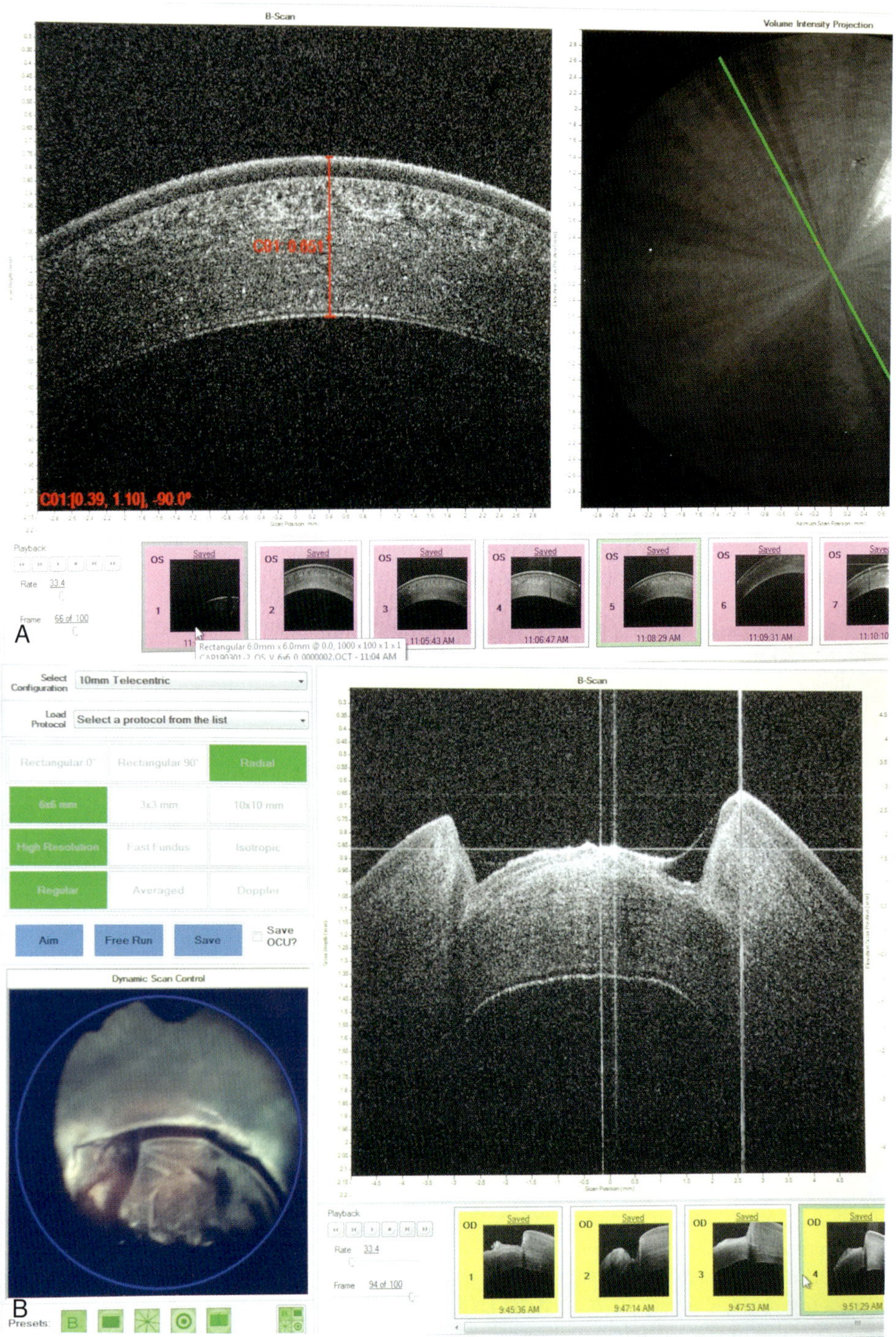

• **Fig. 14.3** **A.** Optical coherence tomography (OCT) screenshot of the axial cornea of an adult female goat. Internal calipers are used to measure the axial corneal thickness (651 µm or 0.651 mm) for this animal. **B.** This imaging modality can be used to assess corneal defects and their response to therapy, such as in this adult horse with a 40–50% depth corneal ulcer.

The small ruminant cornea is comprised of four layers. The anterior, nonkeratinized, stratified, squamous epithelium (epithelium corneae) covers the outermost corneal surface and is continuous with the conjunctival epithelium. The most posterior layer of the anterior epithelium consists of a monolayer of columnar basal cells that lie on a thin basement membrane. The basement membrane of the anterior epithelium is primarily composed of types IV, VI, and VII collagen.[1,2] Several layers of polyhedral, or wing cells, extend anteriorly from the basal cell layer, and anterior to these are numerous layers of nonkeratinized squamous epithelial cells. The basal cells are attached via hemidesmosomes, arranged in a linear manner, to the basal lamina of the basement membrane (lamina limitans).[1,9] The stroma (substantia propria) forms the bulk of the cornea. The stroma is composed of extracellular matrix and a lamellar arrangement of collagen fibrils oriented in parallel lamellae positioned at oblique angles to each other and separated by less than a wavelength of light.[1,21] Interwoven between the collagen fibrils and extracellular matrix are keratocytes. Keratocytes possess cellular extensions that help maintain the stromal lamellae. After a deep corneal injury, keratocytes can differentiate into fibroblasts and contribute to scar formation.[1,2] Descemet's membrane (lamina elastica), located on the posterior aspect of the cornea, is homogeneous and acellular and functions as a protective boundary within the cornea. It is produced throughout life by the corneal endothelium and is made up of types I, III, IV, V, VI, and VIII collagen. Descemet's membrane terminates at the apex of the trabecular meshwork in the area of the limbus.[1,2] The endothelium is a monolayer of flattened polygonal cells lining the most posterior aspect of the cornea. In adult animals, the endothelium rarely undergoes mitosis and has an age-dependent loss of endothelial cells.[1,22,23]

Lens. The lens further focuses light entering the eye to allow for sharp focus of visualized images. The lens is a transparent, biconvex, almost spherical structure that is located posterior to the iris and anterior to the vitreous. It is held in position by the zonular ligaments (zonula ciliaris) that arise from the ciliary epithelium and are composed of fibrillin.[24] Other structures that support the lens include the patellar fossa of the vitreous and the iris. Herbivorous animals have a marginally functional accommodative mechanism resulting in relatively poor near vision.[19]

The lens is transparent and avascular and receives the majority of its nutrients from the aqueous humor. It continues to grow throughout life at a slow, regulated rate because of continued division and differentiation of the lens epithelial cells into lens fiber cells. This growth does not result in an increase in size of the lens but leads to compression of the lens fibers, which are responsible for the reduced transparency which manifests clinically as nuclear sclerosis or cataracts.[1,2]

The lens is enveloped in a basement membrane of primarily type IV collagen. The anterior lens capsule is significantly thicker than the posterior lens capsule and continues to thicken throughout the animal's life.[1,2] The lens capsule is produced by the lens epithelial cells, which are present only on the anterior aspect of the lens. The lens epithelial cell population is made up of three regions. The most central cells are squamous in appearance and rarely undergo mitosis. The cells in the germinative region, which encircles the central epithelium, are more cuboidal in appearance and undergo mitosis at a slow rate. The lens epithelial cells in the equatorial region elongate into lens fiber cells, lose their nuclei by a process called denucleation, and attach at the anterior and posterior lens sutures. The fiber cells are continually being formed—the newest fiber cells are located peripherally and the oldest become the most centralized and compressed lens fibers. Nearly 80% of glucose metabolism in the lens occurs primarily by glycolysis. The tricarboxylic cycle accounts for 5%, the pentose monophosphate shunt accounts for 15%, and the sorbitol pathway accounts for a negligible portion of glucose metabolism.[1,2]

Vitreous. The vitreous (vitreous humor or vitreous body) also refracts light that enters the eye and passes through the lens to focus light on the retina. The vitreous is gel-like and lies posterior to the lens and anterior to the retina. The vitreous is 98% water that is suspended in collagen fibers and glycosaminoglycan matrix. The vitreous body physically holds the retina against the choroid. Continuous turnover of the vitreous does not occur.[1,2]

Sclera. The sclera comprises the posterior 80% of the fibrous tunic. The sclera differs from the cornea in three basic ways: (1) the collagen fibrils of the sclera are irregularly arranged; (2) the scleral epithelium is thicker than the corneal epithelium; and (3) it has small basal cells with scanty cytoplasm.[1,2] Scleral thickness at the entry point of the optic nerve in the sheep is 1.0 to 1.2 mm. It thins at the equator to 0.25 to 0.30 mm and thickens at the corneoscleral junction to 0.4 to 0.5 mm.[1,2] These values have not been determined for goats or cervids.

Vascular Tunic (Tunica Vasculosa Oculi)

The vascular tunic, or uvea, is comprised of the iris, ciliary body, and choroid. These structures are highly vascularized and variably pigmented.[1,2]

Iris. The iris comprises the anterior, and visible portion, of the uvea. It is a muscular diaphragm suspended between the cornea and the lens. It is attached anteriorly to the sclera, at its periphery, by the pectinate ligament and continues posteriorly to fuse with the ciliary body.[25–27] The iris divides the space between the cornea and the lens into the anterior and posterior chambers of the anterior segment. Its central aspect has an aperture, the pupil (pupillae) that changes in size to adjust the amount of light entering the eye and reaching the retina. The muscles that regulate pupil size are the sphincter pupillae and the dilator pupillae. The sphincter muscle is primarily innervated by parasympathetic nerve fibers, while the dilator muscle is innervated by sympathetic nerve fibers. As a result, the pupil constricts (when the animal is in a relaxed state) and dilates (in response to stress) in addition to reacting to increases and decreases in light intensity, respectively. The sphincter muscle lies concentrically near the pupillary margin and the dilator muscle has fibers arranged radially from the sphincter to the ciliary border. The pupil is oval in a horizontal plane in small ruminants and has several round, variably sized black masses at the superior and inferior aspects of the pupillary border called granula iridica (corpora nigra) (Figure 14.4).[1,28,29] The granula iridica are extensions of the posterior pigmented epithelium of the iris. They enhance the effect of pupillary constriction or miosis.[1] In cervids, the pupil is also elongated horizontally, but obvious granula iridica are lacking or are rudimentary (Figure 14.5).

The iris is grossly divided into two regions divided by the collarette. The central region is the pupillary zone, and the peripheral region is the ciliary zone (Figures 14.1A and 14.6A, B). The peripheral half of the ciliary zone contains a circumferential artery, the annular major arterial circle. The major arterial circle is an

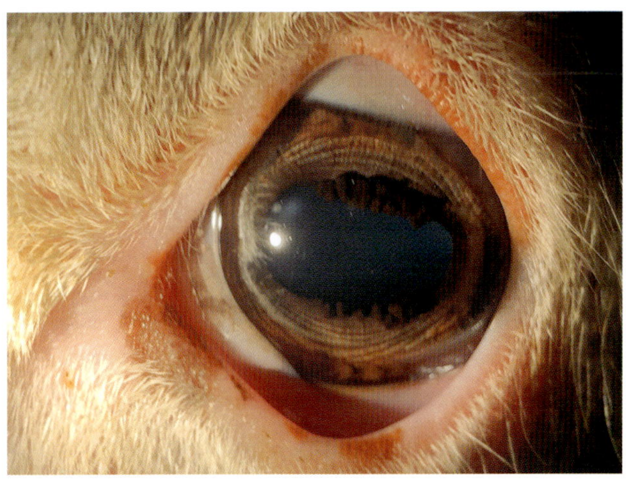

• **Fig. 14.4** Prominent granula iridica are present along both the upper (dorsal) and lower (ventral) pupillary margins in the left eye of this young sheep.

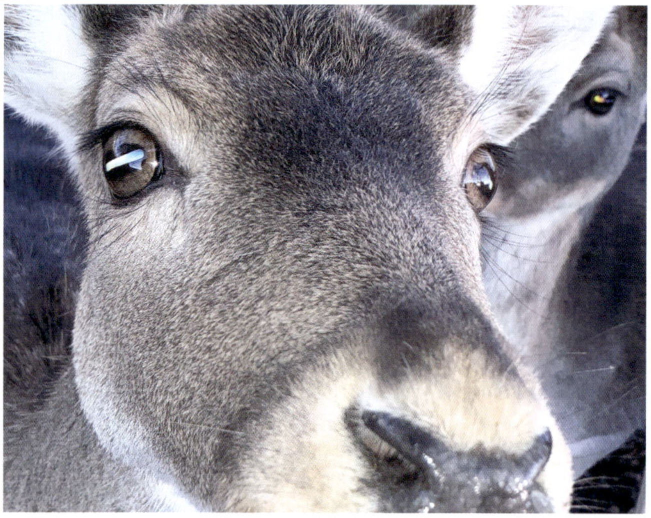

• **Fig. 14.5** The tapetal reflex highlights the horizontally elongated pupil in the right eye of this young fallow deer. Note the lack of granula iridica along the dorsal and ventral pupil margin.

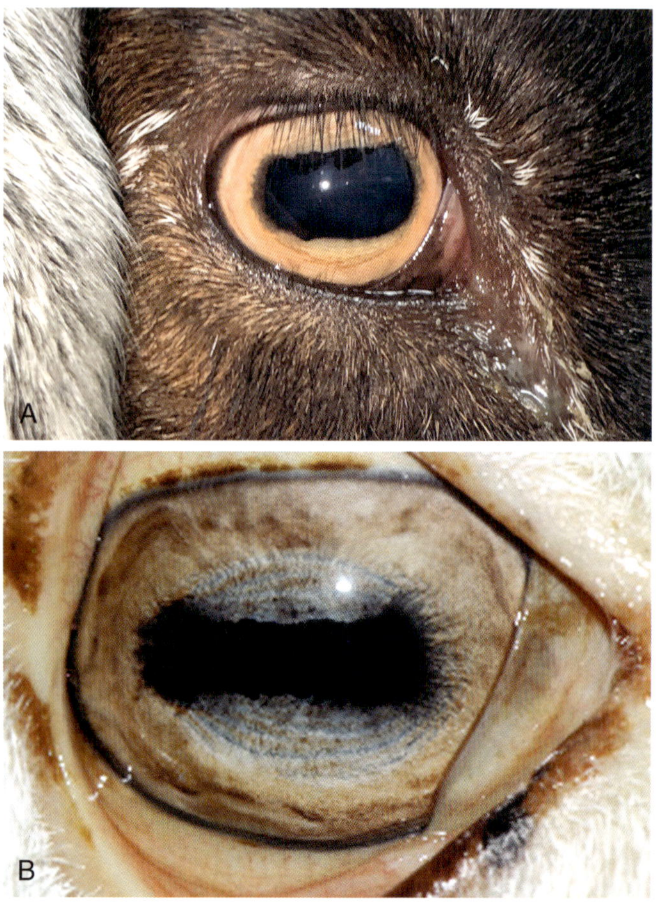

• **Fig. 14.6** **A.** The dark iris collarette represents the pupillary zone and the amber-colored stroma represents the ciliary zone of the anterior surface of the iris in the right eye of this adult goat. **B.** The pupillary zone is made up of the darkly pigmented collarette and the gray areas along the dorsal and ventral aspects of the pupil. The remaining, amber-colored iris represents the ciliary zone in the right eye of this sheep. (Courtesy Dr. Chris Pirie, MSU.)

incomplete circle that originates from the dorsal and ventral branches of the medial and lateral LPCAs. The major arterial circle branches into radial arteries that nourish the rest of the iris. Radial vessels provide venous drainage for the iris. They empty directly into the anterior choroidal circulation.[1,2,28]

The three cellular layers of the iris are the anterior border layer, the middle stroma (which contains the sphincter muscle), and the posterior epithelial layers. The anterior border layer consists of fibroblasts and melanocytes, and their processes form an incomplete layer across the surface of the iris. No continuous layer of epithelium extends across the iris's anterior surface.[1,2] The iris stroma is loosely arranged and consists of fibroblasts, fine collagenous fibers, chromatophores, and melanocytes. Iris color is dependent upon the density of stromal pigmentation. The iris sphincter muscle of sheep, goats, and cervids is probably very similar to that of the horse, another ungulate with an elongated, horizontally orientated pupil.[1,2] In the horse, the iris sphincter lies in the main portion of the central stroma, is covered by the granula iridica, and is parasympathetically innervated.[1,2] The iris dilator muscle is located in the posterior aspect of the iris stroma, is innervated by sympathetic fibers, and is continuous with the pigmented epithelium of the ciliary body. The posterior pigmented epithelium of the iris is continuous with the nonpigmented epithelium of the ciliary body.[1,2] Both the iris dilator muscle and the posterior pigmented epithelium form the granula iridica in herbivores. The size of the dilator muscle in sheep, goats, and cervids is likely similar to that of the horse.[1,2]

Ciliary Body (Corpus Ciliare). The ciliary body is the middle portion of the uvea through which the choroid (posterior uvea) and the peripheral iris (anterior uvea) converge. It consists of two sections: the anterior pars plicata and the posterior pars plana.[1] The pars plicata consists of radial folds called ciliary processes that are "thick and clublike with shallow valleys in herbivores."[30] The ciliary processes stabilize the lens via zonular fibers that extend to the lens equator. In ungulates, the ciliary processes have numerous arterioles and veins within their core. The ciliary processes also have well-developed capillary beds that produce the majority of the aqueous humor.[1,2] The pars plana is the thin, flat portion of the ciliary body that terminates in the pars ciliaris retinae; the junction between the ciliary body and the retina. This portion of the uvea is devoid of vasculature and varies in width because the retina extends further anteriorly, both medially and inferiorly, in most species.[1,2] The ciliary muscles, along with the ciliary processes, comprise the majority of the ciliary body. The ciliary musculature is composed of meridional smooth muscle fibers coursing close to the sclera. This musculature is poorly developed in ungulates, accounting for their poor accommodative ability. Evolution has allowed herbivores to develop large corneas, horizontally oval-shaped pupils, and large anterior chambers for better night vision and good motion detection.[1,2]

Iridocorneal Angle. The iridocorneal angle (ICA) is the most anterior aspect of the ciliary body. The most anterior region of the ICA is the termination of Descemet's membrane.[26] The ICA is bordered by the limbus, the base of the iris, and the ciliary cleft. The ciliary cleft is a triangular region that is the posterolateral extension of the anterior chamber into the ciliary body. Pectinate ligaments are present in the ciliary cleft from the pigmented limbus to the root of the iris.[1,2] The ICA and ciliary musculature of small ruminants are similar to those of cattle. The outflow tract has a large ciliary cleft with prominent spaces of Fontana. The large, semi-oval corneoscleral trabecular meshwork and the uveal trabecular meshwork form a delineated angular aqueous plexus.[26]

The ciliary cleft and pectinate ligaments are smaller in sheep, goats, and cervids than in cattle and horses because of their smaller globe size. Aqueous humor can exit the eye through one of two pathways: the conventional and the unconventional outflow pathway. The majority of aqueous humor exits the eye in most species by the conventional pathway. Specifically, following its production by the ciliary body, aqueous humor passes into the posterior chamber, through the pupil, into the anterior chamber, between the pectinate ligaments, through the trabecular meshwork, into the scleral venous plexus, and then the systemic circulation. Aqueous humor can also exit the eye by a number of ancillary pathways. It can drain anteriorly within the iridal stroma and across the cornea, it can flow posteriorly into the vitreous humor, or it can flow exteroposteriorly along a supraciliary-suprachoroidal space into the adjacent sclera.[1,2] The uveoscleral (unconventional) pathway is the most prominent of the ancillary routes of aqueous drainage. Aqueous humor is absorbed from the ciliary cleft into the anterior face of the ciliary body and diffuses into the sclera and the systemic venous circulation. The percentage of outflow by the uveoscleral pathway has been determined for many species but not for small ruminants. This outflow pathway is thought to be the major aqueous outflow pathway in the horse and may be a major pathway in other ungulates.[1,2,31]

Choroid (Choroidea). The choroid is a dense network of blood vessels and pigmented stroma between the retina and the sclera. The choroid supplies nutrition to the posterior layers of the retina. The total choroidal blood supply far exceeds the need for retinal nutrition and it may also serve as a heat exchange mechanism to prevent the retina from overheating. Morphologically, the choroid can be divided into four layers: suprachoroidea, large vessel layer, medium-sized vessel and tapetum layer, and choriocapillaris. The suprachoroidea is the potential space between the choroidal stroma and is attached loosely to the sclera by the lamina fusca. The LPCAs and nerves travel in the suprachoroidea along the horizontal meridian. The large-vessel layer (lamina vasculosa) is the posterior stromal layer. It has large cavernous vessels, primarily veins, that drain the choriocapillaris and some branches of the SPCA. The medium-sized vessel and tapetum layer are the anterior stromal layer of the choroid. It has smaller vessels connecting the choriocapillaris to the large vessel layer.[1,2] Within this inner stromal layer lies the tapetum. In ungulates, the tapetum is fibrous (tapetum fibrosum) and composed of regularly arranged collagen fibers and occasional fibrocytes. Herbivores are born with mature eyes and well-developed tapeta. Sheep have several hundred layers of well-arranged collagen lamellae.[32] Capillaries penetrate the tapetum at right angles to the collagen lamellae, connecting the choriocapillaris to the medium-sized vessels; when visualized end-on, they are referred to as the "stars of Winslow."[1,2] The choriocapillaris is the single layer of capillaries between the choroidal stroma and the retinal pigmented epithelium (RPE). These capillaries are fenestrated, and external to their endothelium, they have a basement membrane that forms the outermost layer of Bruch's membrane separating the choroid from the RPE.[1,2]

Neural Tunic

The neural tunic is comprised of the retina and optic nerve. Both are derivatives of the forebrain, and both can be visualized during an ophthalmic examination. As a result, changes in their appearance can provide clinical information about that animal's physical status. The retinal vasculature, which originates from the SPCAs, provides the inner retinal layers with the majority of its nutrients, with the vitreous providing the rest. The choriocapillaris is responsible for providing nourishment to the outer retinal layers. The retinal metabolic rate is one of the highest in the body, and therefore, if either the retinal or choroidal vasculature is even marginally compromised, the retina can become ischemic.[1,33]

The retina is comprised of 10 layers, the outermost of which is the RPE; the inner nine layers are known as the sensory retina. The five layers of clinical importance (from posterior to anterior) are as follows: RPE, photoreceptors, inner nuclear layer (bipolar cell nuclei), ganglion cell layer, and the nerve fiber layer (ganglion cell axons).[1,2]

The photoreceptors include the rods and cones. Rods function in dim-light conditions. Cones function in bright light and play roles in color recognition and visual acuity. Rods dominate in sheep, goats, and deer. Photoreceptors are composed of inner and outer segments. The outer segments have rhodopsin embedded in their membranes. Bipolar cells synapse with photoreceptors on one side and with ganglion cells on the opposite side. They transfer the electrical potential generated by the photoreceptors to the ganglion cells. The ganglion cells are the innermost cell layer of the retina. Projecting axons run parallel to the retinal surface in the innermost nerve fiber layer and converge at the optic disc. These axons turn posteriorly to form the optic nerve (CN II). Optic nerve fibers exit the eye through the lamina cribrosa. The highest density of ganglion cells has been determined to be in the area centralis and visual streak of goats.[34] The retina of the goat shows a horizontal visual streak (nasal to temporal) slightly ventral to the optic disc. Additionally, the goat retina also contains an area centralis (circular area of maximal ganglion cell concentration) located temporally and situated close to the optic disc. The goat retina also contains a vertical streak (concentration of ganglion cells) in the upper temporal retina, perpendicular to the horizontal visual streak. There are significant variations in the individual arrangement of both the horizontal and vertical streak in the goat, even between the eyes of the same animal.[34]

The area centralis is the area of maximal cone density and the visual streak is the area of maximal ganglion cell density. The central retina of sheep is similar to that of other mammals with an area centralis and a single visual streak. Goats have an area centralis and also two visual streaks—a horizontal streak and a vertical streak.[34,35] The rod-to-cone ratio for sheep is 30:1 to 40:1.[36] No rod-to-cone ratio has been reported in goats or deer. The retinas of sheep, goats, and deer have two classes of cone pigment, thus providing the requisite retinal basis for dichromatic color vision.[34,35,37,38]

The RPE is a single layer of cells between the sensory retina and the choriocapillaris. It is nonpigmented in the dorsal half of the fundus, allowing the tapetum exposure to light. The primary functions of the RPE are metabolism of retinol for phototransduction and phagocytosis of waste products from the sensory retina. The RPE has tight interepithelial junctions that form part of the blood-retinal barrier.[1]

Sheep, goats, and deer retinae have a holangiotic vascular pattern. In holangiotic retinae, all quadrants of the retina are vascularized with vessels extending from the optic nerve to the periphery. Sheep retinae have three or four major venules and numerous branching arterioles. Occasionally, the superior arteriole and venule wrap around each other. Goat retinae have five to eight primary venules.

The tapetal fundus is roughly triangular; can be yellow, green, to bluish-purple; and is stippled with the stars of Winslow.[39] The dorsomedial tapetal fundus has more pigment than the other

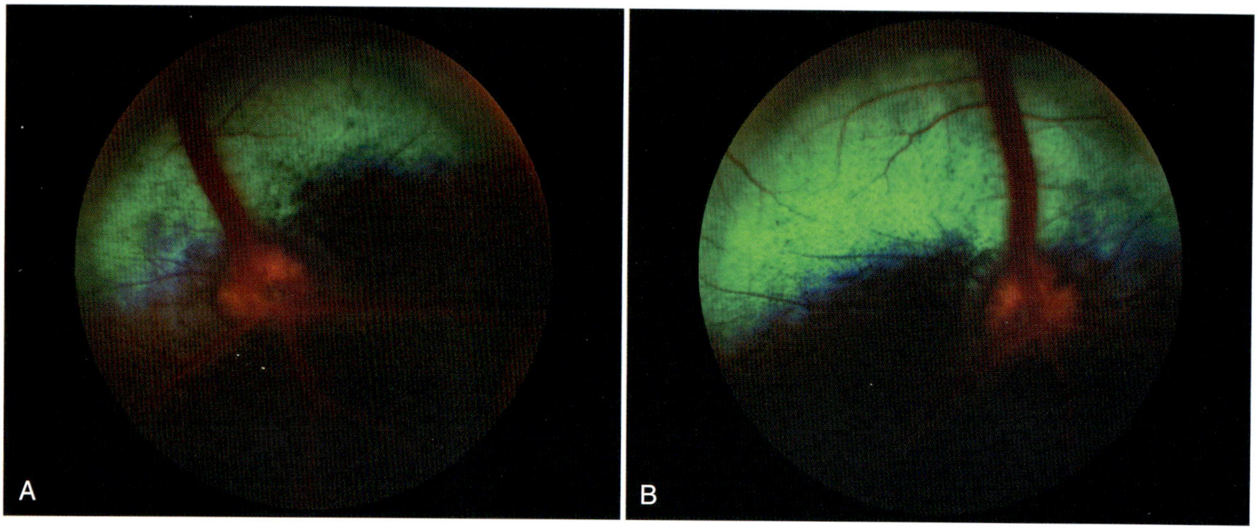

• **Fig. 14.7** **A.** Fundus image of the right eye of a sheep. Note the slightly oval-shaped (kidney bean) optic disc in this young sheep. The four thick and prominent retinal venules extend into the peripheral retina from the optic disc (dorsal, ventromedial, ventral, and ventrotemporal). The dark punctate spots within the tapetum (bright green reflective area dorsal to the optic disc) are the stars of Winslow. **B.** Contralateral fundus image from the same sheep as in Figure 14.7A.

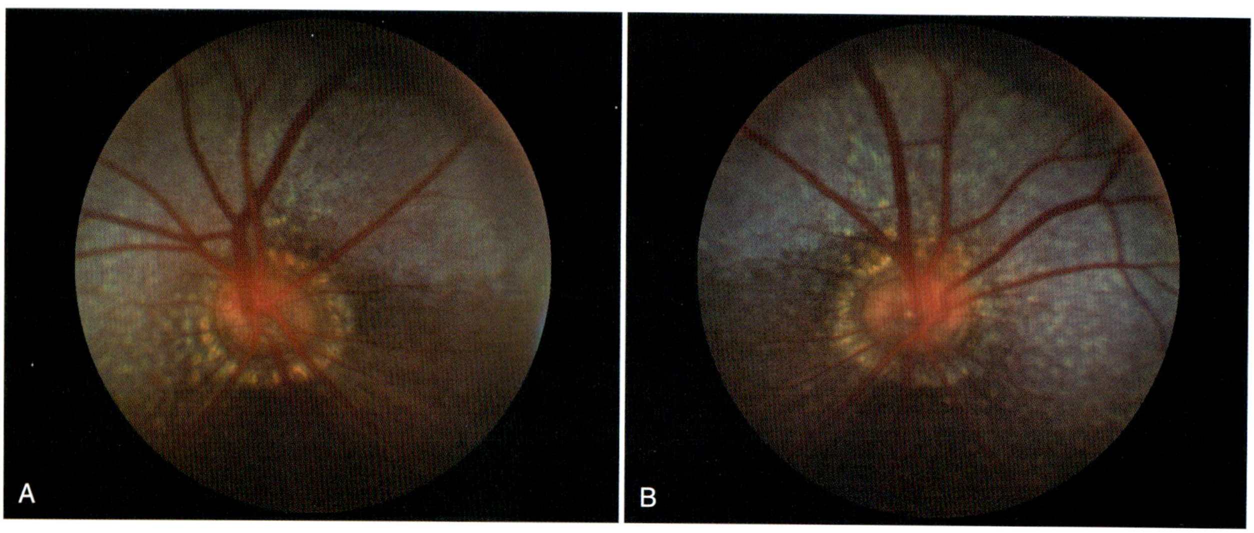

• **Fig. 14.8** **A.** Fundus image of the right eye of a goat. Note the round (circular) optic disc in this adult goat. The four thick and prominent retinal venules extend and branch into the peripheral retina from the optic disc (dorsal, ventromedial, ventral, and ventrotemporal). The dark punctate spots within the tapetum (bright green reflective area dorsal to the optic disc) are the stars of Winslow. **B.** Contralateral fundus image from the same goat as in Figure 14.8A.

sections. The non-tapetal fundus is dark due to the pigment within the RPE and the lack of a tapetal layer over this portion of the fundus. The non-tapetal fundus is located ventral to the tapetal fundus. The tapetal–non-tapetal junction separates the two fundi. In sheep, the optic nerve head is located within the non-tapetal fundus just ventral to this junction. Sheep (Figure 14.7A, B) have a kidney bean–shaped optic disc, and goats (Figure 14.8A, B) have a rounder optic disc that is often located within the tapetal fundus. Goats also have a pigmented ring that surrounds the optic disc.[40] In deer, the optic nerve head is located within the non-tapetal fundus and is horizontally elongated. The temporal and medial ends of the optic nerve head are wider than the center in this species.[41,42]

The optic nerve is composed of the axons of the retinal ganglion cells. The optic nerve head is located ventrolateral to the posterior pole of the globe. It is myelinated in all species; in sheep, goats, and deer, the myelin is maintained as the fibers enter the globe through the lamina cribrosa. The optic nerve head of sheep and goats has a small dark central depression called the physiologic cup or pit. The orbital portion of the optic nerve is enveloped in the thick dura mater and fuses anteriorly with the sclera. Internal to the dura mater is the arachnoid sheath, and within this layer is the pia mater. Herbivores, including sheep, goats, and deer, exhibit more than 80% decussation at the optic chiasm to form the optic tracts. Each optic tract is composed of pupillary and visual fibers. The pupillary fibers travel to the pretectal nucleus to control the pupillary light reflex (PLR), whereas the visual fibers travel to the lateral geniculate nucleus and then to the visual cortex for visual perception.[1,2]

Ophthalmic Examination

Prior to evaluating or examining an individual animal, or group of animals, it is important to obtain a thorough history. The history should pertain not only to the affected individual animal(s) but also to the remainder of the flock or herd. Important, general information that should be obtained include signalment, husbandry, feeding habits, geographic location, recent addition of any new animals, gestation status, past medical history (prior systemic or ocular diseases), and vaccination and deworming status. Specific information that should be obtained pertaining to the specific ailment of the animal(s) in question include duration of current problem, clinical signs associated with ocular disease, and medications and their frequency of administration for the current disease. Additionally, it is important to ascertain the owner's or flock/herd manager's impression of the animal's specific response to therapy. Responses should be subjectively quantified by assigning a limited-scale of attributes (mild, moderate, and severe), which may result in a more accurate impression of the disease progression and subsequent response to therapy, in many instances.[2]

The initial part of any ophthalmic examination should be devoted to observation of the animal(s) from a distance. If the examination is conducted on the farm, it is advisable to observe the animal in its normal habitat as it interacts with the other animals in the flock or herd. Affected animals should be observed from the front; otherwise, subtle differences between both eyes may go undetected. Unilateral blindness may be compensated for, quite well, despite the lateral globe location in small ruminants. An animal may turn its head excessively in an attempt to focus on an object, using its visual eye, when that object lies within the field of view of the eye with compromised visual acuity. If the examiner still harbors doubts concerning vision, he or she can cover each eye individually for better assessment.[2]

The ophthalmic examination (Box 14.1) can be performed under manual restraint in sheep while they are seated on their rumps; goats can stand for the examination. Deer may be examined in a confined space with minimal and light restraint.[43,44] Before touching the head, the examiner should assess the eyes for symmetry in size and position, note the presence of abnormal ocular discharge, observe the eyelids as they pass over the ocular surface, and record any rubbing, blepharospasm, or other abnormalities. The menace test can be used to evaluate the optic nerve (CN II) and facial nerve (CN VII) for the presence of vision and ability to blink, respectively. If the palpebral fissures do not close completely, a palpebral reflex test should be performed by touching the skin around the eye. This test assesses the function of both the trigeminal nerve (CN V) and facial nerve (CN VII). Both pupils should be assessed for size, shape, and symmetry under both light and dark conditions without direct stimulation. Shining a focal bright light source into one eye allows assessment of the direct PLR. After the response from the stimulated eye is observed, the contralateral eye should be quickly evaluated for the consensual pupillary response. The consensual pupillary response is slower and more incomplete compared with the stimulated eye because of unequal crossover of the optic nerve fibers at the optic chiasm. The PLR is a subcortical response that requires normal function of the retina, optic nerve (CN II), midbrain, oculomotor nerve (CN III), and iris sphincter muscle. Cortically blind animals can have a normal PLR. The dazzle response assesses the visual pathway between the optic nerve and the midbrain. A very bright light source directed toward the eye usually causes a bilateral blink or turning of the head away from the light stimulus. This is a subcortical response that reaches the rostral colliculus and also stimulates the facial nucleus to cause the blink reflex. This test is extremely valuable in assessing the prognosis in an eye following a traumatic incident or in which the posterior segment cannot be visualized.[2]

Abnormalities of the orbit can be assessed by palpation of the bones of the orbital rim for fractures and asymmetry or by skull radiography. Difficulty in retropulsing the globe (manually pushing the globes into the posterior orbit through the closed eyelids) may indicate a retrobulbar space-occupying mass or other orbital disease. Difficulty or pain on opening of the mouth may indicate inflammatory orbital disease. Retrobulbar neoplasia usually does not cause pain on opening of the mouth. The involved orbit or globe should always be compared with the contralateral side. The eyelids should be evaluated for entropion or ectropion, complete closure of the palpebral fissures, increased wetness or ocular discharge on the hair adjacent to the eyelid margins, and distichiasis or trichiasis. The patency of the nasolacrimal apparatus can be assessed by determining whether fluorescein dye passes from the lacrimal lake to the nares after it is placed on the globe. If fluorescein dye is not evident at one or both nares, the examiner can use a 22- or 23-gauge cannula attached to a 5-mL syringe filled with sterile saline solution to irrigate the nasolacrimal ducts in an

• BOX 14.1 List of Instruments and Supplies for Ophthalmic Examination

Instruments

- Direct ophthalmoscope and Finoff transilluminator with rechargeable battery handles
- Indirect condensing lenses (14D, 20D, 28D)
- Panoptic ophthalmoscope
- Bright pocket-sized LED flashlight
- Graefe fixation forceps (nonlocking, third eyelid forceps)
- Applanation (Tono-Pen) or rebound (TonoVet) tonometer with tip covers or single-use probes, respectively

Supplies

- Eyewash
- Tropicamide 1% ophthalmic solution
- Proparacaine 0.5% ophthalmic solution
- Fluorescein and Rose Bengal external dye strips
- Schirmer tear test strips
- 1-mL and 3-mL syringes
- 25-G and 30-G needles
  - For application of topical ophthalmic solutions, the needle should be broken off at the hub.
- Lidocaine 2% local anesthetic solution
- Cytobrush or microbrush (collection of cytology samples)
- Glass slides for preparing cytology specimens
- Culturettes (regular tip and mini tip)
- Gauze pads

orthograde direction. This procedure is performed by first applying topical anesthetic (0.5% proparacaine) to the globe and puncta. The distal blunt end of the cannula is inserted into the superior puncta, and saline solution is injected until fluid is seen to exit the inferior puncta. The cannula is then inserted into the inferior puncta and saline solution is gently injected until fluid is seen exiting the distal naris.[2]

The conjunctiva should not be hyperemic, thickened, or edematous (chemosis). Examination for hemorrhage, foreign bodies (especially beneath the nictitating membrane), and lymphoid follicle hyperplasia should be performed. Samples from the conjunctiva for culture and sensitivity, cytology, immunofluorescent antibody (IFA), and biopsy can be obtained in physically restrained animals after the application of topical anesthetic solution. Fluorescein dye should not be applied before sample collection for IFA because it may result in a false-positive result.[45]

The cornea is examined with a focal light source for clarity. A bluish hue is indicative of edema, white opacities may indicate scarring, a yellow-white color is often associated with white blood cell infiltrate, and red is consistent with neovascularization (this condition is generally more prominent at the limbus). Corneal edema can result from injury to the superficial corneal epithelium or corneal endothelium. Corneal ulcers result in focal corneal edema and positive uptake of fluorescein dye. Fluorescein is a hydrophilic dye that binds exposed corneal stroma, but not epithelium or Descemet's membrane. The slit beam on a direct ophthalmoscope can be used to assess the depth of a corneal ulcer by how deeply the beam is projected on the ulcer. If the ulcer is deep and fluorescein dye uptake is not evident, a descemetocele is likely. A perforated corneal ulcer may have aqueous humor draining from the perforation. The iris may also prolapse through the lesion, and along with fibrin, may occlude the perforation. These ulcers should not be manipulated and minimal diagnostics should be performed because surgical intervention is the treatment of choice.

The anterior chamber is evaluated for clarity and depth. Damage to the blood-aqueous barrier allows protein and cells into the aqueous humor, creating turbidity or the Tyndall effect (aqueous flare). The slit beam or the smallest circle on a direct ophthalmoscope can be used to identify aqueous flare. The beam of light is focused directly on the cornea and then observed at 90 degrees to the direction of the beam as it passes through the anterior chamber. There should be no evidence of light absorption within the anterior chamber. Aqueous flare is seen when protein and cells absorb light and the light beam is reflected in the aqueous humor. Iris bombé and intumescent cataracts can cause the anterior chamber depth to appear decreased, and hypermature cataracts can cause the anterior chamber depth to appear increased.[2,40]

The iris is examined for abnormal shape (dyscoria), color, thickness, miosis, or mydriasis inconsistent with the level of ambient light. Dyscoria can result from lens luxation or subluxation, synechia (adhesions), or a mass caudal to or within the iris. Pupil size should be examined in bright and dim light, and the examiner should determine direct and consensual PLRs. The color and thickness of the iris should be compared with the contralateral side; increased iridal thickness may be obvious in cases of cellular infiltrate and anterior uveitis. The granula iridica should be examined for size and symmetry because severe acute or chronic uveitis can cause them to atrophy (Figure 14.9).[2,40]

Intraocular pressure (IOP) in most species is between 15 and 25 mm Hg. The average IOP values in sheep, goats, and deer are summarized in Table 14.1. IOP can be measured in small ruminants using a Tono-Pen applanation or a TonoVet rebound

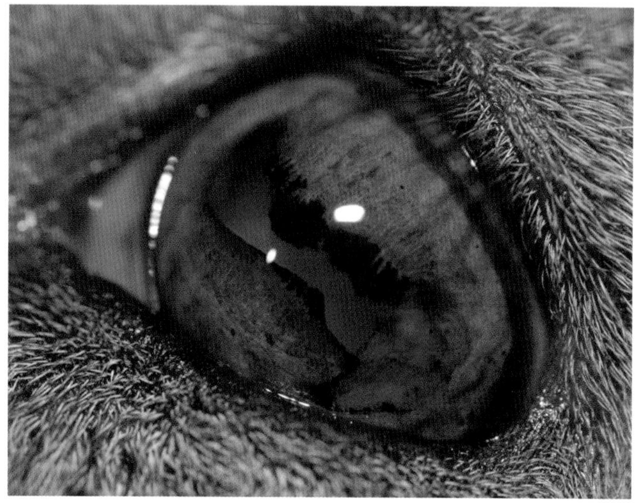

• **Fig. 14.9** Corpora nigra atrophy due to chronic uveitis in a goat. This goat was diagnosed with anterior uveitis of unknown origin. Note the irregular pupil shape (dyscoria) due to posterior synechia (adhesions between the iris and anterior lens capsule) and the fibrin clot within the temporal portion of the anterior chamber.

tonometer. Rebound tonometry using the Tono-Pen is performed by gently tapping the tip of the instrument to the cornea, after the application of a topical anesthetic. The instrument takes a number of readings and then provides the average of those readings in mm Hg. A high reading is consistent with glaucoma. Excessive neck restraint should be avoided during the use of either instrument because this elevates the IOP. Applanation tonometry using the TonoVet tonometer is performed without the use of topical anesthetics. The instrument must be held in the vertical position. The magnetized probe tip is repeatedly projected at the cornea when the examiner depresses the measuring button with their thumb. The IOP is internally calculated by the instrument by evaluating the time required for the probe tip to return to the start position.[46–48]

The lens, vitreous, and fundus are best evaluated through a dilated pupil. The pupil can be dilated with a short-acting topical parasympatholytic such as 1% tropicamide. Time to effect for tropicamide is 10 to 20 minutes, and the effect lasts between 4 and 8 hours.[40] The lens should be evaluated for position and clarity. Nuclear sclerosis is an aging change that does not preclude evaluation of the fundus but must be differentiated from cataracts.

The fundic examination can be performed by either direct or indirect ophthalmoscopy. Direct ophthalmoscopy is performed at a distance of 2 to 3 cm from the patient's eye. The large light circle is used when the pupil is dilated, and the smaller light circles are used when the pupil is not dilated. The instrument is set at either 0 or the red 2 to begin the examination. The numbers are sequentially changed to bring a lesion into focus depending on its location. The disadvantages of direct ophthalmoscopy include the small field of view (approximately 2% of the entire fundus) and difficulty in examining the peripheral fundus. The advantages of direct ophthalmoscopy include greater magnification and the ability to alter the dioptric strength of the ophthalmoscope.[40,49]

Indirect ophthalmoscopy requires a focal light source to be held adjacent to one of the examiner's eyes and an indirect lens (held at arm's length) positioned 2 to 4 cm in front of the patient's eye after the tapetal reflex has been identified. A relatively inexpensive

TABLE 14.1 Intraocular Pressure Values of Small Ruminant Species.[a]

	REBOUND TONOMETRY			APPLANATION TONOMETRY	
Species	Tono-Vet	Tono-Vet-D	Tono-Vet-P	Tono-Pen-XL	Tono-Pen-Avia
[230]**Sheep**					
OS	12.7 ± 3.0				9.8 ± 2.7
OD	11.7 ± 3.3				10.5 ± 2.4
[230]**Goat**					
OS	21.6 ± 5.4				13.0 ± 4.3
OD	24.3 ± 5.6				14.1 ± 4.6
[61]Fallow deer *(Dama dama)*				14.1 ± 2.48	
[61]Mouflons *(Ovis orientalis musimon)*				14.9 ± 2.20	
[61]Ibexes *(Capra ibex)*				13.1 ± 2.43	
[61]Chamois *(Rupicapra rupicapra)*				10.2 ± 2.50	
[46]Adult pygmy goats *(Capra hircus)*					
OS		12.2 ± 1.5	7.9 ± 2.1	10.8 ± 1.8	
OD		11.3 ± 1.4	7.9 ± 1.4	10.8 ± 1.8	
OU		11.8 ± 1.5 (range 9–14)	7.9 ± 1.7 (range 6–12)	10.8 ± 1.7 (range 8–14)	
[16]Barbary sheep or aoudad *(Ammotragus lervia)*			19.5 ± 3.9		
[47]Asian fallow deer *(Dama mesopotamica)*				11.9 ± 3.3	
[47]Eland *(Taurotragus oryx)*				14.6 ± 4.0	
[44] Samba deer *(Rusa unicolor)*				11.4 ± 2.8	
Young animals (<2 years)				(range, 7.5–10.5)	
Adult animal (4–8 years)				(range, 7.5–17.5)	
[43] Brown brocket deer *(Mazama gouazoubira)*				15.3 ± 3.3	
OD				15.1	
OS				15.4	

[a]All values are given in millimeters of mercury (mm Hg). Tono-Vet-D indicates calibrated for the dog, and Tono-Vet-P, unspecific calibration.
OD, Oculus dextra, right eye; *OS*, oculus sinistra, left eye; *OU*, oculus uterque, both eyes.

indirect condensing lens ($50–$75) is effective. The virtual image seen is inverted and reversed. The advantages of using indirect ophthalmoscopy include a larger field of view (approximately 40% of the entire fundus depending on the strength of the lens), which allows the peripheral fundus to be examined more completely, and stereopsis (use of both of the examiner's eyes). Disadvantages include the need for a relatively dilated pupil. Examination in a darkened room and use of a dimmed light source and a 28-diopter lens often allow fundic evaluation without dilation in herbivores through their horizontally oval pupils. Another limitation of indirect ophthalmoscopy is that it requires practice for the examiner to become proficient with the technique. When examining the fundus by indirect ophthalmoscopy, the examiner should move his or her head in the direction that is to be visualized within the fundus. The examiner should have a pattern for examining the fundus beginning with the optic nerve, dividing the fundus into quadrants, and examining each one by evaluating the vessels and color of the tapetal and non-tapetal fundi.[2,40,49]

A viable alternative to both the direct ophthalmoscope and indirect ophthalmoscopy is the PanOptic ophthalmoscope (Welch

Allyn, Inc., Skaneateles Falls, NY). This instrument has the advantage of being used like a direct ophthalmoscope but provides an approximately five times greater field of view. The image appears anatomically correct and the fundus can be examined through a miotic pupil.

Auriculopalpebral Nerve Block

The auriculopalpebral nerve is a branch of the facial nerve and provides motor function to the eyelids.[50] It can be palpated along the dorsal margin of the zygomatic arch. Local anesthesia of the auriculopalpebral nerve results in flaccid eyelids, which facilitates manipulations of the lid and examination of the cornea and conjunctiva, especially in a painful eye. When combined with topical anesthesia (0.5% proparacaine), local anesthesia via the auriculopalpebral nerve block can greatly facilitate additional diagnostic tests and some minor ophthalmic procedures, for example, foreign body removal, corneal or conjunctival sample collection for cytology (Figure 14.10), irrigation of the lacrimal puncta, and subconjunctival injections (Figure 14.11). The auriculopalpebral nerve block is performed by first palpating the nerve over the zygomatic arch and then tenting the skin over the nerve to insert a 22- or 25-gauge needle to the hub (Figure 14.12). A 3-mL syringe with 2% lidocaine or 2% mepivacaine is then attached, and 1 to 1.5 mL of lidocaine is infiltrated subcutaneously around the nerve.[51] Geographic local anesthesia of the eyelids may be useful when performing minor eyelid laceration repairs or for eyelid mass removal. In these situations, a local subcutaneous infiltration of the local anesthetic agent of choice surrounding the area to be treated. Generally, 3 to 4 mL of local anesthetic will provide sufficient analgesia. In small ruminants, the amount of lidocaine 2% used for local anesthetic purposes should remain below the toxic dose (5 mg/kg).[50]

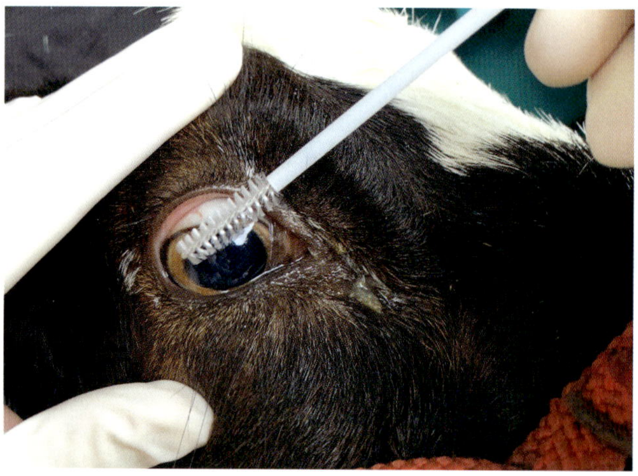

• **Fig. 14.10** Cytology collection using a cytobrush. The examiner maintains contact with the animal using the non-dominant hand to open the eyelid margins.

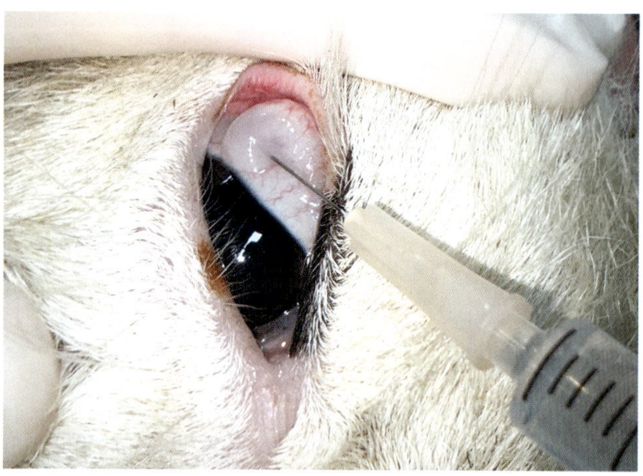

• **Fig. 14.11** The eyelids held open with the examiner's nondominant hand and a 25-gauge needle attached to a 1-mL syringe is used to inject an antibiotic solution into the subconjunctival space.

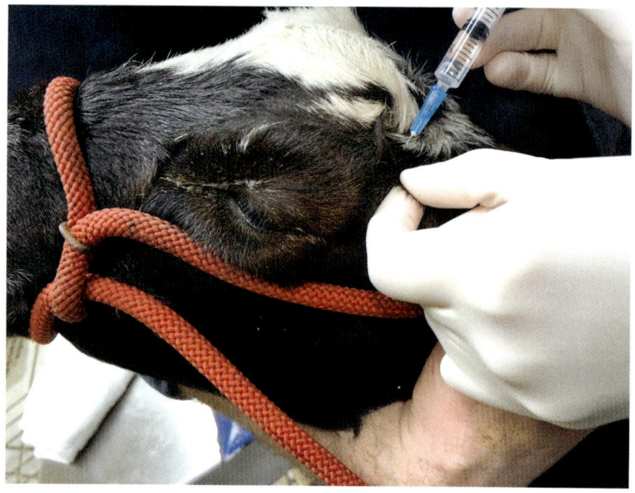

• **Fig. 14.12** Auriculopalpebral nerve block. The auriculopalpebral nerve is palpate over the zygomatic arch. The skin is tented and a 22- or 25-gauge needle is inserted to the hub. 1 to 1.5 mL of lidocaine or mepivacaine is infiltrated subcutaneously around the nerve.

Specialized Diagnostic Tests

Corneoconjunctival Bacterial Culture

Specimens obtained via cotton-tipped applicator or a cytobrush from the conjunctiva, cornea, or third eyelid may be cultured to isolate and identify microorganisms. Aerobic bacterial cultures are valuable for the diagnosis of infectious keratoconjunctivitis in small ruminants. Antibiotic susceptibility testing of bacteria isolated should be used as a guide for therapy.[50]

In clinically normal sheep, 60% of eye swabs were negative for bacterial growth.[52] In sheep, the most commonly isolated bacteria were similar to *Branhamella ovis* (previously *Neisseria ovis*) and were recovered in low numbers. Other frequently isolated organisms were *Micrococcus* and *Streptococcus* species. Less common isolates included *Corynebacterium*, *Acinetobacter*, *Bacillus*, *Staphylococcus*, *Pseudomonas*, *Moraxella*, *Escherichia coli*, and *Pasteurella*.[52–54] In conjunctival swab samples from adult and juvenile goats without ocular disease in the Midwestern United States, *Staphylococcus* and *Streptococcus* spp. were most common. The same study identified age-associated and seasonal variation of bacterial populations and detected the presence of *Moraxella bovoculi* in 40% of adult goats but none of the kids, in which *Staphylococcus equorum* was most commonly identified. These results are similar to previous studies performed in goats.[55,56] The role of *Moraxella* spp. as causative agents of infectious keratoconjunctivitis in small ruminants is not fully understood; however, the bacteria are more frequently isolated from animals with ocular disease than from clinically healthy animals, suggesting either primary or secondary involvement.[57–60] In fallow deer, bacteria were detected in 100% of conjunctival swab samples and were determined to be predominantly gram-positive.[61] Similarly, bacteria were presented in all conjunctival samples of Sambar deer and were predominantly found to be *Staphylococcus* spp. and *Bacillus* spp.[44] A study investigating conjunctival swabs from live-captured and hunter-harvested mule deer detected various gram-positive and gram-negative bacteria including *Staphylococcus* spp. and *Micrococcus* spp. and *Enterobacter* spp., *E. coli*, and *Pseudomonas* spp., respectively, of which some were considered to be environmental contaminants.[62] The same study also identified the presence of *Moraxella bovis* and *Moraxella ovis* in deer without clinical signs of infectious keratoconjuctivits.[62]

Technique. Following the application of topical anesthetic, the upper and lower eyelids are manually retracted and the peripheral edges of the affected conjunctiva or cornea is swabbed using a standard tip or microtip bacterial culturette (e.g., COPAN Transystem swab or BBL CultureSwab, respectively, both made by COPAN Diagnostics, Inc., Corona, CA).[50] Care should be taken to avoid contamination from the palpebral margins. The sample should immediately be placed in the transport tube or plated onto an appropriate growth medium. Corneoconjunctival swabbing ideally should be performed before application of topical anesthetic or fluorescein stain to the eyes. Although topical anesthetic solutions have been reported to have antibacterial effects,[54] culture results obtained from the corneas of 33 dogs, 12 cats, and 19 horses did not differ following the application of saline compared with those obtained following topical anesthesia with 0.5% proparacaine.[63] The additional compliance and post-cytology comfort level of the animal warrant the use of topical anesthesia prior to corneoconjunctival sample collection. Once collected, the sample is submitted to a veterinary microbiology laboratory, with care taken to specify appropriate culture conditions (especially with *Mycoplasma* spp.) for the presumptive clinical diagnosis. Anaerobic bacteria and fungi are rare ocular pathogens in small ruminants.[53] Fungal cultures usually can be obtained using standard culturettes; however, scraping the tissue with a sterile Kimura cytology spatula and placing the sample directly onto fungal culture media may provide even better results.[54]

Corneoconjunctival Cytology

Conjunctival cytologic evaluation is valuable for the diagnosis of infectious keratoconjunctivitis.[50] Corneal cytologic examination is useful in characterizing cellular infiltrates such as bacteria, fungi, and specific types of inflammatory cells. Cell samples obtained from conjunctival scraping also can be submitted for polymerase chain reaction (PCR) testing. Before the procedure is performed, the cornea and conjunctiva should be anesthetized with topical 0.5% proparacaine. An auriculopalpebral nerve block may help to facilitate a quick and efficient sample collection. If conjunctival follicles are present, these areas should be avoided to obtain a more representative sample. Cytologic samples are obtained either by gently scraping the tissue with a spatula or by using a cytobrush (e.g., Care Express Products, Inc., Cary, IL) or regular-size Microbrush (Microbrush International, www.microbrush.com), which is simply rolled over the affected tissue. The cytobrush is inexpensive and very easy to use and creates slides with evenly distributed cells with little crush artifact. Cytologic samples should be very gently rolled or smeared onto a slide and allowed to dry somewhat for 1 or 2 minutes before staining with Diff-Quick, Wright's stain, or Gram stain.[64–68] At least one additional slide should be collected and left unstained for submission to a veterinary clinical pathologist, if required. Viral, mycoplasmal, or chlamydial organisms are poorly identified by Gram staining.[53]

Healthy conjunctiva is characterized cytologically by numerous epithelial cells, occasional lymphocytes, and rare neutrophils. Intracytoplasmic melanin granules may be observed in dark-faced breeds and can be mistaken for bacteria or chlamydial elementary bodies. Goblet cells are more common in animals with subacute to chronic keratoconjunctivitis but can be a normal finding in corneal or conjunctival cytologic preparations. Neutrophils are the predominant cell type seen in acute conjunctivitis, especially of bacterial or viral origin. A few mononuclear cells, multiple bacteria, and degenerating epithelial cells also should be present. Lymphocytes and plasma cells are more typical to chronic infection. Presence of small numbers of eosinophils in otherwise normal sheep probably indicates a local reaction to environmental irritants.[69] A recent study evaluated conjunctival cytology obtained by using a sterile barren interdental brush (Interdental Brush Oral B, Procter & Gamble Brazil, Amazonas, Brazil) from the ventral conjunctival sac of healthy sambar deer *(Rusa unicolor)*.[44] Following sample collection, no macroscopic conjunctival trauma was identified. The conjunctival cytology cell population was characterized by the predominance of columnar epithelial cells containing discrete cytoplasmic pigmentation along with small numbers of squamous pigmented cells and superficial epithelial cells. Additional cells observed were lymphocytes, intact neutrophils, some rare erythrocytes, and bacteria.[44]

Nasolacrimal Irrigation

Signs of nasolacrimal duct obstruction may include moderate to severe epiphora (wet face appearance), especially at the medial eyelid margin (medial canthus), that persists for days to weeks or accumulation of mucus or purulent material, in the absence of obvious ocular lesions or mild conjunctivitis. A presumptive diagnosis of an obstructed nasolacrimal duct is made based on the delayed or absent passage of fluorescein stain from the lacrimal puncta to the nasal punctum (Jones test). Normo-grade irrigation of the nasolacrimal duct is performed after application of a topical anesthetic (0.5% proparacaine). A 5-mL syringe is filled with buffered saline or eyewash solution, and a nasolacrimal cannula or blunted, smooth 20- or 22-gauge stainless steel hypodermic needle is used to cannulate the dorsal and ventral lacrimal puncta, near the medial canthus.[49] Fluorescein stain can be added to the irrigation solution to aid visualization of the fluid passage. In larger patients, a small canine urinary catheter or 3.5F flexible polypropylene catheter (e.g., Tom Cat Catheter, Sherwood Medical Industries, Inc., St. Louis, MO) may be used for normograde and retrograde flushing. In ruminants, the nasal orifice of the nasolacrimal duct is located caudolateral to the alar fold.[8]

Imperforate lacrimal puncta, congenital atresia of the nasal puncta, or agenesis of the distal nasolacrimal duct should be suspected in young animals presented with bilateral nasolacrimal duct obstruction. Surgical intervention and management should follow published guidelines for other ruminants and foals.[49,70]

Treatment Techniques

Cleaning the Eyes and Periocular Tissues

Commercially available eyewash bottles are most appropriate for this purpose. Care must be taken by the examiner to avoid aiming the stream directly at the cornea or holding the bottle tip too close to the surface of the eye, as either may lead to exacerbation of an underlying injury or may directly result in injury to the cornea. Likewise, the tip of the bottle should not touch any ocular or periocular tissues, tear film, mucoid ocular discharge, exudate, or blood owing to the risk of aspirating contaminated fluids back into the eyewash bottle. Mucoid or purulent ocular discharge can be wiped off from the conjunctiva or lid margins with a dry or lightly moistened cotton pad or cotton balls. Gauze pads should not be used around the eyes, as their fibers can easily cause damage to delicate ocular tissues. Care must be taken to avoid contact with the cornea during this process, regardless of the type of materials used.

In preparing periocular tissues before surgery (e.g., tarsorrhaphy, eyelid laceration repair, and third eyelid flap), it is crucial to ensure protection of the globe and avoid causing any additional damage. Application of a sterile artificial tear ointment will help to protect the cornea during general anesthesia. Hair removal near or around the eyes requires particular care and should be done using sharp clipper blades. Repeated lavage using eyewash solution or buffered sterile saline is warranted after clipping to ensure that all hair particles are removed from the ocular surface and conjunctival sac. Povidone-iodine solution (added to sterile saline to obtain a 5% solution) is a useful detergent for periocular skin preparation. Chlorhexidine solutions or scrubs are very irritating to the eye and should be avoided[50] (see Appendix 1).

Topical Medications

Administration of topical eye medications in small ruminants is relatively easy to accomplish when proper restraint has been obtained but can be challenging in a noncooperative animal. In most cases, ophthalmic ointments and solutions can be applied to the eye surface directly from the tube or bottle, respectively. Despite being recommended as an alternative method of application in the past, using a gloved fingertip to smear a ½- to 1-inch strip of ointment across the medial canthus or one of the lid margins not only may result in inadvertent injury, but also, it is a wasteful practice.[71] Use of ophthalmic ointments should be avoided if a deep corneal ulcer or corneal perforation is suspected because such preparations are very irritating to intraocular structures.

Ophthalmic solutions can either be administered directly from the bottle or may be squirted onto the cornea or conjunctiva using a 1-mL syringe with a 26-gauge needle hub (needle broken off after the solution has been drawn up out of the bottle). It is easiest to administer topical ophthalmic solutions or ointments by retracting the eyelids (using the left hand to open the left eyelids and the right hand to open the right eyelids) by placing the index finger on the upper eyelid and the thumb on the lower eyelid (Figure 14.13). The eyelids should be gently retracted (opened) while maintaining constant pressure. Once open, apply the ointment (5-mm strip) or solution (two to three drops) directly to the conjunctiva lining the lower eyelid. A tip to make the application easier is to lightly apply direct pressure to the globe through the upper eyelid with your index finger.

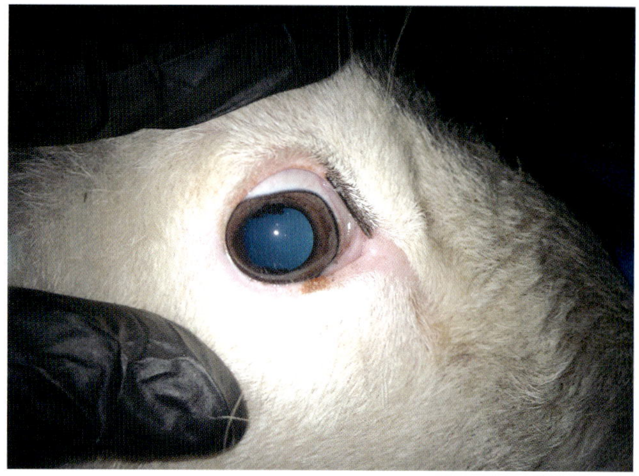

• **Fig. 14.13** Right eye of a young lamb being held open for application of topical ophthalmic medications.

This will push the globe deeper into the orbit, allowing the third eyelid to move across the cornea. The drug can now be applied directly onto the conjunctiva between the third eyelid and lower eyelid. There are two advantages of using this method: (1) the third eyelid blocks the animal's line of sight, so they no longer react (i.e., pull away) to the tube or bottle coming toward their eye; and (2) if contact is made to the tissue with the ointment tube or solution bottle, it will be with the third eyelid and not the cornea, thereby minimizing the risk of inadvertent injury during treatment. Ophthalmic solutions can alternatively be squirted onto the cornea or conjunctiva using a 1-mL syringe with a 26-gauge needle hub (needle broken off after the solution has been drawn up out of the bottle) (Figure 14.14). For this method, the eyelids are held open, as previously described, and the solution is squirted, steadily, but not fast, directly onto the

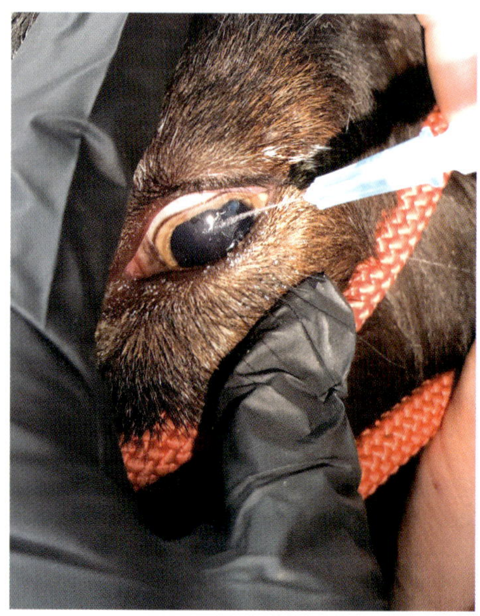

• **Fig. 14.14** Topical ophthalmic solutions being squirted onto the eye using a 1-mL syringe and a 25-gauge needle hub after the needle has been broken off.

cornea from approximately 5 to 10 cm from the eye. This method is generally well tolerated unless excessive pressure is used (rapid application) to squirt the drug onto the cornea, or if the animal is surprised by the stream. This often happens when an attempt is made to squirt the drug onto the eye without manually opening the eyelids. This is not recommended and should be avoided.

The choice of topical eye medication formulation should be based on the specific ocular disease present, product availability, patient demeanor, and ease of treatment for the caretaker. Several ophthalmic medications, either solutions or ointments, are commercially available. Topical ointments have a contact time with the eye of no more than 20 minutes, and even shorter for topical solutions. Ointments are appropriate for eyelid, conjunctival, and corneal disease with no threat of perforation; however, many owners find ointments more difficult to administer, and their use requires a closer proximity to the eye, risking accidental contact with ocular structures. Solutions can be used for eyelid, nasolacrimal, conjunctival, corneal, and anterior intraocular disease. Systemic therapy is required for posterior intraocular disease (chorioretinitis), retrobulbar or orbital disease, severe blepharitis, and severe dacryocystitis. The frequency of topical treatment depends on the specific disease being treated and its severity. A septic corneal ulcer should be treated every 2 to 4 hours; however, prophylactic treatment of a superficial, noninfected corneal ulcer can be appropriately treated every 6 to 8 hours. Anticollagenase drugs for melting corneal ulcers should initially be applied every 1 to 2 hours. In a mild case of uveitis, one dose of atropine may provide mydriasis for several days, whereas in a severe case of uveitis, atropine may be required every 6 hours.[2,49]

Powdered preparations, sprays, insecticides, mastitis preparations, or injectable antibiotics are, in most cases, very irritating to the eyes because of either the carrier type or an acidic or alkaline pH and should be avoided.

Subpalpebral Ocular Lavage System

For safe and reliable delivery of ophthalmic solutions, a single-hole subpalpebral ocular lavage system (SPL) can be a valuable means of providing topical ophthalmic medications. This is especially the case in patients with severe ocular disease requiring frequent medication (q1–q2h), in noncompliant animals, or those with a very painful eye in which direct manipulation and treatment of the eye can be expected to be difficult or uncomfortable.[50] The lavage apparatus is commercially available (Eye Lavage Kit, Mila International, Inc., Erlanger, KY) or can be easily fabricated from polyethylene tubing. Homemade fabrication of an SPL entails cutting a 90-cm-long piece of #190 polyethylene tubing and creating a footplate flange by warming the tube extremity over a match flame until it is softened and then pressing it gently against the flat surface of a scalpel blade.[72]

If necessary, the patient can be sedated before placement of an SPL. An auriculopalpebral nerve block, as previously described, will ease the procedure. The skin at the exit point of the needle tip, in the area of the dorsal to dorsolateral orbital rim, is aseptically prepared and locally anesthetized by infiltrating 2 mL of 2% lidocaine subcutaneously at the site where the needle will exit. Using a 26-gauge needle hub (obtained by breaking off the needle while leaving the hub attached), 0.2 to 0.3 mL of 0.5% proparacaine is sprayed into and across the dorsal conjunctival fornix. If a fabricated SPL is to be used, the lavage tubing is secured into a hub-less needle.

The SPL tubing is attached to a trocar in the commercially available kit. The needle-tubing unit is held in one sterilely gloved hand. To facilitate placement of the trocar through the eyelid while minimizing the risk of iatrogenic injury, a spinal needle catheter sleeve, or the small plastic tube in the Eye Lavage Kit (Mila International, Inc.) can be used as a guide. Not only is the animal's cornea better protected from iatrogenic injury from the trocar, but also the risk of improper placement or inadvertent threading of the SPL tube through the palpebral conjunctiva is all but eliminated. The trocar is then steadily pushed through the fornix of the upper eyelid. Care should be taken to avoid inserting the trocar through the orbital periosteum, as this may result in kinking of the tube, making passage of the medications through the tubing difficult. Once the trocar is approximately 50% exposed through the eyelid, the trocar is grasped in the middle (avoid reaching above the trocar) and the tubing is gently pulled through until the footplate reaches its destination in the dorsal conjunctival fornix. An alternative placement in the lower, medial conjunctival fornix between the eyelid and nictitans has been described in the horse.[73]

Waterproof "butterfly" tape is placed around the tube and sutured to the skin at the lavage exit point from the upper eyelid, to prevent retrograde movement of tubing and footplate and potential damage to the cornea. A 20-gauge, 2-inch intravenous catheter is carefully inserted in the extremity of the polyethylene tubing and then occluded with an injection cap. To avoid tubing damage, the stylet should be retracted 2 to 3 mm from the catheter tip during placement. Additional butterfly suture units are placed along the length of the tubing as needed. To prevent breaks, the remaining free portion of the tubing and catheter is folded (not bent), taped along a wooden tongue depressor or similar light plastic device, and secured to the animal's halter or dorsum. If used to fixate the SPL, the regular halter must be left in place until the ocular condition is improved enough to warrant removal of the SPL.

For each treatment, 0.1 mL of ophthalmic solution is administered through the injection cap of the subpalpebral lavage system. 2 to 3 mL of air should be slowly injected into the catheter following the application of each drug. Care must be taken to avoid rapidly injecting air through the catheter as this will cause significant distress and discomfort to the animal, making subsequent treatments more difficult.

Medications should be given individually as combining some drugs causes precipitates in the tubing[74] and risks diluting the effectiveness of medications. Minor lid swelling can be expected within 48 hours after SPL placement. The swelling must be differentiated with subconjunctival migration of the footplate, which occurs more commonly with small homemade lavage systems, as the footplates are small and firm. Damage to the lavage (e.g., tears and perforations) and loss of the injection cap are common malfunctions associated with the SPL systems. Fortunately, the SPL tubing can be readily spliced using small animal (19- to 21-gauge) intravenous catheters and patience. A tubular stockinette can be placed and fitted around the head of the patient to protect the tubing from getting caught on objects and subsequently torn. Improper placement of the lavage system or loosening of the butterfly sutures can result in corneal ulceration as a consequence of rubbing of the footplate on the cornea. It is therefore essential to check for and correct such technical problems. Loose sutures causing the tubing to slide through the tape butterflies should be repaired immediately, and an improperly placed SPL must be removed and replaced without hesitation in order to avoid severe complications.

Subconjunctival Injections

Subconjunctival injections with antibiotics are meant to provide a drug deposit or an initial high drug concentration locally.[50] They frequently are administered by everting a lid and injecting beneath the palpebral conjunctiva. Depending on the volume injected, a small portion of the drug will leak from the needle tract onto the surface of the eye and mix with the tear film. Local antibiotic concentration may be high initially, but drug persistence over time is expected to be short-lived. Owing to the specifics of eyelid vasculature and lymphatics, the major portion of the injected drug is quickly absorbed into the systemic blood circulation, where it is unavailable for treating the affected globe. Therefore, subconjunctival injections are not recommended for treatment of infectious intraocular diseases in small ruminants.

An alternative and potentially more effective technique consists of injection of nonirritating antibiotics (e.g., procaine penicillin G) under the dorsal or dorsolateral bulbar conjunctiva, using a 25-gauge needle (Figure 14.11). Before injection, proper restraint (physical or chemical), combined with an auriculopalpebral nerve block, is desirable. A few drops of topical ophthalmic anesthetic (e.g., proparacaine) are instilled to improve patient compliance. A total subconjunctival volume of 0.5 mL should be sufficient in most small ruminants. Care must be taken to avoid penetrating the globe; thus, direct visualization of the injection site is essential. Slight hemorrhage at the injection site may occur, and the blood will resorb over a 7- to 10-day period without any long-term consequences. Subconjunctival injection of antibiotics should not be substituted for topical antibiotic administration.[75]

Tarsorrhaphy and Third Eyelid Flap

When protection and support of the cornea are indicated (e.g., with severe corneal ulcer or facial nerve paralysis with subsequent exposure keratitis), a temporary tarsorrhaphy or third eyelid (nictitans) flap procedure can be performed with the use of light sedation, auriculopalpebral nerve block, and topical anesthesia.[50]

Tarsorrhaphy. The placement of a tarsorrhaphy, using horizontal mattress sutures, is useful in cases requiring short-term (a few days to a few weeks) corneal protection.[50,73] Nonabsorbable suture, 3-0 or 4-0, is first placed through a stent (made from a rubber band, intravenous drip set tubing, or button), followed by a partial-thickness bite into the lower eyelid, with the needle entering 3 to 4 mm below the lower eyelid margin and exiting through the center of the eyelid margin through the meibomian gland orifices (Figure 14.15A–C). While the cornea is protected, the suture is continued through the opposite lid margin center and exits the skin in a similar fashion. A second stent is placed, the needle direction is reversed, and the mattress suture is completed by taking a final bite through the lower eyelid stent. Care must be taken to achieve apposition of the lid margins and to avoid inversion (entropion), which could lead to further damage of the cornea. Depending on the size of the palpebral fissure, approximately five to seven horizontal mattress sutures may be necessary to complete the tarsorrhaphy. The lid margins are carefully apposed; then each horizontal mattress is secured in place with surgeons knots. Bow-type knots are not recommended, as they may inadvertently loosen, which may result in significant secondary corneal damage. Care must also be taken to ensure that the knots remain secured. If they come loose, they should be removed or replaced immediately.

Third Eyelid Flap. A third eyelid flap may be used in selected cases of ulcerative keratitis as a temporary ophthalmic bandage.[50] The flap technique is advantageous in that it provides slightly more intimate contact with the cornea than that afforded by a tarsorrhaphy. After administration of a topical anesthetic combined with a local block over the dorsolateral aspect of the upper eyelid, the nictitans is sutured to the dorsolateral fornix of the upper lid with one or two simple interrupted horizontal mattress sutures, with bites spaced accordingly. The preferred suture material is 2-0 or 3-0 nonabsorbable monofilament. In brief, the sutures are preplaced using a curved cutting needle directed through the skin and conjunctiva of the upper eyelid, 1 cm from the lid margin. The upper lid is grasped and pulled away from the globe as the needle is directed out through the palpebral fissure, guarding the cornea. With the third eyelid extended, a partial-thickness horizontal mattress-like bite is taken through the palpebral or front surface of the nictitans, 2 to 3 mm from its free edge. A partial-thickness bite in the cartilage is acceptable so long as it remains on the palpebral surface of the third eyelid. The sutures should not be placed around the base of the T-shaped cartilage or on its caudal or bulbar surface.[72] The suture is completed by passing it back through the palpebral conjunctiva and skin so that the final bite is 2 to 4 mm from the first. An additional suture is preplaced in a similar fashion. Before tying is completed, the sutures are pulled in unison to allow the nictitating membrane to sit as deeply as possible in the dorsal conjunctival fornix, avoiding corneal injury by the suture material. If the flap is to be left in place for several weeks, the sutures should be first placed through stent tubing and tied with surgeons knots, similarly to that just described for tarsorrhaphy. Nonabsorbable sutures should be removed as soon as the ocular disease has resolved.[76]

Tarsorrhaphy and creation of a third eyelid flap are procedures with the primary goal of protecting and supporting the globe.

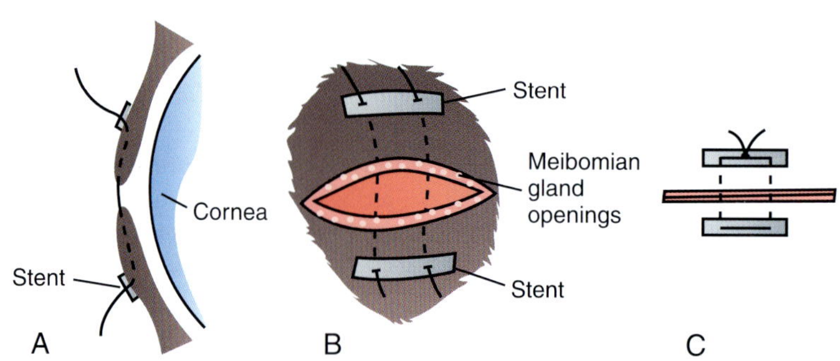

• **Fig. 14.15 A–C.** Placement of temporary tarsorrhaphy sutures and stents.

They should be avoided in cases of melting corneal ulcers, ulcers deeper than three quarters of the corneal stromal thickness, and infected ulcers. Institution of an appropriate primary therapeutic regimen must precede their implementation, and the regimen should continue as needed on the basis of follow-up evaluations.

Housing and Feeding Recommendations

Small ruminants experiencing ocular diseases, regardless of the nature of the condition, must be housed in shaded areas, away from prevailing winds and dusty environments.[50] Ideally, the animals should be fed on the ground. Animals eating hay from an elevated feed trough may further worsen their ocular condition, especially when a deep or melting corneal ulcer is present.

Pathologic Conditions of the Eyelids, Third Eyelid, and Nasolacrimal Duct

Entropion

An inward rolling of the eyelid margin is referred to as entropion. It can affect both the upper and lower eyelids; however, the lower eyelid is more commonly affected. The inward deviation of the eyelid margin allows the eyelashes and/or hairs from the eyelid skin to come in contact with the cornea, thus resulting in significant corneal irritation and discomfort. Entropion is commonly associated with blepharospasm and moderate to severe epiphora. Entropion is a common ocular disease in small ruminants, especially in neonatal lambs.[50,77] In the case of congenital (or primary) entropion, which is relatively common, the lower eyelids are affected bilaterally.[77–81] Secondary (or acquired) entropion may result from trauma, severe dehydration, loss of retrobulbar fat due to emaciation, advanced age, microphthalmia, phthisis bulbi, or painful ocular conditions that cause contraction of the retractor bulbi muscle and blepharospasm.

Clinical Signs. Clinical signs of entropion that may be observed in lambs during the first few weeks of life include blepharospasm, photophobia, rubbing of the eye, epiphora, and keratoconjunctivitis. Epiphora gradually progresses to mucopurulent discharge as the disease progresses and secondary bacterial keratoconjunctivitis develops (Figure 14.16). Secondary entropion is usually unilateral and may affect either the upper or lower eyelid, or both. Animals of any age may be affected by secondary entropion.[2,82]

Treatment. Initial treatment of entropion generally is conservative and involves the administration of topical antibiotic ointments and nonsurgical attempts (e.g., eyelid eversion using temporary "tacking" sutures or Michel-wound-clamps) to evert the affected eyelid(s) (Figure 14.17A–C).[78] Antibiotic ointments should be applied at least every 8 to 12 hours, especially in the early course of the disease. Topical 1% atropine is indicated if severe ocular pain and ciliary spasm are present and should be administered every 12 hours until the pupil is dilated, after which the frequency of administration may be reduced.[76]

Nonsurgical eversion of the affected eyelid may be attempted using a variety of methods, ideally instituted within 48 hours of

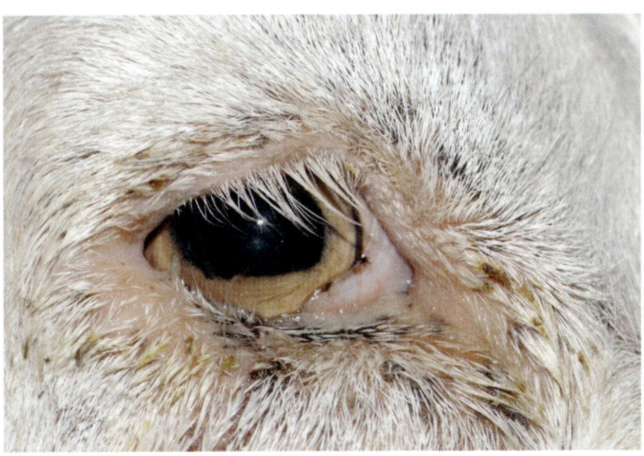

• **Fig. 14.16** Secondary entropion of the right lower eyelid in a goat with keratitis. Note the moderate mucopurulent ocular discharge that developed as a result of chronic corneal irritation and uncontrolled discomfort.

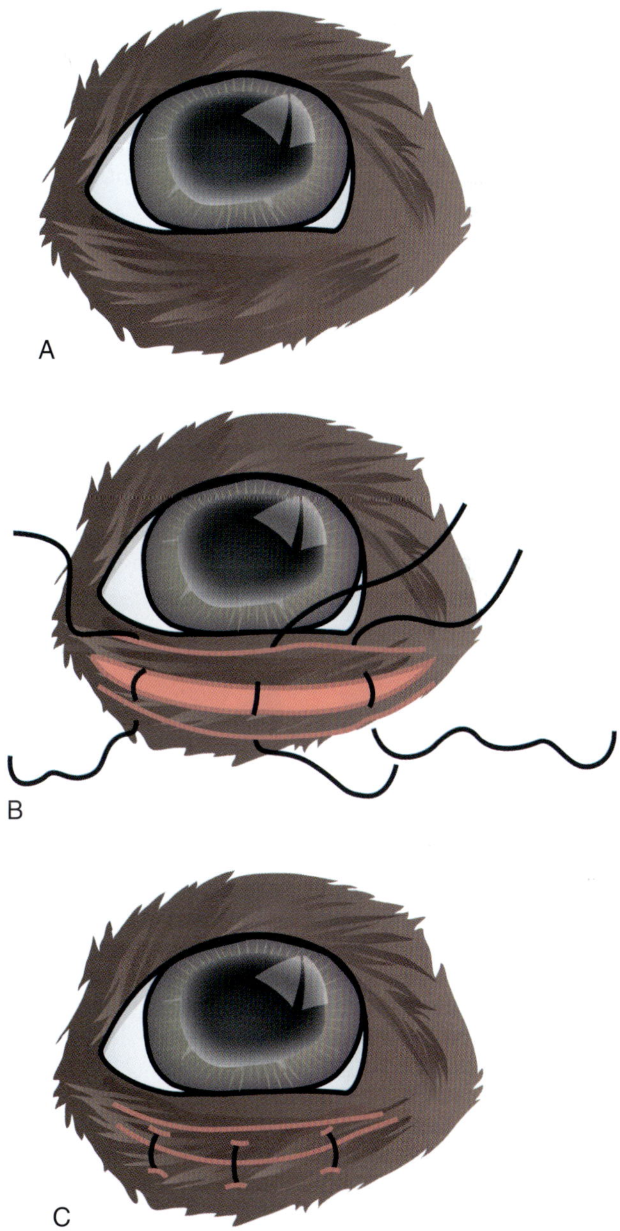

• **Fig. 14.17 A–C.** Nonsurgical correction of entropion in lambs using temporary "tacking" sutures or staples.

birth for best outcome.[2,78–80,82] For economic reasons, entropion in lambs has been treated with subcutaneous injection of benzathine or procaine penicillin to physically alter lid alignment. The injected drug acts as a local irritant that often causes sufficient fibrosis to correct the problem.[80,82] Approximately 1 to 2 mL of penicillin (sufficient to evert the eyelid) is injected in a linear fashion just parallel to the affected eyelid margin.[72] Another method for producing local irritation involves the application of a hemostat on the skin just below and parallel to the eyelid margin for a period of 30 seconds.[82]

Although various correction techniques, including the injection and pinching methods described above, can be successful, the results depend greatly on the frequency and timing of application.[82] Placement of two or three vertical mattress sutures of 2-0 or 3-0 nylon or surgical skin staples (Figure 14.17A–C) is preferred to injection or local irritation techniques by some authors.[50,76,82] Skin staples have the advantage of being easy to apply as well as less traumatic and irritating, with persistence in the tissues for longer than sutures.[83] In most cases, entropion is effectively treated with these nonsurgical methods. Surgical correction should be considered only when temporary eversion techniques have not been successful.[84] Because the condition generally progresses and improves over time, it is strongly recommended to delay permanent surgical correction of entropion to animals of at least 4 to 6 months of age or, ideally, until facial maturity is reached.[83,84]

While suture tacking or wound clip eversion techniques typically resolve entropion in young animals,[72] surgical correction, also referred to as the Celsus-Hotz procedure[85] (Figure 14.18A–D), may be necessary in some cases and is best undertaken with the animal anesthetized and placed in lateral recumbency.[50] After surgical preparation of the area, a crescent-shaped flap of skin is removed from the affected eyelid using a no. 15 scalpel blade. The flap of skin to be removed is first incised 1 to 2 mm distal to the eyelid margin (e.g., at the haired-nonhaired border) and is made 3 to 4 mm wider than the affected area. Placement of a sterile tongue depressor, Jaeger lid plate, or scalpel handle underneath the eyelid in the conjunctival fornix facilitates incision and dissection of the eyelid. A second incision that arcs between the ends of the first incision is made, creating the crescent-shaped skin flap. The skin defect is closed in one layer with a series of small, closely spaced simple interrupted sutures placed perpendicular to the eyelid margins. Closure should begin in the middle of the incision or widest point of the resected tissue and proceed to the edges, to ensure even skin tension across the suture line. Soft, monofilament (nylon), fine (3-0 to 6-0) suture material is recommended. The clinician should take care to tie knots away from the cornea, to prevent irritation. Sutures should be removed in 10 to 14 days. Topical antibiotics should be continued for several days after surgery or until any corneal ulcers have healed. Systemic administration of a nonsteroidal antiinflammatory agent also is indicated to alleviate pain and reduce soft tissue swelling in the postoperative period.[50]

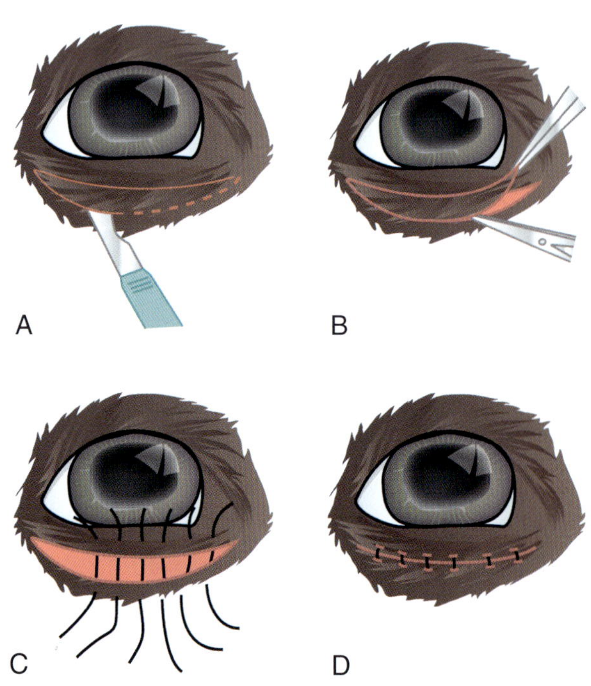

• **Fig. 14.18 A–D.** Celsus-Hotz procedure to correct lower eyelid entropion.

Prevention. Congenital entropion is suspected to be a heritable trait,[86] and affected animals should not be used for breeding purposes.[50] Dusty or windy conditions may contribute to the development of entropion in genetically predisposed animals.[84] The percentage of animals affected by congenital entropion in a flock ranges from 4 to 80%, usually affecting several lambs in the new lamb crop.[87] Female lambs develop entropion more frequently than male lambs do, and the incidence is higher in small pure-bred flocks with only one breeding ram and in breeds with a limited population.[78] By contrast, acquired or secondary entropion normally affects only single animals.[50]

Ectropion

The most common causes of ectropion include iatrogenic overcorrection of entropion and trauma.[50,77,79] Ectropion is relatively rare in small ruminants.[77,79] A congenital upper eyelid eversion has been described in Piebald sheep.[88]

Clinical Signs. Clinical signs of ectropion include drooping of the affected eyelid, epiphora, and exposure keratoconjunctivitis.[50] Some sheep display mild drooping of the eyelids as a normal conformational variation. Mildly affected animals may be predisposed to development of conjunctivitis, but most have no clinical signs of ocular disease.[77]

Treatment. If surgical correction is necessary, a V-to-Y blepharoplasty or eyelid shortening procedure is recommended, using techniques as described for other species.[77,83,85]

Eyelid Trauma

Traumatic injury to the eyelids may result in defects that require surgical reconstruction, especially when involving the lid margins.[50] Minor and major injuries necessitate cleaning, debridement of the wound edges, and primary closure (apposition) of the eyelid tissue. Prompt treatment is essential to avoid distortion, scarring, infection, and loss of eyelid function.[89] Preservation of the eyelid margin is paramount because loss or distortion of this margin may result in inadequate distribution of the precorneal tear film, which may lead to corneal desiccation and fibrosis (scarring) or chronic corneal ulceration. Permanent irritation from disoriented or displaced hairs (trichiasis) may result from eyelid lacerations that are left to heal from second intention or those in which loose eyelid tissue has been excised. The excision of loose or "dangling" eyelid tissue should be avoided, if at all possible.

Surgical preparation must be gentle to prevent further edema. Tissue debridement must be minimal, with freshening of the wound margins (e.g., scraping the laceration edges with a scalpel blade until they are cleaned of obvious debris and exudates), until bleeding is noted.[83] A two-layer tissue closure is recommended. The first layer is in the subcutaneous layer just superficial to the conjunctiva, with care taken not to penetrate the conjunctiva. Braided, absorbable suture (4-0 to 6-0, polyglactin 910) is used to close this layer in a simple continuous pattern. For the second layer, the skin edges are apposed with nonabsorbable (2-0 to 5-0 nylon) sutures in a simple interrupted pattern. A figure-eight suture is ideal at the eyelid margin to provide apposition across the eyelid while keeping the knot away from the lid margin.[89] Topical and systemic antibiotics should be used perioperatively. Standard wound hygiene and application of fly repellent are recommended. The duration of postoperative medical therapy (typically 5–7 days in most patients) varies on a case-by-case basis. Systemic administration of nonsteroidal antiinflammatory drugs and application of warm compress postoperatively may minimize pain and swelling.[83]

Bacterial Blepharitis

Bacterial blepharitis may be caused by *Dermatophilus congolensis*, *Actinobacillus lignieresii*, and *Clostridium novyi*.[2,76,79] *A. lignieresii* infections are characterized by pyogranulomatous nodules with draining tracts. Impression smears of exudate reveal clumps of filamentous gram-negative bacteria and inflammatory cells.[71]

"Bighead" (*C. novyi* infection) usually occurs in rams as a consequence of head trauma during fighting and butting. Affected animals exhibit extensive facial and cervical swelling that may involve the eyelids.[76,79] Blepharoedema may be severe enough to obliterate the palpebral fissure, leading to functional blindness, or may severely impede eyelid function, resulting in exposure keratitis.[79]

Treatment. Prevention of *C. novyi* infection through proper immunization and selective isolation of breeding rams is the most reasonable approach.[2] However, when the disease is diagnosed, systemic antibiotics (e.g., penicillin), antiinflammatory therapy, and supportive treatment for the eyes such as application of topical antibiotic ointments are warranted[79] (see Chapter 16 and Appendix 1).

Viral Blepharitis

Inflammation of the upper and lower eyelids can be associated with numerous pathogens, several of which cause systemic diseases that are likely to affect other body systems. Viral causes of blepharitis in sheep, goats, and cervids include parapoxvirus infections such as contagious ecthyma (orf and sore mouth) and ulcerative dermatosis (lip and leg ulcer), sheep pox and goat pox virus (capripoxiviruses), cervidpoxvirus, and the orbiviruses bluetongue virus and epizootic hemorrhagic disease virus, which are primarily transmitted by *Culicoides* midges (gnats).[2]

Clinical Signs. Lesions of contagious ecthyma are characterized by vesicles or pustules that rapidly progress to proliferative, coalescing, scab-like crusts of the face, especially at the mucocutaneous junctions of the mouth and nose and, less frequently, the eyelids.

Sheep pox virus and goat pox virus are mostly exotic to North America, although goat pox virus has been reported in parts of the United States.[90] The disease affects animals of all ages and causes pyrexia, anorexia, conjunctivitis, rhinitis, and skin lesions on the eyelids. Morbidity and mortality rates are high. The lid lesions first appear as circular (1–3 cm) hyperemic maculas, progress to raised firm papules, and eventually become delicate scabs that can be easily removed.[79] Infections with cervid poxvirus are reported in North American captive and free-ranging cervids with marked cutaneous and, occasionally, systemic signs.[91–94] Clinical signs are similar to those described for sheep and goats, and viral blepharitis and keratoconjunctivitis may occur.

Clinical manifestations of bluetongue are more likely to be observed in sheep than in goats and include blepharitis, blepharoedema, blepharospasm, and conjunctivitis,[77,79] accompanied by pyrexia, oral ulcerations, cyanotic tongue, and abortion in pregnant females. Other ocular lesions associated with this disease include hyperemia and eczema of the adnexal skin and retinal dysplasia.[77]

Treatment and Prevention. There are currently no commercially available ophthalmic antiviral drugs that can be used to treat viral diseases affecting the eyes in veterinary species.[83] Treatment of viral blepharitis in small ruminants is largely symptomatic and involves frequent cleaning of the periocular skin, followed by application of ophthalmic antibiotics to prevent secondary bacterial infection.[77] Symptomatic therapy should include oral or intravenous fluid therapy, systemic or topical nonsteroidal antiinflammatory drugs, and provision of adequate nutrition.

Prevention of viral blepharitis is by strict biosecurity measures, isolation of affected animals, and vaccination if available.

Fungal Blepharitis

Dermatophytosis or ringworm is caused by skin infection with *Microsporum* and *Trichophyton* species. It is uncommon in goats and rare in sheep. Similarly, there are limited reports of clinical dermatophytosis in cervids in the literature.[95–97]

Clinical Signs. Clinical manifestation of dermatophytosis includes facial alopecia and crusting that may affect the eyelids. The lesions often are circular. Pruritus is variable in severity but usually is mild.[2] Young goats are most commonly affected, and cases are most likely to occur during late winter and early spring.[77] Diagnosis may be based on fungal culture, fungal growth on dermatophyte test media (i.e., a DTM plate), and microscopic examination of affected hairs after application of potassium hydroxide (KOH). For fungal cultures, broken hairs at the periphery of the lesions constitute the sample of choice. Dermatophytes are potentially zoonotic, and people should wear gloves when examining and treating infected animals.[2]

Treatment. Fungal blepharitis usually is self-limiting, and most animals recover in the spring with improved pasture conditions. Symptomatic therapy may involve the application of topical antifungal ointments or shampoos.[77]

Parasitic Blepharitis

A variety of ectoparasite infestations can lead to blepharitis either directly through the effects of the parasite itself or indirectly, from the pruritus and consequent self-induced trauma. Chorioptic, psoroptic, or sarcoptic mange may cause intense pruritus but rarely involves only the facial area.[77] Diagnosis is based on clinical signs and confirmed by microscopic examination of skin scrapings. Other external parasites that may cause blepharitis include sheep keds, biting and sucking lice, and ticks.[77,79]

The nematode *Elaeophora schneideri* (arterial worm), a parasite of mule deer and black-tailed deer, may cause disease in small ruminants in the western United States, which has also been described in elk, moose, and white-tailed deer in other areas.[98–101] Following transmission by horseflies, the intermediate host, larval migration, and development result in clinical elaeophoriasis. Larval migration in the leptomeningeal arteries causes ischemic necrosis of brain tissue, resulting in blindness, cerebral signs (see Chapter 13), and sudden death. In surviving animals, lodging of microfilaria in skin capillaries results in clinical signs (sorehead), including facial swelling, blepharospasm, keratoconjunctivitis, alopecia, ulceration, and encrusted lesions of the face. Sorehead most commonly affects adult sheep during the fall and winter.[77,84] Diagnosis is based on consistent presence of clinical signs in animals residing in endemic areas and demonstration of *E. schneideri* microfilaria in skin or conjunctival biopsy specimens.

Treatment. Mite infestations can be treated by ivermectin administration (0.2 mg/kg subcutaneously [SC] at 14-day intervals for two to four treatments), pour-on eprinomectin, insecticide dips, and local application of insecticides as necessary (see Chapter 10). Reported effective treatments for *E. schneideri* infection include piperazine (50 mg/kg PO) and diethylcarbamazine (100 mg/kg PO). The efficacy of ivermectin against this parasite is unknown (see Appendix 1).

Miscellaneous Causes of Blepharitis

Other causes of blepharitis and blepharoedema include photosensitization, solar dermatitis, contact hypersensitivity dermatitis, and cutaneous myiasis.[77,102]

Neoplasia

Neoplasms reported to affect the eyelids of sheep and goats include squamous cell carcinoma, fibroma, fibrosarcoma, melanoma, and papillomatosis.[77,83,102] Pigmented tumors (malignant and benign melanoma, pigmented schwannomas and papillomas) have been reported in red deer *(Cervus elaphus)*[103–105] and fallow deer *(D. dama)*.[106] Involvement of peripheral adjacent lymph nodes or other ocular structures should be determined at time of evaluation. Papillomavirus infection has been documented to cause eyelid warts in sheep and goats.[77,102] Likewise, cutaneous fibromas caused by papillomaviruses are common in cervids, including white-tailed deer and mule deer, and may affect the eyelids.[107,108] In immunocompetent animals, warts generally are fairly benign and self-limiting.

Treatment. Papillomas that interfere with eyelid function or irritate the cornea should be removed.[77] Treatment selection for benign and malignant eyelid neoplasms is determined by the invasiveness of the tumor and its proximity to the eyelid margin and may involve surgical debulking, followed by cryotherapy or local radiofrequency hyperthermia, "block" surgical removal, or CO_2 laser excision. Surgical debulking with adjunct cryotherapy or hyperthermia is a simple, effective, rapid, and affordable approach for use in small ruminants.[50]

Prior to surgical debulking or excision, proper restraint and local anesthesia of the eyelids with 2% lidocaine are recommended.[109] A no. 15 or no. 10 scalpel blade is used to shave as much of the raised portion of abnormal tissue as possible, ideally to the level of the normal skin underneath. If present, significant hemorrhage should be controlled appropriately. In performing cryotherapy, liquid nitrogen is used to freeze the tissues to −30° C at least twice and up to three times, with complete thawing between freeze cycles.[83] A portable nitrous oxide cryotherapy unit with a contact probe is preferred for direct contact with small or pedunculated lesions (less than 5 mm in diameter); however, a spray delivery system with liquid nitrogen may be used with larger, broad-based lesions (greater than 5 mm). Extreme care must be taken to avoid freezing normal ocular and periocular tissues. A piece of Styrofoam cup, shaped according to the area to be protected and coated with sterile ophthalmic lubrication, works well for this purpose.[49,50,83,110] In performing radiofrequency hyperthermia, the surface probes of the unit are used to heat the tissues to 50° C for a period of 30 seconds.[83,111] In horses and cattle with ocular squamous cell carcinoma, the latter technique is not recommended for large tumors (5 cm in diameter or greater) with deep eyelid penetration.[112] Follow-up evaluation is recommended, and retreatment may be necessary in some cases.

Surgical Removal. Selection of the most appropriate surgical approach for en bloc ("block") resection of eyelid neoplasm is based on its size, location, and nature. Surgical resection of small tumors or masses can be performed through an elliptical or tent-shaped incision, as described elsewhere.[72] For removal of larger tumors, a wedge resection or H- or V-to-Y blepharoplasty may be indicated.[83,113] Topical antibiotic ointments should be administered for several days after surgery (see Chapter 10).

No matter which technique is used for treatment of eyelid neoplasms, as much of the tumor as possible should be removed, and margins of the excised tissue should be examined histologically.[50]

Third Eyelid Diseases

Abnormalities of the nictitating membrane are uncommon. Lymphoid follicles of the third eyelid may be very prominent in cases of infectious conjunctivitis, especially if the condition is caused by chlamydial organisms. Carcinomas and adenocarcinomas affecting the third eyelid may be treated by local excision or, preferably, removal of the entire nictitating membrane.[77]

Third eyelid amputation is simple, requiring proper head restraint and use of an auriculopalpebral nerve block coupled with topical anesthetic. In brief, the third eyelid is grasped and fully exteriorized. One or two curved hemostats are clamped across the base of the nictitans, proximal to the lesion. Using a scalpel blade or a sharp pair of scissors, the tissue distal to the hemostat is resected along the clamp. The hemostatic clamps are left in place for at least 2 to 3 minutes for proper hemostasis. If clamps are not used, slight hemorrhage can be anticipated but poses no problem. Closure of the conjunctiva with 5-0 to 6-0 resorbable suture material (polyglactin 910) using a simple continuous pattern will help to prevent secondary orbital infection or seeding of neoplastic cells into the retrobulbar orbit. Microscopic examination of the lesion and its surgical margin is valuable in confirming the diagnosis and establishing a prognosis.[113]

In cases of tetanus (*Clostridium tetani* infection), the third eyelid of affected small ruminants often is prolapsed. Also reported in association with this condition is mild bilateral exophthalmia secondary to retraction of the eyelids.[50]

Thelazia skrjabini was isolated from beneath the asymptomatic nictitating membrane in an adult female white-tailed deer *(Odocoileus virginianus)* in a targeted search for this parasite in a cohort of hunter-killed white-tailed deer and mule deer *(Odocoileus hemionus)* in Alberta, Canada.[114]

Nasolacrimal Duct Disease

Disease of the nasolacrimal duct of sheep most commonly is caused by larvae of the nasal bot *(Oestrus ovis)*. Two species of pharyngeal bot flies (*Pharyngomyia picta* and *Cephenemyia auribarbis*) have been found to parasitize wild red deer *(C. elaphus)* and fallow deer *(D. dama)* in Spain, with *P. picta* larvae being three to six times more prevalent.[115] Normally, the larvae of the nasal botfly mature in the frontal and nasal sinuses until they are sneezed out to complete their life cycle. Occasionally, larvae may aberrantly migrate up the nasolacrimal duct and enter the conjunctival sac, causing local inflammation.

Clinical Signs. Clinical signs of ocular or nasolacrimal infection include epiphora, mucoid or mucopurulent ocular discharge, and conjunctivitis. Affected animals also may exhibit frenzied behavior to avoid adult botflies, stomp, or sneeze and may have a nasal discharge. Finding the larvae in the conjunctival sac is diagnostic.

Treatment. Treatment involves mechanical removal of visible larvae, flushing of the nasolacrimal ducts, and administration of ivermectin (0.2 mg/kg SC). Nasal bot infections are most effectively treated in the fall, when larvae are smaller[77,84] (see Chapter 7 and Appendix 1).

Pathologic Conditions of the Conjunctiva and Cornea

Conjunctival Trauma

Goats, sheep, and cervids have large, prominent eyes that may be traumatized by fencing, feeders, and coarse forage during browsing. Dusty or windy conditions may exacerbate subclinical conjunctivitis.

Clinical Signs. Animals with conjunctival trauma often have conjunctival hyperemia (red and irritated conjunctiva) and/or conjunctival swelling (i.e., chemosis). If the globe appears soft (decreased IOP), the cornea has a wrinkled appearance, or if the anterior chamber is shallow or flat, a scleral or corneal laceration may be present. Careful examination is necessary to prevent further injury. Subconjunctival hemorrhage is often an incidental finding in neonates and is caused by minor trauma during parturition.

Treatment. Uncomplicated cases of conjunctival irritation and minor trauma will likely resolve with a short course (5–7 days) of a topical broad-spectrum antibiotic ointment (e.g., triple antibiotic). The antibiotics are utilized to prevent secondary bacterial infection in addition to providing corneal lubrication.[116]

Corneal Trauma

Corneal trauma has various clinical manifestations and may be caused directly by penetrating foreign bodies or lacerations or from eyelid injuries or neoplasia resulting in secondary ulcerative keratitis. The most common ocular foreign bodies are small particles of plant material that become embedded in the conjunctiva or corneal stroma.

Treatment. Removal of small, superficial foreign bodies is often accomplished with topical anesthesia using 0.5% proparacaine and manual restraint. Initially, small superficial foreign bodies may be dislodged by a strong stream of eye wash aimed directly adjacent to the material to be removed. A thin and powerful stream can be achieved using a 26-gauge needle hub (quickly and repeatedly move the needle back and forth with one hand, while stabilizing the syringe/hub combination with the opposite hand until the needle breaks off at the base of the hub) and 3 mm syringe to spray an exposed edge of the foreign body with a small stream of eye wash. If this method is unsuccessful, an attempt can be made to remove the foreign body using cotton-tipped applicators or ophthalmic forceps. Care must be taken to ensure that the foreign body does not penetrate into the anterior chamber. If that is the case, and the foreign body is dislodged or removed, respectively, aqueous humor may leak from the corneal perforation, putting the eye at risk for further damage to the cornea and secondary intraocular infection (e.g., endophthalmitis). If it is unclear if the foreign body is penetrating or not, referral to an ophthalmologist is recommended.

After foreign body removal, topical broad-spectrum antibiotics should be administered every 6 to 8 hours for several days. Fluorescein dye applied to the corneal surface and evaluated using a cobalt blue filter (direct ophthalmoscope) will confirm corneal reepithelialization (no fluorescein dye uptake can be seen). Nonpenetrating corneal lacerations may be treated as simple corneal ulcers with topical antibiotics and 1% atropine.[116]

Chemical injuries to the cornea and conjunctiva are caused by insecticide dips or sprays, shampoos, disinfectants, or deworming agents inadvertently getting into the eyes. In the case of chemical injuries, immediate lavage with large volumes of isotonic saline or tap water is essential to flush the conjunctival sac and dilute the offending agent. After lavage, the affected eyes should be treated with topical antibiotics (0.1 mL, q4h–q6h) and atropine (0.1 mL q12h–q24h). Additionally, topical autologous serum and/or other anticollagenase preparations such as acetylcysteine, may be beneficial to reduce ongoing corneal degeneration (0.1 mL, q2h–q4h). These lesions may take several weeks to re-epithelialize. Systemic antiinflammatory agents are indicated to control secondary uveitis and to minimize discomfort for the affected animal.[116]

Infectious Keratoconjunctivitis

Infectious keratoconjunctivitis (IKC) (Figure 14.19), also known as "pinkeye," is recognized worldwide as a common contagious disease affecting the eyes of domestic and wild ovids and caprids.[50,117] IKC has also been described as a common disease in Eurasian reindeer *(Rangifer tarandus tarandus)* and has been reported in other deer species, such as mule deer and moose.[59,118–121]

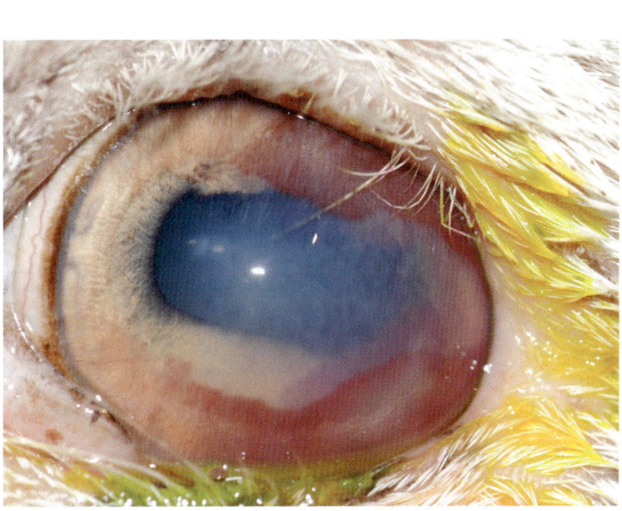

• Fig. 14.19 Keratoconjunctivitis with mild chemosis, epiphora, corneal neovascularization, and secondary (spastic) entropion.

Numerous bacterial agents have been associated with IKC in small ruminants. However, only *Mycoplasma conjunctivae* and *Chlamydophila pecorum* are considered to be the primary etiologic pathogens in sheep and goats.[122–124] In deer, cervid herpesvirus 2 (CvHV2) and other novel herpesviruses appear to be have the greatest role as etiologic agents of IKC.[118,120]

Mycoplasma Keratoconjunctivitis

Mycoplasma species (*M. conjunctivae*, *Mycoplasma mycoides* subsp. *mycoides*, *Mycoplasma capricolum*, *Mycoplasma agalactiae*, and *Mycoplasma arginini*) are important and frequent pathogens causing IKC in domestic sheep and goats (Figure 14.20).[50] Within this group, *M. conjunctivae* appears to be the most commonly isolated pathogen, which has also been associated with disease in free-ranging caprids, in which severe outbreaks have been described.[125] Apparent healthy carriers of *M. conjunctivae* have been described in free-ranging and domestic ovids and caprids, and the pathogen is considered to be endemic in some populations.[126,127] Other clinical syndromes associated with mycoplasmal infection in small ruminants include pleuropneumonia, arthritis, mastitis, and cellulitis.[128]

Clinical Signs. Classic clinical signs of ocular mycoplasmal infections are conjunctival hyperemia, photophobia, blepharospasm, and epiphora, which may become mucopurulent.[50] Clinical signs are commonly observed bilaterally. Corneal neovascularization and opacification beginning at the limbus and central progression may occur in some cases. Occasionally, accompanying conjunctival follicles may be noted. In severely affected animals, findings may include anterior uveitis, corneal ulcers, and temporary or persistent blindness consequent to intense corneal opacity.[117,127,129] Clinical signs of *M. conjunctivae* infection are more common and severe in adult sheep than in lambs.[122,130] Goats are usually less severely affected.[79]

Diagnosis. Diagnosis of mycoplasmal infection is based on clinical signs, IFA staining of conjunctival scrapings, and positive culture of lacrimal secretions, blood, or milk.[77,122] Conjunctival scrapings stained with Giemsa-type stains may reveal basophilic, coccobacillary organisms within the cytoplasm of the epithelial cells (Figure 14.21).[77,122,130] Conjunctival neutrophils, lymphocytes, and plasma cells, as well as necrotic epithelium, also may be observed.[77] Culture results are more likely to be positive when swabs are obtained soon after the onset of clinical signs[130] and placed immediately into *Mycoplasma* transport medium.[122] *M. conjunctivae* also can be detected rapidly with a high level of sensitivity using real-time PCR techniques on conjunctival swab samples.[66]

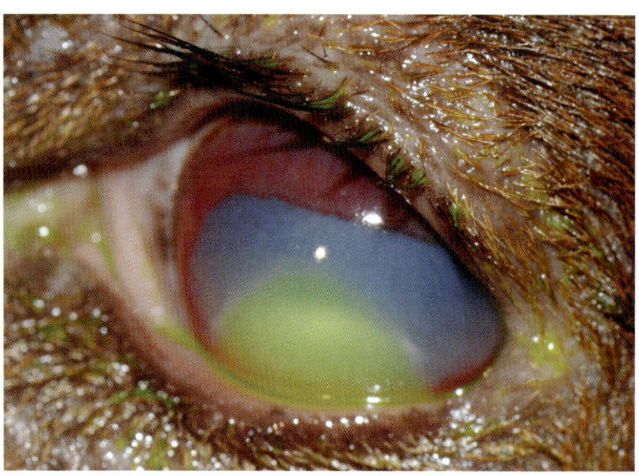

• **Fig. 14.20** *Mycoplasma*-associated keratoconjunctivitis in a goat. Periocular swelling, epiphora, generalized corneal edema with circumlimbal deep corneal neovascularization. Note the fluorescein positive superficial geographic ulcer within the dorsal aspect of the ulcer. This finding indicates an active infectious process.

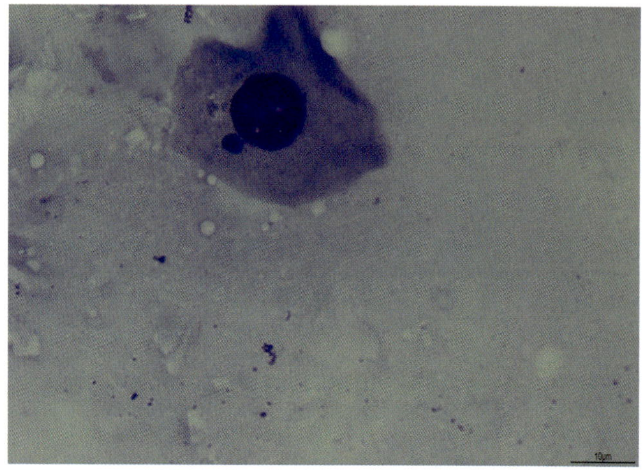

• **Fig. 14.21** Photomicrograph of a conjunctival epithelial cell from the goat in Figure 14.20. Note the basophilic coccobacillary pleomorphic body within the cytoplasm. This finding is consistent with *Mycoplasma* infection. Diff quick, 250× magnification.

Treatment. Many cases of IKC are self-limiting, and the condition may resolve completely within a few weeks without treatment.[131,132] However, immunity to *Mycoplasma*-associated keratoconjunctivitis is poor, and relapses in individual animals and recurrence of outbreaks in flocks are common. The disease can be spread to other flocks or herds by clinically healthy animals, because the organism can persist in the ocular and nasal secretions for 3 to 6 months after apparent clinical recovery from the disease.[122,133] Both systemic and topical antibiotic therapeutic strategies have been proposed, and both may accelerate the recovery period of affected animals.[134,135] Systemic tylosin, oxytetracycline (10–20 mg/kg intramuscularly [IM] or SC), chlortetracycline (80 mg/head/day in the feed), and streptomycin have been found to be effective in vitro against isolates taken from sheep.[135] Topical tetracycline alone (applied at least once a day for 5 or 6 consecutive days)[130] or combined with polymyxin B[134] also is reported to be effective, especially when clinical signs are restricted to the conjunctiva. Subconjunctival administration of oxytetracycline is not recommended because it may cause a severe local inflammatory reaction.[50] If anterior uveitis also is present, atropine sulfate ointments are indicated. A single intramuscular injection of oxytetracycline in lambs experimentally infected with *M. conjunctivae* was successful in improving clinical eye scores; however, it did not clear the bacteria from the ocular secretion.[136] In the face of an outbreak of IKC, the prophylactic use of long-acting oxytetracycline (20 mg/kg every 72 hours IM or SC) may prevent the appearance of clinical signs in other members of the herd or flock[130] (see Appendix 1).

Prevention. Affected animals should be isolated to prevent the spread of disease. Affected herds or flocks often have a history of a recent introduction of new members that were subclinical carriers of *M. conjunctivae*.[122,130] The infection is spread by direct contact with infective ocular secretions, fomites, and face flies.[77,130] Isolation and prophylactic treatment of new addition to the herd or flock have been recommended[77,130] (see Chapters 7 and 16).

Chlamydophila Keratoconjunctivitis

Chlamydophila abortus and *C. pecorum* are two species of the genus *Chlamydophila* (formerly *Chlamydia*) that cause diseases in sheep and goats.[50] Infection with and circulation of *Chlamydophila* spp. has also been reported in different cervine species, but their role as a pathogen is not clear.[137–139] *C. abortus* has affinity for the reproductive tract and represents an important cause of abortion and orchitis in small ruminants.[123] *C. pecorum* commonly is isolated from the digestive tract of ruminants and has been determined to be the cause of keratoconjunctivitis and polyarthritis outbreaks, predominantly in sheep flocks.[53,77,123]

Clinical Signs. Initial ocular manifestations of *Chlamydophila* infection include epiphora, conjunctival hyperemia, and chemosis.[50] As the condition progresses, ocular discharge progresses from mucoid to purulent, inflammation spreads from sclera onto the cornea resulting in corneal neovascularization, and follicle formation in the conjunctiva becomes prominent, which may become chronic.[140,141] Corneal ulceration can occur but is uncommon.[140] Lymphoid follicles appear initially as small, discrete, pale, elevated areas in the conjunctiva that gradually enlarge and coalesce to form pink to red folds in the lower conjunctival fornix. They can protrude as much as 8 to 10 mm to fill the conjunctival fornix and become confluent with the follicles on the surface of the nictitating membrane.[140] Most keratoconjunctivitis cases (approximately 80%) show bilateral and symmetrical lesions.[53,77,140] Clinical signs are generally more severe in lambs compared to adults. Despite the high morbidity (as many as 90% of a lamb crop may become infected), the mortality rate is generally low.[50,53,77] In case of a keratoconjunctivitis outbreak, approximately 25% of affected animals are expected to develop polyarthritis.[142] Due to the similarity in clinical signs, infection caused by *Chlamydophila* in small ruminants can be indistinguishable from that caused by *M. conjunctivae*.[53]

Diagnosis. Early in the disease, microscopic examination of conjunctival scrapings reveals numerous neutrophils with some lymphocytes and plasma cells.[140] Intracytoplasmic chlamydophilic inclusions are basophilic (on Giemsa staining), usually juxtanuclear, and may be found in approximately a third of eye scrapings.[77,122,140,142] Their presence can also be confirmed by IFA testing.[123] The organisms can be cultured from conjunctival scrapings or blood sampled from sheep with keratoconjunctivitis and polyarthritis.[142,143] Organisms are more likely to be found using culture or cytologic methods early in the disease process.[130,144] PCR testing may be used for screening and confirmatory testing.[61,145]

Serologic studies using the complement fixation test (CFT) or enzyme-linked immunosorbent assay (ELISA) assays may also be used to diagnose *Chlamydophila* infection in small ruminants. A four-fold or greater rise between titers in acute and convalescent serum samples (taken 2 weeks apart) identified by CFT may confirm the diagnosis.[122]

Treatment and Prevention. Treatment of *Chlamydophila* infection is as described for mycoplasmal infections. Long-acting systemic and topical tetracycline is reportedly effective.[50,77,122] Parenteral antibiotics should be considered for lambs with *Chlamydophila*-induced keratoconjunctivitis, particularly because of the possibility of polyarthritis as a sequela.[122] To reduce the incidence and severity of clinical disease associated with *Chlamydophila* outbreaks, a recommended regimen is administration of 150 to 200 mg of tetracycline/head/day in the feed.[123] In uncomplicated cases, the disease usually is self-limiting, and recovery can be expected within 2 to 3 weeks[77,140] (see Appendix 1).

Transmission is by direct contact with infective secretions, especially in closely confined animals,[123] and indirectly by insects.[77,140] Recovered animals may shed *C. pecorum* in tears and nasal secretions for several months after the resolution of clinical signs.[77,122] In 8- to 10-month-old lambs, a degree of resistance appears to develop.[140]

Two commercial vaccine products based on a live attenuated temperature-sensitive mutant strain of *C. abortus* are licensed for sheep and goats in several countries. However, there is evidence to suggest that the 1B vaccine strain has been transmitted from vaccinated to naïve animals, causing disease.[146] In the United States, a *Chlamydia psittaci* bacterin is commercially available for aid in the control of ovine enzootic abortion, but its efficacy in preventing keratoconjunctivitis is unknown.

Moraxella ovis Keratoconjunctivitis

The role of *Moraxella ovis* (previously *Branhamella ovis*) as a causative agent for IKC in small ruminants is still unclear. As described earlier, *Moraxella* spp. are often cultured from small ruminants with IKC, but in some reports are isolated as frequently from unaffected animals.[57,147,148] Experimental infection with *Moraxella ovis* did not induce keratoconjunctivitis, even after previous scarification of the cornea,[149] but it is possible that other factors such as strain-specific virulence or coinfection with other pathogens increases the pathogenicity of *Moraxella* spp. *Moraxella ovis* may be opportunistic pathogens contributing to infections by other organisms such as *M. conjunctivae* and *C. pecorum* or may increase the severity of disease.[150–152]

Animals of all ages are susceptible, with those younger than 1 year of age most commonly affected.[151] In clinical cases, bilateral conjunctivitis, epiphora, injected scleral blood vessels, photophobia, and corneal neovascularization occur.[77,150,153] In one report, affected goats also developed 0.5- to 1-mm raised transparent conjunctival follicles.[153] Keratitis is not a common finding of *Moraxella ovis* and may occur only in severe cases.[77,153]

Diagnosis. A predominance of gram negative diplococci on Gram staining of conjunctival scrapings is suggestive of *Moraxella ovis* infection; however, bacterial culture should be used to confirm the diagnosis.[50,150]

Treatment. Affected animals should be treated using parental or topical antibiotics, especially to avoid exacerbation of lesions caused by coinfecting bacteria.[151,154] While *Moraxella* spp. can be treated successfully with a variety of antibiotics, there are differences in antimicrobial susceptibility, and some *Moraxella ovis* may be resistant to oxytetracycline and penicillin.[154] Affected animals should be treated with systemic antibiotics for several days using either long-acting antibiotics such as florfenicol or oxytetracycline or, more frequently, topical antibiotics or short-acting systemic antibiotics (ampicillin or ceftiofur). In one report, injection of procaine penicillin G under the bulbar conjunctiva was successful in treating affected goats.[153] Animals without corneal involvement recover within 48 hours.[150]

Acholeplasma oculi Conjunctivitis

A. oculi has been described as an infrequent ocular and mammary pathogen in sheep and goats.[155–157] Clinical signs of ocular disease include conjunctivitis, keratitis, blepharospasm, epiphora, and pannus.[155,156] Treatment with systemic or topical oxytetracycline may be appropriate in affected animals.

Listerial Keratoconjunctivitis and Uveitis (Silage Eye)

Listeria monocytogenes, the causative organism of listerial encephalitis, septicemia, and abortion, is occasionally associated with ocular disease in small ruminants.[57,158,159] Keratoconjunctivitis and anterior uveitis caused by *L. monocytogenes* infection are associated with the feed of silage, especially baled silage and silage fed in ring feeders, prompting the term "silage eye."[160] The pathogenesis of the disease is poorly understood, but direct exposure of the eye to silage under these feeding conditions is believed to facilitate infection.

Clinical Signs and Diagnosis. Ocular disease is typically not associated with other clinical signs of listeriosis such as neurologic disease or systemic illness. Lesions may be unilateral or bilateral, and clinical signs include catarrhal conjunctivitis, miosis, blepharospasm, moderate to severe ophthalmitis with hypopyon and iridocyclitis, and corneal edema. Bacterial culture or molecular detection of *L. monocytogenes* is used to confirm the diagnosis.[160]

Treatment and Prevention. Successful therapy can be achieved using systemic and/or topical antibiotics and steroids. In one report, topical ophthalmic oxytetracycline alone was ineffective, but when it was combined with parenteral administration of ampicillin, resolution was obtained within 2 weeks of therapy, with no residual corneal scarring.[161] Proper preparation of silage, limiting contact of eyes with silage by changing feed design, and ensuring good nutritional status and housing conditions have been recommended to prevent silage eye.[160]

General Considerations in Management of Bacterial Keratoconjunctivitis

Treatment Options. Most of the bacterial ocular pathogens of small ruminants are susceptible to tetracycline.[50] Combination therapy with long-acting injectable tetracycline (20 mg/kg IM or SC every 72 hours) and an ophthalmic preparation of tetracycline (every 6–8 hours) usually is effective for most bacterial infections.[75] Topical ointments generally are preferred to solutions because of their prolonged contact time and because less drug is likely to be lost in ocular secretions. Subconjunctival injection of antibiotics may be used to achieve initial high concentrations of the therapeutic agent but should not be considered a substitute for application of topical antibiotics.[75] Third eyelid flaps may be used in some cases of ulcerative keratitis as a temporary ophthalmic bandage. In the presence of overt ulcerative keratitis and anterior uveitis, atropine sulfate ointments are recommended. Steroids are contraindicated in cases of corneal ulceration and should be avoided until corneal reepithelialization has occurred.[79]

Removal of ocular discharge is important to prevent blepharitis, periocular dermatitis, and formation of adhesions between the upper and lower lids and to improve the penetration and bioavailability of ophthalmic medications. Removal of exudates or crusts with moistened cotton or gauze, flushing with commercial eye cleaning solutions, and "warm packing" of the eyelids not only improves the patient's comfort but also represent useful and inexpensive add-on therapies for most conjunctival diseases.[50]

Control and Prevention. In epizootic cases of suspected bacterial keratoconjunctivitis, several control measures have been suggested to reduce the spread of disease.[76] Infected animals and animals in direct contact with them should be completely isolated from the rest of the herd or flock for at least 2 weeks, or longer (3–4 weeks) if possible.[50] While in quarantine, clinically affected and exposed animals should be treated and carefully monitored on a daily basis for clinical signs of ocular disease, respectively.

Exposure to environmental irritants such as flies, dust, pollen, and wind should be avoided. Pastures should be mowed to eliminate long-stemmed or rough weeds and grasses. Contaminated stall bedding should be removed, and water troughs and feeders should be cleaned and disinfected. Affected animals may have visual deficits and should either be confined or kept near readily accessible feed and water sources.[50]

Viral Keratoconjunctivitis

CvHV2 has been identified by experimental infection and epidemiologic studies as a primary cause of keratoconjunctivitis in young Eurasian reindeer.[59,162] The disease is characterized by increased lacrimation initially, followed by conjunctivitis and periorbital and corneal edema. In some affected animals, the disease can progress in severity, with the development of corneal ulceration and panophthalmitis leading to permanent blindness.[162] Other alpha- and gammaherpesviruses have been implicated as possible causes of viral keratoconjunctivitis in farmed and free-ranging cervids,[120,163,164] but the role of these pathogens as etiologic agents of cervine ocular disease is less well understood.

As in cattle, malignant catarrhal fever caused by ovine, caprine, or alcelaphine gammaherpesvirus can cause ocular disease in affected deer. Reported eye lesions include conjunctivitis, corneal opacity, and fibrin clots in the anterior eye chamber,[165] accompanied by other systemic clinical signs.

Viral keratoconjunctivitis has been rarely reported in sheep and goats. Severe conjunctivitis, keratoconus, corneal opacification, and blindness were reported in two goats naturally infected with infectious bovine rhinotracheitis virus. The virus was isolated from the nasal secretions of both goats. The goats exhibited clinical signs of respiratory tract disease before ocular involvement was noted, and both recovered.[166] Bluetongue virus infection may cause conjunctivitis, blepharitis, and blepharoedema in sheep[79,167,168] Conjunctival edema and hyperemia are also features in infection of cervids with epizootic hemorrhagic disease virus, a closely related orbivirus.[169]

Mycotic Keratitis

Mycotic keratitis appears to be rare in small ruminants.[79] If fungal elements are cultured or observed in conjunctival scrapings, their presence as possible environmental contaminants should be carefully considered.[50] Fungal cultures should be performed in animals with chronic keratitis, plaque-like corneal growths, or severe keratomalacia, especially if antibiotic and steroidal therapy had been previously administered.[170]

Treatment. Treatment involves the application of topical antifungal agents, such as natamycin, miconazole, itraconazole–dimethyl sulfoxide (DMSO), ketoconazole, or fluconazole.[50] Use of topical miconazole usually is the most cost-effective regimen, and application every 4 to 6 hours is recommended. Superficial keratectomy can be used for both therapeutic and diagnostic purposes.[50]

Parasitic Keratitis

Thelazia californiensis, the eye worm, causes infection in many warm-blooded animals in North America and can be detected in free-ranging deer at high prevalence rates.[62,171] *Thelazia rhodesii* is a parasite of small ruminants in Europe, Asia, and Africa. The nematodes are small, 7 to 18 mm long, and are found in the conjunctival fornix, particularly behind the third eyelid.[79] Infrequently, they may invade the nasolacrimal system. Development of clinical signs of is uncommon.[84,172] Such signs, if present, may include epiphora, conjunctivitis, and subtle blepharospasm in mild cases. With more severe infestation, corneal edema, ulceration, and neovascularization may occur.[172] *O. ovis* larvae can aberrantly migrate into the conjunctiva or nasolacrimal duct of sheep, causing epiphora and conjunctivitis.[84] Keratoconjunctivitis, blepharospasm, and blepharoedema may occur in small ruminants as manifestations of *E. schneideri* infection.[84]

Treatment. *Thelazia* infestation can be removed by irrigation with sterile saline after the application of topical anesthetics.[79] Topical application of an avermectin (e.g., one to two drops of 1% moxidectin for injection) or systemic treatment with avermectins or levamisole should be therapeutic.[170] Face flies and other *Musca* species are intermediate hosts for the parasite, so fly control is essential for reducing the prevalence of infections.[50] Therapy for *O. ovis* and *E. schneideri* is described further on under "Pathologic Conditions of the Eyelid".

Exposure Keratitis

Various etiologies such as listeriosis, otitis media or interna, or trauma can result in facial nerve paralysis or paresis, reducing the ability to blink normally, leading to secondary exposure-related keratoconjunctivitis sicca. This condition can also be caused by locoweed (*Astragalus* and *Oxytropis* species) toxicity, which causes paralysis of the palpebral nerve.[84] Locoweed toxicity also causes marked cytoplasmic vacuolization of the lacrimal gland secretory epithelium. The resultant decrease in tear production further contributes to keratoconjunctivitis sicca, leading to a "dull-eyed" appearance in some affected animals.[173]

Conjunctival Manifestations of Systemic Diseases

The conjunctival membranes are very accessible to physical inspection during an examination and may provide diagnostic clues to many ongoing systemic diseases.[50] Extreme pallor of the conjunctiva may be used for clinical identification of anemic sheep and goats secondary to *Haemonchus contortus* infestation. The severity of the anemia can be scored according to the FAMACHA eye color chart[174] (see Chapters 6 and 16).

Yellow coloration of the conjunctiva and sclera (e.g., icterus) accompanied by weakness, possibly progressing to death, in small ruminants may be due to hemolytic diseases such as copper toxicity, eperythrozoonosis *(Mycoplasma ovis)*, anaplasmosis *(Anaplasma ovis)*, leptospirosis (*Leptospira interrogans* serovar pomona or icterohaemorrhagiae), bacillary hemoglobinuria *(Clostridium haemolyticum)*, and piroplasmosis *(Babesia ovis)*, the last being exotic to the Americas.[50] Icterus also may be a feature of liver diseases such as pyrrolizidine alkaloid toxicity, liver fluke infestation, and infectious hepatitis (e.g., black disease).[50]

Hemorrhages in the conjunctiva are most likely to be traumatic in origin, especially if unilateral. Petechiae or ecchymoses may be observed in patients suffering from gram negative sepsis (as in neonates), severe thrombocytopenia, or warfarin toxicity.[175]

Miscellaneous Disorders of the Eye

Dermoids (choristomas) are ectopic patches of epidermal tissue and can be found on the conjunctiva, limbus, and cornea.[50] Only rare reports exist in small ruminants.[176,177] Dermoids affecting the conjunctiva or palpebral mucosae often are easily removed by sharp dissection with use of topical or regional anesthesia. Corneal dermoids can be surgically removed through a superficial lamellar keratectomy. Regeneration can occur if the entire lesion is not removed.[178] Referral to an ophthalmologist for patients showing regrowth of the lesion is recommended.

Pathologic Conditions of the Uveal Tract and Lens

Uveitis

Clinical Signs. Clinical signs of uveitis may include miosis, photophobia, iris hyperemia, aqueous flare, hypopyon, hyphema, blindness, and fibrin deposition within the anterior chamber (Figure 14.9).[2,40,76,77,79,179]

Aqueous flare (hazy cloudiness of the aqueous humor) is due to breakdown of the blood-aqueous barrier with increased permeability of vessels in the iris and ciliary body, allowing small proteins to pass in the aqueous humor.[83] Hypopyon is due to accumulation of white blood cells, leading to formation of a thick, white layer in the ventral anterior chamber.

Uveitis frequently develops secondary to bacteremia or septicemia and is often observed in neonates with failure of passive transfer.[175] The causative organism usually gains access to the bloodstream through the umbilicus or the gastrointestinal tract if enteritis is present. A thorough physical examination is indicated to identify the origin of the foci of infection and to determine if it has extended to other organs (joints, meninges, and lungs).[175]

Mycoplasma spp. often causes septicemia and systemic disease (pneumonia, mastitis, and polyarthritis) in both neonates and adult animals. The bacterium has been isolated from goats with keratoconjunctivitis and associated iritis.[132] In young goats, *Mycoplasma* infection may result in development of bilateral uveitis with miosis, aqueous flare, and fibrin deposition in the anterior chamber accompanied by polyarthritis.[132] *L. monocytogenes* infections can result in septicemia in 4- to 6-month-old feedlot lambs fed silage-based rations. The affected animals may exhibit clinical signs of uveitis, conjunctivitis, and endophthalmitis, as well as CN deficits.[77,79,84] *E. schneideri* infection ("sorehead") can cause uveitis; however, blepharitis and conjunctivitis are more likely to occur as a result of infection with this bloodborne parasite.[79]

The intracellular protozoan *Toxoplasma gondii* is an uncommon cause of anterior uveitis in small ruminants.[84] In sheep, ocular toxoplasmosis results in nonsuppurative iridocyclitis, involving the iris, ciliary body, and retina.[180] Sheep infected with *Trypanosoma brucei* (an exotic species in the United States) may develop significant keratoconjunctivitis, which is associated with corneal edema and inflammation of the eyelids and panuveitis. Histopathology confirmed a nonpurulent panophthalmitis associated with fibrinous and mononuclear exudate in both the aqueous and vitreous humors, iridocyclitis, choroiditis, retinitis, optic neuritis, and ocular myositis.[181]

Diagnosis and Treatment. The goals of uveitis treatment are to suppress the intraocular inflammation, prevent synechia (adhesions between the iris and cornea [anterior synechia] or between the iris and the anterior lens capsule [posterior synechia]) formation, and identify and treat the underlying cause of the disease. Topical and systemic antiinflammatory drugs (topical corticosteroids [e.g., prednisolone acetate 1% or dexamethasone 0.1%] and systemic nonsteroidal antiinflammatory drugs) are very effective at suppressing intraocular inflammation. Topical atropine is used to prevent synechia formation, to decrease pain by paralyzing ciliary muscle spasm, and to help stabilize the blood-aqueous barrier. Appropriate topical and systemic antibiotics are indicated based on the underlying cause. In septicemic neonates, results of blood culture and sensitivity testing are valuable to determine if antimicrobial agents are indicated. Correction of total or partial failure of passive transfer and use of supportive therapy (e.g., intravenous fluids) are also strongly recommended.[175] Culture of ocular secretions or blood may identify pathogenic *Mycoplasma* or *Listeria* species. Mycoplasmas usually are susceptible to tetracycline, erythromycin, and tylosin.[77,79] Penicillin, tetracycline, or florfenicol generally are effective against *L. monocytogenes*.

Piperazine (50 mg/kg PO) and diethylcarbamazine (100 mg/kg PO) have been reported to be effective treatments against *E. schneideri* infection.[182] Systemic pyrimethamine and sulfadiazine, in combination with topical 10% sulfacetamide, atropine, and steroid ointments, may be effective against ocular toxoplasmosis[79] (see Appendix 1).

Diseases of the Lens

Cataracts. Cataracts are the most common lens abnormality in small ruminants. The majority of cataracts in young animals are suspected to be hereditary.[84] Any opacity in the lens theoretically constitutes a cataract. However, a change associated with aging in the lens that results in a cloudy appearance that does not obstruct visualization of the animal's retina is referred to as nuclear sclerosis. Nuclear sclerosis is a result of compression of the oldest and most central lens material. Cataracts are characterized based on their appearance, anatomical location, and size. The smallest cataracts (less than 5% of the total lens volume) are referred to as incipient. Immature cataracts make up the largest category and range from early immature (6–99%) (Figure 14.22) to late immature (51–99%). Mature cataracts involve the entire lens and are generally bright white in color. After a cataract reaches the mature stage, if it continues to progress, its cortical fibers begin to undergo liquefaction. At this stage, the lens capsule becomes wrinkled and capsular plaques form on the anterior and posterior aspects.[183] Cataracts with an autosomal dominant inheritance have been described in New Zealand Romney sheep.[184] The cataracts were bilateral and the majority of them developed between 2 and 4 months of age; however, some lambs were affected at birth. Congenital, nonprogressive nuclear cataracts that did not result in obvious visual deficits have been observed in sheep and goats.[179] Incipient cataracts and confirmed diabetes mellitus have been reported in twin male lambs.[185] Cataracts also may occur as sequelae to ocular trauma and severe uveitis.[84,179] Any animal with uveitis may develop secondary cataracts, especially in cases of chronic, persistent disease. Septicemia caused by organisms such as *M. agalactiae* can result in uveitis-induced cataracts.[84,179] Intraocular *E. schneideri* infection may cause significant posterior synechia that leads to cataract formation.[186]

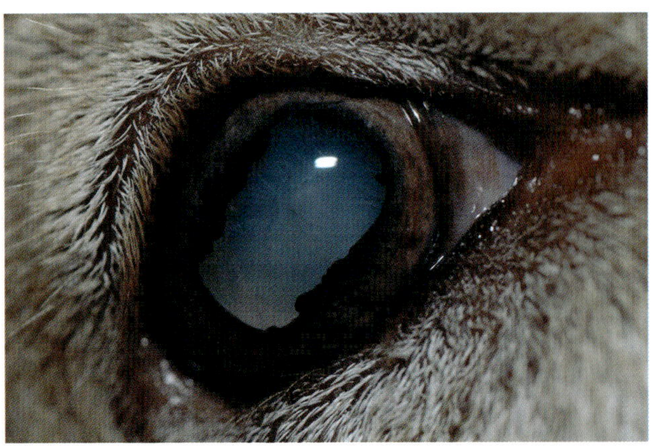

• **Fig. 14.22** Unilaterally immature cataract in an adult goat. The cataract was noted as an incidental finding. The goat did not demonstrate any visual deficits that were obvious to the owner. The cause for this cataract was unknown.

Cataracts have been identified in white-tailed deer *(O. virginianus)*,[176] elk *(Cervus canadensis)*,[187] and in free-ranging moose *(Alces alces)*.[188]

Surgical removal of the lens is the only viable treatment option for cataracts. Animals with cataract secondary to uveitis generally are not good surgical candidates, especially if the disease is active. The client should be referred to an ophthalmologist if he or she wishes to explore the possibility of cataract extraction.[79]

Miscellaneous Conditions Affecting the Lens

Although uncommon, a persistent hyaloid artery remnant may be an incidental finding during ophthalmoscopic examination of small ruminants.[189] The hyaloid artery supplies blood to the lens during fetal development and normally atrophies after birth. Remnants of the hyaloid artery may be seen in as many as 30% of sheep between 1 and 3 years of age, and approximately 40% of goats, in one or both eyes.[189] The remnant of the hyaloid artery appears as a thin, tight linear structure extending from the posterior lens capsule to the optic disc.[189] The point of insertion on the optic disc is referred to as Bergmeister's papilla.

Persistent pupillary membranes (PPMs) have been reported in sheep.[179] The remnants of the embryonic pupillary membrane appear as pigmented strands of iris tissue extending from the iris collarette to the iris stroma (iris to iris PPMs), from the iris collarette to the anterior lens capsule (iris to lens PPMs), or from the iris collarette to the corneal endothelium (iris to cornea PPMs). Mild cases may appear only as small pigmented foci over the anterior lens capsule. Focal opacities may be present in the cornea or on the anterior lens capsule in areas where the PPMs adhere. An essential iris atrophy has been reported in Shropshire sheep.[190] Affected sheep are born apparently normal, but ocular lesions can be seen by 1 to 1.5 years of age. Lesions are bilateral but asymmetric and include partial- or full-thickness holes in the iris stroma and an absent or rudimentary corpora nigra.[190] Pupils are pear shaped and respond sluggishly to light and do not dilate completely following the administration of topical tropicamide. Generally, neither persistent hyaloid remnants, PPMs, or iris atrophy in small ruminants require treatment.[190]

Glaucoma

There is very little information in the available literature pertaining to glaucoma in sheep, goats, or cervids. Glaucoma, in any species, is a neurodegenerative disease that, over time, results in the loss of retinal ganglion cells and, ultimately, blindness.[191] One of the most common risk factors associated with glaucoma in animals is an increase in IOP. Until applanation or rebound tonometry (applanation or rebound) becomes more widely available in small ruminant practices, early detection of glaucoma will remain elusive. Glaucoma is categorized as primary (clinical signs of glaucoma without any identifiable cause) or secondary (clinical manifestation of glaucoma resulting from the presence of an underlying cause, i.e., chronic uveitis).

Topical application of prednisolone acetate, administered every 8 hours, has been shown to cause steroid-induced ocular hypertension in sheep.[192] In that study, the IOP returned to the baseline level over a period of 1 to 3 weeks following discontinuation of the topical prednisolone acetate.[192] The same group of researchers further discovered that a single dose of a gene therapy vector carrying an inducible metalloproteinase human gene can protect against elevation in IOP caused by topical prednisolone acetate application and quickly reduces the elevated IOP caused by topical corticosteroid application.[193]

Glaucoma in small ruminants is associated with ocular inflammatory conditions such as severe keratoconjunctivitis, corneal ulcers, anterior uveitis, ocular trauma, and septicemia.[76,77] Glaucoma develops from a decreased outflow of aqueous humor, which may result from extensive anterior synechia or filtration angle obstruction with inflammatory cells or fibrin.[76,191]

Clinical Signs. Clinical signs of glaucoma include congestion of conjunctival and episcleral blood vessels, epiphora, corneal edema, buphthalmos (enlarged globe), mydriasis, blindness, exposure keratitis, lens luxation, and cataracts.[179]

Treatment. Buphthalmic (enlarged) eyes should be enucleated, especially if exposure keratitis is present or if painful.[76] A silicone intraorbital spherical implant may be placed in some cases if a cosmetic appearance is desired and the animal is unilaterally affected.[179] If the animal retains vision in the affected eye, diode laser cycloablation can be performed to destroy some of the ciliary body epithelial cells, which decreases aqueous humor production. Medical therapy of glaucoma may be attempted and is centered around decreasing aqueous humor production (carbonic anhydrase inhibitors) and minimizing concomitant inflammation.[179]

Pathologic Conditions of the Retina

Infectious Conditions and Related Disorders

Many infectious organisms and septicemic conditions can cause retinitis (retinal inflammation) or retinal changes. Septic neonates and feedlot lambs with listeriosis may develop chorioretinitis.[84] In sheep, toxoplasmosis frequently causes focal retinal necrosis and cyclitis or iridocyclitis.[50,180]

E. schneideri infections in small ruminants can result in retinal disease. Distinct retinal changes associated with this parasite, can be readily observed during ophthalmic examination of the fundus in affected animals.[186] Those changes include diffuse chorioretinal atrophy with proliferation of pigment within the tapetal fundus, attenuation of retinal vasculature, and optic nerve atrophy.[186] The optic discs of affected animals may have an indistinct and hazy outline and may appear edematous (dull, matt) and pale gray.[186] In contrast to elk, affected sheep do not become blind.[186]

Lambs born to dams naturally infected with bluetongue virus, or if a modified live vaccine is administered during the first half of gestation, may develop a necrotizing retinopathy and retinal dysplasia.[194] These lambs have obvious visual impairment and central nervous system defects.[84] Goats and deer are more resistant to bluetongue virus than sheep are.[79,176] Modified live bluetongue vaccine should not be administered to pregnant ewes, but if vaccination is necessary, it should not take place during the first half of gestation.[77]

Scrapie has been shown to be a rare cause of blindness, with affected sheep lacking a menace response and bumping into objects, despite maintaining PLRs.[195] Several raised, and oval-shaped, blister-like lesions were visible scattered throughout the tapetal fundus. The lesions ranged in size from three-fourths to one optic disc diameter.[195] Histology identified the lesions as accumulations of pigmented lipid located between the RPE and photoreceptors in the retina (subretinal space).[195] Finding such lesions in association with chronic weight loss, poor body condition, neurologic signs, wool loss, and pruritus is suggestive of this diagnosis.[195] The presence of prion protein PrPSc can be confirmed in clinical and preclinical ovine cases of scrapie using immunohistochemistry staining of formalin-fixed third eyelid [196,197] or rectoanal mucosa[198] biopsy specimens (see Chapters 13 and 16).[50]

Plant Toxicity

Bracken fern *(Pteridium aquilinum)*, when grazed chronically, causes a progressive retinal degeneration in sheep colloquially called "bright blindness."[199–201] A majority of affected sheep are noted to be blind between September and November,[200] several months after they begin to graze bracken fern.[199] Most sheep are affected between 3 and 4 years of age, and the earliest detectable clinical sign is an increased tapetal hyperreflectivity (shimmering of the tapetal fundus during fundoscopy).[200] Affected sheep are permanently blind but alert. Their pupils are dilated and round, and the PLR is poor.[199,200] Ophthalmoscopic examination may reveal attenuated and narrowed retinal blood vessels that appear more widely separated than normal. In advanced cases, the nontapetal fundus is pale, with small linear cracks and gray foci, and the optic disk may appear pale or grayish-pink.[199,200] Choroidal vessels may be visible in some areas of the fundus.[199] Ptaquiloside, the glycoside present in bracken fern, has been identified as the toxic principal responsible for bright blindness in sheep; however, the exact mechanism of action is unknown.[202] Possible explanations include disturbance in blood circulation secondary to narrowing of the blood vessels[202] and decreased retinal lactate dehydrogenase activity.[200] Platelet and leukocyte counts also are significantly lower in affected sheep.[200] Microscopic lesions are limited to the retina and are characterized by a complete destruction of the outer nuclear layer and photoreceptors.[50,200]

Locoweed (*Astragalus* and *Oxytropis* spp.) toxicity causes marked cytoplasmic vacuolization of the retinal ganglion and bipolar cells, which may result in visual deficits.[173] Blindgrass *(Stypandra imbricata)* toxicity occurs in sheep and goats of Western Australia. Ocular clinical signs include blindness (no PLR, mydriasis) caused by lesions in the photoreceptor layer of the retina, optic nerve, and optic tracts.[203] In southwest Africa, ruminants grazing on *Helichrysum argyrosphaerum* may develop paresis or paralysis and blindness characterized by bilateral mydriasis and papilledema on fundus exam.[204] Cataracts may be observed in affected sheep. The toxic principle of *H. argyrosphaerum* is unknown, but ingestion leads to retinal degeneration and demyelination of the optic nerve.[50,204]

Inherited Retinal Degeneration

Ceroid lipofuscinosis (Batten's disease) is an inherited lysosomal storage disease that causes blindness, ataxia, and tremors in South

Hampshire sheep.[205] Atrophy of the cerebral cortex results in early vision loss, and ceroid lipofuscin pigment accumulation in the retinal cells leads to concurrent retinal dystrophy.[206,207] Decreased retinal function is confirmed with electroretinography.[206,207] Retinal degeneration characterized as a rod-cone dysplasia has been reported in a 4-month old Toggenburg doe.[208] Signs of vision loss including bumping into objects, horizontal nystagmus, poor PLRs, and weight loss were observed after the doe was weaned.

Vitamin A Deficiency

The retina requires a constant supply of vitamin A to maintain vision. Phototransduction is dependent upon vitamin A, and progressive retinal degeneration can develop when insufficient levels of vitamin A are obtained from the animals diet.[19] Rhodopsin initiates the cascade of phototransduction and is made up of opsin (a protein that determines the wavelength of the photon the pigment will absorb) and retinol (a vitamin A derivative).[19] Following photoreceptor light stimulation, rhodopsin undergoes a series of conformational changes and activates transducing activating phosphodiesterase. This activation of phosphodiesterase leads to hyperpolarization in the outer segments of the photoreceptors.[19] Depletion of rhodopsin leads to impaired rod function, which results in diminished vision in low-light situations. Clinically, this manifests as nyctalopia or night blindness in domestic species.[19,83] Ruminants are efficient in converting dietary beta-carotene into vitamin A if they have access to good-quality green forage sources.[50] Vitamin A content is depleted from these forages as they mature in the hay-making process. As a result, the vitamin is no longer available from the hay after several years of storage.[50] Vitamin A is stored in the liver, and hepatic stores may prevent vitamin A deficiency disease for many months if dietary deficiency occurs.[2]

In young calves, vitamin A deficiency induces bony remodeling of the optic canal and thickening of the dura mater, which in turn causes an ischemic necrosis of the optic nerves.[209,210] Remodeling of the optic canal does not occur in skeletally mature animals, and associated blindness probably is caused by retinal degeneration.[209,210]

Clinical Signs. Clinical signs of vitamin A deficiency may not become apparent for at least 3 months in goats[211] and 200 days in sheep[212] if they previously have been grazing good-quality pasture. Under the same conditions of dietary vitamin A deficiency, males apparently are more susceptible than females to the development of clinical signs of deficiency.[210] Nyctalopia is a consistent clinical sign of vitamin A depletion in sheep and goats, along with anorexia and poor body condition.[213,214] Severely affected animals may be completely blind with dilated and unresponsive pupils.[210,213] Ophthalmoscopy reveals papilledema (pale optic disk with an inverted-heart appearance), papillary and peripapillary retinal hemorrhages, and depigmentation of the non-tapetal retina.[210,213] Determination of vitamin A levels in plasma and feed is the most direct method of diagnosing the dietary deficiency.[50]

Treatment. Nyctalopia is reversible with vitamin A replacement. The minimum recommended daily dose of vitamin A for both growing lambs and 60-kg replacement ewes is 50 IU/kg.[215] Pregnant and lactating ewes require 100 IU/kg and 150 IU/kg of vitamin A, respectively.[215] The upper safe dietary limit for sheep and goats has been suggested to be 20,000 IU/kg for a maximum duration of 4 weeks.[215] In affected cattle, the recommended treatment regimen consists of parenteral injection of 440 IU/kg of vitamin A once daily for 3 to 4 days and then 6000 IU/kg every 50 to 60 days until the diet has been enriched.[216] Animals with severe and complete blindness caused by damage to the retina and optic nerves will not regain their vision despite therapy.[210] Allowing free access to green forages or parenterally administering a commercially available vitamin A product usually is preventive in areas in which dry, brown hay is fed for extended periods. In such feeding conditions, inclusion of vitamin A in a feed or mineral supplement is warranted[50] (see Chapter 2).

Blindness

Apparent blindness has been described in severely ill or septicemic animals in association with depression or systemic disease. Evaluation of vision is difficult in neonatal animals because they normally lack a menace response for several days after birth. Blindness can be caused by severe hypoglycemia in kids and lambs or by neurologic diseases such as hydrocephalus, intracranial neoplasia, and any encephalitis, including caprine arthritis-encephalitis, ovine progressive encephalomyelitis (maedi-visna), scrapie, cerebral abscesses, bacterial meningitis, coenuriasis, toxoplasmosis, and aberrant parasite migration (e.g., by larvae of *Parelaphostrongylus tenuis*).[179,217,218] *L. monocytogenes* infections may cause blindness as a sequela of septicemia, which generally causes severe endophthalmitis or, less commonly, meningoencephalitis.[76,218] Other clinical signs of listeriosis are optic neuritis, amaurosis, decreased PLRs, head tilt, and unilateral CN deficits.[218] Pituitary abscesses or neoplasia may lead to blindness if the optic chiasm is compressed. Overeating disease (*Clostridium perfringens* syndrome characterized by ophthalmoscopically type D infection)[219] and hepatic encephalopathy secondary to acute or chronic liver failure may cause blindness and neurologic signs. Diseases causing retinitis or retinal degeneration (e.g., *E. schneideri* infection or bluetongue; intoxication with bracken fern, locoweed, or blindgrass; vitamin A deficiency) may lead to visual impairment. Pregnancy toxemia and ketosis may produce clinically apparent blindness as a consequence of cerebral energy deprivation and swelling.[220] Lightning strike, trauma, and improper use of debudding irons may damage the cerebral cortex, with resultant blindness.[50,77,170,217]

Central blindness is a clinical syndrome characterized by ophthalmoscopically normal eyes, absence of a menace response, and normal PLR bilaterally.[217] Causes of central blindness in sheep and goats include thiamine deficiency, sulfur toxicosis, lead poisoning, and sodium toxicosis or water deprivation (Chapter 13).[50,216]

Ascertaining the animal's signalment, obtaining a complete history, and performing a thorough physical, neurologic, and ophthalmologic examination are warranted to localize the lesion and identify the most likely disorders causing the visual impairment. Diagnostic workup for blindness in small ruminants may include but is not limited to blood glucose level determination (neonates), urinalysis (pregnant doe or ewe), complete blood count, serum chemistry panel, cerebrospinal fluid analysis (for sodium content), cytologic studies and bacterial culture, testing for a significant response to parenteral administration of thiamine (within 12–24 hours), determination of blood lead levels, and computed tomography evaluation. Appropriate treatment should be based on the final diagnosis.[50]

Pathologic Conditions of the Orbit

Exophthalmos

Prominent anterior displacement of the globe (exophthalmos) can be caused by any orbital space-occupying lesion, such as retrobulbar abscesses or neoplasia, especially lymphoma and squamous cell carcinoma. Advanced nasal adenocarcinoma or squamous cell carcinoma may cause exophthalmia and facial asymmetry in sheep and are associated with clinical signs of respiratory disease (e.g., chronic nasal discharge, inspiratory dyspnea, and diminished airflow from the nostrils).[221,222] Orbital cellulitis is rare but may result from periocular puncture wounds, migration of plant awns from the oral cavity, and caseous lymphadenitis–associated abscesses.[2,84]

Cyclopia

Cyclopia in fetal lambs, a developmental anomaly characterized by the presence of only one orbit, has been associated with the consumption of *Veratrum californicum* (skunk cabbage, corn lily, or false hellebore) by ewes on day 14 of gestation.[223,224] The plant grows in the mountain ranges of the Western United States. Other congenital defects attributed to grazing *V. californicum* include anophthalmia, shortening or absence of the maxillary and nasal bones, cebocephalus ("monkey face"), hydrocephalus, and harelip.[223,224] The incidence of congenital deformities may range from 1 to 25% of lambs in flocks grazing pastures contaminated with skunk cabbage.[223] Occasionally, only one lamb of twins is affected.[223,224] Because no treatment is available for affected offspring, prevention is warranted. Examination with a magnifying loupe, ultrasonography, radiography, computed tomography, endoscopy of the upper airways, and cytologic analysis of fine needle aspiration samples or histopathologic examination of tissue biopsy specimens may be appropriate to confirm the cause of exophthalmia. Appropriate treatment should be selected on the basis of the final diagnosis.[50]

Miscellaneous Ophthalmic Problems

Congenital microphthalmia (small eye), along with other ocular defects such as aphakia, aniridia, and optic nerve hypoplasia, may be inherited as an autosomal recessive trait in Texel sheep.[77] Several ocular abnormalities may occur in lambs born to ewes grazing seleniferous pastures, including microphthalmia.[79,225] In addition to microphthalmia, conjunctival cysts, aphakia or displacement of the lens, aniridia or rudimentary iris, and lack of a division between the cornea and sclera have been reported. Some 75% of affected lambs die at birth.[50]

What was initially thought to be bilateral microphthalmia in a 3-day-old male red deer *(C. elaphus)* was diagnosed with complex bilateral ocular dysgenesis. No lens material was found in either eye, and dermoid metaplasia of the primitive lens vesicle was diagnosed on histopathologic evaluation.[226] Microphthalmia and aphakia have also been identified in a small group of white-tailed deer *(O. virginianus)*.[227] A recent survey of 3645 white-tailed deer for congenital ocular abnormalities detected microphthalmia, congenital cataracts, anophthalmia, colobomata, anterior segment dysgenesis, ectopic lacrimal gland tissue, and/or congenital blindness with corneal opacity in 15 affected animals.[176]

Enucleation

Enucleation is indicated for removal of any blind and painful eye, as well as eyes damaged by severe keratitis, perforating injury, glaucoma, and intraocular neoplasia, for which medical therapy is not feasible or effective. Exenteration, involving surgical removal of the entire globe, extraocular muscles, and adnexa, may be necessary in cases of extensive neoplasia. However, transpalpebral or, better even, transconjunctival enucleation can be performed in a much more efficient manner. Regardless of the reason for enucleation, the contralateral eye should be carefully evaluated to ensure normal vision prior to enucleation or exenteration being performed. Systemic peri- and postoperative antibiotics are indicated in cases of significant infectious disease or if the procedure is performed under sedation and local analgesia.

Retrobulbar Anesthesia

Sedation or general anesthesia with local eyelid and retrobulbar anesthesia may be used to facilitate enucleation in small ruminants.[2,51,109,228] Two common retrobulbar anesthesia techniques are the Peterson eye block and the four-point block.[51] Enucleation, or other ophthalmic surgeries, can be facilitated using a retrobulbar block as the optic nerve, extraocular muscles, and sensory innervation of the eye and adnexa are desensitized. The oculomotor (CN III), trochlear (CN IV), maxillary and ophthalmic branches of the trigeminal nerve (CN V), and abducens nerve (CN VI) are all effectively desensitized following retrobulbar anesthesia. A 3.75-cm, 22-gauge, slightly curved (bent) needle may be used to perform retrobulbar anesthesia.[51] Achievement of an acceptable level of local anesthesia is confirmed by corneal desensitization, mydriasis, and lack of globe motility.

Peterson Eye Block. Following aseptic preparation of the injection site with a dilute, aseptically prepared povidone-iodine solution (5%), 2 to 3 mL of local anesthetic (2% lidocaine or mepivacaine) is injected subcutaneously at a point halfway between the lateral canthus and the base of the horn, at the posterior aspect of the supraorbital process and the zygomatic arch.[51] The injection is carried out using an 18- or 16-gauge, ¾-inch needle.[72] A slightly curved, 3- to 4-inch, 18- or 20-gauge needle is then inserted through the skin opening, advanced medially with the concavity of the needle directed caudally and slightly ventrally, along the zygomatic arch.[50,72] The needle tip should then be "walked-off" of the anterior border of the coronoid process of the mandible and advance, without resistance, toward the medial floor of the orbit, approximately 2 to 3 inches. Once the medial orbital floor is contacted, the needle is retracted 2 to 3 mm. Quick aspiration prior to injection of the local anesthetic agent will ensure that the needle has not entered the ophthalmic artery. Approximately 7 to 8 mL of local anesthetic is slowly injected into the retro-orbital space.[50,72]

Four-Point Block. A series of four injections are performed using a 2.5-inch, 20-gauge, slightly curved needle to deposit a local anesthetic agent into the retrobulbar space. Landmarks for the injections are the dorsal, ventral, medial, and lateral edges of the bony orbit. Topical ophthalmic anesthetic (0.5% proparacaine) should be applied and eyelid blocks performed prior to performing the retrobulbar anesthesia in order to desensitize the cornea and conjunctiva and minimize discomfort during the four-point retrobulbar injections.[50,72] The surgeon's index finger should be used to deflect the globe and protect it from the needle as each injection is administered. The clinician palpates the wall of the bony orbit and inserts the needle from the conjunctival fornix until it encounters the apex of the orbit. Approximately 1 to 2 mL of local anesthetic (2% lidocaine or mepivacaine) is injected at each site as the needle is advanced.[2,51,109,228]

Proper needle placement is essential to avoid complications associated with the retrobulbar anesthesia techniques described previously. Although uncommon, retrobulbar hematoma and iatrogenic injury to the globe can occur, especially if the animal moves during the injections. The risk of these complications can be minimized using proper technique and manual or chemical restraint of the animal. Seizure activity resulting from inadvertent injection of lidocaine into the meningeal reflection of the optic nerve has been reported. Although the convulsions associated with this complication are generally self-limiting, they may be fatal.[113]

Subconjunctival and Transpalpebral Enucleation Techniques

Preoperative Considerations. Enucleation may be performed using the subconjunctival or transpalpebral technique. The subconjunctival approach allows for targeted removal of the globe and usually results in less hemorrhage. If a prosthesis is to be placed for a more cosmetic result, the subconjunctival approach should be used.[2,72,228,229] The transpalpebral approach is indicated in cases of significant ocular infection or neoplasia. This method involves the collective removal of the entire globe, conjunctiva, extraocular muscles, and nictitating membrane. If enucleation is to be performed to remove a severely infected and/or ruptured globe, the transpalpebral approach is indicated to reduce surgical contamination.[50]

Transpalpebral Enucleation. After induction of general anesthesia or sedation and retrobulbar anesthesia, the patient is placed into lateral recumbency with the eye to be enucleated toward the surgeon. The affected orbit should be lavaged with a 1:50 dilution of povidone iodine solution and isotonic saline. If a transpalpebral approach is used, the affected eyelids should be sutured closed using a monofilament, nonabsorbable suture material in a simple continuous pattern, prior to clipping and aseptic preparation of the surgical field. A tail of suture should be left at each end of the incision to facilitate manipulation of the eye during surgery. The palpebral skin is incised 3 to 4 mm from the eyelid margins using a no. 15 or no. 10 scalpel blade. Blunt dissection is then performed circumferentially, using curved scissors and proceeding deeply into the eyelids and external to the extraocular muscles. The optic nerve and vessels may be clamped with a curved hemostat, then transected. The orbit should be gently lavaged several times with sterile saline solution containing a broad-spectrum antibiotic. Closure of the remaining soft tissues may be attempted to reduce the orbital dead space and to minimize postoperative sinking of the eyelids; however, this is often difficult in small ruminants because of their rather deep and wide bony orbit. The subcutaneous tissues are closed using absorbable suture (2-0 to 3-0) in a simple continuous or subcuticular pattern. The skin is closed using nonabsorbable suture (2-0) in a simple interrupted pattern. Systemic antibiotics and antiinflammatory drugs should be continued for several days after surgery.

Subconjunctival Enucleation. A subconjunctival approach can be utilized to remove the globe itself, while preserving most of the orbital soft tissue. This method allows for more effective compartmental closure of the orbit, as the periosteum is closed to contain any orbital hemorrhage. The surgical site is prepped as outlined above for the transpalpebral enucleation. An eyelid speculum is placed to facilitate visualization of the globe, and a circumferential conjunctival incision is made approximately 4 to 6 mm posterior to the limbus using small tenotomy scissors. Care must be taken to ensure that the incision incorporates Tenon's capsule, the fibrous bulbar sheath closely apposed to the conjunctiva. The bulbar conjunctiva/Tenon's capsule is then bluntly dissected to expose the extraocular muscle attachments. These muscle attachments are readily located by sliding a muscle hook under their respective scleral attachments. Each isolated extraocular muscle tendon is dissected as close to the sclera as possible, under direct visualization. This results in far less hemorrhage than cutting through the muscle bodies. Following resection of each of the rectus and oblique extraocular muscles, the retractor bulbi muscles, optic nerve, and vessels are sharply dissected using curved or semicurved enucleation scissors. Following removal of the globe, the third eyelid (nictitating membrane) is removed. The eyelid margins are then removed using a no. 15 or no. 10 scalpel blade approximately 4 to 5 mm from the eyelid margins, taking care to ensure that the Meibomian glands and the lacrimal caruncle (medial canthus) are removed in the process. Following removal of the eyelid margins, the remaining conjunctiva is stripped from the eyelid tissue. The periosteum is then closed using absorbable suture (2-0 to 3-0) in a simple continuous pattern. The remainder of the closure is performed as outlined above for the transpalpebral enucleation technique. A modified head bandage may be placed initially to compress the enucleated orbit and decrease postoperative swelling; however, this is generally not necessary. All enucleated eyes should be submitted for histopathologic examination to determine the exact cause of ocular disease.[2,72,228,229]

References

1. Samuelson DA: Ophthalmic anatomy. In Gelatt KN, Gilger BC, Kern TJ, editors: *Veterinary ophthalmology* (vol 1), ed 5, Ames, IA, 2013, John Wiley & Sons, Inc., pp 39–170.
2. Waldridge BM, Colitz CMH: Diseases of the eye. In DG P, editor: *Sheep and goat medicine,* ed 1, Philadelphia, 2002, Saunders, pp 317–339.
3. Bartošová J, Bartoš L, Kotrba R, Ceacero F: Pre-orbital gland opening in farmed red deer (*Cervus elaphus*) during stressful handling, *J Anim Sci* 90:3200–3206, 2012.
4. Bartošová J, Ceacero F, Bartoš L: Pre-orbital gland opening: part of sucking behavior in red deer (*Cervus elaphus*) calves, *J Anim Sci* 90:3207–3212, 2012.
5. Ceacero F, Landete-Castillejos T, Bartosova J, et al: Habituating to handling: factors affecting preorbital gland opening in red deer calves, *J Anim Sci* 92(9):4130–4136, 2014.
6. Rajagopal T, Archunan G: Histomorphology of preorbital gland in territorial and non-territorial male blackbuck *Antelope cervicapra*, a critically endangered species, *Biologia* 66:370–378, 2011.
7. Shively MJ: Integumentary. In Shively MJ, editor: *Veterinary anatomy,* ed 1, College Station, 1984, Texas A & M University Press.
8. Dyce KM, Sack WO, Wensing CJG: The sense organs. In Dyce KM, Sack WO, Wensing CJG, editors: *Textbook of veterinary anatomy,* ed 4, St. Louis, 2010, Saunders Elsevier, pp 332–354.
9. Sisson S, Grossman JD: The sense organs and common integument. In Grossman JD, editor: *The anatomy of domestic animals,* ed 5, Philadelphia, 1953, W. B. Saunders.
10. Gargiulo AM, Coliolo P, Ceccarelli P, Pedini V: Ultrastructural study of sheep lacrimal glands, *Vet Res* 30(4):345–351, 1999.
11. Sinha RD, Calhoun ML: A gross, histologic, and histochemical study of the lacrimal apparatus of sheep and goats, *Am J Vet Res* 27(121):1633–1640, 1966.
12. Brightman AH, Wachsstock RS, Erskine R: Lysozyme concentrations in the tears of cattle, goats, and sheep, *Am J Vet Res* 52(1):9–11, 1991.
13. Gionfriddo JR, Davidson H, Asem EK, Krohne SG: Detection of lysozyme in llama, sheep, and cattle tears, *Am J Vet Res* 61: 1294–1297, 2006.
14. Rehorek SJ, Hillenius WJ, Sanjur J, Chapman NG: One gland, two lobes: organogenesis of the "Harderian" and "nictitans" glands of the Chinese muntjac (*Muntiacus reevesi*) and fallow deer (*Dama dama*), *Ann Anat* 189(5):434–446, 2007.

15. Ribeiro AP, Silva ML, Rosa JP, Souza SF, Teixeira IAMA, Laus JL: Ultrasonographic and echobiometric findings in the eyes of Saanen goats of different ages, *Vet Ophthalmol* 12(5):313–317, 2009.
16. Fornazari GA, Montiani-Ferreira F, de Barros Filho IR, Somma AT, Moore B: The eye of the Barbary sheep or aoudad (*Ammotragus lervia*): reference values for selected ophthalmic diagnostic tests, morphologic and biometric observations, *Open Vet J* 6(2):102–113, 2016.
17. Bayer J: *Augenheilkunde [Ophthalmology]*, ed 3, Wien & Leipzig, 1914, Braumüller.
18. Gilger BC, Ledbetter EC: Diseases and surgery of the canine cornea and sclera. In Gelatt KN, Gilger BC, Kern TJ, editors: *Veterinary ophthalmology* (vol 2), ed 5, Ames, 2013, John Wiley & Sons, Inc., pp 976–1049.
19. Ofri R: Optics and physiology of vision. In Gelatt KN, Gilger BC, Kern TJ, editors: *Veterinary ophthalmology* (vol 1), ed 5, Ames, 2013, John Wiley & Sons, Inc., pp 208–270.
20. LoPinto AJ, Pirie CG, Bedenice D, Ayres SL: Corneal thickness of eyes of healthy goats, sheep, and alpacas manually measured by use of a portable spectral-domain optical coherence tomography device, *Am J Vet Res* 78:80–84, 2016.
21. Maurice DM: The structure and transparency of the cornea, *J Physiol* 136:263–286, 1957.
22. Coyo N, Leiva M, Costa D, Rios J, Peña T: Corneal thickness, endothelial cell density, and morphological and morphometric features of corneal endothelial cells in goats, *Am J Vet Res* 79:1087–1092, 2018.
23. Coyo N, Peña MT, Costa D, Ríos J, Lacerda R, Leiva M: Effects of age and breed on corneal thickness, density, and morphology of corneal endothelial cells in enucleated sheep eyes, *Vet Ophthalmol* 19:367–372, 2016.
24. Mir S, Wheatley HM, Hussels IE, Whittum-Hudson JA, Traboulsi EI: A comparative histologic study of the fibrillin microfibrillar system in the lens capsule of normal subjects and subjects with Marfan syndrome, *Invest Ophthalmol Vis Sci* 39(1):84–93, 1998.
25. Morrison JC, DeFrank MP, van Buskirk EM: Comparative microvascular anatomy of mammalian ciliary processes, *Invest Ophthalmol Vis Sci* 28:1325–1340, 1987.
26. Samuelson DA: A reevaluation of the comparative anatomy of the eutherian iridocorneal angle and associated ciliary body musculature, *Vet Comp Ophthalmol* 6(3):153–172, 1996.
27. Simoens P, De Geest J-P, Lauwers H: Comparative morphology of the pectinate ligaments of domestic mammals, as observed under the dissecting microscope and the scanning electron microscope, *J Vet Med Sci* 58(10):977–982, 1996.
28. LoPinto AJ, Pirie CG, Ayres SL, Bedenice D: Comparison of indocyanine green and sodium fluorescein for anterior segment angiography of ophthalmically normal eyes of goats, sheep, and alpacas performed with a digital single-lens reflex camera adaptor, *Am J Vet Res* 78:311–320, 2016.
29. Rohen JW: [Electronmicroscopic studies on the Granula iridis of Ruminantia (goat, sheep, cow)] Elektronenmikroskopische Untersuchungen über die Granula iridis der Ruminantia, *Albrecht v Graefes Arch klin exp Ophthal* 175:161–173, 1968.
30. Duke-Elder S: *The eyes of mammals in the eye of evolution,* ed 1, St. Louis, 1958, Mosby.
31. Sedacca K, Samuelson D, Lewis P: Examination of the anterior uveoscleral pathway in domestic species, *Vet Ophthalmol* 15(Suppl 1):1–7, 2012.
32. Bellairs R, Harkness LR, Harkness RD: The structure of the tapetum of the eye of the sheep, *Cell Tissue Res* 157(1):73–91, 1975.
33. Gum GG, MacKay EO: Physiology of the eye. In Gelatt KN, Gilger BC, Kern TJ, editors: *Veterinary ophthalmology* (vol 1), ed 5, Ames, 2013, John Wiley & Sons, Inc., pp 171–207.
34. Gonzalez-Soriano J, Mayayo-Vicente S, Martinez-Sainz P, Contreras-Rodriguez J, Rodriguez-Veiga E: A quantitative study of ganglion cells in the goat retina, *Anat Histol Embryol* 26: 39–44, 1997.
35. Schiviz AN, Ruf T, Kuebber-Heiss A, Schubert C, Ahnelt PK: Retinal cone topography of artiodactyl mammals: influence of body height and habitat, *J Comp Neurol* 507:1336–1350, 2008.
36. Braekevelt CR: Retinal photoreceptor fine structure in the domestic sheep, *Acta Anat (Basel)* 116(3):265–275, 1983.
37. Jacobs GH, Deegan II JF, Neitz J: Photopigment basis for dichromatic color vision in cows, goats, and sheep, *Vis Neurosci* 15: 581–584, 1998.
38. Jacobs GH, Deegan JF, Neitz J, Murphy BP, Miller KV, Marchinton RL: Electrophysiological measurements of spectral mechanisms in the retinas of two cervids: white-tailed deer (*Odocoileus virginianus*) and fallow deer (*Dama dama*), *J Comp Physiol A* 174:551–557, 1994.
39. Ollivier FJ, Samuelson DA, Brooks DE, Lewis PA, Kallberg ME, Komáromy AM: Comparative morphology of the tapetum lucidum (among selected species), *Vet Ophthalmol* 7(1):11–22, 2004.
40. Pearce JW, Moore CP: Food animal ophthalmology. In Gelatt KN, Gilger BC, Kern TJ, editors: *Veterinary ophthalmology* (vol 2), ed 5, Ames, 2013, John Wiley & Sons, Inc., pp 1610–1674.
41. D'Angelo GJ, Glasser A, Wendt M, et al: Visual specialization of an herbivore prey species, the white-tailed deer, *Can J Zool* 86: 735–743, 2008.
42. Dukes TW: The ocular fundus of normal white-tailed deer (*Odocoileus virginianus*), *Bull Wildl Dis Assoc* 5:16–17, 1969.
43. Martins BC, Oria AP, Souza AL, et al: Ophthalmic patterns of captive brown brocket deer (*Mazama gouazoubira*), *J Zoo Wildl Med* 38(4):526–532, 2007.
44. Oria AP, Gomes Junior DC, Oliveira AV, et al: Selected ophthalmic diagnostic tests, bony orbit anatomy, and ocular histology in sambar deer (*Rusa unicolor*), *Vet Ophthalmol* 18(Suppl 1):125–131, 2015.
45. da Silva-Curical JMA: Topical fluorescein dye: effects on immunofluorescent antibody test for feline herpesvirus keratoconjunctivitis, *Prog Vet Comp Ophthalmol* 1(2):99, 1991.
46. Broadwater JJ, Schorling JJ, Herring IP, Pickett JP: Ophthalmic examination findings in adult pygmy goats (*Capra hircus*), *Vet Ophthalmol* 10(5):269–273, 2007.
47. Ofri R, Horowitz H, Levison M, Kass PH: Intraocular pressure and tear production in captive eland and fallow deer, *J Wildl Dis* 37(2):387–390, 2001.
48. Ofri R, Horowitz IH, Kass PH: Tonometry in three herbivorous wildlife species. *Vet Ophthalmol* 1:21–24, 1998.
49. Townsend WM: Examination techniques and therapeutic regimens for the ruminant and camelid eye, *Vet Clin North Am Food Anim Pract* 26(3):437–458, 2010.
50. Boileau MJ, Gilmour MA: Diseases of the eye. In Pugh DG, Baird AN, editors: *Sheep and goat medicine,* ed 2, Maryland Heights, MO, 2012, Elsevier Saunders, pp 406–441.
51. Skarda RT: Local and regional anesthetic techniques: ruminants and swine. In Thurmon JC, Tranquilli WJ, Benson GJ, editors: *Veterinary anesthesia,* ed 3, Baltimore, 1996, Williams & Wilkins.
52. Spradbrow PB: The bacterial flora of the ovine conjunctival sac, *Aust Vet J* 44:117–118, 1968.
53. Ramsey DT: Surface ocular microbiology in food and fiber-producing animals. In Howard JL, Smith RA, editors: *Current veterinary therapy, food animal practice,* ed 4, Philadelphia, 1999, WB Saunders, pp 648–651.
54. Whitley RD, Moore CP: Ocular diagnostic and therapeutic techniques in food animals, *Vet Clin North Am Large Anim Pract* 6(3):553–575, 1984.
55. Meekins JM, Apley MD, Lubbers B, Peddireddi L, Rankin AJ: Evaluation of conjunctival bacterial flora in a herd of goats in the Midwestern United States, *Vet Ophthalmol* 20(1):40–45, 2017.
56. Mushi EZ, Binta MG, Chabo RG, Dintwe K: Conjunctival flora of fifty healthy goats in sebele farm, gaborone, Botswana, *J Anim Vet Adv* 6(12):1388–1389, 2007.
57. Akerstedt J, Hofshagen A: Bacteriological investigation of infectious keratoconjunctivitis in Norwegian sheep, *Acta Vet Scand* 45 (1–2):19–26, 2004.

58. Baker JR, Faull WB, Ward WR: Conjunctivitis and keratitis in sheep associated with Moraxella (Haemophilus) organisms, *Vet Rec* 77: 402, 1965.
59. Sanchez Romano J, Mork T, Laaksonen S, et al: Infectious keratoconjunctivitis in semi-domesticated Eurasian tundra reindeer (*Rangifer tarandus tarandus*): microbiological study of clinically affected and unaffected animals with special reference to cervid herpesvirus 2, *BMC Vet Res* 14(1):15, 2018.
60. Wood DR, Watson WA, Hunter D: Conjunctivitis in sheep, *Vet Rec* 77:551, 1965.
61. Kvapil P, Pirs T, Slavec B, et al: Tear production, intraocular pressure and conjunctival bacterial flora in selected captive wild ruminants, *Vet Ophthalmol* 21(1):52–57, 2018.
62. Dubay SA, Williams ES, Mills K, Boerger-Fields AM: Bacteria and nematodes in the conjunctiva of mule deer from Wyoming and Utah, *J Wildl Dis* 36(4):783–787, 2000.
63. Edwards SG, Maggs DJ, Byrne BA, Kass PH, Lassaline ME: Effect of topical application of 0.5% proparacaine on corneal culture results from 33 dogs, 12 cats, and 19 horses with spontaneously arising ulcerative keratitis, *Vet Ophthalmol* 22(4):415–422, 2019.
64. Bonelli F, Barsotti G, Attili AR, et al: Conjunctival bacterial and fungal flora in clinically normal sheep, *Vet Rec Open* 1(1):e000017, 2014.
65. Dagnall GJR: Experimental infection of the conjunctival sac of lambs with *Mycoplasma conjunctivae*, *Brit Vet J* 149(5):429–435, 1993.
66. Giacometti M, Nicolet J, Johansson K-E, Naglic T, Degiorgis M-P, Frey J: Detection and identification of *Mycoplasma conjunctivae* in infectious keratoconjunctivitis by PCR based on the 16s rRNA gene, *J Vet Med B* 46:173–180, 1999.
67. Holzwarth N, Pospischil A, Mavrot F, et al: Occurrence of Chlamydiaceae, *Mycoplasma conjunctivae*, and pestiviruses in Alpine chamois (Rupicapra r. rupicapra) of Grisons, Switzerland, *J Vet Diagn Invest* 23:333–337, 2011.
68. Mayer D, Nicolet J, Giacometti M, Schmitt M, Wahli T, Meier W: Isolation of *Mycoplasma conjunctivae* from conjunctival swabs of Alpine ibex (Capra ibex ibex) affected with infectious keratoconjunctivitis, *J Vet Med B* 43:155–161, 1996.
69. Dagnall GJR: Use of exfoliative cytology in the diagnosis of ovine keratoconjunctivitis, *Vet Rec* 135(6):127–130, 1994.
70. Leiva M, Peña T: Ophthalmic diseases of foals. In Gilger BC, editor: *Equine ophthalmology,* ed 3, Ames, 2017, John Wiley & Sons, Inc., pp 112–150.
71. Moore CP: Diseases of the eye. In Howard JL, editor: *Current veterinary therapy 3: food animal practice,* ed 3, Philadelphia, PA, 1993, WB Saunders.
72. Irby NL: Surgery of the eyes. In *Farm animal surgery,* ed 2, Elsevier, St. Louis, MO, 2017, pp 145–173.
73. Giuliano EA, Maggs DJ, Moore CP, Boland LA, Champagne ES, Galle LE: Inferomedial placement of a single-entry subpalpebral lavage tube for treatment of equine eye disease, *Vet Ophthalmol* 3(2–3):153–156, 2000.
74. Davis JL: Therapeutics in practice: the use of antifungals, *Compendium Equine* 3(3):128–133, 2008.
75. Ramsey DT: Ophthalmic therapeutics. In Howard JL, Smith RA, editors: *Current veterinary therapy, food animal practice,* ed 4, Philadelphia, 1999, WB Saunders, pp 636–638.
76. Moore CP, Whitley RD: Ophthalmic diseases of small domestic ruminants, *Vet Clin North Am Large Anim Pract* 6(3):641–665, 1984.
77. Moore CP, Wallace LM: Selected eye diseases of sheep and goats. In Howard JL, editor: *Current veterinary therapy, food animal practice,* ed 3, Philadelphia, 1993, WB Saunders.
78. Lamprecht H, Pfeiffer A: [Entropion in newborn lambs], *Berl Munch Tierarztl Wochenschr* 102(9):303–310, 1989.
79. Wyman M: Eye diseases of sheep and goats, *Vet Clin North Am Large Anim Pract* 5(3):657–675, 1983.
80. Claine F, Raes M, Leemans J, Muylkens B, Kirschvink N: Monitoring and management of congenital entropion in lambs: a prospective study, *Small Rumin Res* 111:1–5, 2013.
81. Sakul H, Kellom TR: Heritability of entropion in several US sheep breeds, *Small Rumin Res* 23:187–190, 1996.
82. Sakul H, Snowder GD, Hemenway KJ: Evaluation of techniques for correction of entropion in lambs, *Small Rumin Res* 20(2): 187–191, 1996.
83. Maggs DJ: Diseases of the eye. In Smith BP, editor: *Large animal internal medicine,* ed 4, St. Louis, MO, 2009, Mosby Elsevier, pp 1259–1305.
84. Pickett JP: Selected eye diseases of food and fiber-producing animals. In Howard JL, Smith RA, editors: *Current veterinary therapy, food animal practice,* ed 4, Philadelphia, 1999, WB Saunders.
85. Stades FC, van der Woerdt A: Diseases and surgery of the canine eyelid. In Gelatt KN, Gilger BC, Kern TJ, editors: *Veterinary ophthalmology* (vol 2), ed 5, Ames, 2013, John Wiley & Sons, Inc., pp 832–893.
86. Mousel MR, Reynolds JO, White SN: Genome-wide association identifies SLC2A9 and NLN gene regions as associated with entropion in domestic sheep, *Plos One* 10(6):e0128909, 2015.
87. Gelatt KN: Congenital entropion in a Hampshire lamb, *Vet Med Small Anim Clin* 65(8):761, 1970.
88. Littlejohn AI: A Defect of upper eyelid in a flock of piebald sheep, *Vet Rec* 85(7):189–190, 1969.
89. Turner LM, Whitley RD, Hager D: Management of ocular trauma in horses. 2. Orbit, eyelids, uvea, lens, retina and optic-nerve, *Mod Vet Pract* 67(4):341–347, 1986.
90. Smith MC, Sherman DM: Skin. In Smith MC, Sherman DM, editors: *Goat medicine,* ed 2, Ames, IA, 2009, Wiley-Blackwell, pp 23–60.
91. Baughman B, Zhang S, Jin L, et al: Diagnosis of Deerpox virus infection in a white-tailed deer (*Odocoileus virginianus*) fawn, *J Vet Diagn Invest* 23(5):965–970, 2011.
92. Patton JF, Nordhausen RW, Woods LW, MacLachlan NJ: Isolation of a poxvirus from a black-tailed deer (*Odocoileus hemionus columbianus*), *J Wildl Dis* 32(3):531–533, 1996.
93. Sayler KA, Subramaniam K, Jacob JM, et al: Characterization of mule deerpox virus in Florida white-tailed deer fawns expands the known host and geographic range of this emerging pathogen, *Arch Virol* 2018.
94. Williams ES, Becerra VM, Thorne ET, Graham TJ, Owens MJ, Nunamaker CE: Spontaneous poxviral dermatitis and keratoconjunctivitis in free-ranging mule deer (*Odocoileus hemionus*) in Wyoming, *J Wildl Dis* 21(4):430–433, 1985.
95. Wobeser G, Mitcham SA, Saunders JR, Hunt HM: Dermatomycosis (ringworm) in mule deer (*Odocoileus hemionus*), *Can Vet J* 24(10):316–317, 1983.
96. Volmer K, Doll G, Dingeldein W, Herzog A: [Hair alterations in trichophytosis of roe deer—a differential diagnosis for hair parakeratosis], *Tierarztl Prax* 18(1):21–23, 1990.
97. Pal M, Thapa BR: An outbreak of dermatophytosis in barking deer (*Muntiacus muntjak*), *Vet Rec* 133(14):347–348, 1993.
98. Robinson RM, Jones P, Galvin TJ, Harwell GM: Elaeophorosis in sika deer in Texas, *J Wildl Dis* 14(1):137–141, 1978.
99. Couvillion CE, Davidson WR, Nettles VF: Distribution of *Elaeophora schneideri* in white-tailed deer in the southeastern United States, 1962–1983, *J Wildl Dis* 21(4):451–453, 1985.
100. LeVan IK, Fox KA, Miller MW: High elaeophorosis prevalence among harvested Colorado moose, *J Wildl Dis* 49(3):666–669, 2013.
101. Grunenwald CM, Butler E, Wunschmann A, et al: Emergence of the arterial worm *Elaeophora schneideri* in moose (*Alces alces*) and tabanid fly vectors in northeastern Minnesota, USA, *Parasit Vectors* 11(1):507, 2018.
102. Lavach JD: Disorders of the eyelids, conjunctivae, and nasolacrimal system. In Lavach JD, editor: *Large animal ophthalmology,* ed 1, St. Louis, 1990, Mosby, pp 349–354.
103. Vaatstra BI, Munday JS, Morriss PW: Pigmented chin papillomas in red (*Cervus elaphus*) × wapiti (*Cervus canadensis*) stags associated with a novel papillomavirus, *N Z Vet J* 62(2):96–99, 2014.

104. Erdélyi K, Gál J, Sugár L, et al: Papillomavirus-associated fibropapillomas of red deer (*Cervus elaphus*), *Acta Veterinaria Hungarica* 57(2):337–344, 2009.
105. Munday JS, Vaatstra BL, Dunowska M, Laurie RE, Hills S: Genomic characterization of a novel Epsilonpapillomavirus associated with pigmented papillomas in a red deer (*Cervus elaphus*), *Virus Genes* 52(5):633–639, 2016.
106. Hughes KL, Bildfell RJ, Alcantar B: Pigmented tumors in fallow deer (*Dama dama*): 11 cases, *J Vet Diagn Invest* 29(4):483–488, 2017.
107. Sundberg JP, Nielsen SW: Deer fibroma: a review, *Can Vet J* 22(12):385–388, 1981.
108. O'Banion MK, Sundberg JP: Papillomavirus genomes in experimentally induced fibromas in white-tailed deer, *Am J Vet Res* 48(10):1453–1455, 1987.
109. Edmondson MA: Local, regional, and spinal anesthesia in ruminants, *Vet Clin North Am Food Anim Pract* 32(3):535–552, 2016.
110. Tsujita H, Plummer CE: Bovine ocular squamous cell carcinoma, *Vet Clin North Am Food Anim Pract* 26(3):511–529, 2010.
111. Kainer RA, Stringer JM, Lueker DC: Hyperthermia for treatment of ocular squamous cell tumors in cattle, *J Am Vet Med Assoc* 176(4):356–360, 1980.
112. Grier RL, Brewer JWG, Paul SR, Theilen GH: Treatment of bovine and equine ocular squamous cell carcinoma by radiofrequency hyperthermia, *J Am Vet Med Assoc* 177(1):55–61, 1980.
113. Welker B: Ocular surgery, *Vet Clin North Am Food Anim Pract* 11(1):149–157, 1995.
114. Kennedy MJ, Moraiko DT, Treichel B: First report of immature *Thelazia skrjabini* (Nematoda: Thelazioidea) from the eye of a white-tailed deer, *Odocoileus virginianus*, *J Wildl Dis* 29(1): 159–160, 1993.
115. Ruiz I, Soriguer RC, Perez JM: Pharyngeal bot flies (Oestridae) from sympatric wild cervids in southern Spain, *J Parasitol* 79(4): 623–626, 1993.
116. Whitley RD: Ocular trauma. In Smith BP, editor: *Large animal internal medicine,* ed 2, St. Louis, 1996, Mosby.
117. Giacometti M, Janovsky M, Belloy L, Frey J: Infectious keratoconjunctivitis of ibex, chamois and other Caprinae, *Rev Sci Tech Oie* 21(2):335–345, 2002.
118. das Neves CG, Roth S, Rimstad E, Thiry E, Tryland M: Cervid herpesvirus 2 infection in reindeer: a review, *Vet Microbiol* 143(1):70–80, 2010.
119. Dubay SA, Williams ES, Mills K, Boerger-Fields AM: Association of *Moraxella ovis* with keratoconjunctivitis in mule deer and moose in Wyoming, *J Wildl Dis* 36(2):241–247, 2000.
120. Gutierrez JFM, Sondgeroth KS, Williams ES, Montgomery DL, Creekmore TE, Miller MM: Infectious keratoconjunctivitis in free-ranging mule deer in Wyoming: a retrospective study and identification of a novel alphaherpesvirus, *J Vet Diagn Invest* 30(5):663–670, 2018.
121. Taylor SK, Vieira VG, Williams ES, et al: Infectious keratoconjunctivitis in free-ranging mule deer (*Odocoileus hemionus*) from Zion National Park, Utah, *J Wildl Dis* 32(2):326–330, 1996.
122. Hosie BO: Infectious keratoconjunctivitis in sheep and goats, *Vet Ann* 29:93, 1989.
123. Nietfeld JC: Chlamydial infections in small ruminants, *Vet Clin North Am Food Anim Pract* 17(2):301–314, vi, 2001.
124. Trotter SL, Franklin RM, Baas EJ, Barile MF: Epidemic caprine keratoconjunctivitis: Experimentally induced disease with a pure culture of *Mycoplasma conjunctivae*, *Infect Immun* 18(3):816–822, 1977.
125. Mavrot F, Vilei EM, Marreros N, Signer C, Frey J, Ryser-Degiorgis MP: Occurrence, quantification, and genotyping of *Mycoplasma conjunctivae* in wild caprinae with and without infectious keratoconjunctivitis, *J Wildlife Dis* 48(3):619–631, 2012.
126. Fernandez-Aguilar X, Cabezon O, Frey J, et al: Long-term dynamics of *Mycoplasma conjunctivae* at the wildlife-livestock interface in the Pyrenees, *Plos One* 12(10), 2017.
127. Fernandez-Aguilar X, Rossi L, Cabezon O, et al: Infectious keratoconjunctivitis and occurrence of *Mycoplasma conjunctivae* and Chlamydiaceae in small domestic ruminants from Central Karakoram, Pakistan, *Vet Rec* 181(9):237, 2017.
128. Ruffin DC: Mycoplasma infections in small ruminants, *Vet Clin N Am-Food Anim Pract* 17(2):315, 2001.
129. Whitley RD, Albert RA: Clinical uveitis and polyarthritis associated with Mycoplasma species in a young goat, *Vet Rec* 115(9): 217–218, 1984.
130. Greig A: Ovine keratoconjunctivitis, *In Practice* 11(3):110, 1989.
131. Egwu GO, Faull WB, Bradbury JM, Clarkson MJ: Ovine infectious keratoconjunctivitis: a microbiological study of clinically unaffected and affected sheep's eyes with special reference to *Mycoplasma conjunctivae*, *Vet Rec* 125(10):253–256, 1989.
132. McCauley EH, Surman PG, Anderson DR: Isolation of Mycoplasma from goats during an epizootic of keratoconjunctivitis, *Am J Vet Res* 32(6):861–870, 1971.
133. Janovsky M, Frey J, Nicolet J, Belloy L, Goldschmidt-Clermont E, Giacometti M: *Mycoplasma conjunctivae* infection is self-maintained in the Swiss domestic sheep population, *Vet Microbiol* 83:11–22, 2001.
134. Baas EJ, Trotter SL, Franklin RM, Barile MF: Epidemic caprine keratoconjunctivitis: Recovery of *Mycoplasma conjunctivae* and its possible role in pathogenesis, *Infect Immun* 18(3):806–815, 1977.
135. Egwu GO: In vitro antibiotic sensitivity of *Mycoplasma conjunctivae* and some bacterial species causing ovine infectious keratoconjunctivitis, *Small Rumin Res* 7(1):85–92, 1992.
136. Hosie BD, Greig A: Role of oxytetracycline dihydrate in the treatment of mycoplasma-associated ovine keratoconjunctivitis in lambs, *Brit Vet J* 151(1):83–88, 1995.
137. Jelocnik M, Self R, Timms P, Borel N, Polkinghorne A: Novel sequence types of *Chlamydia pecorum* infect free-ranging Alpine ibex (*Capra ibex*) and red deer (*Cervus elaphus*) in Switzerland, *J Wildl Dis* 51(2):479–483, 2015.
138. Tavernier P, Sys SU, De Clercq K, et al: Serologic screening for 13 infectious agents in roe deer (*Capreolus capreolus*) in Flanders, *Infect Ecol Epidemiol* 5:29862, 2015.
139. Liu F, Li JM, Zeng FL, et al: Prevalence and risk factors of brucellosis, chlamydiosis, and bluetongue among sika deer in Jilin Province in China, *Vector Borne Zoonotic Dis* 18(4):226–230, 2018.
140. Hopkins JB, Stephenson EH, Storz J, Pierson RE: Conjunctivitis associated with chlamydial polyarthritis in lambs, *J Am Vet Med Assoc* 163(10):1157–1160, 1973.
141. Wilsmore AJ, Dagnall GJR, Woodland RM: Experimental conjunctival infection of lambs with a strain of *Chlamydia psittaci* isolated from the eyes of a sheep naturally affected with keratoconjunctivitis, *Vet Rec* 127(9):229–231, 1990.
142. Stephenson EH, Storz J, Hopkins JB: Properties and frequency of isolation of chlamydiae from eyes of lambs with conjunctivitis and polyarthritis, *Am J Vet Res* 35(2):177–180, 1974.
143. Storz J, Pierson RE, Marriott ME, Chow TL: Isolation of psittacosis agents from follicular conjunctivitis of sheep, *P Soc Exp Biol Med* 125(3):857, 1967.
144. Cello RM: Ocular infections in animals with PLT (Bedsonia) group agents, *Am J Ophthalmol* 63(5):1270–1273, 1967.
145. Walker E, Jelocnik M, Bommana S, Timms P, Carver S, Polkinghorne A: Understanding the health and production impacts of endemic *Chlamydia pecorum* infections in lambs, *Vet Microbiol* 217:90–96, 2018.
146. Laroucau K, Aaziz R, Vorimore F, Menard MF, Longbottom D, Denis G: Abortion storm induced by the live C-abortus vaccine 1B strain in a vaccinated sheep flock, mimicking a natural wild-type infection, *Vet Microbiol* 225:31–33, 2018.
147. Dagnall GJ: An investigation of colonization of the conjunctival sac of sheep by bacteria and mycoplasmas, *Epidemiol Infect* 112(3):561–567, 1994.
148. ter Laak EA, Schreuder BE, Smith-Buys CM: The occurrence of *Mycoplasma conjunctivae* in The Netherlands and its association

with infectious keratoconjunctivitis in sheep and goats, *Vet Q* 10(2):73–83, 1988.
149. Spradbrow P: Experimental infection of the ovine cornea with *Neisseria ovis*, *Vet Rec* 88(23):615–616, 1971.
150. Bulgin MS, Dubose DA: Pinkeye associated with *Branhamella ovis* infection in dairy goats, *Vet Med Small Anim Clin* 77(12):1791–1793, 1982.
151. Dagnall GJ: The role of *Branhamella ovis*, *Mycoplasma conjunctivae* and *Chlamydia psittaci* in conjunctivitis of sheep, *Br Vet J* 150(1):65–71, 1994.
152. Naglic T, Hajsig D, Frey J, Seol B, Busch K, Lojkic M: Epidemiological and microbiological study of an outbreak of infectious keratoconjunctivitis in sheep, *Vet Rec* 147(3):72–75, 2000.
153. Bankemper KW, Lindley DM, Nusbaum KE, Mysinger RH: Keratoconjunctivitis associated with *Neisseria ovis* infection in a herd of goats, *J Vet Diagn Invest* 2(1):76–78, 1990.
154. Maboni G, Gressler LT, Espindola JP, et al: Differences in the antimicrobial susceptibility profiles of *Moraxella bovis*, *M. bovoculi* and *M. ovis*, *Braz J Microbiol* 46(2):545–549, 2015.
155. Al-Aubaidi JM, Dardiri AH, Muscoplatt CC, McCauley EH: Identification and characterization of *Acholeplasma oculi* spec. nov. from the eyes of goats with keratoconjunctivitis, *Cornell Vet* 63:117–129, 1973.
156. Arbuckle JBR, Bonson MD: The isolation of Acholeplasma oculi from an outbreak of ovine keratoconjunctivitis, *Vet Rec* 106(1):15, 1979.
157. Sadhana OP, Gupta PP, Banga HS, Rana JS: Pathogenicity of *Acholeplasma oculi* for the sheep udder, *Aust Vet J* 70(6):227–228, 1993.
158. Bee DJ: Ovine iritis, *Vet Rec* 132(8):200, 1993.
159. Welchman D, Hooton JK, Low JC: Ocular disease associated with silage feeding and *Listeria monocytogenes* in fallow deer, *Vet Rec* 140(26):684–685, 1997.
160. Erdogan HM: Listerial keratoconjunctivitis and uveitis (silage eye), *Vet Clin North Am Food Anim Pract* 26(3):505–510, 2010.
161. Walker JK, Morgan JH: Ovine ophthalmitis associated with *Listeria monocytogenes*, *Vet Rec* 132(25):636, 1993.
162. Tryland M, Romano JS, Marcin N, et al: Cervid herpesvirus 2 and not *Moraxella bovoculi* caused keratoconjunctivitis in experimentally inoculated semi-domesticated Eurasian tundra reindeer, *Acta Vet Scand* 59(1):23, 2017.
163. Smits SL, Schapendonk CM, van Leeuwen M, et al: Identification and characterization of two novel viruses in ocular infections in reindeer, *Plos One* 8(7):e69711, 2013.
164. Squires RA, Wilson PR, Whelan NC, et al: Alpha and gamma herpesvirus detection in two herds of farmed red deer (*Cervus elaphus*) in New Zealand, *N Z Vet J* 60(1):69–75, 2012.
165. Vikoren T, Li H, Lillehaug A, Jonassen CM, Bockerman I, Handeland K: Malignant catarrhal fever in free-ranging cervids associated with OvHV-2 and CpHV-2 DNA, *J Wildl Dis* 42(4):797–807, 2006.
166. Mohanty SB, Lillie MG, Corselius NP, Beck JD: Natural infection with infectious bovine rhinotracheitis virus in goats, *J Am Vet Med Assoc* 160(6):879–880, 1972.
167. Batten CA, Henstock MR, Bin-Tarif A, et al: Bluetongue virus serotype 26: infection kinetics and pathogenesis in Dorset Poll sheep, *Vet Microbiol* 157(1–2):119–124, 2012.
168. Elbers AR, Backx A, Meroc E, et al: Field observations during the bluetongue serotype 8 epidemic in 2006. I. Detection of first outbreaks and clinical signs in sheep and cattle in Belgium, France and the Netherlands, *Prev Vet Med* 87(1–2):21–30, 2008.
169. Maclachlan NJ, Zientara S, Savini G, Daniels PW: Epizootic haemorrhagic disease, *Rev Sci Tech* 34(2):341–351, 2015.
170. Smith MC, Sherman DM: Ocular system. In Smith MC, Sherman DM, editors: *Goat medicine,* ed 2, Ames, IA, 2009, Wiley-Blackwell, pp 257–273.
171. Beitel RJ, Knapp SE, Vohs Jr PA: Prevalence of eyeworm in three populations of Columbian black-tailed deer in northwestern Oregon, *J Parasit* 60(6):972–975, 1974.
172. English RV, Nasisse MP: Ocular parasites. In Smith BP, editor: *Large animal internal medicine,* ed 2, St. Louis, 1996, Mosby.
173. Van Kampen KR, James LF: Ophthalmic lesions in locoweed poisoning of cattle, sheep, and horses, *Am J Vet Res* 32(8):1293–1295, 1971.
174. Kaplan RM, Burke JM, Terrill TH, et al: Validation of the FAMACHA eye color chart for detecting clinical anemia in sheep and goats on farms in the southern United States, *Vet Parasitol* 123(1–2):105–120, 2004.
175. Rebhun WC: Ocular manifestations of systemic diseases in cattle, *Vet Clin North Am Large Anim Pract* 6(3):623–639, 1984.
176. Clarke LL, Niedringhaus KD, Carmichael KP, Keel MK, Fenton H: Congenital ocular abnormalities in free-ranging white-tailed deer, *Vet Pathol* 55(4):584–590, 2018.
177. LaDouceur EE, Ernst J, Keel MK: Unilateral corneoscleral choristomas (corneal dermoids) in a white-tailed deer (*Odocoileus virginianus*), *J Wildl Dis* 48(3):826–828, 2012.
178. Miller TR, Gelatt KN: Food animal ophthalmology. In Gelatt KN, editor: *Veterinary ophthalmology,* ed 2, Philadelphia, 1991, Lea and Febiger.
179. Lavach JD: Lens, uvea, and glaucoma. In Lavach JD, editor: *Large animal ophthalmology,* ed 1, St. Louis, 1990, Mosby, pp 355–357.
180. Piper RC, Cole CR, Shadduck JA: Natural and experimental ocular toxoplasmosis in animals, *Am J Ophthalmol* 69(4):662, 1970.
181. Ikede BO: Ocular lesions in sheep infected with *Trypanosoma brucei*, *J Comp Pathol* 84(2):203–213, 1974.
182. Pickett JP: Ophthalmic examination techniques for food animals. In Howard JL, Smith RA, editors: *Current veterinary therapy, food animal practice,* ed 4, Philadelphia, 1999, WB Saunders.
183. Colitz CMH, Malarkey D, Dykstra MJ, McGahan MC, Davidson MG: Histologic and immunohistochemical characterization of lens capsular plaques in dogs with cataracts, *Am J Vet Res* 61(2):139–143, 2000.
184. Brooks HV, Jolly RD, West DM, Bruere AN: An inherited cataract in New Zealand Romney sheep, *N Z Vet J* 30(8):113–114, 1982.
185. Mattheeuws D, Derijcke J, Rentiers R, Hoorens J: Diabetes mellitus in two twin male lambs, *Vet Q* 4(3):135–138, 1982.
186. Abdelbaki YZ, Davis RW: Ophthalmoscopic findings in elaeophorosis of domestic sheep, *Vet Med Small Anim Clin* 67(1):69–74, 1972.
187. Kronevi T, Holmberg B, Borg K: Lens lesions in the elk, *Acta Vet Scand* 18(2):159–167, 1977.
188. Kuiken T, Grahn B, Wobeser G: Pathology of ocular lesions in free-living moose (*Alces alces*) from Saskatchewan, *J Wildl Dis* 33(1):87–94, 1997.
189. Rubin LF: Fundus of ox, sheep, and other ruminants and pig. In Rubin LF, editor: *Atlas of veterinary ophthalmoscopy,* ed 1, Philadelphia, 1974, Lea and Febiger.
190. Aguirre G, Greene B, Gross S: Essential iris atrophy in sheep, *proceedings of the American college of veterinary ophthalmologists* 12:84, 1981.
191. Gelatt KN, Brooks DE: The canine glaucomas. In Gelatt KN, editor: *Veterinary ophthalmology,* ed 3, Philadelphia, 1999, Lippincott Williams & Wilkins, pp 701–754.
192. Gerometta R, Podos SM, Danias J, Candia OA: Steroid-induced ocular hypertension in normal sheep, *Invest Ophthalmol Vis Sci* 50:669–673, 2009.
193. Gerometta R, Spiga MG, Borrás T, Candia OA: Treatment of sheep steroid-induced ocular hypertension with a glucocorticoid-inducible MMP1 gene therapy virus, *Invest Ophthalmol Vis Sci* 51:3042–3048, 2010.
194. Silverstein AM, Parshall Jr CJ, Osburn BI, Prendergast RA: An experimental, virus-induced retinal dysplasia in the fetal lamb, *Am J Ophthalmol* 72(1):22–34, 1971.
195. Barnett KC, Palmer AC: Retinopathy in sheep affected with natural scrapie, *Res Vet Sci* 12(4):383–385, 1971.
196. O'Rourke KI, Baszler TV, Besser TE, et al: Preclinical diagnosis of scrapie by immunohistochemistry of third eyelid lymphoid tissue, *J Clin Microbiol* 38(9):3254–3259, 2000.

197. O'Rourke KI, Duncan JV, Logan JR, et al: Active surveillance for scrapie by third eyelid biopsy and genetic susceptibility testing of flocks of sheep in Wyoming, *Clin Diagn Lab Immunol* 9(5): 966–971, 2002.
198. Dennis MM, Thomsen BV, Marshall KL, et al: Evaluation of immunohistochemical detection of prion protein in rectoanal mucosa-associated lymphoid tissue for diagnosis of scrapie in sheep, *Am J Vet Res* 70(1):63–72, 2009.
199. Watson WA, Barlow RM, Barnett KC: Bright blindness. A condition prevalent in Yorkshire hill sheep, *Vet Rec* 77(37):1060–1069, 1965.
200. Watson WA, Barnett KC, Terlecki S: Progressive retinal degeneration (bright blindness) in sheep: a review, *Vet Rec* 91(27):665–670, 1972.
201. Watson WA, Terlecki S, Patterson DSP, Sweasey D, Hebert CN, Done JT: Experimentally produced progressive retinal degeneration (bright blindness) in sheep, *Brit Vet J* 128(9):457–464, 1972.
202. Hirono I, Ito M, Yagyu S, et al: Reproduction of progressive retinal degeneration (bright blindness) in sheep by administration of ptaquiloside contained in bracken. *J Vet Med Sci* 55(6):979–983, 1993.
203. Main DC, Slatter DH, Huxtable CR, Constable IC, Dorling PR: *Stypandra imbricata* ("blindgrass") toxicosis in goats and sheep—clinical and pathologic findings in 4 field cases, *Austr Vet J* 57: 132–135, 1981.
204. Basson PA, Miller ES, Kellerman TS, Albi P, Von Maltitz LJ, Welman WG: Blindness and encephalopathy caused by *Helichrysum argyrosphaerum* DC (Compositae) in sheep and cattle, *Onderstepoort J Vet Res* 42(4):135–148, 1975.
205. Jolly RD, West DM: Blindness in South Hampshire sheep: a neuronal ceroid-lipofuscinosis, *N Z Vet J* 24(6):123, 1976.
206. Graydon RJ, Jolly RD: Ceroid-lipofuscinosis (Batten's disease) sequential electrophysiologic and pathologic changes in the retina of the ovine model, *Invest Ophthalmol Vis Sci* 25:294–301, 1984.
207. Mayhew IG, Jolly RD, Pickett BT, Slack PM: Ceroid-lipofuscinosis (Batten's disease): pathogenesis of blindness in the ovine model, *Neuropathol Appl Neurobiol* 11(4):273–290, 1985.
208. Buyukmihci N: Retinal degeneration in a goat, *J Am Vet Med Assoc* 177(4):351–352, 1980.
209. Hayes KC, Nielsen SW, Eaton HD: Pathogenesis of the optic nerve lesion in vitamin A–deficient calves, *Arch Ophthal* 80(6):777–787, 1968.
210. Paulsen ME, Johnson L, Young S, et al: Blindness and sexual dimorphism associated with vitamin A deficiency in feedlot cattle, *J Am Vet Med Assoc* 194(7):933–937, 1989.
211. National Research Council: Nutrient requirements. In National Research Council, editor: *Nutrient requirements of goats: angora, dairy, and meat goats in temperate and tropical countries,* Washington, DC, 1981, National Academy Press.
212. National Research Council: Nutrient requirements and signs of deficiency. In National Research Council, editor: *Nutrient requirements of sheep,* ed 6, Washington, DC, 1985, National Academy Press.
213. Divers TJ, Blackmon DM, Martin CL, Worrell DE: Blindness and convulsions associated with vitamin A deficiency in feedlot steers, *J Am Vet Med Assoc* 189(12):1579–1582, 1986.
214. Eveleth DF, Bolin DW, Goldsby AI: Experimental avitaminosis A in sheep, *Am J Vet Res* 10(36):250–254, 1949.
215. Commonwealth Scientific and Industrial Research Organisation (CSIRO): *Vitamins, Nutrient requirements of domesticated ruminants,* Melbourne, 2007, CSIRO Publishing.
216. Cebra CK, Loneragan G, Gould D: Vitamin A deficiency. In Smith BP, editor: *Large animal internal medicine: diseases of horses, cattle, sheep, and goats,* ed 4, St. Louis, 2009, Mosby.
217. Collins BK: Neuro-ophthalmology in food animals. In Howard JL, editor: *Current veterinary therapy, food animal practice,* ed 3, Philadelphia, 1993, WB Saunders.
218. Miller PE: Neurogenic vision loss. In Howard JL, Smith RA, editors: *Current veterinary therapy, food animal practice,* ed 4, Philadelphia, 1999, WB Saunders.
219. Uzal FA, Songer JG: Diagnosis of *Clostridium perfringens* intestinal infections in sheep and goats, *J Vet Diagn Invest* 20(3):253–265, 2008.
220. Smith MC: Polioencephalomalacia in goats, *J Am Vet Med Assoc* 174(12):1328–1332, 1979.
221. Rings DM, Rojko J: Naturally occurring nasal obstructions in 11 sheep, *Cornell Vet* 75(2):269–276, 1985.
222. Johnson R, Coy CH, Perry RL, Trapp A, Mullaney TP: Nasal squamous-cell carcinoma in a sheep, *Mod Vet Pract* 63(11): 897–900, 1982.
223. Binns W, James LF, Shupe JL, Everett GA: A congenital cyclopian-type malformation in lambs induced by maternal ingestion of a range plant, *Veratrum californicum, Am J Vet Res* 24:1164–1175, 1963.
224. Binns W, Shupe JL, Keeler RF, James LF: Chronologic evaluation of teratogenicity in sheep fed *Veratrum californicum, J Am Vet Med Assoc* 147(8):839–842, 1965.
225. Rosenfeld I, Beath OA: Congenital malformations of eyes of sheep, *J Agric Res* 75(3):93–103, 1947.
226. Gelmetti D, Bertoletti I, Giudice C: Bilateral complex microphthalmia with intraocular dermoid cyst in a neonate red deer (*Cervus elaphus*), *J Wildl Dis* 46(3):961–965, 2010.
227. Fulton AB, Albert DM, Buyukmihci N, Wyand DS, Stone WB: Spontaneous anophthalmia and microphthalmia in white-tailed deer, *J Comp Pathol* 87(4):557–568, 1977.
228. Schulz K: Field surgery of the eye and para-orbital tissues, *Vet Clin North Am: Food Anim Prac* 24(3):527–534, vii, 2008.
229. Hartley C, Grundon RA: Diseases and surgery of the globe and orbit. In Gilger BC, editor: *Equine ophthalmology,* ed 3, Ames, 2017, John Wiley & Sons, Inc., pp 151–196.
230. Peche N, Eule JC: Intraocular pressure measurements in cattle, sheep, and goats with 2 different types of tonometers, *Can J Vet Res* 82:208–215, 2018.

15

Diseases of the Mammary Gland

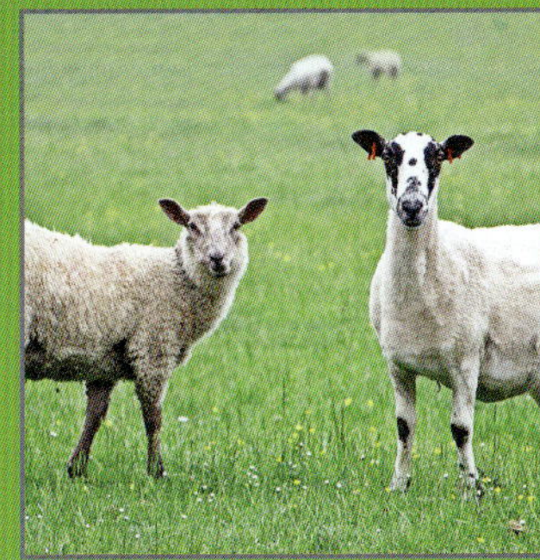

PAUL J. PLUMMER, KELLY M. STILL BROOKS, AND MISTY A. EDMONDSON

Growth in the small ruminant dairy industry is driving the need for more sheep- and goat-specific research and tailored application of milk quality principles and practices to small ruminant production settings. Intramammary infections (IMIs) in dairy operations result in significant economic losses to the producer. Mammary health is critical to young stock performance in food and fiber herds and to overall wellbeing in small ruminants kept as pets.

Normal Anatomy of the Mammary Gland

The mammary structure of the sheep and goat consists of two functionally and anatomically separate glands (halves), each with one teat; four teats are typically observed in cervids. Each half is supported by a medial and a lateral suspensory ligament. In turn, these ligaments branch off as secondary laminae that enter and support the gland tissue. The medial suspensory ligaments are adhered together and run on midline from the prepubic symphysial tendon to the abdominal tunic. The intramammary groove is formed where the medial suspensory ligaments meet the skin of the ventral udder. The elastic medial ligament should hold the udder high and tight to the abdominal wall above the level of the hocks. Heritability of the medial suspensory ligament conformation is 0.33,[1] and breeding programs should specifically select against a pendulous udder in order to minimize the risk or trauma and mastitis. The lateral suspensory ligaments run deep to the skin and superficial to the mammary neurovascular and lymphatic structures. The draining supramammary (superficial inguinal) lymph node is located at the dorsocaudal aspect of each gland. The main arterial supply to the udder is from the external pudendal arteries, which emerge from the inguinal rings and can be readily identified by their tortuous path. The paired external pudendal veins, paired branching subcutaneous abdominal veins, and paired perineal veins drain the udder and the supramammary lymph nodes. The gland is innervated by the genitofemoral nerve with superficial contributions from the lumbar cutaneous nerves (cranially) and from the mammary branch of the pudendal nerve (caudally).

Each half of the udder consists of multiple gland lobes that drain into six to nine milk ducts.[2] These ducts coalesce to form a gland cistern, which in turn drains into the teat cistern. Furstenberg's ring, an annular venous structure, forms the demarcation between udder and teat. As in cattle, the teat wall consists of five layers: mucosa, vascular connective tissue, circular and longitudinal muscular layers, and epithelium. A 0.5- to 1.0-cm streak canal at the distal end of the teat connects the teat cistern to the teat orifice and is identified proximately by the rosette of Furstenberg. The streak canal is an important anatomic and physiologic barrier to the udder with its keratin-producing squamous epithelial cell lining and muscular teat sphincter.

Production and Component Benchmarks

Species and operation type significantly influence various aspects of lactation. Dairy goats typically are milked for a 305-day lactation with a 60-day dry period, in a regimen similar to that for dairy cattle. In commercial operations, it is common for kids to be hand-reared on pasteurized milk or milk replacer in order to allow the sale of more milk and in some cases to minimize risk of vertical transmission of pathogens. In smaller or hobby dairy goat operations, kids may be allowed to nurse. Dairy sheep have a much steeper lactation curve of approximately 5 months, similar to that for sheep and goats in meat and fiber operations. A common practice in dairy sheep operations is to dam-raise the lambs for the first 1 to 2 months and then switch over to machine milking for commercial milk production; the suckling and suckling-to-milking periods offer some unique challenges with regard to mastitis control. Farm-raised white-tailed deer operations may use either hand rearing or allow nursing, or in some cases a combination of approaches based on the sex of the fawn. Hand rearing has the potential benefit of acclimating the deer to more human contact but requires significant labor and time. Nutrition, mastitis, and reproduction are the major factors influencing production in all herd types (see Chapters 2 and 8).

Milk volume and composition differ among the dairy species. Compared with milk from goats and cows, sheep milk is highest in fat (7.62%), proteins (6.21%), caseins, and other solids.[3] As a result, rennet coagulation time is shortened and curd firmness and yield are typically improved during cheese production. However, dairy sheep produce less milk volume per lactation period, and genetic potential differs significantly between European and U.S. lines. As a rough average, the East Friesian breed produces approximately 1000 lb of milk per lactation, and the Lacaune lait breed, evaluated on an as-milked basis (excluding milk used to dam-rear the lambs), produces around 650 lb per lactation. Cervid milk is much higher in fat (8.3–22.5%) and protein (10.3–11.9%) and lower in lactose (2.2–3.8%) than milk of domestic ruminants.[4]

Goat milk frequently is suggested for cow milk–intolerant children and adults; 40% of people who cannot digest cow milk will be able to tolerate goat milk.[3] Digestibility is facilitated by smaller fat globules and a higher proportion of short-chain fatty acids, such as the appropriately named caproic, caprylic, and capric acids.[3] Dairy goats produce more milk volume than that typical for sheep, with component percentages falling between those of cattle and sheep. Production volume and components are significantly influenced by breed, herd, and individual genetic potential. Miniature breeds produce a smaller volume of milk with higher fat and protein content. The average milk production in Wisconsin herds for 2008 was 1288 lb/doe, with the top four herds averaging 1510 lb/doe.[5] By comparison, the 2009 "honor roll" members of the California Dairy Herd Improvement Association (DHIA) produced as much as 2717 lb/doe and 603 lb/doe for standard and miniature breed dairy goats, respectively.[5] In many commercial operations, milk production of greater than 2000 lb during the first lactation is selected for higher production typical in subsequent lactations.

In the standard European breeds, a 3.8% fat content is typical.[3] Among the top California operations, fat contents as high as 4.9% and 6.9% were recorded for standard and miniature breeds.[6] In one high-volume operation, however, the result of a butterfat test was very low at 2.7%. As in cow milk, milk fat in goat milk can be suppressed by highly fermentable diets (with a carbohydrate-to-forage ratio greater than 2:1), subacute ruminal acidosis, and heat stress. Increasing dietary forage and offering free-choice buffers (e.g., bicarbonate) will help raise measured butterfat content. In the standard European breeds, protein averages 2.9%.[3] Among the top California operations, protein ranged from 2.61 to 3.96% and 3.91 to 5.0% in the standard and miniature breeds, respectively.[6] Unlike cow milk, the fat in goat milk does not readily rise to the top while sitting, making it essentially naturally homogenized, due to the smaller size of the fat globule.

Somatic Cells

In small ruminants, normal increases in somatic cell counts (SCCs) are associated with increased parity, days in milk, stressors, and onset of estrus, as well as with infection. The contribution of these factors is compounded in a seasonally producing herd. In a survey of 71 U.S. goat dairies, 65% did not meet grade A standards near the end of their lactation cycle,[7] and many had difficulty meeting grade B standards of 1.5 million cells/mL. Apocrine milk production in small ruminants, in contrast to merocrine milk synthesis in cattle, complicates SCC determination because some testing methods will miscount normal DNA-free cytoplasmic droplets; goats produce 10 times more cytoplasmic droplets than sheep does.[8] The Levowitz-Weber stain used for cattle SCC determinations does not adequately differentiate between leukocytes and cytoplasmic droplets.[8] Direct microscopic counts using the pyronin Y methyl green stain is specified by the U.S. reference standard for small ruminant milk, but staining methods and technician competency may vary by laboratory.[8,9] With Fossomatic techniques, counts are in good agreement with the reference standard.[7,9] Due to the difficulty in collection, SCCs are not generally monitored or measured in cervids.

Normal somatic cell populations also differ dramatically between the species. Neutrophils are the most common leukocyte in both the infected and uninfected caprine mammary gland, making up 74 to 80% of the cell population in late lactation.[10] By comparison, the noninfected ovine mammary gland cell population is comparable to that in cattle, being largely composed of macrophages (45 to 85%), with fewer neutrophils (10 to 35%), lymphocytes (10 to 17%), and epithelial cells (2 to 3%); neutrophil numbers increase during infection and are highly correlated with SCC.[8,10]

The degree to which infection directly correlates with SCC is controversial. Some workers suggest that IMI status is the major variable factoring into SCC.[10,11] In one goat dairy, however, although SCC increased with IMI prevalence, 90% of SCC variability related to factors other than mastitis.[12] In both species, higher SCCs in early and midlactation are more likely to indicate infection than equivalent counts in late lactation,[2,10] and repeated tests, or comparative samples between udder halves, are more informative than single test points.[10] SCC also is moderately heritable, estimated at approximately 0.11 to 0.15 in the larger sheep breed databases. French Lacaune breeders are trying to reduce SCC through selective breeding.[10]

Bacterial Pathogens

Bacterial pathogens responsible for clinical and subclinical mastitis in small ruminants are well characterized. Sporadic cases of clinical mastitis most frequently are caused by *Staphylococcus aureus*, coagulase-negative *Staphylococcus* spp., *Arcanobacterium pyogenes*, *Corynebacterium*, *Pasteurella* spp., and *Pseudomonas* spp.[10] Outbreaks of clinical mastitis most frequently involve *S. aureus*, *Streptococcus* spp. (*Streptococcus uberis*, *Streptococcus agalactiae*, and *Streptococcus suis*), and opportunists such as *Aspergillus*, *Pseudomonas*, *Burkholderia*, and *Serratia*.[10] Similar pathogens are presumed to cause clinical mastitis in cervids. Additionally, mastitis due to disseminated *Trueperella pyogenes* and *Mycobacterium bovis* infections have been reported in North American white-tailed deer.[13,14]

Numerous studies have identified coagulase-negative *Staphylococcus* spp. as, by far, the most important cause of subclinical mastitis in both the sheep (78%) and goat (71%). *Staphylococcus epidermidis* and *Staphylococcus caprae* are isolated most frequently, although other species are commonly identified.[9,10] Shedding of coagulase-negative staphylococci often is cyclic, in inverse proportion to SCC elevation, and may be missed on single culture. From 60 to 80% of cultured strains of coagulase-negative staphylococci are hemolytic. Hemolytic strains, and *S. epidermidis* as a species, tend to cause very high elevations in SCC, whereas other coagulase-negative staphylococcal species may not be obviously associated with an elevated SCC.[10] *S. aureus* is the second most frequently isolated subclinical mastitis agent in the sheep (4%) and goat (8%), whereas *Streptococcus* spp. and *Corynebacterium* are less frequently identified.[10] Unlike dairy cattle, gram negative bacteria are infrequent causes of mastitis in the sheep (3%) and goat (8%).[10] This difference is likely due to the difference in fecal consistency between small ruminants and cattle, resulting in less contamination of the teat end by feces containing gram negative organisms. Although rarely involved in mastitis, *Listeria* and *Salmonella* spp. are worth mentioning owing to their zoonotic potential; *Listeria* can be shed from clinically normal udders.[2]

Functional Abnormalities and Therapies

Congenital Abnormalities

Supernumerary Teats. The normal conformation of the udder in both sheep and goats includes the presence of two teats, one on each half of the udder; however, some animals may be identified with three to six teats. Dairy breed organizations (for both goats and sheep) often identify supernumerary teats as a serious disqualification in both sexes and prohibit the surgical removal and subsequent registration of purebred animals with extra teats. In meat animals and unregistered stock, less emphasis is placed on teat conformation, and many meat breed animals have supernumerary teats. In some instances, breeders have even advocated the selection of meat breed replacement animals that have four "clean" teats (i.e., fully and separately developed) as a means of increasing productivity.

As with many conditions in goats and sheep, a variety of lay terms have emerged to describe specific supernumerary teat conformations. A *clean* teat is a single normally shaped teat with a single teat orifice located at the end of the teat. Teats are then further classified as *functional* or *nonfunctional*, based on the presence of a single teat orifice and the ability to produce and excrete milk from that teat. Nonfunctional teats have the potential to interfere significantly with nursing if associated with a separate milk gland that is not drained by the primary teat; in our experience, the presence of such teats can lead to udder asymmetry with a slightly increased risk of mastitis. *Cluster* teats are multiple teats in close proximity to each other but remaining distinctly independent (i.e., not split or bifid). In some instances, two teats will be fused for some or all of their length. These fused teats may have either one or two teat orifices. If the fused portion accounts for less than 50% of the teat length, the teats are referred to as *split*, whereas teats that are fused for the entire length often are referred to as *fishtailed*. Both teat types have been referred to as *bifid* teats. In rare instances, more than two teats may be fused together; such large, conglomerate teats are referred to as "Christmas tree" teats because of their multibranched appearance. Animals with supernumerary teats also may have supernumerary mammary glands—a condition referred to as *hypermastia*.

As mentioned earlier, most dairy breed organizations prohibit the registration of animals with more than two clean functional teats. The breed registry requirements for meat breeds vary widely by registry. The American Boer Goat Association (ABGA) allows registration of animals with up to two functional teats per side (for a total of four) and also allows split teats (in which 50% or more of the teat is separate), with clean teats being preferable. The ABGA considers cluster teats and fishtail teats to be disqualifications.

Bifid (split or fishtailed) teats, when present, sometimes can be associated with and drain two distinct and noncommunicating portions of the mammary gland. In such instances, a thin membranous division along the full length of the teat cistern may be visualized with ultrasonography of the distal teat. For this examination, a 7.5-MHz or higher-resolution probe will provide images of reasonable quality. Use of a probe standoff will facilitate better-quality images; in field situations, submerging the teat in a plastic container of water will suffice for this purpose. For this technique, a small plastic flat-sided storage container is filled with water and then lifted to the ventral portion of the udder, with the teat submerged in the middle of the container. Coupling gel can then be applied to the probe and the side of the container, and the teat is imaged in the middle of the water bath through the side of the container. In the presence of a membranous division of the teat cistern, a distinct variable-thickness hyperechoic division will be seen extending down the length of the teat cistern dividing the two teats. This finding is of greatest clinical significance when one of the teat cisterns lacks a teat orifice. In such cases, this portion of the gland cannot be emptied of milk and may remain swollen and painful until the gland atrophies, which can take prolonged periods in high-producing animals.

From a production standpoint, the presence of supernumerary teats poses significant management problems. Most obviously, because the milking machine claws have only two teat cups, the presence of more than two functional teats constitutes a practical problem in getting the animals milked. Furthermore, the presence of a split or bifid teat precludes proper placement of the inflation and renders milking by mechanical means impossible on that teat. These issues are less important in meat production operations; nevertheless, supernumerary teats can complicate initial attempts at nursing by newborn lambs or kids, with cluster teats in particular presenting significant challenges for offspring trying to latch on to a functional teat.

Although detailed studies of the inheritance of supernumerary teats in small ruminants are not available, a genetic mode of inheritance has been recognized. Consequently, attention to the teat structure in breeding males and females should be of high priority, and animals with unacceptable teat conformation should be culled. Surgical correction of supernumerary teats, especially those classified as a disqualification, does not address the genetic inheritance of this condition and only prolongs and increases the prevalence of this defect in the breeding population.

Weeping Teats and Teat Wall Cyst. In some animals selected for high milk production, milk-secreting tissue may be present in the wall of the teat. Three outcomes are possible relative to the milk produced by such tissue:

1. In some instances, the milk passes through local pores into the teat cistern, with no clinical evidence of presence of this tissue.
2. Alternatively, the milk can pass through skin pores in the external epithelial surface of the teat and be released onto the skin surface, resulting in a "weeping teat." Because the muscular orifice typical of the teat streak canal is absent, this tissue may be prone to development of retrograde bacterial infections and localized mastitis. Clinically, animals with weeping teats are easily identified by the presence of milk on the lateral external surface, particularly at the time of milking. Owners of affected animals also may report that during hand-milking, their hands become wet with milk. Apart from the aesthetic downside of these lesions and the very occasional associated mastitis, they generally do not pose significant health problems for affected animals. The use of silver nitrate sticks to cauterize these weeping pores has been reported[2]; however, this procedure may potentially lead to the development of a teat cyst, as described later in this chapter.
3. Finally, if no porous passage exists for the milk to move out of the teat wall, a teat wall cyst will develop to contain the accumulating milk. In such cases, the cyst can be readily identified clinically by detection of a focal fluctuant swelling in the teat wall.

Teat wall cysts may be as small as a couple of millimeters in diameter up to 1 to 2 cm in diameter. Ultrasonographic evaluation of the teat (as just described for bifid teats) will readily identify a hypoechoic fluid-filled structure located in the teat wall.

Aspiration of the cyst, performed using aseptic technique, will confirm the diagnosis.[2] In some instances, presence of the cyst may lead to difficulty in placing the teat cup on the teat; however, this problem generally is of limited importance. Perhaps more significant is the occasional teat cyst that results in deformation of the mucosal wall of the teat cistern with consequent functional outflow obstruction of milk through the teat canal. In such cases, ultrasonography-guided aspiration of the cyst may restore milk flow, and surgical resection of the teat cyst can be performed if warranted.

Poor Suspensory Ligament Support. The mammary gland is supported by three primary attachments: the two lateral suspensory ligaments and the medial suspensory ligament located between the two halves of the udder and oriented in the axis parallel to the animal's body. These three suspensory ligaments provide the support necessary to hold the udder up tight against the body wall, where it is less likely to be injured. In cases where these suspensory ligaments do not provide sufficient support, the udder will be carried in a more pendulous fashion with excessive movement and swinging during locomotion. One commonly used rule of thumb is that ideally the udder should be held above the level of the hock in lactating sheep and goats, while cervids generally have smaller and higher-held udders.

Poor support of the udder contributes to a variety of potential problems for both the doe or ewe and her offspring. Excessively low carriage of the udder often makes it difficult for newborn lambs or kids to find the teats, because by nature, they tend to look up at the base of the udder. Furthermore, as the lambs and kids grow older, a normal nursing posture becomes impossible when teats are close to the ground. In the doe, poor udder support predisposes the animal to injury, bruising, and mastitis. Pendulous udders can experience significant trauma associated with swinging while the animal runs, or more directly when either the females' penmates step on a portion of the udder or teat or from injury incurred in a drop chute. Pendulous udders also are more prone to damage during dog attacks or from barbed wire or horns of other animals. With regard to mastitis, the low carriage of the mammary system exposes it to more fecal and environmental contamination from the bedding and predisposes affected animals to some forms of mastitis, including coliform mastitis.

Poor udder conformation generally is considered to be an inherited genetic defect and should be negatively selected for in breeding programs, for the health of both the females and their offspring. Commercially available nylon mesh udder supports are available when warranted. Alternatively, a mastectomy provides a long-term solution if the animal is being kept as a pet. Because these animals should not be bred, the absence of an udder will not be of significant concern with regard to raising offspring.

Uneven or Asymmetric Udder. Asymmetric udders or uneven udders can occur as both a congenital and an acquired condition. In rare instances, the suspensory ligaments of the udder are attached in an asymmetric fashion, which results in a "twisted" appearance of the udder in relation to the main body axis. In dairy goats, it is relatively common for does to have an asymmetric udder associated with uneven milk production. This situation may be present from the time of parturition or may develop over the course of the lactation period. In some cases, this finding may be associated with a subclinical infection with coagulase-negative staphylococci on the side with less milk production, so milk culture of each half performed separately is suggested. If the condition occurs as a herd-level problem, a thorough evaluation of the milking system should be conducted in addition to individual animal milk cultures. Milking system cleaning and disinfection practices should be evaluated, as well as milking claw design and placement during milking. In our own practice, we have observed a herd-level problem with asymmetric udders associated with placement of milking claws from the side, resulting in differential milking rates from the halves and, consequently, differential milk production.

Physiologic Abnormalities

Agalactia. *Agalactia* is the absence of milk production in an animal that should be producing milk. The two most common causes of this condition in domesticated small ruminants are systemic disease and mastitis. Cervid lactogenesis is especially sensitive to environmental and nutritional cues. In animals with severe systemic disease and decreased feed intake, milk production will drop dramatically and, in some cases, will cease altogether. A good physical examination often will identify the specific systemic disease, and treatment should be focused on correction of the underlying issue. If the duration and extent of the systemic disease are limited in duration and severity, the animal may return to some level of milk production for the remainder of the lactation. If, however, the insult is severe, milk production may not be salvageable for that lactation. A syndrome known as "contagious agalactia" associated with mastitis may be caused by any of several members of the *Mycoplasma* genus. Many of the organisms considered in the etiology of this syndrome are not routinely found in the United States and are considered the agents of foreign animal diseases; however, *Mycoplasma* spp. have been identified as a significant cause of mastitis in some U.S. operations and can be associated with decreased or absent milk production. In clinical practice, the presence of agalactia with evidence of abnormal mammary gland secretions or texture should result in inclusion of mastitis (due to any of the organisms discussed later) on the differential diagnosis list.

Udder Edema. Udder edema is a common finding in recently fresh animals, especially primiparous goats and sheep. Careful evaluation of an enlarged mammary gland is indicated to differentiate between mastitis and edema. In mastitis, the gland often will be enlarged, may be either very warm or very cold to the touch, may be painful, and typically expresses milk with an abnormal-looking texture or color or with an odor. In edema of other causes, the clinical presentation also will include mammary gland swelling, but the milk will be normal. Considerations in the differential diagnosis for udder edema should include trauma, hypoproteinemia, recent parturition (fresh doe or ewe), and dependent edema. A less obvious but nonetheless important possibility is hypoproteinemia associated with intestinal parasitism. In one herd, udder edema was the first clinical sign of hypoproteinemia and resolved after appropriate therapy for the parasitic infection (see Chapter 6).

In most cases, uncomplicated udder edema resolves without treatment in recently fresh animals. Correction of the primary cause of hypoproteinemia generally will result in clinical resolution when this is the cause of udder edema. Diuretics such as furosemide can be considered if the udder edema poses a significant risk for trauma or is seen to impede locomotion; however, extra-label drug usage requirements would be important considerations in that decision.

Precocious Udder. Precocious udder can occur in all small ruminant species but most commonly is observed in nulliparous dairy goats with high genetic potential for production. In these animals, the mammary gland development occurs before breeding or is excessive for the stage of gestation in bred animals. The presence of a precocious udder generally is not cause for concern; however, the udder should be evaluated for texture, heat, and pain which may be indicative of a mastitis. If heat and pain suggest the presence of an infection, expression of some secretions for bacterial culture often is possible, but the benefit of this procedure must be weighed against the decreased mammary gland protection associated with removing the keratin plug from the teat streak canal. Precocious udders may be asymmetric but should be soft and pliable on palpation. If an infection is confirmed, antimicrobial therapy may be indicated. Although intramammary infusion of an appropriate drug for mastitis therapy may be considered, the very small size of the streak canal may preclude infusion without significant trauma. In such cases, systemic therapy with an antimicrobial with good volume of distribution may be a more effective option. In either case, emphasis on appropriate drug withdrawal protocols is important because most producers are not accustomed to scenarios involving antimicrobial-associated milk withdrawals at the time of parturition.

Gynecomastia. *Gynecomastia* refers to the abnormal development of a mammary system and milk secretion in a male. Three different causes have been identified in small ruminants, particularly goats. In two published reports, the animals had evidence of sex chromosome abnormalities, one with Y chromosome deletions and the other with sex chromatin in the neutrophils.[15,16] Gynecomastia also has been reported to occur as the consequence of a familial predisposition associated with high milk production in the maternal line. It is speculated that the affected animals may have higher baseline production of prolactogenic hormones that lead to the abnormal mammary gland development.[17] Similarly, animals with endocrine imbalances associated with adrenal tumors may exhibit gynecomastia.[18] Finally, excessive mechanical stimulation of the teats associated with simulated milking or nursing appears to be sufficient to elicit mammary gland development with secretion of small volumes of milk.[17]

In many cases of short-term gynecomastia, the fertility of the buck may not be affected; nevertheless, a full breeding soundness exam is always warranted. When the mammary gland is excessively large, it may interfere with normal cooling of the testicles, with the potential for decrease in or loss of fertility.[17] With abnormalities involving the sex chromosomes, the affected animal generally is infertile.

Obstructions to Flow

Blind Half. Severe damage to the mammary gland associated with mastitis (bacterial or viral) or trauma may result in fibrosis of the secretory tissue and the loss of function in one or both halves of the mammary gland. In such cases, the mammary gland typically appears atrophied and no milk can be expressed from the gland. The situation may resolve spontaneously at the time of the next parturition or may be present for the remainder of the animal's life. Anecdotally, some practitioners also have utilized chemical (chlorhexidine or iodine) means of "killing" one half of an udder in cases of chronic non-treatable mastitis; however, no published reports have evaluated the safety of this procedure, and the potential exists for adulterated milk from the untreated gland. In naturally occurring cases of "blind halves," no therapy is required, and the prognosis for returning to normal full production is moderate to guarded.

Hard Milker. In some animals, the small size of the streak canal in the teat severely limits flow of milk through the orifice; animals with this condition are routinely referred to as "hard milkers." This problem may be the result of genetic inheritance of small streak canals or due to trauma or irritation associated with teat end lesions. In severe cases, any of several types of teat knife or bistoury can be used to expand the streak canal opening. The instrument is placed through the streak canal and then removed in such a fashion as to cut the internal portion of the streak canal while minimally cutting the external portion of the canal. This procedure should be performed while the udder is full, to assist in assessing the teat opening size. A second or third cut may need to be performed in severe cases. After surgery, the teat ideally should be milked every 20 minutes for 2 hours and then every hour until the next day. Owners should be warned that milking will become more difficult over the next 2 to 3 days owing to swelling, but the surgery should not be repeated until at least 1 week later, when a true assessment of the success can be determined. This procedure does carry significant risk of inducing a mastitis or chronic teat leakage if the surgeon is overly aggressive. In the authors' experience, some does with small but milkable teat orifices tend to have lower SCCs; however, no controlled studies have been performed to determine the role of teat canal size in relation to mastitis and SCC. In commercial herds that wish to keep hard milkers due to their genetic potential or lower SCC, one could consider milking all affected animals in a single group to reduce parlor dysfunction associated with having a single slow milking animal in a group.

Teat Spider and Lactoliths. Another consideration in the differential diagnosis with animals that are difficult to milk is the presence of a so-called teat spider or one or more lactoliths. Unlike with tight streak canals, these conditions result in difficult milking as a consequence of partial or intermittent blockage of the canal from abnormal tissue or by calcified concretions. Tissue-associated blockage often is secondary to formation of a mass on a pedunculated stalk that allows its free movement—the *teat spider*. A concretion termed a *lactolith* may form within the teat cistern, starting from a particulate nidus or teat gargot, and grow to the point that it can occlude flow through the teat canal. Typically, blockage occurs at the top of the streak canal by a ball valve mechanism.

In cases of blockage, palpation of the teat often will reveal a firm pea-size mass that may be movable in the teat cistern. Ultrasound examination can be performed as described in the "Diagnostic and Therapeutic Procedures" section and can reveal the presence of a tissue mass extending from the mucosa surface of the teat cistern. With this type of lesion, two basic forms of therapy have been used: (1) various forms of teat knives can be introduced through the streak canal and used to macerate the teat spider so that it can be removed in smaller portions[19] and (2) alternatively, a surgical thelotomy may be performed to remove the mass. Anesthetic block is obtained with local infiltration of lidocaine in a circumferential pattern at the base of the teat. For the procedure, a 3- to 4-cm-long incision is made parallel to the length of the teat. A teat cannula should be passed through the streak canal and used to protect the mucosa of the opposite side of the teat cistern during entry. The mucosa surrounding the lesion should be undermined and its edges apposed with monofilament suture[19] to prevent excessive granulation tissue from developing and occluding the teat cistern. The submucosa and intermediate layer are closed in a continuous horizontal pattern using resorbable monofilament suture, and the skin is closed with simple interrupted sutures.

Common Surgeries of the Teat and Udder

Teat Laceration Repair. The first step in repair of any teat laceration is to consider the prognosis for return to function. Several factors influence the prognosis, including laceration severity (partial thickness versus full thickness), laceration site, direction of laceration (parallel versus perpendicular to teat axis), and involvement of complex anatomic structures (streak canal or annular ring). With a full-thickness laceration that penetrates either the teat cistern or gland cistern, the risk of mastitis or elevated SCC is significant. An additional risk with these lesions is the potential for postoperative development of teat fistulas. The likelihood of successful laceration repair generally increases as the laceration moves closer to the base of the teat and when the laceration is oriented parallel to the teat axis.

Preoperatively the animal can be sedated if necessary, and a ring block with 2% lidocaine is performed around the base of the teat, with care taken to avoid the circumferential vein and the teat and gland cistern. If the laceration is full-thickness, some clinicians also place a tourniquet at the base of the teat to minimize interference with surgical visualization by milk from the teat. If necessary, the wound should be surgically debrided, with preservation of as much tissue as possible. Full-thickness lacerations should be closed in three layers.[19] First, the submucosa is closed using a continuous horizontal pattern that does not penetrate the mucosa, followed by closure of the intermediate layer using a similar pattern, best accomplished with 4-0 monofilament synthetic absorbable suture introduced by a swaged-on taper needle. Finally, the skin is closed using 4-0 or 3-0 monofilament suture in a simple interrupted pattern. Postoperatively, the patient should not be subjected to mechanical milking or hand-milking for at least 10 days. Instead, the milk should be passively removed from the teat cistern using a teat cannula. Intramammary antibiotics should be given every other day during this time, and the mammary gland should be closely monitored for signs of mastitis.

Teat Fistula Repair. Teat fistulas that develop after teat lacerations increase the risk for mastitis in that gland of the udder. Because they do not have a streak canal or sphincter, they are open to retrograde movement of bacteria and often are associated with elevated SCCs or mastitis. When surgical correction of the fistula is warranted, the lesions should be allowed to heal until the fistula is well demarcated and easily visible. The teat should be anesthetized as described previously; then an elliptical incision is made along an axis parallel to that of the teat and around the perimeter of the fistula. Care is taken to minimize the width of the elliptical tissue removed so as to retain as much normal skin as possible for closure. The incision is closed as described for the full-thickness teat laceration.

Mastectomy. Radical mastectomy is a treatment for mammary conditions such as gangrenous mastitis not responsive to medical treatment, precocious udder that exhibits inappropriate lactation, or other localized mammary disease. Goats with gangrenous mastitis present with clinical signs of a discolored (dark) udder that is cold, painful, and swollen. The milk usually is blood-tinged. Most animals are affected at 10 to 15 days after kidding. Medical treatment is seldom successful, and chronic mastitis frequently is the end result.[20] Mastectomy has proved to be a safe and effective treatment to allow good quality of life in pet animals or in genetically valuable animals to be used as embryo donors, or in natural dams of offspring to be hand-raised.[21]

A radical mastectomy is performed with the animal in dorsal recumbency under general anesthesia (Figure 15.1). This positioning allows access to more skin for closure with minimal tension. Some veterinary surgeons prefer an elliptical skin incision. The inverted cloverleaf skin incision, however, allows dissection of the skin away from the mammary tissue and identification of the vasculature to allow ligation of the vessels to prevent hemorrhage (Figure 15.2). The arterial blood supply to the mammary gland arises from the external pudendal and perineal arteries. The blood drains from the gland by way of the external pudendal and perineal veins as well as the large subcutaneous abdominal vein. The mammary tissue can be bluntly dissected off the external rectus sheath by fanning of the operator's hand under the glandular tissue. The skin closure is then done in an X shape, with latex drains placed subcutaneously exiting away from the incision line (Figure 15.3). The dissection leaves abundant dead space, which should be ablated as much as possible by tacking the subcutaneous tissue to the external rectus sheath with absorbable sutures.

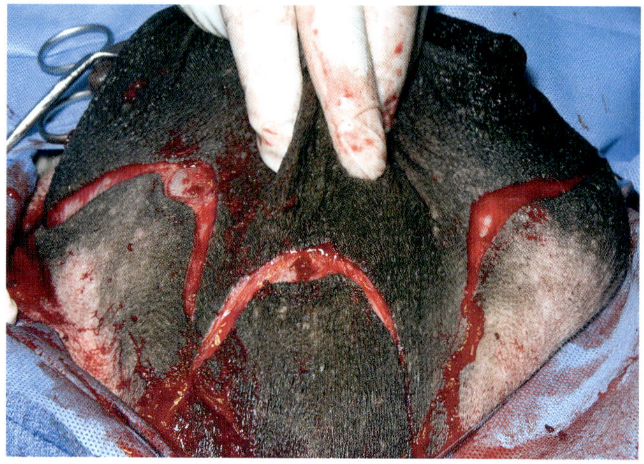

• **Fig. 15.1** Three lines of the four that make up the inverted cloverleaf skin incision for mastectomy in a 4-year-old pygmy doe. This view is from the rear, with the animal in dorsal recumbency. The teats are being held adjacent to each other by an assistant's gloved hand. (Courtesy Dr. A.N. Baird, Purdue University.)

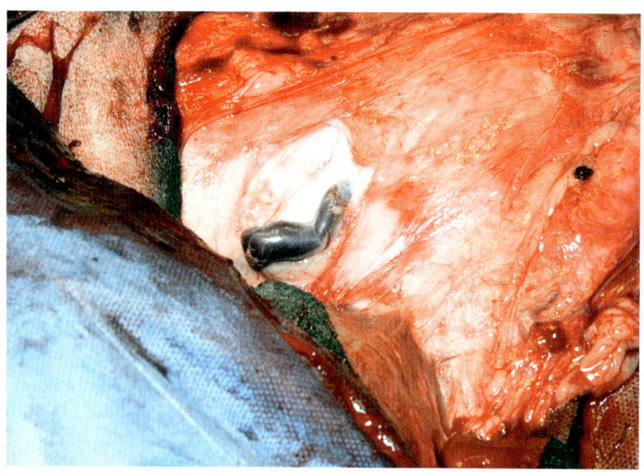

• **Fig. 15.2** The external pudendal vein near the right inguinal ring, in the doe shown in Figure 15.1. In this caudal view, the skin has been dissected to the *left* and the mammary tissue is to the *right*. (Courtesy Dr. A.N. Baird, Purdue University.)

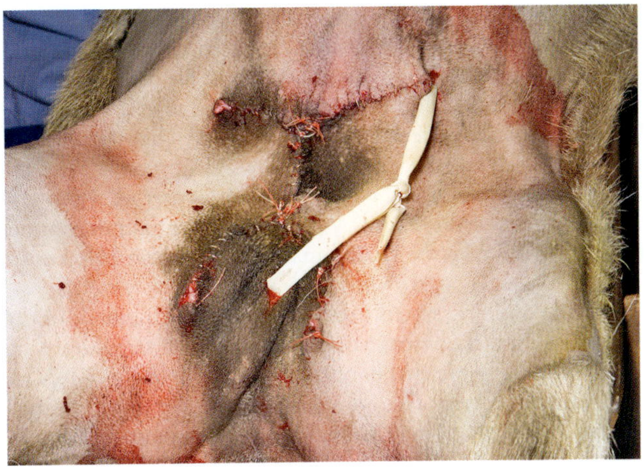

• **Fig. 15.3** X-shaped skin closure after mastectomy in the doe with a latex drain in place. The view is from the right side of the doe with her rear to the right. (Courtesy Dr. A.N. Baird, Purdue University.)

Partial mastectomy may be performed in the case of unilateral disease. The partial mastectomy is done through an elliptical incision around the teat of the affected gland. Partial mastectomy is technically more difficult to perform because of collateral circulation and different dissection required. Care must be taken in the dissection not to compromise the gland to be left intact.[22]

An alternative to radical mastectomy in does with gangrenous mastitis is ligation of the mammary vasculature in conjunction with the amputation of the teat. This surgical approach allows drainage of the glandular discharge and, ultimately, avascular necrosis of the udder. When compared with a traditional radical mastectomy, this method was described as quicker to perform, less expensive, and less stressful to the goat.[23] However, the sloughing udder may not be cosmetically pleasing to the owner.

Ligation of the External Pudendal Artery. The patient with severe gangrenous mastitis may be an unsatisfactory anesthetic risk. In such cases, one option is to ligate the external pudendal artery and vein as they exit the inguinal canal. This procedure can be performed with use of mild sedation and local anesthesia with the animal in lateral recumbency. After ligation of these vessels, the absorption of toxins from the mammary gland is limited, and the mammary gland will atrophy because the external pudendal artery is the primary vascular supply for the mammary gland of sheep, goats, and cervids.[19]

For this procedure, the animal is placed in lateral recumbency, and the area external to the inguinal canal is infiltrated with 2% lidocaine. A skin incision is made over the region and blunt dissection is used to identify the inguinal canal with both the external pudendal artery and vein exiting it. Each vessel is triple-ligated and incised, leaving two ligatures on the cardiac side. The dead space is minimized using several layers of subcutaneous sutures, and the skin is closed in a routine fashion. The clinician also may consider teat amputation after this surgery, in order to facilitate drainage of the mammary gland.[19]

Mastitis: Diagnostic Approach and Techniques

Herd Milk-Quality Investigation

Mastitis is an "economic, hygienic, and legal" problem for producers.[10] Although the incidence of small ruminant clinical mastitis typically is less than 5% per year,[9,10] problem herds may have clinical mastitis rates of 30 to 50%. The prevalence of subclinical mastitis in the average herd is very high, especially during late lactation, when chronic infections are at their highest prevalence.[10] Mastitis in small ruminants, especially the goat, often persists through the lactation and dry periods, and reinfection is common. Self-cure rates for subclinical mastitis during the dry period are 35 to 67% in the ewe and 20 to 60% in the doe.[10] New infections are associated with the first third of lactation, the start of machine milking, and the suckling-to-milking transition.[10] Mastitis control programs should focus on hygiene, the milking system and process, dry-off protocols, and culling. Culling often is the best recommendation for animals with clinical mastitis and for those with subclinical disease that do not respond to dry therapy (Figure 15.4).[2,10]

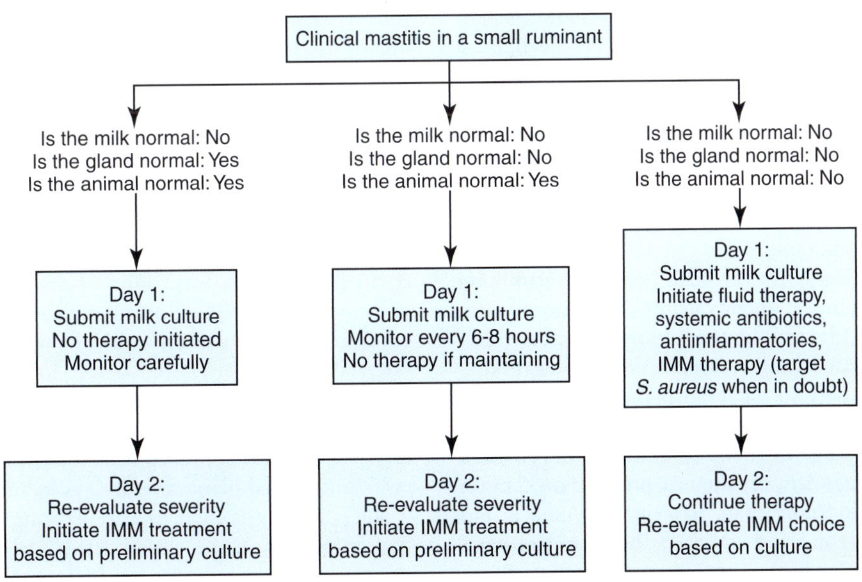

• **Fig. 15.4** Flow chart for clinical mastitis in a small ruminant. *IMM*, .

Prevention and Control

Hygiene. Skin flora and IMIs are the main reservoir for staphylococcal and streptococcal pathogens. Infections are spread and established during milking or nursing, and nursing of two or more offspring increases the risk of clinical mastitis in dam-reared systems.[10] Although supporting evidence for their use is minimal, udder hygiene practices common to cattle dairies are encouraged in sheep and goat dairy operations.[2] The dry, pelleted form of small ruminant feces facilitates good udder hygiene scores; this is especially important at milking, when the teats must be clean and dry. Teat-dipping is recommended, especially "post-dipping," which can reduce the incidence of new IMI by 30 to 40% and also improve bulk tank SCCs[8]; in goat herds, use of individual or single-use towels also can reduce IMI rates.[24] These effects are most obvious during early lactation and in herds with high levels of IMI. If the producer is unwilling to adopt routine teat-dipping, strategic application of teat dips during the high-risk periods is a reasonable compromise.[2,8,24] Teat dip solutions should be clean and changed regularly, with use of potable water to avoid contamination with *Pseudomonas* and *Serratia*.[10] Intramammary infusions should be applied with good aseptic technique and minimal cannula insertion. Splitting or sharing antibiotic infusion tubes between teats is not recommended, but if it is done, the healthy half should be infused first.[2,10] Any teat injury (e.g., lacerations, frostbite, orf infections, and teat end hyperkeratosis) increases the opportunity for pathogen colonization.

Farm hygiene and general herd management practices can have a direct effect on udder health. Bedding areas should be kept clean and dry to prevent coliform invasion. Moldy feed and bedding may introduce fungal pathogens.[1] Strict attention should be paid to stocking density; poor air ventilation and increased humidity associated with overcrowding will result in high airborne bacterial counts and a more favorable cutaneous environment for pathogens. There is some evidence to the role of nutrition in reducing clinical and subclinical mastitis, specifically ensuring that adequate levels of vitamin A and E and selenium are provided in the prepartum and lactating ration and that animals are managed to avoid prepartum ketosis.[25,26] Similarly, there is reasonable evidence that parasitic infections increase the risk of mastitis through relative depletion of energy stores and increased incidence of ketosis.[27]

Milking Processes. Milking practices and the milking system may have a critical impact on udder health by causing mechanical insult or by providing bacterial reservoirs in dirty equipment. Producers are advised to implement a milking order whereby primiparous and nonmastitic animals are milked first. This strategy will decrease major (clinical) mastitis rates among first-lactation animals and decrease minor (subclinical) mastitis rates among multiparous animals.[10] Milking insult cumulatively increases end-of-lactation bulk tank SCCs.[10]

Milking practices that should be avoided include overmilking and undermilking, claw removal under vacuum, and vigorous udder massage or stripping. Overmilking will promote teat end hyperkeratosis and subsequent bacterial colonization; undermilking can increase udder sensitivity to bacterial pathogens.[10] In dairy cattle, milkout and milk letdown are directly influenced by the teat prep process and timing. In sheep or goats, however, milk letdown is not closely dependent on the teat preparation process because most of the milk (more than 50% in dairy sheep and 80% in goats) is stored in the gland cistern, rather than the gland alveoli.[2,28] Impact events such as claw removal under vacuum, vigorous udder massage, and machine stripping transmit mastitis through retrograde entry of infected milk and surface bacteria into the teat.[10] Overmilking in commercial operations is often due to a relatively high number of animals in the parlor with short milking times and minimal help. When teat end keratosis is observed, particular attention should be paid to how the parlor is managed and to whether the first animals having units placed on them are being overmilked while the milker is prepping and placing the remainder of the units. Although uncommon in commercial goat dairies, the use of automatic take-offs can help control some of this issue.

Machine milking systems should optimize equipment to production levels, teat conformation, and operation size. Ideal small ruminant milking systems have not been fully characterized, and it is likely that current recommendations will continue to evolve. Institution of a program of annual system inspection and maintenance is a reasonable and often-overlooked step. Detailed information on how to perform a system inspection is published by the National Mastitis Council (NMC) as well as other sources. Inflations should be inspected and replaced before visible wear caused by time, milking, and sanitation processes. Suggested replacement frequencies include every 1000 to 1500 milkings and annually (for rubber inflations) and on alternating years (for silicone inflations)[1] and as often as every 60 days.[2] The milking system should be cleaned twice daily by a clean-in-place (CIP) system using appropriate detergents, sanitizers, and water temperatures. A blacklight exam can identify milkstone or protein deposits missed by the cleaning program; further information on CIP processes is published by the NMC.

Most milking system mechanical recommendations are based on data from dairy cattle. Milk lines should be constructed with sufficient size and slope to avoid milk slugging. Low-line systems that permit lower and more consistent teat end vacuum are preferred in small ruminant dairies.[2,24] Low teat end vacuum pressures of 11.5 to 12 mm Hg are appropriate for small ruminant low-line systems[2]; slightly higher teat end vacuum pressure is necessary in high-line systems. Unnecessarily high vacuum pressure will cause teat end hyperkeratosis and increased SCCs.[10] System vacuum requirements are similar to those for cattle dairies. Line system requirements can be calculated by summing a base of 30 cubic feet per minute (CFM) plus 1.5 CFM/milking unit and 3 to 4 CFM in reserve; bucket systems require a base of 10 CFM plus 1 CFM/unit. Current recommendations for pulsation rate are 70 to 100 pulsations/minute, with milk-to-rest ratios ranging from 50:50 to 70:30[2]; these are at the higher end of cattle-specific recommendations. Pulsation rates are often set similar to cattle or slightly higher with as high as 90 per minute being used in some operations.

Dry-Off. The dry period permits udder involution and colostrum development before the next lactation cycle. If well managed, it is an excellent opportunity to improve udder health and cure existing IMIs. Institution of dry-off should be prompted by decreased milk production or increased bacterial or somatic cell concentration or should coincide with the next kidding date. Generally, it is considered better for udder health to abruptly cease milking than to gradually decrease milking frequency; however, some studies in nursing ewes have failed to demonstrate a difference.[29] This approach is facilitated by decreasing the doe's or ewe's nutritional plane several days in advance of the dry date.

Dry therapy is used to cure existing infections or to prevent new infections in the close post-dry period; the former is more important in sheep and goats.[30] Animals with IMIs that persist through the dry period despite appropriate treatment should be culled.[10] Intramammary dry treatments significantly improve mastitis cure rates in the ewe (65 to 95.8%) and doe (50 to 92.5%) in comparison with untreated control animals[10,30]; coagulase-negative staphylococcal infections are more responsive to dry therapy than are *S. aureus* infections.[11] In herds with a low prevalence of subclinical mastitis (30 to 40% or less), selective treatment of only infected animals or halves is a reasonable approach; otherwise, all animals should be dry-treated.[9–11,30] In *Mycoplasma*-free herds, goats with multiple individual SCCs (iSCCs) greater than 2 million cells/mL probably are infected with *S. aureus* (with sensitivity of 100% and specificity of 74%) and should be dry-treated or culled.[9,10] Unless steps are taken to prevent new IMI in the following lactation period, dry-treated animals will lose their udder health advantage by 75 to 100 days in milk.[8,11] Given the importance of antibiotic stewardship, blanket dry treatment should only be used when a sufficient medical rationale can be articulated. Otherwise, selective therapy should be used with decisions based on individual animal history, examination, and risk.

Parenteral dry therapy is theoretically an option in meat and fiber herds but should only be used after consideration of routine antibiotic stewardship concepts. It is not advised in dairy operations, however, because antibiotics that achieve effective concentrations in the gland are associated with prolonged milk residues. Limited evidence suggests that two or more injections of parenteral medication may be needed to achieve mastitis cure rates above those in control animals.[10] Several studies show a positive effect of extra-label tilmicosin on udder texture, bacterial shedding, and preweaned lamb performance when administered to ewes[10,31]; tilmicosin should not be used in goats owing to reports of adverse events. Additionally, the benefit of using a broad-spectrum, medically important antibiotic for these limited medical benefits should be weighed.

Clinical trials are unavailable for several other drugs that theoretically should be effective in the mammary gland. Both tulathromycin (2.5 mg/kg subcutaneously in a one-time dose) and florfenicol (20 to 25 mg/kg intravenously or intramuscularly [IM] twice a day) are legal for extra-label drug use under the Animal Medicinal Drug Use Clarification Act (AMDUCA) in the United States. Tiamulin (25 mg/kg IM twice daily) is not available in an injectable form in the United States, and the labeled swine feed and water additives are not legal for extra-label use. Other drugs that are not labeled or recommended for food animal use in the United States include the aminoglycosides tobramycin and apramycin, along with two fluoroquinolones (enrofloxacin and norfloxacin) that cannot be legally used extra-label in the United States.[10]

Three nonantibiotic dry period interventions are teat sealants, mastitis vaccination, and vitamin E and selenium supplementation. Vitamin E and selenium supplementation may decrease SCC in the following lactation.[2,10] Teat sealants are available in either external (e.g., Stronghold) or internal (Orbeseal) formulations. Research in dairy cattle demonstrates that appropriately applied teat sealants help prevent new IMIs during the critical dry-off and precalving weeks.[32] Although sheep and goats are less susceptible to acquiring new infections during the dry period, these products may help in certain herds for which the environment is less than optimal. External sealants may require multiple applications—once at dry-off and repeated applications from 10 days before parturition until kidding or lambing. The internal sealant should last through the dry period and will need to be stripped out at the first milking.[32] Early milk from animals treated with internal sealants will appear clotty and mastitic but will not cause a positive reaction on the California mastitis test (CMT). External sealants may be the better choice in herds that dam-rear the young, unless personnel will be available at parturition to vigorously strip out the sealant material before nursing can begin.

Staphylococcal and coliform mastitis vaccines are available. Several *S. aureus* vaccinations have been used in small ruminants with variable success. They are most effective in decreasing the severity but not the frequency of mastitis and may be of value if gangrenous mastitis prevention is the goal, rather than reduction in herd infection prevalence and decreased SCCs.[2] A commercially available vaccine in Europe has shown efficacy at decreasing subclinical carriage of coagulate-negative *Staphylococcus* while also decreasing the severity of acute gangrenous *S. aureus* mastitis. There is hope that this vaccine may have approval for marketing in the United States in the near future. The coliform J5 cattle vaccine originally was modeled in goats. This vaccine did reduce shedding and clinical signs in experimental infection.[2] In general, coliform mastitis is not a significant problem in small ruminant herds, and when counts are elevated, hygienic practices should be evaluated first.

Elevated Bulk Tank Bacterial Counts

Elevated bulk tank bacterial counts indicate poor milk quality and create an economic crisis for the producer when in excess of legal limits (U.S. Pasteurized Milk Ordinance [PMO] Grade A, more than 100,000 colony-forming units [CFUs]/mL; PMO Grade B, more than 300,000 CFUs/mL). The first step is to determine the bacterial source: mastitis, dirty udders, dirty equipment, or poor milk cooling. The standard panel of bulk tank bacteriologic tests includes the standard plate count (SPC), preliminary incubation (or preincubation) count (PIC), lab-pasteurized count (LPC), and coliform count (Table 15.1). The SPC regulatory test is a measure of the total bacteria in the milk flora and generally is nonsensitive to source. Unlike with infections in cattle, very high elevations in SPCs do occur with high herd prevalence of staphylococcal IMI. Clinical laboratories that are more accustomed to reading cattle milk cultures may report growth of coagulase-negative staphylococci as "nonsignificant"; in small ruminants, culture of these organisms is very significant. The PIC is performed on milk that has been incubated at 55° F for 18 hours before plating and counting; this test selects for psychrotrophic bacteria, and the PIC is an indicator of on-farm sanitation and milk cooling problems. The LPC is performed on milk that has been subject to pasteurization temperatures and times in the lab before plating and counting; this test selects for thermoduric bacteria, and an increased LPC is an indicator of poorly cleaned milking equipment, biofilm development, and occasionally dirty udders. The coliform count is performed by plating milk on selective media and is an indicator of dirty udders (elevated but relatively lower levels), poor equipment sanitation (high levels), or possibly coliform mastitis (rare in the small ruminant). It is important that the bulk tank sample was correctly obtained; a sanitized dipper should be used to draw a 2-oz sample from the top of a tank that has been thoroughly agitated for 10 minutes.

The results of these tests will direct the remainder of the diagnostic investigation (see Figure 15.4). Consistently high coagulase-negative *Staphylococcus* counts in these test is highly suggestive of a IMI source as these organisms. Scores indicative of mastitis necessitate follow-up individual cultures in order to isolate the pathogen(s) and identify infected animals. Improved mastitis

TABLE 15.1 **Standard Bulk Tank Bacteriologic Test Panel: Significance of Results.**

Procedure/Result (cfu/mL)	Mastitis	Dirty Udder	Dirty Equipment	Poor Cooling
SPC > 10,000	Possible	Possible	Possible	Possible
SPC > 100,000	Possible (especially in small ruminants)	Unlikely	Possible (more likely in cattle)	Possible (more likely in cattle)
LPC > 200–300	Unlikely	Possible	Possible, more likely	Unlikely (can occur under certain circumstances)
PIC high versus SPC (> 3–4 × SPC or > 50,000)	Unlikely	Possible	Possible, more likely	Possible, more likely
SPC high/no increase in PIC	Possible	Unlikely (can occur under certain conditions)	Possible	Unlikely (can occur under certain conditions
Coliform count high (> 25–50)	Possible (rare, especially in small ruminants)	Possible	Possible	Unlikely (can occur under certain conditions)

Murphy, S. 1997. Raw milk bacteria tests: SPC, PIC, LPC and coliform count - what do they mean for your farm? pp. 34-42 in Proceedings for the National Mastitis Council 1997 Regional Meeting. Syracuse, NY. in:- RAW MILK BACTERIA TESTS – Standard Plate Count, Preliminary Incubation Count, Lab Pasteurization Count and Coliform Bacteria Counts & SOURCES AND CAUSES OF HIGH BACTERIA COUNTS – AN ABREVIATED REVIEW –.

controls, selective therapy, and removal of individual animals from the main milking string may be necessary. Milking procedures and udder cleanliness scores should be examined if dirty animals are implicated. Problems with equipment sanitation require a thorough inspection of the entire milking and CIP system. Any gasket or rubber components should be closely inspected, the CIP process and chemicals should be reviewed, and the cleaning water should be tested. The farm's milking equipment supplier can be a welcome asset in this investigation. If inadequate cooling or holding temperatures are suspected, submersible temperature data loggers such as the HOBO (Onset, Bourne, Massachusetts) can track milk temperatures between milk shipments.

Elevated Bulk Tank Somatic Cell Counts

Some commercial milk processors pay a premium or deduct from the base price based on low or high SCC, respectively. Unfortunately, a high bulk tank SCC often is ignored until a regulatory violation occurs. Such problems often arise late in the lactation cycle, when making substantial changes can be very difficult. Although nonpathologic increases in SCC are unavoidable, especially in goats, it is possible to influence SCC by controlling subclinical mastitis. Focusing on the annual average bulk tank SCC will help control for lactation-stage confounding factors and identify herd-level IMI. A strong correlation (r^2 = 0.845) between the annual average bulk tank SCC and persistent subclinical mastitis has been documented in ewes. Each 100,000 cell/mL–step increase in average bulk tank SCC equals a 2.5% increase in flock IMI prevalence (e.g., 250,000 cells/mL = 16% prevalence; 1 million cells/mL = 35% prevalence).[1] Although interpretation of SCC in goats is more complex, a survey of 155 French goat dairies demonstrated a similar association: bulk tank SCC of 750,000 cells/mL = 30% (± 12%) prevalence; 1 million cells/mL = 39% (± 8%) prevalence; and 1.5 million cells/mL = 51% (± 8%) prevalence.[10] For these reasons, elevations in bulk tank SCC should be treated as an udder health problem until proven otherwise.

In cattle, high bulk tank SCCs typically are broken down into "cow versus herd" and "new versus chronic" classification categories. High iSCCs are tallied, and a 15% threshold is used to separate out herd issues from a few very high-level shedders. If it is a herd problem, then the percentage of new infections (10% threshold) is used to classify chronicity; new problems often are due to lapses in milking technique or hygiene (Schukken Y, personal communication, 2009). Although this approach has not been validated in small ruminants, the theory should translate. Most often, chronic, herd-level IMI is observed in small ruminants.

iSCCs and production records should be obtained to identify the heaviest contributors to the tank and likely candidates for individual cultures. While interpretation of individual goat SCC scores is imprecise, individual ewe SCC scores greater than 1,000,000 are indicative of mastitis and counts between 500,000 and 1,000,000 are suspect and should be cultured.[33] Whole-herd CMT testing is a cheaper but less informative option. Bulk tank aerobic and *Mycoplasma* cultures should be performed. If these tests support subclinical mastitis, individual culture specimens should be obtained in all animals with the top 50% SCCs; ideally, all animals would be tested. Milking processes and dry therapy should be closely reviewed, as discussed earlier. Nonphysiologic, noninfectious causes of elevated individual or bulk tank SCCs include feeding the Guatemalan avocado leaf (20 g of fresh leaf/kg of body weight) and very recent intramammary infusions.[2]

Milk-Quality Crisis Intervention

Because a majority of bulk tank SCC and bacterial violations occur in late lactation, one rapid but temporary solution is to identify and remove the highest-contributing animals through milk diversion, treatment, or dry-off. These animals can be identified by calculating and ranking the contribution to the tank for each herd member; current iSCC or quantitative bacterial counts and production volumes are needed. The per-animal contribution to the tank can be estimated by multiplying the iSCC or bacterial counts by production volume after first converting to matching units. This "Band-Aid" approach will allow the producer to maintain the maximum possible production while quickly meeting regulatory standards. If the underlying disease issues are not addressed, a rapid return to elevated herd counts can be expected. In one 138-head goat dairy, the bulk tank bacterial counts were reduced from 1 million CFUs/mL to as low as 6000 CFUs/mL simply by removing 13 animals from the main milking string/line.

Considerations in Responsible Antibiotic Therapies and Residue Avoidance

Important considerations in medicating dairy animals include bioavailability in the udder and residue avoidance. Route of administration (systemic or intramammary) and drug type will influence both factors. Generally, an antibiotic that easily crosses into mammary tissue after systemic administration will persist in the milk for an extended period. Because very few drugs are labeled for small ruminants in the United States, proper extra-label use under AMDUCA guidelines should be followed. Drugs prohibited from extra-label use (e.g., enrofloxacin [Baytril], phenylbutazone, chloramphenicol, and metronidazole) should not be used in sheep and goats in the United States. Future restrictions on extra-label cephalosporin use exist for cattle; however, minor species including all small ruminants are exempt from the extra-label cephalosporin ban. Given that almost all IMI antibiotics available are cephalosporins, this exemption is critical to the treatment of mastitis in small ruminants. Although gentamicin is legally allowed, the American Association of Small Ruminant Practitioners supports a voluntary ban on the use of this drug in ruminants because of extremely long tissue-withdrawal times.

One significant challenge with extra-label drug use is calculating an appropriate withdrawal period. Several studies have documented increased milk residues from cattle intramammary products used in goats,[2,10] and goats that are dry less than 2 months are at increased risk for dry-therapy residues.[2] General recommendations include at least doubling the label withdrawal period.[2] The European Union requires a 7-day withdrawal period for all extra-label lactating intramammary therapy regimens and a 14-day withdrawal for nonlactating intramammary therapy regimens.[10] Clearance of systemic penicillin is highly variable in the goat, and residue testing should be performed before the milk is returned to the tank.[2] The Food Animal Residue Avoidance Databank (available at www.farad.org) can be consulted for specific pharmacokinetic and residue concerns. More information on AMDUCA and extra-label drug use is available on the American Veterinary Medical Association website (www.avma.org/reference/amduca/amduca1.asp).

Diagnostic and Therapeutic Procedures

California Mastitis Test. The CMT is widely used in the United States as a rapid "animal-side" assay that can be used in conjunction with clinical signs to identify mastitis. The basis for this test is lysis of somatic cells by the CMT reagent to precipitate the DNA and proteins contained in the cells. Consequently, the development of a change in viscosity of the reagent when it is added to milk is directly related to the relative number of somatic cells. Based on the viscosity change, the sample can be semiquantitatively scored to allow for sample comparison and to facilitate communication of the severity. In the United States, the scale in common use ranks the samples from "trace" to "+++." Concurrent to evaluating the change in viscosity, the CMT reagent also contains a pH indicator that will turn from blue to yellow in acidic milk.

Owing to the higher SCCs in dairy goats relative to dairy cattle and the seasonal variability in SCCs in the fall, the interpretation of CMT results in goats is more complicated than in cows. With clinical mastitis, the test will clearly show evidence of a change and provides additional support for a diagnosis. The more complicated situation arises in trying to interpret "trace" or "+" reactions in animals that have no clinical signs of mastitis. For this reason, the CMT may be best used to evaluate trends in animals or to compare the results for one half of the udder with those for the other half. Demonstration of a clear difference in the test results between halves of the udder would provide good support for an increased SCC in one side and may require further diagnostic investigation including, but not limited to, a more thorough physical exam, milk culture, and SCC. The CMT also may provide a reasonably low-cost screening test to evaluate each of the animals in a herd with high bulk tank SCCs or bacterial counts. Of note, however, if an animal with a very high SCC contributes only a small amount of milk to the bulk tank, its contribution may involve a lower total number of cells than that contributed by a very heavy milker shedding moderate levels of cells or bacteria. Therefore, the one downside of using the CMT as a screening test for bulk tank problems is that it does not allow for specific quantitation and subsequent "percent contribution" calculations, which provide the most useful data in these situations.

To perform the CMT, equal amounts of milk and CMT reagent are added to individual wells of the CMT paddle and swirled while scoring. The paddles are made of white plastic that allow for easy visualization of "stringing" with even small changes in viscosity. The results should be read quickly and will change with prolonged incubation. The paddle should be rinsed with clean water between uses (Figure 15.5).

Somatic Cell Count Testing. Monthly measurement of individual animal SCCs is a sensitive and easy method of identifying subclinical mastitis cases in dairy herds. Such testing often is performed as part of a monthly DHIA testing plan; however, very few producers use the data to fullest potential. The results are reported back as either an actual count or a linear score that is logarithmically derived from the actual count. Perhaps one of the easiest ways to utilize these data is to monitor for animals that have a linear score above a preselected "trigger score" or have had a significant jump in linear scores from the previous test point. These animals should be identified and "pulled" for further evaluation by physical exam and milk culture. Use of a CMT in these animals may help identify if one half is worse than the other, to focus diagnostic testing, with expected cost savings if separate milk cultures are to be performed for each half. Application of these techniques to herd-level problems is discussed in the earlier "Diagnostic and Therapeutic Procedures" section. There is evidence that log-transformed somatic-cell scores can be used to indirectly select ewes for traits conferring resistance to IMI and improved milk quality parameters.[34]

One important consideration with use of SCC testing is that some automated SCC methods developed for cattle are not valid when applied in dairy goats. Unlike cattle, goats produce milk by apocrine secretion, which results in the release of a large quantity of nonnucleated cellular debris in the milk. If this debris is enumerated by the automated cell counter as a true somatic cell, it will result in a falsely elevated count. For this reason, SCCs in

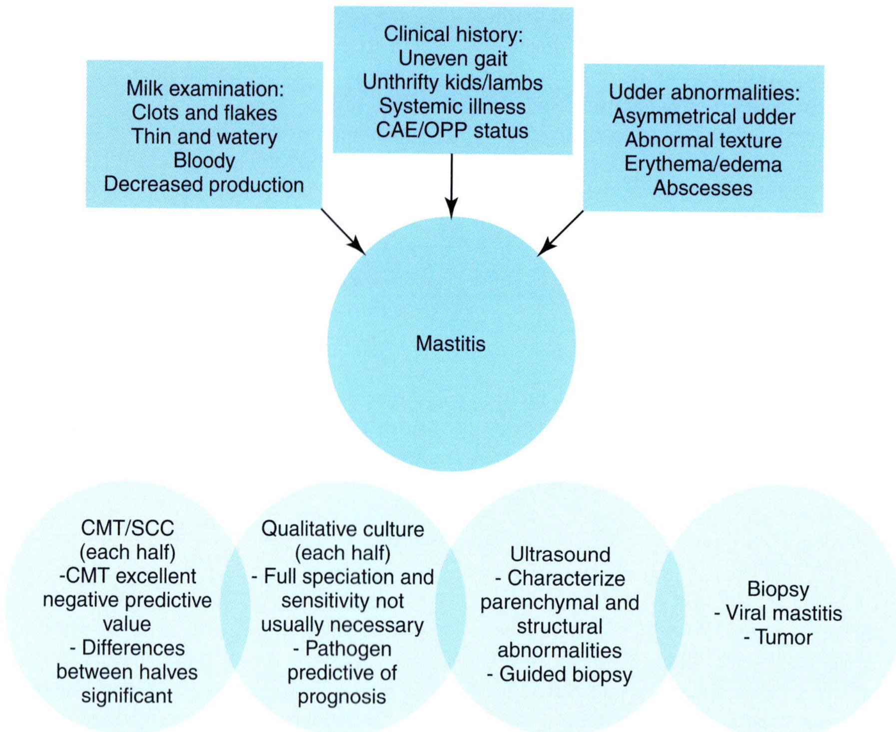

• **Fig. 15.5** Flow chart for individual animal mastitis investigation. *CAE*, Caprine arthritis-encephalitis; *CMT*, California mastitis test; *OPP*, ovine progressive pneumonia; *SCC*, somatic cell counts.

dairy goats are most accurate when performed with a dye procedure that monitors for nuclear staining. The Pasteurized Milk Ordinance requires that such a technique, the pyocyanin green assay, be used for all regulatory purposes associated with dairy goat milk.

Milk Culture and Antibiotic Susceptibility Testing. Milk cultures provide a cheap and cost-effective means of confirming a clinical mastitis, driving therapy, and determining the potential sources for infection. Cultures should be obtained before the initiation of antimicrobial therapy and should be collected in a sterile fashion. The teat should be thoroughly disinfected with teat dip and then cleaned with isopropyl alcohol. Care should be taken to prevent recontamination of the sample or of the teat by the collector's hands. A sterile milk vial should be used for sample collection; after the cap is removed, the tube should be held close to horizontal to prevent contaminates from falling into the tube during collection. An important consideration is whether the sample should be collected as a composite sample of the two halves or as a "half" sample with independent samples taken from each side. If one half of the udder is clearly more affected then the other, an independent sample of the effected side probably is warranted. In instances in which no clear differences are observed between the udder halves, the decision may be more difficult. Individual samples ideally should be collected from each half, although culture cost must be weighed against the potential added benefit. In many cases, the results of the halves are not the same, often with one side being culture-negative and the other culture-positive. Recognition of such differences will help focus intramammary therapy to the affected side, with some drug cost savings realized from not having to treat both sides (Table 15.2).

After collection, the milk samples should be rapidly cooled to minimize overgrowth of contaminates and then sent to the laboratory for testing. If the samples will not be inoculated within 24 hours, freezing the samples until processing may be considered. The effect of freezing on bacterial recoverability has been evaluated and apparently is negligible, especially with *S. aureus*, which may be more readily identified *after* freezing—an effect probably mediated by cellular rupture and release of intracellular organisms. Also of clinical importance is the identification of likely suspects among possible etiologic pathogens, because this consideration may have significant implications for sample submission. For instance, if involvement of *Mycoplasma* spp. is suspected, this possibility needs to be noted on the submission form and a separate *Mycoplasma* culture requested in addition to the standard aerobic culture. In cases in which the clinician is familiar with the herd and knows what microorganisms are common in the herd, rapid culture screening that does not speciate the organisms may be sufficient to drive clinical decision-making to maximize cost savings. In such cases, for example, knowing that the organism is gram positive and looks like either a "strep" or a "staph" may be all that is needed. On-farm culture systems that use combinations of selective media have been developed to allow producers to perform their own milk cultures but do require some training and supervision to be fully effective.

Milk cultures ideally should be collected and submitted in all cases of clinical mastitis and when significant changes in SCC are observed during monthly testing. Recent data suggest that many animals with subclinical mastitis may freshen, so routine screening of recently fresh animals in herds in which significant subclinical mastitis is present may be considered. Farm records should be kept with the culture information, to permit trend evaluation and identification of common organisms, which can be used to drive therapy decisions during the wait for culture results.

TABLE 15.2 Treatment Recommendations Based on Milk Culture Results in Small Ruminants.

Bacterial Culture Result	Treatment Recommendations	
No growth	*If not sick*: No antibiotics; monitor for disease progression	*If sick (fever, off feed, dehydrated)*: Antiinflammatories, IV or oral fluids if warranted for dehydration; monitor often for progression of disease
Coagulase-negative staphylococci	*If not sick*: IMM lactating antibiotics; milk last; record culture result in record; monitor closely for recurrence	*If sick (fever, off feed, dehydrated)*: IMM lactating antibiotics, fluid therapy if warranted; monitor often for progression of disease
Staphylococcus aureus	*If not sick*: Immediately segregate animal and milk last; consider culling; extended IMM therapy is an option but need to monitor culture status; monitor for disease progression	*If sick (fever, off feed, dehydrated)*: Treat aggressively (rapid deterioration is possible): IV fluid therapy, IMM lactating therapy with drug effective against staphylococci and NSAIDs; consider teat amputation, pudendal artery ligation, or mastectomy in genetically valuable animals if systemic illness progresses; monitor often for progression of disease
Coliform	*If not sick*: IMM antibiotics with high CFU count (consider use of IMM preparation with adequate coliform activity, possibly ceftiofur hydrochloride IMM preparation); monitor low CFU counts; monitor for disease progression	*If sick (fever, off feed, dehydrated)*: Treat aggressively (possible rapid deterioration): IV or oral fluid therapy, systemic antibiotics with good gram negative activity, IMM antibiotics with high CFU count, NSAIDs; monitor for progression of disease

CFU, Colony-forming unit; *IV*, intravenous; *NSAID*, nonsteroidal antiinflammatory drug.

In most instances, treatment decisions have already been made before the results of antibiotic sensitivity testing, which often takes 48 hours after sample submission, become available. Determining sensitivity patterns may be helpful in driving treatment decisions on future cases, particularly when common trends in the isolated organisms are observed. An additional important consideration is that only a limited number of drugs have mammary-specific minimum inhibitory concentration cutoff points for testing; thus, reported sensitivity findings need to be interpreted in light of the drug distribution and locally attainable concentrations. A point worthy of emphasis is that no drugs are currently labeled for use in mastitis of sheep, goats, or cervids—hence, all such regimens constitute extra-label drug use and must follow the guidelines provided by AMDUCA.

When herd-level problems are identified, the use of bulk tank milk cultures also may be worthwhile. These cultures provide a herd-level view of potential pathogens and of the relative extent of mastitis issues in the herd. Bulk tank milk culture samples should be collected only after the tank has been agitated for a minimum of 5 minutes and should be taken from the top of the tank using a sterile dipper.[35] Samples should not be collected at the outlet of the tank. The primary bulk tank culture method used is the SPC, which enumerates culturable bacteria per milliliter of bulk tank milk. It also provides some speciation and an estimate of relative numbers of different bacterial classes, which can assist in identifying what pathogens are present in the herd and what organisms predominate in the sample. Knowledge of the most prevalent organisms can help identify the likely source of the problem, because the organisms that cause subclinical mastitis (commonly coagulase-negative staphylococci) typically do not overlap with the organisms commonly associated with poor sanitation of the milking system.

Two additional bulk tank milk culture techniques, the LPC and the PIC, can be used for further evaluation of the types of organisms present. For the LPC, the bulk tank milk sample is subjected to a simulated pasteurization process. This test is used to identify thermophilic organisms (those that survive and replicate in hot conditions), which often are associated with improper sanitation and cleaning of the milking system or pipeline. Elevations in LPC should trigger further evaluation of the milking system, replacement and cleaning of pipeline gaskets, and evaluation of the cleaning protocols. The second test is the PIC, which allows a moderate-temperature incubation period before an SPC is performed. This test identifies organisms that may be associated with milk spoilage as well as organisms that will overgrow if the bulk tank is not cooling appropriately and rapidly. Bulk tank cultures can also be used to assess the herd status of contagious organisms such as *S. aureus* and *Mycoplasma*. As with standard milk culture, the laboratory needs to be made aware if *Mycoplasma* culture is needed at the time of sample submission.

Ultrasound Examination. Mammary gland ultrasonography is most helpful in identifying lesions associated with the teat cistern, streak canal, or teat wall.[36] Details of its use for this purpose are provided in the sections discussing those topics. Ultrasonography also can be utilized to evaluate focal swellings of the mammary gland associated with abscessation of the supramammary lymph nodes; elevated length (> 9.5 mm), depth (> 6.7 mm), and ellipse area (> 11.7 mm^2) of the supramammary lymph node is a sensitive (92–96%) through non-specific (50–62%) indicator of subclinical mastitis in ewes.[37] The procedure is best performed with a 7.5- to 10-MHz linear or curvilinear probe and a latex standoff. Use of a standoff permits higher-resolution imaging of superficial structures, particularly of the teat. Alternatively, the teat can be submerged into a plastic container holding water and the probe used to image it through the container wall, creating an inexpensive standoff (Figure 15.6). Endoscopic examination of the teat has been described using a 2.7-mm rigid endoscope under local anesthesia and strict aseptic conditions.[33]

Biopsy. In cases in which other diagnostic modalities fail to provide sufficient evidence of a specific cause mastitis, mammary gland biopsy may be considered. This procedure should not be used to evaluate routine mastitis cases and should instead be reserved for complex cases in which definitive diagnosis both is necessary and will drive treatment decisions. Complications of udder biopsies include iatrogenic mastitis, production of blood tinged milk, and udder edema.

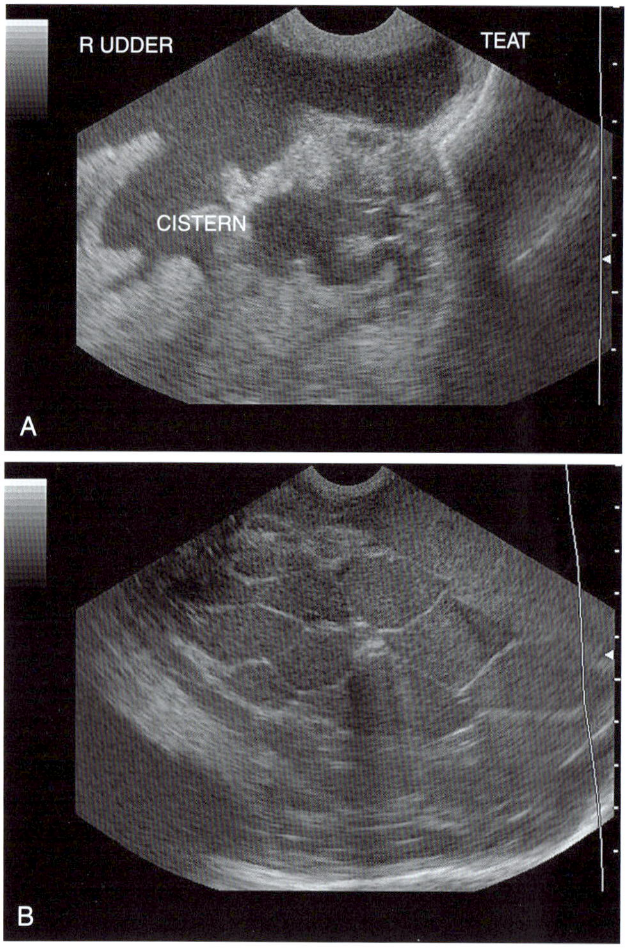

• **Fig. 15.6 A.** Ultrasound image of the right mammary gland obtained from a 3-year-old LaMancha cross goat, demonstrating the normal appearance of the udder in a lactating goat. The cistern has an echogenic appearance in which the anechoic milk accumulates and is directed toward the teat. The milk usually is seen to swirl during real-time examination. This image was obtained using a 7-MHz microconvex transducer. Dorsal is to the *left*. **B.** Ultrasound image of the mammary gland of a 4-year-old pygmy doe with chronic mastitis of 1 year's duration. Fibrin strands of adhesions, in response to the chronic inflammation, appear as hyperechoic lines throughout the gland cistern. The normal gland cistern should appear as a cavity containing anechoic milk. This image was obtained using a 7-MHz microconvex transducer. The adhesions were confirmed by gross examination after mastectomy in this goat. (Courtesy Dr. Debra Baird, Purdue University.)

Biopsy is best performed using a 16- to 18-gauge spring-loaded biopsy needle. In our experience, the automated feature of these biopsy needles allows more reliable collection and results in higher-quality biopsy specimens. Generally, the skin is prepared using sterile technique and the needle is introduced through the skin into the area of interest. Of note, with some styles of instruments, the biopsy tray will extend 1 to 2 cm past the needle with deployment. The biopsy instrument should therefore not be advanced too deep to miss the desired biopsy area. Ultrasound-assisted or -guided biopsy allows for sampling a target area when localized lesions are present. The biopsied material can be used for bacterial culture, viral isolation, and histopathologic analysis when needed. In one report, the biopsy was performed by passing a Tru-Cut needle through the streak canal and up into the mammary gland parenchyma.

Mastitis Pathogens

Clinical Mastitis. Although clinical mastitis constitutes a small percentage of mastitis cases in small ruminants, usually less than 5%, it frequently is the form of mastitis that the producer is most aware of.[10] Clinical signs of mastitis include hard and swollen glands, enlarged supramammary lymph nodes, and possibly fever. Milk from affected glands may have an "off" color, contain flakes or clots, or be thinner or thicker than normal. Lameness or abnormal gait may be observed in some animals because of pain in the affected gland. Clinical mastitis usually is limited to sporadic cases, but occasional herd outbreaks have been observed.[38–40] Even with treatment, clinical mastitis can become subclinical mastitis in many cases and clinical cure is not synonymous with bacteriological cure. When possible, best outcomes are typically achieved through early treatment with an effective drug.

Several different organisms have been implicated in small ruminant clinical mastitis. The most common cause of clinical mastitis in both dairy and meat production systems is *S. aureus.*[10] *Mannheimia haemolytica* is also a significant primary cause of clinical mastitis in meat production systems.[41] Other organisms that have been implicated include coagulase-negative staphylococci, *Enterobacteria* spp., *Pseudomonas* spp., *A. pyogenes, Streptococcus* spp., *Bacillus* spp., mycoplasmas, and fungal organisms.[10]

Coliform Mastitis. Although coliforms are very common in clinical mastitis in dairy cattle, these organisms are not a common cause of clinical mastitis in small ruminants. Coliforms account for between 1.4% and 14.2% of reported cases.[42–44] Coliforms, mainly *Escherichia coli* and *Klebsiella*, have been isolated in cases of small ruminant clinical mastitis. Both organisms are gram negative rods and form large gray or yellow, colonies. The relatively lower incidence of coliform mastitis in small ruminants probably is due to the difference in fecal consistency between small ruminants and cattle. The drier feces of small ruminants contribute to less fecal contamination of the udder. Coliform mastitis is most common in periparturient does.

Clinical Signs Clinical signs of coliform mastitis include fever, elevated heart rate, swelling, and heat and pain in the affected gland.[45] Although coliforms are not the predominant species associated with this disorder, they have been isolated in clinical cases.[44] Coliforms can cause an endotoxin release that leads to severe systemic illness in the affected animal. Many of the clinical signs of coliform mastitis are associated with release of lipopolysaccharides and the systemic response to these endotoxins.

Treatment Treatment of coliform mastitis must be aimed at elimination of the organism as well as supportive care of the patient. Intramammary and systemic antibiotics may be indicated. Controversy exists regarding the benefit of antibiotic therapy in cases of coliform mastitis. It is believed that the bacteria are cleared from the udder very quickly and that a majority of the clinical signs constitute a reaction to the endotoxin release; intramammary antibiotics may therefore be of little benefit.[46] Some research has shown a benefit from systemic antibiotics. Systemic antibiotics may be helpful in cases with evidence of septicemia. Therefore, treatment with systemic antibiotics should be considered in cases in which the animal is systemically ill. Supportive care includes administration of antiinflammatory agents, such as nonsteroidal antiinflammatory drugs (NSAIDs), and intravenous fluid support (see Chapter 3 and Appendix 2). It is important to evaluate the hydration status of the patient when NSAID dosages are determined. Dehydration increases the potential for nephrotoxic effects of NSAIDs. Until the hydration status is corrected, the dose of NSAIDs should be reduced to decrease the chance of damage to the kidneys.

Prevention. Coliform mastitis is an environmental disease, so prevention strategies should be aimed at the environment. Care should be taken to provide dry, clean bedding, and teats should be dried thoroughly after milking. Efforts also should be made to prevent teat end injuries as well, because teat injuries may predispose affected animals to the development of coliform mastitis.

Bluebag (Gangrenous Mastitis). Bluebag is a form of acute mastitis characterized by ischemic necrosis of the udder causing discoloration of the udder. The most common bacterium isolated in gangrenous mastitis is *S. aureus*.[44,47] *M. haemolytica*, *Clostridium* spp., and the coliforms also have been isolated in cases of gangrenous mastitis.[44] In one study, *S. aureus* was isolated in 60% of cases.[46] Gangrenous mastitis typically is seen during lactation but occasionally appears during the last week of gestation as well.

Clinical Signs. Clinical signs of gangrenous mastitis begin with change in the teat or udder floor becoming cool and edematous. The affected animal also may become lame. Animals with gangrenous mastitis often will develop a fever and have a decreased appetite as well. Eventually, the udder progresses in appearance from a reddish to a blue discoloration, and the secretions become watery and red. Occasionally, gas bubbles may be present as well. In some cases, death may occur within 24 hours of onset of clinical signs. If the animal survives the initial stage of infection, a demarcation line will form on the udder, and the affected portion of the udder will slough. Supramammary lymph nodes also will become enlarged, edematous, and hemorrhagic. Histopathologic exam of the affected tissues reveals proliferation of the connective tissue and thrombosis and necrosis of groups of lobules.[47]

Treatment. Treatment of gangrenous mastitis varies depending on the severity of the infection. Early cases can be treated with antiinflammatory agents, systemic antibiotics, and fluid support. As cases progress and a larger portion of the udder becomes necrotic, surgical removal of the affected udder may be required. Surgical removal can be accomplished through a surgical mastectomy or by vascular ligation and teat amputation.[23] The case-fatality rate is high with gangrenous mastitis, especially in cases left untreated.

S. aureus Mastitis. *S. aureus* is the most common cause of clinical mastitis in small ruminants, accounting for 11 to 65.3% of the cases.[42–44] This organism is a gram positive coccus that occurs in clumps or pairs. It forms large colonies that are surrounded by a zone of incomplete hemolysis and up to 2 mm of complete hemolysis (Figure 15.7). Most but not all isolates exhibit such double-zone hemolysis.

Clinical Signs. The clinical presentation in *S. aureus* mastitis ranges from severe gangrenous mastitis to subclinical mastitis. Acute infections manifest with a swollen, hot, and painful udder half accompanied by systemic illness. Chronic infections are associated with decreased production accompanied by induration and abscess formation within the udder.[2] Subclinical infections are extremely difficult to treat and should be considered contagious.

Control. *S. aureus* is thought to be transmitted primarily through milking. The organism resides in microabscesses in chronically infected animals, which then serve as a source of infection for other members of the herd or flock. *S. aureus* mastitis can be very difficult to cure, with documented resistance to streptomycin (48–87%) and up to 30% resistance to penicillin and ampicillin.[48] All culture-positive animals should either be culled or milked last to prevent spread to flock- or herdmates. *S. aureus* is shed intermittently, so a single negative culture does not mean

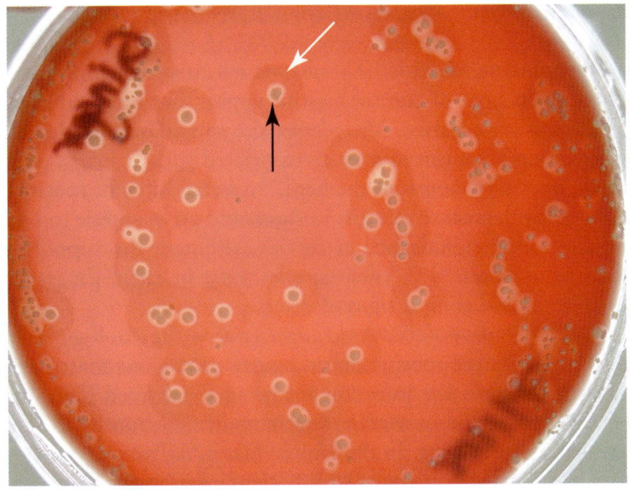

• **Fig. 15.7** Characteristic double-zone hemolysis of *Staphylococcus aureus*. *Black arrow* shows the complete hemolysis zone; *white arrow* shows the incomplete hemolysis zone.

that an animal is truly clear of the organism. Before an animal can be returned to the main milking string, negative results on serial cultures and persistently low SCCs must be documented. *S. aureus* milk should be pasteurized before it is fed to kids or lambs, because diarrhea, pneumonia, and even death have been reported in kids and lambs consuming infected milk.[2] Recently, a commercial biofilm matrix polysaccharide vaccine (VIMCO, HIPRA, Spain) has been licensed in Europe for control of *S. aureus* mastitis in small ruminants.

Mannheimia Mastitis. *M. haemolytica* is a common cause of mastitis in sheep and occasionally has been isolated from goat's milk. This organism is a gram negative bipolar rod that forms medium, gray-tinged, transparent colonies on blood agar. Hemolysis also can be seen on blood agar. *M. haemolytica* probably is transmitted by suckling kids or lambs, where it often is found as part of the normal flora of the upper respiratory tract.[49,50] Clinical signs can mimic those of *S. aureus* mastitis, so this infection should be a consideration in the differential diagnosis for bluebag.

Pseudomonas Mastitis. *Pseudomonas* is a gram negative rod that forms granular and dry-appearing colonies of a variety of colors. The source of *Pseudomonas* may be contaminated water or teat dips, old pitted inflations on the milking machine, and wet bedding. Case presentations range from subclinical to gangrenous mastitis.[40,51] Affected animals show clinical signs of systemic disease such as inappetence, fever, and depression, in addition to a firm, swollen, painful udder. Culling of infected and carrier animals is recommended; however, aggressive therapy may be successful.[52] When this organism is cultured from a mastitis specimen, careful attention should be paid to the water in the parlor and the teat dip as a possible source.

T. pyogenes Infection. *T. pyogenes* (previously known as *A. pyogenes*) is a small gram-negative rod that grows slowly on blood agar and forms very small "peach fuzz" colonies. *T. pyogenes* infections are associated with multiple abscesses in the udder. *T. pyogenes* infections are more severe in nonlactating animals than in lactating animals. With chronic infection, culling is advised. If no evidence of spread to any other organs is found, amputation of the affected teat or gland can be performed.[2]

Other Species Associated With Clinical Mastitis. Additional species that have been isolated in clinical mastitis cases include

Streptococcus spp., *Micrococcus* spp., *Corynebacterium* spp., and *Bacillus* spp.[43,52,53]

Mycoplasma Mastitis. *Mycoplasma* mastitis frequently is suspected when signs of clinical mastitis appear, but repeated bacterial cultures are negative. *Mycoplasma* also should be considered as the infecting organism in mastitis associated with arthritis, pneumonia, or conjunctivitis in the herd.[54] Several different species of *Mycoplasma* that cause mastitis in sheep and goats appear to be of limited clinical significance in cervids, although the supporting literature is sparse.[55,56] These species vary in their geographic distribution and clinical signs of disease.

Mycoplasma agalactiae. *M. agalactiae* is the etiologic agent associated with the specific disease entity contagious mastitis. At present, *M. agalactiae* infection is rare in the United States but commonly is found in Mediterranean countries, Europe, Middle East, and South Africa. In the United States, *M. agalactiae* mastitis is a reportable disease. Clinical signs of contagious mastitis include septicemia with localization in the udder, joints, or eyes. The organism is shed in the milk, urine, feces, and ocular and nasal discharge for months, which can be a source of infection for other animals in the flock or herd.[10] Transmission of *M. agalactiae* is through ingestion or inhalation. Environmental contamination can occur and can be a source of infection as well.

Mycoplasma Mycoides Subsp. Mycoides (Large Colony). *M. mycoides* subsp. *mycoides* (large colony) has been identified in cases of mastitis in the United States, Israel, and Europe.[38,44,54,57–60] This species is associated with respiratory disease as well.[54] It also has been classified by some workers as a cause of contagious agalactia. The disease associated with the organism occurs frequently in Europe.

Mycoplasma Putrefaciens. *M. putrefaciens* has been associated with outbreaks of mastitis, agalactia, abortion, and arthritis in California, Europe, and the Middle East.[2,45] *M. putrefaciens* also has been identified in cases of subclinical mastitis characterized by fibrosis or palpable inflammation within the udder with no visible changes in the milk. This organism does not always cause fever in affected animals.

Other Mycoplasmas. Several other *Mycoplasma* species have been described in association with mastitis. *M. mycoides* subsp. *capri* and *M. mycoides* subsp. *capricolum* have both been implicated in cases of mastitis in goats in France. Experimental infections with *M. mycoides* subsp. *capricolum* resulted in severe clinical mastitis in does, manifesting with thick yellowish secretions, increased somatic cells, agalactia, and enlarged lymph nodes. Pneumonia, polyarthritis, and keratoconjunctivitis also were observed in the nursing kids. *Mycoplasma arginini* has been associated with purulent mastitis in does in India but usually is considered nonpathogenic.

Clinical Signs. Clinical signs of *Mycoplasma* mastitis develop within 5 to 7 days of infection. Affected animals usually are in early lactation. Early signs of *Mycoplasma* mastitis seen during the septicemia stage include decreased appetite and depression. Some animals also will be unwilling to follow the herd. The septicemic stage is followed by development of purulent mastitis and agalactia. The secretions initially are watery but quickly become thick and lumpy. A very rapid decrease in milk production with progression to agalactia within 2 to 3 days may be seen. Affected udders may return to production in subsequent lactations. Mycoplasma does not always affect both halves of the udder. In cases in which young animals are ingesting the affected milk, pneumonia and polyarthritis may develop in the young stock. Mortality rates can reach up to 20% if the disease is left untreated. Carrier animals can be found in herds or flocks and can act as a source of infection to the rest of the herd or flock. Several *Mycoplasma* species have been cultured from the external ear canals of goats and sheep and may be a reservoir for the organism in carrier animals.[61] In addition, ear mites have been suggested as a potential vector for spread between animals because large numbers of mycoplasmas have been isolated from ear mites, which easily pass between animals.[61] *Mycoplasma* mastitis also can occur in conjunction with outbreaks of respiratory disease, arthritis, or abortion.[61,62] Death can be seen during the acute stage of the disease.

Diagnosis. Mycoplasma mastitis can be suspected when blood agar cultures are negative in face of a clinical mastitis outbreak or when SCCs are elevated with no cause. Special cultures must be performed to diagnose *Mycoplasma*, so *Mycoplasma* cultures must be specifically requested from the diagnostic lab. In addition to milk samples, joint fluid, ocular swabs, ear swabs, blood, liver, spleen, feces, and urine can all be potential samples for culture. Polymerase chain reaction (PCR) assay is available and may speed diagnosis of *Mycoplasma* infection. Serologic testing using a commercially available enzyme-linked immunosorbent assay (ELISA) is available in Europe but is not widely available or utilized in the United States at this time.

Histopathologic examination reveals marked interstitial inflammation with mononuclear leukocytes seen around acini and ducts. Additionally, mononuclear cells and desquamated epithelial cells also may be seen within the ducts. Immunohistochemistry or Giemsa staining may identify the organism.

Treatment. Treatment of *Mycoplasma* mastitis generally is ineffective. Antibiotics that typically are effective against mycoplasmas can be tried but may induce carrier status in affected animals, and their use entails very extended milk withdrawal periods. Slaughter or culling of affected animals is recommended unless *Mycoplasma* is endemic in the herd or flock. In such situations, anti-*Mycoplasma* treatment is recommended for all animals in the herd or flock.

Control. *Mycoplasma* usually is introduced into the herd or flock through a carrier animal that has subclinical disease. If available, serologic testing may be used to determine the herd status.[63] In vaccinated herds, such testing is unable to differentiate between infected and vaccinated animals.[63] In dairy herds, bulk tank cultures can be a starting point to determine if *Mycoplasma* is present in the herd or flock. Outbreaks may occur months to years after the introduction of a carrier animal. This time lag reflects the potential for intermittent shedding of mycoplasmas. Stress can trigger shedding of the organism. Reported risk factors for *M. agalactiae* infections have included introduction of outside rams, improper cleaning of milking equipment, and leaving the young animals on the dams.[64]

In herds or flocks in which *Mycoplasma* is present, any affected animals should be either culled or segregated.[38] The decision to cull or to segregate should be based on the prevalence of the organism within the herd or flock. In addition, the use of common udder towels should be avoided, and individual single-use towels should be instituted. With *M. agalactiae* infection, environmental contamination is an important transmission factor. *M. agalactiae* is shed in urine and feces, so it is important to remove bedding and disinfect stalls. Because *Mycoplasma* organisms lack a cell wall, they appear to be susceptible to most routine disinfectants.

Several vaccinations have been developed but are not commercially available at this time.[65] The vaccines appear to protect against clinical disease, but carrier states can still develop despite vaccination. Therefore, vaccination should be used only as part of a complete prevention program. Vaccination may complicate the interpretation of serologic test findings, because such tests are unable to differentiate between vaccinated animals and infected animals.

Fungal Mastitis. Although uncommon, fungal mastitis does occur and usually is the result of prolonged antibiotic use. A variety of organisms have been implicated, including *Candida albicans, Aspergillus fumigatus, Aspergillus terreus, Cryptococcus albidus, Cryptococcus neoformans, Yersinia pseudotuberculosis, Nocardia* spp., *Rhodotorula glutinis,* and *Geotrichum candidum.* Clinical signs of fungal mastitis include purulent mammary secretions, induration of the affected gland, fever, and weight loss.[66] Generally, treatment is not recommended owing to the lack of approved drugs for use in food-producing species.

Subclinical Mastitis

Subclinical mastitis is a significant cause of elevated SCC and decreased production levels in small ruminants. Subclinical disease accounts for a majority of mastitis cases in a flock or herd and is a common cause of high bacterial counts or SCCs. Identification of animals affected by subclinical mastitis is much more difficult than recognition of those with clinical mastitis. In subclinical mastitis, few outward signs emerge to indicate the presence of a problem. Occasionally, the affected milk may have a slightly "off" color and may contain clots or blood, but frequently, the affected milk may be completely normal in appearance. Some producers will note a decrease in production levels for an animal subsequently found to have subclinical mastitis. Detection of subclinical mastitis may require some additional testing such as with CMT or by SCC.

Bacterial Subclinical Mastitis. The most common cause of subclinical mastitis in most herds or flocks will be bacterial in origin. Coagulase-negative staphylococci have been implicated as the leading cause of subclinical mastitis, with prevalence rates of 71% and 78%, respectively, in goats and sheep.[1] The second most common reported cause of subclinical mastitis is *S. aureus,* with reported prevalence rates of 8% in goats and 4% in sheep.[10] Subclinical *S. aureus* infections may start as clinical mastitis, which subsequently progresses to chronic, subclinical mastitis.

Coagulase-Negative Staphylococci A variety of species have been implicated in causing subclinical mastitis, including *S. epidermidis, S. caprae, Staphylococcus haemolyticus, Staphylococcus simulans, Staphylococcus lugdunensis, Staphylococcus chromogenes,* and *Staphylococcus warneri.*[67–71] *S. epidermidis* and *S. caprae* are the most common isolates (Figure 15.8). These subclinical infections tend to persist through the lactation cycle and are more common in older does and with later lactation. Coagulase-negative staphylococci commonly are found on the skin or in the environment. An ongoing debate concerns the clinical significance of infections due to coagulase-negative staphylococci.[68,71] Overall, the economic importance is unclear, because these infections do not cause severe illness or major production losses. A high prevalence of these infections is seen in many dairy goat herds.

Coagulase-Positive Staphylococci. *S. aureus* is the most common coagulase-positive staphylococcal isolate in subclinical mastitis. Many of these subclinical cases started as clinical mastitis, which did not resolve completely because the organism was not fully eradicated from the udder. Chronic *S. aureus* mastitis can be very difficult to clear, and any culture-positive animals either should be culled from the milking herd or should be milked last to decrease the potential to spread the organism to other animals in the herd. Only after multiple negative cultures and a low SCC have been obtained should an animal be returned to the main milking string.

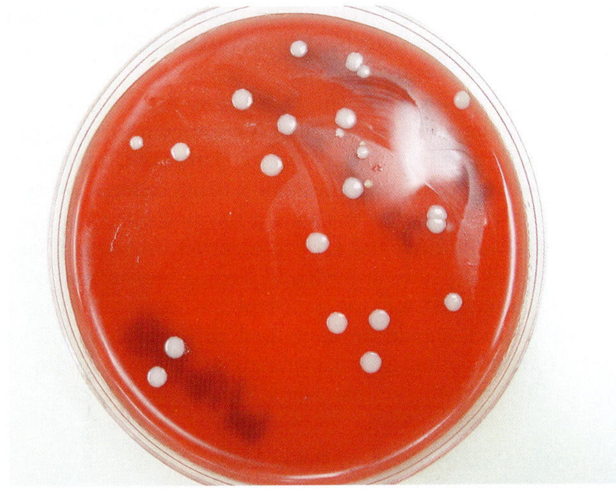

• **Fig. 15.8** Typical appearance of nonhemolytic staphylococci. Often, these are coagulase-negative staphylococci.

Streptococcus spp. Streptococci also have been isolated in cases of subclinical mastitis. Prevalence rates range between 1.1% and 6.8% of subclinical mastitis cases.[43,44,52,53] With the exception of *S. agalactiae,* these organisms are environmental contaminants and should be treated as such.

Retroviral Mastitis. The caprine and ovine retroviruses that are the agents of caprine arthritis-encephalitis (CAE) and ovine progressive pneumonia (OPP), respectively, both can be the cause of subclinical mastitis. Although mastitis may not be the primary clinical sign observed with each of these infections, the mastitis caused by these viruses can significantly affect the productivity of the doe or ewe.

Retroviral mastitis commonly is referred to as "hard udder" or "hard bag." It is an interstitial mastitis that frequently is recognized at the time of parturition. The primary clinical manifestation in interstitial mastitis is a firm udder with loose overlying skin. No edema in the skin, heat, or erythema is noted. At the start of lactation, the affected animal may produce little to no milk, but milk production may gradually increase over the first couple of weeks after parturition. Any milk that is produced will be normal in appearance but will have significantly elevated cell counts. Evidence of systemic illness is lacking in affected animals. Supramammary lymph nodes also may be enlarged. Firmness also may be noted in the udder of does or ewes that are milking normally. In addition, affected animals may show signs of arthritis or respiratory problems.

Diagnosis of retroviral mastitis includes a physical exam to rule out other potential causes such as metritis, udder edema, or teat obstruction. Biopsy of the affected udder also can be done antemortem but frequently is done at necropsy. Histopathologic changes that may be observed include an accumulation of mononuclear cells (lymphocytes, macrophages, and plasmacytes) in the parenchyma and around the ducts. Occasionally, these cells will be organized into lymphoid follicles. The cellular infiltrations can compress ducts or protrude into ducts. Lobular atrophy and prominent corpora amylacea also have been reported. CAE or OPP testing can be done on either the herd level or in individual animals. Testing options include ELISA, agar gel immunodiffusion (AGID) testing, and PCR testing. Additionally, bacterial and mycoplasmal cultures should be done to rule out bacterial mastitis.

Unfortunately, no treatment is available for CAE or OPP. Therefore, culling of affected animals is recommended. Cortisone injections can be given 2 days before parturition to decrease clinical signs and make the animals more comfortable. Control of CAE and OPP is aimed at eradicating the viral infection within the herd or flock. CAE and OPP prevention programs include removal of kids or lambs at birth and feeding heat-treated colostrum and pasteurized milk or milk replacer. Biannual testing of the herd or flock should be done, and all seropositive animals culled. Another option is to dam-raise kids or lambs on known CAE- or OPP-negative animals (see Chapter 16).

Zoonotic Pathogens of Raw Milk

Because of today's growing interest in raw milk products, the veterinarian should be aware of the potential risks associated with raw milk consumption. At present, raw milk sales are allowed in 30 states, and efforts are ongoing in several other states to legalize the sale of raw milk. Proponents of raw milk availability cite higher nutritional qualities, increased nutritional benefits, and better taste as reason for consumption of raw milk. Little research has been able to document improved nutritional values and benefits of raw milk. Opponents of raw milk cite the public health implications for requiring pasteurization. Since the implementation of the Pasteurized Milk Ordinance, a majority of reported milk-associated foodborne illnesses have been associated with consumption of raw milk products. Between 2000 and 2008, 12 outbreaks associated with consumption of raw unpasteurized milk were reported, compared with only two documented outbreaks associated with pasteurized milk consumption.[72] Especially in consideration of the quantity of raw versus pasteurized milk consumed, these data show the significantly higher rate of foodborne illnesses associated with raw milk consumption.

Several foodborne pathogens have been identified and isolated from raw milk. The most commonly identified organisms that are studied further for clinical significance are *Campylobacter jejuni*, Shiga toxin–producing *E. coli*, *Listeria monocytogenes*, and salmonellae. Several surveys have been done to evaluate the incidence of these organisms in bulk tank milk from cattle dairies. A summary of the reported findings found that the incidence of these organisms varies significantly between surveys.[72] Several studies also have looked directly at the incidence of these organisms in goat or sheep milk; isolates have included *C. jejuni*, *L. monocytogenes*, *Salmonella*, and *E. coli*.[73–78] In these reports, the most common isolate is *S. aureus*, with 7 to 43% of samples culturing positive for *S. aureus*.[74–77,79] In addition to these foodborne pathogens, several other potentially zoonotic organisms can be found in unpasteurized milk and milk products, including *Coxiella burnetii*, *Brucella melitensis*, *Mycobacterium tuberculosis*, and *M. bovis*, all of which do not show up on routine milk culture and require additional diagnostic testing.[80] In investigations of potential foodborne pathogens in raw milk, it is important to consider the source of such organisms. Although several of these organisms are shed directly into the milk, other organisms find their way into the milk through fecal contamination of the product at the time of or after milking. Depending on the organism involved, detection and control methods will vary depending on the potential source of the organism. An important point is that several of these organisms are shed intermittently, so negative bulk tank cultures may not reflect the microbiologic reality, and the occurrence of a single fecal contamination event can infect a tank.

Home pasteurization can be performed to reduce the incidence of foodborne pathogens in milk or milk products used for home consumption. As specified in the Pasteurized Milk Ordinance, pasteurization can be performed by heating the milk to a temperature of 161° F for 15 seconds. Several other combinations of heat and time, as set forth in the Pasteurized Milk Ordinance, also are effective.

References

1. Wiggans GR, Hubbard SM: Genetic evaluation of yield and type traits of dairy goats in the United States, *J Dairy Sci* 84(Suppl 1): E69–E73, 2001.
2. Smith M, Sherman D: Mammary System. In Smith M, Sherman D, editors: *Goat medicine,* ed 2, Ames, IA, 2009, Wiley-Blackwell.
3. Jandal JM: Comparative aspects of goat and sheep milk, *Small Rumin Res* 22(2):177–185, 1996.
4. Silver H: Deer milk compared with substitute milk for fawns, *J Wildl Manage* 25(1):66–70, 1961.
5. Dietman P, Tranel L: *The Wisconsin Goat Dairy Profitability Project: 2007 and 2008 Results for a select Group of Wisconsin Goat Dairies.* 2009, Wisconsin Farm Center, Wisconsin Department of Agriculture, Trade and Consumer Protection.
6. Association CDHI: Honor roll. 2009. Available at: http://caldairygoats.com/cdhiagoats.htm. Accessed February 1, 2010.
7. Droke EA, Paape MJ, Di Carlo AL: Prevalence of high somatic cell counts in bulk tank goat milk, *J Dairy Sci* 76(4):1035–1039, 1993.
8. Paape MJ, Poutrel B, Contreras A, Marco JC, Capuco AV: Milk somatic cells and lactation in small ruminants, *J Dairy Sci* 84(Suppl 1):E237–E244, 2001.
9. Contreras A, Sierra D, Sánchez A, et al: Mastitis in small ruminants, *Small Rumin Res* 68(1–2):145–153, 2007.
10. Bergonier D, de Cremoux R, Rupp R, Lagriffoul G, Berthelot X: Mastitis of dairy small ruminants, *Vet Res* 34(5):689–716, 2003.
11. Poutrel B, de Cremoux R, Ducelliez M, Verneau D: Control of intramammary infections in goats: impact on somatic cell counts, *J Anim Sci* 75(2):566–570, 1997.
12. Wilson DJ, Stewart KN, Sears PM: Effects of stage of lactation, production, parity and season on somatic cell counts in infected and uninfected dairy goats, *Small Rumin Res* 16(2):165–169, 1995.
13. O'Brien DJ, Fitzgerald SD, Lyon TJ, et al: Tuberculous lesions in free-ranging white-tailed deer in Michigan, *J Wildl Dis* 37(3): 608–613, 2001.
14. Turnquist SE, Fales WH: Disseminated *Actinomyces pyogenes* infection in a free-ranging white-tailed deer, *J Vet Diagn Invest* 10(1):86–89, 1998.
15. Panchadevi S, Pandit R: Milking males—two case studies, *Indian Vet J* 56:590–592, 1979.
16. Rieck G, Hohn H, Loeffler K, Marx D, Bohm S: Gynakomastie bei einem Ziegenbock. II: Zytogeneticsche Befunde: X)/XY—Mosaik mit variablen Deletionen des Y-Chromosoms, *Zuchthyg* 10:159–168, 1975.
17. Wooldridge A, Gill M, Lemarchand T, Eilts B, Taylor H, Otterson T: Gynecomastic and mammary gland adenocarcinoma in a Nubian buck, *Can Vet J* 40(9):663–665, 1999.
18. Lofstedt R, Laarveld B, Ihle S: Adrenal neoplasia causing lactation in a castrated male goat, *J Vet Int Med* 8:382–384, 1994.
19. Fubini S, Ducharme N, editors: *Farm animal surgery,* ed 1, St. Louis, 2004, Saunders.
20. Peer FU, Bhattacharyya HK: Studies on caprine gangrenous mastitis, *Indian J Small Rumin* 13(1):92–94, 2007.
21. Cable CS, Peery K, Fubini SL: Radical mastectomy in 20 ruminants, *Vet Surg* 33(3):263–266, 2004.
22. Youssef H: Mastectomy as a radical treatment for some prevalent udder affections in goats in Al-Gasseem, *Assuit Vet Med J* 41: 181–193, 1999.

23. El-Maghraby H: Comparison of two surgical techniques for mastectomy of goats, *Small Rumin Res* 40(3):215–221, 2001.
24. East NE, Birnie EF, Farver TB: Risk factors associated with mastitis in dairy goats, *Am J Vet Res* 48(5):776–779, 1987.
25. Barbagianni MS, Mavrogianni VS, Katsafadou AI, et al: Pregnancy toxaemia as predisposing factor for development of mastitis in sheep during the immediately post-partum period. *Small Rumin Res* 130:246–251, 2015.
26. Koutsoumpas A, Giadinis N, Petridou E, et al: Consequences of reduced vitamin A administration on mammary health of dairy ewes, *Small Rumin Res* 2013;110:120–123.
27. Mavrogianni VS, Papadopoulos E, Spanos SA, et al: Trematode infections in pregnant ewes can predispose to mastitis during the subsequent lactation period, *Res Vet Sci* 96(1):171–179, 2014.
28. Caja G, Such X, Roval M: *Udder Morphology and Machine Milking Ability in Dairy Sheep*. Paper presented at: 6th Great Lakes Dairy Sheep Symposium 2000; University of Wisconsin–Madison.
29. Petridis IG, Mavrogianni VS, Fragkou IA, et al: Effects of drying-off procedure of ewes' udder in subsequent mammary infection and development of mastitis, *Small Rumin Res* 110(2):128–132, 2013.
30. Fox LK, Hancock DD, Horner SD: Selective intramammary antibiotic therapy during the nonlactating period in goats, *Small Rumin Res* 9(3):313–318, 1992.
31. Croft A, Duffield T, Menzies P, Leslie K, Bagg R, Dick P: The effect of tilmicosin administered to ewes prior to lambing on incidence of clinical mastitis and subsequent lamb performance, *Can Vet J* 41(4): 306–311, 2000.
32. Godden S: *Use of External and Internal Teat Sealants to Prevent New Intramammary Infections During the Dry Period*. In Extension UoW, ed. Available at: dysci.wisc.edu/uwex/brochures/brochures/GoddenTreatSealants.pdf.
33. Fragkou IA, Boscos CM, Fthenakis GC: Diagnosis of clinical or subclinical mastitis in ewes, *Small Rumin Res* 118(1):86–92, 2014.
34. Rupp R, Bergonier D, Dion S, et al: Response to somatic cell count-based selection for mastitis resistance in a divergent selection experiment in sheep, *J Dairy Sci* 92(3):1203–1219, 2009.
35. Murphy S: *Raw milk bacterial tests—standard plate, preliminary incubation, lab pasteurization and coliform counts—sources and causes of high bacteria counts*, Ithaca, NY, 2004, Quality Milk Production Services, p 704.
36. Franz S, Floek M, Hofmann-Parisot M: Ultrasonography of the bovine udder and teat, *Vet Clin North Am Food Anim Pract* 25:669–685, 2009.
37. Hussein HA, El-Khabaz KAS, Malek SS: Is udder ultrasonography a diagnostic tool for subclinical mastitis in sheep? *Small Rumin Res* 129:121–128, 2015.
38. Kinde H, DaMassa AJ, Wakenell PS, Petty R: Mycoplasma infection in a commercial goat dairy caused by *Mycoplasma agalactiae* and *Mycoplasma mycoides* subsp. mycoides (caprine biotype), *J Vet Diagn Invest* 6(4):423–427, 1994.
39. Yeruham I, Schwimmer A, Friedman S, et al: Investigation and control of mastitis outbreaks caused by Pseudomonas aeruginosa in a sheep flock and a goat herd, *Berl Munch Tierarztl Wochenschr* 118(5–6):220–223, 2005.
40. Sela S, Hammer-Muntz O, Krifucks O, Pinto R, Weisblit L, Leitner G: Phenotypic and genotypic characterization of *Pseudomonas aeruginosa* strains isolated from mastitis outbreaks in dairy herds, *J Dairy Res* 74(4):425–429, 2007.
41. Arsenault J, Dubreuil P, Higgins R, Belanger D: Risk factors and impacts of clinical and subclinical mastitis in commercial meat-producing sheep flocks in Quebec, Canada, *Prev Vet Med* 87 (3–4):373–393, 2008.
42. Suarez VH, Busetti MR, Miranda AO, Calvinho LF, Bedotti DO, Canavesio VR: Effect of infectious status and parity on somatic cell count and California mastitis test in pampinta dairy ewes, *J Vet Med B Infect Dis Vet Public Health* 49(5):230–234, 2002.
43. Lafi SQ, al-Majali AM, Rousan MD, Alawneh JM: Epidemiological studies of clinical and subclinical ovine mastitis in Awassi sheep in northern Jordan, *Prev Vet Med* 33(1–4):171–181, 1998.
44. Mork T, Waage S, Tollersrud T, Kvitle B, Sviland S: Clinical mastitis in ewes; bacteriology, epidemiology and clinical features, *Acta Vet Scand* 49:23, 2007.
45. Dhondt G, Burvenich C, Peeters G: Mammary blood flow during experimental *Escherichia coli* endotoxin induced mastitis in goats and cows, *J Dairy Res* 44(3):433–440, 1977.
46. Hogan J, Larry Smith L: Coliform mastitis, *Vet Res* 34(5):507–519, 2003.
47. Abu-Samra MT, Elsanousi SM, Abdalla MA, et al: Studies on gangrenous mastitis in goats. *Cornell Vet* 78(3):281–300, 1988.
48. Gelasakis AI, Mavrogianni VS, Petridis IG, Vasileiou NGC, Fthenakis GC: Mastitis in sheep—the last 10 years and the future of research, *Vet Microbiol* 181(1):136–146, 2015.
49. Scott MJ, Jones JE: The carriage of *Pasteurella haemolytica* in sheep and its transfer between ewes and lambs in relation to mastitis, *J Comp Pathol* 118(4):359–363, 1998.
50. Gougoulis DA, Kyriazakis I, Tzora A, Taitzoglou IA, Skoufos J, Fthenakis GC: Effects of lamb sucking on the bacterial flora of teat duct and mammary gland of ewes, *Reprod Domest Anim* 43(1): 22–26. 2008.
51. Leitner G, Krifucks O: *Pseudomonas aeruginosa* mastitis outbreaks in sheep and goat flocks: antibody production and vaccination in a mouse model, *Vet Immunol Immunopathol* 119(3–4):198–203, 2007.
52. Hall SM, Rycroft AN: Causative organisms and somatic cell counts in subclinical intramammary infections in milking goats in the UK, *Vet Rec* 160(1):19–22, 2007.
53. Ndegwa EN, Mulei CM, Munyua SJ: Prevalence of microorganisms associated with udder infections in dairy goats on small-scale farms in Kenya, *J S Afr Vet Assoc* 72(2):97–98, 2001.
54. Rodriguez JL, Poveda JB, Oros J, Herraez P, Sierra MA, Fernandez A: High mortality in goats associated with the isolation of a strain of *Mycoplasma mycoides* subsp. *mycoides* (large colony type), *Zentralbl Veterinarmed B* 42(10):587–593, 1995.
55. Behymer D, Jessup D, Jones K, Franti CE, Riemann H, Bahr A: Antibodies to nine infectious disease agents in deer from California, *J Zoo Wildl Med* 20(3):297–306, 1989.
56. Dudek K, Bednarek D, Szacawa E, Ayling RD: Screening of the Cervidae family in Poland for Mycoplasma species, *J Vet Res* 60(4): 399–402, 2016.
57. DaMassa AJ, Brooks DL, Adler HE: Caprine mycoplasmosis: widespread infection in goats with *Mycoplasma mycoides* subsp *mycoides* (large-colony type), *Am J Vet Res* 44(2):322–325, 1983.
58. Bar-Moshe B, Rapapport E: Observations on *Mycoplasma mycoides* subsp. *mycoides* infection in Saanen goats, *Isr J Med Sci* 17(7): 537–539, 1981.
59. East NE, DaMassa AJ, Logan LL, Brooks DL, McGowan B: Milkborne outbreak of *Mycoplasma mycoides* subspecies mycoides infection in a commercial goat dairy, *J Am Vet Med Assoc* 182(12): 1338–1341, 1983.
60. Blikslager AT, Anderson KL: *Mycoplasma mycoides* subspecies mycoides as the cause of a subauricular abscess and mastitis in a goat, *J Am Vet Med Assoc* 201(9):1404–1406, 1992.
61. DaMassa AJ, Brooks DL: The external ear canal of goats and other animals as a mycoplasma habitat, *Small Rumin Res* 4: 85–93, 1991.
62. DaMassa AJ: Recovery of *Mycoplasma agalactiae* from mastitic goat milk, *J Am Vet Med Assoc* 183(5):548–549, 1983.
63. Corrales JC, Esnal A: Contagious agalactia in small ruminants, *Small Rumin Res* 68(1–2):154–166, 2007.
64. Al-Momani W, Nicholas RA, Janakat S, Abu-Basha E, Ayling RD: The in vitro effect of six antimicrobials against *Mycoplasma putrefaciens*, *Mycoplasma mycoides* subsp. *mycoides* LC and *Mycoplasma capricolum* subsp. *capricolum* isolated from sheep and goats in Jordan, *Trop Anim Health Prod* 38(1):1–7, 2006.
65. de la Fe C, Assuncao P, Saavedra P, Tola S, Poveda C, Poveda JB: Field trial of two dual vaccines against *Mycoplasma agalactiae* and *Mycoplasma mycoides* subsp. *mycoides* (large colony type) in goats, *Vaccine* 25(12):2340–2345, 2007.

66. Jensen HE, Espinosa de los Monteros A, Carrasco L: Caprine mastitis due to aspergillosis and zygomycosis: a pathological and immunohistochemical study, *J Comp Pathol* 114(2):183–191, 1996.
67. Valle J, Piriz S, de la Fuente R, Vadillo S: Staphylococci isolated from healthy goats, *Zentralbl Veterinarmed B* 38(2):81–89, 1991.
68. Deinhofer M, Pernthaner A: *Staphylococcus* spp. as mastitis-related pathogens in goat milk, *Vet Microbiol* 43(2–3):161–166, 1995.
69. Ariznabarreta A, Gonzalo C, San Primitivo F: Microbiological quality and somatic cell count of ewe milk with special reference to staphylococci, *J Dairy Sci* 85(6):1370–1375, 2002.
70. Moroni P, Pisoni G, Antonini M, et al: Subclinical mastitis and antimicrobial susceptibility of *Staphylococcus caprae* and *Staphylococcus epidermidis* isolated from two Italian goat herds, *J Dairy Sci* 88(5):1694–1704, 2005.
71. Leitner G, Merin G: Changes in milk composition as affected by subclinical mastitis in goats, *J Dairy Sci* 87(6):1719–1726, 2004.
72. Oliver SP, Boor KJ, Murphy SC, Murinda SE: Food safety hazards associated with consumption of raw milk, *Foodborne Pathog Dis* 6(7):793–806, 2009.
73. Harris N, Kimball T: *Campylobacter jejuni* enteritis associated with raw goat's milk, *Am J Epidemiol* 126(2):179–186, 1987.
74. Little C, De Louvois J: Health risk associated with unpasteurized goats' and ewes' milk on retail sale in England and Wales. A PHLS Dairy Products Working Group Study, *Epidemiol Infect* 122(3): 403–408, 1999.
75. Foschino R, Invernizzi A: Microbial composition, including the incidence of pathogens, in goat milk from the Bergamo region of Italy during a lactation year, *J Dairy Res* 69(2):213–225, 2002.
76. Muehlherr JE, Zweifel C, Corti S, Blanco JE, Stephan R: Microbiological quality of raw goat's and ewe's bulk-tank milk in Switzerland, *J Dairy Sci* 86(12):3849–3856, 2003.
77. Almeida G, Figueiredo A, Rola M, et al: Microbiological characterization of randomly selected Portuguese raw milk cheeses with reference to food safety, *J Food Prot* 70(7):1710–1716, 2007.
78. Desenclos JC, Bouvet P, Benz-Lemoine E, et al: Large outbreak of *Salmonella enterica* serotype paratyphi B infection caused by a goats' milk cheese, France, 1993: a case finding and epidemiological study, *BMJ* 312(7023):91–94, 1996.
79. D'Amico DJ, Groves E, Donnelly CW: Low incidence of foodborne pathogens of concern in raw milk utilized for farmstead cheese production, *J Food Prot* 71(8):1580–1589, 2008.
80. Lejeune JT, Rajala-Schultz PJ: Food safety: unpasteurized milk: a continued public health threat, *Clin Infect Dis* 48(1):93–100, 2009.

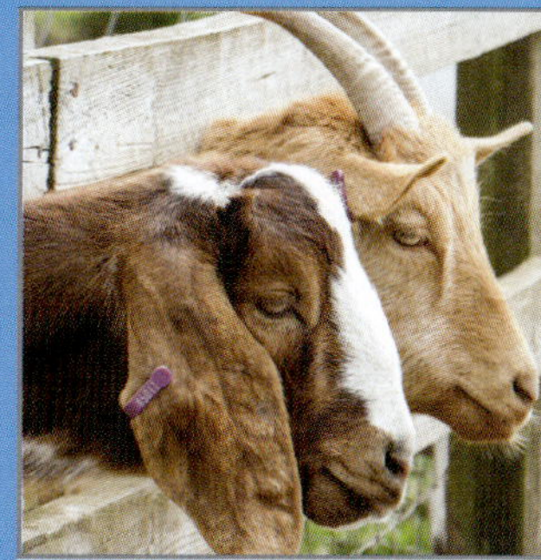

16

Diseases of the Hematologic, Immunologic, and Lymphatic Systems (Multisystem Diseases)

BENJAMIN W. NEWCOMER, CHRIS CEBRA, MANUEL F. CHAMORRO, EMILY REPPERT, MARGARET CEBRA, AND MISTY A. EDMONDSON

In this chapter, multisystemic diseases are discussed in small ruminants (sheep, goats, and cervids). These include diseases of the hematologic, immunologic, and lymphatic systems. In general, species will be discussed together, but when pertinent data are available, each species will be considered separately. The terms "cervid" and "deer" have been used interchangeably in parts of this chapter by the authors.

Basic Hematology

An adequate volume of blood for hematologic and biochemical analysis is best obtained from the jugular vein. A docile animal may be restrained in a standing position or tipped up (sheep only) with the head turned away from the jugular vein to be used. Wilder ones, such as some cervids, may require restraint devices or chemical sedation. Ideally, the animal should be restrained by someone other than the blood collector, although the same person may be able to both restrain a sheep and collect blood if the animal is tipped up or a halter is used (see Chapter 1). The animal should be at rest, with minimal excitement. The collector parts or clips the wool or hair to visualize the jugular vein and then uses the hand not holding the needle to apply digital pressure proximally just above the thoracic inlet to block blood movement through the vein. The vessel may take a second or more to distend after pressure is applied. The collector may then use the needle-bearing hand to "strum" the vessel and cause the blood to oscillate. If in doubt about whether the distended vessel is the jugular vein, the collector can release the hand placing pressure on the vessel and observe whether the distended vessel disappears; if it does, the distended vessel was probably the jugular vein. The collector should avoid vessels that pulsate because these are likely to be the carotid arteries. The area should be cleaned with alcohol or other disinfectant, water, or a clean, dry gauze sponge. An 18- or 20-gauge, 1- to 1.5-inch needle is usually adequate to collect blood from an adult, whereas a 22-gauge needle may be used in a neonate. The skin of adults or males may be thicker and more difficult to penetrate with the needle. A syringe or evacuated tube attached to a Vacutainer (Becton Dickinson Inc., Rutherford, NJ) can be used to collect blood. The needle should be plunged through the skin into the vein at an approximate 30-degree angle. The blood should not come out of the vessel in pulsatile waves; this is suggestive of an arterial stick. After aseptically obtaining an adequate volume of blood, the collector removes the needle and releases the pressure on the vessel near the thoracic inlet. Pressure should be applied to the site of puncture for a minute or more to prevent extravascular leakage of blood and hematoma formation. The blood should be carefully transferred to a vial containing the appropriate anticoagulant to prevent red blood cell (RBC) rupture. Goat erythrocytes are small and particularly prone to hemolysis. To minimize this problem, goat blood should be collected with a needle and syringe, not a Vacutainer. White blood cell (WBC) differential distribution, individual blood cell staining characteristics, and morphology may be assessed by microscopic examination of a stained blood film. The differential distribution provides more information than total WBC count because inflammatory conditions in artiodactyls often result in a shift in neutrophil populations toward more degenerate, toxic, or immature forms without changing the overall WBC count.[1] The preferred anticoagulant for a complete blood count (CBC) is ethylenediaminetetraacetate (EDTA), and tubes should be filled to ensure the proper blood-to-anticoagulant ratio. Blood samples should be processed as soon as possible after collection. If a delay is anticipated, the blood sample should be refrigerated (4° C) and an air-dried blood smear should be made because prolonged contact of blood with EDTA causes changes in WBC morphology and the separation of some RBC parasites. Blood can be refrigerated for 24 hours and still yield an accurate CBC.

A reference range for hematologic data for sheep and goats is provided in Table 16.1 (see Appendix 2, Tables 1 and 2). Goats tend to have a low mean corpuscular volume (MCV) because of their small erythrocytes. Sheep and goats younger than 6 months old tend to have lower hematocrit, RBC count, hemoglobin, and

TABLE 16.1 Normal Hematologic Parameters for Sheep and Goats.

Parameter (Units)	Adult Sheep	Adult Goat
Hematocrit (%)	27–45	22–36
Hemoglobin (g/dL)	9–15.8	8–12
Red blood cell count ($\times 10^6/\mu L$)	9–17.5	8–17
Mean corpuscular volume (fL)	28–40	15–26
Mean corpuscular hemoglobin concentration (g/dL)	31–34	29–35
Platelet count ($\times 10^5/\mu L$)	2.4–7.0	2.8–6.4
Total white blood cell count ($/\mu L$)	4000–12,000	4000–13,000
Segmented neutrophils ($/\mu L$)	1500–9000	1400–8000
Band neutrophils ($/\mu L$)	0	0
Lymphocytes ($/\mu L$)	2000–9000	2000–9000
Monocytes ($/\mu L$)	0–600	0–500
Eosinophils ($/\mu L$)	0–1000	0–900
Basophils ($/\mu L$)	0–300	0–100
Total plasma protein (g/dL)	6.2–7.5	6.0–7.5
Fibrinogen (mg/dL)	100–600	100–500

plasma protein concentrations, as well as a higher total WBC count. Neonates often have a high hematocrit at birth that decreases with colostral ingestion. Lactating animals may have decreased hematocrits, RBC counts, and hemoglobin concentrations. Animals grazing at high altitude (mountain goats and Bighorn sheep) tend to have increased RBC counts, hematocrits, and hemoglobin concentrations.

Interpreting hematologic changes in cervids is more complex. Restraint method affects a variety of parameters in non-acclimated individuals. Physical restraint yields red cell counts and hematocrit and hemoglobin concentrations that are 20 to 40% higher than animals immobilized chemically.[2,3] Neutrophil, lymphocyte, monocyte, and total white cell counts are also 70 to 100% higher in physically restrained cervids (see Appendix 2, Tables 1 and 2).

Adult deer also have seasonal variations in their hemogram. Red cell numbers and related values are highest during midsummer and late winter.[3] White cells, especially neutrophils, are also highest in midsummer, and platelet counts are highest in spring and fall. These changes may relate to diet or to seasonal activities, such as antler growth and rutting conflicts, which increase the chance of trauma.

Red cell stickling has also been reported in a variety of deer species. This appears to relate to a mutation in hemoglobin's β-globin component, similar to the disorder in people, but no pathologic role has been described.[4]

Additional Hematologic Assessments

Bone Marrow Aspiration

Bone marrow aspirates and core biopsy samples taken from sites of active erythropoiesis can be useful to evaluate erythrocyte production and determine the cause of anemia and other hemogram abnormalities. The sites of biopsy include the sternebrae, femur, and ileum. The procedure should be done under chemical sedation or anesthesia (see Chapter 18). The area over the biopsy site is clipped and surgically prepared; the sampler should wear sterile gloves to maintain asepsis. Aspirates can be obtained by inserting a sterile needle attached to a 3- or 6-cc syringe containing one or two drops of EDTA through the bone and into the bone marrow. Drawing back on the syringe plunger several times may aid in the procurement of an acceptable sample; such a sample may consist of as little as 0.5 mL of bone marrow. If the sample is going to be processed immediately, no anticoagulant is required. Core biopsies are obtained using a Jamshidi or Westerman-Jensen biopsy needle. The skin is incised with a scalpel and the biopsy needle is inserted into the bone and turned several times to obtain a core sample. More than one site may be used. The sampler then closes the skin with sutures or staples. Biopsy samples are preserved by placing them in 10% neutral buffered formalin solution. Impression smears can be made from these samples by gently rolling them on a clean glass slide before placing them in the formalin solution. Information obtained from bone marrow samples includes subjective data regarding cell density, megakaryocyte numbers, abnormal cells, maturation patterns of RBCs and WBCs, and the ratio of erythroid to myeloid cells. Prussian blue stain can be used on bone marrow to demonstrate iron stores. Bone marrow aspirates and biopsies are painful and invasive procedures. Therefore, animals should be placed on antibiotics and antiinflammatory drugs prophylactically.

Blood Cultures

Blood cultures can be useful in diagnosing bacteremia in an intermittently or persistently febrile animal or one with numerous sites of organ infection. Ideally, the clinician should obtain the sample before instituting antimicrobial therapy. However, if this is impossible, antimicrobial therapy should be discontinued 48 to 72 hours before sampling. Samples should be taken before and during febrile episodes. The jugular vein is most commonly used to attain a blood culture. As described previously, the skin over the jugular vein should be clipped and surgically prepared. The person collecting the blood sample should wear sterile gloves and use a sterile needle and syringe. Blood samples should be placed immediately in a blood culture flask. The chances of attaining a positive culture from bacteremic animals increase with the size of the sample up to about 30 mL, but adding more than the recommended amount to any single culture vial may overwhelm the capacity of the specialized antibiotic-absorbing resins within the flasks. The clinician should change the needle on the sample syringe after collecting the blood and before putting the sample in the culture medium. Samples should be refrigerated until they can be sent to a diagnostic laboratory, where aerobic and sometimes anaerobic cultures are made.

The FAMACHA System of Assessing Anemia

As an alternative to hematologic testing, comparing conjunctival color to swatches on a standardized FAMACHA chart has been used as a rapid and inexpensive assessment of anemia in whole flocks, primarily to assess the impact of *Haemonchus contortus* and other blood-sucking parasites.[5,6] Results from a number of trials have yielded fair to good sensitivity to packed cell volume and *H. contortus* load in both sheep and goats. Similar to body condition scoring systems, it is essential to calibrate assessors to ensure consistency when using this system.[7] Also, some breeds read differently on the cards, and use of an electronic color analyzer, while more expensive and less field-friendly, may detect anemia earlier (see Chapter 6, Figure 6.4A, B, and Chapter 19).[8] Easy use of this technique in deer is limited by their intractability and has not been reported.

Changes in the Hemogram

The most common and significant abnormality of the hemogram is anemia. Anemia occurs most commonly after blood loss, hemolysis, or chronic disease. Blood loss is usually covert and commonly caused by gastrointestinal or external parasites. Overt blood loss is usually caused by major trauma such as that caused by dog bites, severe lacerations, male rivalry fighting, or complications of castration or dehorning. CBC values appear normal immediately after acute blood loss. However, after a few hours of fluid redistribution, anemia and hypoproteinemia are evident. Evidence of red cell regeneration (macrocytosis, reticulocytosis, and nucleated red cells) should appear within a day or two of the blood loss.

Hemolysis occurs most commonly after ingestion of toxic plants, RBC parasitism, intravenous (IV) injection of hypotonic or hypertonic agents, contact with bacterial toxins, water intoxication, or immune-mediated destruction of opsonized erythrocytes. Ingested toxins include sulfur compounds from onions and *Brassica* plants (kale and canola),[9–12] nitrates, nitrites, and copper.[13–16] Except for that caused by copper, hemolysis usually occurs within a day or two after ingestion. Copper toxicosis can occur after acute overingestion but more commonly is seen in animals that are chronically overfed copper and suffer some stressful event. Goats are more tolerant of excess copper than sheep are, and certain breeds of sheep, particularly the Suffolk, are highly sensitive to copper toxicosis (see Chapters 2 and 5).

Hemolytic bacterial toxins include those from *Clostridium perfringens* type A, *Clostridium haemolyticum*, and *Leptospira interrogans.*[17,18] Intraerythrocytic parasites include *Anaplasma* species, *Mycoplasma (Eperythrozoon)* species, and *Babesia* species.[19–23] Immune-mediated RBC destruction is very uncommon except with parasitemia, the administration of certain drugs (penicillin), or bovine colostrum to small ruminant neonates.[24] Rapid reduction of plasma osmolality can lead to osmotic lysis of erythrocytes. This can occur locally as a sequela to rapid IV injection of hypotonic substances or after ingestion of a large quantity of water following a period of water deprivation and dehydration (water intoxication). Selenium and copper deficiency have also been associated with Heinz body anemia.[25]

Parasite infestation, opsonization, and ingestion of toxic plants typically cause extravascular hemolysis. In these cases, damaged erythrocytes are removed by cells of the reticuloendothelial system, resulting in anemia, pallor, weakness, depression, icterus, and dark urine. Bacterial toxins, changes in plasma osmolality, and copper toxicosis cause intravascular hemolysis, resulting in the additional signs of hemoglobinemia and hemoglobinuria. Other signs such as fever, neurologic symptoms, and sudden death may be seen with specific diseases. Signs of regeneration should be seen on the hemogram 1 to 2 days after the onset of hemolysis.

Anemia that is not related to the loss or destruction of erythrocytes usually results from a lack of production and thus are nonregenerative. Although mild forms may exist in pregnant sheep and goats and those deficient in vital minerals (e.g., iron, selenium, copper, and zinc), the most common cause of nonregenerative anemia is chronic disease. Under these conditions, iron is sequestered in an unusable form in the bone marrow; staining a marrow sample with Prussian blue stain reveals large iron stores, differentiating this disease from iron-deficiency anemia. The causes of anemia of chronic disease are numerous and include infectious conditions (e.g., pneumonia, foot rot, and caseous lymphadenitis), malnutrition, and environmental stressors.[1]

Treatment of Anemia

Most anemia does not require treatment. Unless loss of RBC mass is rapid and severe, the animal is usually able to compensate to the decreased oxygen-carrying capacity by decreasing activity. It is important to remember in this regard that anemia often first becomes apparent to the manager of a flock or herd when animals appear overly stressed or die during movement or handling.

If possible, the cause of the anemia should be addressed. This can involve trying to control internal and external parasites, changing the diet, and treating infectious diseases. Maintaining adequate hydration is essential in animals with intravascular hemolysis to avoid hemoglobin-induced renal tubular damage. Specialty compounds such as molybdenum salts, such as ammonium molybdate, and sulfur or penicillamine for copper toxicosis[16] and methylene blue (15 mg/kg in a 4% solution in 5% dextrose or normal saline intravenously) for nitrate toxicity are usually too expensive or difficult to be used on a flock-wide basis but may be useful in valuable individual animals. Veterinarians should be aware that methylene blue is no longer approved for use in food-producing animals.

Animals with severe acute blood loss or hemolysis may benefit from a whole blood transfusion. Because transfusion reactions are rare and strong erythrocyte antigens have not been identified in small ruminants (including cervids), almost any donor of the same species is acceptable for a first transfusion. Cross-matching can be done to ensure compatibility, which becomes more important if the animal receives more than one transfusion. Blood should be withdrawn aseptically from the donor and collected by a bleeding trocar into an open flask or by a catheter into a special collection bag. Blood should be mixed at a 7.5:1 ratio with acid-citrate dextrose, or 9:1 with 2% sodium citrate, or another suitable anticoagulant and administered through a filtered blood administration set. If the jugular vein is not accessible, blood may be infused into the peritoneal cavity, but the slower absorption from that site makes it less effective for treating acute blood loss. The first 15 to 30 minutes of administration should be slow. If no reaction is seen (fever, tenesmus, tachypnea, tachycardia, and shaking), the rate may be increased. Transfused erythrocytes may only survive a few days, and therefore, the original cause of the anemia must be addressed.[1]

Changes in the Leukogram

Peripheral WBCs include granulocytes (neutrophils, eosinophils, and basophils) and mononuclear cells (lymphocytes and monocytes). Immature forms of neutrophils and lymphocytes may be seen during severe inflammatory diseases. Abnormalities of the neutrophil line are usually the best cellular evidence of inflammation in small ruminants, and inflammation is almost always a sequela of infection. An increase in neutrophil numbers and their proportional contribution to the total WBC count is usually seen in mild gram positive, subacute, or chronic bacterial infections. Animals with more severe disease may exhibit high or normal counts, but a greater proportion of the neutrophils will have toxic changes or be immature forms (band cells, metamyelocytes, or myelocytes). In severe, acute inflammation and many diseases caused by gram negative bacteria, a temporary reduction in neutrophil numbers is observed, often with a concurrent shift toward more toxic or immature forms.

If the animal survives the peracute disease, neutropenia should resolve over 3 to 4 days, first through an increase in immature cells, and later through a mature neutrophilic response. Another important cause of increased total and relative neutrophil counts is stress (or glucocorticoid administration), which inhibits neutrophil margination and extravasation and thereby increases the number of these cells in the midstream blood.

Increases in eosinophil counts are usually related to exposure to eukaryotic parasites. Decreases are rarely of clinical significance and may be part of the stress response. Idiopathic allergic-type reactions also are indicators of pathology but are very rare. Increases in basophils are rarely clinically significant.

Increases in lymphocyte counts often reflect chronic inflammatory disease such as that seen with internal abscesses. In rare cases, lymphocytosis may consist of abnormal, blast-type cells and indicate a lymphoproliferative neoplasm. Lymphopenia is an important part of the stress response; nevertheless, the clinician must keep in mind that many diseases stimulate a stress response. Therefore, lymphopenia and neutrophilia may represent either stress or inflammation, and an examination of neutrophil morphology and plasma fibrinogen concentrations may be useful in distinguishing the two situations. A high fibrinogen concentration, toxic changes, and high counts of immature neutrophils indicate inflammation under those circumstances. Blood monocyte counts also may indicate stress or chronic inflammation. The difficulties in interpreting individual cell count abnormalities highlight the importance of obtaining a differential WBC count and description of cellular morphology in assessing sick sheep and goats.

Leukogram abnormalities are rarely given specific treatment. It is far more common and useful to use the information from the leukogram to develop a plan to treat the disease responsible for the abnormality.

Assessment of the Lymphatic System

Palpation of external lymph nodes is part of the thorough physical examination. Lymph nodes that can be found in normal sheep and goats include the submandibular, prescapular, and prefemoral nodes. None of these should be prominent or painful on palpation. Additional nodes that may be palpated occasionally in normal animals include the parotid, retropharyngeal, supramammary, perirectal, and popliteal nodes. Internal lymph nodes that may be identified during specialized diagnostic procedures include the mediastinal, mesenteric, and other abdominal nodes.

Enlargement of lymph nodes may be focal, multifocal, or generalized. Identification of a single enlarged superficial node does not always rule out a multifocal or generalized disorder because the status of the internal nodes often cannot be determined. Enlargement generally indicates either inflammation or neoplasia. Inflammatory enlargement is generally related to an associated disease with an infectious component. Small ruminants are particularly sensitive to lymph node–based infections (e.g., caseous lymphadenitis), so the search often does not extend beyond aspirating or draining the lymph node itself. Neoplastic enlargement almost always results from lymphosarcoma.

Diseases of the Lymphatic System

Lymphosarcoma

Pathogenesis. Neoplastic transformation of a member of the lymphocyte cell line leads to unregulated clonal expansion of that cell. The cause of transformation is usually unknown; in rare cases, especially in flock outbreaks in sheep, it can be linked to exposure to the bovine leukemia virus, which has occurred experimentally and as a result of the administration of whole blood *Anaplasma* vaccines. Whether the bovine leukemia virus can induce lymphosarcoma in goats and cervids is still unclear. Multicentric lymphosarcoma has been reported sporadically in white-tailed deer *(Odocoileus virginiatus)* and other deer, but bovine leukemia virus infection has not been diagnosed in cervids.[26]

In one study of neoplastic diseases affecting goats from 1987 to 2011, lymphoma was identified as the most common neoplasm, accounting for 17.7% of the assessed tumors.[27] In contrast to other species such as cattle, sheep, and horses, lymphomas in goats are predominantly T-cell lymphomas affecting the mediastinum. A recent study attempted to classify the type of lymphoma affecting 15 goats. Using immunohistochemistry (IHC), it was determined that 73% (n = 11) of affected goats had T-cell lymphoma and only 27% (n = 4) had B-cell lymphoma.[28] Proliferation of T or B lymphocytes leads to mass lesions and infiltration of viscera. These changes cause physical obstruction (to breathing, blood flow, urination, defecation, etc.), ulceration of mucosal surfaces (blood loss, bacterial invasion), immune system dysfunction, organ failure, and generalized malaise and cachexia. Tissue masses may be internal or visible on external examination.

Clinical Signs. Clinical signs in affected animals vary according to the type of lymphoma (T- or B-cell) and the location of the masses. T-cell lymphomas in goats are usually localized in the thoracic cavity and/or neck, suggesting thymic origin or homing.[27] In contrast, B-cell lymphomas tend to have a multicentric distribution.[27] Lymphoma in small ruminants usually presents with non-specific signs that can mimic other respiratory or gastrointestinal conditions. Slowly progressive weight loss is the most common finding. In some cases, generalized peripheral lymphadenopathy and expansile masses are noted[29]; at first, they usually are presumed to be caseous lymphadenitis abscesses. Progressive chemosis and exophthalmos have been reported in a sheep and a goat with multicentric B-cell lymphoma.[29,30] Most masses form at the sites of internal or external lymph nodes. In sheep, masses in the brain, skin, joint, and lymphoid tissue have been reported.[30] Leukemia is rare. The most common abnormalities are those of chronic disease and cachexia and include nonregenerative anemia and hypoalbuminemia. Bone marrow examination may reveal clonal expansion of lymphoid precursor cells.

In cervids, lymphadenopathy and multifocal masses affecting the heart, blood vessels, kidney, urinary bladder, and peritoneum have been reported.[31] A more recent report described a subcutaneous maxillary mass in a 13-year-old captive-born, female white-tailed deer.[26] The mass was diagnosed as focal lymphosarcoma with local metastasis.

Diagnosis. History and clinical signs are important in the diagnosis of lymphoma in small ruminants. Age of affected animals ranges from 2 to 18 years and no gender or breed predisposition has been reported.[29] Final diagnosis of affected animals is achieved through necropsy, histopathology, and IHC. Lesions seen at necropsy include homogeneous white to tan masses that bulge on the cut surface. They may be small or large. Less commonly, diffuse paleness of the reticuloendothelial organs is noted. Microscopic examination of these tissues reveals infiltrates of abnormal cells of the lymphocyte line.

Prevention. Avoiding exposure to the bovine leukemia virus and restricting the use of instruments to one animal between cleaning procedures may help prevent the spread of lymphosarcoma. In most animals, however, this neoplasm appears to develop spontaneously.

Failure of Passive Transfer

Pathogenesis. Lambs, kids, and fawns are born with functional lymphocytes that can produce endogenous immunoglobulin. These cells develop the ability to respond to foreign antigens in the fetus during mid to late gestation. Because of a lack of in utero exposure, however, basal concentrations of immunoglobulin are very low at birth. These cells therefore are naïve to foreign antigens and unable to develop protective immunity through specific cell-mediated and immunoglobulin production. Additionally, as with other ruminants, no transplacental passage of maternal immunoglobulin to fetal sheep, goats, and fawns occurs. Lambs, kids, and fawns depend exclusively on intestinal absorption of maternally derived colostral antibodies, immune cells (T-lymphocytes), and other immune factors to provide a ready supply of specific immunity and allow opsonization of pathogens for the first months of life.

Adequate passive transfer requires delivery of a sufficient quantity of good-quality colostrum (immunoglobulin G [IgG] concentration in mg/mL) into the gastrointestinal tract, as well as adequate absorption of antibodies (timely) from the colostrum into the blood. However, the amount of maternal colostrum produced by the dam, and its composition, as well as the ability of the newborn to stand and nurse in a timely manner, can be affected by several factors. Colostrum IgG concentration and volume of production can be influenced by breed, age, nutrition, body condition score (BCS) at parturition, and vaccination status of the dam. The IgG concentration in colostrum samples from ewes of different breeds can vary between 60 and 125 mg/mL.[32] One study demonstrated that primiparous ewes with low BCS (< 2.75) at lambing produced less colostrum compared with multiparous ewes with similar BCS. Additionally, ewes with higher BCS (> 2.75) tended to produce higher volumes of colostrum compared with ewes with lower BCS.[32] Another study suggested that undernutrition of ewes during late gestation can affect colostrum quality and immune development and function in newborn lambs.[33] It has been suggested that at least 30 g of total IgG should be fed to newborn lambs and kids during the first 24 hours of life to reach adequate transfer of passive immunity. Adequate transfer of passive immunity in small ruminant neonates has been suggested as serum IgG levels at 24 hours of life of ≥ 15 mg/mL. One study indicated that lambs that nurse low-quality colostrum (IgG < 30 mg/mL) had lower serum IgG concentrations compared with lambs that that nurse colostrum of higher quality (IgG > 110 mg/mL), indicating that the concentration of IgG in colostrum is a determining factor for the presentation of failure in the transfer of passive immunity.[34] Other factors such as pregnancy toxemia, gastrointestinal parasitism, excess of iodine intake during pregnancy, and inadequate vaccination of the dam can result in poor colostrum synthesis and quality.[35]

Timely consumption of maternal colostrum during the first hours of life is essential to achieve adequate transfer of passive immunity. In small ruminants, cells of the small intestine are able to internalize and transfer IgG into the blood during the first 24 hours of life; however, the absorption efficiency of IgG is higher during the first 6 to 12 hours of life.[32,36] Factors associated with the neonate, such as weakness, inability to stand, and congenital abnormalities, will prevent timely nursing of maternal colostrum and lead to failure of passive transfer (FPT). Litter size and body weight (BW) of the kid(s) have also been correlated with inadequate absorption of IgG from colostrum. One study demonstrated that litter sizes of three light goat kids (< 2.8 kg BW) or more had significantly lower mean serum IgG levels at 24 hours of life when compared with litter sizes of one or two heavier kids (9.85 versus 18.30 mg/mL, respectively).[37] This suggests that special attention and monitoring should be paid to multiple fetus gestation as the risk of FPT under these circumstances at kidding is higher; however, the quality of colostrum, amount ingested, and adequacy of absorption are rarely monitored by small ruminant producers in natural or artificial rearing systems. The use of monitoring tools to evaluate colostrum quality and IgG absorption is common in modern dairy cattle operations, and these tools are readily available for small ruminant production systems. Recent reports have presented the use of %Brix in maternal colostrum and neonate serum and its positive correlation with serum total proteins (STPs) at 24 hours as effective monitoring tools of FPT in lambs and goat kids.[38–40] The use of STP has also been used to monitor colostrum deficiency intake in mule deer fawns[41]; however, adequate values of serum IgG for cervid neonates have not been established yet.

Inadequate colostrum intake and low serum IgG at 24 to 48 hours of life have been consistently associated with higher morbidity and mortality rates in lambs, goat kids, and fawns. One study reported that 46% of lamb mortality between 24 hours and 5 weeks of age can be attributed to FPT.[42] Another study suggested that colostrum deficiency and low serum IgG in goat kids resulted in higher mortality rates at weeks 10 and 12 of life due to chronic infections with *Pasteurella multocida* and *Escherichia coli*.[43] Other reports demonstrated that 45% of lambs with a serum IgG of < 6 mg/mL at 24 hours died before 3 weeks of age compared with only 5% of the lambs with a serum IgG of > 6 mg/mL at 24 hours.[34] In a previous report, mule deer *(Odocoileus hemionus)* fawns with a STP of ≤ 5 g/dL between days 1 and 7 of age developed diarrhea and died before 17 days of age compared with fawns with STP > 5 g/dL.[41] In a more recent report, a 7-day-old Formosan sambar deer *(Rusa unicolor swinhoei)* with a history of colostrum deprivation died due to severe suppurative meningitis caused by *E. coli* infection.[44]

In addition to immunoglobulins, colostrum also contains large quantities of fat-soluble vitamins that do not cross the placenta. The most important of these are vitamins A, D, and E, which are important in bone development and the immune or inflammatory response. Neonates that have not ingested enough colostrum are likely to be deficient in these vitamins.

Diagnosis. History of dam dystocia, inadequate colostrum nursing, complete colostrum deprivation, and signs of undernourishment or sepsis in the first few days after birth are usually a presumptive indication of failure in the transfer of passive immunity. A high prevalence of diarrhea and respiratory disease in neonates should prompt investigation and evaluation of passive transfer of immunity in affected herds or flocks. Owners occasionally evaluate lambs or kids for adequate intake by picking up the animal and holding it at ear level, while carefully cradling the head and neck, and then shaking the abdomen to hear milk in the abomasum; however, this is not a reliable indication of adequate transfer of passive immunity. A definitive diagnosis of FPT can be made by direct laboratory measurement (single radial immunodiffusion [SRID]) of IgG in serum at 24 hours of life. Although some practitioners use the value of IgG used in dairy calves (10 mg/mL), others have suggested an IgG value < 15 mg/mL to establish the presence of FPT in small ruminants.[45]

Numerous semiquantitative methods of estimating IgG are available and are easy to use in sheep, goats, and cervids. The most common is the measurement of serum total solids or STP values at 24 hours of life through an optical refractometer. The STP at 24 hours of life in a well-hydrated animal has demonstrated correlation with serum IgG in calves, lambs, and goat kids. Studies in goat kids indicated that an STP between 5.3 and 5.4 g/dL was associated with adequate transfer of passive immunity.[39,40] Another study demonstrated FPT in lambs with STP values < 4.5 g/dL at 24 hours of life.[32] A study in mule deer suggested that fawns with an STP ≤ 5 g/dL had inadequate colostrum intake and FPT. Recently, the measurement of %Brix in maternal colostrum and serum with a digital Brix refractometer has become an alternative method to evaluate colostrum quality and FPT in dairy operations. Colostrum %Brix > 22% and serum %Brix > 8.4% have been associated with adequate transfer of IgG in calves and goat kids.[39] Other qualitative methods to assess the transfer of passive immunity in large animals include various agglutination (glutaraldehyde), precipitate assays (sodium sulfate), and measurement of γ-glutamyl transferase (GGT) in serum. These methods may be relied on to give an overall flock assessment of adequacy of passive transfer, but they are rarely accurate enough to provide definitive information on individual animals.

Treatment. FPT is not in itself pathologic, but it greatly increases the neonate's susceptibility to infectious diseases. The amount of colostrum absorbed across the gut decreases with time, especially in animals that have been ingesting other proteins (e.g., the casein in milk); it also decreases with illnesses that decrease gastrointestinal function. Neonatal small ruminants should receive at least 4 g of IgG/kg of BW or ideally 30 g of total mass of IgG from a good-quality colostrum source (> 50 mg/mL of IgG) during the first hours of life.[32] Other authors recommend an intake of 180 to 210 mL of colostrum/kg during the first 18 hours of life.[46] In artificial rearing systems or lamb feedlots, feeding of colostrum every 6 hours until 24 hours of life is recommended.[47] When same species' maternal colostrum is unavailable, goat colostrum or bovine colostrum/colostrum replacers or are a good alternative; however, hemolysis has been reported in lambs receiving cattle colostrum.[48] One study demonstrated that there was no difference in serum IgG levels of lambs that received the same volume of sheep or goat colostrum at birth.[47] Another study demonstrated that lambs that received 250 mL of a bovine colostrum replacer at birth in addition to 250 mL of stored sheep colostrum at 6 hours of life had higher serum %Brix values at 24 hours and had less incidence of disease during the preweaning period compared with lambs that received the same volume of stored sheep colostrum at birth and at 6 hours of life.[38] Since IgG absorption cannot be extended more than 24 hours after birth, administration of an oral colostrum source is the best treatment in the immediate postpartum period in still-healthy neonates. After the window for immunoglobulin absorption has closed, plasma, serum, or whole blood administered by the IV or intra-peritoneal route is the best way to raise the neonate's blood immunoglobulin concentrations. Adult donor plasma contains approximately 2.5 to 3.5 g of immunoglobulin/dL, so administration of a volume equivalent to 10% of BW or a dose of 20 to 40 mL/kg has been recommended for the treatment of large animal neonates. If plasma is used instead of colostrum, administration of vitamins A, D, and E also may be beneficial.

If colostrum and plasma are unavailable or cost-prohibitive, "closing" the gut as quickly as possible with milk, maintaining high standards of hygiene, and possibly administering prophylactic antibiotics offer the greatest prospects for preventing infectious disease. Vaccination of the neonate or the administration of antitoxin hyperimmune serum should not be considered protective but may be of value.

Prevention. Prevention of FPT should be based on the establishment of an adequate colostrum program managing the previously mentioned factors that affect production, quality, and absorption of maternal colostrum components in lambs, goat kids, and fawns. Ensuring colostral quality is best done through good nutrition, health care, and vaccination of dam (see Chapters 2 and 19). Administration of vaccines 6 weeks before parturition, followed in 2 weeks with a booster, provides the highest quantity of protective immunoglobulin in the colostrum. Antepartum leakage is rarely the problem in small ruminants that it is in horses and cattle. However, in a flock or herd environment, still-pregnant dams may steal babies from other sheep or goats. To prevent such theft and the resultant loss of colostrum by the "adopted" neonate, owners may choose to keep pregnant animals separate from those that have already delivered. If complete separation is not possible, the dam and her offspring should be allowed to bond with each other in a private pen ("jug" or "crate") for at least 24 hours before being placed back with the flock. Clipping excessive wool or mohair from around the perineal area and udder before lambing or kidding, expressing the teats to ensure they are not plugged, and having extra colostrum available when pregnant females are placed in jugs or crates are other good preventive measures.

Uncomplicated Neonatal Diarrhea

Etiology and Pathogenesis. Uncomplicated diarrhea in lambs, goat kids, and fawns may be caused by infectious agents such as viruses, bacteria, and protozoa. In goat kids and elk calves, metabolic causes of diarrhea have been described.[49,50] Group B and A rotavirus, enterotoxigenic *E. coli* K99, *Cryptosporidium parvum*, and other *Cryptosporidium* spp. have been commonly identified as causal agents of diarrhea in small ruminant neonates.[51–54] With recent advances in diagnostics and metagenomics of the enteric environment of large animals, novel viruses have been identified as potential causal agents of diarrhea in lambs and goat kids. Adenovirus, Astrovirus, Calicivirus, Coronavirus, and Picornavirus have been identified in feces of diarrheic lambs and goat kids[55]; however, their role in the pathogenesis of neonatal diarrhea is still uncertain. These organisms differ from the agents of complicated diarrhea in that they do not invade beyond the gut wall or result in systemic toxemia (see Chapter 5). Additional causes of diarrhea reported in goat kids and elk include lactose intolerance and hypernatremia, respectively.[49,50] Less frequently, bacteria such as *C. perfringens*, *Clostridium difficile*, and attaching and effacing *E. coli* have been associated with complicated diarrhea in small ruminant neonates.[54,56]

The net result of such an infection is that a large volume of water and electrolytes are lost into the bowel due to malabsorptive, hypersecretory, or hyperosmolar processes. If enough fluid and electrolytes are lost, dehydration and metabolic acidosis arise, inducing systemic clinical signs of depression and weakness in association with diarrhea. In goats, this clinical entity is one component of the floppy kid syndrome.

Clinical Signs. Profuse, watery, yellowish-green to brown diarrhea without fever is the hallmark clinical sign. With severe dehydration and acidosis, affected lambs, kids, and fawns become weak and dull and lack appetite.[50–52] Excessive salivation and loss of suckle reflex have also been reported in affected lambs and kids.[51,52] Mucous membranes become tacky, and skin tenting times are prolonged. Shock signs may develop. Physical assessment often must take the place of clinicopathologic analysis in affected neonates.

Mild, nonclinically complicated diarrhea is characterized by profuse diarrhea with minimal systemic signs. The affected animal is bright and alert, with minimal skin tenting, and can stand and eat readily, with a strong suckle reflex. It is less than 5% dehydrated, with a blood pH of 7.35 to 7.50, and bicarbonate deficit is minimal.

Moderate uncomplicated diarrhea is characterized by profuse diarrhea in a dull but responsive animal. Skin tenting is prolonged, but eye luster is normal. The affected animal is able to stand and eat but eats slowly and has a weak suckle reflex. The head typically is held down. It is 5 to 7% dehydrated, with a blood pH of 7.10 to 7.25 and a bicarbonate deficit of 5 to 8 mEq/L. Severe uncomplicated diarrhea is characterized by profuse diarrhea. The affected animal is dull and minimally responsive, with a very long skin tent time and dull, sunken eyes. It can stand only with assistance and prefers to stay in sternal recumbency with its head up. The animal eats very slowly, if at all, and has a minimal suckle reflex. It is 8 to 10% dehydrated, with a blood pH of 6.90 to 7.10 and a bicarbonate deficit of 10 mEq/L.

Very severe uncomplicated diarrhea is characterized by profuse diarrhea and profound weakness. The animal's skin remains tented for more than 1 minute, and its eyes are very sunken and dull. It is nonresponsive with no suckle response. It is unable to maintain sternal recumbency, lying on its side instead. The animal is 10 to 12% dehydrated, with a blood pH of 6.8 to 7.0 and a bicarbonate deficiency of 15 to 20 mEq/L.

Epidemiology. Morbidity and mortality of uncomplicated diarrhea in small ruminants and fawns vary depending on the cause. Reports of rotaviral diarrhea in newborn lambs indicate morbidity rates between 50% and 100% and mortality rates between 0 and 10%[51,52]; however, one study reported a 50% case fatality rate in lambs affected with types B and A rotavirus diarrhea.[52] Another study reported mortality rates between 10% and 30% in lambs and kids affected with *C. parvum* diarrhea.[57] Most of infectious agents associated with uncomplicated neonatal diarrhea in small ruminants are shed by adult animals and older lambs/kids around stressful events such as lambing/kidding and extreme weather conditions. One study reported that pregnant does shed 7 to 10 times more oocysts during the 3 weeks around kidding compared with other time periods.[58] Additionally, poor husbandry/hygiene of lambing/kidding sheds, fecal soiling, flock size (> 200 animals), lambing/kidding season (winter/spring), and the presence of *C. perfringens* type A in feces have been suggested as potential risk factors for uncomplicated diarrhea in small ruminant neonates.[58–60]

Clinical Pathology. The leukogram should be normal or show abnormalities compatible with stress. Serum biochemical or blood gas analysis may reveal evidence of intestinal malabsorption, electrolyte loss, metabolic acidosis (hypoglycemia, hyponatremia, hypochloremia, hyperkalemia, low bicarbonate, and increased anion gap), and dehydration (hyperalbuminemia and increased blood urea nitrogen [BUN] and creatinine). In contrast with the common leukogram and biochemical abnormalities found in calves, lambs, and goat kids with uncomplicated diarrhea, elk calves with diarrhea develop leukocytosis, hyperchloremia, and hypernatremia (serum Na > 153 mEq/L).[50] Additionally, increased anion gap, BUN, creatinine, and albumin concentrations have been reported in affected elk calves.[50]

Diagnosis. A presumptive diagnosis may be based on the characteristic history and clinical signs. Response to conservative treatment also is supportive of this diagnosis. Identification of the specific causative agent is less important than proper treatment of affected animals; however, feces or intestinal contents from affected animals can be submitted for electron microscopy, reverse-transcription polymerase chain reaction (PCR), and cell culture immunofluorescent assays to identify viruses.[51–53] Additionally, intestinal tissue can be submitted for IHC for rotavirus and *C. parvum.*[53,57] Feces of affected animals can also be submitted for enzyme-linked immunosorbent assay (ELISA), Ziehl-Neelsen staining technique, light or fluorescence microscopy, sugar flotation, and auramine or fluorescent antibody staining for the diagnosis of *C. parvum* infection.[60] Fecal culture to determine a bacterial cause is recommended.

Treatment. The immediate goals of treatment are rehydration, replacement of lost electrolytes, and restoration of acid-base balance as these are usually the leading causes of death in affected neonates. Less immediate goals are provision of nutrition and replacement of ongoing losses. The aggressiveness of treatment is dictated by the severity of the condition, as well as economic considerations.[61]

1. *Rehydration*: Calculate the percent dehydration and use to calculate fluid requirements for a 24-hour period.
   Example: 10% dehydration in a 3-kg lamb:
   Dehydration: 0.1×3 kg $\times$ 1 kg/L = 0.3 L or 300 mL.
   Maintenance: 100 mL/kg/day = 0.3 L or 300 mL.
   Total fluids to replace in 24 hours = 0.6 L or 600 mL
   Fluid loss due to dehydration (300 mL in this case) should be replaced during the first 4 hours and the rest can be replaced in the next 20 hours.
2. *Replace lost electrolytes*: Sodium, chloride, and bicarbonate are lost roughly in proportion to extracellular fluid (ECF) in the acute phase of diarrhea (1–2 days) in untreated animals. Potassium tends to be increased in this phase due to the presence of metabolic acidosis and care should be taken when selecting fluids containing potassium to treat affected animals at this time. In chronic cases of diarrhea, and especially in cases where the owner/producer has given oral milk replacer or electrolyte supplements/replacements to affected animals before veterinary evaluation, the serum concentration of sodium, potassium, and bicarbonate might be variable or increased. Special care should be taken in these cases when selecting fluids to treat affected animals as the risk of causing hypernatremia is higher.[61] In cases of diarrhea in elk calves, hypernatremia is common, and fluids should be selected accordingly.[50] In the majority of cases, initial replacement of sodium, chloride, and bicarbonate with fluids containing proper composition is recommended.[61]
3. *Restore the acid-base balance*: Estimate bicarbonate deficit by blood gas analysis (24 mEq, as measured), serum bicarbonate concentration, or physical assessment. In calves, clinical signs of posture, demeanor, and presence of absence of suckle reflex can be used to estimate base deficit, and this might be applied for small ruminant neonates. Briefly, diarrheic neonates that are alert, are standing, and have a suckle have a bicarbonate deficit < 8 mEq; those that are depressed, are sternal recumbent, and have no suckle have a bicarbonate deficit between 8 and 10 mEq; and those that are severely depressed, laterally recumbent, no suckle animals have a bicarbonate deficit > 15 mEq.[61] After calculating the bicarbonate deficit, calculate the whole body need of bicarbonate using the following formula:

Bicarbonate needs = $0.6 \times$ bicarbonate deficit (mEq) $\times$ BW (kg)

Example: Assessment suggests a bicarbonate deficit of 16 mEq bicarbonate in a 3-kg, comatose lamb with prolonged skin tenting (0.6 is the multiplier for ECF in a neonate): 0.6 × (16 mEq) × 3 kg = 29 mEq bicarbonate. Commercial IV 8.4% sodium bicarbonate solutions contain 1 mEq of bicarbonate per milliliter and could be added directly to IV fluids in severely dehydrated and acidotic animals.[61]

Therefore, the immediate goal is to provide 300 mL of fluid and 29 mEq of bicarbonate to this lamb in a formulation that resembles normal ECF. Fluids can be given by various routes. Selection of route of administration of fluids depends on degree of dehydration, presence or not of a strong suckle reflex, and degree of depression. Neonates with advanced degrees of dehydration, depression, and absence of suckle reflex will benefit from IV fluid therapy. In contrast, neonates with mild dehydration and active suckle reflex can be effectively treated with oral electrolytes[61]; however, if oral fluids have not produced an improvement within 2 to 4 hours, IV treatment should be strongly considered. Other routes such as subcutaneous, intra-peritoneal, and intra-osseous can also be used for fluid administration to neonates.

Routes

Oral

- *Advantages*: Oral fluids are inexpensive (nonsterile) and easy to give. They are less likely to cause fatal arrhythmias or neurologic disease than IV fluids.
- *Disadvantages*: An animal receives a maximum of its gastric volume (5% of BW), and good gastric motility is required. Oral fluids may not be well absorbed by a damaged gut. Absorption also is slow.

Intravenous

- *Advantage*: This method allows rapid correction of all deficits, even in moribund animals.
- *Disadvantages*: It is expensive (sterile), requires venous access, and can rapidly lead to overcorrection.

Subcutaneous

- *Advantages*: This method does not require venous access or good gut motility.
- *Disadvantages*: It is expensive (sterile), and the fluids may not be well absorbed in very dehydrated animals. Absorption is not as quick as by IV administration. Animals should be given only hypotonic or isotonic fluids.

Intra-peritoneal

- *Advantages*: This method does not require venous access or gut motility. Fluids are absorbed quickly by this route.
- *Disadvantages*: It is expensive (sterile) and can cause peritonitis. Isotonic fluids are best used in this route. Only a limited volume can be given.

Many commercial oral electrolyte solutions for neonatal ruminants are available; however, not all of them fulfill the requirements to adequately replace fluids and electrolytes in neonatal ruminants with diarrhea. Oral electrolyte solutions must contain enough sodium (90–110 mEq), provide agents that increase absorption of water (glycine, glucose, and acetate), provide an alkalinizing agent (bicarbonate, propionate, acetate, and citrate; acetate has demonstrated best results), and an energy source (glucose).[61] The amount of carbohydrates might vary and is usually higher in "high-energy" solutions specifically used for severely affected neonates that are not eating and develop negative energy balance. Less carbohydrate is needed in less severely affected animals because they are usually eating some and are less likely to have severe negative energy balance. Fluids to be avoided include medicated milk replacers and unbuffered saline solutions.

IV treatment should be provided with a sterile commercial product. Such preparations typically contain 25 to 30 mEq/L of base. Additional sodium bicarbonate solution or sterile powder can be added to fluid therapy based on the bicarbonate deficit (1 mEq/mL of 8.4% solution and 12 mEq of bicarbonate/g of powder, respectively). The bicarbonate deficit should be over the first 4 hours.

After deficits are replaced, the following continued treatments and adjuncts may be considered:

1. Continued administration of fluids (oral rather than IV, if possible) to replace ongoing losses:
   - Oral electrolytes at a volume equal to 5% of the BW per feeding can be given; the number of feedings can be increased from two (normal) to three to six per day.
   - IV fluids can be continued at twice the maintenance fluid rate until appetite is restored.
   - More bicarbonate may be necessary.
2. Consideration of addition of milk to the treatment regimen:
   - Milk or milk replacers should be added to the therapy of neonates with diarrhea. They provide nutrition to the affected neonate, preventing negative energy balance and promoting intestinal healing.
   - Care should be taken to NOT mix oral electrolyte solutions with milk or milk replacers in the same container as the concentration of sodium and overall osmolarity of the solution can dramatically increase, leading to hypernatremia or other metabolic abnormalities.
   - Milk or milk replacers should be given in small volumes (~20% of total requirements) but at a higher frequency (every 3–6 hours) to avoid overloading the abomasum and intestine of affected animals. Lambs fed milk lose less weight with scours.
   - Free water helps prevent hypernatremia.
   - Milk is a good potassium source (see Chapter 3).

Elk Deer Calves. Elk deer calves commonly develop diarrhea with hypernatremia (serum Na > 153 mEq/L) compared with other large animal neonates, where hyponatremia is more common.[50] Therefore, administration of oral electrolyte solutions designed for other ruminants (calves, lambs, and kids) should be avoided in these animals. A dilution (1:2 or 1:4) of commercially available bovine calf electrolyte solutions to reduce sodium content is recommended for the treatment of elk calf diarrhea.[50] The use of lactated Ringer's solution, which has a low sodium concentration in addition to a very low reduction rate of serum sodium (< 1.7 mEq/L/hour) has been advocated in the fluid therapy of hypernatremic elk calves with diarrhea.[50]

Additional Therapy. Dextrose (2.5–5%) solutions can be added to the fluid therapy of hypoglycemic animals. The use of nonsteroidal antiinflammatory drugs (NSAIDs) in neonatal ruminants with diarrhea is controversial due to the risk of renal damage and abomasal ulceration; however, in cases of diarrhea complicated by septicemia or endotoxemia, NSAIDs should be used to reduce the effects of systemic inflammation. Flunixin meglumine at a dose of 1.1 to 2.2 mg/kg is the only NSAID approved for food animal use. Similarly, the use of oral or systemic antibiotics in cases of uncomplicated diarrhea is controversial due to its potential effect on the intestinal microbiota and development of bacterial resistance; however, their use is warranted in the presence of septicemia or endotoxemia in addition to diarrhea. In these cases, β-lactams such as oral amoxicillin or systemic ceftiofur are usually good choices. The effect of mucosal protectants and probiotics in cases of diarrhea is unknown in small ruminant neonates, and their use is left to practitioners based on their own experiences (see Appendix 1).

Prevention. Prevention of uncomplicated diarrhea in small ruminant neonates is based primarily on the timely feeding of adequate amounts of good quality maternal colostrum or colostrum replacer (see "Failure of Passive Transfer" section). Vaccination of dams with antigens of common infectious agents associated with uncomplicated neonatal diarrhea before parturition has demonstrated to be effective increasing colostrum immunity and prevention of diarrhea in lambs.[62] Maintenance of adequate husbandry and hygiene conditions in lambing/kidding sheds or barns is necessary to reduce neonatal exposure to infectious agents normally shed in feces of dams during parturition such as rotavirus and *C. parvum*.

Other Causes of Weakness and Depression in Neonates

Ruling out infectious causes of depression and weakness is difficult, and clinicians often do well to assume that an infectious disease is contributing to clinical signs when making treatment decisions. However, several noninfectious systemic disturbances also can depress neurologic and muscular function. Successful treatment often requires identification and correction of each of these disturbances. Among the more common abnormalities leading to depression in neonates are hypoxemia, metabolic or respiratory acidosis, hypothermia, hyperthermia, hypoglycemia, dehydration, azotemia, and some electrolyte imbalances.

Hypothermia and hyperthermia can easily be diagnosed by measuring body temperature with a rectal thermometer. Hypothermia is far more common and can result from weakness, shock, and environmental stress. Cold, windy weather or tube feeding with cold milk replacer or fluids can lead to a rapid drop in core body temperature, especially in neonates that are small or weak or have been inadequately licked off or were rejected by their dams. Strong, vigorous neonates usually are protected by heat produced during muscular activity and are able to seek food and shelter. Clinical signs appear when the rectal temperature drops to 98° F (36.7° C) or below. Protection from wind and cold such as with an individual ewe jug or pen, heat lamps (positioned far enough away so as not to burn the neonate), hot water bottles, blankets, and administration of warm fluids is helpful in treating and preventing hypothermia. Shearing the ewe before lambing is of value because it forces the ewe to seek shelter. If this management technique is used, care should be taken to avoid inducing severe hypothermia in the dam.

Environmental hyperthermia is much less common than fever in neonates. Therefore, treatment for infectious diseases in young animals with high temperatures usually is warranted. Providing cool shelter with good ventilation, minimizing stressful events, ensuring adequate fluid intake, and shearing the adults are the best defenses against environmental heat stress.

Hypoglycemia also is easy to diagnose with the aid of an inexpensive, portable glucose meter. Lambs and kids typically develop hypoglycemia under the same circumstances as those leading to hypothermia. Administering 50 mL/kg of dextrose (approximately 3.5 fl oz/lb, or 5% of BW) in warm milk replacer or 1 mL/kg of 50% dextrose, by either the IV or oral route (diluted to 5% dextrose), should provide ample energy to correct hypoglycemia. IV administration may be necessary if gut motility is absent. Follow-up treatment may be necessary if the neonate does not regain its appetite.

Except during severe conditions, normal lambs and kids should be able to maintain normal body core temperature. They should therefore be examined for an underlying disorder if they exhibit signs of hypothermia or hyperthermia. Clinicians and owners should not assume that warming and feeding a cold, weak neonate will always correct the problem.

Hypoxemia is much more difficult to diagnose. Portable blood gas meters for arterial analysis and radiography units for thoracic imaging are available but are still not in common use in small ruminant practice. For those reasons, hypoxemia usually is underdiagnosed. Hypoxemia can result from prematurity or dysmaturity, infection, depression or weakness (decreased ventilation), meconium aspiration, bullous emphysema, hernias, and other thoracic fluid or tissue masses. It is likely to be a contributing factor in illness and death in most weak neonates younger than 3 days of age. Such animals benefit from the provision of supplemental oxygen, either through a nasal insufflation tube or by oxygen tent. In addition to its direct effect on general wellbeing and behavior/attitude, hypoxemia at birth leads to poor gut function and subsequent poor colostral absorption. Many animals that exhibit FPT and subsequent sepsis had a previous bout of hypoxemia.

Azotemia, metabolic acidosis, and electrolyte imbalances are difficult to diagnose without clinicopathologic analysis. Therefore, these problems are best treated in animals showing signs of dehydration with the administration of a balanced, physiologic electrolyte solution. Metabolic acidosis usually is accompanied by either obvious evidence of bicarbonate loss (diarrhea) or severe dehydration. However, neither of these conditions is present with floppy kid syndrome. This descriptive title is applied to muscle weakness, anorexia, and depression in kids observed in the first 2 weeks of life. By its strictest definition, *floppy kid syndrome* refers to metabolic acidosis with a high anion gap without dehydration or any known cause in young kids that were normal at birth. A variety of disorders and conditions have been proposed as the cause of metabolic acidosis without dehydration, including intestinal fermentation of milk in well-fed kids with subsequent absorption of volatile fatty acids, transient neonatal renal tubular acidosis, and lactic acidosis secondary to toxic impairment of cardiovascular function. Overgrowth of *C. perfringens* type A often is suggested as a source of the toxin. With a high anion gap, a pathologic condition that leads to overproduction of an organic acid is more likely than one that leads to bicarbonate loss. The disease can occur in individual animals or in outbreaks; although parity of the dam and number of offspring have not been associated with this metabolic disturbance, aggressively feeding kids are more likely to suffer from milk fermentation or clostridial overgrowth. An infectious etiology appears to be more likely in herds displaying an increased incidence of this metabolic disturbances as the kidding season progresses. The disease also is reported to be more common in meat goats than in dairy goats. The prevalence can vary tremendously from year to year in a single flock or region. A similar disease has been reported in calves and llama crias, and lambs are likely to be susceptible under the right conditions.

Because blood gas analysis and exclusion of other diseases often are impractical, the term *floppy kid syndrome* frequently is used by owners to refer to any kid that is weak and does not have an overt, organ-specific sign (e.g., diarrhea). Different pathologic processes are grouped together by their common clinical endpoint (as with "thin ewe syndrome"), and the veterinarian is charged with determining the etiology in a specific flock. Most possible causes are found in the previous list of conditions that cause weakness and depression in neonates. Among these entities, sepsis and hypoxemia are the most important items and therefore must also be considered possible causes of floppy kid syndrome. Treatment and prevention of floppy kid syndrome currently follow the same lines as for treatment and prevention of neonatal sepsis or enteritis. Spontaneous recovery of animals with floppy kid syndrome may occur. However, in valuable kids, quick assessment of blood chemistry and base deficits will allow requisite correction of electrolyte and blood pH abnormalities with 1.3% sodium bicarbonate.[63]

Diseases Caused by Tissue-Invading Clostridia

Tissue-invading clostridia are large, straight, gram positive rods that are 3 to 10 μm in length. *C. perfringens* and *C. haemolyticum* are smaller bacteria, and *Clostridium novyi*, *Clostridium chauvoei*, and *Clostridium septicum* are larger. The bacteria grow best under anaerobic conditions and produce waste gases. Clostridia bear spores, which may be the only viable form in the environment (soil and decomposed organic matter). Identification of these spores within bacteria on microscopic examination is useful to identify clostridia, but it is not diagnostic of disease. Spores in *C. perfringens* are central and do not affect the shape, whereas most other species have the spore toward one end and appear slightly club shaped.

Clostridia cause infectious, noncontagious disease. The bacteria inhabit the intestinal tract and are present in the feces of ruminants. Small numbers of organisms in their dormant spore form also may reside in tissues such as liver and skeletal muscle. They can be isolated from soil, where most are thought to have short life spans. Soil concentrations are highest in locations recently contaminated with ruminant feces, especially crowded, overused facilities such as feedlots and lambing sheds. Environmental contaminations are associated with cool, damp times of the year such as late winter and spring.

The concentration of organisms and their toxins found in the feces, gut contents, and internal organs of most adult ruminants usually is small. Competition and peristalsis prevent overgrowth in the gut, and aerobic conditions prevent overgrowth in other tissues in live animals. However, rapid overgrowth and tissue invasion ensue after death, making rapid postmortem examination essential to ascertain whether clostridial organisms are responsible for the death. Pathogenic clostridial organisms all produce heat-labile protein exotoxins. Most make a variety of toxins, and the relative contribution of each toxin to the disease state is not known.

Enteric Infections

C. perfringens is a normal commensal of the intestinal tract of clinically healthy large animals, including cervids; however, the number of bacteria and their toxin production within the intestine usually remain low due to peristalsis and normal homeostasis.[64] *C. perfringens* is classified into five biotypes (A, B, C, D, and E) based on the production of four major exotoxins, namely alpha (CPA), beta (CPB), epsilon (ETX), and iota (ITX); however, the production of more than 16 different exotoxins in various combinations has been associated with these bacteria, including perfringolysin O (PFO), enterotoxin (CPE), and beta2 toxin (CPB2).[64] The different biotypes of *C. perfringens* cause different diseases in relation with the exotoxins they produce. The major effect of the phospholipase/sphingomyelinase CPA, produced by all *C. perfringens* biotypes, is cell lysis and hemolysis, and its role on intestinal disease of large animals is not well understood. However, this toxin has been associated with hemolytic disease and hemorrhagic enteritis in large animals; CPB, produced by *C. perfringens* types B and C, is a trypsin-labile toxin associated with necrotizing enteritis and enterotoxemia in large animal neonates; ETX, produced by *C. perfringens* types D and B, is a trypsin-activated necrotizing toxin associated to vasculitis, edema, and necrosis of the CNS and enterotoxemia; and ITX, another trypsin-activated necrotizing toxin produced by *C. perfringens* type E, has also been associated to intestinal disease in small ruminants.[64,65] *C. perfringens* types C and D are considered the most important types in veterinary medicine as they can cause disease in most farm animals.[66] Severe clinical disease due to bacteria sporulation and massive toxin production only occurs when the normal intestinal environment and microbial balance are disrupted in affected individuals. Decreased peristalsis and poor ruminal and abomasal function have also been proposed as factors that contribute to disease presentation. Weather and handling stresses, feed changes, and an overabundance of high-energy feeds such as milk, bakery products, and cereal grains might promote bacteria overgrowth and exotoxin synthesis and release. Additionally, other enteric infections that disrupt the mucosal border may increase systemic absorption of toxins and promote severe disease.

C. perfringens type A Disease

C. perfringens type A is a normal inhabitant of the intestinal tract of large animals and is ubiquitous in the environment (soil). One study reported *C. perfringens* type A as the most common isolate among other clostridia from healthy young lambs.[67] *C. perfringens* type A has been associated with a fatal hemolytic syndrome in younger lambs and cattle but not goats ("yellow lamb disease"),[66,68] acute hemorrhagic enteritis and hemolytic enterotoxemia in cattle (hemorrhagic bowel/jejunal syndrome) and goats,[66,69,70] and intestinal hemorrhage and splenomegaly in farmed deer.[71,72] Risk factors for infection have not been established; however, high soluble carbohydrate diets and high BCSs have been associated with clinical disease.[69,70,72] This disease occurs most commonly in lambs 2 to 6 months old. Under favorable conditions, the organisms proliferate and cause a corresponding increase in alpha toxin production. The alpha toxin (CPA), in synergy with the beta2 toxin (CPB2), is responsible for hemolytic crisis, vasculitis, and gastrointestinal lesions. The clinical course usually is less than 24 hours.

Clinical Signs. In most cases, sudden death or history of found dead is common. Clinical signs observed usually include weakness, depression, fever or hypothermia, icterus, anemia, hemoglobinuria, tachypnea, colic, hemorrhagic diarrhea or absence of feces, and terminal recumbency.[66,69,70–72] Adult animals also are susceptible to hemolytic disease and vasculitis caused by *C. perfringens* type A infection.[66] Fatal abomasitis and rumenitis in neonates and juveniles also have been blamed on *C. perfringens* type A, but the rapid postmortem proliferation of the organism makes substantiation of this claim difficult.[73] Morbidity in a flock is lower than for many of the other enteric clostridial diseases, but the mortality rate is very high.

Diagnosis. The most characteristic clinicopathologic change is neutrophilic leukocytosis with a left shift. Other evidence of systemic toxemia (metabolic acidosis, azotemia, and increases in liver and muscle enzymes) also may be seen. Laboratory evaluation reveals evidence of intravascular hemolysis. Necropsy in sheep, goats, and cervids usually reveals evidence of hemolysis, pallor, jaundice, hemoglobinuria, hyperemic and edematous intestines, splenomegaly, gastrointestinal serosal and mucosal hemorrhage, and multifocal internal petechial hemorrhages.[66,69,70–72] The isolation of *C. perfringens* type A from necropsied animals is not itself diagnostic. Definitive diagnosis can be made based on identification of the alpha toxin and the absence of other toxins by ELISAs or older, live animal assays. More recently, multiplex PCR techniques are replacing immunodiffusion assays for the identification of a specific toxin-producing gene isolate, typing of bacteria, and demonstration of toxins or toxin genes.[74] Gut content and intestinal samples collected from freshly dead animals make the most meaningful samples for diagnosis.[74]

Treatment. Administration of high doses (> 30,000 IU/kg BID) of penicillin and *Clostridium* antitoxin (10–20 mL subcutaneously [SC] or orally [PO]) is the mainstay of treatment, although animals may die acutely before therapies can be instituted.

Prevention. A conditionally licensed toxoid against the clostridial alpha toxin is available for cattle in the United States. A recent report demonstrated that a new vaccine including recombinant CPA, CPB, and ETX was effective at inducing protective antibodies to *C. perfringens* biotypes in cattle, sheep, and goats. This could be an alternative for the prevention of morbidity and mortality caused by *C. perfringens* type A. Prevention efforts should focus on environmental hygiene and avoiding gut conditions favorable for proliferation of the organism (high content of soluble carbohydrates in the diet). Because this type appears to survive better in soil than other types, preventing ingestion of soil may be important in preventing disease.

C. perfringens Type B and C Disease

C. perfringens types B and C occur in the soil and the animals' housing environment and can be shed by asymptomatic individuals. The reported geographic range of both diseases is limited (type B to the United Kingdom and South Africa and type C to the United Kingdom, Australia, and North America), even though infection with *C. perfringens* type C appears to occur worldwide. These organisms cause very similar diseases called *lamb dysentery* and *hemorrhagic enterotoxemia*, respectively. Very young lambs and kids (1–4 days to 2–3 weeks of age) are usually affected due to the presence of trypsin inhibitors in colostrum.[75] Older animals may become susceptible as a result of overwhelming infection or trypsin inhibition by some soy and sweet potato products or temporary suppression of pancreatic trypsin production (Struck in adult sheep). With both diseases, the beta toxin (CPB) is a required pathophysiologic factor, and inactivation of this toxin after maturation of pancreatic trypsinogen secretion is what commonly limits the susceptible population to neonatal animals. The cytolytic and necrotizing effects of the beta toxin (CPB), in synergy with the beta2 toxin (CPB2), cause necrosis and ulceration of the intestinal mucosa and are translocated into circulation, causing severe toxemia and death.[75] The diseases initially affect lambs and kids younger than 3 days of age, with illness occasionally occurring in older lambs. The incidence of disease in lambs and kids can be around 15 to 30%, with a case fatality rate of 100%. High stocking density in lambing areas, cold weather, single-born lambs, and high milk production of dams have been suggested as potential risk factors for type B and C enterotoxemia.[76] Because of management practices in young animals and age-related vulnerability, fecal contamination of teats, hands, and equipment that enter the mouths of the neonates (orogastric tubes and nipples) is a major cause of infection.

Clinical Signs. Severely affected animals or those at the beginning of an outbreak usually are found dead. Less acutely affected animals expel initially yellow, fluid feces that progressively become brownish and/or hemorrhagic. Feces may also contain flecks of blood and show splinting of the abdomen, especially when handled, along with signs of colic and feed refusal. The clinical course usually is short, and the disease is almost always fatal. One study reported acute abdominal pain, hemorrhagic diarrhea, and death within 24 hours of experimental oral inoculation of three goat kids with a field strain of *C. perfringens* type C.[75] Dehydration, anemia, and severe weakness are also common clinical signs in affected animals. Terminal convulsions and coma occasionally are noted, especially in outbreaks in the United States. *C. perfringens* type C in older sheep causes the disease known as "struck." Affected animals usually are found dead or with signs of toxemia. Specific antemortem signs of gastrointestinal disease are rare. Specific antemortem signs of gastrointestinal disease are rare. Clinical pathology changes observed in these animals include neutrophilic leukocytosis with a left shift. Additional evidence of systemic toxemia (metabolic acidosis, azotemia, and increases in liver and muscle enzymes) also may be seen.

Necropsy Findings. Postmortem examination reveals focal hemorrhagic ulcers (up to 2.5 cm in diameter) in the small intestine (mostly in the ileum) with type B infection and diffuse reddening with hemorrhage and necrosis of the abomasum and the entire segments of the intestine with type C infection. Type C infections in ruminants can also present with generalized peritonitis, subendocardial and subepicardial hemorrhages, and hemorrhagic lymph nodes. Animals that die very rapidly may exhibit minimal or no gross abnormalities of the intestine. A similar syndrome of type C enterotoxemia has been previously reported in a sika deer *(Cervus nippon)*.[72] Sudden death, severe hemorrhagic gastritis including forestomach and abomasum, and catarrhal enteritis was observed in the affected animal.

Diagnosis. Diagnosis of these diseases is made by identification of characteristic history, clinical signs, postmortem lesions, and positive toxin assays. Because the beta toxin is very labile, negative toxin assays are less significant than negative assays for presence of other tissue-invading clostridia. The isolation of *C. perfringens* type B or C from necropsied animals is not itself diagnostic. Immunodiffusion assays or multiplex PCR of intestinal contents for specific isolate and beta toxin (CPB) identification are recommended to obtain final diagnosis (see "Diagnosis" in "*C. perfringens* type A" section).

Treatment. If the infection is identified early in the disease course, high doses of oral and parenteral penicillin and *C. perfringens* C and D antitoxin may be of benefit. IV fluids and antiinflammatory agents may be indicated as well. Usually, the condition is not recognized early enough, and animals are found dead or dying.

Prevention. A beta toxoid is available in the United States and other countries. It usually is packaged with an epsilon toxoid. The best protection is achieved by vaccinating pregnant dams twice, with the second dose administered approximately 3 to 4 weeks before lambing or kidding and annual booster. Deer does should receive double the dose of sheep as low antibody responses to clostridia have been reported in these animals.[77,78] Vaccination of pregnant dams is directed to increase specific colostrum antibodies to protect neonates. Juveniles also should be vaccinated twice or three times at 2 months, 3 months, and 4 months. Adults, including males, should receive an annual booster. In the face of an outbreak, the lambing area should be moved to a different place. Additionally, vaccination of dams and newborns with a beta toxoid and administration of *C. perfringens* C and D antitoxin can be carried out in the face of an outbreak to reduce morbidity and mortality.

C. perfringens Type D Disease

C. perfringens type D produces epsilon toxin (ETX), which is responsible for causing type D enterotoxemia in sheep, goats, calves, and deer.[79,80] Other common names for the disease include "overeating disease" or "pulpy kidney disease." The disease has a worldwide distribution and occurs primarily in suckling lambs of 1 to 10 weeks of age, although it has also been reported in weaned lambs up to 10 months of age and adult sheep. The disease is also common in grazing goats and deer. The prevalence of disease has been reported from 1.49 to 3.14%, with a 100% case fatality rate in feedlot lambs.[81] One study on proportional distribution of goatherd mortality in the province of Quebec, Canada, reported a 17.1% mortality of goats to *C. perfringens* type D enterotoxemia.[82] The disease is more common in feedlot lambs after they enter the lot. Tail docking, castration, and other management interventions are thought to decrease the incidence of this disease by temporarily decreasing appetite. The disease also affects unvaccinated adult sheep, even without any history of stressors or feed changes. Sudden changes in the diet are the main predisposing factor in goats. The disease can occur in vaccinated goats, as vaccination has not demonstrated to be completely protective in this species.[83,84]

C. perfringens type D is normally found in the gastrointestinal tract of healthy ruminants, but the acid environment of the abomasum and continuous peristalsis help to keep numbers of bacteria and levels of toxin production low. However, under specific conditions such as overingestion of high-energy feeds (milk, grain, and lush pasture), excess of fermentable starches in the intestine, and intestinal stasis, the organism proliferates rapidly, producing lethal quantities of epsilon toxin. These conditions are usually triggered in well-conditioned, fast-growing animals that are on a highly nutritious diet. The epsilon toxin, once produced, acts locally, causing increasing gut permeability and widespread tissue damage. Epsilon toxin and other exotoxins are then absorbed through the intestinal tract into systemic circulation and transported to the brain, lungs, and kidneys, causing increased endothelial permeability, perivascular edema, and generalized necrosis.[79,83] The characteristic increased vascular permeability and perivascular edema in the kidney and brain are responsible for the name of "pulpy kidney disease" and "focal symmetric encephalomalacia."

Clinical Signs. The course of the disease is usually very short (0.5–12 hours), so sudden or spontaneous death is a common clinical sign across affected small ruminant species.[80,84–86] Natural disease caused by *C. perfringens* type D differs between sheep and goats, possibly because of a difference in relative local and systemic actions of the epsilon toxin, although experimental models have demonstrated that both species develop similar lesions.[84,87,88] In sheep, systemic actions of the toxin leads to mostly neurological signs such as dullness, depression, ataxia, trembling, stiff limbs, opisthotonus, convulsions, frothy mouth, and rapid death. In goats, actions of the toxin appear to be more localized to the intestinal tract, causing enterocolitis, colic, diarrhea, dehydration, and occasional neurological signs.[85,86]

Necropsy Findings. Postmortem findings in sheep are characterized by edema of the brain, lungs, and heart in addition to hydropericardium.[89] Edema of the kidneys (pulpy kidney lesion) is inconsistent. Sheep usually demonstrated minor and inconsistent intestinal changes.[89] Other lesions reported in cattle and deer include hemorrhages on the epicardium, thymus, and diaphragm and petechial hemorrhages in the jejunal mucosa.[80,90] Necropsy lesions reported in goats include pseudomembranous enterocolitis with mucosal ulceration, as well as fibrin, blood clots, and watery contents in the bowel lumen. Evidence of systemic toxemia, including multifocal petechial and ecchymotic hemorrhage, proteinaceous exudates in body cavities, pulmonary edema, hydropericardium, and cerebral malacia with perivascular cuffing, have also been reported in goats and affected deer.[80,84,87,88,91]

Clinical Pathology. Characteristic clinicopathological changes include pronounced hyperglycemia and glucosuria, which are considered a hallmark of *C. perfringens* D enterotoxemia.[86] Additionally, neutrophilic leukocytosis with a left shift and evidence of systemic toxemia (metabolic acidosis, azotemia, and increases in liver and muscle enzymes) also may be seen.

Treatment. In general, the course of disease is too acute for the establishment of any treatment. However, as with infections with types B and C, if the disease is identified early in the disease course, high doses of oral and parenteral penicillin in addition to *Clostridium* C and D antitoxin may be of benefit. IV fluids and antiinflammatory agents may be indicated as well.

Prevention. Vaccination of pregnant ewes with two doses of toxoid, with the second dose given 3 to 4 weeks before lambing, and adequate ingestion of colostrum are the best methods of protecting newborn lambs. Vaccination of older lambs should occur before exposure to diets rich in carbohydrates (grain—feedlot settings) or lush pastures. In these cases, lambs should be vaccinated twice or three times around 2, 3, and 4 months of age. Males and adult females that are not part of the breeding program may be vaccinated annually. Vaccination has been shown to protect goats from experimental disease, but clinical evidence suggests that well-vaccinated goats are still susceptible to developing clostridial enteritis. The toxoids may not protect against local action of the toxins in the goat, which appears to play a greater role in their disease than it does in the sheep.[84,87,88] More frequent vaccination (every 6 months) in goats is suggested to increase protection. The adjuvant present in some multivalent clostridial vaccines may cause subcutaneous reactions that may lead to abscess formation. In the face of an outbreak, immediate mass administration of C and D antitoxin (200 IU/kg) in addition to vaccination is recommended.[92]

Nonenteric Clostridial Infections

C. novyi, *C. septicum*, *C. chauvoei*, and *C. sordelli* have been identified as causal agents of severe muscle, liver, and abomasal necrosis in small ruminants and cervid species.[66,93–95] These organisms are usually present in the soil and environment and in the gastrointestinal tract and liver of healthy ruminants.[66] Pathogenesis is usually facilitated by trauma of affected tissues, local multiplication of the organism, local and systemic damage by exotoxin production, and ultimately death.[66,96] Four types of *C. novyi* have been described, A, B, C, and D. *C. novyi* type C is considered nontoxigenic and therefore is not associated with disease. *C. novyi* type A produces alpha toxin and is associated with wound infections and myonecrosis in cases of "bighead" and "malignant edema." *C. novyi* type B produces alpha and beta toxins and is associated with infectious necrotic hepatitis or "black disease."[97,98] The temporal and geographic distributions of black disease resemble those of fascioliasis, with the highest incidence of disease in milder, moister months in many countries. Black disease is less common in sheep than in cattle and is rare in goats.[66,96] *C. novyi* type D *(C. haemolyticum)* produces beta toxin and is associated with bacillary hemoglobinuria (red water disease). *C. septicum* produces alpha toxin and is associated with malignant edema and necrotic abomasitis (Braxy). *C. chauvoei* produces alpha and beta toxins and is associated with severe myonecrosis observed in blackleg and *C. sordelli* produces a hemolytic toxin associated with myonecrosis in cases of malignant edema and blackleg.[96,97]

Black Disease

Pathogenesis. Spores of the organism shed in feces of carrier animals contaminate the environment and are ingested with feed/grass and stored within Kupffer cells.[97,98] Liver damage caused by migrating liver fluke larvae (*Fasciola hepatica*, *Fasciola gigantica*, and *Cysticercus tenuicollis*) create perfect ischemic conditions that induce germination of *C. novyi* type B spores and toxin synthesis and production.[97,98,99] The alpha toxin is necrotoxic and causes liver necrosis and diffuse damage of the vascular system.[98] The beta toxin is produced in smaller amounts and contributes to vascular damage and systemic toxemia. Infective organisms also may be brought into the liver by the flukes.

Clinical Signs. The course of disease from first illness to death is short and never lasts more than a few hours in sheep. Therefore, peracute or sudden death is not uncommon in this species. Well-nourished adult sheep between 2 and 4 years are more commonly affected. The disease course is a little longer (1–2 days) in cattle and deer.[66,95] Affected sheep are debilitated, fail to keep up with the flock, and exhibit generalized weakness, sternal recumbency, separation, and anorexia. Tachypnea and tachycardia may be seen; high fever (105–107° F) occurs early in the disease. Clinical signs observed in cattle, goats, and deer are similar and may include severe depression, anorexia, abdominal distention, colic, ruminal stasis, and lateral recumbency.[66,94,95,99,100,101] A report of black disease in a forest reindeer *(Rangifer tarandus fennicus)* described serosanguinous discharge from mucocutaneous orifices (nostrils and anus), periorbital edema, and nystagmus in addition to other clinical signs.[95]

Necropsy Findings. Necropsy might be difficult due to rapid autolysis of tissues in affected animals. Severe venous congestion usually darkens the underside of the skin of affected animals, giving this disease its common name of "black disease." Fluid in the pericardial sac, pleural space, and peritoneal cavity is usually present.[66] Endocardial and epicardial hemorrhages are a common finding. The liver is swollen and congested and on its diaphragmatic surface presents pale foci of coagulation necrosis; however, solid organs such as liver and kidneys could be in an advanced state of autolysis. Characteristic lesions of black disease in the liver are single or multiple yellow to white areas (1–2 cm in diameter) of necrosis surrounded by a bright hyperemic zone.[102] A recent report of black disease in a reindeer described moderate amounts of dark red thoracic and pericardial fluid, edema of the lungs and upper respiratory tract, swollen spleen, and several well-circumscribed areas of black discoloration in the liver.[95]

Diagnosis. The most characteristic clinicopathological change is neutrophilic leukocytosis with a left shift. Additional evidence of systemic toxemia (metabolic acidosis, azotemia, and increases in liver and muscle enzymes) also may be seen; however, diagnosis of black disease is based on characteristic history (endemic liver fluke areas), clinical signs, and postmortem findings and testing. An impression smear of the margins of the liver might reveal large numbers of gram positive rods, but this is not definitively diagnostic. Anaerobic culture of *C. novyi* from typical liver lesions, in addition to demonstration of the alpha/beta toxins from peritoneal fluid or liver (fresh—refrigerated), through ELISA or PCR is required to establish final diagnosis.[98,100] The use of fluorescent antibody and IHC for the identification of *C. novyi* on liver impression smear samples or other liver (formalin-fixed) samples have also been described.[95,100]

Treatment and Prevention. Treatment is rarely possible because of the fulminant clinical course of the disease; however, if treatment is attempted, high doses of penicillin G sodium (20,000–40,000 IU/kg) IV every 6 hours or oxytetracycline 10 mg/kg IV every 12 hours should be initiated. Supportive care, including IV fluids, nutritional support, and stress reduction, may be beneficial. In the face of an outbreak, vaccination of the whole herd/flock should be initiated immediately.

Efforts to control fluke infestation constitute the most effective approach to prevention of this disease. Administration of multivalent clostridial vaccines containing *C. novyi* is highly effective. Animals should be vaccinated every 6 months starting around 2 to 3 months of age and before parturition as protective immunity is short lived. In flocks at high risk for developing this disorder, a booster vaccine given 1 month before expected fluke exposure may provide additional protection.[99,100] Deer should be vaccinated in the same fashion as sheep but double the vaccine dose for sheep should be used for these animals as they do not develop a strong antibody response to commercially available multivalent vaccines.[77,78] Efforts to eliminate the organism from soil and environment are usually unrewarding but carcasses of animals dying from the disease should be burned, deeply buried, or removed from the premises.

Bacillary Hemoglobinuria (Red Water Disease)

Pathogenesis. *C. novyi* type D *(C. haemolyticum)* is the etiologic agent associated with red water disease. *C. haemolyticum* is similar to other clostridial species in its life cycle and appears to thrive on alkaline soils and pastures with standing water. The disease tends to be seasonal occurring at times of high larval fluke migration. Similar to *C. novyi* B, *C. haemolyticum* colonizes the livers of healthy animals and proliferates after liver damage, including damage caused by migrating flukes (*F. hepatica*, *Fascioloides magna*, *Dicrocoelium dendriticum*, and *C. tenuicollis*), liver abscessation (*Fusobacterium necrophorum* or *Trueperella pyogenes*), or damage incurred during liver biopsy.[100,103] Under ischemic conditions of the liver, spores of *C. haemolyticum* germinate and produce high amounts of beta toxin. The beta toxin causes localized hepatic necrosis and after reaching circulation induces severe intravascular hemolysis and damage of the capillary endothelium.[103] Intravascular hemolysis leads to rapid anemia and death due to anoxia. The disease is seen worldwide and is more commonly reported in sheep than in goats. Bacillary hemoglobinuria has been reported in a free-ranging elk calf *(Cervus elaphus roosevelti)* found dead in the southwest of the state of Washington, United States.[104]

Clinical Signs. Bacillary hemoglobinuria usually affects well-nourished animals older than 1 year of age.[105,106] In most cases, the disease is per-acute and sudden dead or found dead is the only sign.[103] In cases where signs are recognized antemortem, affected animals appear weak, depressed, and febrile (104–106° F); blood or blood-tinged froth may be present in the nostrils; rectal bleeding and bloody feces may be present; and severe hemoglobinuria (dark red, port wine-colored urine) is usually observed.[105,106] Blood appears thin and watery and mucous membranes are pale and icteric. Heart and respiratory rates are high and become much higher with any sort of effort or stress. Other terminal signs include bloat and the presence of blood in the nostrils, mouth, vagina, and rectum. Death occurs within hours to a few days after onset of clinical signs.[100]

Necropsy Findings. Gross lesions include jaundice of mucous membranes and tissues and subcutaneous petechial/ecchymotic hemorrhages, edema, and emphysema. Marked autolysis of internal organs might prevent identification of typical lesions. Dark red urine is present in the bladder.[102] Lymph nodes and spleen are congested and hemorrhagic. Hemorrhagic abomasitis and enteritis might occur, as well as the presence of hemoglobin-stained transudate in pleural and peritoneal cavities and pericardial sac. Pulmonary edema is common. The pathognomonic lesion is the ischemic hepatic infarcts ranging from 5 to 30 cm in diameter with a hyperemic interface with healthy liver tissue.[100,102]

Diagnosis. Clinicopathological abnormalities usually include anemia, leukocytosis with mature neutrophilia, and degenerative left shift (immature forms of neutrophils and toxic changes) often is present.[106,107] Serum biochemical evaluation may reveal increased levels of liver enzymes such as sorbitol dehydrogenase, GGT, aspartate aminotransferase, and increased indirect total serum bilirubin.[105–107] Presumptive diagnosis can be made on history, clinical sigs, clinicopathological abnormalities, and postmortem findings; however, similar to black disease, final diagnosis should be based on anaerobic culture of *C. novyi* from typical liver lesions in addition to demonstration of the beta toxins from peritoneal fluid or liver (fresh—refrigerated) through ELISA or PCR techniques.[98,100,104,106] The use of fluorescent antibody and IHC for the identification of *C. novyi* on liver impression smears or other liver (formalin-fixed) samples has also been described.[95,100] More recently, a PCR assay for the detection of *C. novyi* type D in cattle has been reported.[107]

Treatment and Prevention. Treatment is rarely possible because of the fulminant clinical course of the disease; however, if treatment is attempted, high doses of penicillin G sodium (20,000–40,000 IU/kg) IV every 6 hours or oxytetracycline 10 mg/kg IV every 12 hours should be initiated. Supportive therapy should include the administration of IV fluids, blood transfusions, and antiinflammatory agents. Efforts to control liver flukes and prevent other causes of liver damage are most important. Administration of multivalent clostridial vaccines containing *C. novyi* is highly effective. Animals should be vaccinated every 6 months starting around 2 to 3 months of age and before parturition as protective immunity is short lived. In flocks at high risk for developing this disorder, a booster vaccine given 1 month before expected fluke exposure may provide additional protection.[100] Deer should be vaccinated in the same fashion as sheep, but double the vaccine dose for sheep should be used as these animals as they do not develop a strong antibody response to commercially available multivalent vaccines.[77,78] Efforts to eliminate the organism from soil and environment are usually unrewarding but carcasses of animals dying from the disease should be burned, deeply buried, or removed from the premises.

Bighead

Pathogenesis and Clinical Signs. Fecal and soil contamination of wounds received during fighting (head-butting) or dehorning (disbudding) leads to proliferation of *C. novyi* type A in damaged head and neck tissues.[100] Accumulation of secreted toxins leads to swelling, edema, serohemorrhagic exudates, and local tissue necrosis. Wounds appear and smell gangrenous. Systemic toxemia may affect internal organs, leading to the death of the animal. *C. sordelli* causes identical disease.

Diagnosis. Laboratory analysis may reveal an increase in enzymes of muscle or liver origin as well as neutrophilic leukocytosis with many immature and toxic neutrophils. Postmortem findings include local necrosis around the injury site. Diagnosis usually is made by characteristic clinical signs and lesions.

Treatment. Wound management (disinfection, debridement) and administration of high doses of penicillin G sodium (20,000–40,000 IU/kg) IV every 6 hours are important treatment considerations.

Prevention. Ram management may aid in the prevention of head-butting wounds. Vaccination with multivalent clostridial toxoids starting around weaning time (3–6 months of age) and with annual boosters also may be helpful. In flocks with a high prevalence of this disorder, a booster vaccine given to rams 1 month before the breeding season and to ewes/does before parturition may provide additional protection.[100]

Malignant Edema and Braxy

Pathogenesis. *C. septicum* is the most important agent in the pathogenesis of malignant edema and braxy. In the case of malignant edema, other tissue-invasive clostridia (*C. chauvoei*, *C. sordelli*, and *C. perfringens* A) have also been associated with this disease, and mixed infections are common. The pathogenesis of infection is often similar to that seen with bighead and blackleg: soil or fecal clostridial invasion of a contaminated wound. In sheep and goats, this disease has been reported following lambing/kidding, after shearing of tail docking.[100] *C. septicum* can also invade the abomasal lining of lambs, causing severe hemorrhagic, necrotic abomasitis known as braxy.[108] Activation of dormant bacteria in previously damaged tissue (myositis/abomasitis) similar to that seen in clostridial necrotic hepatitis also occurs.[108] In both cases (malignant edema and braxy), bacterial toxins precipitate local tissue necrosis and systemic toxemia. The alpha, beta, gamma, and delta toxins produced by *C. septicum* are lecithinase, deoxyribonuclease, hyaluronidase, and hemolysin, respectively. Commonly affected sites of malignant edema include castration, dehorning, and injection sites; the umbilicus; and the postpartum uterus.[100] Factors that promote braxy have not been identified, although it usually affects weaned and yearling lambs in the winter after ingestion of frozen feedstuffs implicated as initial causes of abomasitis.[100,108] Both forms of the disease have worldwide distribution and are described more in sheep than in goats.[100,108]

Clinical Signs. Malignant edema is characterized by local lesion (wound) or regional pain characterized by swelling and edema that progressively becomes tense and dark (skin). High fever, signs of shock/toxemia, and frothy exudation of the wound are usually present. Evidence of subcutaneous gas production is less common in this infection than in blackleg. Uterine infection may cause a fetid vaginal discharge. Death occurs within hours to a few days after onset of clinical signs.[100] Braxy usually causes death before any abnormalities are noted. On rare occasions, signs of sudden onset of illness with high fever, abdominal distention, depression, colic, and recumbency may be seen before death.[100]

Diagnosis. Characteristic clinicopathologic changes include neutrophilic leukocytosis with a left shift. A decrease in WBC and RBC counts also is possible because of the leukocidal and hemolytic effects of the toxins. Additional evidence of systemic toxemia (metabolic acidosis, azotemia, and increases in liver and muscle enzymes) also may be seen. Examination of a Gram-stained smear from the edematous swelling(s) or wound swabs could give an early diagnosis. One study reported the successful use of a PCR assay for the identification of bacteria associated with malignant edema in cattle, sheep, and other ruminants.[109] Postmortem changes with malignant edema include dark red, swollen muscle filled with hemorrhagic, proteinaceous exudate and little or no gas. With braxy, the abomasal wall is hemorrhagic and necrotic. Both diseases are associated with rapid postmortem decomposition of the carcass.

Treatment and Prevention. Wound management and the rapid administration of high doses of penicillin (penicillin G sodium at 20,000–40,000 IU/kg IV every 6 hours) are important in treating malignant edema. Local treatment consists of surgical incision of the affected area to provide drainage and irrigation with peroxide. Injection of penicillin directly into or in the periphery of the lesions may help. Ancillary treatments such as IV fluids, antiinflammatory agents (e.g., flunixin meglumine, 2 mg/kg IV), and nutritional support may be necessary. Maintenance of good hygiene during procedures such as lambing, tail docking, shearing, castration, obstetric manipulation, and administering injections is helpful in preventing malignant edema. Multivalent clostridial toxoids may provide some protection and should be given annually to animals at risk for the disorder.[110]

Blackleg

Pathogenesis. Several species of clostridial organisms can cause myonecrosis in small ruminants.[93,111,112] The disease is acute to per-acute, has a short course of duration, and is usually fatal. *C. chauvoei*, *C. septicum*, and *C. sordelli* are commonly involved with clostridial myonecrosis in ruminants.[111–113] Blackleg can be enzootic in some areas or farms because of increased bacterial contamination and occurs more commonly in the warm months of the year.[113–115] Animals between 4 months and 3 years of age can be affected.[111,112] *C. chauvoei* is the most important cause of blackleg. *C. sordelli* tends to be involved in the myonecrosis of older feedlot animals.[112] These organisms are found in the soil and can gain access to muscles after translocation from the gastrointestinal tract and liver into systemic circulation. Additionally, direct inoculation of the organisms by penetrating wounds or intramuscular injections has been suggested. Local tissue trauma, wounds, unsanitary procedures (i.e., shearing, tail docking, and castration), umbilical infection (neonates), or vaginal trauma from lambing can create perfect conditions for the germination of clostridial spores inducing rapid toxin synthesis and production.[113] In some cases, bacterial proliferation appears to occur in a site distant from the original wound (i.e., fetal infections after shearing of a ewe and myocardial necrosis in cattle and sheep).[113] Bacterial toxins cause severe local tissue necrosis, systemic toxemia, and ultimately death. As with braxy, several other strains of tissue-invasive clostridia can cause this disease and mixed infections are common.

Clinical Signs. Clostridial myonecrosis usually progresses rapidly and sudden death or history of found dead is not uncommon.[111–113] Clinical signs in animals who are still alive include local to regional painful, edematous swelling most commonly in the limbs or trunk muscles. Skin of the affected area can become discolored and crepitus; however, in affected sheep, subcutaneous edema and gaseous crepitation are uncommon and cannot be felt before death.[111] Other signs might include stiff gait, lameness, fever, and signs of shock. In cases where the infection occurred through a wound, there is extensive local damage and malodorous serosanguinous fluid discharge. *C. chauvoei* also causes uterine infection and severe gangrenous mastitis in postparturient ewes.[111,113] In these cases, uterine and mammary infections may cause fetid vaginal and mammary discharge, respectively. Death often occurs within 12 to 36 hours after onset of clinical signs.

Necropsy Findings. Rapid tissue autolysis is not uncommon in animals that succumb to clostridial myonecrosis. Blood-stained fluid and froth can be observed discharging from nostrils and anus. In small ruminants and especially sheep, affected muscle areas are more localized and deeper, brown to black discoloration is present, the subcutaneous edema is not as severe, and, although there is gas present, is not in such large amounts as in cattle. In cases of infection from skin wounds, the area demonstrates subcutaneous edema, swelling, and underlying muscle discoloration. In cases of infection through the urogenital tract, typical lesions are found in the perineal area, vagina, uterus, and fetus. Lung congestion, fibrinohemorrhagic pleuritis, pericarditis, myocardial damage, and bloat are also common findings.[111,112]

Diagnosis. It is rarely possible to obtain samples for clinicopathological analysis due to the per-acute course of the disease. If samples can be obtained, common findings include neutrophilic leukocytosis with a left shift. A decrease in WBC and RBC counts also is possible because of the leukocidal and hemolytic effects of the toxins. Additional evidence of systemic toxemia—metabolic acidosis, azotemia, and increases in liver and muscle enzymes—also may be seen. Presumptive diagnosis can be made from history, characteristic clinical signs, and gross pathology findings; however, aspirates or tissue specimens from affected muscles for direct smear examination, fluorescent antibody testing, or anaerobic culture are required for definitive diagnosis.[111,112] A multiplex PCR is available for identification of pathogenic clostridia on fluid and tissue samples.[109]

Treatment and Prevention. Aggressive antibiotic therapy (e.g., penicillin G sodium or potassium penicillin at 20,000–40,000 IU/kg IV every 6 hours), in combination with surgical debridement of affected tissues (fasciotomy), and supportive care (nutritional support, IV fluids, and antiinflammatory agents) are important within the treatment plan for clostridial myositis. Prognosis for treatment of all types of clostridial myositis cases is usually guarded to poor and depends on the duration and extension of the lesions. Maintaining excellent hygiene during invasive procedures such as castration, obstetric manipulation, shearing, tail docking, and administering injections is helpful in preventing blackleg. Multivalent clostridial toxoids may provide some protection and should be given to all animals starting at weaning time, before parturition, and annually.[114,115]

Diseases Caused by Noninvasive Clostridia

Both tetanus and botulism are important diseases in small ruminant medicine. These two diseases are covered elsewhere in this book (see Chapters 5, 11, 13, 19, and 20).

Juvenile and Adult Sepsis

Pathophysiology

Older animals are generally more resistant to sepsis than neonates because they have larger amounts of circulating antibodies. However, this resistance can be overwhelmed by aggressive bacteria, or loss of immune function can allow invasion by opportunistic bacteria. Malnutrition, parasitism, transport, overcrowding, other diseases, extreme weather conditions, and other stressors are the major causes of immune suppression.

Clinical Signs

Sepsis may produce peracute, acute, or chronic disease signs. Peracute signs include fever, injected mucous membranes (including the sclera), tachycardia, tachypnea, dyspnea, swollen joints, lameness, splinting of the abdomen, weakness, depression, anorexia, recumbency, seizures, coma, and sudden death. Acute signs are similar, except that they persist for a longer period and therefore are more likely to be noticed. Chronic signs usually result from the partial clearance of infection after an acute episode, which may be clinical or inapparent.

Gram Negative Sepsis

Pathogenesis. Gram negative bacteria and their toxins gain access to the blood from a site of proliferation or destruction. The most important toxin is endotoxin, a group of lipopolysaccharide molecules that reside within the wall of the bacteria. Bacteria or endotoxins incite a systemic inflammatory response, chiefly through activation of host macrophages and stimulation of host cytokine release. These cytokines cause inflammation, produce leukocyte recruitment, increase capillary permeability, induce fever through stimulation of the hypothalamus, and have regional or diffuse vasomotor effects.

Because the ruminant gut has a plentiful population of gram negative bacteria, it is implicated as the source of most cases of gram negative sepsis. Grain overload causes a die-off of the normal gram negative ruminal flora, ulcerative enteric disease allows invasion of bacteria or absorption of their toxins, and ingestion of pathogens provides a suitable place for proliferation and route for invasion of the body. Gram negative sepsis caused by opportunistic organisms is best recognized in immunocompromised neonates but also can be seen in stressed or immunocompromised animals of all ages. *E. coli* is commonly found in fecal material, *Klebsiella pneumoniae* is found in feces and wood products, *F. necrophorum* lives in the gastrointestinal tract and in soil and invades through compromised gastric mucosa or foot-rot lesions, and *Pseudomonas aeruginosa* is commonly found in water and wash solutions.

Primary pathogens are most common in adults. Although some coliform bacteria may fit into this category, by far, the most important genus is *Salmonella.* Sources of *Salmonella* infection are numerous and include carrier animals of the same species, cattle, rodents, birds, other animals, environmental contamination, and possibly feedstuffs. Only one serotype of *Salmonella* is specifically adapted to sheep *(Salmonella abortus ovis)*, and it is not found in North America. No strain is known to be host-adapted to goats or cervids. Therefore, all infections in sheep, goats, and cervids have the potential to spread to and from other species, including humans. Serotypes of *Salmonella* that have caused important infections in sheep or goats include *Salmonella typhimurium*, *Salmonella dublin*, and *Salmonella montevideo.* Most of these infections lead to bacteremia with mild systemic signs, followed by abortion. *S. dublin* and *S. typhimurium* tend to cause more illness in adults because of fibrinonecrotic enteritis.

Clinical Signs. Affected animals can exhibit anything, from mild depression with a low-grade fever to shock. Common signs include fever, tachycardia, tachypnea, depression with slow or absent eating and drinking, weakness or recumbency, and injection or cyanosis of mucous membranes. Organ-specific signs may betray the source or at least the primary location of the infection. Fetid discharge may be seen with metritis or abortion; dyspnea and abnormal lung sounds may be seen with pulmonary infection; and bloat, ruminal atony, abdominal distention, and diarrhea may be seen with gastrointestinal infections.

Diagnosis. The most common abnormality identified on a CBC with peracute gram negative sepsis is panleukopenia. Over the course of several days, this condition may resolve, first through an increase in immature neutrophils and later through an increase in mature neutrophils and restoration of lymphocyte counts. Very immature cells, severe toxic changes, and persistence of neutropenia suggest a poor prognosis. Serum biochemical changes often reflect the severity of the condition. The greater the evidence of shock or tissue damage, the worse the prognosis. Metabolic acidosis with a large anion gap and azotemia suggest advanced disease. Necropsy findings include diffuse evidence of inflammation, including pulmonary congestion, and polyserositis with body cavity exudates. Hemorrhagic pneumonia or fibrinonecrotic enteritis may be seen and reflect the source of bacterial invasion. In all cases, diagnosis is best confirmed by bacteriologic culture of body tissues or fluids. In the live animal, culture of blood, feces, or tracheal fluid yields the best results. When several animals are infected, environmental samples (including feed, water, and bedding) should be tested for the presence of the bacteria. Bacteriologic culture of aborted fetuses or placentas frequently yields heavy growth of the organism.

Prevention. Maintaining overall good health and hygiene is the best means of preventing gram negative sepsis. Antiendotoxin bacterins are available for cattle in the United States, but their use in small ruminants has been too limited to assess their efficacy. During a flock outbreak, the use of autogenous bacterin may help prevent the spread of disease on a farm.

Important Bacterial Causes of Sepsis

Actinobacillus seminis is a gram negative bacillus or coccobacillus that affects primarily the male and female reproductive tracts. Infection causes posthitis, epididymitis, and orchitis in rams and metritis and abortion in ewes. Other sites of infection, including rare occurrences of chronic sepsis, also are possible. Serologic tests are much more useful for identifying infected flocks than infected individuals within flocks. Definitive diagnosis depends on bacteriologic culture of the organism and differentiation of it from *Brucella ovis.* The bacillus is common in sheep in some parts of the world but is uncommon in North American sheep and goats.

T. pyogenes is best known as an abscess-forming bacterium because of the thick pus formed in response to infection by it and the fibrinous response it elicits. It occasionally also causes sepsis. Its association with chronic sepsis lends credence to the belief that *Trueperella* is often a secondary invader that colonizes tissues damaged by another bacterium (see Chapter 10).

Bacillus anthracis is a large, gram positive, anaerobic bacillus that causes anthrax. It forms spores under aerobic conditions (such as on culture plates) but rarely does so when oxygen tensions are low, as in carcasses. The organism affects most mammals, with herbivores being most susceptible. It is usually carried from one area to another by shedding or dying animals and also can multiply in alkaline, nitrogenous soils. Periods of heat and intermittent flooding promote overgrowth of the organism. *B. anthracis* spores may be inhaled or ingested; in rare cases, the bacillus itself may be spread by biting flies. After local replication, the organism gains access to the blood, where it multiples readily. Large numbers of the organisms colonize the spleen. *B. anthracis* secretes a holotoxin made of edema factor), protective antigen, and lethal factor. This toxin impairs phagocytosis, increases capillary permeability, and inhibits clotting. Splenic engorgement, generalized edema, circulatory shock, and bleeding diathesis are the most common lesions and signs of anthrax. Generalized infection should be considered uniformly fatal. Death may occur before or within hours of initial recognition that the animal is sick. Prophylactic antibiotic treatment of healthy animals (oxytetracycline 10 mg/kg IV SID) may decrease spread and mortality during outbreaks. The disease is reportable in many areas. Local forms of anthrax also occur, most commonly after transmission through a skin wound or fly bite. Local heat, pain, swelling, and necrosis are seen first, and the generalized syndrome often follows.

Treatment for Sepsis (Adult and Juvenile)

Bacterial organisms are rarely identified before important treatment decisions must be made. Therefore, treatment should follow general principles and have a wide spectrum of efficacy. Antimicrobial drugs are the cornerstone of treatment. In meat- or milk-producing animals, the veterinarian must be careful to use drugs within label directions or have a rational plan for extra-label drug use. The issue of extra-label drug use is especially important in small ruminants and cervids because very few pharmaceutical products have been licensed for them in North America.

Unless a specific organism is suspected (clostridiosis or anaplasmosis), a single antibiotic or combination of antimicrobial drugs to provide a broad spectrum of coverage should be selected. Penicillins, macrolides, tetracyclines, and cephalosporins all provide effective coverage against gram positive pathogens. The newer third-generation cephalosporins are effective against many systemic and enteric gram negative pathogens. The gram negative pathogens of the respiratory tract are often sensitive to other classes of antibiotics. Macrolides and tetracyclines also are effective against *Mycoplasma* species and rickettsial organisms.

NSAIDs are almost always beneficial in severe infectious conditions because of their antiinflammatory, antipyretic, and anti-endotoxic effects. They are likely to be more effective than corticosteroids because they provide benefits without suppressing the immune response. All such drug use should be considered extra-label and administered accordingly with appropriate withdrawal times established. Specific antisera are available for some of the clostridial diseases and may be beneficial if given before widespread tissue necrosis has occurred. Severely compromised animals should be treated with fluids for shock (see Chapter 3).

Zoonotic Infections

Contagious Ecthyma

The most common zoonotic disease risk posed by exposure to small ruminants is orf, also known as contagious ecthyma in animals (see Chapter 10). The disease is caused by an epitheliotropic poxvirus and is transmitted to humans by direct contact with infected animals. Skin trauma is a significant risk factor for transmission in both humans and animals. In humans, erythematous macules or papules appear at the site of infection 2 to 3 days following exposure. The infection is generally self-limiting in immunocompetent individuals with complete healing occurring within 8 weeks.

Reproductive Pathogens

Brucella Melitensis. Apart from contagious ecthyma, the greatest risk of zoonotic disease from small ruminants is due to pathogens typically found in the reproductive tract that are transmitted to humans through contact with aborted fetuses, the placenta, or birthing fluids or through the consumption of raw or improperly pasteurized dairy products. *B. melitensis* is more common in goats than sheep (see Chapter 8). Swine, cattle, and other ruminants are common hosts. Infection in animals usually causes inapparent mammary infection and abortions; infection in humans is characterized by undulant fever, myalgia, and fatigue.

Coxiella Burnetii. C. burnetii is a rickettsial organism that is an important cause of abortion in sheep and goats (see Chapter 8). Wildlife and farm-raised deer may serve as reservoir hosts for infection in other ruminants and humans.[116] Infection is a documented cause of reproductive failure in farmed deer and prolonged shedding of the organism is an important source of environmental contamination.[117] In addition to abortion, newly infected sheep and goats occasionally have mild, transient fevers. *C. burnetii* is far more important as the cause of Q fever in humans, who become infected after inhaling particles, handling contaminated animals, or coming into contact with contaminated body fluids (uterine fluid, milk) from infected animals. Infection in humans may be asymptomatic, present with flu-like symptoms, or, in the chronic form, present as granulomatous hepatitis, osteomyelitis, or bacterial endocarditis.

Chlamydophila spp. *Chlamydophila abortus* (previously *Chlamydia psittaci*) is an obligate intracellular parasite and the cause of enzootic abortion of small ruminants (see Chapter 8). *Chlamydophila pecorum* may cause polyarthritis and keratoconjunctivitis (see Chapter 14) in sheep and goats. Transmission between animals and to humans most commonly occurs through direct contact with infected tissues or materials. Infection in humans results in an acute febrile syndrome or respiratory symptoms. Chlamydial diseases are more commonly reported in sheep than in goats. Chlamydial diseases are suspected to cause disease in other species, including deer. Recent serologic evaluation of wild ungulates identified multiple species of deer with antibodies against several Chlamydial species.[118] The clinical significance of serological infection in these species remains undetermined.

Francisella Tularensis. *F. tularensis* is more common in sheep than goats. The organism has many hosts, of which the most important are wild rabbits and rodents. It can contaminate water sources. Transmission to sheep is usually through biting arthropods that have previously fed on an infected wild mammal. Acute or chronic sepsis may be seen, with more widespread and severe disease occurring in sheep with poor immune function. At necropsy, the disease is characterized by military foci of necrosis in the liver, and less commonly in the lymph nodes, spleen, and lungs. Most cases in humans result in acute onset of flu-like symptoms a few days after exposure.

L. interrogans. Pathogenesis. *Leptospira* spp. are spirochete bacteria that live in moist environments. Their survival time outside of hosts is usually short, so their most important reservoirs are the kidneys of infected animals, especially rodents. Infected animals shed the organisms through urine and most other body fluids. Organisms enter new hosts through mucous membranes and skin breaks and cause bacteremia. Signs of sepsis range from inapparent to severe, with more severe signs predominating in neonates. Intravascular hemolysis may result. In animals that survive the acute stage, infection may localize in sites such as the kidneys, eyes, and fetoplacental unit. Abortion may occur a month or more after acute signs first become evident while renal shedding may occur for several months. Leptospirosis is zoonotic. In most cases, infections in humans are asymptomatic and self-limiting. However, in approximately 10% of cases, severe, and potentially fatal, systemic disease may develop, including jaundice, renal failure, and pulmonary hemorrhage.

Clinical Signs Acute leptospirosis causes signs of sepsis, including fever, depression, dyspnea, exercise intolerance, weakness, and death (see Chapter 12). Additionally, many affected animals show signs of intravascular hemolysis such as anemia, icterus, and hemoglobinuria.

Diagnosis Evidence of intravascular hemolysis such as anemia, hyperbilirubinemia, hemoglobinuria, and hemoglobinemia is suggestive of this disease. In chronic infection, non-specific inflammatory changes and azotemia may be seen. Animals dying in the acute hemolytic stage are likely to have dark, discolored urine, bladder, and kidneys. Spirochetes can be identified on dark-field microscopy of fresh urine or plasma from infected animals and may be cultured with special techniques. In animals with less severe infection, a rise in antibody titers can be used to support a diagnosis of leptospirosis.

Prevention Numerous vaccines are available for sheep. Because protection is serotype specific, it is important to vaccinate against common serotypes in the area. *Leptospira pomona* is the most consistent isolate from sheep and goats; *Leptospira hardjobovis* is the predominate serovar in deer.[119] Vaccination immunity is thought to be short lived; boosters should be given at least twice a year in endemic areas. Vaccination of deer against serovars *Hardjobovis* and *Pomona* has been associated with decreased urine shedding and increased growth rate in young animals.[120]

Listeria Monocytogenes

Pathogenesis. *L. monocytogenes* causes disease with similar frequency in sheep and goats (see Chapter 13). The organism is a common soil and fecal contaminant. It also proliferates in silage that is not properly acidified and in rotting, woody debris. Risk of exposure depends on the feed and environment of the animals. Environmental and fecal contamination is a more common source than silage in small ruminants overall because most sheep and goats throughout the world are not fed silage. Infection in humans almost always results from ingestion of contaminated food products or unpasteurized milk.

Clinical Signs. Nervous system dysfunction and abortion are the most common manifestations of the disease. Animals with the brainstem form of the disease display signs reflective of cranial nerve dysfunction, including drooped ears or eyelids, decreased facial sensation, and deviated nasal septum. A head tilt and circling may be present; in advanced cases of the disease, the animal is recumbent. Clinical signs are mainly unilateral, occasionally bilateral, according to the nerve nuclei affected.

Diagnosis. Antemortem diagnosis of listeriosis is difficult. A presumptive diagnosis is made based on history, clinical signs, and potential response to treatment. Histopathologic identification of microabscesses in the brainstem and culture of the organism from affected tissues can be used to confirm the diagnosis.

Pasteurella and Pasteurella-Like Infections

P. multocida

Pathogenesis. *P. multocida* is a small, gram negative, bipolar, ovoid rod that inhabits the pharynx of healthy ruminants. It can survive in soil and water for varying amounts of time after contamination with ruminant nasal secretions. Healthy ruminants shed *P. multocida* much more frequently than *Mannheimia haemolytica.* Disease occurs when bacteria colonize the lower respiratory tract or enter the blood. Risk factors for pulmonary and systemic infection include viral or mycoplasmal respiratory diseases, temperature extremes, respiratory tract irritants, transport, overcrowding, changes to higher-energy feeds, and handling stress. These factors are thought to both increase bacterial replication in the airway and suppress mechanisms to clear the infection. Pasteurellosis is a major problem in feedlot sheep but less common in small breeding or hobby flocks. Pasteurellosis also is a significant disease in certain wild small ruminants such as bighorn sheep.

Direct spread of the organism between animals occurs with nasal contact, and indirect spread occurs after contact with infected nasal secretions. The organism persists in the environment for longer periods during warm, moist weather. *P. multocida* produces a polysaccharide capsule that inhibits phagocytosis and an endotoxin that contributes to clinical signs. The major disease caused by *P. multocida* is pneumonia (see Chapter 7). However, *Pasteurella* spp. also are capable of entering the blood to cause septicemia in young lambs and hemorrhagic septicemia in adults. Occasionally, focal infections such as septic arthritis and mastitis are found.

Clinical Signs. Clinical signs of pneumonic and septicemic pasteurellosis include severe depression, bilateral purulent nasal discharge, coughing, diarrhea, anorexia, high fever, and edema of the head, neck, and brisket. The disease course can be short with septicemic pasteurellosis and is usually more insidious with *P. multocida* pneumonia. *Pasteurella* mastitis is characterized by the bluebag condition or gangrene of the udder.

Diagnosis. Inflammatory changes in the leukogram and hyperfibrinogenemia are the most frequent abnormalities. With severe disease and in the septicemic form, immature neutrophils may predominate over mature cells. Inflammation of the intestine and abomasum also may be seen. Hemorrhage and fibrin are usually absent or less prominent than in pneumonia caused by *M. haemolytica.* Samples for bacteriologic culture are usually obtained postmortem. Blood or tracheal fluid may be obtained before death if the value of the animal warrants it.

M. haemolytica

M. haemolytica is a gram negative rod that is a common commensal inhabitant of the tonsils of young animals. Disease is much more frequently described in sheep than in goats and occurs when the organism gains access to the lower respiratory tract.

Clinical Signs and Diagnosis. The most common syndrome is enzootic pneumonia, which is seen in young lambs and their dams (see Chapter 7). Hemorrhagic bronchopneumonia is the major lesion and respiratory signs predominate. Gangrenous mastitis (bluebag) is seen in some of the dams, presumably after they have been nursed by infected offspring. Factors that promote respiratory disease, including viral infections, airborne irritants, high stocking density, and stress, are thought to promote invasion of the lower airway by these bacteria.

Bibersteinia trehalosi

B. trehalosi is a gram negative rod that is a commensal inhabitant of the upper respiratory tract (see Chapter 7). Disease is much more frequently described in sheep than in goats and occurs when the organism gains access to the lung or blood. Replication occurs in the lung and systemic toxemia or bacteremia resulting in septicemic pasteurellosis. Septicemic pasteurellosis is a significant cause of mortality in young lambs and in some farms is the leading cause of death in the age group.

Clinical Signs. Septicemic pasteurellosis occurs most commonly in weaned lambs, often following some form of stress such as transport, marketing, or weaning itself. The course of the disease is relatively rapid, and animals may be found dead within 6 hours without showing premonitory clinical signs. When observed, clinical signs include depression, recumbency, and signs of toxemia.

Diagnosis. Septicemic pasteurellosis should be suspected when presented with a dead, recently weaned, sheep with a recent history of stress. Diagnosis is best confirmed by typical lesions at necropsy and culture of the organism from bodily tissues. Demonstration of *B. trehalosi* in nasal swabs is of limited value due to the high prevalence of upper respiratory tract colonization in healthy lambs. At necropsy, there may be no evidence of pneumonia, but blood-stained foam can be found in the upper respiratory tract. Ulceration of the pharynx and esophagus is commonly present as is subcutaneous hemorrhage of the neck and thorax.

Prevention. Treatment is difficult due to the rapid course of disease. Efforts should be made to minimize stressors, particularly during and following weaning, and to manage management factors that may contribute to the disease. Vaccination with *Pasteurella* bacterins is rarely effective at controlling natural outbreaks of disease.

Other Bacterial Causes of Disease

Common Abscess-Forming Bacteria

Pathophysiology. Abscess-forming bacteria are usually able to survive phagocytosis and thereby avoid destruction by cells of the immune system. Alternatively, they invoke such an inflammatory response that the host body "walls off" the entire region with fibrous tissue. Abscesses may occur locally, frequently after a wound infection, or at numerous or distant sites from the point of infection. For abscesses to occur at the latter sites, the organism must travel either by way of the blood or within leukocytes. Disease characterized by multifocal or internal abscesses usually results from a low-grade, transient event of bacteremia.

The best known and most important abscess-forming bacterium in small ruminants is *Corynebacterium pseudotuberculosis*, the gram positive, facultative anaerobic coccobacillus that causes caseous lymphadenitis. Infection is usually maintained in a flock by infected animals that spread the organism to others through purulent material draining from open abscesses. The organism is very hardy, so infection can occur through direct contact or indirect contact with contaminated common instruments and facilities. Infection is usually introduced into a flock through acquisition of an infected animal, although it also can occur when a naive flock is moved into a contaminated area. Horses, cattle, and humans also are minor hosts. Infection is thought to occur after ingestion, inhalation, or wound contamination. Except for lower respiratory tract invasion, a surface break is thought to be necessary. Contaminated shears, tail-docking knives, and emasculators readily spread the organisms through a flock. Abscesses can form at the site of invasion or more commonly at the site of the local lymph node.

Clinical Signs. Clinical signs of external abscesses include surface swellings and draining lesions. Drainage may be intermittent and usually consists of thick, yellow-white purulent material. Internal abscesses are more difficult to diagnose. Thoracic masses may cause inspiratory dyspnea or occlude venous return to the heart. Abdominal lesions may cause tenesmus, stranguria, and occasionally colic. The most common sign of internal abscesses is weight loss with or without intermittent fever. Common external sites include the submandibular or retromandibular space and the preinguinal, prefemoral, and supramammary lymph nodes. Head and neck lesions are more common in goats, whereas sheep have a more even distribution of cranial and caudal lesions, presumably as a result of shearing wounds. External infections rarely cause clinical illness beyond the draining abscess, although some degree of cachexia may be present.

Diagnosis. Diagnosis is often made by the characteristic lesions with their thick, nonmalodorous pus. Bacteriologic culture provides a definitive diagnosis, which may be important for flock management. Serologic tests have been developed to identify carrier animals and may be useful if the manager wishes to eliminate infection from the flock.

Treatment. Treatment is often unrewarding: antibiotic sensitivity profiles do not reflect the degree of protection afforded the organisms within the abscesses. Long-term treatment with antibiotics and drainage of any compromising masses may lead to some degree of resolution, but internal abscesses are likely to persist.

Prevention. Prevention through the use of vaccines has been attempted. Vaccines appear to reduce the severity of the disease but do not completely prevent infection. Moreover, live attenuated bacterins lead to de facto infection of all vaccinated animals and therefore should not be used in naïve flocks.[121]

Other abscess-forming bacteria are most important as differential diagnoses for caseous lymphadenitis. *T. pyogenes* is another wound contaminant that affects focal areas or regional external lymph nodes. It also commonly colonizes damaged internal tissues such as postpneumonic lungs, postacidotic livers, and damaged feet and heart valves. It is thought to be ubiquitous and poorly invasive in ruminants and therefore does not have the same flock significance as *C. pseudotuberculosis*. Flocks with outbreaks of this infection often have suboptimal management. *F. necrophorum* causes similar disease and often coinfects with *T. pyogenes*. It is generally more necrotizing and leads to greater systemic signs of acute illness, including death. *F. necrophorum* also produces fetid pus, whereas *T. pyogenes* usually does not. *Rhodococcus equi* is a rare cause of pulmonary abscesses in sheep.

Numerous small, coalescent, nodular skin abscesses may result from *Pseudomonas pseudomallei* infection (melioidosis). Infection usually occurs after the sheep or goat is bitten by an insect that previously fed on an infected rodent. This organism is found in many subtropical regions, including the Caribbean, but is not reported in North America.

Fusobacterium Infections

F. necrophorum causes or is associated with a variety of diseases in sheep and is likely to cause many similar diseases in goats. It is best known as a cause of foot rot and hepatic abscesses and appears to be important in lip-leg ulceration. It is an enteric gram negative anaerobe and as such can cause gram negative sepsis after entrance of the bacteria or its toxins into the circulation. *F. necrophorum* has a poor ability to invade healthy tissue. However, it readily colonizes regions damaged by trauma, persistent moisture, and infection. In addition to endotoxin, the bacterium produces leukocidal and cytolytic toxins that form zones of necrosis around bacterial colonies. This tissue necrosis and the foul-smelling waste gases produced by the bacteria are characteristic of necrobacillosis, or *F. necrophorum* infection. Clinical signs include necrotic, fetid lesions, usually of the mouth or feet, that can cause ingestion or lameness problems. Efforts to maintain good hygiene are helpful in preventing fecal contamination. Additionally, preventing trauma to foot and mouth tissues through good surface choices and proper pasture drainage is important.

Yersiniosis

Pathogenesis. *Yersinia* spp. are gram negative bacteria. *Yersinia enterocolitica* and *Yersinia pseudotuberculosis* both have many mammalian and avian hosts, including humans, and cause clostridial enteritis–like disease in goats. Rodent and bird hosts may be important reservoir populations for infections in domestic animals. Kids younger than 6 months develop enteritis, bacteremia, and diarrhea that is watery but not bloody. Severe toxemia and sudden death can occur. Older kids and flocks with chronic exposure tend to have less severe acute disease. Instead, chronic diarrhea and weight loss are seen, usually in association with gut wall and abdominal abscesses. Sheep, deer, and wild ungulates are rarely affected.

Clinical Signs. Signs of enteritis or sepsis predominate in acute disease, whereas signs of wasting are more common in chronic disease.

Diagnosis. Evidence of acute or chronic inflammation is provided by blood work. Characteristic necropsy lesions include numerous microabscesses in the gut wall and mesenteric lymph nodes, as well as other evidence of enteritis or sepsis. Culture of lesions and demonstration of a rising antibody titer are diagnostic.

Prevention. Avoiding exposure to sources and maintaining overall flock health are helpful in preventing losses due to yersiniosis.

Mycobacterial Disease

Pathogenesis. *Mycobacteria* are small, aerobic, straight or curved pleomorphic rods with thick lipid cell walls. They can be stained with acid-fast stains and are usually gram positive. The bacteria live within infected animals of many mammalian species and survive for several years in warm, moist environments. Infection occurs after ingestion or inhalation. An identifying characteristic of the mechanism of infection by *Mycobacteria* is the bacteria's ability to survive within macrophages by preventing fusion of phagosomes and lysosomes. The organisms are carried to local lymphatic vessels or lymph nodes, where they form granulomas. As they enlarge, granulomas may develop necrotic or mineralized centers surrounded by macrophages and giant cells. Disease can be local, regional, or generalized, depending on the distance the organism is carried from the original site of infection. Granulomatous pneumonia, enterocolitis, and lymphadenitis are the most common local and regional forms of the disease.

Organisms from ruptured granulomas may be spread in contaminated respiratory secretions and feces. Mycobacterial infections of all types are uncommon in North American sheep, goats, and cervids, and these species are considered to be relatively resistant to infection. *Mycobacterium bovis* is the most common organism associated with ovine tuberculosis in other countries (see Chapter 7), but *Mycobacterium avium* is more common in the United States. The most common mycobacterial infection is Johne's disease (paratuberculosis) caused by the etiologic agent *M. avium* subsp. *paratuberculosis* (see Chapter 5). *Mycobacterium tuberculosis* is rare in the United States. Mycobacterial infections are reportable in most parts of the United States. Some debate is ongoing about human susceptibility to *M. avium* subsp. *paratuberculosis*; the other organisms are known to be pathogenic in people.

Clinical Signs. The most common clinical sign is emaciation. Diarrhea may be seen terminally in both tuberculosis and paratuberculosis. The disease is insidious, with signs becoming more apparent over several weeks to months. Respiratory signs may be seen, especially with infection by *M. bovis* or *M. avium* subsp. *paratuberculosis*.

Diagnosis. Reports of clinicopathologic abnormalities are rare. Hypoalbuminemia and hypoproteinemia are likely to be common with chronic enterocolitis caused by either tuberculosis or paratuberculosis. The most common necropsy lesions seen in tuberculosis are nodular lesions of the lung, liver, lymph nodes, spleen, and intestines. Histologic evaluation reveals the nodules to be granulomas with giant cells and acid-fast organisms. Frequently, the center of the lesion is necrotic and mineralized. Intestinal lesions appear to be more common than pulmonary lesions in goats. The lesions of paratuberculosis are centered around the ileocecocolic junction and the adjacent mesentery. The regions may appear normal or be notably thickened. Thickening of bowel or nodular infiltrates of lung or liver may be detected antemortem using imaging modalities, such as ultrasonography or computed tomography. Postmortem diagnosis is made by identifying characteristic lesions and culturing the organisms. Antemortem diagnosis of tuberculosis is best achieved by observing the reaction to intradermal injection of tuberculin with or without comparative injection of purified protein derivatives of *M. bovis* and *M. avium* subsp. *paratuberculosis*. All tuberculosis testing should be done in accordance with local regulations. Antemortem diagnosis of Johne's disease can be achieved by fecal culture of the organism, but this test takes several weeks to months to complete and is far less reliable in sheep or goats than cattle, with a sensitivity as low as 0.08. Serologic tests (e.g., ELISA) appear to be sensitive and specific for Johne's disease in animals demonstrating clinical disease rather than preclinical infection. Serologic detection of clinical Johne's disease in cervids has been shown to be highly sensitive and specific while the sensitivity of fecal culture is low in both sheep and goats. The recommended organism detection method in both species is fecal PCR.[122] Fecal or milk PCR can be used on pooled samples for flock identification and to type the organism.

Prevention. Tuberculosis should not be endemic in flocks in the United States because positive animals are quarantined or destroyed. Preventing exposure to wild ruminants and other possible sources is crucial. Except in goat flocks raised for the production of milk that is to be sold unpasteurized, testing is uncommon, so animals are usually not identified until they develop overt disease. Paratuberculosis is much more common and may be maintained in flocks by carrier animals. No effective treatment is available for either disease, nor should any be encouraged because efforts should be concentrated on eliminating infection from the flock or herd. Vaccination of sheep is used extensively in Australia to control paratuberculosis. Prolonged vaccination has been shown to decrease fecal shedding in infected animals over time.[123]

Nonhemotropic Mycoplasmal Diseases

Pathogenesis. *Mycoplasma* spp. are very small, simple bacteria that parasitize cells of higher species. They are common inhabitants of mucous membranes and can have either a commensal or pathogenic relationship with the host. Transmission between animals is most likely through direct or indirect contact with body fluids from infected animals, inhalation of respiratory droplets, and arthropod vectors. Common sites for superficial infection include the ocular membranes, lung, mammary gland, and female reproductive tract. The organisms can also enter the blood and cause septicemia, abortion, pleuritis, and polyarthritis. Flare-ups often occur during times of crowding and during parturition, when neonates can spread the organisms from the mother's mouth to her udder and in turn become infected by ingesting contaminated milk.

The most important mycoplasma species in the United States are *Mycoplasma conjunctivae*, *Mycoplasma capricolum*, and the less pathogenic *Mycoplasma ovipneumoniae*. They are most commonly associated with keratoconjunctivitis, acute or chronic sepsis, and pneumonia, respectively. *M. conjunctivae* and *C. abortus* are the most common causes of pinkeye in North American small ruminants. *Mycoplasma* spp. are thought to inhibit tracheal ciliary function and thus may have a role similar to viruses in "shipping fever pneumonia" in facilitating lower respiratory tract invasion by primary bacterial pathogens. Many of the major pathogenic serotypes found in other countries (some of which cause severe pleuropneumonia without the participation of another bacteria), including *Mycoplasma mycoides* subsp. *mycoides*, *Mycoplasma mycoides* subsp. *capri*, *Mycoplasma agalactiae*, and strain F38, are not found in or have been eradicated from North America

Clinical Signs. Keratoconjunctivitis, mastitis, exudative vulvovaginitis, fever, cough, dyspnea, exercise intolerance, abortion, lameness, swollen joints, neonatal death, and depression may all be seen with mycoplasma infections.

Diagnosis. No specific clinical pathologic findings occur with these diseases. Mycoplasma infection should be suspected in sheep and goats with severe exudative pleuropneumonia in some parts of the world. Mycoplasma can be identified by bacteriologic culture or staining of exudates. Examiners must take care in interpreting positive cultures from body surfaces because nonpathogenic mycoplasma are common.

Prevention. Vaccines against mycoplasmal infections are available in some parts of the world, but not in the United States. Providing fly control, preventing stress and overcrowding, and isolating sick animals from healthy ones may help prevent the spread of disease.

Blood and Tissue Parasites

Anaplasma ovis, *Mycoplasma ovis*, and *Babesia* spp.

Pathogenesis. *A. ovis* and *M. ovis* are small bacteria that lack cells walls and parasitize erythrocytes. These and similar organisms have undergone recent reclassification following molecular analysis. Other species of hemotropic mycoplasmas may affect sheep and cervids.[116] The organisms are spread from animal to animal by insect or mechanical vectors. Known arthropod vectors for *A. ovis* include ticks and horseflies; other biting flies may be more important with *M. ovis* infection. Hypodermic needles and equipment used for tail-docking, castrating, or disbudding animals may be important in iatrogenic transmission. After being introduced into a naive host, the organisms proliferate, and the number of red cells infected increases rapidly until an effective immune response begins 1 to 2 weeks later. A similar proliferation of organisms may occur in chronically infected animals after temporary immune suppression. The humoral and cellular immune responses against *A. ovis* lead to opsonization of parasitized erythrocytes and their removal by cells of the reticuloendothelial system; *M. ovis* infection is thought to cause more intravascular hemolysis. The result in both cases is hemolytic anemia.[117] The protozoon parasites *Babesia ovis* and *Babesia motasi* have similar life cycles and cause similar diseases, but they have been eradicated and are reportable in the United States. *Babesia* spp. affecting small ruminants are generally less pathogenic than are their bovine counterparts.

Animals surviving acute hemolytic crisis reduce the parasites to low numbers but rarely clear the infection completely; they serve as sources of infection for other animals. Sheep and goats are susceptible to infection by either organism; goats generally appear to be more resistant to the development of severe parasitemia and clinical signs.

Clinical Signs. Signs present during hemolytic crises include fever, weakness, pale mucous membranes, and pigmenturia. Urine discoloration results from increased amounts of bilirubin in most cases, although hemoglobinuria may be seen in some sheep with *M. ovis* infection. Icterus is usually present only after the acute hemolytic crisis. Clinical signs are exacerbated during times of stress, and infection is often first noted when the animals are moved or handled. Chronically infected animals may appear clinically normal, may have recrudescence of infection after stress, or may display signs of ill-thrift such as poor body condition and fleece. Babesiosis occasionally causes concurrent central neurologic signs.

Diagnosis. The major clinical laboratory finding is regenerative anemia with detection of the intraerythrocytic bodies. Chronically infected sheep often have high counts of nucleated erythrocytes. Because *M. ovis* consumes glucose, hypoglycemia and metabolic acidosis may be detected, especially in blood samples that are not processed immediately. Diagnosis is by identification of the organisms on blood smears. Special stains are available to make the organisms more visible. Postmortem lesions include pallor or icterus of membranes and splenomegaly. Some evidence of vasculitis, including edema or exudates in body tissues or cavities, may be seen with *M. ovis* infection.

Treatment. *Mycoplasma* spp. and *Anaplasma* spp. are sensitive to tetracycline antibiotics. Babesiosis is more difficult to treat. Effective drugs include diminazene, pentamidine, and imidocarb dipropionate. Supportive care for all blood parasite infections includes whole blood transfusions, nutritional support, and administration of fluids.

Prevention. Prevention in most cases involves maintaining low levels of parasites rather than eliminating them entirely. This method ensures continual stimulation of the immune response, whereas eradication often leaves the animal susceptible to another bout of acute infection. Vector control can also be important in management of the disease.

Anaplasmataceae of WBCs

Pathogenesis. Two organisms belonging to the *Anaplasmataceae* family, *Ehrlichia ovis* and *Anaplasma phagocytophilum*, infect ovine WBCs, causing fever, immune suppression, and some organ damage. *A. phagocytophilum* is the causative agent of tick borne fever in sheep and granulocytic anaplasmosis in horses, dogs, and humans. The organism is transmitted by ticks (*Ixodes* spp.) and maintained in the environment by asymptomatic carrier animals. The distribution and incidence of disease is seasonal with the life cycle of the tick. The organism infects cells of the granulocytic lineage, leading to severe persistent neutropenia and acute lymphopenia. Fever occurs 1 to 2 weeks after infection, lasts as long as 2 weeks, and occasionally relapses. Chronic infection is common. Spleen, lung, liver, and kidney tissue may show some damage because of immune destruction of infected cells, but organ-specific signs are usually the result of secondary infection. Secondary bacterial joint infections in lambs infected with *A. phagocytophilum* develop debilitating lameness known as tick pyemia.

E. ovis causes fever (benign ehrlichiosis) 1 to 2 weeks after infection. Because of this organism's predilection for mononuclear cells, the degree of immunosuppression and subsequent importance of this disease are much less than for *A. phagocytophilum* infection.

Diagnosis. Specific diagnosis is best made by identifying darkly stained bodies at the periphery of granulocytic cells, as well as occasional large bodies deep within the cytoplasm of some cells. Stained bodies also can be seen on the periphery of mononuclear cells from a blood smear during the acute febrile stage or in tissues during chronic infection. Serologic tests are available for detection of *Anaplasmosis*. The available cELISA is incapable of distinguishing species of anaplasma and serologic results must be interpreted appropriately, and the species confirmed by PCR.

Both infections affect sheep and goats (*A. phagocytophilum* also affects many other ruminants, including white-tailed deer), but neither has been reported in North America. A recent study demonstrated that sheep are capable of being experimentally infected with a human isolate *A. phagocytophilum*. Interestingly, the sheep did not develop clinical disease.[118] Such findings suggest that sheep could serve as asymptomatic carriers and potential reservoirs for humans. *A. phagocytophilum* is widespread in northwestern Europe, including the United Kingdom, Scandinavia, and India, and *E. ovis* is found mainly in countries bordering the Indian Ocean. In spite of documented seropositive status of animals, there have been no reports of sheep or goats naturally infected with *A. phagocytophilum* in the United States developing clinical disease.

Treatment and Prevention. Treatment and prevention efforts should focus on reducing vectors and bacterial counts during vector season. Both organisms are susceptible to treatment with tetracycline.

Trypanosomiasis

People and animals can become infected with trypanosome protozoa. The trypanosomes can complete their developmental cycle only in tsetse flies (*Glossina* species). Trypanosomes multiply in blood, tissues, and body fluids of their vertebrate hosts and are transmitted between vertebrate hosts in the saliva of blood-sucking flies as they feed. The trypanosome species that are known to infect goats and sheep include *Trypanosoma congolense*, *Trypanosoma vivax*, *Trypanosoma brucei* subsp. *brucei*, *Trypanosoma evansi*, and *Trypanosoma simiae*.

Pathogenesis. After entering through the skin, trypanosomes reach the bloodstream by way of the lymphatic system. The parasites multiply, and the prepatent period lasts for 10 to 14 days after infection. The infection is characterized by periods of parasitemia, followed by the absence of parasites. This pattern of infection occurs because of antigenic variation: Trypanosomes vary the antigenic nature of their glycoprotein surface coat to evade the host's immune system. This immune system–evasive maneuver prolongs infection and is responsible for chronic disease. Some trypanosomes tend to invade extravascular spaces, such as the ocular aqueous humor and cerebrospinal fluid. The pathogenicity of trypanosomes varies with the different host species. Trypanosomes may produce a hemolysin early in the course of the disease that causes anemia in the host. Later, increased phagocytic activity results in massive erythrocyte destruction.

Clinical Signs. The clinical signs are variable and non-specific and depend on the speed of onset of anemia and the degree of organ impairment. Entire herds may be affected. All aspects of production are impaired—fertility, birth weight, lactation, weaning weight, growth, and survival. Trypanosomiasis may predispose the animal to the development of other diseases that mask the underlying trypanosome infection.

Trypanosomiasis may be acute, subacute, or chronic, with chronic infection occurring most commonly. Acute disease often causes abortion. Dairy goats may show a sudden drop in milk production. Depression, anorexia, and a stiff gait may be present. Physical examination reveals tachycardia, tachypnea, and a slight fever. Hyperemic mucous membranes and excessive lacrimation may be noted. Affected animals often become recumbent and anorexic and die within 1 to 3 weeks of onset of clinical signs. If the animal survives, progression to the subacute phase, characterized by listlessness, weight loss, enlargement of superficial lymph nodes, and a dull, dry hair coat, may occur. In such cases, auscultation findings are similar to those in other forms of acute cardiac disease, as well as pale mucous membranes and a pronounced jugular pulse. The animal may linger for several weeks or months, or the chronic form of the disease may develop. Affected animals show ill-thrift: dull and dry hair coat, inelastic skin, lethargy, emaciation, peripheral lymphadenopathy, pale mucous membranes, and exercise and stress intolerance. Death may occur many months or even years after infection and usually results from congestive heart failure. Subclinical trypanosomiasis causes acute episodes when animals are stressed by inadequate nutrition, increased production demands, or concurrent disease.

Diagnosis. Diagnosis is difficult because the parasitemia is intermittent, clinical signs are non-specific, and infection is not always synonymous with disease. A PCR assay is gaining acceptance as the most sensitive diagnostic modality, but not all infected animals exhibit clinical disease. Although a tentative diagnosis of pathologic trypanosomiasis can be made on the basis of history, clinical signs, and the presence of appropriate vectors, a definitive diagnosis requires identification of trypanosomes on a fresh blood smear, a Giemsa-stained blood smear, or less commonly, a lymph smear. Examination of the buffy coat of centrifuged blood with darkfield phase-contrast spore illumination is the most sensitive direct microscopic method and is useful when parasite numbers are low. Pathogenic trypanosomes must be distinguished from more ubiquitous, nonpathogenic species particularly common in cattle, such as *Trypanosoma theileri*. Repeated blood sampling in individual animals often is necessary, because as noted, parasitemia is intermittent. The diagnosis is supported by evidence of anemia on a CBC. Indirect diagnostic methods include an indirect fluorescent antibody test and the ELISA. These tests are less helpful for diagnosis of a single clinical case but are useful in assessment for herd infection. Both *T. congolense* and *T. brucei* readily infect rats and mice, and detection of these pathogens can be used to diagnose the infection indirectly.

Treatment. Treatment consists of the use of trypanocidal agents and supportive care. Animals with acute, subacute, and subclinical disease respond better to treatment than those with chronic disease because of the irreversible damage to hematopoiesis associated with chronic infection. With most trypanocides, the therapeutic index is low and varies with the host species.

Trypanocide efficacy also varies with the species of trypanosome present; resistance to agents is common. Some trypanocides are irritating to the skin and may cause severe inflammation at the injection site.

In sheep and goats with *T. brucei* infection, the trypanocide of choice is diminazene aceturate, which should be used at a higher dosage rate (7 mg/kg given intramuscularly [IM] or SC) than that recommended for cattle. Protection after trypanocide use usually lasts 2 to 4 months, depending on the season. Animals must be rested before and after treatment. Supportive care consists of providing fluids, an environment conducive to rest, good nutrition, and possibly blood transfusions.

Prevention. Vector control, stress and nutrition management, and selection of trypanosome-tolerant breeds of sheep and goats all help control or prevent trypanosomiasis. No vaccine is available. Animals can be treated with insecticides (pyrethroids) to prevent bites by tsetse flies and other flies. Control is accomplished by strategic use of trypanocides during the peak season. Continued parasitologic and clinical surveillance is essential to determine the efficacy of control measures.

Sarcocystis spp. and *Neospora caninum*

Pathogenesis. *Sarcocystis* spp. are protozoon parasites that have a two-host life cycle. Sexual reproduction occurs in the bowel of a carnivore (mainly dogs and wild canids) after the carnivore ingests cysts in the muscles of sheep, goats, and cervids. Sporocysts are passed in the carnivore's feces and later ingested by a sheep, goat or cervid. The sporocysts hatch in the ruminant gut and invade the vascular endothelium during three phases of asexual reproduction. After the third phase (approximately 8 to 10 weeks after ingestion), merozoites enter the ruminant's muscle tissue and encyst. Clinical signs are uncommon but can occur during the stages of reproduction and muscle invasion of the host. *N. caninum* has a similar life cycle and causes similar disease, except that it appears more likely to cause abortion and affect the central nervous system.

Clinical Signs. Most infections are asymptomatic. However, if a large number of sporocysts are ingested, tissue damage may occur during the intestinal, vascular, and muscle stages of the *Sarcocystis* life cycle. Fever, lameness or a stiff gait, reluctance to move, and diarrhea may be seen. Central neurologic signs (blindness, changes in mentation, and seizures) may occur if the organisms invade the brain or interrupt blood flow to it. Abortion can occur as early as 4 weeks after ingestion. With severe chronic infections, emaciation and anorexia are seen.

Diagnosis. The most characteristic abnormality is an increase in muscle enzyme activity in the blood. Anemia is common and may result from extravascular hemolysis. Cerebrospinal fluid may show mild mononuclear pleocytosis or may appear normal. On necropsy, muscles may display pale streaks or macroscopic cysts throughout. Other evidence of vasculitis includes hemorrhagic serosal surfaces, body cavity fluids, and lymphadenopathy. Microscopic or ultrastructural examination of affected tissues should reveal the presence of organisms. Specific antibody tests are available and do not cross-react with *T. gondii* antibodies. Blood antibody titers often peak around the onset of clinical signs and should be markedly higher than baseline values. Antibody preparations also are available for identification of organisms in tissue preparations.

Treatment. Sheep infected with *Sarcocystis* species can be treated with salinomycin (200 ppm in complete feed), monensin (0.5–1 mg/kg PO), or amprolium (25–40 mg/kg PO). Drugs such as sulfadiazine or trimethoprim (25–44 mg/kg IM SID), pyrimethamine (0.5–1 mg/kg PO SID), and clindamycin have shown some success in treating *Neospora* infections. These treatments are off-label and thus are governed by regulations regarding extra-label drug use.

Prevention. Preventing contamination of feedstuffs with the feces of infected carnivores and preventing ingestion of raw meat by carnivores are most important, but these measures may not be possible in flocks handled with dogs or those living on range land. Anticoccidial drugs appear to decrease the chance of clinical disease.[119]

T. gondii

Pathogenesis. *T. gondii* is a protozoon parasite with a life cycle very similar to *Sarcocystis*, except that the definitive host is the cat and that a wider range of mammalian and avian species, including humans, appear to be capable of acting as intermediate hosts. Sporocysts are infective a few days after passage in cat feces, and most ruminants are infected by eating feed contaminated with cat feces. People can become infected by ingesting raw meat or milk from infected animals.

Abortion, stillbirth, and neonatal death are the most common forms of clinical disease in sheep and goats, and *Toxoplasma* should be considered one of the most common causes of perinatal losses in small ruminants (see Chapter 8). Abortion usually occurs during the final month of pregnancy. Fever, vasculitis-induced disease, and neurologic disease are less common manifestations.

Clinical Signs. Beyond abortion, clinical disease is rare in adults and resembles systemic sarcocystosis. Clinical signs include fever, dyspnea, depression, and anorexia. Neurologic signs are more common than with *Sarcocystis* infection, especially in lambs and kids infected in utero.

Diagnosis. No specific laboratory abnormalities are associated with toxoplasmosis. Nodular lesions similar to sarcocysts may be seen in various tissues, including the brain. Aborted or stillborn fetuses may appear normal except for histologic lesions in the brain, liver, or lung, but more commonly fetuses are macerated. The placenta is usually abnormal, with gross and microscopic evidence of necrosis of the cotyledons. Microscopic identification of the organism in body tissues is the most common means of diagnosis. Serologic tests also are available.

Treatment and Prevention. Drugs similar to those used to treat *Neospora* may be effective against *Toxoplasma.* Preventing contamination of feeds with cat feces and preventing ingestion of dead animals by cats are the most important ways of stemming the spread of this organism. Both methods are likely to be difficult in most flocks. Direct spread from one animal to another is rare.

Acute Viral Diseases

Bluetongue

Etiology. Bluetongue is an acute viral disease of domestic and wild ruminants caused by an RNA virus in the genus *Orbivirus* and family *Reovirus*; it is transmitted by the insect vector *Culicoides varipenniis* in North America and other *Culicoides* species in other countries. Six of the 24 serotypes of the virus are found in the United States. Of the domestic ruminants, sheep are most severely affected. Goats and cattle rarely develop acute disease.

Clinical Signs. Bluetongue disease has two different manifestations—reproductive problems (see Chapter 8) and acute vasculitis of several organ systems. With vasculitis, a spiked fever often precedes depression, anorexia, and rapid weight loss. Leukopenia is present. Affected animals may develop edema of the lips, tongue, throat, ears, and brisket. Other signs include excessive salivation and hyperemia or cyanosis of the oral mucosa, including the tongue (hence the name *bluetongue*). Affected sheep often produce profuse serous nasal discharge that soon becomes mucopurulent and produces crusts and excoriations around the nose and muzzle. Oral lesions progress to petechial hemorrhages, erosions, and ulcers. Pulmonary edema is often severe, and pneumonia may develop. Skin lesions can progress to localized dermatitis. Affected sheep may exhibit stiffness or lameness because of muscular changes and laminitis. Cyanosis or hemorrhagic changes of the skin of the coronet can extend into the horny tissue. After recovery, a definite ridge in the horn of the hoof may be present for many months. In severe cases, the hoof sloughs. Mortality varies widely. In Africa, the virus is much more virulent than in the United States, and mortality ranges from 2 to 30%. The reproductive or teratogenic form of the disease varies greatly with strain, host, and environmental factors. Teratogenic effects include abortions, stillbirths, and weak, live "dummy lambs." Congenital defects may include hydranencephaly.

Diagnosis. In parts of the world where the disease is common, the diagnosis is usually based on clinical signs alone. The virus can be isolated from blood, semen, or tissues (spleen and brain from aborted fetuses). Viral isolation from blood obtained during the viremic state is the most definitive means of diagnosis. Serologic evaluation involves two types of viral antigen groups called *P7* and *P2*. The former is found in all bluetongue viruses, and the latter determines the serotype. Sera are commonly tested with complement fixation, agar gel immunodiffusion (AGID), or one of several ELISA tests. A competitive ELISA is considered the best serologic test for detecting group antibodies to bluetongue virus. A direct fluorescent antibody test is available. Molecular tests (e.g., PCR) for bluetongue have recently become available and are extremely sensitive and specific. They can be useful for distinguishing serotypes. Other clinicopathologic signs that aid in diagnosis include leukopenia during the early febrile stage of the disease and an increase in serum CK corresponding to the latter phase of muscle stiffness and lameness.

Treatment. Treatment is non-specific and consists of nursing care. Because of the reluctance of animals to eat, they should be fed a gruel of alfalfa pellets by stomach tube or encouraged to eat soft feeds and green grass. Broad-spectrum antimicrobials are often used to treat secondary pneumonia and dermatitis. Animals should be kept on soft bedding with good footing. Water and shade should be readily available. NSAIDs are commonly used.

Prevention. The *Culicoides* vector is difficult to eliminate, so animals should be kept indoors during periods of peak gnat activity (dusk and early evening). Owners should attempt to eliminate gnat breeding grounds such as overflowing watering troughs and shallow septic systems and should limit exposure of sheep to gnats with the use of repellent sprays.

Modified live vaccines based on local strains and serotypes are available in some parts of the world. Some cross-protection among serotypes does occur. The vaccine should be administered at least 2 weeks before breeding season to prevent teratogenic effects. Vaccinated breeding rams may have a slight risk of decreased fertility. Lambs can be vaccinated in the face of an outbreak. Pregnant animals cannot be vaccinated with modified live vaccines. Sheep that have recovered from an attack of bluetongue are solidly resistant for months to infection by the same viral strain and to some other viral types. Active immunity in sheep requires both humoral and cellular immunity.

Epizootic Hemorrhagic Disease

Etiology. Epizootic hemorrhagic disease virus (EHDV) is an orbivirus belonging to the family *Reoviridae*. The virus is structurally related to bluetongue virus, and the pathogenesis and clinical signs of disease resulting from these two viral infections are very similar. At least seven distinct serotypes of EHDV are recognized, although formal classification of serotypes has yet to be finalized. Only two serotypes (EHDV1 and EHDV2) have historically circulated throughout North America, and those serotypes are largely considered to be endemic in almost all areas of the United States, with the exception of the northeast and arid areas of the southwest. However, in 2006, EHDV6 was isolated from surveillance efforts in dead white-tailed deer.[124] Since then, EHDV6 has been increasingly identified from both surveillance samples and clinical cases and is also believed to be endemic in several regions.[125]

Pathogenesis. Epizootic hemorrhagic disease (EHD) is a noncontagious disease that is transmitted by the *Culicoides* biting midges. *Culicoides sonorensis* is the primary vector of EHDV in the United States, although other species are also suspected to transmit the disease based on the geographic distribution of clinical cases, although this has yet to be formally shown. Due to the vector-borne route of transmission, peak incidence of the disease is closely associated with peak vector population, namely, in the late summer and fall of the year.

Although capable of infecting a wide range of wild and domestic ruminants, EHDV is largely a pathogen of wild cervids, particularly white-tailed deer. Episodes of clinical disease are less common in mule deer, pronghorn antelope, and bighorn sheep and have lower morbidity and mortality. Sheep are only rarely infected with the virus and goats appear to be resistant to the virus. Cattle are commonly infected based on seroprevalence surveys, but overt clinical disease is uncommon. As a rule, infection in livestock is usually asymptomatic except for periodic epidemics. The last major EHD epidemic in the United States occurred in 2012 and affected a variety of captive and wild ruminant species.[126] In endemic areas, seroprevalence in cervids and other ruminants is high, but clinical disease is not commonly seen. Conversely, where seroprevalence is low, introduction of the virus results in widespread infection, where morbidity and mortality can reach 90% and 60%, respectively.

Following transmission of the virus by biting midges, EHDV replicates in the endothelial cells of the lymphatics surrounding the site of the bite. A primary viremia allows for systemic spread of the virus and secondary replication in lymph nodes throughout the body and the spleen. Viremia is important for disease propagation and generally lasts no more than 3 weeks following infection, although the virus can occasionally be isolated from deer infected 50 days previously. Antibodies to EHDV are first detected 10 to 14 days following infection but are not always capable of completely neutralizing the infection. Thus, it is possible to find both neutralizing antibodies and live virus in the same animal. Passive antibodies in fawns can be found up to approximately 4 months of age. As in adults, antibodies in fawns may not protect from infection but generally protect from severe clinical signs.

Clinical Signs. Clinical disease in white-tailed deer can be peracute, acute, or chronic. The course of the peracute syndrome of diseaseis relatively short, with death often occurring within 36 hours of infection, with or without the presence of clinical

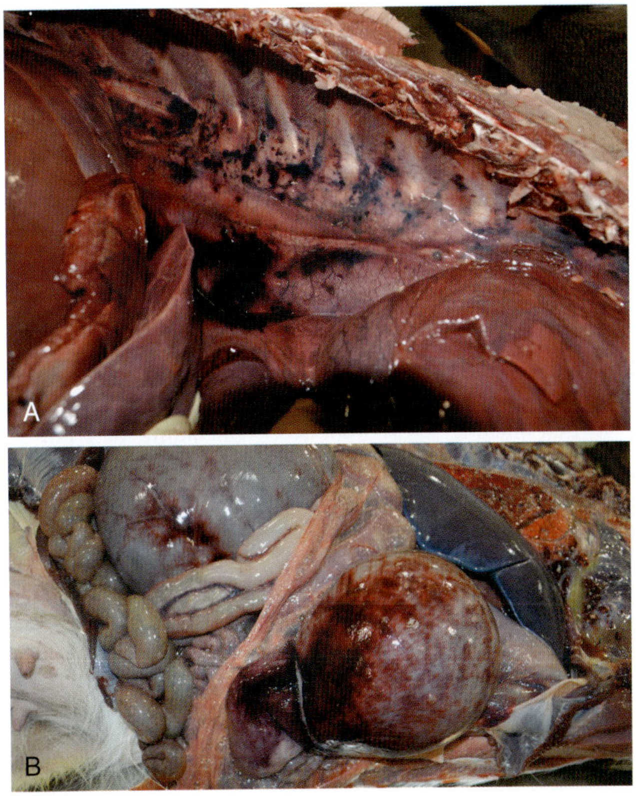

• **Fig. 16.1** **A.** The lungs of the adult pen-raised, white-tailed deer, have been retracted to reveal to ecchymoses on the ventral surface of the "ribcage." Petechiae and ecchymoses can occur anywhere within the carcass in cases of epizootic hemorrhagic disease (EHD), but common locations are on the epicardium, on the pleural surface the ribs, subcutaneously, and on the surface of the spleen. **B.** Ecchymoses over the surface of the reticulum (bottom right of photo) and the surface of the rumen (left side of photo). In addition to EHD, this deer also had bronchopneumonia (fibrin overlying consolidated lung can be seen in the far right of photo). (Courtesy Dr. Kelley Steury, Auburn, AL.)

signs. When present, clinical signs include severe edema of the head and neck, swelling of the tongue and conjunctiva, anorexia, fever, weakness, and respiratory distress. Hemorrhagic diatheses are not present antemortem but may occur after death. In contrast, in the acute form of the disease, the clinical signs of the peracute form are accompanied with bleeding throughout body tissues (Figure 16.1A, B). Ulcers may be evident in the oral cavity and throughout the upper gastrointestinal tract, forestomachs, and abomasum. Case fatality rates are high for both the peracute and acute forms. Deer that recover after several weeks of illness are said to suffer from the chronic form of the disease. Signs of previous illness may include breaks or rings in the hoof horn due to interrupted growth and synthesis leading to lameness, sometimes severe. Ulceration and scarring of the rumen and gastrointestinal tract may result in loss of body condition despite a seemingly normal appetite and ample nutrition. Widespread evidence of vasculitis may be observed histopathologically.

Diagnosis. The gold standard for EHDV diagnosis is virus isolation. Demonstration of neutralizing antibodies to EHDV reference strains is evidence of previous infection but may be of limited value in endemic areas where seroprevalence levels are expected to be high. Also, all potentially suspected serotypes must be used when testing the sample, thereby increasing the time and cost involved with the test. Continued research and refinement of molecular techniques, including PCR, are ongoing and are attractive due to the short turnaround times and the potential for high throughput of samples. However, it is important to remember that a positive result using molecular techniques does not equate to the presence of infectious virus, and thus, interpretation of results must be done with caution.

Control. Control of EHD is difficult and relies on a combination of disease surveillance, vector control, and potentially, vaccination. Eradication of vector-borne diseases from endemic areas is difficult and time-consuming, and thus, disease control is likely more attainable than strict eradication. Vector control is more important in the late fall and summer, when populations are at peak levels and viral transmission is more likely. Midge-proofed housing and the treatment of animals with pyrethroid insecticides have been attempted but may be logistically challenging and have yet to have been demonstrated efficacious. Vaccine availability in North America is limited, but inactivated autogenous vaccines have been developed from isolates obtained from ill or recently diseased animals. Autogenous vaccines are tested for purity but not necessarily for efficacy. Vaccine usage must be approved by the U.S. Department of Agriculture prior to administration.

Peste des Petits Ruminants (Pseudorinderpest)

Etiology. Peste des petits ruminants (PPR) is an acute or peracute, febrile, often fatal disease of ruminants caused by a virus in the family *Paramyxoviridae* and genus *Morbillivirus.* Sheep are less susceptible than goats and white-tailed deer. Cattle are only subclinically infected, and some wild ungulates, as well as camels, appear to suffer the occasional epizootic. The virus (PPRV) is serologically related to the virus that causes rinderpest. Geographically, the virus is found throughout Northern Africa, the Middle East, and adjacent regions of Asia, with possible movement into southern Africa and Europe noted.

Pathogenesis. The main route of infection is respiratory, and PPR is spread by airborne droplets. All secretions and excretions of infected animals are contagious throughout the course of the disease, but no carrier state exists. The virus targets lymphoid tissue. Lymphocytes are destroyed in germinal centers in lymph nodes, Peyer's patches, tonsils, splenic corpuscles, and cecal lymphoid tissue. Immunosuppression results from lymphoid destruction. Lymphocytes are partially replaced by plasma cells, macrophages, an eosinophilic acellular matrix, and occasionally neutrophils. The epithelial lining of the mouth and digestive tract is highly vulnerable to the PPRV. With the loss of the alimentary tract mucosa, weight loss and diarrhea become severe. The incubation period is usually 2 to 6 days, with up to 10 days possible.

Clinical Signs. The clinical disease produced by PPRV in sheep and goats closely resembles that of rinderpest, but the course is much more rapid. With the acute form, sheep and goats typically display an abrupt rise in temperature to 104° to 106° F (40°–41° C). Within a few days, infected animals develop nasal and lacrimal discharge, depression, thirst, anorexia, and leukopenia. Congestion of the conjunctival and other mucous membranes occurs, followed by serous and mucopurulent exudates. Sheep and goats develop oral erosions with necrotic foci, which results in excessive salivation. Diarrhea that may be profuse but rarely hemorrhagic develops within 2 to 3 days and is accompanied by abdominal pain, tachypnea, emaciation, and severe dehydration. Bronchopneumonia, particularly that caused by *Pasteurella* spp., may be a terminal sequela. Death usually occurs 5 to 10 days after the onset of fever. Pregnant sheep or goats with PPR may abort.

Diagnosis. A presumptive diagnosis of PPR can be made on the basis of clinical, pathologic, and epizootiologic findings. The diagnosis can be confirmed by isolating the virus from blood or tissues, including lymph nodes, tonsils, spleen, and lung. Immunocapture ELISA or PCR may be used to detect infection several days before the development of clinical disease. Most serologic tests (complement fixation or AGID) cannot differentiate between PPR and rinderpest. Characteristic postmortem findings include necrotic stomatitis that is generally confined to the inside of the lower lip and adjacent gum, the cheeks near the commissures, and the ventral surface of the free portion of the tongue. Abomasal erosions are often present. In the small intestine, Peyer's patches are markedly affected, particularly in the first portion of the duodenum and terminal ileum. The large intestine may be severely affected. Lesions occurring near the ileocecal valve, at the cecocolic junction, and in the rectum are often described as *zebra stripes* that indicate areas of congestion along the folds of the mucosa.

Treatment and Prevention. Infection with PPRV has no specific treatment. Mortality can be reduced by supportive care, including the administration of antimicrobial and antiinflammatory agents, as well as nutritional support. In the United States, state and federal veterinarians should be notified if PPRV is suspected. Methods used to eradicate rinderpest are useful in the eradication and control of PPR. All sick sheep and goats and those exposed should be slaughtered and disposed of by burning, burying, or rendering. The premises should be decontaminated, and the area quarantined. Sheep and goats can be protected against PPR by immunization with rinderpest vaccines or by the simultaneous administration of PPR hyperimmune bovine serum and virulent PPRV.[127]

Louping Ill

Pathogenesis. Louping ill is a tickborne disease caused by a flavivirus. It affects mainly lambs but occasionally also affects other livestock species and infrequently affects deer, camelids, and humans. Transmission is most common during tick season, and *Ixodes ricinus* is thought to be the most important infective host.

Many sheep clear the infection after a few days of fever and viremia, but others develop severe, fatal viral encephalitis. The virus is shed in many secretions, including milk, which is an important source of infection for other animals (and humans). The severity of the disease depends on herd immunity because previous exposure gives long-lasting immunity. Colostrum from immune females is protective for the neonate. High antibody titers also appear to shorten the duration and level of viremia and thereby prevent invasion of the central nervous system. Naïve flocks may have fatality rates as high as 60%.

Clinical Signs. High biphasic fever, anorexia, and depression are seen in most infected sheep. Lambs may die quickly before illness is noted. Some sheep also develop central neurologic signs, including hyperexcitability, muscle tremors, and rigidity. Abnormal coordination and muscle activity may cause sheep to move with a bounding gait (hence the name *louping ill*).

Diagnosis. The condition has no characteristic gross lesions. Microscopic examination of animals with neurologic signs reveals evidence of viral meningoencephalitis. Diagnosis is made by history (based on location, signs, and time of year), the identification of characteristic lesions, virus isolation, or fluorescent antibody staining of fresh brain tissue. A demonstrated increase in specific antibody titers in survivors strongly suggests the presence of this infection.

Prevention. Vaccines are available in endemic areas to control infection. Vector control during tick season also is important. Lambing season should also be timed so that lambs have high colostral antibody protection at the time of exposure to ticks.

Foot-and-Mouth Disease and Vesicular Stomatitis

Pathogenesis. Foot-and-mouth disease is caused by a highly contagious picornavirus and has been eradicated from the United States. Vesicular stomatitis is caused by a rhabdovirus and is intermittently eradicated from the United States. Both diseases are highly contagious, nearly indistinguishable from each other clinically, and reportable. Foot-and-mouth disease has a broad host range that includes most hoof stock (including pigs but not horses) and several other mammalian species. Vesicular stomatitis also affects many species of hoof stock, including both pigs and horses. Sheep and goats are relatively less susceptible than cattle, particularly to vesicular stomatitis.

The viruses are spread by aerosol and mechanical vectors and primarily colonize skin or mucous membranes. Milking machines, flies, birds, and humans all may be important mechanical vectors. Vesicular stomatitis tends to remain at the site of infection, and colonization is facilitated by damage to the skin. Oral mucous membranes, coronary bands and interdigital skin, and teat-end skin are common sites of lesions. Vesicular stomatitis outbreaks in the United States tend to occur in the summer or fall and end with the first killing frost.

Viremia plays more of a role with foot-and-mouth disease. The virus is present in most body tissues and fluids in infected animals and can be transmitted through milk, meat, bone, and hide products; semen; equipment that pierces the skin; and biting arthropods. It also tends to spread through the circulation from the site of infection to other susceptible tissues, including the sites of vesicular stomatitis, as well as to the nasal cavity, mammary glandular epithelium, and ruminal pillars.

The basic lesion for both diseases are the vesicles that form in the oral cavity and on the teats and coronary band. The vesicles quickly rupture and may not be visualized before forming erosions. Ruptured vesicles leave deep erosions on the skin or mucous membranes and appear to cause pain. Tissue damage and inflammation are often compounded by secondary bacterial infection, which can cause greater morbidity and mortality than the original viral infection. Morbidity is related to feed refusal, increased recumbency, and secondary infections of the mouth, udder, and feet.

Clinical Signs. Sheep and goats usually develop minor lesions, if any, and are more important in many outbreaks as transport or multiplying hosts than as primary clinical cases. However, identification of lesions should raise suspicion of this disorder. In the worst cases, vesicles, erosions, and ulcers are seen at target sites. They may appear mildly inflamed and erythematous; if they are infected, they may appear severely inflamed with hemorrhage and necrosis. Other signs vary according to the location and severity of the lesions. Lingual and buccal lesions cause salivation, dysphagia, and feed refusal. Foot lesions, which are the most common clinical manifestation in small ruminants, cause lameness and recumbency. Teat lesions cause reluctance to be milked or nursed and a decrease in production. Fever also may be seen early in the disease, when vesicles are most apparent. The fever then usually abates, and vesicles are replaced by erosions or ulcers. Abortion may occur, especially with foot-and-mouth disease, and is probably related to the fever rather than to fetal infection. The disease is usually self-limiting; most animals recover within 2 to 3 weeks. Shedding of the virus causing vesicular stomatitis is thought to subside soon after healing of lesions. Foot-and-mouth disease virus may be shed for as long as 6 months, and all body secretions and tissues should be considered contagious, including milk, semen, meat, and offal. Both viruses have zoonotic potential and cause a disease in humans that resembles mild influenza. The diseases are self-limiting, but people can shed the viruses in sufficient quantities to infect other animals.

Diagnosis. No characteristic clinicopathologic changes are reported for either virus. Gross lesions resemble those seen before death and include vesicular, erosive, and ulcerative lesions of the mouth, feet, and teat ends; foot-and-mouth disease also causes lesions of the mammary gland and ruminal epithelium. Microscopic findings include hydropic degeneration of cells of the stratum spinosum of the epidermis without inclusion bodies. Secondary bacterial infection may lead to deeper ulcers and complicate identification of the viral etiology of these lesions. Myocarditis lesions may be seen with some forms of foot-and-mouth disease.

A presumptive diagnosis may be made by identifying characteristic lesions during a season and in an area at risk for one of these infections. In North America, bluetongue should be considered as an important differential diagnosis for ulcerative oral lesions in sheep. A confirmed diagnosis of foot-and-mouth disease is achieved by a combination of virus isolation (from vesicles), IHC, and serology by regulatory officials. Identifying the source of infection also is very important. Diagnosis of vesicular stomatitis is achieved by complement fixation or fluorescent antibody staining of virus in vesicular fluid or detection of a rise in antibody titers. Flocks with either of these diseases in the United States are subject to quarantine and possible destruction (especially for foot-and-mouth disease).

Prevention. Meticulous personal hygiene and avoidance of contact with new animals are important during outbreaks to prevent spread between flocks. Vaccines against foot-and-mouth disease are available in many parts of the world, but not in the United States. Most nations slaughter or quarantine affected animals. Vaccines against vesicular stomatitis are available and are most commonly used if the risk of outbreak is high, but vaccination does not prevent infection or shedding. Good hoof and teat care and soft feeds may help prevent spread of the virus by providing a healthy, intact barrier against invasion.

Sheep and Goat Pox

Pathogenesis. Sheep and goat pox are caused by two closely related poxviruses. Some strains are infective to both sheep and goats; most are species specific. They are maintained in populations by infected animals, and transmission occurs by aerosol or direct or indirect contact. Flies may play an important role as mechanical vectors in some flocks. Viruses remain infective in the environment for as long as 6 months.

After infection, viremia and inflammation of the oral, nasal, and ocular mucous membranes occur. Erythematous papular pox lesions appear a few days later. Severity varies according to strain pathogenicity, breed susceptibility, and immune status. Mild infections are characterized by lesions concentrated in the non-wooled or hairless regions of the skin. Severe infections produce lesions throughout the oral cavity, respiratory tract, and peritoneal cavity. Secondary infection is common with the severe form and mortality is high. If the animal survives, lesions heal in 3 to 4 weeks. Both diseases have been eradicated from the United States and are reportable. People can develop mild disease on exposure to these viruses.

Clinical Signs. Fever, inappetence, conjunctivitis, and upper respiratory signs are seen in the initial stages. Pox lesions are visible shortly thereafter. Secondary infection can lead to a variety of more serious signs indicative of respiratory disease, sepsis, and shock.

Diagnosis. Characteristic pox lesions are highly suggestive of this disease. Microscopic analysis reveals eosinophilic intracytoplasmic inclusion bodies, acantholysis, and pustule formation within the epidermis and occasionally the dermis. Viral particles may be seen on ultrastructural examination. Gross and microscopic lesions are characteristic with the severe form, but mild disease may produce mild lesions that are difficult to differentiate from other viral diseases that cause oral proliferative or ulcerative lesions. Virus can be isolated from blood or tissues (mainly skin) during the acute viremic stage and identified by antibody staining of more chronic lesions. Serologic tests are available to detect rising titers in convalescent animals.

Treatment and Prevention. No specific treatment is available for sheep or goat pox. Antibacterial drugs may be useful to treat secondary infection. Judicious use of insecticides and confinement of affected animals may prevent spread. Vaccines are available in some countries, but not in the United States. Infected flocks are placed under quarantine or destroyed in regions where the diseases are not endemic. These viruses are difficult to eradicate from flocks because of their environmental persistence and the constant supply of susceptible hosts.

Chronic Viral Diseases

Caprine Arthritis-Encephalitis Virus Infection

Caprine arthritis-encephalitis virus (CAEV) is an enveloped, single-stranded retrovirus in the *Lentivirus* genus. Like other retroviruses, CAEV integrates into the host chromosomal DNA before replicating. The virus is able to remain latent or undergo sporadic bouts of productive viral replication. CAEV is closely related to ovine lentiviruses.

Clinical Signs. Clinical disease may be evident in only 10% of goats from a CAEV-infected herd at any given time. As many as 85% of seropositive goats may be clinically normal. CAEV produces four clinical syndromes: encephalomyelitis, arthritis, interstitial pneumonia, and indurative mastitis. The pattern of disease usually varies with age. Arthritis is generally seen in sexually mature goats, whereas encephalomyelitis is generally seen in kids 2 to 4 months old. Interstitial pneumonia and indurative mastitis are more common in adult goats. Some goats suffer from a wasting disorder characterized by poor body condition and rough hair coat.

Diagnosis. A presumptive diagnosis of CAEV can be made on the basis of history and clinical signs suggestive of one or more of the syndromes. In general, ELISA tests are better for detecting disease in an individual animal because the sensitivity of the test is higher than that of the AGID, whereas the AGID is better for herd screening that requires high specificity. With the AGID test, false negatives may occur in goats that have not yet seroconverted to recent infection. Individual goats may take months or years to seroconvert or may never do so. Parturition or advanced stages of disease also may contribute to a false-negative result. False positives may occur in goats younger than 90 days old that have colostral antibodies. For this reason, it is often suggested that kids be at least 6 months old before they are tested. PCR testing has high specificity and sensitivity and can detect infection within a day of exposure. Other less commonly used tests include a Western blot to detect antibodies and a Northern blot to look for mitochondrial RNA. Because of the limitations in interpreting serologic results, CAEV-induced disease can only be definitively diagnosed by identification of characteristic lesions from examination of biopsy specimens or postmortem viral isolation.

Treatment. No specific treatments are available for any of the syndromes associated with CAEV. Young goats suffering from encephalomyelitis may benefit from physical therapy if they are recumbent, and bottle feeding may help maintain hydration and caloric intake. Antibiotics may be beneficial to goats affected with interstitial pneumonia or mastitis if secondary bacterial infection is present. Generally, the prognosis is poor for the encephalitic form and guarded for the other forms.

Prevention. Prevention of CAEV is crucial because infection is lifelong. Infected colostrum and milk are the most important sources of infection. Newborn kids should be prevented from ingesting colostrum from infected does and should instead be fed pasteurized goat's milk or milk from CAEV-negative goats. All goats in a herd should undergo serologic testing twice yearly; seropositive goats should be segregated or culled to prevent direct contact between infected and uninfected animals.

Ovine Progressive Pneumonia Virus Infection

Ovine progressive pneumonia (OPP) is an ultimately fatal retroviral disease that causes chronic, progressive, debilitating inflammatory conditions of the lungs (United States) and central nervous system (other parts of the world). It also is called *maedi-* (mæði is Icelandic for "shortness of breath") *visna* (meaning "wasting"). The virus is a member of the *Lentivirus* genus of retroviruses and is closely related to CAEV. Recombination between OPP and CAE viruses has been observed.[128]

The virus primarily affects sheep and rarely goats and has been identified worldwide, except in Australia and New Zealand. The disease has a long incubation period and protracted clinical course.

Pathogenesis. Only sheep older than 2 years of age are affected by OPP virus (OPPV). The virus is spread by direct contact, probably in respiratory and salivary secretions, and by excretion in the milk and colostrum. Transplacental transfer is of minor importance. Virus is excreted by animals that exhibit clinical signs and asymptomatic animals. Infection is established in the monocyte and macrophage cell line and spread by these cells to the lungs, lymph nodes, choroid plexus, spleen, bone marrow, mammary gland, and kidneys. Like CAEV, OPPV evades the cellular and humoral immune system of the host by incorporation of its provirus in host DNA, low-grade replication of virus only when monocytes differentiate into macrophages (restricted replication), and production of antigenic variants that are not neutralized by existing antibodies. Continual antigenic stimulation of the host by low-grade replication of OPPV results in chronic inflammation and resultant lymphoid proliferation in various target tissues. The virus may prevent B lymphocytes from differentiating into plasma cells in lymph nodes and may thereby impair immunoregulation. Seroconversion occurs within 2 to 3 weeks after infection.

Clinical Signs. In the United States, serologic surveys reveal infection rates of between 30 and 67% but rarely is more than 5% of a flock lost to OPPV. Icelandic, Texel, Border Leicester, and Finnish Landrace appear to be susceptible sheep breeds. More resistant sheep breeds include Rambouillet, Suffolk, and Columbia.

Various clinical syndromes are associated with OPPV and include wasting (thin ewe syndrome), dyspnea occasionally with a dry cough, pneumonia, mastitis ("hard bag"), posterior paresis, arthritis, and vasculitis. In North America, pneumonia and indurative aseptic mastitis are common sequelae of infection. Coinfection with the Jaagsiekte virus (the cause of pulmonary adenomatosis) worsens respiratory signs. Visna, the neurologic form, is more common in goats. Over the course of up to a year, subtle signs such as a head tilt or hindlimb weakness progress to gross incoordination, whole body tremors, and rarely more profound cranial nerve signs.

Diagnosis. A presumptive diagnosis can be made on the basis of clinical signs, poor response to treatment, characteristic postmortem findings, and serologic testing. Definitive diagnosis requires PCR or isolation of the virus from WBCs (buffy coat of whole blood sample) or tissues. Less expensive and faster serologic tests include AGID, ELISA, and an indirect immunofluorescence test. The AGID test is frequently used as a flock screening test, but the ELISA is more sensitive on an individual basis and can detect antibodies earlier in the course of the disease. As with CAEV, false negatives and false positives are possible.

Characteristic postmortem lesions include generalized wasting and firm, noncollapsing lung or firm, mottled mammary glands, both with regional lymphadenopathy. Microscopic evaluation of those tissues reveals interstitial non-septic, mononuclear cell infiltrates, although these may be complicated by secondary infections. Histopathology of nervous tissue reveals meningoleukoencephalitis.

Treatment. No effective treatment is available for OPPV. Supportive therapy that includes appropriate husbandry and control of secondary infection with antibiotics may prolong life for a few weeks or months but, ultimately, the disease is fatal. Because of the poor prognosis and risk of exposure of naive animals to clinical disease, long-term treatment is not recommended.

Prevention. The only known method of preventing OPPV infection in a flock is to prevent exposure to the virus. Management practices that help decrease the incidence of horizontal transmission include disinfection of milking equipment, dehorning instruments, and tail docking and castration tools before use and between animals. Contaminated feed and water also are potential routes of infection and should not be shared among infected and uninfected animals. Serologic testing and separation or culling of seropositive animals may help reduce infection. Although OPPV can readily be isolated from ewe colostrum, colostral transmission of OPPV has not been definitively established. However, many prevention guidelines recommend that offspring from infected dams be separated from the dam before they nurse and then be fed cow colostrum and artificially reared. Quarantine and serologic testing of flock additions before placing them with the current flock and purchase of sheep only from OPPV-free flocks are important to prevent the introduction of new infections. Because of the potential cross-species spread, all precautions taken for sheep also apply to contact goats. Serologic testing should be performed at least annually in a flock until two consecutive negative test results are obtained.

Border Disease Virus

Border disease virus (BDV) is in the genus *Pestivirus* and family *Flaviviridae*, which also includes the two genotypes of bovine viral diarrhea virus (BVDV) and classical swine fever virus. It rarely causes disease in adults and is most important as a cause of in utero infection of lambs and kids. The condition gets its name from the fact that it was first reported in sheep along the Welsh border of the United Kingdom. Other names such as "hairy shakers" and "fuzzy lamb disease" refer to some of the clinical signs seen in affected newborns. It is important to recognize that although BDV is genetically distinct from the two types of BVDV, sheep and goats also are susceptible to some strains of BVD.

Pathogenesis. Horizontal transmission of BDV occurs through contact with secretions and excretions of body fluids and tissues from infected animals. The virus crosses intact mucous membranes and can spread rapidly through a flock. The major reservoir is the persistently infected sheep or goat. These reservoirs are usually asymptomatic, congenitally infected, and often seronegative animals that shed large quantities of virus. These may be residents of a flock with an ongoing problem or bought in as replacement animals to a naïve flock. Some cross-infection from other species is possible, particularly from cattle.

Adult, immunocompetent sheep rarely show any signs of acute infection. However, if a pregnant ewe or doe is infected, the virus may be transmitted vertically to the embryo or fetus. Depending on the stage of gestation, embryonic or fetal infection may have different outcomes ranging from embryonic reabsorption to normal birth. These infections are the most important aspect of border disease.

The major organ system targeted by BDV is the fetal central nervous system. The hallmark lesion is hypomyelination, or degeneration of oligodendroglial cells. Three factors contribute to this lesion. The first is direct viral damage. The second is viral-induced inhibition of the thyroid gland that causes decreased secretion of thyroid hormones. In the absence of these hormones, a resultant lowered concentration of a specific nucleotide in the central nervous system also contributes to the hypomyelination. The third factor is altered immune function. The virus causes the host to produce a virus-specific delayed hypersensitivity reaction that causes inflammation in the central nervous system. It also causes immunosuppression. Death often results from opportunistic conditions such as parasitism, diarrhea, and bronchopneumonia.

Clinical Signs. Clinical signs depend on the time during gestation when the fetus or embryo is exposed to the virus. Clinical signs also may vary in severity from animal to animal because different fetuses develop competent immune systems at different times. If the fetus or embryo is exposed to the virus within 45 days of conception, it dies and is resorbed or aborted. These losses are not usually noticed by the flock manager. The principal manifestation in the flock is a large number of open ewes and a small lamb crop. Infection of the fetus between days 45 and 80 of gestation causes damage to rapidly growing systems such as the skin and nervous, lymphoid, thyroid, and skeletal systems. Congenital malformations are seen at birth. Lambs have abnormal fleece characteristics (hairy rather than woolly in consistency), small stature, domed heads, shortened legs, and dark pigmentation of the skin, particularly on the dorsal aspect of the neck. The lamb may exhibit tonic-clonic tremors ("hairy shakers") when awake, which may prevent standing or suckling. Most of these lambs die within a few days of birth. If they survive, the hair changes disappear in 9 to 12 weeks and the central nervous system signs resolve by 20 weeks. Goats infected at this time have similar symptoms except that they rarely exhibit hair coat changes. If kids are infected before day 80 of gestation and are still viable, they may become persistently infected and immunologically compromised. They are small at birth and generally weak.

Typical outbreaks of border disease cause abortions and birth of weak lambs in the first year as the virus rapidly spreads throughout a susceptible flock and then insignificant losses in the succeeding years as adult sheep develop immunity. However, if new naïve ewes are introduced in the flock, substantial losses may occur in perpetuity.

Diagnosis. Border disease viral antigens can be demonstrated in abomasum, pancreas, kidney, thyroid, skin, and testicle tissues from aborted fetuses and persistently infected animals using fluorescent antibody tests. However, IHC on ear notch samples is not considered as reliable for detecting persistently infected small ruminants as it is for cattle. The virus can be isolated, or viral antigen detected by ELISA, from serum, heparinized whole blood, and tissue taken from brain, spinal cord, spleen, and bone marrow from affected lambs. Whole blood is better than serum if colostral antibodies are likely to be high; serum is an adequate sample in neonates and juveniles that have not suckled.

Antibodies to the virus may be quantified by serum neutralization, AGID, and complement fixation with hyperimmune BVD antiserum. Serologic tests are useful to detect exposure in late-gestation (after day 80) neonates and unvaccinated animals but may be confounded by colostral antibodies in suckling neonates, previous exposure, and vaccination in older animals. Any titer in a presuckling neonate indicates in utero exposure, whereas a serum neutralization titer of 1:20 to 1:320 suggests infection in adults. The presence of specific antibodies in the cerebral spinal fluid suggests BDV infection. Negative presuckling serologic tests do not rule out exposure because persistently infected lambs tend to be immunotolerant to the BDV and therefore are born without an antibody titer. These animals may subsequently develop a titer that is indistinguishable from that of a normal animal. Although persistently infected animals do not respond immunologically to the strain of the virus they carry, they may respond to other strains of the virus, including vaccine strains.

As with BVD, PCR assays are gaining popularity for the detection of BDV in fluids and tissue samples. These assays appear to be superior to other techniques, except in autolyzed tissues. Real-time PCR may also be used to differentiate BDV from BVD and to type isolates.

Gross postmortem findings include hydranencephaly, porencephaly, microcephaly, cerebellar hypoplasia, abnormal rib curvature, brachygnathia, doming of the frontal bones of the skull, narrowing of the distance between the orbits, shortening the crown-to-rump length, shortening of the diaphyseal length, retention of secondary hair fibers, and abnormal skin pigmentation. The major histopathologic changes include hypomyelination and hypercellularity of the white matter. Glial cells appear normal.

Treatment. No treatment is available for border disease infection. Supportive care may include assistance in nursing and standing for affected lambs, provision of good bedding and solid footing, and treatment of secondary opportunistic infection.

Prevention. Control is primarily achieved by eliminating persistently infected carrier animals from the flock and preventing the addition of new carrier animals. This is easiest in a closed flock but especially difficult in small ruminant flocks because of the frequent desire to import new genetics. To identify carriers, virus isolation must be performed on every animal in the flock; carrier animals must be culled. Additionally, all unborn animals must be considered potential carriers and should be tested at birth. An alternative solution in hobby flocks is to arrest breeding activity until all animals have been shown to be free of infection. New animals should be quarantined and tested before admission to the flock. Herd screening with the ear skin biopsy test using fluorescent antibody staining to detect virus is less expensive and more convenient than the whole blood virus isolation test.

The role of vaccination in preventing infection is still unclear. No vaccine against BDV is available, but some reports suggest that BVDV vaccines for cattle may be helpful for sheep at risk. However, these vaccines have proven to be more effective at preventing clinical disease in vaccinated animals than in preventing in utero infection because they do not prevent transient viremia. Vaccination decreases viremia and fetal infection but does not eliminate them. Therefore, vaccines play a role in decreasing economic loss but do not replace culling of carrier animals as the major method of control.

Scrapie

Another member of the slow infection group of diseases of small ruminants is scrapie. It is an afebrile, chronic, progressive degenerative disorder of the central nervous system of sheep and occasionally of goats (see Chapter 13). Scrapie is caused by a prion and, as such, is one of the transmissible spongiform encephalopathies.

Sheep (and goats and mouflon to a lesser degree) are the natural hosts for scrapie. Clinical signs often do not usually appear until animals are 2 years old, and animals as old as 5 years may exhibit clinical disease. Both vertical and horizontal transmission have been demonstrated experimentally in sheep and goats. Abnormal scrapie protein has been identified in milk, urine, and seminal plasma of sheep up to 20 months prior to the development of clinical signs. Also, new evidence from deer with chronic wasting disease, a similar disorder, suggests that infective prions are excreted in the saliva and feces well before the development of clinical signs. These new revelations may help explain horizontal transmission of infection.

Clinical Signs. The onset of scrapie is insidious. Initially, sheep show subtle changes in behavior such as mild apprehension, staring or fixed gaze, failure to respond to herding dogs, and boldness around humans. Several months later, the animals become intolerant of exercise and develop a clumsy, unsteady gait and floppy ears. Later, the sheep develop itchy skin that causes them to rub themselves excessively against firm, immobile objects (origin of the name *scrapie*). This leads to excoriations and wool damage. There is a general decline in body condition and coordination.

Diagnosis. Histologically, the only consistent lesions are degenerative changes in the central nervous system consisting of bilaterally symmetric vacuolation of the neurons in the brainstem and spinal cord with accompanying spongy degeneration. As a preclinical test, IHC may be performed in lymphoid tissue from the tonsils, third eyelid, or rectoanal mucosa, but none of these methods is foolproof. CWD is discussed in Chapters 13, 19, and 20.

References

1. Morris DD: Anemia. In Smith BP, editor: *Large animal internal medicine*, ed 2, St Louis, 1996, Mosby.
2. Cross JP, Mackintosh CG, Griffin JF: Effect of physical restraint and xylazine sedation on haematological values in red deer (*Cervus elaphus*), *Res Vet Sci* 45:281, 1988.
3. Gaspar-López E, Landete-Castillejos T, Estevez JA, Ceacero F, Gallego L, García AJ: Seasonal variations in red deer (*Cervus elaphus*) hematology related to antler growth and biometrics measurements, *J Exp Zool A Ecol Genet Physiol* 315:242, 2011.
4. Esin A, Bergendahl LT, Savolainen V, Marsh JA, Warnecke T: The genetic basis and evolution of red blood cell sickling in deer, *Nat Ecol Evol* 2:367, 2018.
5. Vatta AF, Letty BA, van der Linde MJ, van Wijk EF, Hansen JW, Krecek RC: Testing for clinical anaemia caused by *Haemonchus* spp. in goats farmed under resource-poor conditions in South Africa using an eye colour chart developed for sheep, *Vet Parasitol* 99(1): 1–14, 2001.
6. Kaplan RM, Burke JM, Terrill TH, et al: Validation of the FAMACHA eye color chart for detecting clinical anemia in sheep and goats on farms in the southern United States. *Vet Parasitol* 123 (1–2):105–120, 2004.
7. Reynecke DP, van Wyk JA, Gummow B, Dorny P, Boomker J: Validation of the FAMACHA© eye colour chart using sensitivity/specificity analysis on two South African sheep farms, *Vet Parasitol* 177(3–4):203–211, 2011.
8. Moors E, Gauly M: Is the FAMACHA chart suitable for every breed? Correlations between FAMACHA scores and different traits of mucosa colour in naturally parasite infected sheep breeds, *Vet Parasitol* 166(1–2):108–111, 2009.
9. Selim HM, Yamato O, Tajima M, Maede Y: Rumen bacteria are involved in the onset of onion-induced hemolytic anemia in sheep, *J Vet Med Sci* 61(4):369–374, 1999.
10. McPhail DB, Sibbald AM: The role of free radicals in brassica-induced anaemia of sheep: an ESR spin trapping study, *Free Radic Res Commun* 16(5):277–284, 1992.
11. Smith RH: Kale poisoning: the brassica anaemia factor, *Vet Rec* 107 (1):12–15, 1980.
12. Van Kampen KR, James LF, Johnson AE: Hemolytic anemia in sheep fed wild onion (*Allium validum*), *J Am Vet Med Assoc* 156(3): 328–332, 1970.
13. Maiorka PC, Massoco CO, de Almeida SD, Gorniak SL, Dagli ML: Copper toxicosis in sheep: a case report, *Vet Hum Toxicol* 40(2): 99–100, 1998.
14. Soli NE, Froslie A: Chronic copper poisoning in sheep. I. The relationship of methaemoglobinemia to Heinz body formation and haemolysis during the terminal crisis, *Acta Pharmacol Toxicol (Copenh)* 40(1):169–177, 1977.
15. Todd JR: Chronic copper toxicity of ruminants, *Proc Nutr Soc* 28(2):189–198, 1969.
16. Hidiroglou M, Heaney DP, Hartin KE: Copper poisoning in a flock of sheep. Copper excretion patterns after treatment with molybdenum and sulfur or penicillamine, *Can Vet J* 25(10):377–382, 1984.
17. Decker MJ, Freeman MJ, Morter RL: Evaluation of mechanisms of leptospiral hemolytic anemia, *Am J Vet Res* 31(5):873–878, 1970.
18. Smith BP, Armstrong JM: Fatal hemolytic anemia attributed to leptospirosis in lambs, *J Am Vet Med Assoc* 167(8):739–741, 1975.
19. Overås J: Studies on *Eperythrozoon ovis*—infection in sheep, *Acta Vet Scand Suppl* 28(Suppl 28):1, 1969.
20. Sutton RH: *Eperythrozoon ovis*—a blood parasite of sheep, *N Z Vet J* 18(8):156–164, 1970.
21. Sutton RH, Jolly RD: Experimental *Eperythrozoon ovis* infection of sheep, *N Z Vet J* 21(8):160–166, 1973.
22. Neimark H, Hoff B, Ganter M: *Mycoplasma ovis* comb. nov. (formerly *Eperythrozoon ovis*), an epierythrocytic agent of haemolytic anaemia in sheep and goats, *Int J Syst Evol Microbiol* 54(Pt 2): 365–371, 2004.
23. Hornok S, Meli ML, Erdos A, Hajtós I, Lutz H, Hofmann-Lehmann R: Molecular characterization of two different strains of haemotropic mycoplasmas from a sheep flock with fatal haemolytic anaemia and concomitant Anaplasma ovis infection, *Vet Microbiol* 136(3–4):372–377, 2009.
24. Nappert G, Shepherd G, Archer J, Haines D, Naylor JM: Bovine colostrum as a cause of hemolytic anemia in a lamb, *Can Vet J* 36(2):104–105, 1995.
25. Suttle NF, Jones DG, Woolliams C, Woolliams JA: Heinz body anaemia in lambs with deficiencies of copper or selenium, *Br J Nutr* 58(3):539–548, 1987.
26. Larsen RS, Carpenter JW, Kennedy GA, Morales N: Maxillary lymphosarcoma in a white-tailed deer (*Odocoileus virginianus*), *J Wildl Dis* 38:611–615, 2002.

27. Löhr CV: One hundred two tumors in 100 goats (1987–2011), *Vet Pathol* 50:668–675, 2013.
28. Kiser PK, Löhr CV: Lymphoma classification in goats, *Vet Pathol* 54:611–619, 2017.
29. Valentine BA, Stieger-Vanegas S, Brown SR, Tornquist SJ, Young K: Exophthalmos due to multicentric B-cell lymphoma in a goat, *Can Vet J* 52:1350–1352, 2011.
30. Rushton JO, Thaller D, Krametter-Froetscher R: Ocular involvement of multicentric malignant B-cell lymphoma in a ewe. A case report, *Tierarztl Prax Ausg G Grosstiere Nutztiere* 45:182–186, 2017.
31. Cosgrove GE, Satterfield LC, Nettles VF: Neoplasia. In Davidson WR, Hayes FA, Nettles VF. Kellog FE, editors: *Diseases and parasites of white-tailed deer*, Miscellaneous Publication No. 7. Tall Timbers Research Station, Tallahassee, Florida, pp. 62–71, 1981.
32. Alves AC, Alves NG, Ascari IJ, et al: Colostrum composition of Santa Inês sheep and passive transfer of immunity to lambs, *J Dairy Sci* 98:3706–3716, 2015.
33. Chadio S, Katsafadou A, Kotsampasi B, et al: Effects of maternal undernutrition during late gestation and/or lactation on colostrum synthesis and immunological parameters in the offspring, *Reprod Fertil Dev* 28:384–393, 2016.
34. McGuire TC, Regnier J, Kellom T, Gates NL: Failure in passive transfer of immunoglobulin G1 to lambs: measurement of immunoglobulin G1 in ewe colostrums, *Am J Vet Res* 44:1064–1067, 1983.
35. McGovern FM, Magee DA, Browne JA, MacHugh DE, Boland TM: Iodine supplementation of the pregnant dam alters intestinal gene expression and immunoglobulin uptake in the newborn lamb, *Animal* 10:598–606, 2016.
36. Castro-Alonso, A, Castro N, Capote, J, et al: Short communication: apoptosis regulates passive immune transfer in newborn kids, *J. Dairy Sci* 91:2086–2088, 2008.
37. Castro N, Capote J, Morales-Delanuez A, Rodríguez C, Argüello A: Effects of newborn characteristics and length of colostrum feeding period on passive immune transfer in goat kids, *J Dairy Sci* 92:1616–1619, 2009.
38. Berge AC, Hassid G, Leibovich H, Solomon D, Haines DM, Chamorro MF: A field trial evaluating the health and performance of lambs fed a bovine colostrum replacement, *J of Anim Res and Nutri* 3:1–4, 2018.
39. Oman RE, Streeter R, Taylor J, Gilliam L, Dawson L: Use of a digital Brix refractometer to estimate serum immunoglobulin in goat kids. *J Int Med* 32(6):2200, 2018. doi:10.1111/jvim.15319.
40. O'Brien JP, Sherman DM: Field methods for estimating serum immunoglobulin concentrations in newborn kids, *Small Rumin Res* 11:79–84, 1993.
41. Parkinson DE, Ellis RP, Lewis LD: Colostrum deficiency in mule deer fawns: identification, treatment and influence on neonatal mortality, *J Wildl Dis* 18:17–28, 1982.
42. Sawyer M, Willadsen CH, Osburn BI, McGuire TC: Passive transfer of colostral immunoglobulins from ewe to lamb and its influence on neonatal lamb mortality, *J Am Vet Med Assoc* 171:1255–1259, 1977.
43. Pisarska A, Stefaniak T, Poplawski M, et al: Transfer of maternal passive immunity to kids in goat herd, *Pol J Vet Sci* 5:251–255, 2002.
44. Shyu CL, Lin CC, Hsuan SL, Chiou SH, Chan JP: Suppurative meningitis in a 7-day-old Formosan sambar deer (*Cervus unicolor swinhoei*) caused by *Escherichia coli*, *Can Vet J* 51:308–310, 2010.
45. Hunter AG, Reneau JK, Williams JB: Factors affecting IgG concentration in day-old lambs, *J. Anim. Sci* 45:1146–1151, 1997.
46. Mellor DJ, Murray L: Effects of maternal nutrition on udder development during late pregnancy and on colostrum production in Scottish Blackface ewes with twin lambs, *Res Vet Sci* 39:230–234, 1985.
47. Hernández-Castellano LE, Morales-delaNuez A, Sánchez-Macías D, et al: The effect of colostrum source (goat vs. sheep) and timing of the first colostrum feeding (2h vs. 14h after birth) on body weight and immune status of artificially reared newborn lambs, *J Dairy Sci* 98:204–210, 2015.
48. Winter A: Bovine neonatal pancytopenia and anaemia in lambs caused by feeding cow colostrum, *Vet Rec* 168:84, 2011.
49. Weese JS, Kenney DG, O'Connor A: Secondary lactose intolerance in a neonatal goat, *J Am Vet Med Assoc* 217:372–375, 2000.
50. Carmalt JL, Baptiste KE, Naylor JM: Hypernatremia in neonatal elk calves: 30 cases (1988–1998), *J Am Vet Med Assoc* 216:68–70, 2000.
51. Theil KW, Grooms DL, McCloskey CM, Redman DR: Group B rotavirus associated with an outbreak of neonatal lamb diarrhea, *J Vet Diagn Invest* 7:148–150, 1995.
52. Theil KW, Lance SE, McCloskey CM: Rotaviruses associated with neonatal lamb diarrhea in two Wyoming shed-lambing operations, *J Vet Diagn Invest* 8:245–248, 1996.
53. Galindo-Cardiel I, Fernández-Jiménez M, Luján L, et al: Novel group A rotavirus G8 P[1] as primary cause of an ovine diarrheic syndrome outbreak in weaned lambs, *Vet Microbiol* 149:467–471, 2011.
54. Muñoz M, Alvarez M, Lanza I, Cármenes P: Role of enteric pathogens in the aetiology of neonatal diarrhoea in lambs and goat kids in Spain, *Epidemiol Infect* 117:203–211, 1996.
55. Martella V, Decaro N, Buonavoglia C: Enteric viral infections in lambs or kids, *Vet Microbiol* 181:154–160, 2015.
56. Arroyo LG, Rousseau JD, Staempfli HR, Weese JS: Suspected *Clostridium difficile*–associated hemorrhagic diarrhea in a 1-week-old elk calf, *Can Vet J* 46:1130–1131, 2005.
57. Ozmen O, Yukari BA, Haligur M, Sahinduran S: Observations and immunohistochemical detection of Coronavirus, *Cryptosporidium parvum* and *Giardia intestinalis* in neonatal diarrhoea in lambs and kids, *Schweiz Arch Tierheilkd* 148:357–364, 2006.
58. Castro-Hermida JA, Delafosse A, Pors I, Ares-Mazás E, Chartier C: *Giardia duodenalis* and *Cryptosporidium parvum* infections in adult goats and their implications for neonatal kids, *Vet Rec* 157:623–627, 2005.
59. French NP, Berriatua E, Kaya G, Morgan KL: Case control study of diarrhoea and faecal soiling in two- to six-month-old lambs, *Vet Rec* 143:408–412, 1998.
60. Giadinis ND, Symeoudakis S, Papadopoulos E, Lafi SQ, Karatzias H: Comparison of two techniques for diagnosis of cryptosporidiosis in diarrhoeic goat kids and lambs in Cyprus, *Trop Anim Health Prod* 44:1561–1565, 2012.
61. Smith G, Bertchold J: Fluid therapy in calves, *Vet Clin North Am FA Pract* 30:409–427, 2014.
62. Altmann K, Mukkur TK: Passive immunisation of neonatal lambs against infection with enteropathogenic *Escherichia coli* via colostrum of ewes immunised with crude and purified K99 pili, *Res Vet Sci* 35:234–239, 1983.
63. Rowe JD, East NE: Floppy kid syndrome (metabolic acidosis without dehydration in kids), *Proceedings of the 1998 Symposium on the Health and Disease of Small Ruminants Western Veterinary Conference*, Las Vegas, Nev, 1998.
64. Uzal FA, Vidal JE, McClane BA, Gurjar AA: *Clostridium perfringens* toxins involved in mammalian veterinary diseases, *Open Toxinology J* 2:24–42, 2010.
65. Kim HY, Byun JW, Roh IS, et al: First isolation of *Clostridium perfringens* type E from a goat with diarrhea, *Anaerobe* 22:141–143, 2013.
66. Songer JG: Clostridial enteric diseases of domestic animals, *Clin Microbiol Rev* 9:216–234, 1996.
67. Mignaqui AC, Marcellino RB, Ronco T, et al: Isolation and molecular characterization of *Clostridium perfringens* from healthy Merino lambs in Patagonia region, Argentina, *Anaerobe* 43:35–38, 2017.
68. McGowan B, Moulton JE, Rood SE: Lamb losses associated with *Clostridium perfringens* type A, *J Am Vet Med Assoc* 133:219–221, 1958.
69. Dennison AC, VanMetre DC, Callan RJ, Dinsmore P, Mason GL, Ellis RP: Hemorrhagic bowel syndrome in dairy cattle: 22 cases (1997–2000), *J Am Vet Med Assoc* 221:686–689, 2002.
70. Dray T: *Clostridium perfringens* type A and beta2 toxin associated with enterotoxemia in a 5-week-old goat, *Can Vet J* 45:251–253, 2004.

71. Embury-Hyatt CK, Wobeser G, Simko E, Woodbury MR: Investigation of a syndrome of sudden death, splenomegaly, and small intestinal hemorrhage in farmed deer, *Can Vet J* 46:702–708, 2005.
72. Sato Y, Matsuura S: Gastric mucormycosis in a sika deer (*Cervus nippon*) associated with proliferation of *Clostridium perfringens*, *J Vet Med Sci* 60:981–983, 1998.
73. Jelinski MD, Ribble CS, Chirino-Trejo M, Clark EG, Janzen ED: The relationship between the presence of *Helicobacter pylori*, *Clostridium perfringens* type A, *Campylobacter* spp, or fungi and fatal abomasal ulcers in unweaned beef calves, *Can Vet J* 36:379–382, 1995.
74. Meer RR, Songer JG: Multiplex PCR method for genotyping *Clostridium perfringens*, *Am J Vet Res* 58:702, 1997.
75. Garcia JP, Beingesser J, Fisher DJ, et al: The effect of *Clostridium perfringens* type C strain CN3685 and its isogenic beta toxin null mutant in goats, *Vet Microbiol* 157:412–419, 2012.
76. Sayeed S, Uzal FA, Fisher DJ, et al: Beta toxin is essential for the intestinal virulence of *Clostridium perfringens* type C disease isolate CN3685 in a rabbit ileal loop model, *Mol Microbiol* 67:15–30, 2008.
77. Alexander TL, Buxton D, Buxton D: Clostridial diseases, In Alexander TL, Buxton D, editors: *Management and diseases of deer*, ed 2, 1994, Veterinary Deer Society, pp 121–123.
78. Mackintosh CG: Vaccines for control, prevention and eradication of disease in farmed deer, In *Proceedings of a deer course for veterinarians*, deer branch of the New Zealand veterinary association, Vol. 9, 1992, Methuen, MA, pp 92–97.
79. Fernandez-Miyakawa ME, Sayeed S, Fisher DJ, et al: Development and application of an oral challenge mouse model for studying *Clostridium perfringens* type D infection, *Infect Immun* 75:4282–4288, 2007.
80. English AW: Enterotoxaemia caused by *Clostridium perfringens* type D in farmed fallow deer, *Aust Vet J* 62:320, 1985.
81. Salman MD, Dargatz DA, Kimberling CV, Reif JS, Hopper GE: Rates of diseases and their associated costs in two Colorado sheep feedlots (1985–1986), *J Am Vet Med Assoc* 193:1518–1523, 1988.
82. Debien E, Hélie P, Buczinski S, Lebœuf A, Bélanger D, Drolet R: Proportional mortality: a study of 152 goats submitted for necropsy from 13 goat herds in Quebec, with a special focus on caseous lymphadenitis, *Can Vet J* 54:581–587, 2013.
83. Uzal FA, Kelly WR, Morris WE, Bermudez J, Biasón M: The pathology of experimental *Clostridium perfringens* type D enterotoxemia in sheep, *J Vet Diagn Investig* 16:403–411, 2004.
84. Uzal FA, Kelly WR: Enterotoxaemia in goats: a review, *Vet Res Comm* 20:481–492, 1996.
85. Uzal FA, Songer JG: Diagnosis of *Clostridium perfringens* intestinal infections in sheep and goats, *J Vet Diagn Invest* 20:253–265, 2008.
86. Ali Nasir A, Younus M, Rashid A, et al: Clinico-pathological findings of *Clostridium perfringens* type D enterotoxaemia in goats and its hemolytic activity in different erythrocytes, *Iran J Vet Res* 16:94–99, 2015.
87. Uzal FA, Kelly FA: Experimental *Clostridium perfringens* type D enterotoxemia in goats, *Vet Pathol* 35:142, 1998.
88. Blackwell TE: Clinical signs, treatments, and postmortem lesions in dairy goats with enterotoxemia: 13 cases (1979–1982), *J Am Vet Med Assoc* 200:214, 1992.
89. Garcia JP, Adams V, Beingesser J, et al: Epsilon toxin is essential for the virulence of *Clostridium perfringens* type D infection in sheep, goats, and mice, *Infect Immun* 81:2405–2414, 2013.
90. Filho EJF, Carvalho A, Assis, RA, et al: Clinicopathologic features of experimental *Clostridium perfringens* type D enterotoxemia in cattle, *Vet Pathol* 46:121–123, 2009.
91. Uzal FA, Fisher DJ, Saputo J, et al: Ulcerative enterocolitis in two goats associated with enterotoxin- and beta2 toxin-positive *Clostridium perfringens* type D, *J Vet Diagn Invest* 20:668–672, 2008.
92. Odendaal MW, Visser JJ, Botha WJ, Prinsloo H: The passive protection of lambs against *Clostridium perfringens* type D with semi-purified hyperimmune serum, *Onderstepoort J Vet Res* 55:47–50, 1988.
93. Armstrong HL, Macnamee JK: Blackleg in deer, *J Am Vet Med Assoc* 117:212–214, 1950.
94. Mackintosh C, Haigh JC, Griffin F: Bacterial diseases of farmed deer and bison, *Rev Sci Tech* 21:249–263, 2002.
95. Voigt K, Dagleish MP, Finlayson J, Beresford G, Foster G: Black disease in a forest reindeer (*Rangifer tarandus fennicus*), *Vet Rec* 165: 352–353, 2009.
96. Hjerpe CA: Bovine vaccines and herd vaccination programs, *Vet Clin North Am Food Anim Pract* 6:167–260, 1990.
97. Hatheway CL: Toxigenic clostridia, *Clin Microbiol Rev* 3:66–98, 1990.
98. Busch C, Schömig K, Hofmann F, Aktories K: Characterization of the catalytic domain of Clostridium novyi alpha-toxin, *Infect Immun* 68:6378–6383, 2000.
99. Hamid ME, Mohamed GE, Abu Samra MT, Hamad AA: First report of infectious necrotic hepatitis (black disease) among Nubian goats in Sudan, *Rev Elev Med Vet Pays Trop* 44:273–275, 1991.
100. Songer JG: *Clostridium novyi* (myonecrosis, black disease, and bacillary hemoglobinuria) and *Clostridium septicum* (braxy) infections, In Anderson DE, Rings DM editors: *Current veterinary therapy food animal practice*, ed 5, St Louis, MO, 2009, Saunders Elsevier, pp 58–61.
101. Hamid ME, Mohamed GE, Abu Samra MT, Hamad AA: First report of infectious necrotic hepatitis (black disease) among Nubian goats in Sudan, *Rev Elev Med Vet Pays Trop* 44:273, 1991.
102. Stalker MJ, Hayes MA: Liver and biliary system. In *Pathology of domestic animals*, vol 2, ed 5, St Louis, MO, 2007, Saunders Elsevier, pp 297–388.
103. Olander HJ, Hughes JP, Biberstein EL: Bacillary hemoglobinuria: induction by liver biopsy in naturally and experimentally infected animals, *Pathol Vet* 3:421, 1966.
104. Bender LC, Hall PB, Garner MM, Oaks JL: Bacillary hemoglobinuria in a free-ranging elk calf. *J Zoo Wildl Med* 30:293–296, 1999.
105. Vine N, Fayer J, Harwood D: Bacillary hemoglobinuria in dairy cows, *Vet Rec* 159:160, 2006.
106. Randhawa SS, Sharma DK, Randhawa CS, Gill BS, Brar RS, Singh J: An outbreak of bacillary haemoglobinuria in sheep in India, *Trop Anim Health Prod* 27:31–36, 1995.
107. Takagi M, Yamato O, Sasaki Y, et al: Successful treatment of bacillary hemoglobinuria in Japanese Black cows, *J Vet Med Sci* 71: 1105, 2009.
108. Ellis TM, Rowe JB, Lloyd JM: Acute abomasitis due to *Clostridium septicum* infection in experimental sheep, *Aust Vet J* 60:308–309, 1983.
109. Sasaki Y, Yamamoto K, Kojima A, Norimatsu M, Tamura Y: Rapid identification and differentiation of pathogenic clostridia in gas gangrene by polymerase chain reaction based on the 16S-23S rDNA spacer region, *Res Vet Sci* 69:289–294, 2000.
110. Eustis SL, Bergeland ME: Suppurative abomasitis associated with *Clostridium septicum* infection, *J Am Vet Med Assoc* 178:732, 1981.
111. Glastonbury JR, Searson JE, Links IJ, Tuckett LM: Clostridial myocarditis in lambs, *Aust Vet J* 65:208–209, 1988.
112. Uzal FA, Paramidani M, Assis R, Morris W, Miyakawa MF: Outbreak of clostridial myocarditis in calves, *Vet Rec* 152:134–136, 2003.
113. Williams BM: Clostridial myositis in cattle: bacteriology and gross pathology, *Vet Rec* 100:90, 1977.
114. Troxel TR, Burke GL, Wallace WT, et al: Clostridial vaccination efficacy on stimulating and maintaining an immune response in beef cows and calves, *J Anim Sci* 75:19–25, 1997.
115. Reed GA, Reynolds L: Failure of *Clostridium chauvoei* vaccines to protect against blackleg, *Aust Vet J* 53:393, 1977.
116. Ruiz-Fons F, Rodriguez O, Torina A, et al: Prevalence of *Coxiella burnetti* infection in wild and farmed ungulates, *Vet Microbiol* 126(1–3):282–286, 2008
117. Gonzalez-Barrio D, Almeria S, Caro MR, et al: *Coxiella burnetii* shedding by farmed red deer (*Cervus elaphus*), *Transbound Emerg Dis* 62(5):572–574, 2015.

118. Salinas J, Caro MR, Vicente J, et al: High prevalence of antibodies against Chlamydiaceae and *Chlamydophila abortus* in wild ungulates using two "in house" blocking-ELISA tests, *Vet Microbiol* 135 (1–2):46–53, 2009.
119. Ayanegui-Alcerreca MA, Wilson PR, Mackintosh CG, et al: Regional seroprevalence of leptospirosis on deer farms in New Zealand, *N Z Vet J* 58(4):184–189, 2010.
120. Subharat S, Wilson PR, Heuer C, et al: Growth response and shedding of *Leptospira* spp. in urine following vaccination for leptospirosis in young farmed deer, *N Z Vet J* 60(1):14–20, 2012.
121. Hagan WA, Bruner DW, Timoney JF: *Corynebacterium pseudotuberculosis*. In Hagan WA, Bruner DW, Timoney JF, editors: *Hagan and bruner's microbiology and infectious diseases of domestic animals,* ed 8, Ithaca, NY, 1988, Comstock Publishing.
122. Sweeney RW, Collins MT, Koets AP, et al: Paratuberculosis (Johne's disease) in cattle and other susceptible species, *J Vet Intern Med* 26(6):1239–1250, 2012.
123. Reddacliff L, Eppleston J, Windsor P, et al: Efficacy of a killed vaccine for the control of paratuberculosis in Australian sheep flocks, *Vet Microbiol* 115(1–3):77–90, 2006.
124. Allison AB, Goekjian VH, Potgieter AC, et al: Detection of a novel reassortant epizootic hemorrhagic disease virus (EHDV) in the USA containing RNA segments derived from both exotic (EHDV-6) and endemic (EHDV-2) serotypes, *J Gen Virol* 91 (Pt 2):430–439, 2010.
125. Ruder MG, Johnson D, Ostlund E, et al: The First 10 Years (2006–15) of Epizootic hemorrhagic disease virus serotype 6 in the USA, *J Wildl Dis* 53(4):901–905, 2017.
126. Stevens G, McCluskey B, King A, et al: Review of the 2012 Epizootic hemorrhagic disease outbreak in domestic ruminants in the United States, *PLoS One* 10(8):e0133359, 2015.
127. Hagan WA, Bruner DW, Timoney JF: Peste des petits ruminants. In Hagan WA, Bruner DW, Timoney JF, editors: *Hagan and bruner's microbiology and infectious diseases of domestic animals,* ed 8, Ithaca, NY, 1988, Comstock Publishing.
128. Pisoni G, Bertoni G, Puricelli M, et al: Demonstration of coinfection with and recombination by caprine arthritis-encephalitis virus and maedi-visna virus in naturally infected goats, *J Virol* 81(10): 4948–4955, 2007.

17 Diseases of the Cardiovascular System

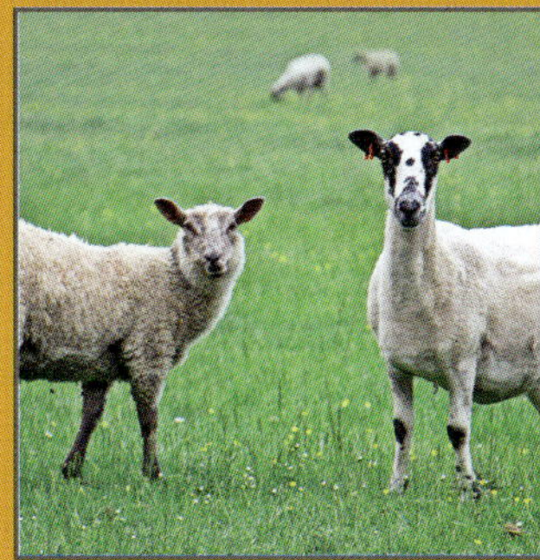

DANIEL K. NEWHARD†, JENNA E. BAYNE, AND THOMAS PASSLER

Examination of the Cardiovascular System

History

Thorough information about history and signalment helps to formulate an accurate differential diagnosis list and guides appropriate treatment. Breed, sex, use, and age can be predisposing factors to cardiovascular disease. For example, while clinical signs of cardiovascular disease in neonatal or juvenile patients are most likely caused by congenital heart disease, acutely developed clinical signs in adult animals suggest an acquired disease. The onset and duration of clinical signs help to distinguish cardiac from noncardiac conditions. Most conditions caused by left-sided cardiac decompensation have an acute onset. In contrast, noncardiac etiologies are more likely associated with chronic respiratory clinical signs. On the other hand, right-sided cardiac decompensation is typically more chronic, and associated clinical signs such as ascites and peripheral edema may be present for a longer duration. History of travel, feed, and housing environment are important since many environmental factors can lead to cardiovascular disease (plant and nutritional toxicities, nutritional deficiencies, and endemic infectious diseases). Information about the presence and nature of clinical signs in other herd members may suggest the presence of a common source or an infectious etiology.

Visual Examination

Visual examination of the animal can provide important information about cardiovascular health. The animal should be observed for overt signs of cardiovascular compromise, such as tachypnea, dyspnea, coughing, exercise intolerance, weakness, collapse, nasal discharge, abdominal distention, and peripheral edema. Interaction of the small ruminant with the examiner, handler, or other animals of the herd can suggest disease severity. Animals with severe cardiac disease, such as those in respiratory distress, may be disorientated and stop interacting with the surrounding environment. The size and growth rate of the animal should be noted, as neonatal or juvenile animals with significant cardiovascular disease tend to be smaller than their healthy cohorts. Cardiac cachexia is common in animals with significant cardiac disease, and body condition score and musculature should be noted. Occurrence of similar clinical signs in multiple herd members should be noted as they may suggest a common etiological source (feed or environmental toxicity, nutritional deficiency, or infectious disease).

Cardiac Auscultation

Cardiac auscultation allows detection of heart rate and rhythm, heart murmurs, and presence of pericardial disease. With some individual variation, the heart extends from the third to the fifth intercostal space. Prior to auscultation, both hemithoraces should be palpated simultaneously for the point of maximal intensity (PMI) at which the heartbeat is palpated most strongly. In normal animals, the PMI is located on the left hemithorax at the level of the mitral valve, which represents the apex of the heart. This usually coincides with the left fourth intercostal space. Certain cardiac conditions causing right-sided pathology (pulmonic stenosis, tetralogy of Fallot, and pulmonary hypertension) can shift the PMI to the right hemithorax. The semilunar valves are auscultated cranially and dorsally to the PMI on the left hemithorax, usually around the third intercostal space. This area represents the base of the heart. Palpation of the base of the heart is important for detection of congenital cardiac defects such as semilunar valve pathology, atrial septal defects (ASDs), and ventricular septal defects. An arterial pulse should be palpated simultaneously with cardiac auscultation, if possible. Systole coincides with the arterial pulse, so concurrently palpating an arterial pulse may aid in matching auscultation abnormalities (heart murmurs and/or irregular rhythms) with the appropriate phase of the cardiac cycle.

There are four main heart sounds: S1, S2, S3, and S4. S1 and S2 are the two heart sounds that can be auscultated most reliably, but S3 and S4 may not be present or may not be heard unless hemodynamic or pathologic processes are present. Tensing and closure of the atrioventricular valve (AV) apparatuses lead to the generation of the first heart sound, S1. This sound is usually heard most loudly over the left apex, coinciding with the mitral valve. Tensing and closure of the semilunar valves generate the S2 heart sound, coinciding with the end of ventricular systole. S3 and S4 cannot be auscultated in most ruminants, but when present, cardiac pathology should be suspected. These sounds are referred to as gallop sounds and occur during diastole. S3 is generated by rapid ventricular filling at the beginning of diastole and is

†Deceased

associated with ventricular systolic dysfunction with dilation of the affected ventricle. S4 is generated by atrial contraction, with blood entering a noncompliant or dilated ventricle. S4 is most often heard in animals with significant ventricular diastolic dysfunction, such as those with restrictive cardiomyopathy or constrictive pericarditis.

Muffled Heart Sounds. The heart sounds can be dampened, or muffled, when attenuated by structures between the stethoscope and the heart. While blood transmits vibrations generated by the heart very well, other fluids, tissues, air, and bone attenuate cardiac vibrations. Body habitus and age can affect the acoustics of the heart sounds. Large depositions of adipose tissue, thick skin, and thick musculature can attenuate heart sounds. Fluid between the stethoscope and the heart, such as subcutaneous edema, pleural effusion, and pericardial effusion, can muffle heart sounds. Gas accumulation, associated with subcutaneous emphysema, pneumothorax, and pneumopericardium, can muffle heart sounds. Similarly, abnormal soft tissue structures or solidification of tissues, such as cutaneous or subcutaneous masses, pulmonary masses, pneumonia, pulmonary edema, pulmonary abscesses or granulomas, and pulmonary hemorrhage can lead to attenuation of heart sounds.

Cardiac Murmurs. Cardiac murmurs are auditory vibrations caused by turbulent and/or high-velocity blood flow within the heart or great vessels. Flow velocity, vessel size, and blood viscosity have an impact on the generation of heart murmurs. The timing of a murmur can be systolic, diastolic, or continuous. Systolic murmurs are present at the start of or within the S1 to S2 interval. Diastolic murmurs are present at the start of or within the interval from S2 to the subsequent S1 sound. Simultaneous palpation of the arterial pulse aids in distinguishing systolic and diastolic murmurs. Peripheral arterial pulses can help determine hemodynamic status. Depending on the size of the animal, the femoral, transverse facial, and brachial arteries are the most appropriate peripheral arteries for palpation in ruminants. The femoral artery is located in the inguinal region of the pelvic limbs within the femoral triangle and is often the most consistently palpable peripheral artery in sheep.[1] The transverse facial artery crosses superficially over the ramus of the mandible and is palpable midway between the ventral aspect of the mandible and the temporomandibular joint.[2] The brachial artery may be palpable along the midline on the medial aspect of the brachium of the thoracic limbs.[2] The arterial pulse occurs with systole, and murmurs heard concurrently with palpation of the arterial pulse are systolic. A diastolic murmur is heard between palpated arterial pulses. A continuous heart murmur is one heard throughout all of systole and diastole, with no clear demarcation between the two phases of the cardiac cycle. To-and-fro murmurs are uncommon but can be confused with continuous heart murmurs. To-and-fro murmurs have a systolic and diastolic component, either from the same valve or two different cardiac lesions during the same cardiac cycle, and can occur with severe infective valvular endocarditis, which can cause turbulent blood flow in systole and significant aortic regurgitation during diastole.

Murmurs can be divided into physiologic (functional) and pathologic categories. Physiologic murmurs are present in hyperdynamic states, usually due to increased cardiac output. These conditions include pain, excitement, fever, pregnancy, lactation, anemia, and iatrogenic fluid overload. Physiologic murmurs are usually mild to moderate in intensity, systolic, and heard most loudly over the left base since they are caused by increased velocity across the semilunar valves during systole. The location of the heart murmur suggests the area of the heart affected. While apical murmurs include those associated with the AVs, basilar murmurs include those associated with the semilunar valves or sometimes with atrial and ventricular septal defects. A congenital defect is most likely the cause of a murmur in neonatal or juvenile animals (Table 17.1), whereas acquired cardiac disease is more likely in adult animals with a newly developed murmur (Table 17.2).

Pathology of one or both of the AVs can cause an acquired apical systolic heart murmur. Valvular endocarditis most commonly affects the AVs, especially the tricuspid valve leaflets in small ruminants and cervids.[1,3–5] Although endocarditis of either valve can alter the morphology and function of the valve, a murmur may or may not be present. In sheep and deer, endocarditis may be associated with polyarthritis, with *Erysipelothrix rhusiopathiae* and *Streptococcus* species having been isolated in sheep.[3] The vegetative lesions may become sufficiently severe to cause right-sided congestive heart failure (CHF), but despite the presence of clinical signs of valvular endocarditis, cases may not be diagnosed until postmortem examination.[1,4,5] Acquired basilar systolic heart murmurs can be associated with endocarditic lesions on either of the semilunar valves, with the aortic valve being most commonly affected.[6] If sufficiently severe, significant aortic regurgitation can occur, causing a diastolic murmur as well. Calcification of the semilunar valve cusps may be associated with ingestion of plants with high 1,25 dihydroxycholecalciferol concentrations,[7,8] which, while rare in small ruminants and cervids, should prompt a nutritional analysis when encountered.

TABLE 17.1 Congenital Cardiac Lesions and Their Associated Heart Murmurs and Natural Outcomes in Small Ruminants and Deer.

Lesion	Murmur Side	Murmur Location	Murmur Timing	Natural Outcome[a]
Ventricular septal defect*	Right > left	Base > Apex	Systolic	L-CHF
Tetralogy of Fallot	Left	Base	Systolic	R-CHF, polycythemia
Patent ductus arteriosus	Left	Base	Continuous	L-CHF
Mitral valve dysplasia	Left	Apex	Systolic	L-CHF
Tricuspid valve dysplasia	Right	Apex	Systolic	R-CHF
Atrial septal defect*	Right > left	Base	Systolic	L-CHF

*, Left-to-right shunting; *L-CHF*, left-sided congestive heart failure; *R-CHF*, right-sided congestive heart failure
[a]Represents most severe form of each condition; patients with mild or moderate forms may be asymptomatic.

TABLE 17.2 Acquired Cardiac Lesions and Their Associated Heart Murmurs and Natural Outcomes in Small Ruminants and Deer.

Lesion	Murmur Side	Murmur Location	Murmur Timing	Natural Outcome[a]
Tricuspid valve degeneration/endocarditis	Right	Apex	Systolic	R-CHF
Aortic valve endocarditis[b]	Left	Base	Systolic	L-CHF
Aortic valve calcification	Left	Base	Systolic	L-CHF
Mitral valve degeneration	Left	Apex	Systolic	L-CHF

L-CHF, left-sided congestive heart failure; *R-CHF*, right-sided congestive heart failure.
[a]Represents most severe form of each condition; patients with mild or moderate forms may be asymptomatic.
[b]Severe aortic valvular endocarditis may also cause a diastolic murmur due to severe aortic insufficiency.

Auscultating Arrhythmias. In addition to evaluating for heart murmurs, cardiac auscultation also provides valuable information regarding the cardiac rhythm. Premature ectopic beats can be heard and substantiated via concurrent arterial pulse palpation. During premature ectopic beats, there is usually an arterial pulse deficit associated with that beat. Although auscultation and arterial pulse palpation can diagnose premature ectopic beats, these alone cannot differentiate atrial from ventricular premature beats—an electrocardiogram is required to make this distinction.

Bradyarrhythmias can be caused by electrolyte imbalances and structural pathology to the cardiac conduction system. Alterations in calcium, potassium, and magnesium are the electrolytes that tend to have the strongest effect on cardiac rhythm. Changes to the conduction system can be due to fibrosis and/or infiltrative disease (infection, inflammation, and neoplasia).

Tachycardia can be caused by excitement, stress, fever, pain, hypovolemia, electrolyte derangements, toxins, systemic disease (gastrointestinal disease, infection, or inflammation), anemia, and primary cardiac disease. A thorough history of travel and environmental factors (toxins in feed, exposure to toxic plants, etc.) should be recorded. As with bradyarrhythmias, blood electrolyte concentrations should be measured when persistent or paroxysmal tachycardia is present. In animals with clinical signs associated with an arrhythmia (episodic weakness, lethargy, or syncope), it is recommended to auscultate for prolonged periods of time, because some arrhythmias, especially tachyarrhythmias, can be paroxysmal and easily missed during abbreviated auscultation. Once electrolyte derangements are ruled out in patients with a bradyarrhythmia or tachyarrhythmia, echocardiography is warranted to assess the potential for structural cardiac disease. If echocardiography does not demonstrate overt structural disease, measuring serum cardiac troponin I (cTnI) is recommended (see later), as myocarditis can cause significant arrhythmias.

Pericardial Friction Rubs. Pericardial friction rubs are extra sounds created by the rubbing together of the parietal and visceral pericardial layers. In normal animals, the movement of these layers is inaudible. When the layers are inflamed, they no longer interact smoothly and friction is created. This results in audible sounds, which can occur in synchrony with the heartbeat, during both phases of respiration, and/or between breaths. Occurrence between breaths differentiates pericardial from pleural friction rubs, which are auscultated only during respiration. The most common cause of pericardial friction rubs in small ruminants is infectious pericarditis, but noninfectious inflammatory and idiopathic pericarditis can occur.

Peripheral Arterial Pulses

The locations for peripheral arterial pulse palpation were previously discussed. Decreased cardiac output and systemic hypotension are common causes of weak arterial pulses. Obstructive lesions, such as thrombi or tumors, can also cause weak or absent arterial pulses. In cases of weak arterial pulses occurring secondary to decreased cardiac output or hypotension, all palpable peripheral arterial pulses are expected to be weak, as these conditions affect the cardiovascular system as a whole.

Hyperdynamic pulses, also called bounding or "water-hammer" pulses, are caused by conditions causing a larger difference between the systolic and diastolic pressure. Hyperdynamic pulses occur most commonly with diseases causing a significant decrease in diastolic pressures, such as patent ductus arteriosus (PDA), significant aortic insufficiency, and the hyperdynamic phase of shock.

Pulsus paradoxus describes an abnormally large decrease in cardiac output and peripheral pulse strength during the respiratory cycle in cases of cardiac tamponade and constrictive pericarditis. Normally, preload to the right side of the heart increases slightly during inspiration, which decreases flow to the left side of the heart. This causes a decrease in systemic cardiac output during inspiration. This pattern is reversed during expiration, causing an increase in cardiac output and peripheral pulse strength.

As previously discussed, peripheral arterial pulse deficits can be palpated during ectopic beats. Because of the abbreviated interval between the normal beat and subsequent premature beat, diastolic filling is decreased. This leads to decreased cardiac output during the following systolic phase, creating an arterial pulse deficit during the ectopic beat.

Mucous Membranes

Evaluation of the mucous membranes can be performed to assess hydration and perfusion status. It also provides information on potential clinicopathologic abnormalities, such as anemia or icterus. Mucous membranes most commonly evaluated include the buccal, scleral, conjunctival, and vulvar or preputial mucous membranes.

Capillary Refill Time. Capillary refill time (CRT) helps to assess perfusion, although it is somewhat insensitive for determining cardiac output and tissue perfusion status accurately. CRT can be decreased in patients in hyperdynamic states, and the mucous membranes may appear injected due to peripheral vasodilation.

Causes include those of both benign and malignant etiologies, such as excitement, stress, fever, and hyperdynamic shock. In these conditions, concurrent tachycardia would be expected. CRT can be prolonged in patients with decreased tissue perfusion and hypodynamic shock. Since CRT can be insensitive as a one-time diagnostic measurement, serial evaluation of CRT may be more useful in determining the efficacy of treatment.

Pale Mucous Membranes. Pale mucous membranes usually indicate anemia or decreased tissue perfusion. White mucous membranes are suggestive of significant anemia and/or significantly decreased tissue perfusion.

Dark Mucous Membranes. Dark red or muddy mucous membranes can signify polycythemia. Right-to-left shunts should be considered in young patients with polycythemia, as chronic hypoxia associated with these shunts stimulates increased release of erythropoietin. Severe polycythemia may cause petechiae and ecchymosis of the mucous membranes. Methemoglobinemia causes the mucous membranes to become brown in color.

Icteric Mucous Membranes. Icteric, or yellow-colored, mucous membranes are caused by the accumulation of bilirubin. Prehepatic, hepatic, and posthepatic causes of hyperbilirubinemia should be considered, although prehepatic (hemolysis) causes are most common in small ruminants.[9] Icterus develops once bilirubin exceeds 2 mg/dL.[10]

Cyanotic Mucous Membranes. Cyanosis (blue or purple coloring of the mucous membranes) is indicative of decreased concentrations of oxygenated hemoglobin. The degree of cyanosis is dependent on the concentration of deoxyhemoglobin, and cyanosis usually occurs only once deoxyhemoglobin concentrations exceed 5 g/dL. Animals with significant anemia cannot develop cyanosis due to an insufficient amount of hemoglobin. Cyanosis can be categorized as central or peripheral. Central cyanosis is caused by arterial hypoxemia and usually presents as generalized cyanosis. In this condition, all mucous membranes (those of the cranial and caudal aspects of the body) are expected to be cyanotic. Causes include right-to-left shunts, ventilation-perfusion mismatch, diffusion impairment, hypoventilation, and inspiration of air with low oxygen concentrations. A right-to-left PDA classically causes "differential cyanosis," with the mucous membranes of the head being normal in color, while the mucous membranes of the caudal half of the body (vulvar or preputial) are cyanotic. A congenital cardiac defect causing right-to-left shunting should be considered in any neonatal or juvenile patient that has persistent hypoxemia despite supplemental oxygen therapy.

Peripheral cyanosis refers to the cyanosis of the distal extremities, including the limbs and ear pinnae. Peripheral cyanosis is caused by pooling of blood in the venous system and/or decreased arterial blood flow. Decreased arterial blood flow is most often caused by significantly decreased cardiac output (valvular regurgitation and/or cardiac dysfunction), local vasoconstriction (during hypothermia and states of shock), and arterial obstruction (thromboembolism and neoplasia). Unlike patients with central cyanosis, those with peripheral cyanosis are expected to have normal arterial oxygen saturation. Since some causes of peripheral cyanosis can lead to regional arterial hypoxemia, peripheral blood collection at affected sites may lead to inaccurate results. These results provide the local arterial oxygen saturation but may not represent systemic saturation. Therefore, peripheral arterial blood sampling should be performed from an unaffected area in patients with peripheral cyanosis, if possible.

Hydration Status

Hydration status can also be assessed by evaluating the mucous membranes. Dry and tacky mucous membranes are often associated with at least 5 to 7% dehydration. Assessing the hydration status based on mucous membrane quality is subjective and may not accurately represent the severity of dehydration. Therefore, other clinical indications of dehydration should be evaluated concurrently (see Chapter 3).

Venous Pressures

Jugular venous pulses, ascites, and peripheral edema can all be caused by increased venous pressures. Among cardiogenic causes, pericardial disease, *cor pulmonale*, tricuspid valve disease, right ventricular dysfunction, left-sided cardiac disease, and arrhythmias can lead to right-sided CHF.

Chronic inflammation of the pericardium, due to chronic infection, neoplasia, or chronic pericardial and pleural effusions, can lead to constrictive pericarditis. Constrictive pericarditis has a profound effect on diastolic filling and, when compromised, severely affects cardiac output. Since the heart cannot fill appropriately, constrictive pericarditis often leads to right-sided CHF.

Cor pulmonale is defined as right-sided cardiac disease secondary to pulmonary pathology. Various pulmonary pathologies can lead to pulmonary hypertension, which then leads to right-sided cardiac remodeling. All causes of pulmonary pathology leading to pulmonary hypertension, except those associated with left-sided cardiac disease, can be categorized under cor pulmonale. Pneumonia, pulmonary vasculitis, parasitic infestation, neoplasia, pulmonary thromboembolism, chronic hypoxia, and chronic lower airway disease can all cause cor pulmonale.[8,11] Identifying cor pulmonale is important so that appropriate treatment for pulmonary pathology, as well as supportive care for the cardiac changes, is initiated.

Left-sided cardiac disease can lead to right-sided CHF. Reactive pulmonary arterial vasoconstriction occurs with significant left-sided cardiac disease, causing pulmonary hypertension. Therefore, left-sided cardiac disease should be considered in any patient with signs of right-sided CHF.

Bradyarrhythmias and tachyarrhythmias can both lead to increased venous pressures and subsequent right-sided CHF. Chronic bradycardia can lead to cardiomegaly due to a reduction in cardiac output from the right side of the heart, increasing intracardiac pressures, and preventing appropriate cardiac filling from the systemic venous system. Tachycardia can lead to right-sided CHF by not allowing appropriate diastolic filling time. Thus, venous return to the heart is compromised and decompensation occurs. Controlling the underlying arrhythmia is imperative in adequately controlling fluid accumulation in these circumstances.

Jugular Venous Pulses. The presence and quality of jugular venous pulses can be used to assess venous pressures. In normal, standing animals with the head held in a neutral position, jugular venous pulsations can be detected extending one third up the neck. Jugular pulsations that extend greater than one third up the neck toward the mandible are an indication of increased venous pressures. Jugular venous pulsations should not be assessed if the head is held in a lowered position, which causes venous pooling. While the lack of a jugular pulses suggests hypovolemia, an obvious jugular pulse may not be noticeable in some normal patients. In normal animals, central venous pressure decreases slightly during inspiration. This phenomenon is absent in cases of constrictive pericarditis because intrathoracic pressure changes during the respiratory cycle are not translated to the cardiac chambers. Therefore, venous pressure actually increases during inspiration, causing pronounced jugular pulses during inspiration. This is termed *Kussmaul's sign* and is indicative of constrictive pericarditis.

Ascites. Ascites caused by primary cardiovascular disease occurs due to increased hepatic sinusoidal hydrostatic pressures, which can damage the endothelium, increase membrane permeability, and lead to effusion. Hepatic sinusoids have a fenestrated, discontinuous endothelium and lack a typical basement membrane, which predispose to increased permeability.[10] Abdominal ballottement and/or ultrasonography can be performed to determine if ascites is present. Once ascites is confirmed, a hepatojugular reflex test can be performed as a quick method to determine if ascites is due to increased intravascular hydrostatic pressure (right-sided CHF). The hepatojugular reflex test is performed by applying compression to the abdomen in a cranial direction (toward the liver) and holding the compression for 20 to 30 seconds. If the ascites is due to increased intravascular hydrostatic pressure, the increased pressures in the abdomen increase intravascular hydrostatic pressure in the jugular veins, causing engorgement and potentially abnormal pulsation of the jugular veins. Ascites secondary to increased intravascular hydrostatic pressure can compromise venous return from the gastrointestinal organs. Gastric and/or intestinal edema can be present, which can lead to nausea, gastroenteritis, and even malabsorptive/maldigestive conditions. Significant ascites also pushes the diaphragm cranially and can impair appropriate respiratory function. When ascites is caused by other etiologies (metabolic conditions, vasculitides, lymphatic abnormalities, peritonitis, etc.), caution must be exercised if drainage is considered, since depletion of fluids, proteins, and electrolytes can occur rapidly.

Peripheral Edema. While often associated with noncardiac conditions, such as intestinal parasitism, peripheral edema is a common sign of right-sided CHF, and all of the cardiac and pericardial causes previously discussed should be considered when peripheral edema is present. The edema usually accumulates in gravity-dependent areas, such as the distal limbs, submandibular region, ventral thorax, ventral abdomen, and prepuce. As described earlier, cor pulmonale and left-sided cardiac disease can manifest as right-sided CHF; therefore, primary pulmonary pathology and left-sided cardiac disease should be considered in animals with peripheral edema.

Pleural Effusion. Pleural effusion can be caused by right-sided CHF but may not always cause clinical signs. A significant amount of pleural effusion can cause tachypnea and dyspnea, but in most cases, a subclinical volume is detected and other clinical signs and physical examination findings are used to determine a potential etiology. Many noncardiac etiologies may also cause of pleural effusion, and additional diagnostic tests are recommended to determine the most likely cause.

Left-Sided Congestive Heart Failure

Left-sided CHF occurs due to increased left atrial pressure and subsequent increased pulmonary capillary hydrostatic pressure. In the early stages of pulmonary edema, fluid remains in the interstitial space, but as the disease progresses, alveolar flooding can occur. This allows edema to leak into the airways and presents as oral and/or nasal discharge. Clinical signs associated with pulmonary edema in small ruminants include tachypnea, dyspnea, coughing, and oral and/or nasal discharge. This discharge can be clear, serosanguinous, foamy, and/or mucoid. As discussed, significant left-sided cardiac disease can manifest as right-sided CHF, so jugular venous pulses, ascites, and peripheral edema may be present. Causes of left-sided CHF include those of congenital and acquired origin. Congenital diseases leading to left-sided cardiac decompensation include abnormalities associated with the aortic valve and mitral valve, atrial or ventricular septal defects, and PDA. Acquired cardiac diseases leading to left-sided cardiac decompensation include infective valvular endocarditis and myocarditis of various etiologies.

Cardiogenic Weakness, Exercise Intolerance, and Syncope

Significantly decreased cardiac output can cause weakness, exercise intolerance, and syncope. Cardiac conditions leading to these signs include arrhythmias, pulmonary hypertension, and systemic hypertension. Syncope is defined as a transient loss of consciousness due to decreased perfusion to the brain. Episodic weakness and "presyncope" are terms sometimes used when animals are ataxic, and may even collapse, but never completely lose consciousness. Syncope can mimic neurologic disease. Seizure-like activity, such as paddling, opisthotonos, urination, and defecation can be seen in cardiogenic syncope as well as with primary neurologic diseases. If the episode is not witnessed by the examiner, an accurate history of the event is crucial. Primary neurologic seizures usually include a postictal phase, with animals showing prolonged disorientation and/or ataxia. A postictal phase is not expected in animals with cardiogenic syncope. As a caveat, prolonged cerebral hypoperfusion due to decreased cardiac output can cause direct neurologic side effects, mimicking a postictal phase. Neurocardiogenic (vasovagal) syncope and myotonia congenita (fainting goat syndrome) can also mimic cardiogenic syncope, although the latter is often associated with a stiff gait and generalized muscle contractions immediately prior to occurrence.[8]

Myocarditis

Myocarditis can be caused by multiple etiologies, including infectious, immune mediated, toxic, neoplastic, and idiopathic. The inflammation can cause arrhythmias and/or cardiac dysfunction (systolic and diastolic) via disruption of the cardiac electrical conduction system and structural damage to the myocytes, respectively. Although history, electrocardiographic (ECG), and/or echocardiographic findings may suggest myocarditis, a definitive diagnosis requires myocardial biopsy. Thus, it is difficult to obtain a diagnosis with routine, noninvasive tests. Because of this, the use of biomarkers has become more frequent in these species. Cardiac biomarkers allow noninvasive diagnosis of cardiac abnormalities, with plasma cTnI concentrations being used most often for the detection of myocarditis. cTnI is specific to the myocardiocytes and is released into circulation with myocardial cell injury or necrosis, which occurs with myocarditis. cTnI assays have been validated in small ruminant and cervid species, with concentrations less than 0.02 ng/mL considered normal in healthy adult animals of these species.[12–15] cTnI is increased in small ruminants with congenital cardiac defects and myocarditis of various etiologies and can increase during routine and complicated pregnancies and parturition for both the dam and offspring.[14–17] The age of the animal should be taken into consideration when interpreting cTnI concentrations, as levels are increased in newborn goat kids.[14] Due to the apparent differences in reference ranges in age groups, life stages, and species, cTnI concentrations should be compared to appropriately matched controls when possible. Plasma cTnI concentrations can provide valuable information as to the presence of myocarditis but do not insinuate a specific cause of the myocarditis. Therefore, ancillary diagnostic tests should be used in combination with plasma cTnI concentrations to determine a specific cause.

Electrocardiography

ECG records the electrical potentials generated by the heart and is useful in diagnosing cardiac arrhythmias and conduction disturbances. Electrodes can be adhered to the animal via alligator clips, small (21–23 gauge) needles, or electrode pads. When using needles, the needle should be inserted through the dermis, or deeper, for appropriate securement. The use of alcohol and conductive gel on each electrode is recommended. Shaving the skin at the attachment location of each electrode reduces artifacts and improves accuracy of tracings. ECG tracings can be recorded in the right lateral or standing positions, as body position has not been shown to result in significant changes on the ECG.[18]

There are two common methods for acquiring ECG recordings based on positioning of the electrodes: the base-apex lead method and the six-lead method using bipolar standard and augmented unipolar limb leads (Figure 17.1). Using the base-apex lead method, lead I usually shows the best tracing, but there is some individual variation. For the six-lead method, the electrodes are usually placed just proximal to the elbow and stifle joints, but they can be moved proximally or distally on the limbs to reduce artifacts. The method of ECG recording affects the amplitudes and durations of the ECG waveforms (Figure 17.2).[19] In sheep and goats, the P wave is usually positive in lead II but can be negative in normal animals, and the T wave is usually of opposite polarity of the major QRS deflection.[18,20] Respiratory sinus arrhythmia is common in goats, with occasional instances of second-degree AV block type 1 and wandering pacemaker, suggesting that vagal tone is dominant in this species.[18,21]

Age, breed, and species should be considered when evaluating intervals, amplitudes, and durations of the ECG waveforms. Although mostly similar, there are some significant differences in ECG parameters between sheep and goats.[20] Age has a strong influence on ECG parameters in sheep and goats and affects the heart rate, PR interval, QT interval, QRS amplitude, and T-wave amplitude being dependent on age.[18,22] There is also considerable variation between breeds, especially in the QRS pattern. This normal variation is thought to be due to differences in topographic anatomy of the heart within the thorax, position of the heart related to the limbs, variability of the size and shape of the heart, and subtle changes in the mechanism of ventricular activation. P-wave polarity and morphology can also vary, as positive, inverted, and notched P waves have been reported in normal sheep and goats.[20,23] Because of these differences, it is recommended that the practitioner use species-, age-, and breed-matched reference ranges for all ECG parameters recorded.

ECG Intervals and Waveforms. Each waveform on the ECG represents activation of specific areas or chambers of the heart, as discussed in the following.

P wave—represents atrial depolarization; firing of the sinoatrial node is not detected on the surface ECG.

PR interval—corresponds to conduction through the bundle of His.

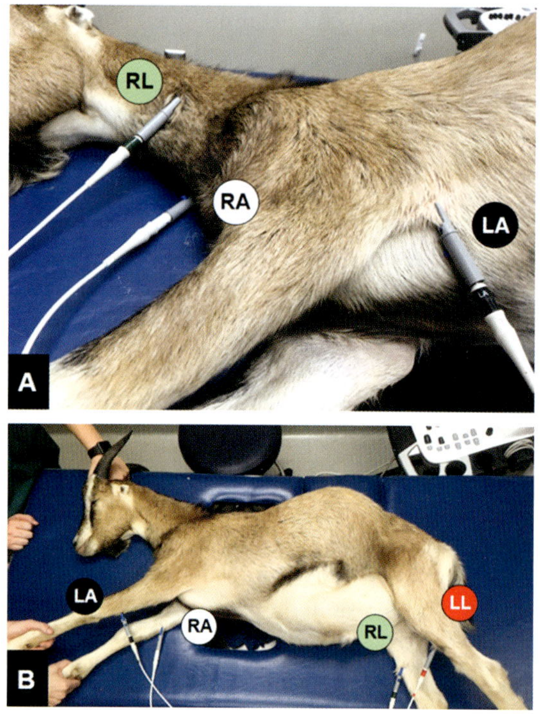

• **Fig. 17.1 A.** Electrode placement for the base-apex lead configuration in an awake, 1-year-old LaMancha buck in right lateral recumbency. Positive electrode (left arm, *LA*) is placed at the level of the apex beat on the left thorax, the negative electrode (right arm, *RA*) is placed in the right jugular furrow in the caudal third of the neck, and the third electrode (right leg, *RL*, or left leg, *LL*) is placed remotely from the heart. **B.** Electrode placement for the limb lead configuration in the same goat. Positive electrode is placed on the left thoracic limb, the negative electrode is placed on the right thoracic limb, the red electrode (*LL*, left leg) is placed on the left pelvic limb, and the green electrode (*RL*, right leg) is placed on the right pelvic limb.

QRS complex—represents ventricular depolarization and is variable within and between species and breeds.

T wave—represents ventricular repolarization.

QT interval—represents electrical systole. This occurs just before mechanical systole as seen on echocardiography.

Chamber Enlargement on ECG. The following ECG changes are suggestive of cardiac chamber enlargement, but additional diagnostic imaging (e.g., thoracic radiographs, echocardiography) is recommended to confirm suspicion of underlying cardiomegaly based on ECG recordings.

P wave

Increased amplitude—right atrial enlargement; termed *P pulmonale*

Prolonged duration—left atrial enlargement; termed *P mitrale*

R wave

Increased amplitude—left ventricular enlargement

Prolonged duration—may represent left ventricular enlargement or left bundle branch block depending on the degree of prolongation

Conduction Disturbances on ECG. Disturbances in conduction, such as bundle branch block and AV block, can be recorded on ECG. Since the majority of these changes are due to underlying disease, additional diagnostic tests (e.g., echocardiography, cTnI levels) are recommended to aid in determining the etiology.

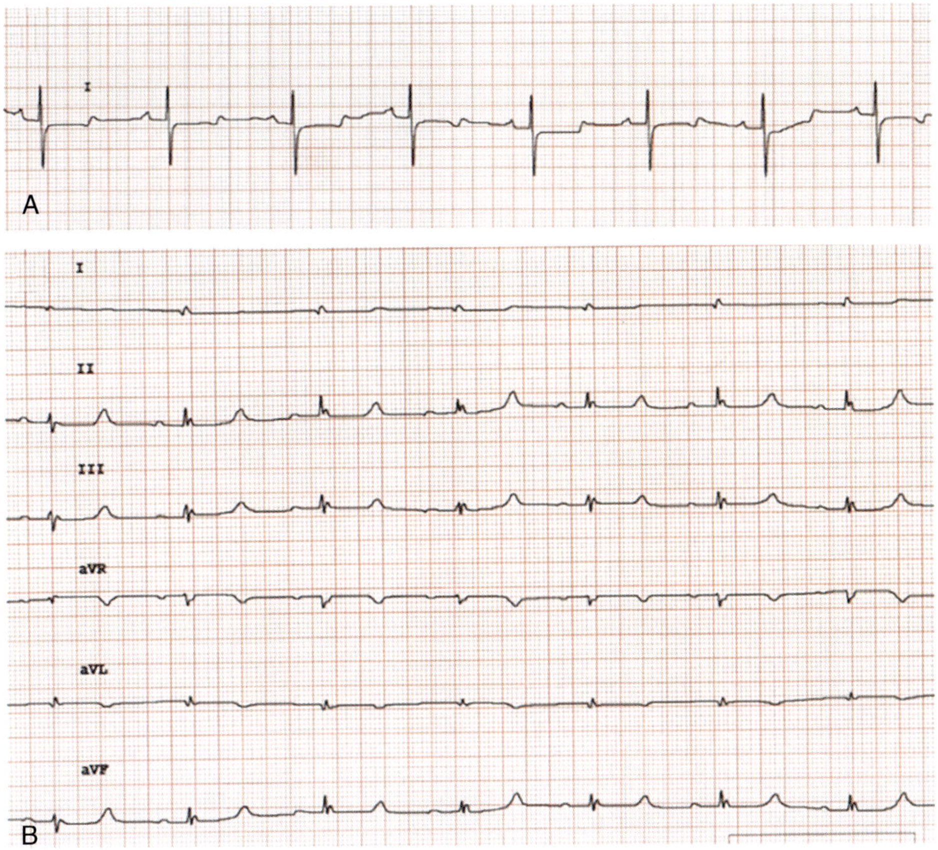

• **Fig. 17.2** **A.** Normal base-apex electrocardiogram (ECG) recording from lead I in a 1-year-old LaMancha buck in right lateral recumbency. **B.** Normal limb lead ECG recording from the same goat. Both tracings are recorded at 50 mm/second and 20 mm/mV.

Bundle Branch Block. The His bundle splits into the left and right bundle branch. Delayed or complete absence of conduction through one of the branches results in ECG changes. Regardless of the side affected, bundle branch block results in prolongation of the QRS complex. In other species, a positive or negative net deflection of the prolonged QRS complex determines if the bundle branch block is left sided or right sided, respectively, which is difficult to assess in small ruminants due to the high variability of the QRS morphology on ECG tracings. However, detection of a prolonged QRS complex warrants further investigation. Causes of bundle branch block usually involve infiltrative disease (infectious, inflammatory, or neoplastic) and/or significant cardiomegaly.

Atrioventricular Block. AV block can be due to delayed conduction or complete absence of conduction through the AV node and/or bundle of His. There are three degrees of AV block. First-degree AV block and second-degree AV block type 1 are often associated with increases of the vagal tone, which can be normal. Second-degree AV block type 2, high-grade second-degree AV block, and third-degree AV block are usually associated with cardiac pathology and should be further evaluated with echocardiography and cTnI levels.

First-degree AV block—prolongation of the PR interval. Conduction through the AV node and bundle of His is present, but delayed.

Second-degree AV block—signal is intermittently not conducted through the AV node and/or bundle of His, as denoted by a P wave without an associated QRS complex. There are three categories of second-degree AV block.

Second-degree AV block type 1 (Mobitz type 1, Wenckebach)—the PR interval prolongs in consecutive beats prior to a blocked P wave. This diagnosis requires that there are at least two consecutively conducted P waves with associated QRS complexes prior to the blocked P wave.

Second-degree AV block type 2 (Mobitz type 2)—the PR interval remains constant in the consecutive beats prior to the blocked P wave. This diagnosis also requires that there are at least two consecutively conducted P waves with associated QRS complexes prior to the blocked P wave.

High-grade second-degree AV block—conducted P waves with associated QRS complexes are present in combination with nonconducted P waves, but there are not two consecutively conducted P waves prior to the conduction block, so a description of type 1 or type 2 AV block cannot be assigned.

Third-degree AV block—complete AV dissociation is present. No P waves are conducted, and an escape rhythm is usually present. None of the QRS complexes are associated with any of the P waves.

Arrhythmias

Bradyarrhythmias. ECG evaluation of a bradycardic animal is essential in determining the electrophysiologic cause and appropriate treatment. ECG can distinguish bradyarrhythmias such as sinus bradycardia, AV block, and atrial standstill. In most cases, the blocked P waves in AV block cannot be auscultated, so ECG is helpful in determining their presence. Atrial standstill is denoted by the absence of P waves with an escape rhythm (either junctional or ventricular in origin). There are two types of atrial standstill: transient atrial standstill (sinoventricular) and persistent atrial standstill. Transient atrial standstill, also termed sinoventricular rhythm, is often caused by electrolyte disturbances, specifically hyperkalemia; therefore, measuring serum electrolyte concentrations is recommend in animals with this arrhythmia. Correction of electrolyte abnormalities is the treatment of choice. Persistent atrial standstill involves primary pathology of the atrial tissue and not has been reported in small ruminants.

Tachyarrhythmias. Auscultation of a tachyarrhythmia cannot determine the cause alone; therefore, ECG is used to determine whether the arrhythmia is supraventricular (arising from above the AV node) or ventricular. The QRS morphology of supraventricular tachyarrhythmias usually mimics that of the normal sinus beats, but the QRS morphology of ventricular tachyarrhythmias is often wide and bizarre, suggesting ventricular origin without use of the normal conduction system. Distinguishing a supraventricular from ventricular tachyarrhythmia is essential for appropriate treatment. Infiltrative disease and cardiomegaly may lead to supraventricular and ventricular tachyarrhythmias, and additional diagnostic tests are warranted if either of these arrhythmias is detected. Figure 17.3 shows an ECG recording from an adult sheep in which an irregular rhythm was auscultated. The average heart rate is 110 bpm, but the ECG shows an atrial rate of 300 bpm, consistent with a supraventricular tachycardia. The tachycardic atrial rate and subsequent AV block could not be detected on auscultation alone, highlighting the importance of utilizing an ECG in animals with an arrhythmia.

Echocardiography

Echocardiography provides a rapid, noninvasive assessment of cardiac chamber structure and function, valve morphology and competency, blood flow velocity through the heart, and intracardiac lesions. The pericardium and pericardial space can also be readily evaluated. Echocardiography can be performed with the animal in the standing position or in lateral recumbency and can be performed from both sides of the chest. For improved contact between the skin and transducer, clipping of the hair is often necessary. The exposed skin should be sprayed with alcohol, and coupling gel should be applied to the transducer to optimize image quality. For most small ruminants and deer, a 5-MHz phased-array transducer should provide adequate images, but a 6- or 7-MHz phased-array transducer may be sufficient for smaller animals (< 10 kg). For thorough evaluation, both long-axis and short-axis views should be obtained. Right-sided parasternal views are often easier to obtain than those on the left hemithorax, so they will be discussed briefly. The best imaging window is often 2 to 3 cm dorsal to the olecranon in the 4th and 5th intercostal spaces.[24] Because of the cranial location of the heart, the right thoracic limb needs to be pulled cranially or abducted to allow appropriate positioning of the transducer. For long-axis views, the marker on the transducer should be pointed toward the animal's shoulder, approximately 45 degrees from horizontal. Four-chamber long-axis images can be obtained from this view, as shown in Figure 17.4. Short-axis (transverse) views are obtained by rotating the probe clockwise and pointing the marker toward the animal's elbow. Transverse images of the left ventricle and associated papillary muscles, left atrium and aorta, and main pulmonary artery and its associated branches are obtained by fanning the probe from the apex toward the base of the heart. Detailed orientation of the transducer and structures obtained for each view are discussed elsewhere.[24]

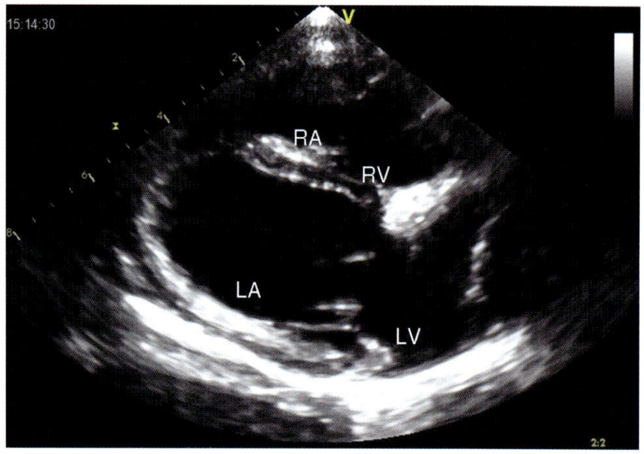

• **Fig. 17.4** Two-dimensional right parasternal long-axis four-chamber view in a 1-year-old LaMancha buck showing the normal left atrium (LA), left ventricle (LV), right atrium (RA), and right ventricle (RV).

Different echocardiographic modalities can be used to evaluate certain cardiac parameters. B-mode (most often two-dimensional imaging), M-mode (motion-mode), spectral Doppler (pulsed-wave and continuous wave Doppler), and color Doppler are the most commonly used modalities. Two-dimensional imaging is used to evaluate the structure and function of the cardiac chambers and structure of the cardiac valves. M-mode is used to evaluate cardiac chamber size, systolic function, and wall thickness.

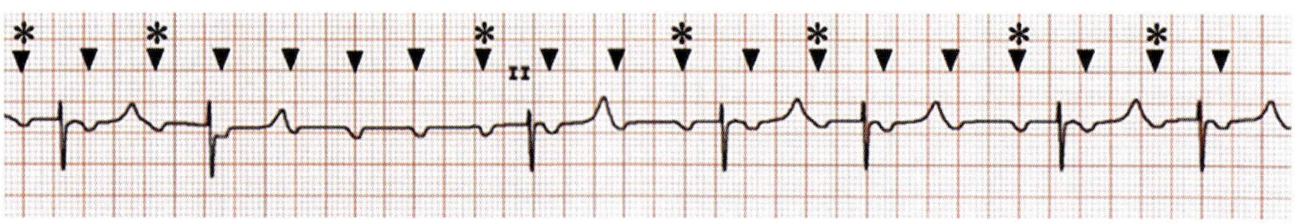

• **Fig. 17.3** Base-apex electrocardiogram (ECG) tracing of an atrial tachycardia with high-grade second-degree AV block in an adult sheep. The P waves in the tracing are negative and denoted by the *arrowheads*. Conducted P waves are denoted by *asterisks*. The atrial (P-P) rate is 300 bpm. The average ventricular (R-R) rate is 100 bpm (instantaneous rate = 46 to 130 bpm). There is variable AV conduction, ranging from 2:1 to 5:1 AV conduction. The PR interval varies, consistent with Wenckebach periodicity, which is a normal electrophysiologic response to the atrial tachycardia. Paper speed = 50 mm/sec; amplitude = 10 mm/mV. (Courtesy Dr. Rebecca Legere, Auburn University.)

Spectral Doppler is most often used to record blood flow velocity across cardiac valves or intracardiac shunts, and color Doppler is used to detect blood flow and its direction through cardiac chambers and across valves.

Echocardiography is useful in diagnosing congenital and acquired cardiac disease. Although heart murmur characteristics can suggest specific cardiac lesions, echocardiography is the only noninvasive diagnostic modality to provide a definitive diagnosis. Two-dimensional imaging can be used to detect the location, type, and extent of congenital and acquired defects, while spectral and color Doppler can be used to assess the velocity, direction, and turbulence of blood flow across lesions and valves. The usefulness of echocardiography in diagnosing congenital cardiac disease is highlighted in Figure 17.5, showing an ASD in a 9-month-old doeling that presented for respiratory distress. Two-dimensional imaging was used to visualize the lesion in Figure 17.5A, and color Doppler was used to determine the direction of flow across the lesion, as seen in Figure 17.5B. An example of diagnosing acquired disease via echocardiography is presented in Figure 17.6, which shows a myocarditic lesion in a 3-week-old Anglo-Nubian doeling that was presented for fever. There is limited literature on echocardiographic parameters in sheep and goats, but species-specific and breed-specific reference ranges are available for two-dimensional, M-mode, and pulsed-wave parameters in small ruminants.[24–27] Evaluation of echocardiographic parameters in goats during pregnancy, lactation, and the dry period has also been performed.[28]

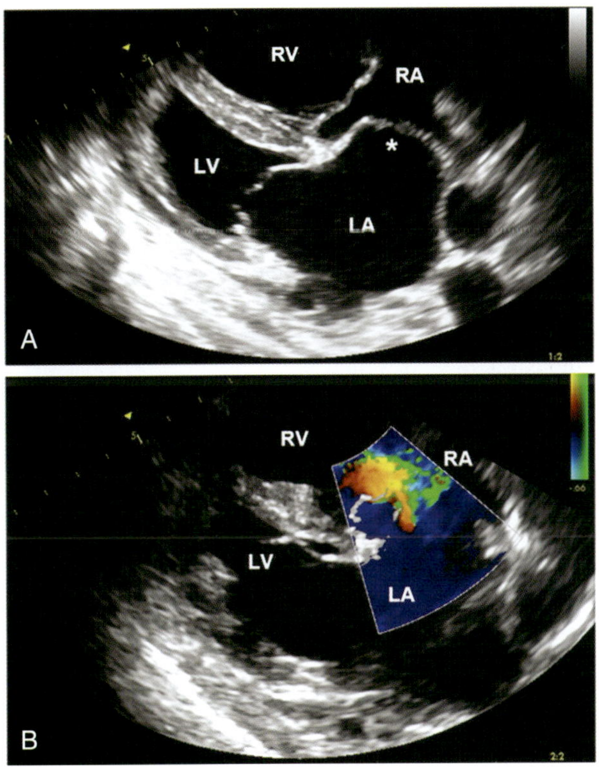

• **Fig. 17.5. A.** Two-dimensional right parasternal long-axis view showing an interatrial septal abnormality *(*)* in a 9-month-old doeling presenting for respiratory distress. Note the atrial septal aneurysm bowing toward the right atrium. Given the aneurysmal dilation and central location of the defect within the interatrial septum, a patent foramen ovale is most likely, but a secundum atrial septal defect cannot be excluded. The right ventricle is moderately dilated. **B.** Same view with color Doppler interrogation, showing left-to-right flow across the interatrial septal defect from the left atrium into the right atrium. *LA*, Left atrium; *LV*, left ventricle; *RA*, right atrium; *RV*, right ventricle.

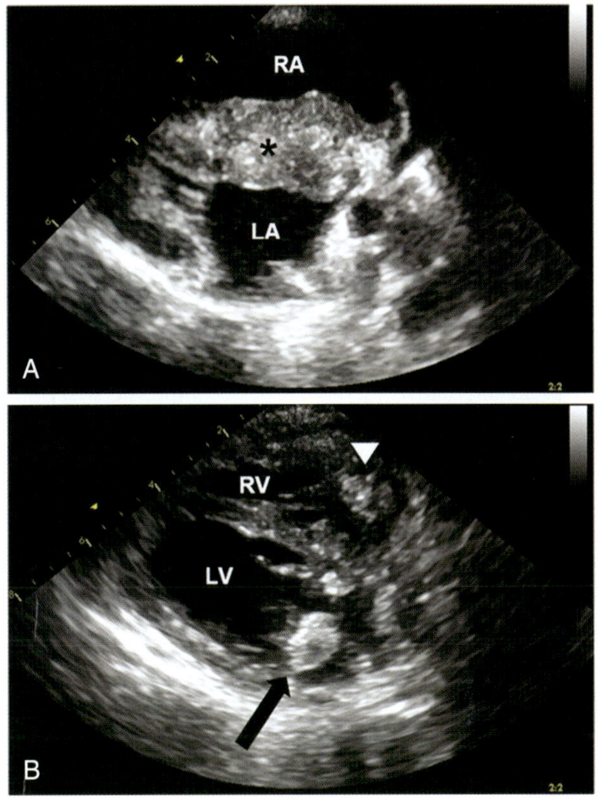

• **Fig. 17.6 A.** Two-dimensional right parasternal long-axis view highlighting the interatrial septum *(*)* in a 3-week-old Anglo-Nubian doeling presenting for fever. The interatrial septum is extremely thickened and heteroechoic with irregular margins. A premortem diagnosis of suppurative myocarditis was made based on endomyocardial biopsies. **B.** A similar echocardiographic view from the same doeling 2 months later, showing resolution of the lesion in the interatrial septum, but extension of the lesion to the mitral *(black arrow)* and tricuspid *(white arrowhead)* valves. *LA*, Left atrium; *RA*, right atrium; *LV*, left ventricle; *RV*, right ventricle.

Cardiopulmonary Resuscitation

Evidence-based consensus guidelines on cardiopulmonary resuscitation (CPR) in veterinary medicine are available.[29,30] Preparedness and prevention include routine training and ready availability of drugs and equipment necessary to perform CPR. When available, monitoring devices such as ECG and capnography should be used. Early recognition and quick, standardized assessment of the high-risk animal is critical. Evaluation of the airway, breathing, and circulation (ABCs) identifies animals in cardiopulmonary arrest (CPA), and CPR should be started immediately even if CPA cannot be definitively confirmed.[30] Basic life support includes chest compressions and ventilation. The main goals of chest compressions are to (1) restore pulmonary elimination of CO_2 and O_2 uptake by providing pulmonary blood flow and (2) deliver O_2 to tissues by providing systemic arterial blood flow.[30] Use of drug therapy during resuscitation must follow and not precede nor impact performance of ventilation and chest compression efforts. Administration by venous or intra-osseous routes is preferable. Use of vasopressors (e.g., epinephrine), parasympatholytics (e.g., atropine), antiarrhythmics (e.g., lidocaine), intravenous fluids, and alkalinizing agents (e.g., bicarbonate) may be indicated during CPA. Reversal agents should be used where appropriate (e.g., naloxone, yohimbine, and atipamezole) (see Appendix 1 and Chapter 18).[30]

Chest Compressions

The animal is placed in lateral recumbency. In mature animals, a two-hand technique, with the hands placed directly over the heart, should be performed. In lambs, kids, or fawns, a one-hand technique with the hand wrapped around the sternum over the heart is an alternative method. Chest compressions should be one-third to one-half the width of the chest and at a rate of 100 to 120 compressions per minute, regardless of animal size or species. The person's elbows are locked, and shoulders are directly above the hands. Compressions are delivered without interruption in cycles of 2 minutes—pauses of 2 to 5 seconds every 2 minutes allow switching of personnel to avoid fatigue and to obtain ECG recordings. Excessive pauses between compressions should be avoided.[30]

Ventilation

If possible, the animal should be intubated with a cuffed endotracheal tube. Ventilation and chest compressions occur simultaneously. A low minute ventilation is adequate during CPR because pulmonary blood flow is reduced. Goals include a ventilation rate of 10 breaths/minute, a short inspiratory time of approximately 1 second, and a tidal volume of approximately 10 mL/kg. Hyperventilation should be avoided. Mouth-to-nose ventilation can be performed if intubation is not possible. Pressure over the esophagus should be applied to maximize air movement into the trachea rather than the esophagus. Compressions and mouth-to-nose breaths should occur at a ratio of 30 compressions to two breaths, continued for 2-minute cycles.[30]

Monitoring

Capnography allows assessment of end-tidal CO_2 ($ETCO_2$), which can be a useful indicator of chest compression efficacy, as $ETCO_2$ is proportional to pulmonary blood flow when minute ventilation is held constant. Very low $ETCO_2$ values during CPR (e.g., < 10–15 mm Hg) are associated with a reduced likelihood of resuscitation success.[30] Common ECG arrest rhythms observed in dogs and cats are asystole, pulseless electrical activity, and ventricular fibrillation.

Congenital Cardiac Diseases

A description of congenital cardiac lesions with associated murmurs and natural outcomes for each is listed in Table 17.1. Ventricular septal defects (VSDs) are the most common congenital cardiac abnormality in kids, lambs, and probably deer. Both perimembranous and muscular VSDs have been reported, and the perimembranous form is more common.[31–33] Because the left ventricular pressures are greater than the right ventricular pressures, ventricular septal defects shunt blood from left to right. The perimembranous location of the defect allows blood to immediately flow to the lungs via the main pulmonary artery, causing pulmonary overcirculation. If severe enough, this can lead to left-sided CHF. The associated heart murmur is right sided, is systolic, and can be apical or basilar, depending on the orientation of blood flow. Right-to-left shunting, or Eisenmenger's physiology, occurs if significant right-sided pathology is present, which increases right ventricular pressures above those of the left ventricle. This allows deoxygenated blood to bypass the lungs, potentially leading to cyanosis and polycythemia.

Tetralogy of Fallot has been reported in kids and lambs and, similar to right-to-left shunting VSDs, can cause cyanosis and polycythemia.[17,33] Tetralogy of Fallot is characterized by a perimembranous VSD, dextropositioned (or over-riding) aorta, pulmonic stenosis, and secondary right ventricular concentric hypertrophy. The VSD and dextropositioned aorta allow deoxygenated blood to flow into the aorta, causing the cyanosis and polycythemia.

Although rare, cases of PDA have been reported in ruminants, which, in contrast to other species, are not expected to have PDA after birth. Therefore, a continuous murmur in a neonatal ruminant should always be considered to be abnormal.[34] PDA leads to significant volume overload to the lungs and left side of the heart, ultimately leading to left-sided CHF. Dysplasia of the mitral and tricuspid valve has been described. Ebstein's anomaly, which is a form of tricuspid valve dysplasia with apical displacement of the tricuspid valve annulus, was reported in two kids.[35] This is associated with a right-sided, apical, systolic heart murmur. ASDs have been reported and are usually present concurrently with other congenital cardiac defects.[31,35] An ASD can cause a heart murmur, but the heart murmur(s) associated with concurrent cardiac defects usually camouflage those of the ASD.

Treatment of congenital cardiac defects varies depending on the defect. Left-sided CHF, regardless of cause, can be treated with diuretics (e.g., furosemide 0.5–1 mg/kg intravenously [IV]). Treatment of left-sided CHF secondary to a PDA or hemodynamically significant VSD is often futile, as diuretics have poor long-term control of the associated volume overload. Surgical ligation or interventional closure of a PDA can be performed but is often foregone in ruminants due to associated costs, possibility of heritability, or likely cardiac-related death prior to correction. Animals with significant right-to-left shunts are not responsive to oxygen therapy and succumb to the condition or are euthanized due to poor quality of life and grave prognosis. Phlebotomy can be performed in polycythemic animals, but this often does not provide long-term control of the disease.

Acquired Cardiac Diseases

Pericardial Diseases

Pericarditis

Etiology and Pathophysiology. Pericarditis can be classified as either primarily effusive, constrictive, or a combination of both. Inflammation between the parietal and visceral layers of the pericardium results in the accumulation of serous or fibrinous inflammatory exudate. A common cause in cattle is the advancement of a reticular foreign body through the cranial wall of the reticulum and diaphragm into the pericardium, carrying bacteria into the pericardium and causing traumatic reticulopericarditis (hardware disease). Hardware disease is rare in small ruminants but has been reported in sheep, goats, and deer.[36–39] More common causes of pericarditis include hematogenous spread of bacteria during septicemia or extension of disease within the thorax.[40] Other causes of pericarditis include external wounds and neoplastic effusions.[41]

Regardless of etiology, pericarditis results in decreased cardiac distensibility and increased ventricular end-diastolic pressures. This impairs the ability of the heart to fill during diastole, which reduces venous return to the heart and increases atrial pressures. Overall, the myocardial perfusion is reduced, resulting in decreased ventricular contractility, stroke volume, and cardiac output. Decreases in arterial pressures and renal blood flow result. Compensatory mechanisms (increased heart rate, vasoconstriction, and sodium retention) initially ameliorate the condition, but failure to maintain cardiac output eventually leads to circulatory collapse.

Clinical Signs. Affected animal may be febrile and demonstrate signs of thoracic pain, such as standing with abducted elbows, grunting, and breath-holding.[36,42] Non-specific but consistent signs include anorexia, depression, and loss of body condition. Clinical signs depend on the time course and volume of fluid accumulation within the pericardium. Sudden death is a possible development. Depending on the severity of cardiac tamponade, jugular distention and edema of the submandibular, brisket, and ventral abdomen may be apparent, along with other signs of CHF.[42] On auscultation, the most consistent signs of pericarditis include tachycardia due to cardiac compression and muffled heart sounds. Abnormalities in heart sounds reflect the fluid characteristics within the pericardial space. A large amount of serous fluid results in splashing or gurgling sounds, with alternating loud and quiet heartbeats. The presence of fibrinous exudate results in rubbing, squeaking, or scratching sounds. The characteristic "washing machine murmur" in cases of traumatic pericarditis results from accumulation of fluid and gas in the pericardium.[42] Lung sounds may be dampened, or absent ventrally, and more pronounced dorsally.

Diagnosis. Ultrasonography is the method of choice for imaging pericardial effusion.[43] In cases with significant amounts of pericardial effusion, ultrasound equipment used for pregnancy diagnosis in ambulatory practice (high-frequency linear probe) may be sufficient to visualize abnormal fluid and to guide sampling. On ultrasound examination, the fluid surrounding the heart can appear anechoic to echogenic, the pericardium is thickened, and the presence of echoic strands of fibrin may be noticed. The presence of hyperechoic pinpoint echoes corresponds to gas, indicating the presence of anaerobic bacteria. Significant pericardial effusion causing cardiac tamponade can result in right ventricular diastolic collapse and right atrial collapse. ECG findings associated with pericarditis include decreased amplitude of the QRS complexes, electrical alternans, and S-T segment elevation or slurring. A right axis deviation may be noted using the standard limb leads.[44,45]

Ultrasound-guided pericardiocentesis (further described under treatment) allows collection of samples for cytological characterization and bacterial culture (aerobic and anaerobic), as well as fungal and virus isolation, if indicated. Cytological changes suggestive of infectious pericarditis in cattle include a straw-colored to blood-tinged, foamy, and malodorous fluid; an increased protein concentration (> 3.5 g/dL); and an increased white blood cell count ($> 2500/\mu L$) comprised mainly of neutrophils.[46] Thoracic radiographs may demonstrate apparent cardiomegaly and obstruction of the cardiac silhouette, vena cava, and diaphragm. Dorsal displacement of the trachea and interstitial pneumonia may also be noted. In hardware cases, radiographs of the reticulum, diaphragm, and caudal thorax may be useful in the visualization of metallic foreign bodies.[42] Clinicopathologic changes are non-specific and may include evidence of hemoconcentration, mild anemia, leukocytosis with an absolute neutrophilia or lymphopenia, and hyperfibrinogenemia. Hypoalbuminemia and hyperglobulinemia may be present. Mild increases in liver enzymes, creatinine, bilirubin, and serum urea nitrogen are frequently seen.[42] Myocardial biomarkers may be increased, but the usefulness of cardiac troponins for distinguishing between pericarditis and other cardiac, thoracic, and systemic diseases is limited.[47]

Treatment. Traumatic pericarditis has a poor prognosis, and euthanasia should be considered. In cattle, several therapeutic options are described for the treatment of traumatic reticulopericarditis. Conservative treatments may entail the administration of a magnet and long-term antibiotics, as well as the removal of a foreign body by rumenotomy to prevent further migration, but this is rarely curative. More intensive therapies include (1) pericardiocentesis and pericardial lavage, (2) pericardiotomy, pericardial lavage, and placement of pericardial drain, and (3) fifth rib resection, pericardiostomy, and daily pericardial lavage until wound closure by secondary intention. Ultrasound-guided placement of chest tubes within the pericardial sac should be performed under heavy sedation and local anesthesia or general anesthesia. Surgical interventions require general anesthesia. The reader is directed elsewhere for detailed descriptions of the surgical procedures.[48–51] Regardless of the method used, pericardial drainage rarely results in full return of normal heart function. All therapeutic options carry a guarded to poor prognosis, are for salvage purposes, and can be cost-prohibitive.[49–51] Prognosis for nontraumatic pericarditis is also guarded. Identification and treatment of concurrent systemic disease (e.g., septicemia) are critical, and treatment of the potentially resulting restrictive pericarditis may require surgical intervention.

Aspiration and drainage of pericardial fluid are performed most often on the left side in large animals, in the fifth or sixth intercostal space, near but dorsally to the level of the costochondral junction to avoid the cranial epigastric vessels. This is best and most safely performed with ultrasound guidance.[48] If the amount of pericardial fluid is minimal, an 18- to 14-gauge over-the-needle catheter (with extension tubing and a three-way stopcock) can be used to aspirate fluid for diagnostic purposes. When a large amount of fluid is present, a large-bore trocar catheter is more suitable to facilitate drainage. The site is surgically prepared, blocked with local anesthesia, and a stab incision is made in the skin. Introduction of the catheter should be near the cranial aspect of the rib to avoid the intercostal neurovascular structures, which course along the caudal aspect of each rib. The catheter is advanced slowly until a popping sensation is felt as it penetrates the parietal pericardium. As fluid fills the catheter, the catheter is advanced over the trocar into the pericardial space until only several centimeters of it remains externally or until the heart is felt beating at the tip of the catheter, at which point the catheter is retracted slightly. The catheter is secured using a Chinese finger-tie suture and is either clamped off or left open with a one-way Heimlich valve affixed.[52] The rate of pericardial fluid drainage should be controlled to minimize the effect of fluid shifts and hemodynamic decompensation. ECG monitoring throughout the procedure is useful for detecting the development of arrhythmias. If observed, the depth of the catheter should be decreased. Administration of diuretics before pericardiocentesis is contraindicated—by decreasing preload, diuretics decrease cardiac filling and can precipitate cardiogenic shock. When indicated, diuretic use should be reserved until after pericardial drainage.[53] Pericardial lavage is beneficial to remove infectious organisms, inflammatory cells, and fibrin and can be performed once to twice daily using balanced polyionic fluids. Following pericardial lavage, intrapericardial instillation of antimicrobials (sodium penicillin, ceftiofur, ampicillin, or ticarcillin) may be considered. Sodium penicillin is preferable to potassium penicillin to avoid arrhythmias. Indwelling pericardial catheters are typically maintained for 1 to 3 days.[52] Intravenous treatment with systemic broad-spectrum antibiotics is indicated, ideally based on bacterial susceptibility. Systemic antibiotics should be administered for several days to weeks. Nonsteroidal antiinflammatories should be used to control pain and inflammation (e.g., flunixin meglumine 1.1 mg/kg, IV, q12–24h).

Prevention. Prevention of septicemia involves good nutrition and colostrum management and adequate husbandry and vaccination practices. Forages and feed should be free of foreign objects and debris. Routine use of magnets in small ruminants is typically not indicated but may be used in at-risk flocks or herds.

Diseases of the Myocardium

Cardiotoxic Plants

Various plants contain plant-defensive compounds that can cause cardiovascular toxicity in ruminants. Free-ranging species and animals with access to abundant forage and browse are less likely to ingest sufficient amounts to cause toxicity. A greater risk of consumption exists during periods of forage scarcity or when toxic plants or seeds are blended in hay and concentrates. Clinical signs caused by cardiotoxic plants vary, depending on the affected species, toxic principle, and ingested amount. In addition to sudden death, a common clinical sign of cardiotoxicity, affected animals may show other signs of cardiovascular, neurologic, and enteric disease. Table 17.3 lists cardiotoxic plants reported to cause disease in small ruminants and/or deer, and the associated pathophysiology and clinical signs are discussed here.

Avocado—Avocado trees are cultivated in tropical and subtropical regions around the world. Toxicity is associated with the Guatemalan varieties. While Guatemalan × Mexican hybrids (Hass) are also toxic, the Mexican varieties are not.[54] Leaves are the most toxic plant part, but fruit, stems, and seeds are also toxic. Sufficient consumption leads to myocardial degeneration with associated clinical signs of weakness, dyspnea, tachycardia, tachypnea, peripheral edema, and cardiac arrhythmia.[54] In addition to cardiac disease, consumption of avocado leaves may also cause a non-infectious mastitis in goats.[55]

Cardiac Glycosides—Worldwide, a wide variety of plant genera produce cardiac glycoside compounds (cardenolides or bufadienolides) that are associated with either acute or chronic toxicity in livestock.[56,57] Clinical signs are caused by toxic effects on the autonomous nervous system, heart, and gastrointestinal system. Cardiac glycosides inhibit cellular Na^+K^+ATPase transport pumps, resulting in decreased potassium and increased sodium concentrations in affected cells. Increased intracellular sodium causes an increase in intracellular calcium affected by the cellular Na^+Ca^{2+} exchanger. Electrolyte disturbances, in conjunction with an increased vagal tone, result in impaired cardiac conduction, bradycardia, and dysrhythmia with poor cardiac output and function. Cardiac glycosides are present in all plant parts and remain toxic in dried leaves.[57] Consumption of relatively small amounts of plant material may cause acute cardiac toxicity, for example, 0.110 g/kg to

TABLE 17.3 Plants Associated With Cardiovascular Disease in Small Ruminants and Deer.

Group	Common Name	Latin Name	Toxic Principle	Reports of Cardiotoxicity in:
	Avocado	*Persea americana*	Persin	Sheep and goats[54,164]
	Canary grass	*Phalaris* spp.	Tryptamine alkaloids	Sheep[60,62]
	Coffee weed	*Senna (Cassia) occidentalis*	Dianthrone	Sheep and goats[64,65]
	Cottonseed	*Gossypium* spp.	Gossypol	Sheep and goats[67,69]
Plants containing cardiac glycosides	Common Oleander Yellow oleander	*Nerium oleander* *Thevetia peruviana*	Oleandrine, other cardenolides	Sheep and goats[58,165]
	Foxglove	*Digitalis purpura*	Digitoxin, other cardenolides	Sheep and captive red deer[166,167]
	Lily of the valley	*Convallaria majalis*	Convallatoxin, other cardenolides	
	Dogbane (Indian hemp)	*Apocynum cannabinum*	Cymarin	
	Milkweed	*Asclepias* spp.	Calactin, and cardenolides	
	Hellebore	*Helleborus* spp.	Hellebrin, helleborin, and others	
	Jimsonweed	*Datura stramonium*	Tropane alkaloids atropine, hyoscyamine, and scopolamine	Sheep and goats[168]
Plants containing grayanotoxins	Laurels	*Kalmia* species	Grayanotoxins	Sheep and goats[169]
	Rhododendron azalea	*Rhododendron* spp.	Grayanotoxins	Sheep and goats[71,72]
	Yew	*Taxus* spp.	Taxine alkaloids	Sheep, goats, fallow deer, moose, and roe deer[73–76,170]

0.330 g/kg body weight (BW) of dried oleander leaves resulted in rapid development of clinical signs and death in experimentally exposed sheep and goats.[58,59] Clinical signs of intoxication include lethargy, abdominal pain, rumen stasis and distention, diarrhea, polyuria, dyspnea, tachypnea, bradycardia, dysrhythmia, and death.[56,58,59]

Canary Grass—Grasses of the genus *Phalaris* have been associated with neurologic disease (see Grass staggers, Chapter 13) and sudden death caused by cardiac failure in sheep and, less commonly, cattle. Cardiac failure may occur as part of two distinct syndromes, termed "cardiac sudden death" and "PE-like sudden death."[60,61] The indole alkaloids responsible for *Phalaris* staggers do not cause sudden death, during which peracute ammonia toxicity was detected.[62,63] The pathophysiology of canary grass poisoning likely involves multiple toxic principles, and cardiac failure may occur with or without clinical signs of neurologic disease.

Coffee Weed—*Senna occidentalis* and sicklepod *(Senna obtusifolia)* commonly grow in disturbed soils, such as corn and soybean fields, but are also found in pastures and along roadways. While the entire plant is toxic when consumed, seeds are of greatest concern when they contaminate crops during harvest. Dianthrone, the toxic principle of *Senna*, is a myotoxin that causes a mitochondrial myopathy in a dose-dependent fashion.[64] Degeneration of skeletal and cardiac muscles result in clinical signs of muscular weakness, tremors, recumbency, myoglobinuria, and death. The effects of *Senna* poisoning appear to be irreversible, and affected animals often die or are euthanized within 30 days.[65]

Cottonseed—Gossypol is a yellow polyphenolic pigment of cotton, which is concentrated in seed glands. The concentration of gossypol varies among cotton varieties and ranges from 0.02 to 6.64%.[66] Gossypol is present in whole cottonseed and cottonseed meal, especially when oil has been extracted by solvent extraction. Protein binding in the rumen reduces the risk of toxicity, which is therefore more common in monogastric species and young ruminants. The risk of toxicity is influenced by the dietary content of protein, iron, selenium, calcium, and vitamin E, and toxic effects on reproductive function and hematologic parameters may occur without overt clinical signs.[67,68] Toxicity of gossypol is cumulative, and clinical signs typically occur weeks or months after introducing cottonseed byproducts into the diet. For example, daily intake of approximately 400 mg of free gossypol per animal for 3 months resulted in CHF in three of five dairy goats.[67] Lambs receiving 409 mg per day of free gossypol died within 30 days.[69] Gossypol has multiple toxic effects on tissues, and cardiotoxicity is associated with the production of reactive oxygen species and lipid peroxidation.[66] Clinical signs include anorexia, dyspnea, cough, and peripheral edema and may be mistaken as respiratory disease.

Grayanotoxin—Some plants in the family *Ericaceae*, including azalea, mountain laurel, rhododendron, and others, produce grayanotoxins, which are found in all parts of the plant, with greatest concentrations in the leaves. Leaves are toxic when fresh or dried, and poisoning of small ruminants commonly occurs following exposure to yard clippings. In ruminants, ingestion of 0.1 to 0.2% of plant material may be toxic. Grayanotoxins bind to voltage-dependent sodium channels and increase the influx of sodium ions and, secondarily, calcium ions into excitable cells such as nerve, heart, and muscle cells.[70] Clinical signs develop rapidly following exposure[71,72] and include lethargy, signs of abdominal pain, vomiting, ataxia, head-pressing, convulsion, cardiac dysrhythmias, and death. Most clinical signs resolve within 24 hours, but signs of neurologic disease and aspiration pneumonia may be prolonged.[70]

Yew—Several species of the genus *Taxus* are associated with toxicity in ruminants. All plant parts, with exception of the nontoxic red berry (aril) containing toxic seeds, are poisonous to ruminants. Yew poisoning has been reported in small ruminants, and only small amounts of leaves are necessary to cause toxicity (2.5 g of leaves/kg BW for sheep and 12 g of leaves/kg BW for goats).[56,73,74] Yew poisoning has also been reported in captive and free-ranging deer.[75,76] However, there are apparent species and breed-specific tolerances to yew intoxication, and yew is browsed extensively by some deer populations.[77,78] The variation in tolerance to yew consumption among ruminants may be result of ruminal or hepatic adaption following exposure to sublethal doses.[75,79] Yew contains various cardiotoxic alkaloids, of which taxine A and B are the most important cardiotoxins. Taxines inhibit sodium and calcium channels of cardiomyocytes, causing dysrhythmia, AV blockade, bradycardia, and cardiac arrest. Sudden death is the most common clinical sign and occurs within 24 hours of consumption, but dyspnea, muscle tremors, and collapse may be observed.[56]

Treatment. Following removal of the source of toxicity, treatment consists mainly of supportive therapy. Oral administration of activated charcoal ($\geq$ 2 g/kg BW) and mineral oil or magnesium sulfate reduce toxin absorption and enhance excretion. A rumenotomy may be performed in cases of recent exposure. Intravenous or oral fluid therapy is recommended, but volume overload should be prevented. Intravenous lidocaine (loading dose of 1 to 2 mg/kg, followed by CRI of 1–2 mg/kg/h) can be administered to control cardiac arrhythmias. Atropine (0.05–0.1 mg/kg, slow IV to effect) is used to treat bradycardia and AV block. Propranolol (0.25–1 mg/kg IV), a beta-adrenergic receptor blocking agent, can be administered to treat tachycardia.

Prevention. Plant-associated toxicities can be prevented by provision of good forage in adequate quantities, proper disposal of hedge clippings, and avoidance of potentially toxic plants when preparing hay, silage, or green chop.

Ionophore Toxicity

Etiology and Pathophysiology

Ionophores are commonly used feed additives in ruminant and poultry diets and enhance growth and feed efficiency, prevent rumen acidosis, avoid fog fever, or control coccidia. Commercially available ionophores include monensin, salinomycin, lasalocid, laidlomycin, narasin, and maduramycin. Ionophore toxicity has been reported in many mammalian and avian species, including sheep, goats, and deer, but sensitivity to toxicity varies between species and ionophores.[80] Cases of ionophore toxicity are typically caused by errors during feed mixing but may be associated with accidental or deliberate access to feed formulated for a less sensitive species. In one report, litter from poultry fed maduramicin resulted in chronic ionophore toxicity in cattle and sheep.[81] Ionophores bind and transport monovalent or divalent cations along concentration gradients across biological membranes. Normally, ion gradients across cell membranes are tightly controlled by specialized transport complexes, such as Na^+-K^+-ATPase and Ca^{2+}-Mg^{2+}-ATPase, but during ionophore toxicity, control of physiologic ion gradients is lost.[82] Exertion of cation efflux complexes, ATP depletion, and effects of increased Ca^{2+} on cellular and mitochondrial metabolism result in reduced cellular function and cell death. Highly excitable cells, including those of the myocardium, skeletal muscles, gastrointestinal tract, and nervous tissues, are especially sensitive to the effects of ionophores, and clinical signs are associated with damage to these cells. Damage to cardiac myocytes results in degenerative cardiomyopathy and CHF with reduced cardiac function and output. The renin-angiotensin-aldosterone system is activated in response to reduced cardiac output and increases afterload by increasing arterial resistance.[9] This compensatory response in combination with reduced cardiac function leads to pulmonary edema, a common clinical and postmortem finding in affected ruminants.[83,84]

Clinical Signs. Clinical signs of ionophore toxicity in ruminants vary depending on the ingested dose and type of ionophore and may develop peracutely to acutely after consumption of toxic doses in feed. While sudden death without premonitory signs is possible in cases of severe overdosing,[83] clinical signs of acute intoxication typically develop within 24 hours of initial exposure. Animals not dying following acute exposure or those exposed to lower doses are likely to have clinical signs for several weeks to months, characterized by ill-thrift, decreased growth rates, muscular weakness, and, potentially, sudden death from cardiac failure. Feed refusal is often an initial clinical sign; however, lower toxic doses do not appear to prevent consumption.[85–87] Typical clinical signs of acute intoxication include lethargy, muscle weakness, stiff and stilted gait, recumbency, abdominal pain, diarrhea, salivation, clear nasal discharge, dyspnea, and moist coughing.[84,85,87,88] Incoordination, opisthotonos, convulsive seizures, and other neurologic signs may be observed in some affected animals. Further examination may reveal tachycardia, pulmonary edema, rumen hypomotility, dehydration, and congested mucous membranes. Cardiac arrhythmias, jugular distention, jugular pulses, peripheral edema, and cardiac murmurs as result of ventricular dilatation may be signs of cardiac failure in some cases.[9,86]

Diagnosis. Ionophore toxicity should be suspected when signs of inappetence, musculoskeletal damage, and cardiac insufficiency with postmortem findings of rhabdomyolysis and cardiomyopathy are observed, especially when they occur shortly after a feed change. The diagnosis is confirmed by analysis of feed (0.5–1 kg), gastrointestinal contents, and liver samples.[89] Blood work reflects damage to skeletal and cardiac muscles (elevated concentrations of cTnI, creatine kinase [CK], and lactate dehydrogenase [LDH]) and kidneys (elevated blood urea nitrogen and creatinine concentration), erythrocyte fragility, and reduced serum potassium and calcium concentrations.[9,90] An ECG may reveal supraventricular tachycardia or other arrhythmias, with absence of the P-wave, large, deformed QRS complexes, and significant tachycardia.[88] Echocardiography may reveal evidence of a dilated cardiomyopathy and decreased myocardial function.[9] Typical postmortem findings include pulmonary edema; pleural, pericardial, and peritoneal effusion; cardiac dilation; presence of pale streaking and hemorrhages on skeletal and cardiac muscles; and cardiac petechiation. Histologically, cellular necrosis and fibrosis in myocardium, skeletal muscles, liver, and kidney are detected.

Treatment. Specific treatments for ionophore toxicity are not available. Severely affected animals should be euthanized. Following removal of the offending feed, symptomatic therapy may include careful fluid therapy to correct dehydration and electrolyte imbalances, while preventing fluid overload. Oral administration of activated charcoal may help to reduce ionophore absorption. Affected animals should be kept in a quiet environment or stall-rested, as sudden cardiac failure is possible in animals recovered from acute intoxication. Administration of diuretics (e.g., furosemide) and antiarrhythmic drugs (e.g., quinidine) may improve clinical signs, but their long-term benefit in cases of ionophore toxicity has not been demonstrated.

Prevention. Ionophores are apparently safe for small ruminants and deer when correctly dosed; therefore, prevention is based on correct formulation and offering medicated feeds only to the intended species. Ionophore toxicity may be potentiated by various antibiotics, including tiamulin, oleandomycin, chloramphenicol, erythromycin, and sulfonamides, and concurrent administration should be avoided.

Nutritional Myodegeneration (White Muscle Disease)

Etiology and Pathophysiology

Nutritional myodegeneration, also called white muscle disease (WMD), weak calf syndrome, or stiff lamb disease, is a myodegenerative disease of the skeletal and cardiac muscles due to deficiencies in selenium, vitamin E, or both.[91,92] WMD occurs in most livestock species, including sheep and goats, as well as deer.[93] It typically affects young, rapidly growing animals and often those born to dams fed selenium-deficient diets during gestation. In utero development of WMD is possible, resulting in abortion or neonatal death.[94] Two distinct clinical syndromes are observed: a cardiac form and a skeletal form.

Normal cellular metabolism results in the generation of free radicals and peroxides that are scavenged by antioxidants. Selenium is an essential trace element, often incorporated into proteins as the amino acid selenocysteine, an integral component of selenoproteins. The selenoprotein family includes at least 25 proteins that are involved in multiple physiologically processes. This includes the selenoenzyme glutathione peroxidase (GSH-Px), a biologic antioxidant.[95] Another important antioxidant is vitamin E (i.e., α-tocopherol), which is involved in the prevention of peroxide formation from fatty acids. Deficiencies of selenium and vitamin E result in the destruction of cell membranes and proteins. In skeletal and cardiac muscles, free radical–mediated rhabdomyolysis occurs.[96] Many animals deficient in selenium and/or vitamin E exhibit no evidence of nutritional myodegeneration, and sometimes both nutrients must be deficient to cause clinical signs.

Clinical Signs. The cardiac and skeletal forms of WMD are associated with peracute to subacute disease. Severe cardiac decompensation and sudden death in neonatal lambs and kids may be observed within hours of birth with the cardiac form.[97] Clinical signs of the cardiac form are caused by myocardial, diaphragmatic, and intercostal muscle damage and include profound weakness, recumbency, lack of suckle reflex, dyspnea, tachypnea, and foamy or blood-tinged nasal discharge. Death may occur within 24 hours. An irregular, rapid heart rate and a cardiac murmur may be present. Animals that survive the cardiac form may fail to thrive due to permanent myocardial damage, and myodegeneration of skeletal muscles may be observed later in life.[98]

Diagnosis. Antemortem evaluation of selenium and vitamin E status can be performed in whole blood, plasma, and serum. Plasma concentrations of vitamin E are preferred. Plasma selenium concentrations are impacted by recent administration of mineral products or changes in the diet. Whole blood concentrations of selenium or glutathione peroxidase analysis (an indirect measure of selenium) reflect long-term selenium status, as these include measurement of selenium incorporated into intracellular selenoproteins over the previous several months.[99] Testing should include whole blood selenium concentrations and plasma vitamin E concentrations. Liver samples can be used to evaluate body stores of selenium. Ration analysis may help support a herd diagnosis.[100] Non-specific clinicopathologic findings suggestive of WMD include significant increases in CK, aspartate aminotransferase, and LDH. Evidence of dehydration and myoglobinuria may be present. Under experimental conditions, selenium-deficient lambs demonstrated progressive ECG changes, which included an elevation of S-T segment and an increase in T-wave amplitude.[101]

At necropsy, grossly visible lesions include white streaks in muscle fibers and pale areas associated with acute coagulative necrosis, chronic fibrosis, or mineralization of the myocardium. Chronic passive congestion of the liver and congestion and edema of the lungs may be present. Histopathologic changes reflective of cardiocytic injury include myofibrillar lysis and sarcoplasmic vacuolation and granule formation, along with nuclear enlargement and proliferation.[102] With increasing disease severity, contraction band necrosis and mineralization of myocardial lesions are observed.[102]

Treatment. The cardiac form of WMD carries a poor to grave prognosis, despite appropriate treatment and supportive care. Both oral and injectable vitamin E products are available. Injectable selenium and vitamin E preparations should be used.[97] The vitamin E content of combination supplements is insufficient to correct vitamin E deficiency. The risk of selenium toxicity should be stressed to producers, as accidental oversupplementation is a common cause of selenium toxicosis.[103] In lambs, the LD_{50} for intramuscularly administered sodium selenite has been reported to range from 0.45 to 1 mg of Se/kg BW. Signs of selenium toxicity include cardiovascular collapse, with development of pulmonary edema, hydrothorax, and hydropericardium.[104]

Prevention. Prevention is based on proper supplementation of the dam either by salt mix or by total ration supplementation (0.1–0.3 ppm selenium in the diet). During late gestation, use of injectable selenium and vitamin E products may be necessary, which should be administered at least one month prior to parturition[105] (see Chapters 2 and 11).

Parasitic Myositis and Myocarditis

Sarcocystis

Sarcocystis, a protozoan parasite, has an obligatory prey-predator life cycle with asexual stages developing in the intermediate host (e.g., sheep, goat) and sexual stages developing in the definitive host (e.g., carnivore).[106] Numerous sarcocystis species have been described in domestic livestock and wildlife species. Generally, host specificity is greater for the intermediate host than the definitive host. While generally nonpathogenic in the definitive host, sarcocystis species may be pathogenic or nonpathogenic for intermediate hosts. Sheep are intermediate hosts for five sarcocystis species: *Sarcocystis tenella*, *Sarcocystis arieticanis*, *Sarcocystis gigantea*, *Sarcocystis medusiformis*, and *Sarcocystis mihoensis.* Goats are intermediate hosts for three species: *Sarcocystis capracanis*, *Sarcocystis hircicanis*, and *Sarcocystis moule.*[107] Depending on geographic location, the prevalence of sarcocystis can be very high.[107] Sheep and goats become infected by ingesting sporocysts shed in the feces of infected definitive hosts. Merogony and cyst formation (asexual reproduction) take place in the intermediate host, and gametogony (sexual reproduction) and sporogony take place in the definitive host. Initial stages in the intermediate host affect the vascular endothelium, followed by the production of sarcocysts in muscle, which are comprised of the infective bradyzoite stage. Carnivores are infected by consuming tissues containing mature sarcocysts.[106] In intermediate hosts, clinical signs typically occur during the acute phase, during which the parasite multiplies in blood vessels. The presence of edema and hemorrhage may be observed in multiple organs. In chronic phases, lesions are restricted to muscle, consisting of nonsuppurative myositis and degeneration of sarcocysts. Common sites involve the tongue, esophagus, diaphragm, and heart. Both microscopic and macroscopic lesions are possible, depending on sarcocystis species.[108] Condemnation of carcasses due to macroscopic sarcocysts is of economic importance worldwide.[109] Diagnosis can be obtained by light microscopy of tissues.[110] Detailed ultrastructural descriptions of pathological changes and differentiation of sarcocystis species occurs by electron microscopy and molecular techniques (see Chapter 6).[111,112]

Cysticercosis

Cysticercus ovis is the intermediate stage of the canine cestode, *Taenia ovis*, with sheep and goats representing intermediate host species. Domestic dogs and, to a lesser extent, wild canids are the definitive hosts, becoming infected by ingestion of viable cysticerci in infected sheep or goat meat.[113] In the definitive host, the adult tapeworm resides in the intestinal tract and produces eggs, which are passed in the feces and are immediately infective. Sheep and goats are infected by ingestion of contaminated pasture and feedstuffs with feces from dogs actively shedding *T. ovis* ova. Larvae hatch within the ruminant gastrointestinal tract and subsequently migrate to form tissue cysts in skeletal and cardiac muscles.[114] Cysticerci in muscle lesions are infective to canids at approximately 6 to 8 weeks of development in the intermediate host and remain infective for approximately 4 to 8 weeks.[115] Most infections of sheep and goats are clinically inapparent and are detected at harvest. The appearance of tissue lesions prompts the common name: sheep measles. Maturation and subsequent degeneration of cysts, approximately 7 to 10 weeks after ingestion, can result in clinical signs that depend on the affected muscles. Signs may include sudden death, gait deficits, chewing abnormalities, and ill-thrift.[116] *T. ovis* does not appear to be zoonotic but is of significant economic consequence due to carcass condemnation. *T. ovis* is not known to infect cervids. However, infections with cysticerci of *T. ovis krabbei* were reported in red deer, roe deer, fallow deer, reindeer, and caribou. *T. ovis krabbei* possesses a similar sylvatic cycle to *T. ovis*, with foxes and wolves, and less commonly, domestic dogs as the main definitive hosts.[117]

Diagnosis. Infection is most commonly found at necropsy or harvest, by the presence of multiple, white, 3- to 10-mm-long ovoid lesions in heart, diaphragm, and skeletal muscles. The gross appearance of tissue cysts changes with time, beginning as cystic lesions and degenerating into caseous nodules over several weeks postinfection. Chronic lesions may become calcified. Skeletal and cardiac muscle cysts due to *T. ovis krabbei* in deer are similar in appearance.[118] Historical information may include exposure to infected guardian/stock dogs or wild canids. Changes in ECG have been described in lambs with cardiac involvement under experimental challenge conditions. These included sinus tachycardia and arrhythmias, atrial fibrillation or dissociation, a pathologic Q deflection, decreased amplitude of the R wave, and inversion of the T wave.[116]

Prevention. Treatment of cysticerci tissue cysts is neither cost-effective nor practical in large production settings. The effects of praziquantel and mebendazole on cysts of *Echinococcus granulosus*, *Taenia hydatigena*, and *T. ovis* have been evaluated in sheep. If clinical signs necessitate the treatment of individual cases, use of praziquantel (50 mg/kg, subcutaneously) could be attempted, but efficacy is limited when tissue cysts are numerous.[119] Therefore, mitigation of risk factors and minimizing exposure is the mainstay of cysticercosis control. Efforts should include reducing infection in guardian and stock/companion dogs with routine use of anthelmintics effective against *Taenia* species (e.g., praziquantel). New dogs should be treated with a cestocide at least 1 week prior to entry onto the farm and should not have access to carcasses. Treatment of guardian dogs with a cestocide should occur prior to pasture turnout and retreatment occurring every 5 weeks in order to eliminate patent infections (as the prepatent period is 6 weeks).[120] Dead livestock should not be fed to guardian dogs, and carcasses should be properly disposed of by burial, composting, or incineration (see Chapters 6 and 20).[121]

Endocardial and Vascular Diseases

Vegetative Endocarditis

Etiology and Pathophysiology

Infectious endocarditis is rare in small ruminants and has a poor prognosis. Only a few cases of infectious endocarditis in sheep and goats are reported,[5,122,123] and even fewer are available for cervids.[3,124] Therefore, discussions of pathogenesis and recommendations for diagnostics, treatment, and prognosis are commonly extrapolated from horses and cattle. Acquired endocarditis may be inflammatory, infectious, degenerative, traumatic, or idiopathic in etiology. Risk factors for the development of endocarditis include disturbed blood flow (e.g., congenital heart defects), endothelial injury, hemostatic dysfunction, and bacteremia allowing colonization of the endocardium.[125] Chronic active infections, such as rumenitis, liver abscesses, mastitis, and metritis, with sustained or intermittent bacteremia, are believed to predispose ruminants to bacterial endocarditis. In small ruminants and cervids, *E. rhusiopathiae*, *Mannheimia haemolytica*, *Listeria* spp., and *Streptococcus* spp. were reported as causative pathogens of infectious endocarditis. While the right AV is presumably most commonly affected, involvement of all heart valves has been reported.[3,122,123] Vegetative lesions interfere with the proper functioning of the valve and result in cardiac dysfunction, either impairing ejection of blood by obstruction or by valvular insufficiency. Valve incompetence can eventually result in CHF (discussed earlier).[5,126] Depending on the valve involved, sequelae may include pulmonary venous hypertension and left-sided heart failure (with aortic and mitral regurgitation) or elevated central venous pressure and right-sided heart failure (with tricuspid regurgitation). In ruminants, right-sided heart failure is most common. Fragmentation and septic embolization are common, resulting in infarction and abscess formation at distant sites such as the lung, liver, kidney, and joints.[126]

Clinical Signs. The clinical signs of bacterial endocarditis are insidious, and specific signs of heart disease are not frequently observed early during disease. Advanced cases may have signs of severe debilitation and CHF. Based on limited case reports, recognition of bacterial endocarditis in small ruminants is likely to occur late in the disease when evidence of heart failure is present.[5,123] Historical information may include previous treatment for chronic inflammatory processes. Clinical criteria to assess sensitivity and specificity of different clinical findings and ancillary tests are described in cattle with bacterial endocarditis.[127] Clinical signs may include intermittent fever, reduced appetite, weight loss, poor body condition score, polyarthritis, lameness, and evidence of thoracic pain, as well as evidence of CHF (e.g., exercise intolerance, tachycardia, respiratory distress, cough, jugular distention and pulsation, subcutaneous edema, and ascites).[128] The absence of an audible murmur should not preclude a diagnosis of bacterial endocarditis, as cardiac auscultation can lack sensitivity and specificity, with $< 60\%$ of cattle with bacterial endocarditis having an audible murmur at presentation.[129]

Diagnosis. Diagnosis of bacterial endocarditis can prove difficult. Physical examination with detailed cardiac auscultation is critical, as most small ruminants are evaluated in the field without access to additional diagnostic tools. Loud, pounding heart sounds should prompt the clinician to listen carefully for a murmur.[126] The presence of systolic heart murmurs over the left or right heart apex or diastolic murmurs over the left base are suggestive of valve incompetence. A heart murmur in a sheep or goat with concurrent clinical signs of bacterial endocarditis has a high positive predictive value.[126] Evidence of CHF further strengthens a presumptive diagnosis of bacterial endocarditis. However, ancillary diagnostic methods are required to confirm a presumptive diagnosis. These include echocardiography and bacteriological blood culture.[129,130]

A complete echocardiographic examination is both sensitive and specific for the diagnosis of vegetative endocarditis. Two-dimensional echocardiography can detect lesions, dysfunction, or insufficiency of the heart valves and provide assessment of ventricular function. Detection is limited to lesions measuring at least 2 to 3 mm in size. M-mode ultrasonography may help detect chamber enlargement and a decrease in left ventricular shortening fraction. Color flow, pulse wave, or continuous wave Doppler ultrasound evaluation may be useful to help quantify the severity of valve regurgitation.[130]

Bacteriologic culturing of blood samples in suspected cases of bacterial endocarditis is of diagnostic and therapeutic value. Periodic emboli arising from the infected endocardium are common in bacterial endocarditis. Ideally, blood is collected during febrile episodes and before antibiotic administration. For example, three venous blood samples, collected aseptically from separate venipuncture sites, are collected during a 1- to 2-hour period.[131] Culture and antimicrobial susceptibility results should be used in the selection of antibiotic treatment. Use of molecular techniques to identify potential infectious microorganisms involved in endocarditis is becoming more common in livestock species.[132]

Non-specific clinicopathological findings may include nonregenerative anemia, neutrophilia with or without a left shift, hyperglobulinemia, and hyperfibrinogenemia suggestive of chronic infection.[127,133] Radiographic changes associated with bacterial endocarditis in small ruminants have not been reported but may include generalized or focal cardiac enlargement and evidence of embolic pneumonia.

Treatment. Treatment of bacterial endocarditis requires long-term administration of antibiotics. Bactericidal antibiotics with good tissue penetration should be administered for a minimum of 4 to 6 weeks, up to several months.[131] Serial evaluation of clinicopathologic parameters, blood culture, and echocardiographic measurement of endocardial lesions help with decisions regarding continued therapy and the likelihood of disease resolution. The decision to treat bacterial endocarditis should be weighed against the likelihood of treatment failure, a protracted convalescence with consideration of animal welfare, costs incurred by prolonged drug administration, lengthy drug withdrawal periods, and the possibility that the carcass is deemed unfit for human consumption at harvest. Even with prolonged antibiotic therapy, treatment of bacterial endocarditis carries a poor to grave prognosis (see Appendix 1).[126,131,134]

Shock

Etiology and Pathophysiology

Shock is defined as inadequate cellular energy production, which most commonly results from poor tissue perfusion and decreased oxygen delivery. Hypoperfusion and tissue hypoxia can be caused by inappropriate vascular tone, leaky vasculature, pooling of blood within capacitance vessels, or reduced cardiac output or a combination thereof. If left untreated, the resulting multiorgan dysfunction can progress to multiorgan failure.[135–138] Numerous causes and pathophysiological mechanisms are involved in shock, and a detailed description is beyond the scope of this chapter. Functional classifications of shock include hypovolemic shock (loss of intravascular volume), distributive shock (maldistribution of vascular volume), cardiogenic shock (failure of the cardiac pump), metabolic (derangement of cellular metabolism), and hypoxic causes (e.g., severe anemia).[136] Common causes of shock in ruminants include severe dehydration, electrolyte and acid-base disturbances, anemia, sepsis, overwhelming bacterial infections, myocarditis, and cardiovascular anomalies.

Clinical Signs. Physical assessment of the circulatory system allows assessment of global perfusion. A diagnosis of shock is made based on physical examination, which should be performed serially during the monitoring and treatment of shock.[139] Perfusion parameters include mentation, temperature of extremities, heart rate, peripheral pulse quality, CRT, mucous membrane color, jugular fill, and urine production. Additional parameters of dehydration assessment include skin tent turgor, eyeball recession, and dryness of mucous membranes.[140,141] Examination includes careful auscultation of the heart and lungs, which should be performed repeatedly during treatment to detect subtle changes suggestive of pulmonary dysfunction, fluid overload, or continuing failure to respond to resuscitation efforts. Body temperature is also evaluated, with both hypothermia and hyperthermia (primary hyperthermia and true fever) common. Clinical signs commonly observed in ruminants with shock include weakness, depression or obtunded mention, decreased urination and defecation, pale or cyanotic mucous membranes, and alterations in respiration. Depending on the inciting cause, a moderate to severe degree of dehydration may be present. Monitoring devices, such as blood gas analysis, blood pressure, pulse oximetry, and point-of-care tests (e.g., L-lactate) may provide useful data to the clinician.

Diagnosis. Diagnosis is made by characteristic clinical exam findings and supported by clinicopathologic abnormalities. Clinicopathologic data may reflect the inciting cause as well as the extent of organ injury due to ongoing shock. In-house analyses should include packed cell volume, serum total protein, blood smear evaluation, urine dipstick, and urine-specific gravity quantification.[141] The severity of dehydration or anemia should be interpreted in conjunction with clinical examination findings. Use of handheld meters for blood glucose and L-lactate can be helpful, the former particularly useful in neonatal lambs and kids.[142,143] When possible, a complete blood cell count and serum biochemistry should be performed. Severe inflammatory or infectious states (septic or maldistributive shock) may cause neutropenia with the presence of immature neutrophils. Disseminated intravascular coagulopathy may be present, evidenced by thrombocytopenia and low fibrinogen concentrations (in the case of fibrinolytic states). Changes on serum biochemistry may include metabolic acidosis, azotemia, and alterations in blood glucose. Increases in liver enzymes may be due to a primary disease or can reflect impaired perfusion of the liver.[141] In cases of presumptive sepsis, blood culture may be useful in finding a definitive diagnosis. Other measurements of tissue perfusion, oxygen delivery, and cardiac output include: central venous pressure, mean arterial pressure, urine output, pulse oximetry, venous and arterial blood gas analyses, and echocardiography and pulmonary artery catheterization to determine cardiac output indices.[144,145] However, routine use of these monitoring tools in sheep and goats are limited.

Treatment. The treatment goals for shock therapy include early recognition of shock and the restoration of tissue perfusion and oxygen delivery. Therapy for all forms of shock, except cardiogenic shock, is based on the administration of intravenous fluids to restore effective circulating volume and tissue perfusion. Delivery of fluids by subcutaneous or oral routes is ineffective in animals with shock. Current guidelines in veterinary critical care medicine favor the fluid challenge method.[146,147] This entails the use of isotonic crystalloids given as fluid boluses with the serial appraisal of clinical parameters for goal directed endpoints and, if warranted, the continuation of fluid therapy and additional treatments (e.g., vasopressors). The goals of resuscitation are the rapid correction of hypovolemia and the reversal of clinical signs of shock, as seen with improvement in perfusion parameters (as discussed earlier). Additional goals include the correction of hypotension, tachycardia, oliguria, and hyperlactatemia. Treatment of dehydration requires more time but should be part of the clinical assessment. Once resuscitation efforts have been achieved, intravenous fluid therapy is continued as needed to address maintenance requirements and ongoing losses. The maximum bolus rate (shock rate) of 90 mL/kg/h is often stated in the veterinary literature; however, other authors recommend lower rates (e.g., 30–50 mL/kg/h) to prevent overhydration and hypertension.[148] Importantly, perfusion parameters should be reassessed repeatedly following administration of boluses (e.g., 10–20 mL/kg administered over 20–30 minutes) with additional boluses as needed. Typically, one to three boluses are necessary, and a fourth bolus is rarely required.[146] In addition to isotonic crystalloids, hypertonic saline (7–7.5%) can be administered at a rate of 4 mL/kg IV.[149] If appropriate, plasma or whole blood transfusions may be used to treat failure of passive transfer, anemia, endothelial dysfunction during sepsis/SIRS, or other causes of reduced oncotic pressure. Use of commercial colloid products in sheep and goats is rare, but recommendations made for other species apply. Colloids can be administered at a rate of 3 to 5 mL/kg but should not exceed 10 mL/kg/day due to the risk dose-dependent coagulopathies.[150] Importantly, ongoing hemorrhage must be controlled, as resuscitative efforts exacerbate bleeding if present. If hemorrhage is uncontrollable, hypotensive resuscitation is warranted. If animals remain hypotensive despite intravascular volume resuscitation (i.e., a full shock dose has been administered without significant improvement), vasopressor or inotrope therapy may be required to treat myocardial dysfunction. Commonly used vasopressors include catecholamines (e.g., epinephrine, norepinephrine, and dopamine) and positive inotropic drugs (e.g., dobutamine).[151] Additionally, corticosteroids may be used as adjunct pressor agents. Resuscitation in the case of cardiogenic shock requires special attention, as these animals are very prone to the development of pulmonary edema, dyspnea, and the untoward effects of stressful handling. If tolerated, supplemental oxygen therapy via nasal cannula or facemask should be provided. Furosemide can be used at a dose of 1 to 2 mg/kg IV every 6 to 12 hours. Greater doses (up to 8 mg/kg) or an increased frequencies of administration (i.e., every 1–2 hours) may be required until respiratory characteristics improve.[152] Electrolytes should be monitored when using diuretics at high doses or for prolonged periods.[153,154] During resuscitation therapy, monitoring for volume overload is of utmost importance, especially in animals at risk for fluid overload and pulmonary edema (e.g., hypoproteinemia/hypoalbuminemia and renal insufficiency). Clinical signs of fluid overload include increased respiratory rates, subtle changes on thoracic auscultation, presence of serous ocular and nasal discharge, subcutaneous edema, and deterioration of mentation.[155] Further details about fluid therapy can be found in Chapter 3. Other treatments for primary disease processes, such as antimicrobials, antiinflammatory drugs, and antitoxins as well as basic supportive care should be administered, as indicated (see Chapter 3).[156]

Heartwater (Cowdriosis)

Etiology and Pathophysiology

Heartwater is a tick-borne, rickettsial disease of various wild and domestic ruminants in sub-Saharan Africa and islands in the Indian Ocean and the Caribbean caused by *Ehrlichia ruminantium* (formerly *Cowdria ruminantium*). The genus *Ehrlichia* shares the family Anaplasmataceae with four other rickettsial genera including *Anaplasma*, *Neoehrlichia*, *Neorickettsia*, and *Wolbachia*. Several tick species in the genus *Amblyomma* serve as vector for *E. ruminantium*, including *Amblyomma hebraeum* (bont tick) in southern Africa, *Amblyomma lepidum* in eastern Africa, and *Amblyomma variegatum* (tropical bont tick) in sub-Saharan Africa and island of the Indian Ocean and Carribean.[157] Other tick species appear to be suitable vectors, raising concerns that the disease could spread to currently unaffected areas, including Central, North, and South America. Heartwater is one of the most important diseases of African livestock, and the disease is most severe in introduced animals, hampering efforts of genetically improving production parameters of indigenous breeds. In endemic areas, severe heartwater occurs in nonindigenous sheep and goat breeds and in introduced Rusa (Timor) deer and chital (Axis deer), but the disease is possible in various other ruminants, including white-tailed deer, either by natural or experimental infection.[158,159]

After the transmission of *E. ruminantium* by infected ticks, the organism replicates in cells of the mononuclear phagocyte system in regional lymph nodes, followed by hematogenous dissemination and invasion of vascular endothelial cells of many organs, including the brain. Increased vascular permeability leads to fluid accumulation in body cavities, tissue edema, and corresponding clinical signs. The outcome of infection and severity of clinical signs depend on various host and pathogen-associated factors, such as genetic susceptibility, immune status, age, and pathogenic genotype of the organism. Animals surviving infection may be carriers for extended periods of time.

Clinical Signs. After an incubation time of 7 to 35 days (14 days on average), infection with *E. ruminantium* may result in peracute, acute, or subacute disease.[160,161] Peracute disease is uncommon but can occur in nonindigenous goat breeds and is characterized by sudden death preceded by paroxysmal convulsions or, occasionally, diarrhea. In the more common acute form, clinical signs include fever, listlessness, respiratory signs such as moist coughing and dyspnea, lowered head position, and progressive neurologic signs. Neurologic signs include incoordination, ataxia, dysmetria, hyperesthesia, behavioral changes, chewing movements, licking of the lips, lateral recumbency, paddling, opisthotonos, and seizures. The subacute from is characterized by prolonged pyrexia and milder respiratory and neurologic signs, from which affected animals may recover with 1 to 2 weeks.[160,161]

Diagnosis. Postmortem findings include severe hydropericardium and hydrothorax, ascites, pulmonary edema, presence of frothy serous foam in the airways, and brain edema.[161] Giemsa or CAM's quick staining allows visualization of the organism by light microscopy in the cytoplasm of endothelial cells in smears of brain tissue or tissue sections from brain or kidney. The organism can also be detected in tissue samples or blood by polymerase chain reaction, loop-mediated isothermal amplification, or culture on ruminant endothelial cells.[160,162] Various serological tests for *E. ruminantium* are available, but results should be interpreted carefully, due to cross-reactivity with other bacteria in the family Anaplasmataceae and low antibody titers in some infected animals.[160]

Treatment. Antibiotic treatment and prevention rely on tetracyclines, and different treatment regimens have been recommended (e.g., 5–10 mg/kg tetracycline IV or intramuscularly [IM] every 12–24 hours or two doses of 20 mg/kg oxytetracycline IM or subcutaneously [SC] on two successive days). Treatment should be initiated during the febrile stage of the disease to prevent additional organ damage and worse prognosis.[8,160]

Prevention. Prevention of heartwater is based on tick control, use of resistant (indigenous) breeds in endemic areas, preventative use of tetracyclines, and vaccination. While successful control of *A. variegatum* has been possible on some Caribbean islands, control or eradication of *Amblyomma* is difficult and impractical under many field conditions due to the development of resistance to acaricides and need for regular handling of animals. Long-acting acaricides are a valuable replacement for long-practiced plunge dipping. Strategic tick control aims at reducing tick numbers, while maintaining a low level of challenge and, thus, immunity. Regular or preventive use of tetracycline antibiotics is expensive and likely results in the development of antibiotic resistance. Newly introduced animals may be treated with multiple doses of tetracycline as described previously. Inactivated, attenuated, and recombinant vaccines have been developed, but a highly efficacious vaccine that is protective against all immunotypes of the genetically diverse pathogen is still needed.[160,163]

References

1. Scott PR: Cardiovascular system. In Scott PR, editor: *Sheep medicine*, ed 2, Boca Raton, FL, 2015, CRC Press, pp 145–148.
2. Mansour M, Wilhite R, Rowe J: *Guide to ruminant anatomy: dissection and clinical aspects*, Hoboken, NJ, 2017, John Wiley & Sons, Inc.
3. Badger SB: Infectious epiphysitis and valvular endocarditis in a red deer (*Cervus elaphus*), *N Z Vet J* 30(3):17–18, 1982.
4. Crilly JP, Morrison LR, Scott PR: Endocarditis and ventricular wall abscessation in a vasectomised Herdwick ram, *Vet Rec Case Rep* 3(1):e000178, 2015.
5. Scott PR, Sargison ND: Extensive ascites associated with vegetative endocarditis and Sarcocystis myositis in a shearling ram, *Vet Rec* 149(8):240–241, 2001.

6. Geisel O: Zur Pathologie der Ziegenaorta, *Vet Pathol* 10(3): 202–218, 1973.
7. Braun U, Mitchell K, Schramm S, Nogler S, Hatt J, Malbon A: Ultrasonographic findings in two sheep with enzootic calcinosis, *Schweiz Arch Tierheilkd* 158(12):827–832, 2016.
8. Smith MC, Sherman DM: *Goat medicine,* ed 2, Ames, IA, 2009, Wiley Blackwell.
9. Cebra C, Cebra M: Diseases of the cardiovascular system. In Pugh DG, Baird AN, editors: *Sheep and goat medicine,* ed 2, Maryland Heights, MO, 2012, Elsevier Saunders, pp 503–516.
10. Brown DL, Van Wettere AJ, Cullen JM: Hepatobiliary system and exocrine pancreas. In Zachary JF, editor: *Pathologic basis of veterinary disease,* ed 6, St. Louis, MO, 2017, Elsevier, pp 412–470.
11. Gay CC, Richards WP: Cor pulmonale and atrial fibrillation in goats as a sequel to pneumonia, *Aust Vet J* 60(9):274–275, 1983.
12. Boesch JM, Boulanger JR, Curtis PD, et al: Biochemical variables in free-ranging white-tailed deer (*Odocoileus virginianus*) after chemical immobilization in clover traps or via ground-darting, *J Zoo Wildl Med* 42(1):18–28, 2011.
13. Boesch JM, Gleed RD, Erb HN, Solter PF: Laboratory validation of a point-of-care cardiac troponin I assay for use in white-tailed deer *(Odocoileus virginianus), J Zoo Wildl Med* 46(3):468–475, 2015.
14. Tharwat M, Al-Sobayil F, Al-Sobayil K: The cardiac biomarkers troponin I and CK-MB in nonpregnant and pregnant goats, goats with normal birth, goats with prolonged birth, and goats with pregnancy toxemia, *Theriogenology* 78(7):1500–1507, 2012.
15. Tharwat M, Al-Sobayil F, El-Sayed M: Cardiac troponin I in healthy newborn goat kids and in goat kids with cardiac nutritional muscular dystrophy, *Acta Vet Hung* 61(4):442–453, 2013.
16. Karapinar T, Eroksuz Y, Beytut E, Sozdutmaz I, Eroksuz H, Dabak M: Increased plasma cardiac troponin I concentration in lambs with myocarditis, *Vet Clin Pathol* 41(3):375–381, 2012.
17. Neuwald EB, Soares FA, Dreyer CT, et al: Increase in cardiac troponin I in a lamb with Tetralogy of Fallot, *J Vet Med Sci* 75(10): 1371–1373, 2013.
18. Szabuniewicz M, Clark DR: Analysis of the electrocardiograms of 100 normal goats, *Am J Vet Res* 28(123):511–516, 1967.
19. Fakour S, Mokhber Dezfuli MR, Nadalian MG, Rezakhani A, Lotfollah Zadeh S: Electrocardiographic parameters of Markhoz goat using base apex lead and six standard limb leads, *Iran J Vet Res* 14(3):241–244, 2013.
20. Ahmed JA, Sanyal S: Electrocardiographic studies in Garol sheep and Black Bengal goats, *Res J Cardiol* 1:1–8, 2008.
21. Pogliani FC, Birgel Junior EH, Monteiro BM, Grisi Filho JHH, Raimondo RFS: The normal electrocardiogram in the clinically healthy Saanen goats, *Pesquisa Veterinária Brasileira* 33:1478–1482, 2013.
22. Sudhakara RB, Sivajothi S: Electrocardiographic studies in different age groups of Nellore cross-breed sheep, *Int Clin Pathol J* 6(1): 30–32, 2018.
23. Schultz RA, Pretorius PJ, Terblanche M: An electrocardiographic study of normal sheep using a modified technique, *Onderstepoort J Vet Res* 39(2):97–106, 1972.
24. Hallowell GD, Potter TJ, Bowen IM: Reliability of quantitative echocardiography in adult sheep and goats, *BMC Vet Res* 8:181, 2012.
25. Leroux AA, Farnir F, Moonen ML, Sandersen CF, Deleuze S, Amory H: Repeatability, variability and reference values of pulsed wave Doppler echocardiographic measurements in healthy Saanen goats, *BMC Vet Res* 8:190, 2012.
26. Leroux AA, Moonen ML, Farnir F, et al: Two-dimensional and M-mode echocardiographic reference values in healthy adult Saanen goats, *Vet Rec* 170(6):154, 2012.
27. Szalus-Jordanow O, Czopowicz M, Witkowski L, et al: Reference intervals of echocardiographic measurements in healthy adult dairy goats, *PLoS One* 12(8):e0183293, 2017.
28. Olsson K, Hansson A, Hydbring E, von Walter LW, Haggstrom J: A serial study of heart function during pregnancy, lactation and the dry period in dairy goats using echocardiography, *Exp Physiol* 86(1): 93–99, 2001.
29. Fletcher DJ, Boller M, Brainard BM, et al: RECOVER evidence and knowledge gap analysis on veterinary CPR. Part 7: clinical guidelines, *J Vet Emerg Crit Care (San Antonio)* 22(Suppl 1):S102–S131, 2012.
30. Fletcher DJ, Boller M: Chapter 3—cardiopulmonary resuscitation. In Silverstein DC, Hopper K, editors: *Small animal critical care medicine,* ed 2, St. Louis, 2015, W.B. Saunders, pp 11–17.
31. Bisaillon A, DeRoth L, Roy R: Congenital cardiac anomalies in a lamb, *Vet Pathol* 19(6):718–720, 1982.
32. Gendron A: A ventricular septal defect in an axis deer, *J Zoo Anim Med* 6(2):28–28, 1975.
33. Parry BW, Wrigley RH, Reuter RE: Ventricular septal defects in three familially-related female Saanen goats, *Aust Vet J* 59(3):72–76, 1982.
34. Jafari Dehkordi A, Hoseini F: Patent ductus arteriosus in a lamb: a case report, *Vet Res Forum* 7(1):85–88, 2016.
35. Gardner SY, Reef VB, Palmer JE, Reimer JM, Sweeney RW: Echocardiographic diagnosis of an anomaly of the tricuspid valve in a male pygmy goat, *J Am Vet Med Assoc* 200(4):521–523, 1992.
36. Abo-Shehada MN, Al-Rawashdeh O, Al-Natour M: Traumatic pericarditis in an Awassi lamb, *Br Vet J* 147(1):78–81, 1991.
37. Akkoc A: Traumatic reticulopericarditis in a Saanen goat, *Turk J Vet Anim Sci* 31(4):283–285, 2007.
38. Baydar E, Kulualp K, Eroksuz Y, Karapinar T, Eroksuz H: Traumatic reticuloperitonitis in a flock of sheep, *J Appl Anim Res* 44(1): 311–314, 2016.
39. Foreyt WJ, Leathers CW: Traumatic reticulopericarditis in a mule deer, *J Wildl Dis* 22(3):446, 1986.
40. Williamson MM, Pettifer JK, Mccoy RJ, Taylor T, Kennedy J, Ross AD: Pleuropneumonia and pericarditis in a goat with isolation of *Mycoplasma mycoides* subspecies *mycoides* large colony, *Aust Vet J* 85(4):153–155, 2007.
41. Braun U, Hagen A, Pusterla N, Caplazi P: Echocardiographic diagnosis of a cardiac fibrosarcoma in the right atrium of a sheep, *Schweiz Arch Tierheilkd* 137(5):187–192, 1995.
42. Braun U: Traumatic pericarditis in cattle: clinical, radiographic and ultrasonographic findings, *Vet J* 182(2):176–186, 2009.
43. Buczinski S: Cardiovascular ultrasonography in cattle, *Vet Clin North Am Food Anim Pract* 25(3):611–632, 2009.
44. Freestone JF, Thomas WP, Carlson GP, Brumbaugh GW: Idiopathic effusive pericarditis with tamponade in the horse, *Equine Vet J* 19(1):38–42, 1987.
45. Robinson JA, Marr CM, Reef VB, Sweeney RW: Idiopathic, aseptic, effusive, fibrinous, nonconstrictive pericarditis with tamponade in a standard bred filly, *J Am Vet Med Assoc* 201(10):1593–1598, 1992.
46. Radostits OM, Gay CC, Hinchcliff KW, Constable PD: Diseases of the pericardium. In Radostits OM, Gay CC, Hinchcliff KW, Constable PD, editors: *Veterinary medicine: a textbook of the diseases of cattle, horses, sheep, pigs, and goats,* ed 10, Philadelphia, PA, 2007, Saunders Elsevier, pp 430–432.
47. Mellanby RJ, Henry JP, Cash R, Ricketts SW, Bexiga JRD, Mellor DJ: Serum cardiac troponin I concentrations in cattle with pericarditis, *Vet Rec* 161(13):454–455, 2007.
48. Ducharme NG, Desrochers A, Mulon P-Y, Nichols S: Chapter 13—surgery of the bovine (adult) respiratory and cardiovascular systems. In Fubini SL, Ducharme NG, editors: *Farm animal surgery,* ed 2, St. Louis, MO, 2017, Elsevier, pp 193–222.
49. Ducharme NG, Fubini SL, Rebhun WC, Beck KA: Thoracotomy in adult dairy cattle: 14 cases (1979–1991), *J Am Vet Med Assoc* 200(1):86–90, 1992.
50. Mason TA: Suppurative pericarditis treated by pericardiotomy in a cow, *Vet Rec* 105(15):350–351, 1979.
51. Rings DM: Surgical treatment of pleuritis and pericarditis, *Vet Clin North Am Food Anim Pract* 11(1):177–182, 1995.
52. Jesty SA: Chapter 123—pericardial disease. In Sprayberry KA, Robinson NE, editors: *Robinson's current therapy in equine medicine,* ed 7, St. Louis, 2015, W.B. Saunders, pp 516–520.

53. Nelson OL, Ware WA: Pericardial effusions. In Bonagura J, Twedt D, editors: *Kirk's current veterinary therapy XIV,* St. Louis, MO, 2009, Saunders, pp 825–831.
54. Grant R, Basson PA, Booker HH, Hofherr JB, Anthonissen M: Cardiomyopathy caused by avocado (Persea americana Mill) leaves, *J S Afr Vet Assoc* 62(1):21–22, 1991.
55. Craigmill AL, Seawright AA, Mattila T, Frost AJ: Pathological changes in the mammary gland and biochemical changes in milk of the goat following oral dosing with leaf of the avocado (Persea americana), *Aust Vet J* 66(7):206–211, 1989.
56. Constable PD, Hinchcliff KW, Done SH, Grünberg W: Yew (*Taxus* spp.) toxicosis. In Constable PD, Hinchcliff KW, Done SH, Grünberg W, editors: *Veterinary medicine—a textbook of the diseases of cattle, horses, sheep, pigs and goats,* ed 11, St. Louis, MO, 2017, Elsevier, pp 699–700.
57. Knight AP, Walter RG: Plants affecting the cardiovascular system. In Knight AP, Walter RG, editors: *A guide to plant poisoning of animals in North America*, Jackson, WY, 2002, Teton NewMedia.
58. Barbosa RR, Fontenele-Neto JD, Soto-Blanco B: Toxicity in goats caused by oleander (*Nerium oleander*), *Res Vet Sci* 85(2):279–281, 2008.
59. Adam SE, Al-Yahya MA, Al-Farhan AH: Response of Najdi sheep to oral administration of *Citrullus colocynthis* fruits, *Nerium oleander* leaves or their mixture, *Small Rumin Res* 40(3):239–244, 2001.
60. Gallagher CH, Koch JH, Moore RM, Steel JD: Toxicity of *Phalaris tuberosa* for sheep, *Nature* 204:542–545, 1964.
61. Bourke CA, Rendell D, Colegate SM: Clinical observations and differentiation of the peracute *Phalaris aquatica* poisoning syndrome in sheep known as 'polioencephalomalacia-like sudden death'. *Aust Vet J* 81(11):698–700, 2003.
62. Bourke CA, Carrigan MJ, Dixon RJ: Experimental evidence that tryptamine alkaloids do not cause *Phalaris aquatica* sudden death syndrome in sheep, *Aust Vet J* 65(7):218–220, 1988.
63. Bourke CA, Colegate SM, Rendell D, Bunker EC, Kuhn RP: Peracute ammonia toxicity: a consideration in the pathogenesis of *Phalaris aquatica* 'polioencephalomalacia-like sudden death' poisoning of sheep and cattle, *Aust Vet J* 83(3):168–171, 2005.
64. Lopes DI, Sousa MG, Ramos AT, Maruo VM: Cardiotoxicity of *Senna occidentalis* in sheep (*Ovis aries*), *Open Vet J* 6(1):30–35, 2016.
65. El Sayed NY, Abdelbari EM, Mahmoud OM, Adam SE: The toxicity of *Cassia senna* to Nubian goats, *Vet Q* 5(2):80–85, 1983.
66. Gadelha IC, Fonseca NB, Oloris SC, Melo MM, Soto-Blanco B: Gossypol toxicity from cottonseed products, *Sci World J* 2014:231635, 2014.
67. East NE, Anderson M, Lowenstine LJ: Apparent gossypol-induced toxicosis in adult dairy goats, *J Am Vet Med Assoc* 204(4):642–643, 1994.
68. El-Mokadem MY, Taha TA, Samak MA, Yassen AM: Alleviation of reproductive toxicity of gossypol using selenium supplementation in rams, *J Anim Sci* 90(9):3274–3285, 2012.
69. Morgan S, Stair EL, Martin T, Edwards WC, Morgan GL: Clinical, clinicopathologic, pathologic, and toxicologic alterations associated with gossypol toxicosis in feeder lambs, *Am J Vet Res* 49(4):493–499, 1988.
70. Jansen SA, Kleerekooper I, Hofman ZL, Kappen IF, Stary-Weinzinger A, van der Heyden MA: Grayanotoxin poisoning: 'mad honey disease' and beyond, *Cardiovasc Toxicol* 12(3):208–215, 2012.
71. Black DH: Rhododendron poisoning in sheep, *Vet Rec* 128(15): 363–364, 1991.
72. Puschner B, Holstege DM, Lamberski N: Grayanotoxin poisoning in three goats, *J Am Vet Med Assoc* 218(4):573–575, 527–578, 2001.
73. Coenen M, Bahrs F: Animal nutrition for veterinarians—actual cases—lethal intoxication of goats by branches of yew withdrawn from a Garden, *Dtsch Tierarztl Wochenschr* 101(9):364–367, 1994.
74. Rae CA, Binnington BD: Yew poisoning in sheep, *Can Vet J* 36(7):446–446, 1995.
75. Handeland K, Vikoren T, Josefsen TD, Madslien K, Valdecanas B, Uhlig S: Yew (*Taxus*) intoxication in free-ranging cervids, *PLoS One* 12(12), 2017.
76. Wacker R: Yew (*Taxus-baccata*) poisoning in fallow deer, *Tierarztl Umsch* 38(4):264-&,1983.
77. Angus KW: Plant toxicity apparent low toxicity of yew for roe deer *(Capreolus capreolus*), *Vet Rec* 166(7):216–216, 2010.
78. Scott WA: Apparent low toxicity of yew in muntjac deer and Soay sheep, *Vet Rec* 166(8):246–246, 2010.
79. Weaver JD, Brown DL: Incubation of European yew (*Taxus baccata*) with white-tailed deer (*Odocoileus virginianus*) rumen fluid reduces taxine A concentrations, *Vet Hum Toxicol* 46(6):300–302, 2004.
80. Poppenga RH: Feed additives. In Smith BP, editor: *Large animal internal medicine,* ed 5, Saint Louis, MO, 2015, Elsevier Mosby, pp 1609–1611.
81. Bastianello SS, Fourie N, Prozesky L, Nel PW, Kellermann TS: Cardiomyopathy of ruminants induced by the litter of poultry fed on rations containing the ionophore antibiotic, maduramicin. II. Macropathology and histopathology, *Onderstepoort J Vet Res* 62(1):5–18, 1995.
82. Kart A, Bilgili A: Ionophore antibiotics: toxicity, mode of action and neurotoxic aspect of carboxylic ionophores, *J Anim Vet Adv* 7(6): 748–751, 2008.
83. Ashrafihelan J, Eisapour H, Erfani AM, Kalantary AA, Amoli JS, Mozafari M: High mortality due to accidental salinomycin intoxication in sheep, *Interdiscip Toxicol* 7(3):173–176, 2014.
84. Jones A: Monensin toxicosis in 2 sheep flocks, *Can Vet J* 42(2): 135–136, 2001.
85. Glover GJ, Wobeser G: Monensin toxicity in a captive white-tailed deer (*Odocoileus-virginianus*), *J Zoo Anim Med* 14(1):13–16, 1983.
86. Hall JO: Ionophores. In Plumlee, Konnie H: *Clinical veterinary toxicology,* St. Louis, MO, 2004, Mosby, pp 120–127.
87. Nation PN, Crowe SP, Harries WN: Clinical signs and pathology of accidental monensin poisoning in sheep, *Can Vet J* 23(11):323–326, 1982.
88. Agaoglu ZT, Akgul Y, Keles I, Ugras S, Aksoy A, Cinar A: Accidental salinomycin intoxication of Angora goats in Turkey, *Small Rumin Res* 45(2):159–161, 2002.
89. Roder JD, McCoy CP: Ionophore toxicoses. In Howard JL, Smith RA, editors: *Current veterinary therapy: food animal practice,* ed 4, Philadelphia, PA, 1999, W.B. Saunders Company, pp 244–245.
90. Deljou M, Aslani MR, Mohri M, Movassaghi AR, Heidarpour M: Clinical, laboratory and pathological findings in sub-acute monensin intoxication in goats, *Vet Res Forum* 5(3):161–167, 2014.
91. Logan EF, Rice DA, Smyth JA, Ellis WA: Weak calf syndrome and parenteral selenium supplementation, *Vet Rec* 126(7):163–164, 1990.
92. Maas J, Bulgin MS, Anderson BC, Frye TM: Nutritional myodegeneration associated with vitamin E deficiency and normal selenium status in lambs, *J Am Vet Med Assoc* 184(2):201–204, 1984.
93. Pourliotis K, Giadinis ND, Sofianidis G, et al: Congenital nutritional myodegeneration (white muscle disease) in a red deer (*Cervus elaphus*) calf, *N Z Vet J* 57(4):244–247, 2009.
94. Hamliri A, Olson WG, Johnson DW, Kessabi M: Evaluation of biochemical evidence of congenital nutritional myopathy in two-week prepartum fetuses from selenium-deficient ewes, *Am J Vet Res* 51(7):1112–1115, 1990.
95. Hosnedlova B, Kepinska M, Skalickova S, et al: A summary of new findings on the biological effects of selenium in selected animal species—a critical review, *Int J Mol Sci* 18(10):pii: E2209, 2017.
96. Bostedt H, Schramel P: The importance of selenium in the prenatal and postnatal development of calves and lambs, *Biol Trace Elem Res* 24(2):163–171, 1990.
97. Cawley GD, Bradley R: Sudden death in calves associated with acute myocardial degeneration and selenium deficiency, *Vet Rec* 103(11): 239–240, 1978.
98. Ewan RC, Baumann CA, Pope AL: Effects of selenium and vitamin E on nutritional muscular dystrophy in lambs, *J Anim Sci* 27(3): 751–756, 1968.
99. Hidiroglou M: Trace elements in the fetal and neonate ruminant: a review, *Can Vet J* 21(12):328–335, 1980.

100. Ammerman CB, Miller SM: Selenium in ruminant nutrition: a review, *J Dairy Sci* 58(10):1561–1577, 1975.
101. Godwin KO: Electrocardiograms of lambs in selenium deficiency, *Nature* 209(5027):1030–1031, 1966.
102. Kennedy S, Rice DA: Histopathologic and ultrastructural myocardial alterations in calves deficient in vitamin E and selenium and fed polyunsaturated fatty acids, *Vet Pathol* 29(2):129–138, 1992.
103. Gabbedy BJ: Toxicity in sheep associated with the prophylactic use of selenium, *Aust Vet J* 46(5):223–226, 1970.
104. Amini K, Simko E, Davies JL: Sudden death associated with myocardial contraction band necrosis in Boer goat kids, *Vet Pathol* 48(6):1212–1215, 2011.
105. Cawley GD, McPhee I: Trials with a long acting parenteral selenium preparation in ruminants: sheep, *Vet Rec* 114(23):565–566, 1984.
106. Dubey JP, Lindsay DS: Neosporosis, toxoplasmosis, and sarcocystosis in ruminants, *Vet Clin North Am Food Anim Pract* 22(3): 645–671, 2006.
107. Amairia S, Amdouni Y, Rouatbi M, Rjeibi MR, Awadi S, Gharbi M: First detection and molecular identification of Sarcocystis spp. in small ruminants in North-West Tunisia, *Transbound Emerg Dis* 65(2):441–446, 2018.
108. Hu JJ, Liu TT, Liu Q, et al: Prevalence, morphology, and molecular characteristics of *Sarcocystis* spp. in domestic goats (*Capra hircus*) from Kunming, China, *Parasitol Res* 115(10):3973–3981, 2016.
109. Borji H, Parandeh S: The abattoir condemnation of meat because of parasitic infection, and its economic importance: results of a retrospective study in north-eastern Iran, *Ann Trop Med Parasitol* 104(8):641–647, 2010.
110. Landsverk T, Gamlem H, Svenkerud R: A sarcocystis-like protozoon in a sheep with lymphadenopathy and myocarditis, *Vet Pathol* 15(2):186–195, 1978.
111. Haziroglu R, Guvenc T, Tunca R: Electron microscopical studies on cysts of *Sarcocystis arieticanis* within cardiac muscle of naturally infected sheep, *Parasitol Res* 89(1):23–25, 2003.
112. Al Quraishy S, Morsy K, Bashtar AR, Ghaffar FA, Mehlhorn H: *Sarcocystis arieticanis* (Apicomplexa: Sarcocystidae) infecting the heart muscles of the domestic sheep, *Ovis aries* (Artiodactyla: Bovidae), from K. S. A. on the basis of light and electron microscopic data, *Parasitol Res* 113(10):3823–3831, 2014.
113. Jenkins DJ, Urwin NA, Williams TM, Mitchell KL, Lievaart JJ, Armua-Fernandez MT: Red foxes (*Vulpes vulpes*) and wild dogs (dingoes (*Canis lupus dingo*) and dingo/domestic dog hybrids), as sylvatic hosts for Australian *Taenia hydatigena* and *Taenia ovis*, *Int J Parasitol Parasites Wildl* 3(2):75–80, 2014.
114. Ransom BH: Cysticercus ovis, the cause of tapeworm cysts in mutton, *J Agric Res* 1(1):15–57, 1913.
115. Sutton RJ: Observations on experimental infections of dogs with *Taenia ovis*, *Res Vet Sci* 17(2):200–203, 1974.
116. Kostov I, Georgieva D: [Changes in the ECG telemetry of lambs infected with *Cysticercus ovis*], *Vet Med Nauki* 22(6):56–61, 1985.
117. Al-Sabi MN, Chriel M, Holm E, Jensen TK, Stahl M, Enemark HL: Reappearance of *Taenia ovis* krabbei muscle cysts in a roe deer (*Capreolus capreolus*) in Denmark after 60+ years, *Vet Parasitol* 196(1–2):225–229, 2013.
118. Flueck WT, Jones A: Potential existence of a sylvatic cycle of *Taenia ovis* krabbei in Patagonia, Argentina, *Vet Parasitol* 135(3–4):381–383, 2006.
119. Heath DD, Lawrence SB: The effect of mebendazole and praziquantel on the cysts of *Echinococcus granulosus*, *Taenia hydatigena* and *T. ovis* in sheep, *N Z Vet J* 26(1–2):11–15, 1978.
120. DeWolf BD, Poljak Z, Peregrine AS, Jones-Bitton A, Jansen JT, Menzies PI: Development of a Taenia ovis transmission model and an assessment of control strategies, *Vet Parasitol* 198(1–2): 127–135, 2013.
121. DeWolf BD, Peregrine AS, Jones-Bitton A, Jansen JT, Mactavish J, Menzies PI: Distribution of, and risk factors associated with, sheep carcass condemnations due to *Cysticercus ovis* infection on Canadian sheep farms, *Vet Parasitol* 190(3–4):434–441, 2012.
122. Aslani MR, Ebrahimi Kahrisangi A, Baghban F, Kazemi A, Heidari M, Salehi N: Endocarditis associated with *Erysipelothrix rhusiopathiae* in a fat-tailed ram, *Iran J Vet Res* 16(3):310–312, 2015.
123. LaHue N, Parish S: *Mannheimia haemolytica* vegetative endocarditis in a Suffolk wether, *Can Vet J* 56(5):484–485, 2015.
124. Eskens U, Zschock M: [Erysipelas in the roe deer—a case report], *Tierarztl Prax* 19(1):52–53, 1991.
125. Peddle G, Sleeper MM: Canine bacterial endocarditis: a review, *J Am Anim Hosp Assoc* 43(5):258–263, 2007.
126. Power HT, Rebhun WC: Bacterial endocarditis in adult dairy cattle, *J Am Vet Med Assoc* 182(8):806–808, 1983.
127. Bexiga R, Mateus A, Philbey AW, Ellis K, Barrett DC, Mellor DJ: Clinicopathological presentation of cardiac disease in cattle and its impact on decision making, *Vet Rec* 162(18):575–580, 2008.
128. Buczinski S, Rezakhani A, Boerboom D: Heart disease in cattle: diagnosis, therapeutic approaches and prognosis, *Vet J* 184(3): 258–263, 2010.
129. Buczinski S, Tsuka T, Tharwat M: The diagnostic criteria used in bovine bacterial endocarditis: a meta-analysis of 460 published cases from 1973 to 2011, *Vet J* 193(2):349–357, 2012.
130. Mohamed T, Buczinski S: Clinicopathological findings and echocardiographic prediction of the localisation of bovine endocarditis, *Vet Rec* 169(7):180, 2011.
131. Dowling PM, Tyler JW: Diagnosis and treatment of bacterial endocarditis in cattle, *J Am Vet Med Assoc* 204(7):1013–1016, 1994.
132. Agerholm JS, Jensen TK, Agger JF, Engelsma MY, Roest HI: Presence of *Coxiella burnetii* DNA in inflamed bovine cardiac valves, *BMC Vet Res* 13(1):69, 2017.
133. Porter SR, Saegerman C, van Galen G, et al: Vegetative endocarditis in equids (1994–2006), *J Vet Intern Med* 22(6):1411–1416, 2008.
134. Constable P: Treatment of bacterial endocarditis in cattle, *J Am Vet Med Assoc* 199(3):299–301, 1991.
135. Brown AJ, Mandell DC: Chapter 39—cardiogenic shock. In Silverstein DC, Hopper K, editors: *Small animal critical care medicine*, ed 2, St. Louis, 2015, W.B. Saunders, pp 210–213.
136. de Laforcade A, Silverstein DC: Chapter 5—shock. In Silverstein DC, Hopper K, editors: *Small animal critical care medicine*, ed 2, St. Louis, 2015, W.B. Saunders, pp 26–30.
137. Hardaway RM: Cellular and metabolic effects of shock, *J Am Vet Med Assoc* 175(1):81–86, 1979.
138. Kinoshita G, Washizu M, Motoyoshi S, Breznock EM: The effect of hypovolemic shock and reperfusion on the hepatic oxygen supply-uptake relationship in the dog, *J Vet Med Sci* 57(4):697–702, 1995.
139. Hackett TB: Chapter 2—physical examination and daily assessment of the critically ill patient. In Silverstein DC, Hopper K, editors: *Small animal critical care medicine*, ed 2, St. Louis, 2015, W.B. Saunders, pp 6–10.
140. Rudloff E: Chapter 57—assessment of hydration. In Silverstein DC, Hopper K, editors: *Small animal critical care medicine*, ed 2, St. Louis, 2015, W.B. Saunders, pp 307–311.
141. Divers TJ, Norton J: Shock and systemic inflammatory response. In Orsini JA, Divers TJ, editors: *Equine Emergencies - Treatment and Procedures*, St. Louis, MO, 2014, Elsevier Saunders, pp 565–572.
142. Kaynar O, Karapinar T, Hayirli A, Baydar E: Reliability of the Lactate Scout point-of-care instrument for the determination of blood L-lactate concentration in sheep, *Vet Clin Pathol* 44(4): 559–563, 2015.
143. Pichler M, Damberger A, Schwendenwein I, Gasteiner J, Drillich M, Iwersen M: Thresholds of whole-blood beta-hydroxybutyrate and glucose concentrations measured with an electronic hand-held device to identify ovine hyperketonemia, *J Dairy Sci* 97(3): 1388–1399, 2014.
144. Hutchinson KM, Shaw SP: A review of central venous pressure and its reliability as a hemodynamic monitoring tool in veterinary medicine, *Top Companion Anim Med* 31(3):109–121, 2016.

145. Marshall K, Thomovsky E, Johnson P, Brooks A: A review of available techniques for cardiac output monitoring, *Top Companion Anim Med* 31(3):100–108, 2016.
146. Balakrishnan A, Silverstein DC: Chapter 60—shock fluids and fluid challenge. In Silverstein DC, Hopper K, editors: *Small animal critical care medicine,* ed 2, St. Louis, 2015, W.B. Saunders, pp 321–327.
147. Butler AL: Goal-directed therapy in small animal critical illness, *Vet Clin North Am Small Anim Pract* 41(4):817–838, vii, 2011.
148. Smith GW, Berchtold J: Fluid therapy in calves, *Vet Clin North Am Food Anim Pract* 30(2):409–427, vi, 2014.
149. Constable PD: Hypertonic saline, *Vet Clin North Am Food Anim Pract* 15(3):559–585, 1999.
150. Glover PA, Rudloff E, Kirby R: Hydroxyethyl starch: a review of pharmacokinetics, pharmacodynamics, current products, and potential clinical risks, benefits, and use, *J Vet Emerg Crit Care (San Antonio)* 24(6):642–661, 2014.
151. Silverstein DC, Beer KA: Controversies regarding choice of vasopressor therapy for management of septic shock in animals, *J Vet Emerg Crit Care (San Antonio)* 25(1):48–54, 2015.
152. Harada K, Ukai Y, Kanakubo K, et al: Comparison of the diuretic effect of furosemide by different methods of administration in healthy dogs, *J Vet Emerg Crit Care (San Antonio)* 25(3):364–371, 2015.
153. Patel A, Smith FG: Dose-dependent cardiovascular, renal, and endocrine effects of furosemide in conscious lambs, *Can J Physiol Pharmacol* 75(9):1101–1107, 1997.
154. Smith FG, Sener A, Hyland P: Chronic furosemide treatment alters renal responses to furosemide in conscious lambs, *Pediatr Nephrol* 14(10–11):916–921, 2000.
155. Boesch JM, Gleed RD, Gagne JW, Ortved K, Dykes NL, Horne WA: Acute noncardiogenic pulmonary edema in an anesthetized Nubian goat kid, *Vet Anaesth Analg* 36(6):567–573, 2009.
156. Keir I, Dickinson AE: The role of antimicrobials in the treatment of sepsis and critical illness-related bacterial infections: examination of the evidence, *J Vet Emerg Crit Care (San Antonio)* 25(1):55–62, 2015.
157. Anonymous. *Heartwater*, 2007. Available at: http://www.cfsph.iastate.edu/FastFacts/pdfs/heartwater.pdf. Accessed 4 June 2018.
158. Peter TF, Burridge MJ, Mahan SM: *Ehrlichia ruminantium* infection (heartwater) in wild animals, *Trends Parasitol* 18(5):214–218, 2002.
159. Vachiéry N, Marcelino I: Heartwater. In *Manual of diagnostic tests and vaccines for terrestrial animals,* Paris, France 2008, OIE World Organisation for Animal Health, Available at: http://www.oie.int/standard-setting/terrestrial-manual/access-online/. Accessed 1 June 2018.
160. Allsopp BA: Heartwater—*Ehrlichia ruminantium* infection, *Rev Sci Tech* 34(2):557–568, 2015.
161. Stoltsz H: Heartwater. *AfriVIP.* 2013. Available at: http://www.afrivip.org/education/livestock/high-impact/vector-borne-diseases/heartwater/2013/materials. Accessed 4 June 2018.
162. Nakao R, Stromdahl EY, Magona JW, et al: Development of loop-mediated isothermal amplification (LAMP) assays for rapid detection of *Ehrlichia ruminantium, BMC Microbiol* 10:296, 2010.
163. Constable PD, Hinchcliff KW, Done SH, Grünberg W: Heartwater (cowdriosis). In Constable PD, Hinchcliff KW, Done SH, Grünberg W, editors: *Veterinary medicine—a textbook of the diseases of cattle, horses, sheep, pigs and goats,* ed 11, St. Louis, MO, 2017, Elsevier, pp 2031–2033.
164. Parton K, Bruere AN: Plant poisoning of livestock in New Zealand, *N Z Vet J* 50(3 Suppl):22–27, 2002.
165. Ada SE, Al-Yahya MA, Al-Farhan AH: Acute toxicity of various oral doses of dried *Nerium oleander* leaves in sheep, *Am J Chin Med* 29(3–4):525–532, 2001.
166. Corrigall W, Moody RR, Forbes JC: Foxglove (*Digitalis purpurea*) poisoning in farmed red deer (*Cervus elaphus*), *Vet Rec* 102(6):119–122, 1978.
167. Maclean A: Suspected foxglove poisoning in sheep, *Vet Rec* 79(25):817–818,1966.
168. Eldirdiri NI, Wasfi IA, Adam SEI, Edds GT: Toxicity of *Datura stramonium* to sheep and goats, *Vet Hum Toxicol* 23(4):241–246, 1981.
169. Marsh CD, Clawson AB: Mountain laurel (*Kalmia latifolia*) and sheep laurel (*Kalmia angustifolia*) as stock-poisoning plants, *United States Department of Agriculture* 1930 (Technical Bull. No. 219.).
170. Handeland K: Acute yew (Taxus) poisoning in moose (*Alces alces*), *Toxicon* 52(7):829–832, 2008.

18

Anesthetic and Pain Management

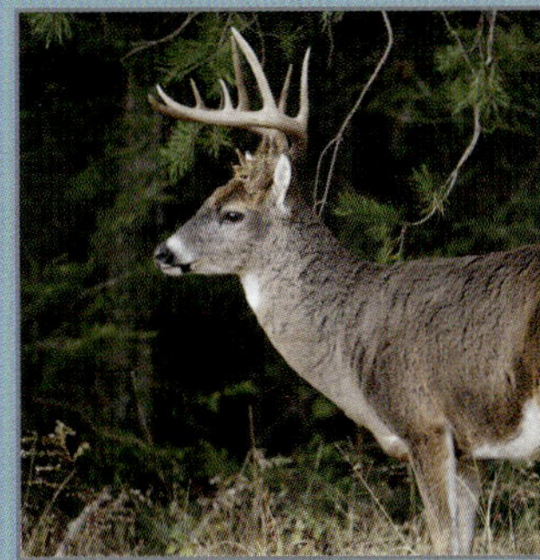

ANN B. WEIL AND A.N. BAIRD

Introduction

General anesthesia in sheep and goats has many similarities to the process used for large ruminants, with the exception that it is generally easier to induce and manage recumbency. The anatomy and physiology of small ruminants are similar enough to cattle to make many techniques comparable and often procedures can be accomplished with sedation and local anesthesia. Food- and fiber-producing animals like sheep and goats are also popular pets, so proper anesthetic care is needed for several of the more common procedures and problems with small ruminant husbandry. There is little information in the literature concerning the anesthesia of goats compared with that of sheep due to the popularity of sheep as a model for biomedical research. Sheep and goats are similar enough that most of the recommendations in this chapter can be applied to both species. Cervids will be discussed separately. Pain assessment and management should always be taken into account when working with all species. A balanced anesthesia technique is useful to provide optimal conditions for surgery, including good muscle relaxation, unconsciousness, and analgesia. Small ruminants and cervids may be anesthetized with injectable agents alone, or injectable anesthetics combined with inhaled anesthetics for maintenance. Rarely is inhalant anesthetic alone utilized in adults.

There are very few anesthetic drugs approved for use in small ruminants, which are classified as a minor species according to Food and Drug Administration definitions. As thiobarbiturates are the only approved drug in sheep, and only one anesthetic is approved in goats (ophthalmic proparacaine), the majority of anesthetic and analgesic drugs are used in an extra-label fashion (ELDU) in small ruminants.[1] Modern inhaled anesthetics have little cumulative effect on milk or meat residues, but other drugs such as analgesics, sedatives, and injectable anesthetics may be part of the anesthetic plan. The Food Animal Residue Avoidance Databank is an excellent resource for advice on extra-label drug use in food animal species, providing up-to-date advice on milk and meat withdrawal times when anesthetic drugs are used. Some of the information available is summarized in Table 18.1.[1–3] Proper preanesthetic preparation of small ruminants is crucial to success if a general anesthetic technique is necessary. Despite their small size or stature, adult small ruminants are subject to the same concerns of regurgitation, aspiration, and bloating as large ruminants. When planning general anesthesia for elective procedures, adult small ruminants should be fasted for 12 to 18 hours and water deprived for 8 to 12 hours in order to decrease the size of the rumen and reduce the risk of aspiration.[4] Almost all drugs used in an anesthetic protocol will reduce gastrointestinal motility. Normal eructation is hampered by general anesthesia and lateral or dorsal recumbency, thus promoting the tendency to bloat. Increased abdominal size and pressure can make ventilation more difficult, especially if there is no means to provide assistance. Pulmonary functional residual capacity may be better preserved when ruminants are fasted prior to anesthesia.[5] Neonatal small ruminants are prone to hypoglycemia and so are not fasted if nursing. If an emergency anesthesia is required and the animal cannot be fasted, then care must be taken to avoid regurgitation and aspiration of fluid at the time of induction and intubation.

Venous catheterization is very helpful prior to general anesthesia. Small ruminants and cervids have a prominent and easy-to-catheterize external jugular vein. Either side of the neck may be utilized, although the esophagus does run down the left side of the neck. If the jugular vein is not accessible, the cephalic veins can be utilized, although it is much more difficult to maintain a catheter for postanesthetic use. Venous catheters are easier to place and have less stress imposed on the animal if preanesthetic sedation is used. Sedatives may be administered intramuscularly to avoid damaging the vein prior to catheterization. Muscles of the hind limb (semimembranosus, semitendinosus) or the epaxial muscles may be used for intramuscular drug administration. A 16-gauge catheter is usually sufficiently sized for small ruminants and cervids. A sterile prep should be used if the catheter is intended to be in place for several days.

Intubation of small ruminants is advised when general anesthesia is performed in order to protect the airway from the aspiration of rumen contents. Passive regurgitation of rumen contents can occur any time during the course of general anesthesia as the cardia relaxes, while lightly anesthetized ruminants experience active regurgitation when intubation is attempted.[4] Intubation can be challenging in these species, especially in goats. The tracheal size of ruminants tends to be smaller than that of other species, so a sheep or goat would have a smaller tracheal diameter than a foal or dog of comparable size. Small ruminants have a narrow oral cavity with a larynx positioned well behind a large tongue. Strips of gauze can be used to hold the mouth open instead of an

TABLE 18.1 The FARAD Recommended Withdrawal Interval for Sheep and Goats for Single and Multiple Treatments of Anesthetic Drugs[a] (see Appendix 1).

Drug	Dose (mg/kg)	Meat Withdrawal Interval (Days)	Milk Withdrawal Interval (Hours)
Acepromazine	Up to 0.13 IV	7	48
Aspirin Aspirin	Typical use 100 PO	1 1	24 24
Butorphanol	0.02 to 0.05 SC or IV	2	72
Detomidine Detomidine	Up to 0.08 IM, IV 0.05 to 0.08 IV	3 7	72 72
DMSO	Not specified	4	96
Guaifenesin	Up to 100 IV	3	48
Flunixin Meglumine	0.5–1 mg/kg IV	10	72
Ketamine	Up to 2 IV; 10 IM	3	48
Ketoprofen	Up to 3.3 IV, once daily for 3 days	7	24
Lidocaine with epinephrine	Infiltration, epidural	1	24
Phenylbutazone	5, every other day	6 to 8 months	
Ultra-short-acting barbiturate	Thiamylal, up to 5.5 Thiopental, up to 9.4	1	24
Tolazoline	2 to 4 IV	30	NA
Xylazine	0.016 to 0.1 IV 0.05 to 0.3 IM 0.3 to 2.0 IM	10	120
Xylazine	0.1 to 0.3	5	72
Yohimbine	Up to 0.3 IV	7	72

DMSO, Dimethyl sulfoxide; *FARAD*, Food Animal Residue Avoidance Databank; *IM*, intramuscularly; *IV*, intravenously; *PO*, per os; *SC*, subcutaneously.
[a]Whenever using unapproved pharmacologics in animals intended for meat or milk production, the clinician should check with federal authorities concerning proper withdrawal times.

assistant's fingers for safety reasons as well as making more room in the oral cavity to visualize the larynx. It is more difficult to open the mouth fully to visualize the larynx than it is in dogs and cats. The tongue should be gently pulled forward and to one side of the mouth. It is common to find the epiglottis entrapped by the soft palate upon induction of general anesthesia. The use of a laryngoscope is very helpful to improve conditions for successful intubation. The tip of the laryngoscope blade should be placed underneath the epiglottis and pushed down to bring the larynx forward and assist in visualization.

Other techniques that aid in intubation include the use of a guide tube or stylet. A polypropylene canine urinary catheter (10F, 22 inches) can be passed between the arytenoid cartilages with the help of a laryngoscope. The stylet should be two to three times the length of the endotracheal tube. Depending on the length of the endotracheal tube to be used, a stylet of sufficient length must sometimes be "crafted" by joining two or more urinary catheters together. Once the guide tube has been gently placed within the trachea, the endotracheal tube can be slid over the guide tube. This helps with visualization, as the guide tube is much smaller than the endotracheal tube and is easier to inspect for proper placement. Goats are generally a bit more difficult to visualize the larynx and intubate than sheep. Care should be taken to ensure that the animal is at an appropriate depth of anesthesia: too deep a plane may result in apnea in a patient that is difficult to intubate and gain control of the airway. Too light a plane of anesthesia can make intubation impossible and will stimulate the larynx. Repeated attempts at intubation with repetitive stimulation of the larynx can increase the likelihood of regurgitation and fluid may flood the pharynx. It is helpful to keep suction equipment available for this situation. All ruminants should be held in sternal recumbency until intubation is accomplished and the cuff of the endotracheal tube is sufficiently inflated to prevent aspiration of fluid. The endotracheal tube should be quickly secured in place with a gauze tie or tape and then the cuff inflated. The cuff should be inflated enough to protect the lungs from aspiration of secretions and gastric contents, but not excessively inflated so that the tracheal mucosa is damaged from overpressure.[6] The cuff of the endotracheal tube should contain sufficient air (or be an exact fit) to enable the anesthesia provider to use an airway pressure of 20 cm H_2O when ventilating the animal.

Premedications

Premedication of sheep and goats facilitates catheter placement and reduces stress to the animal. These drugs may also be a source of analgesia, depending on the drug selected. Premedications may be administered intramuscularly or intravenously, but intramuscular use is generally easier to administer and results in a less intense drug effect of longer duration. Care must be taken in animals that have a thick fleece that the drug actually goes into the muscle and not the fiber. Premedication choices for small ruminants include phenothiazines, benzodiazepines, opioids, guaifenesin, and sometimes alpha-2 agonists. Small ruminants are, in general, easier to physically restrain than larger ruminants.

Most of the time, a combination of drugs will result in better clinical effects than the use of a single agent. The combination of tranquilizers or sedatives with an opioid is called neuroleptanalgesia.[7] Lower drug doses can be used because of the synergism of effect when drugs are combined. This has the benefit of improved sedation or analgesia while minimizing and reducing undesirable side effects like cardiovascular depression, because you can lower doses of drugs that have a greater impact on the cardiovascular system. Please see Table 18.2 for drug doses.

Phenothiazines and Butyrophenones

Acepromazine and azaperone are two tranquilizers that can be useful in small ruminant and cervid chemical restraint protocols. Acepromazine is the most common phenothiazine tranquilizer in veterinary medicine and is readily available. Azaperone is classified as a butyrophenone. They have very similar clinical effects. Acepromazine is a dopamine antagonist. Acepromazine does not have an analgesic effect, and the heavy sedation produced by drugs like the alpha-2 agonists should not be expected from the use of this drug. Doses that have been recommended in sheep and goats range from 0.03 mg/kg to 0.05 mg/kg, which may increase the risk of regurgitation during anesthesia.[8] Nonetheless, acepromazine can be useful to calm patients and facilitate catheter placement, while enabling the use of lower doses of other drugs to induce and/or maintain anesthesia. Side effects like hypotension and reduced cardiac output are minimized when low doses are used. Respiratory depression is minimal with this drug. There is no antagonist for acepromazine.[9] Azaperone (0.2 mg.kg) is labeled for swine but is a neuroleptic drug that can be used to reduce stress while translocating deer.[10] Zuclopenthixol acetate (1 mg/kg) can provide up to 4 days of tranquilization, and deer treated with this drug demonstrated decreased flight distance, decreased stress, and improved feed and water consumption.[11]

TABLE 18.2 Preanesthetic and Sedative/Analgesic Drug Dosages for Sheep and Goats (see Appendix 1).

Preanesthetic Drug	Dosage for Sheep (mg/kg)	Dosage for Goats (mg/kg)
Acepromazine	0.03–0.05 mg/kg IV 0.05–0.1 mg/kg IM	0.01–0.05 IV 0.05–0.1 mg/kg IM
Butorphanol	0.05–0.2 mg/kg IV	0.05–0.2 mg/kg IV
Buprenorphine	0.005–0.1 IV or IM	0.005–0.1 IV or IM
Detomidine	0.003–0.01 IV, IM	0.003–0.01 IV, IM
Diazepam	0.1–0.5 IV, IM	0.1–0.5 IV, IM
Fentanyl	0.01 IV	0.01 IV
Guaifenesin	≤1 mL/kg of 5% solution	≤1 mL/kg of 5% solution
Midazolam	0.1–0.5 IV, IM	0.1–0.5 IV, IM
Morphine	0.05–0.5 IV, IM	0.05–0.5 IV, IM
Xylazine	0.01–0.02 IV standing 0.1–0.2 IV recumbent 0.2–0.3 IM	0.01–0.02 IV standing 0.05–0.1 IV recumbent 0.1–0.3 IM

IM, Intramuscularly; *IV*, intravenously.

Sources: Lin HC, Caldwell F, Pugh DG: Anesthetic management. In Pugh DG, Baird N, editors: *Sheep & Goat Medicine*, ed 2, St. Louis, MO, 2012, Elsevier; Valverde A. Treatment of acute and chronic pain in ruminants. In Egger CM, Love L, Doherty T, editors: *Pain Management in Veterinary Practice*, Ames, 2014, John Wiley & Sons; Riebold TW: Ruminants. In Grimm, KA, Lamont LA, Tranquilli, WJ, Greene, SA, Robertson, SA, editors: *Veterinary Anesthesia and Analgesia: The Fifth Edition of Lumb and Jones*, Ames, IA, 2015, John Wiley & Sons.

Benzodiazepines

Benzodiazepines available to veterinarians include diazepam, midazolam, and zolazepam. Zolazepam is part of a proprietary mixture (Telazol; distributed by Zoetis, Kalamazoo, Michigan; Made in Spain) and is not readily available as a single agent. Diazepam and midazolam are both controlled substances and subject to appropriate controlled-drug handling, as are the opioid drugs. Both drugs are useful sedatives in small ruminants, as they produce predictable sedation without the excitement sometimes seen in other species. Midazolam is a water-soluble benzodiazepine and as such is better suited for intramuscular administration than diazepam. Diazepam is an insoluble drug that is formulated in a propylene glycol vehicle: administration of this drug intramuscularly will result in drug effect, but it is not as well absorbed from the muscle and is a painful injection. Diazepam should not be mixed with drugs other than ketamine in the same syringe as precipitation will readily occur. In addition to their utility as sedatives in small ruminants, benzodiazepines are anticonvulsants with minimal cardiovascular depression associated with their use. This is a distinct advantage, as their use with other drugs will result in less cardiovascular depression from other drugs. They do not promote arrhythmias. They are excellent muscle relaxants. The effects of benzodiazepines may be antagonized by flumazenil. It is rare for this to be necessary in small ruminants. A benzodiazepine is frequently used along with dissociative anesthetics in order to provide muscle relaxation. In a study that examined the optimum dose of midazolam for sedation in goats, it was reported that 0.6 mg/kg of midazolam administered intramuscularly produced the maximum level of sedation 20 minutes postinjection.[12] The same dose given intravenously (IV) produced maximum hypnosis in 5 minutes. Increasing the IV dose to 1.2 mg/kg resulted in an increased reflex suppression and longer duration of effect.[12] The author (AW) has used doses of 0.2–0.5 mg/kg IV or intramuscularly (IM) with good effect for sedation, especially if combined with an opioid.

Guaifenesin

Guaifenesin is a centrally acting muscle relaxant that acts on the internuncial neurons of the spinal cord.[13] It has mild sedative properties and provides very little analgesia.[14] Although most commonly used in equine anesthesia, it can be a helpful addition to anesthetic protocols for small ruminants and cervids. Five percent solutions are most commonly commercially available and most appropriate for use in ruminants, as red blood cell lysis can occur with 10% solutions of guaifenesin. Guaifenesin can be used as part of a premedication plan or it can be used with anesthetic agents like ketamine as a vehicle to maintain general anesthesia in a total IV anesthesia (TIVA) plan. Commonly, a guaifenesin solution is given rapidly in a large volume compared to most drugs. Many anesthesia providers will use a pressurized bag or bottle if they are accustomed to using it in horses. Care must be taken when using the solution in small ruminants that an inadvertent overdose is not given. This author (AW) recommends no more than 1–2 mL/kg be administered prior to induction in small ruminants. The use of a catheter is highly recommended, as the solution is quite irritating if administered perivascularly.

Opioids

Commonly used opioids in small ruminants include butorphanol, nalbuphine, morphine, fentanyl, and buprenorphine. This class of drug is important to consider for meeting the analgesic needs of animals. Most injectable anesthetics, with the exception of the dissociative anesthetics (ketamine or tiletamine), do not contribute an antinociceptive effect to a balanced anesthetic or sedative protocol. Opioids provide excellent supraspinal analgesia of variable potency depending on the receptor type activated. Opioids are classified primarily via receptor type: "full" agonists act mostly on the mu receptor. Partial agonists such as buprenorphine act on the mu receptor but do not turn on all the mu receptors to their full effect or do not turn on all of the receptors. Agonist-antagonist drugs like butorphanol or nalbuphine are kappa receptor agonists and mu receptor antagonists.[15] Butorphanol remains a mainstay of large animal analgesia due to its relative lack of side effects compared to the full opioid agonists in these species. Nonetheless, significant pain in small ruminants may require treatment with a full mu agonist opioid such as morphine or fentanyl. Opioids may be administered IM, IV, or via a continuous-release patch (fentanyl). They are not very bioavailable when administered orally due to first pass metabolism by the liver.

All of these opioids can be useful sedatives in small ruminants, especially if they are combined with other drugs or if the animal is very young, very old, or debilitated. Full mu receptor opioids like morphine can contribute to dysphoria in large animal species. This can manifest as an increase in movement and locomotor activity, as well as excitement or agitation. Kappa agonist opioids such as butorphanol or nalbuphine are much less likely to cause this effect. However, they have less analgesia associated with their use as well. Opioids also cause respiratory depression, although this is rarely a reason not to use them in an animal that needs analgesia. Opioids can cause bradycardia (via a stimulation of vagal tone) without a reduction in cardiac contractility, which makes them useful in debilitated animals as the bradycardia is rarely necessary to treat. One side effect of concern is the reduction of gastrointestinal motility that they can produce. This can lead to increased chance of regurgitation and aspiration due to a reduction in rumen motility. Morphine can last 4 to 6 hours in the goat, where butorphanol may last 1 to 3 hours. Buprenorphine can provide analgesia of up to 6 hours' duration, depending on the dose used.[16]

Opioids may be reversed by drugs that are mu antagonists/kappa agonists like butorphanol or nalbuphine. The opioid effects may also be antagonized by pure antagonists like naloxone or naltrexone, which have no agonistic activity. Naltrexone has a longer duration of action than that of naloxone, which may make it preferable for cervid use in order to avoid renarcotization when highly potent opioids have been used.[10]

Alpha-2 agonists

Alpha-2 agonists are among the strongest conventional sedatives available to veterinarians. They cause sedation by their action on presynaptic alpha-2 receptors within the central nervous system.[17] Alpha-2 agonists currently available include xylazine (labeled for use in equine and cervidae), detomidine and romifidine (equine label), medetomidine, and dexmedetomidine. Dexmedetomidine carries a small animal label and has the most specificity for the alpha-2 receptor. Xylazine has mixed alpha-1 and -2 adrenergic activity as well as a local anesthetic effect. These drugs can be administered intramuscularly as well as intravenously. They are also used within the central nervous system for epidurals or spinal anesthesia. Xylazine remains the most popular and practical alpha-2 adrenergic agonist in large animal practice. Ruminants are very sensitive to the effects of xylazine, with goats appearing to be more sensitive than sheep.[8]

Alpha-2 agonists produce dose-dependent cardiovascular depression. Xylazine reduces cardiac contractility as well as stimulates a vagally mediated bradycardia. It tends to have a biphasic effect on blood pressure, as initially alpha-receptors within the peripheral vasculature are stimulated to produce vasoconstriction and a rise in blood pressure. Eventually, stimulation of alpha-2 receptors within the central nervous system causes an inhibition of norepinephrine release with resulting hypotension. More alpha-2-specific drugs like medetomidine or dexmedetomidine tend to hold the vasoconstriction phase longer. This increase in systemic vascular resistance and afterload leads to a reduction in cardiac output even at low or micro doses. Other side effects of alpha-2 agonists include sweating (in species that can sweat), increased urine production (due to an inhibition of antidiuretic hormone), and hyperglycemia (insulin resistance).[18] Hence, these drugs should be used with caution in animals that have cardiac disease or urinary tract obstruction. Alpha-2 agonists like xylazine can also have an oxytocin like effect.[18] The use of xylazine in ruminants in the last trimester of pregnancy should be avoided, if possible, in order to avoid premature parturition.

Alpha-2 agonists provide excellent analgesia as well as sedation. They also produce profound reductions in gastrointestinal motility and excellent muscle relaxation. Respiratory depression may be significant depending on the dose used. Sheep can exhibit pulmonary edema and a reduced oxygenation when given an alpha-2 adrenergic agonist. This effect has been reported with xylazine, clonidine, detomidine, medetomidine, dexmedetomidine, and romifidine.[19–23] This effect appears to be highly breed and/or individual animal specific. The mechanism behind alpha-2–related pulmonary edema and hypoxemia appears to be multifactorial: it may be related to direct alpha-2 receptor activation on vascular and bronchial smooth muscle, causing bronchospasm and vasospasm as well as alpha-2 receptor activation on platelets, causing transient platelet aggregation with pulmonary microembolism; pulmonary intravascular macrophage activation may be followed by cytokine and inflammatory mediator release. Nonetheless, rapid IV injection of alpha-2 adrenergic agonists should be avoided in sheep unless oxygen is provided. Alpha-2–related hypoxemia is worsened by general anesthesia as postural changes and central nervous system depression also contribute to the problem.[22]

Small ruminants are considered relatively sensitive to the effects of xylazine. They tolerate higher dosing than do large ruminants like cattle but have more sensitivity than camelids or equines. The use of an antagonist should be considered when an individual has an undesirable reaction to an alpha-2 agonist or has received an overdose. Alpha-2 antagonists include yohimbine, tolazoline, idazoxan, and atipamezole. Yohimbine has weak anti-alpha-2 activity. Tolazoline is a non-specific alpha-2 antagonist.

Atipamezole is the most specific alpha-2 antagonist and should be used when highly alpha-2-specific agonists like dexmedetomidine, medetomidine, or detomidine have been used. Pulmonary edema from alpha-2 adrenergic agonist administration can be prevented by antagonists like atipamezole, tolazoline, and idazoxan, but not yohimbine.[24–26] The use of antagonists can be helpful in shortening recovery time and decreasing the undesirable side effects of alpha-2 agonists. However, reversal of alpha-2 adrenergic agonists should not be considered an innocuous procedure: excitement, sympathetic nervous stimulation, and cardiovascular stimulation can occur. Selection of reversal agent and dose should be made by taking into consideration the alpha-2 agonist used, the dose given, and the time elapsed since drug administration. Tolazoline has been associated with negative outcomes in several species, including llamas and calves.[27,28] When using reversal agents, best practice may be to use the lowest dose needed to titrate for arousal and avoid high doses administered intravenously.

Anticholinergics

Ruminants produce a lot of saliva during sedation and general anesthesia. However, the use of anticholinergics like atropine or glycopyrrolate as premedications to try to "dry up" this process is not recommended. High doses of anticholinergics are required to achieve this, and they produce tachycardia and mydriasis and result in more viscous secretions that tend to occlude airways.[16,29–32] Anticholinergics also reduce intestinal motility, leading to a buildup of gas in the rumen, making the occurrence of tympany more likely. The use of low-dose anticholinergic therapy for treatment of intraoperative bradycardia is discussed in the section on anesthetic complications.

Injectable Anesthetics

The use of premedications (previously mentioned in this chapter) will reduce the amount of injectable and inhaled anesthetics necessary to achieve a balanced general anesthesia technique. With the exception of the alpha-2 agonists, all premedications have less cardiovascular and respiratory depression than general anesthetic agents do. Injectable anesthetic agents available for use in small ruminants include barbiturates, dissociative anesthetics, propofol, and alfaxalone. Table 18.3 lists the dosages for induction agents in sheep and goats.

TABLE 18.3 Induction Agents for Sheep and Goats (see Appendix 1).

Anesthetic Agent	Dosage for Sheep (mg/kg)	Dosage for Goats (mg/kg)
Alfaxalone	2 IV	
Ketamine	2–7.5 IV 10–15 IM	2–10 IV 10–15 IM
Propofol	4–6 IV for unsedated 2–4 IV if sedated	4–6 IV for unsedated 2–4 IV if sedated
Telazol	2–4 IV	2–4 IV

IM, Intramuscularly; *IV*, intravenously.

Sources: Riebold TW: Ruminants. In Grimm KA, Lamont LA, Tranquilli WJ, Greene SA, Robertson SA, editors: *Veterinary Anesthesia and Analgesia: The Fifth Edition of Lumb and Jones*, Ames, IA, 2015, John Wiley & Sons; Lin HC, Caldwell F, Pugh DG: Anesthetic Management. In Pugh DG, Baird N, editors: *Sheep & Goat Medicine*, ed 2, St. Louis, MO, 2012, Elsevier; Dzikiti TB. Intravenous anaesthesia in goats: a review. *J S Afr Vet Assoc* 84 (1), 1-8, 2013.

Barbiturates

Thiobarbiturates, once the mainstay of general anesthesia in most species, are now very difficult to acquire and are no longer in common use.

Dissociative Anesthetics

Ketamine and tiletamine (Telazol) are two dissociative anesthetics available for use in small ruminants and cervids. They are administered intramuscularly or intravenously. Their ease of administration and relative safety profile make them a practical choice for small ruminant general anesthesia. Ketamine is often combined with a benzodiazepine such as diazepam or midazolam to reduce undesirable side effects like seizure-like activity and muscle rigidity.[33] Tiletamine comes already combined with zolazepam in the proprietary mixture known as Telazol. Telazol has the advantage of a smaller volume of administration than a ketamine/diazepam mixture and tends to have a longer duration of action in most species. Telazol can produce delayed recovery in many species. Ketamine is almost always combined with a sedative or tranquilizer. This may be an alpha-2 adrenergic agonist, a benzodiazepine, and/or an opioid. Most commonly, this will be xylazine or a benzodiazepine. Higher doses of ketamine given intramuscularly (10–15 mg/kg IM) can last about 45 minutes following xylazine administration (0.1–0.2 mg/kg IM) in sheep or about 15 minutes for a smaller dose of ketamine (3–5 mg/kg) given intravenously.[4,18]

Dissociative anesthetics stimulate endogenous release of catecholamines by the sympathetic nervous system. As such, they are considered indirectly supportive of the cardiovascular system by increasing heart rate, stroke volume, cardiac output, and systemic blood pressure. If the patient is unable to release endogenous catecholamines, then dissociative anesthetics are negative inotropes similar to other injectable anesthetics.[34,35]

Ketamine produces a characteristic respiratory pattern called apneustic breathing. Apneustic breathing is a breath-holding pattern whereby the animal will hold its breath for a period of time and then take several shallow breaths. The apneustic breathing pattern of ketamine is striking in equine and feline anesthesia but appears less apparent in small ruminants.[4] All injectable anesthetics should be considered respiratory depressants, which reduce ventilation, but the dissociative anesthetics tend to support spontaneous ventilation well in most species. It is the authors' opinion that ketamine is not as likely to induce apnea as propofol or alfaxalone.

Ketamine is also used as part of a pain management protocol. It is an *N*-methyl-D-aspartate (NMDA) antagonist, which helps reduce central sensitization in the dorsal horn of the spinal cord. NMDA receptors are recruited during nociceptive processing and utilize excitatory neurotransmitters like glutamate to increase processing of nociceptive information leading to "wind up."[36] Ketamine is used to decrease this nervous system trafficking and is one of the few anesthetics noted to have an analgesic effect. Ketamine should not be used as the sole analgesic agent in a pain management program.

Although dissociative anesthetics remain a practical mainstay for anesthesia in small ruminants and cervids, one disadvantage is that they cannot be reversed. When drug combinations are made with opioids, benzodiazepines, and alpha-2 agonists, it is recommended that reversal of the other drugs should not occur until the side effects of the dissociative anesthetic (muscle rigidity, trembling, etc.) have time to dissipate.

Propofol

Propofol is a nonsteroidal, nonbarbiturate injectable anesthetic. It has a high volume of distribution and very rapid metabolism and clearance, with extrahepatic sites of metabolism.[34] It provides a rapid and smooth induction that easily facilitates intubation in the goat.[37] Propofol causes a reduction in systemic vascular resistance and reduces arterial blood pressure and cardiac output.[38,39] It causes dose-dependent depression of ventilation with transient cyanosis in patients that are not preoxygenated.[40] A comparison of the use of propofol, thiopental, or ketamine in goats showed that recovery times (times to recovery of the swallowing reflex and to standing) were significantly shorter and side effects (apnea, regurgitation, hypersalivation, and tympany) were less common when propofol was used as the induction agent compared to ketamine or thiopental.[41] A quicker recovery was attributed to the improved clinical performance in this study. None of the animals in this study received a premedication, so higher doses of injectable anesthetics were used than when injectable anesthetics typically are given after sedatives or tranquilizers. Like most injectable anesthetics, propofol does not provide any analgesia.

The pharmacokinetic and pharmacodynamics profile of propofol makes it ideal for TIVA use as recovery is rapid once the continuous rate infusion is discontinued. More information about TIVA is given at the end of this section.

Alfaxalone

Alfaxalone is a steroid general anesthetic that works on the GABA neurotransmitter in the central nervous system. It is similar to propofol in many regard, as it has a rapid onset of action, rapid redistribution, and a short terminal half-life.[42,43] When alfaxalone has been used in sheep at 2 mg/kg, there are minimal adverse effects and an uneventful recovery.[44] There is little information concerning the use of alfaxalone alone in goats—previous work is based on saffan, when alfaxalone was combined with alfadolone and solubilized in a 20% polyethoxylated castor oil (Cremorphor-EL).[45,46] The present formulation of alfaxalone is labeled for dogs and cats and does not cause the histamine-related problems associated with the old drug formulation.

Injectable Combinations for Chemical Restraint and/or General Anesthesia

Various combinations of the previously mentioned drugs can be administered IM, IV, or SC (subcutaneously) in order to produce sedation or short-acting general anesthesia. Many practical injectable anesthetic protocols are based on the combination of an alpha-2 agonist, opioid, and dissociative anesthetic like ketamine or Telazol. The use of alpha-2 agonists must be considered with caution in sheep and goats but is an essential component to cervid anesthesia or sedation. Sheep and goats have a good sedative effect to benzodiazepines compared to horses or small animals, so the use of an alpha-2 agonist can be omitted. Tables 18.2 through 18.4 list some drugs that can be used in combinations to provide injectable anesthesia or to induce animals for intubation and subsequent maintenance with inhalant. The addition of a small dose of ketamine to sedative protocols is a technique called a ketamine "stun." It can be a useful addition to add more patient cooperation as it adds more analgesia and dissociative sedation to a protocol. Patients may appear awake yet oblivious to their surroundings and procedures being performed.[47]

Total Intravenous Anesthesia

IV injectable anesthetics are commonly used in veterinary medicine to achieve intubation, while inhaled anesthetics are often used to maintain anesthesia. IV injectable anesthetics may also be used to maintain anesthesia, especially in situations where inhaled anesthesia is not practical or possible, such as field or farm anesthesia or magnetic resonance imaging for research animals. The advantages of IV anesthesia include rapid onset of action and low cost, as well as reduction in environmental contamination and human exposure. Disadvantages to the use of TIVA could include the cost of an infusion pump in order to provide a consistent constant rate infusion and the tendency for drugs to have an accumulative effect over time with a potential delay in recovery.[48]

Injectable anesthetics are usually administered as an IV bolus to fill the volume of distribution of the central compartment, followed by a lower amount of drug to maintain an effective plasma concentration of drug for the duration of the planned procedure.[49,50] The maintenance phase can be handled by giving intermittent boluses of drug or by administering the drug at a constant rate. The constant rate infusion tends to maintain a more consistent plane of anesthesia over time, eliminating the "peaks and trough" in the plasma concentration of a drug. Most anesthetic procedures of 1 hour or greater may be more easily controlled by using a constant rate infusion. A constant rate infusion can be maintained with a fluid pump, syringe-driver pump, or simply a fluid bag spiked with the necessary drugs and administered at a calculated rate. A buretrol can be used for a smaller volume of drug. Nonetheless, a venous catheter and intubation of the patient are optimal for this type of anesthesia. Hypoxemia can be expected in sheep, goats, or cervids anesthetized and maintained on ambient air, so oxygen supplementation is warranted.

Ideal TIVA drug combinations would be stable in solution, have good effect as an anesthetic agent, have a rapid onset of action, have few deleterious side effects, and would clear the body rapidly without accumulation.[48] Recovery should be predictable and smooth, without excitement. Drugs available for use in TIVA protocols include propofol, alfaxalone, ketamine, opioids, and benzodiazepines. Alpha-2 agonists are useful for adding excellent analgesia and muscle relaxation but can be associated with significant cardiovascular depression and hypoxemia in sheep and goats. If alpha-2 agonists are added, the dosages should be much lower than those associated with equine combinations. Table 18.4 shows drug combinations available for use as TIVA in sheep and goats.

Inhalants

Modern inhaled anesthetic agents include isoflurane, sevoflurane, and desflurane. Halothane is no longer available. Isoflurane and sevoflurane are more practical for veterinary use than desflurane, with isoflurane the most widely used veterinary inhalation

TABLE 18.4 Intravenous Anesthetics and Adjuncts for Maintenance of Anesthesia in Sheep and Goats (see Appendix 1).

Drug	Infusion Rate (mg/kg/h)
Propofol	12–36
Ketamine	1.8–3
Fentanyl	0.005–0.30
Midazolam	0.1–0.9
Lidocaine	≤6 (after 2 mg/kg loading dose)
Guaifenesin (1 L) mixed with 1–2 g ketamine ± 100 mg xylazine	1–2.2 mL/kg/h to effect

Sources: Lin HC, Caldwell F, Pugh DG: Anesthetic management. In Pugh DG, Baird N editors: *Sheep & Goat Medicine*, ed 2, St. Louis, MO, 2012, Elsevier; Riebold TW: Ruminants. In Grimm, KA, Lamont LA, Tranquilli, WJ, Greene, SA, Robertson, SA editors: *Veterinary Anesthesia and Analgesia: The Fifth Edition of Lumb and Jones*, Ames, IA, 2015, John Wiley & Sons; Dzikiti TB. Intravenous anaesthesia in goats: a review. *J S Afr Vet Assoc* 84 (1), 1-8, 2013.

anesthetic in North America.[51] General anesthesia using inhalant drugs requires the use of an anesthetic machine. The inhaled drugs are metered into the system with the use of a precision vaporizer, which is calibrated for one inhalant only. They are usually administered with oxygen as the carrier gas in veterinary medicine. This has the advantages of providing oxygen support and a means of ventilation. The modern inhalants require very little metabolism and are eliminated from the body by being exhaled from the lungs, so recovery is usually rapid depending on the duration of the anesthetic period. Disadvantages of using inhalant anesthesia include the cost of equipment and the expertise required, as well as being somewhat cumbersome to use in a non-hospital situation.

Both isoflurane and sevoflurane support vital organ blood flow well and can be considered relatively friendly to the cardiovascular system. Inhalants do cause some reduction in cardiac contractility and are potent vasodilators, both of which contribute to a reduction in systemic blood pressure and cardiac output. Vasodilation will also contribute to hypothermia in thin patients with prolonged anesthetic periods. Inhalants cause profound respiratory depression, especially isoflurane. Muscle relaxation is proportional to the vaporizer setting. Sevoflurane is more insoluble than isoflurane, which means that mask induction and recovery from anesthesia are quicker. The comparison in induction and recovery times in healthy animals may not be very noticeable. Sevoflurane is significantly more expensive than isoflurane.

MAC stands for minimal alveolar concentration of inhaled anesthetic and is a measure of potency. One MAC unit will keep 50% of a population from responding with purposeful movement to a supramaximal stimulus. It usually requires 1.5 units for a surgical plane of inhaled anesthesia. The MAC for isoflurane for sheep is 1.58%[52] and for goats is 1.2% to 1.4%.[53,54] The MAC for sevoflurane in the goat is 2.3%.[55] It is important to note that the use of premedication drugs and injectable anesthetics will reduce the amount of inhaled anesthetic needed to maintain the animal.

Inhalants are administered via the respiratory system; as such, they require either intubation of the trachea or can be given by a tight-fitting face mask or a device such as a laryngeal mask airway. Mask induction is not recommended in adult small ruminants, however tempting their small size would make it appear. The risk of aspiration of rumen contents and the relative difficulty in intubating these species make it a more prudent choice to sedate with premedication and induce with injectable anesthetics prior to maintenance with either inhalant anesthetics or additional injectable anesthetics. Mask induction is a reasonable alternative for neonates that require general anesthesia and are still essentially monogastric in function.

A small animal anesthesia machine can be used for small ruminants less than 60 kg. A larger sized canister for chemical CO_2 absorbent is needed for larger animals.

Monitoring

General anesthesia and sedation greatly impact the central nervous system, the cardiovascular system, and the respiratory system. Monitoring the depth of anesthesia centers around these body systems. Routine central nervous system monitoring in veterinary medicine tends to rely on basic information like eye position, palpebral and corneal reflexes, lack of purposeful movement, etc. Monitoring of anesthetized animals should be continuous, and a careful record of events, drug doses and physiological parameters maintained. Positioning of ruminants is a key component to safe anesthetic practice. It is important to keep in mind the effect that recumbency has on anesthetized large animals, even small ruminants. Sternal recumbency is the most desirable position, but often it is not feasible for surgery. Nonetheless, all ruminant patients should be returned to sternal recumbency as soon as possible for recovery purposes. All ruminants continue to produce a significant amount of saliva while undergoing sedation or anesthesia. Whenever possible, the unintubated patient should be positioned so that the saliva runs out of the mouth rather than accumulating in the back of the pharynx. This can be achieved by propping the head up while pointing the mouth down.

Assessment of depth of anesthesia in small ruminants can be challenging, as they do not display some of the easier-to-evaluate depth indicators in other species. If in doubt, anesthetic depth should be reduced until obvious signs of lightness such as muscle tension, movement, swallowing, etc., are re-established. The palpebral reflex disappears with minimal depth of anesthesia, and rotation of the eye is not as useful an indicator of depth of anesthesia in small ruminants as it is in horses and cattle.[4] The corneal reflex should be maintained in all species, small ruminants and cervids included. Please see the section on cervid anesthesia for monitoring comments specific to those species.

The cardiovascular system can be monitored by assessing heart rate, mucous membrane color, capillary refill time, pulse quality, and blood pressure. The heart rate for sheep and goats varies with age. Juveniles will have a heart rate of 90 to 130 beats/min, which will decrease with maturity.[4]

Hypotension is a very common complication in the anesthetized patient, especially when the patient is maintained with inhalant anesthetics. Ruminants in general tend to maintain a higher systemic blood pressure than horses or small animals. Blood pressure is simple to measure in the anesthetized patient and is very helpful to monitor depth of anesthesia and overall patient welfare. It is used as an estimate of tissue perfusion. Hypotension is generally defined as a mean arterial pressure less than 60 mm Hg. Inhalant anesthetics, such as isoflurane or sevoflurane, contribute to hypotension by vasodilation and reduction of cardiac output. When hypotension is present in the anesthetized patient, there is concern that vital organs and tissues are not receiving sufficient oxygen to support their needs.

Blood pressure monitoring is a simple method of detecting and controlling hypotension. Blood pressure can be monitored by direct or indirect means.[56] Direct blood pressure monitoring utilizes a catheter placed in a peripheral artery and is connected via fluid-filled tubing to a transducer, which converts the pressure wave to an electronic signal. Direct arterial pressure monitoring is considered a more accurate method of blood pressure measurement than the indirect, cuff-based methods. Indirect methods include Doppler technology, which measures systolic blood pressure, or the oscillometric monitors, which measure the oscillation or movement of the vessel wall. Both are dependent on the cuff selected for accuracy. The width of the cuff should be 40% of the circumference of the limb. Too large a cuff will result in a blood pressure reading that is lower than actual and too small a cuff will give a reading that is too high. The oscillometric units will give systolic, mean, and diastolic blood pressure numbers. It is important to remember that the indirect methods are not as accurate as direct measurement but are very helpful to monitor trends. Correlation between the two methods (indirect versus direct) is not always good in ruminants, so an arterial catheter is recommended if blood pressure monitoring is critical.[57] The cuff of an oscillometric blood pressure monitor can be placed on the limb (usually forelimb) of a small ruminant. The median auricular artery is most commonly used for arterial catheter placement if direct blood pressure measurement is desired.

Respiratory Monitoring

All anesthetized patients hypoventilate under general anesthesia. Hypoventilation is an insidious problem, as most veterinarians and technicians assume that an adequate respiratory rate and respiratory efforts equate to adequate alveolar ventilation and gas exchange. The amount of gas exchanged with each breath (tidal volume) has two components: dead space gas and alveolar ventilation.[58] Dead space gas is the air that is in the conducting airways and is not available for gas exchange. It tends to remain relatively constant and is the first gas in and out of the mouth or nasal passages, trachea, and other conducting units of the respiratory tree. Therefore, when tidal volume decreases (which inevitably happens under general anesthesia) and dead space gas remains the same, alveolar ventilation must decrease. Hypoventilation can be confirmed by observing end-tidal CO_2 values greater than 45 mm Hg and by observing less frequent respiratory efforts. Spontaneously breathing respiratory rates are usually 20 to 40 breaths/min in sheep and goats.[4] Ruminants have a decreased tidal volume compared with other species.[59]

A capnometer is a useful piece of equipment for respiratory monitoring. Capnometry is the measurement and numerical display of CO_2 during the respiratory cycle. These are instruments designed to continuously and noninvasively evaluate the end-tidal (end of exhalation) level of carbon dioxide respired by a patient. A "capnograph" is the machine that records a graphic display with its characteristic waveform, while "capnogram" is the term used for the actual waveform. The level of CO_2 and the shape of the resultant wave form can be extremely useful in evaluating the respiratory status of a patient.[60] Its primary use is to assess ventilation; it does not give any information about oxygenation. The American Society of Anesthesiologists (ASA) now recommends capnometry coupled with pulse oximetry as the standard of care for respiratory monitoring of anesthetized patients.

The partial pressure of end-tidal CO_2 (expiratory plateau) should be between 35 and 45 mm Hg. Carbon dioxide is produced in the body by cellular metabolism and then transported via blood to the lungs to be eliminated. Hypoventilation leads to higher-than-normal arterial partial pressure levels of CO_2. Slightly high levels of CO_2 can benefit an anesthetized patient as it stimulates the sympathetic nervous system to release endogenous catecholamines, which help support cardiovascular function.[61,62] However, very high levels of CO_2 will lead to acidosis, narcosis, arrhythmias, and myocardial failure. Anesthesia produces generalized central nervous system depression and the medullary respiratory center may not respond to higher levels of CO_2 with increased ventilation. Some patients may be very sensitive to the respiratory depression imposed by general anesthesia. These patients may experience respiratory arrest without intervention (intermittent positive pressure ventilation [IPPV]) by the anesthetist. An airway pressure of 12 to 15 cm of H_2O is commonly used as a guideline for IPPV. Ruminants may require higher airway pressure to maintain adequate ventilation because of the effect of the rumen on abdominal pressure as well as reduced functional residual capacity in the thorax. Physical problems that may exacerbate hypoventilation include obesity, pregnancy, and positioning in surgery (perineal stands, etc.). These patients will require more intervention and ventilation support. Patients who have thoracic masses or noncompliant chests may require higher airway pressure in order to provide adequate ventilation. This needs to be assessed on an individual basis.

Capnometry is very useful to determine correct intubation, especially in species that are difficult to intubate. Esophageal intubation should not produce detectable levels of CO_2. Low levels of end-tidal CO_2 ($\leq$35 mm Hg) may be a result of hyperventilation. It can also be seen with hypothermia, excessive anesthetic depth, or the use of paralytic muscle relaxants. Pulmonary systemic or pulmonary circulation is a significant cause of low end-tidal CO_2 levels. Patients experiencing cardiac arrest will have precipitous drops in CO_2, and capnometry can be very helpful in establishing the effectiveness of CPR.

Hypoxia/hypoxemia can be a complication of general anesthesia, especially in the equine but also in small ruminants and cervids when certain conditions prevail. Five major causes of hypoxemia or low arterial oxygen tensions (PaO_2) include (1) low inspired oxygen concentration; (2) hypoventilation, especially when FIO_2 = 21% (room air); (3) barriers to diffusion, e.g., pneumothorax and pulmonary edema; (4) ventilation-perfusion mismatch; and (5) right-to-left shunt (physiologic).[63]

Low inspired oxygen concentration can occur with equipment failures and errors, most commonly when someone forgets to turn on the oxygen flow meter or delivers too low a flow for the size of the animal, not meeting metabolic oxygen requirements. It also occurs when endotracheal tubes become kinked or occluded with blood/secretions. A common manifestation of this occurrence is the patient who appears to be "waking up" or is at too light a depth. Hypoxemia will cause a ventilatory drive when PaO_2 levels are less than 50 to 60 mm Hg and the gasping behavior of the severely hypoxemic patient can mimic arousal.

Hypoventilation can be a reason for low oxygen tensions even if the patient is breathing 100% oxygen if the hypoventilation is severe. The fact that most anesthetized patients breathe 100% oxygen helps prevent this problem, since hypoventilation is such a common problem in the anesthetized patient. Oxygen supplementation should be considered in patients undergoing injectable anesthesia, even if inhalant anesthetic is not used or the patient is not intubated, as breathing room air can lead to prolonged recovery and other adverse consequences when cerebral blood flow and oxygen delivery are compromised during a general anesthetic. Sheep positioned in lateral recumbency may experience a reduction in PaO_2 even without chemical restraint.[64]

Problems such as pneumothorax or pulmonary edema create barriers to the diffusion of respiratory gases. Oxygen is usually affected first, since CO_2 is about 20 times more soluble than oxygen. Pulmonary edema, pleural effusion, and pneumothorax should be corrected as much as possible prior to general anesthesia. Occasionally, occult conditions will manifest during the course of general anesthesia and must be handled during the procedure. Ventilation/perfusion mismatch and right-to-left pulmonary shunting do occur in small ruminant anesthesia but do not tend to be as frequent a problem as in the anesthetized horse. The administration of PEEP, or positive end expiratory pressure, can be helpful in the hypoxemic patient as it increases alveolar participation and may recruit collapsed alveoli.

Patient oxygenation can be monitored via pulse oximetry or blood gas analysis. Pulse oximetry is more frequently used, as it is economical, noninvasive, continuous, and easy to put on the patient. The probe is placed on a nonhaired, nonpigmented area of the body that is thin. This can prove to be a challenge in some ruminants. In small ruminants and cervids, the tongue is the most commonly used area for pulse oximetry, although the ear, prepuce, or vulva can be used as well. However, the pulse oximeter has some limitations in the information that it provides. It measures the amount of hemoglobin that is saturated with oxygen (SpO_2) and will usually give you a pulse rate as well. The hemoglobin oxygen dissociation curve illustrates the relationship between hemoglobin saturation and the partial pressure of oxygen. A saturation of 90% corresponds to a partial pressure of oxygen of 60 mm Hg, which is defined as hypoxemia. A saturation of 99% to 100% can correspond with an O_2 saturation of 90 to 500 mm Hg—a vast range that is dependent on the inspired concentration of O_2. In veterinary medicine, most anesthetized patients breathe 100% oxygen, so we normally expect to see PaO_2 in the 200 to 300 mm Hg range. Pulse oximetry is also prone to problems with the probe—prolonged contact will cause some decrease in tissue perfusion and cause the probe to stop reading. This can lead to the anesthetist disregarding a low SpO_2 reading when the patient is actually experiencing a desaturation event.

When inhalant anesthesia is used, a balanced isotonic electrolyte solution should be administered intravenously at a rate of 5 to 10 mL/kg/h. An initial rate of 10 mL/kg/h can be useful when small ruminants have been water deprived prior to the anesthetic event. Dextrose can be added to the electrolyte solution at a concentration of 2.5% or 5.0% when pediatric patients undergo anesthesia. The vasodilation produced by inhalant anesthesia will accelerate heat loss in small ruminants, so an external heat source like a circulating water pad or forced air warmer is useful to help maintain normothermia.

Ruminants tend to recover quietly from general anesthesia, without the emergence delirium or excitement seen frequently in other species. They should be placed in sternal recumbency for recovery to minimize the chance of bloat or ruminal distension. As in other species, the endotracheal tube should be removed when the animal can swallow and protect the airway. Care should be taken to remove the tube straight out of the mouth, as it is easy to snag the endotracheal tube cuff on the sharp edges of the molars if the tube is pulled sideways. Likewise, care should be taken to protect the tube from chewing as the sharp molars can easily sever the endotracheal tube. When extubating a ruminant, it is useful to leave the endotracheal tube cuff partially inflated in order to remove any accumulated fluid or debris from the airway or pharyngeal area, thus avoiding aspiration of rumen contents or saliva just after extubation.

Pain Assessment and Management

Pain assessment and management in food animals should be part of basic veterinary and husbandry activities.[65] It is simple to expect that animals experiencing surgery will need analgesia, but we have a long way to go before there is a straightforward way to assess pain in prey species such as small ruminants and cervids. An estimate of the severity of the pain condition must be made based on clinical signs, physiological parameters, behavior, and empathy.[65] Small ruminants are timid prey species that exhibit minimal signs of pain when compared to small carnivores or other species. Behavioral responses of sheep to painful husbandry practices have been assessed by teams of researchers in Scotland and New Zealand and consist of restlessness, rolling, jumping, tail wagging, lip curl, trembling, and abnormal postures when lying down or standing.[66] One can expect that sheep may tolerate severe injury without overt signs of pain or distress.[67] Pain can also cause cessation of rumination, inappetence, lack of water intake, or facial expression changes. Goats are more likely than sheep or cattle to vocalize in response to pain, but even less is known about behavioral responses to pain in this species. Staffieri et al. (2009) investigated perioperative analgesic protocols in goats and modified a pain assessment scoring system to include flock behavior as well as movement and animal comfort.[68]

Drugs used for analgesia in small ruminants and cervids have been discussed previously in this chapter under premedications prior to general anesthesia or as part of an injectable anesthetic protocol. Evidence for the systemic use of opioids in sheep and cattle comes from pain models using cutaneous thermal and mechanical stimulation.[69] Butorphanol, fentanyl, buprenorphine, and meperidine have proven to be effective analgesics for thermal noxious stimulation when given intravenously.[70–74] Fentanyl and meperidine (to a lesser extent) were considered effective when a pressure or mechanical stimulus was applied.[71,72]

Opioids can also be administered epidurally or intrathecally—more information about their use when administered in this manner can be found in the section on regional techniques. Dosages for individual analgesic agents can be found in Table 18.5.

Commercially available fentanyl patches have been evaluated in small ruminants, as sheep are a common model in orthopedic biomedical research. Their use can be considered in individual animals experiencing severe injury or significant surgical pain. The careful application of a transdermal patch results in consistent plasma levels of fentanyl for at least 40 hours postapplication.[75] Transdermal patches should be applied for an estimated dose of 2 μg/kg/h depending on animal size and patch size. They should be applied to the animal prior to surgery—one study suggests that the ideal time may be 24 to 36 hours prior to orthopedic surgery.[76] Transdermal patches continuously release fentanyl, and good skin contact is needed in order to produce consistent plasma fentanyl levels. Care must be taken not to heat the patch-skin interface (warming devices used in the operating room) so as to not prematurely increase the amount of fentanyl released from the patch. The effects of transdermal patch application have been considered superior to buprenorphine when evaluated in a double-blinded pain study.[77]

TABLE 18.5 Doses of NSAIDs and Analgesics for Sheep and Goats (see Appendix 1).

Drug	Dose	Duration (hours)
Opioids		
Buprenorphine	0.005–0.01 mg/kg SC	6
	0.005–0.1 mg/kg IV, IM	8–12
Butorphanol	0.05–0.2 mg/kg	1–3
Fentanyl	0.01 IV 0.001–0.005 mg/kg/h CRI 50 µg/h patch	1–2 5–12
Meperidine	5 IM	0.25–0.5
Morphine	0.05–0.5 IV, IM 0.1 mg/kg epidural	1–6 6–12
NSAIDs		
Aspirin	50–100 mg/kg PO	12–24
Carprofen	2 mg/kg PO, SC, IV	24
Diclofenac	1 mg/kg IV, IM	
flunixin meglumine	1 mg/kg IV	12
Ketoprofen	2 mg/kg IV	12
Meloxicam	0.5 mg/kg IV 2 mg/kg PO loading dose, then 0.5 mg/kg subsequently 0.5 mg/kg IV 2 mg/kg PO loading dose, then 1 mg/kg daily PO	8: goats 24: goats 12: sheep 24: sheep

CRI, Constant rate infusion; *IM*, intramuscularly; *IV*, intravenously; *NSAID*, nonsteroidal anti-inflammatory drug; *PO*, per os; SC, subcutaneously.

Sources: Lin HC, Caldwell F, Pugh DG: Anesthetic Management. In Pugh DG, Baird N, editors: *Sheep & Goat Medicine*, ed 2, St. Louis, MO, 2012, Elsevier; Riebold TW: Ruminants. In Grimm KA, Lamont LA, Tranquilli WJ, Greene SA, Robertson SA, editors: *Veterinary Anesthesia and Analgesia: The Fifth Edition of Lumb and Jones*, Ames, IA, 2015, John Wiley & Sons; Valverde A. Treatment of acute and chronic pain in ruminants. In Egger CM, Love L, Doherty T, editors: *Pain Management in Veterinary Practice*, Ames, 2014, John Wiley & Sons.

A study looking at the use of a transdermal fentanyl patch in the goat showed that a 50 µg/h patch placed on the neck of 40-kg goats resulted in bioavailability that exceeded 100% due to the recycling of highly lipid soluble fentanyl through the ruminosalivary cycle.[78] This may result in adverse side effects like excessive sedation, dysphoria, respiratory depression, ileus, and inappetance. This may suggest that lower doses of fentanyl patches should be used in goats versus sheep. A commercially available transdermal fentanyl solution labeled for the dog was used in research sheep in an effort to find a product that could be easily applied and provide long-lasting plasma levels of fentanyl to sheep undergoing orthopedic surgery. Several doses were evaluated and adverse effects noted at all doses.[79]

Nonsteroidal Antiinflammatory Drugs

NSAIDs, or nonsteroidal antiinflammatory drugs, can be used in the perioperative period in combination with sedatives, local anesthetics, and general anesthesia. They are among the most important drugs used in all species of animals as they possess both analgesic and antiinflammatory properties. They are drugs that inhibit cyclooxygenase (COX) enzymes, lipoxygenase, and thromboxane enzymes. COX acts on arachidonic acid to release prostaglandins and other mediators of inflammation; thus, NSAIDs play an important role in reducing inflammatory mediators.[1] They have the advantage of providing excellent analgesia, both peripherally and centrally (spinal cord) without adding sedation and central nervous system depression.[80] They are easy to administer parenterally and have a convenient dosing schedule. They also have high bioavailability when administered orally. Caution should be taken with dosing and use of the drugs when the animal is hypovolemic, in renal failure, neonatal, or debilitated.

Some of the most common NSAIDs used in ruminants are flunixin meglumine, ketoprofen, aspirin, meloxicam, and carprofen.[81] NSAIDs are often described by the specificity of the COX inhibitory action. Flunixin meglumine is a COX-1 inhibitor approved for use in beef and lactating dairy cattle to treat fever and inflammation associated with respiratory disease, mastitis, or endotoxemia. It is used in sheep and goats, but meat and milk withdrawal times are not as established as in cattle. Meloxicam, a COX-2 inhibitor, is given at 0.5 mg/kg IV every 8 hours to goats or at 0.5 mg/kg orally every 24 hours following a loading dose of 2 mg/kg orally.[81] A study comparing the pharmacokinetics of meloxicam between sheep and goats determined that meloxicam is metabolized at different rates between the two species, with goats metabolizing the drug faster than sheep.[82] A single dose of 0.5 mg/kg IV was used and the elimination half-life in sheep was determined to be 10.85 hours compared to 6.73 hours in goats, with both species having a small volume of distribution. The study extrapolated an effective plasma target concentration of 0.73 µg/mL from previous studies in horses and concluded that meloxicam should be administered every 12 hours in sheep and every 8 hours in goats to achieve plasma levels considered to be analgesic.[81,82] Oral administration of meloxicam in goats has been shown to have a high bioavailability (79%) and a half-life of nearly 11 hours.[83] The bioavailability of meloxicam in sheep has been found to be 72%. Oral dosing of 2 mg/kg loading dose, followed by 1 mg/kg daily administration, has been recommended in sheep.[84]

The smaller body size of sheep and goats makes the use of meloxicam or carprofen more economically reasonable than its use in cattle, especially for those small ruminants that are pets. As the use of phenylbutazone is prohibited in female dairy cattle older than 20 months, the use of this drug in dairy goats or sheep should be avoided.[81]

Local Anesthetics

Local anesthetics are readily available for use in small ruminants and deer. They have the distinct advantage of providing anesthesia without sedation or hypnosis. When combined with sedation, the use of local or regional techniques may help avoid general anesthesia and recumbency. They can be administered directly in the vicinity of the surgical site or they can be administered in a perineural technique for regional anesthesia in order to accomplish surgery without general anesthesia. Alternately, they may be used in the anesthetized patient to reduce the need for general anesthesia and promote cardiovascular stability. Lidocaine may be given systemically in order to manage arrhythmias, augment intestinal motility, improve analgesia, and reduce requirements for general anesthetics.[85]

Most local anesthetics are weakly basic tertiary amines with a hydrophilic end, a lipophilic end, and an intermediate hydrocarbon chain. Local anesthetics are classified based on the structural components of the drug into the amide group and the esters group. Lidocaine is the prototype for the amide group, and most modern and commonly used local anesthetics belong to this class. They are usually available as acid solutions of water soluble salts. The acid salt is neutralized in the tissue, liberating the base which is the part of the drug that penetrates the cell membrane. Because of this, local anesthetics are less effective in inflamed tissues with lower pH because there is less drug liberated under these conditions.[86]

All local anesthetics work by blocking sodium ion channels during nerve transmission. They act mainly on voltage-gated $Na+$ channels but also block voltage-dependent $K+$ and Ca^{2+} channels, but with lower affinity.[87–91] Local anesthetics produce reversible conduction blockade of impulses along central and peripheral pathways. Lidocaine is the agent most likely to affect motor function as well as sympathetic activity and sensory function.

Three common local anesthetics used by large animal veterinarians include lidocaine, mepivacaine, and bupivacaine. Lidocaine has a fast onset time, moderate duration, and moderate toxicity. The duration of plain lidocaine is approximately 1 hour.[92] Mepivacaine is very similar to lidocaine in onset and action with a slightly longer duration of effect (up to 2 hours), probably because it is associated with less vasodilation.[90] Bupivacaine is a longer-acting drug (3–10 hours) with a reportedly slower onset time (20–30 minutes).[92] Bupivacaine is the most cardiotoxic of the local anesthetics and should never be used systemically. It is useful when sensory blockade accompanied by minimal motor dysfunction is desired.[85] Lidocaine is used systemically for its antiarrhythmic effect, as well as for its analgesic and promotility effects on the gastrointestinal tract in many species.

While local and regional anesthesia is considered by many to be a safer option than general anesthesia, it is important to remember that local anesthetics can be toxic, both systemically and locally. The central nervous system may be the first system to be affected. Signs of toxicity include sedation, tremors, and/or twitching, and these signs may progress to seizures.[93] Seizure is frequently the first sign seen by veterinarians. There is no evidence to suggest that patients with epilepsy are at greater risk for seizure when local anesthetics are used. The cardiovascular system is also greatly impacted as local anesthetics slow the conduction rate and reduce excitability (hence their antiarrhythmic effect) and decrease myocardial contractility.[86,94] Local anesthetics also cause vasodilation peripherally, which can reduce cardiac output. The vasodilation that they produce can also reduce the duration of their effect. Epinephrine can be added to local anesthetics as a vasoconstrictor to increase the duration of effect. Epinephrine (1:200,000 to 1:50,000) at concentrations of 5–20 μg/mL can be added to the local anesthetic solution. The addition of epinephrine to lidocaine can increase the duration of effect from 1 hour to 3 hours.[86] Epinephrine should not be combined with local anesthetics when used to ring block extremities, teats, or other areas where vascular compromise may be a concern.

Local administration of these drugs can produce tissue reactivity and inflammation. They can also cause allergic reactions both peripherally and systemically. Sheep and especially goats are considered relatively sensitive to the toxic effects of local anesthetics. Regional techniques should be performed with a maximum dose of 6 mg/kg of lidocaine or mepivacaine and 1.5–2.0 mg/kg of bupivacaine to decrease the chance of toxicity.[85] The drugs can be diluted if a larger volume is desired for the block. An accurate body weight is helpful in calculating the dose needed, especially in young lambs and goats. Chondrotoxicity is a concern when using local anesthetics for an intraarticular block. Local anesthetic toxicity has been demonstrated in vivo and in vitro in both human and animal cartilage.[95–99] Bupivacaine in particular has been shown to be quite chondrotoxic. The marked chondrotoxicity shown by bupivacaine and lidocaine is due to necrosis rather than apoptosis.[97] Evidence suggests that there is a greater risk of chondrolysis with a longer exposure to local anesthetics rather than a single injection and that mepivacaine appears to be the least toxic at this time.[85,97]

Regional Techniques

Cornual Blocks

A cornual block is used in sheep and goats undergoing a dehorning procedure. In the goat, the cornual branch of the zygomaticotemporal nerve is blocked (as in calves) as well as the cornual branch of the infratrochlear nerve. It is not necessary to block the second cervical nerve, as is recommended in cosmetic dehorning of adult cattle.[16,69] In order to perform the block, 1–3 mL of lidocaine can be placed at each of the two sites, depending on the size of the animal, using a 20- or 22-gauge, 1.5-inch needle. To block the zygomaticotemporal nerve, the needle is inserted along the lateral edge of the frontal bone between the lateral canthus of the eye and lateral base of the horn, about 1 inch in front of the base of the horn. The cornual branch of the infratrochlear nerve is blocked by inserting the needle halfway between the medial canthus of the eye and the medial base of the horn (Figure 18.1). General anesthesia may be preferred in very young individuals to avoid toxicity or in individuals with very large horns to provide better anesthetic and surgical conditions. A regional technique may be combined with general anesthesia for optimal analgesia in those circumstances.

Eye Blocks

A regional block of the globe can be used to facilitate analgesia/anesthesia for enucleation. Local anesthetic drops such as tetracaine or proparacaine can be used on the cornea to anesthetize the cornea for foreign body removal or to assist with analgesia or diagnostics in the case of corneal ulcers. The oculomotor, trochlear, abducens, ophthalmic, and maxillary nerves should be blocked. Lidocaine or bupivacaine can be used.

Retrobulbar or Four-Point

A 20- or 22-gauge, 1.5-inch needle can be used for small ruminants.[69] The needle is inserted into the back of the orbit at 12:00, 3:00, 6:00, and the 9:00 clock positions. One to three milliliters per site of lidocaine or diluted local anesthetic is used in small ruminants. The needle can be curved so that penetration of the globe is avoided.

Peterson and Eyelid

A 20- or 22-gauge, 1.5- or 2.5-inch needle can be used for small ruminants.[69] The needle is inserted perpendicular to the notch

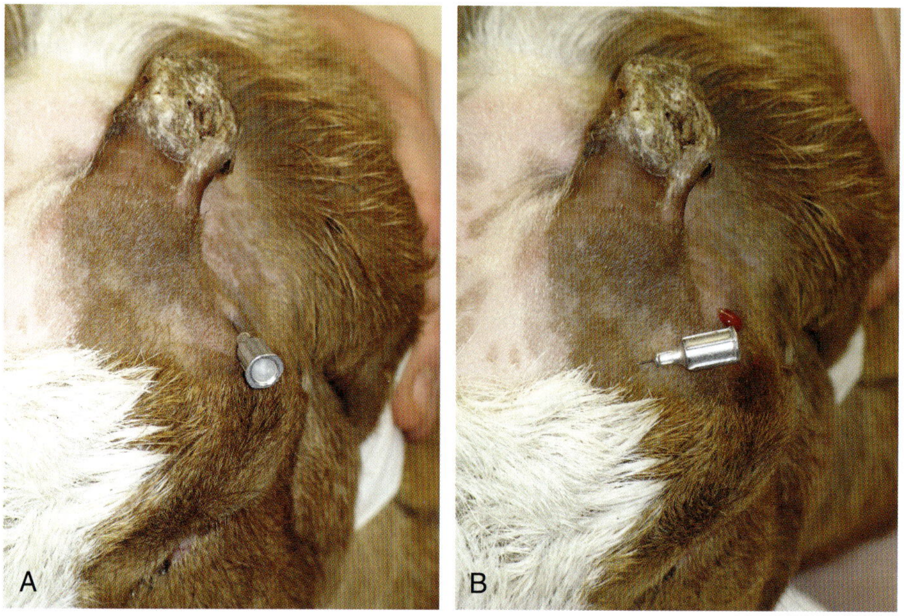

• **Fig. 18.1** Needle placement for cornual block for subcutaneous injection of local anesthetic midway between the lateral canthus of the eye and the lateral base of the horn **(A)** and another midway between the medial canthus of the eye and the medial base of the horn **(B)**.

between the zygomatic arch and the supraorbital process until it reaches the coronoid process of the mandible. Then, the needle is directed cranially to bypass the coronoid process until it strikes the bone of the orbit behind the eye. Three to seven milliliters of lidocaine can be used in small ruminants. In order to desensitize the eyelid, the auriculopalbebral branch of the facial nerve must be blocked. The needle is inserted subcutaneously along the caudal border of the zygomatic arch for 2 to 3 inches. The eyelids can also be infiltrated around the edges. Two to three milliliters of lidocaine can be used.

Paravertebral Blocks

Proximal and distal paravertebral blocks can be performed in small ruminants, although they are not frequently utilized. To perform a proximal block, a 20-gauge, 1.5-inch needle can be used to anesthetize the flank area (T13, L1, L2 spinal nerves).[16,69] The needle is inserted perpendicular to the skin about 2 inches lateral to the dorsal spinous process until it strikes the cranial edge of the transverse process behind the nerve to be blocked. The needle is walked off cranially until it penetrates the intertransverse ligament to block the ventral branch. Then, the needle is withdrawn to the level of the ligament to block the dorsal branch. Two to four milliliters of lidocaine can be used for the ventral branch and 1 mL for the dorsal branch in small ruminants.

A distal paravertebral block is performed by inserting a 20-gauge, 1.5-inch needle perpendicular and ventral to the lateral distal edge of the transverse processes of L1, L2, and L4 to block the ventral branches of T13, L1, and L2 spinal nerves.[16,69] The dorsal branches are blocked when the needle is withdrawn and redirected dorsally. Two to four milliliters of lidocaine can be used for the ventral branch and 1 mL for the dorsal branch in small ruminants.

Epidural and Subarachnoid Analgesia and Anesthesia

Injection of various analgesics and/or local anesthetics can be made epidurally or intrathecally to provide regional anesthesia and analgesia of variable intensity and duration, depending on the agents selected. Epidural administration of drugs can be made either cranially at the lumbosacral junction (L6–S1) or caudally at the sacrococcygeal junction or first intercoccygeal space (Figure 18.2). Administration of drugs in the lumbosacral space will provide

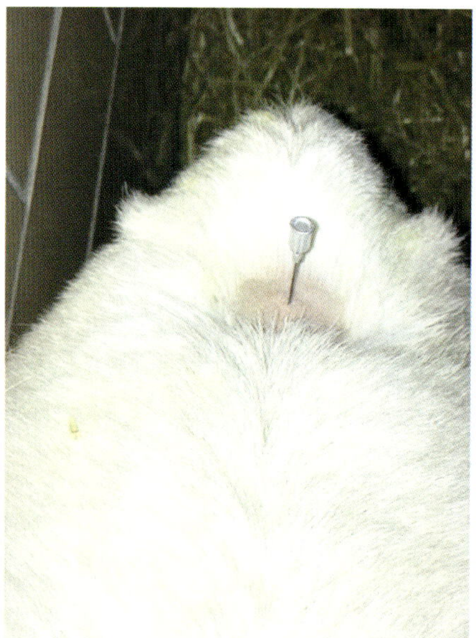

• **Fig. 18.2** Needle placement in a standing goat for a sacrococcygeal junction epidural injection.

regional anesthesia or analgesia to the abdomen and pelvis. Administration in the sacrococcygeal junction will provide anesthesia/analgesia to the skin and viscera in the middle sacral area, skin and adjacent tissue of the perineum, and the inner aspect of the thigh and tail. The subarachnoid space is smaller than the epidural space, so if cerebrospinal fluid is encountered while performing an epidural, a smaller volume of drugs should be administered. Spread of epidurally administered medications depend on the dose of the drug administered and the total volume of drug given. An increased or diluted volume of drugs can be used if one desires to "push" the epidural higher. Conversely, a smaller volume and lower dosage of drugs can concentrate the effect to the pelvis. Doses and volumes should be reduced to two thirds of what is recommended by body size for pregnant animals. Larger doses and volumes of a drug may have the potential to cause more adverse effects. Usually, the desired outcome of epidural or intrathecal anesthesia is a loss of sensation; however, there is also the potential to have sympathetic nervous system blockade with resulting hypotension or a loss of motor function. See Table 18.6 for doses of epidurally administered agents.

In order to perform a cranial or lumbosacral epidural, the animal should be positioned in sternal recumbency or standing. The site for injection can be palpated as a depression at the intersection of the dorsal midline and a line drawn between the cranial borders of the iliac wings. The area on the dorsal midline should be clipped and prepared with sterile technique. A 20- or 22-gauge needle, 1.5 or 2.5 inches, may be used. The needle is inserted perpendicularly in the lumbosacral space, which is located slightly caudal to a line that joins the cranial border of the wing of the ilium. The needle should be inserted through the skin and the hub of the needle filled with saline. The needle is inserted further until the "pop" of the needle is felt penetrating the interarcuate ligament. The negative pressure of the epidural space should suck the fluid out of the hub of the needle—this is frequently described as the "hanging drop" technique. The drug can be slowly injected without resistance to the injection. If a local anesthetic is given in the lumbosacral space, the animal will not be able to remain standing.

Injection of the sacrococcygeal or intercoccygeal site is technically easier than the lumbosacral site. A similar hanging drop technique may be used with the needle placed at a 10- to 15-degree angle to perpendicular in the space on the midline.[16] Often, the hanging drop does not work as well in small ruminants as other species and one must depend on ease of injection to validate proper placement of the needle. Caudal epidural block will permit the animal to remain standing but is not indicated for anesthesia of the udder or male genitalia.[16]

Several classes of drugs can be used to provide analgesia in the epidural or the subarachnoid space. Local anesthetics have been traditionally used because of their low cost and availability, but opioids, alpha-2 agonists, and ketamine can also be used within the central nervous system. It is important to keep in mind that any drug injected into the epidural space will have systemic effects, as the epidural space is lined with blood vessels. The use of opioids produces analgesia without loss of motor function. Epidurally administered morphine can provide analgesia up to 24 hours in many species due to its hydrophilic nature and tendency to stay within the epidural space. Xylazine has local anesthetic activity in addition to its alpha-2 agonist effects and is popular for caudal epidurals in mares. Studies have compared the use of buprenorphine (a partial mu agonist opioid) and lidocaine intrathecally in goats with the use of lidocaine and xylazine.[68] The analgesia lasted longer and was accompanied by less adverse effects with respect to sedation and cardiovascular function.[68]

TABLE 18.6 Epidural/Subarachnoid[a] Drug Dosages for Use in Sheep and Goats (see Appendix 1).

Drug	Dosage (mg/kg)	Duration (hours)
Lidocaine	0.1–2	1–2
Bupivicaine	1.5–1.8	3–4
Ketamine	0.5–2.5	1–2
Morphine	0.1 (dilute to 3–5 mL total volume with sterile saline)	6–12
Xylazine	0.05–0.1 (dilute to 2–3 mL total volume with sterile saline)	1–2
Buprenorphine	0.005	3

[a]Use one-half the dose or the low end of the dosage range if administering drugs into the subarachnoid space.

Sources: Staffieri F, Driessen B, Lacitignola, et al: A comparison of subarachnoid buprenorphine or xylazine as an adjunct to lidocaine for analgesia in goats, *Vet Anaesth Analg* 36:502–511, 2009; Valverde A, Doherty TJ. Anesthesia and analgesia in ruminants. In: Fish R, Danneman PJ, Brown M, et al, editors: *Anesthesia and Analgesia in Laboratory Animals*, ed 2, London, 2008, Academic Press.

Intraarticular Blocks

Intraarticular lidocaine plus bupivacaine has been shown to be effective in relieving postoperative pain in sheep undergoing stifle arthrotomy.[100] The authors used lidocaine preoperatively (2 mL) and bupivacaine postoperatively (2 mL) with analgesia lasting 3 to 7 hours after surgery. Bupivacaine has been shown to have some chondrotoxicity, which should be taken into consideration when considering the use of this drug in an intraarticular manner.[85,97] In goats, 0.75 mg/kg of intra-articular bupivacaine before stifle arthrotomy provided up to 100 minutes of analgesia but did not reduce the need for postoperative analgesics.[101] Mepivacaine has been shown to be the least chondrotoxic local anesthetic in common use.[97]

Testicular Blocks

Anesthesia to the spermatic cord and testicle can be provided by local anesthetics in conjunction with sedation or general anesthesia or on its own. For complete anesthesia of the surgical site, the scrotal skin and spermatic cord must be blocked. Local anesthetic can be injected directly into the center of the testicle until the testicle feels firm, so that the local anesthetic will migrate up the spermatic cord. Another option is to pull the testicle down and inject local anesthetic directly into the tissues in the area of the spermatic cord. It is important to remember the size of the animal and an appropriate dose-up to 6 mg/kg of lidocaine for sheep and goats. The skin of the scrotal incision can be infiltrated as well.[102]

Regional IV Block (Bier)

IV regional anesthesia can be performed in small ruminants when anesthesia of a distal extremity is desired. The technique requires the placement of a tourniquet and an IV catheter distal to the tourniquet. The animal is placed in lateral recumbency and sedation is generally recommended, as tourniquet use is associated with some pain. A distal venous catheter is placed, then a tourniquet applied proximal to the site of injection, tight enough to occlude arterial flow to the limb. An Esmarch rubber bandage can also be used to exsanguinate the limb. The tourniquet should remain in place for the duration of the procedure, but procedures of less than 1 hour are recommended for this technique. Lidocaine (10–20 mL) is the most common local anesthetic used for this block as it will be released systemically when the tourniquet is removed.[16] Bupivacaine should not be used due to its cardiovascular toxicity.

Complications of General Anesthesia

Complications of general anesthesia in any species often center around the body systems most affected. Reduction of cardiac output can be expected, with some individuals experiencing excessive bradycardia, hypotension, cardiovascular decompensation, and/or collapse. Atropine or glycopyrrolate can be given if the heart rate is excessively low. The use of an anticholinergic in order to "dry up" or reduce salivation and respiratory secretions is usually not recommended or necessary. While ruminants do not suffer hypotension as easily as other species under general anesthesia, occasionally, systemic mean arterial pressure is less than 70 mm Hg. If hypotension does occur, the depth of anesthesia should be checked to see if the animal could require less inhaled anesthetic. A fluid challenge of 5 mL/kg intravenously can be administered. Colloidal products like Vetstarch may be given in cases of significant hypotension or if the animal has low plasma proteins. Sympathomimetic drugs like dobutamine or ephedrine can be used if hypotension is not relieved by vaporizer management and fluid therapy. Animals undergoing strictly injectable anesthetic are less likely to by hypotensive. Table 18.7 contains drug dosages for use with anesthetic complications.

Respiratory embarrassment and compromise are very common, with large animal species particularly affected. Ruminants are particularly at risk due to the volume of fluid in the rumen. This increases abdominal pressure, which can translate to increased thoracic pressure through the diaphragm, leading to a reduction in functional residual capacity and hypoventilation. When ruminants are induced on an emergency basis, without water deprivation to reduce the size and volume in the rumen, aspiration of rumen fluid is possible with the risk of aspiration pneumonia. Every effort should be made to intubate animals as efficiently as possible with a minimum of laryngeal manipulation, which makes it more likely to stimulate regurgitation. The animal should be maintained in sternal recumbency to protect the airway until intubation and endotracheal tube cuff inflation.

As previously discussed in this chapter, sheep can experience significant hypoxemia with all alpha-2 agonists like xylazine, detomidine, or medetomidine. For this reason, the authors prefer not to use an alpha-2 agonist in valuable or pet individuals. Pulmonary edema can also be observed when alpha-2 agonists have been administered. Furosemide at 2 mg/kg IV can be given if signs of pulmonary edema are exhibited and supplemental oxygen administered.

If rumen tympany should occur while the animal is undergoing general anesthesia, a stomach tube should be passed through the esophagus into the rumen in order to relieve the gas pressure. Particular attention needs to be paid to the animal's ability to ventilate if rumen tympany occurs. Antagonism of sedative drugs like alpha-2 agents can be considered as soon as possible after the procedure in order to relieve the effects of sedation and decreased GI motility.

TABLE 18.7 Antagonists and Emergency Drugs for Use in Sheep and Goats (see Appendix 1).

Drug	Dosage (mg/kg)
Atipamezole	0.05 IV
Atropine	0.06–0.1 IV
Calcium borogluconate solutions-23%	0.5–1 mL/kg/h IV
Doxapram	5–10 IV
Dobutamine	0.005–0.010 mg/kg/h IV
Dopamine	0.002–0.015 mg/kg/min IV
Ephedrine	0.02–0.06 IV
Epinephrine	0.02–0.2 IV
Flumazenil	0.1–1 IV
Furosemide	1–2
Glycopyrrolate	0.002–0.005 IV 0.005–0.01 IM
Naloxone	0.01–0.02 IV to effect
Naltrexone	0.05–0.1 SC
Yohimbine	0.1–0.3 IV 0.3–0.5 IM

IM, Intramuscularly; *IV*, intravenously.

Example Anesthetic Protocols

Goats With Urinary Tract Obstruction

For a 25-kg pygmy goat with urethral obstruction:

1. Premedication: Use a combination of butorphanol 0.2 mg/kg with midazolam or diazepam 0.2 mg/kg IV or IM
2. Preoxygenate with 3 L/min of 100% oxygen by face mask
3. Induce with 2.2 mg/kg ketamine IV followed by 2 mg/kg propofol to effect for intubation
4. Intubate and maintain with isoflurane, small animal machine
5. Fluid therapy: Plasmalyte A or Normosol-R 5 mL/kg/h if serum K+ is within normal limits
   a. Use non-K+-containing fluid (normal saline) if hyperkalemia is present
6. Can repeat butorphanol if needed postoperatively
7. Morphine/lidocaine cranial epidural

Ovine Caesarean Section

1. Sedate ewe with 0.2 mg/kg butorphanol + 0.2 mg/kg diazepam or midazolam
2. Line block infiltration with lidocaine
3. Oxygen therapy via face mask

Cervid Anesthesia

There is an increasing frequency of need for veterinarians to anesthetize hoof stock. There is a huge variety of deer worldwide, and it is beyond the scope of this chapter to discuss each species in detail. Therefore, emphasis will be placed on white-tailed deer and elk and general practices discussed. Game-farmed deer and elk may require chemical restraint in order to accomplish some husbandry practices and treat injured animals. Capture of both wild and domesticated deer must be carefully planned, as prolonged periods of chase or stressful handling will increase the likelihood of hyperthermia and trauma and capture myopathy. Elective procedures should be planned for the cool part of the day whenever possible.[103] Captive deer should be fasted for 24 hours prior to a planned procedure.[103] Anesthetic planning will depend on the availability of equipment and the skill of the personnel involved. Game-farming situations may have squeeze or drop-floored chutes available to physically restrain animals. Free-ranging deer may be captured with net guns, drive nets, or clover traps. Nonetheless, the animal should spend the least amount of time in physical or chemical restraint, and sedation of animals may help reduce stress and improve working conditions. Mature white-tailed deer weigh between 60 and 150 kg and mature elk weigh between 230 and 318 kg.[104] Intranasal administration of drugs like xylazine can be used to reduce stress.[105] This technique can be used in deer that have been captured by physical means and produces reliable sedation and stress reduction in elk (1.5–2 mg/kg).[106] The technique can be utilized by attaching a venous catheter (2–3 inches length) to a syringe in order to spray the drug further up the nasal cavity. Onset of sedation can be expected in 1 minute and can be antagonized with yohimbine. It is very important to keep deer as calm as possible as the sedative effects of any drug can be overridden with stress and excitement. One rule of thumb is that dosing of sedatives should be on the "high side," as underdosing cervids leads to longer induction times and greater likelihood of capture myopathy. Animals can be partially reversed once recumbent if needed. Table 18.8 contains anesthetic dose information as well as antagonist dosages.

There are many drugs that can be utilized—some are commonly available to large-animal veterinarians and some, such as the potent narcotics, are more difficult to obtain. Opioid availability in general may be a concern. North American cervids like white-tailed deer and elk can be anesthetized with a variety of combinations of opioids, alpha-2 agonists, dissociative anesthetics and tranquilizers. Sedation and anesthesia of deer and elk can be a challenge, depending on whether the animal is accustomed to human contact or is completely wild. If excitement can be avoided, then xylazine is a practical and less expensive sedative in these species. Cervids are prone to the same complications of sedation and anesthesia as other ruminants, so steps must be taken to avoid hypoxemia, rumen tympany, and regurgitation. Recumbent sedation can be accomplished in farmed white-tailed deer with 2–3 mg/kg xylazine administered intramuscularly.[103] American elk require approximately 1 mg/kg xylazine IM to produce recumbent sedation.[106] Once the drug has been injected, the animal should be left alone until it assumes lateral or sternal recumbency with its head down. The animal should be approached with caution, as animals that appear to be heavily sedated can rouse suddenly without warning. The chance of sudden arousal can be minimized by injecting 1–2 mg/kg ketamine intravenously into the jugular vein.[103] This can be repeated as necessary at 10- to 15-minute intervals. The effects of the xylazine can be antagonized with yohimbine (0.1–0.2 mg/kg) or with tolazoline (2–4 mg/kg).[103] Alpha-2 antagonists can be administered half intravenously and half intramuscularly.

TABLE 18.8 Drug Dosages for White-Tailed Deer and Elk (see Appendix 1).

Drug	Dosage (mg/kg)
Deer	
Xylazine	2–3 IM
Ketamine	1–2 IV
Butorphanol	0.02–0.05
Combined: xylazine	1.5 IM
Telazol	3 IM
Elk	
Xylazine	1
Telazol	2
Antagonists	
Yohimbine	0.1–0.2 (1/2 IV, 1/2 IM)
Tolazoline	2–4

Source: Caulkett N, Arnemo JM: Cervids (deer). In West G, Heard D, Caulkett N, editors: *Zoo Animal & Wildlife Immobilization and Anesthesia*, ed 2, Ames, IA, 2014, John Wiley & Sons.

Other injectable combinations can be utilized in farmed or free-ranging deer. Xylazine can be combined with Telazol to capture wild deer.[107,108] American elk require 1 mg/kg xylazine with 2 mg/kg Telazol, while deer take 1.5 mg/kg xylazine plus 3 mg/kg Telazol.[104] There is predictably more variation in drug response in free-ranging deer. Drug combinations with less volume are easier to administer via dart. Telazol has advantages over ketamine in that it requires less drug volume for effect. Free-range deer and elk are at greater risk of complication than captive animals. Drug requirements tend to be higher and there is some risk associated with remote delivery. Some protocols that can be used are listed in Table 18.7. Guaifenesin and ketamine ± xylazine can be used to maintain injectable anesthesia, similar to its use in other ruminants, if a jugular catheter has been placed. Venous access can be achieved by cannulating the jugular, cephalic, or saphenous veins.

Fawns may be easier to handle and sedate than adult animals. Protocols suitable for small ruminants can be adapted for use with fawns. They can be premedicated with diazepam (0.2 mg/kg IV) and butorphanol (0.05 mg/kg IV) and then mask induced with inhalant or induced with 2 mg/kg IV ketamine.[103] Dextrose at 2.5% should be added to crystalloid fluids.

Positioning of anesthetized cervids is important for optimal animal care. Deer should be positioned in sternal recumbency with the head and neck extended to improve airway patency and help any saliva to drain from the mouth rather than accumulate in the pharynx. Intubation is recommended for animals undergoing a lengthy anesthetic process but can be difficult in large deer and elk. Their long and narrow head makes it difficult to open the mouth and visualize the larynx. Use of a long flat laryngoscope blade is recommended for optimum success, as well as a stylet or guide tube. It is helpful to have the flange of the laryngoscopy

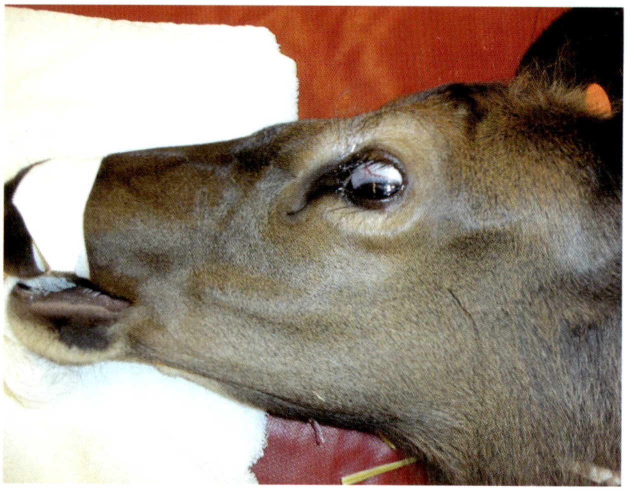

• **Fig. 18.3** Ventral strabismus in an anesthetized deer which is indicative of an appropriate plane of surgical anesthesia.

blade removed to improve the visibility of the larynx and maneuverability within the oral cavity. The epiglottis in deer is long and mobile, making intubation more difficult as well. The author (AW) has occasionally intubated large elk digitally, in a similar fashion to large cattle. Once intubated, cervids can be maintained with additional injectable anesthetics or with inhalant anesthesia and oxygen. Isoflurane or sevoflurane can be used, but isoflurane is more economical at this time. Deer weighing less than 100 kg can be maintained on a small animal anesthesia machine with an oxygen flow rate of 50 mL/kg/min. Vaporizer concentration should be expected to be lower with the concomitant administration of injectable anesthetics but may have to be increased as the injectable drugs wear off. If inhaled anesthetics are used, then an isotonic crystalloid fluid should be administered at 5–10 mL/kg/h.

Monitoring of anesthesia will depend on equipment availability and the working conditions (Figure 18.3). Deer can be expected to develop hypoxemia when anesthetized, so the ability to monitor oxygenation with a pulse oximeter can be critical. Supplemental oxygen should be administered in order to maintain saturation ≥95%. Pulse oximeters will also report a heart rate. All general anesthesia promotes hypoventilation, so anesthetized deer can be expected to hypoventilate, making supplemental oxygen even more helpful. If the animal is being maintained with inhaled anesthesia, IPPV can be used to combat hypoventilation. Blood pressure can be measured with an oscillometric monitor and an adult (human) cuff placed around the forelimb. Most cervids experience hypertension while anesthetized, so blood pressure can be expected to be higher than in horses or small animals. The auricular artery can be used to obtain samples for blood gas analysis.

Body temperature is very important to monitor in anesthetized hoof stock as deer are prone to hyperthermia and hypoxemia. Rectal temperature should be monitored every 5 to 10 minutes as deer are prone to hyperthermia.[109,110] Rectal temperatures greater than 40° C are a cause of concern, and the animal should be actively cooled. Body temperature greater than 41° C should be treated as an emergency and the authors recommend administering an antagonist and allowing it to recover as quickly as possible.[103] Hyperthermia in the face of hypoxemia is a critical concern, as hyperthermia increases metabolic oxygen demand.

Velvet antler removal is a common surgical procedure in farmed deer. A lidocaine ring block technique can be used to provide local anesthesia and analgesia, thus decreasing the need for prolonging sedation or general anesthesia. Lidocaine without epinephrine is used to infiltrate the tissues around the base of the antler at a dose rate of 1 mL/cm of pedicle circumference.[111]

Acknowledgments

The authors acknowledge the work of Hui-Chu Lin, Fred Caldwell, and D.G. Pugh in this chapter of the previous edition of this text.

References

1. Lin HC, Caldwell F, Pugh DG: Anesthetic Management. In Pugh DG, Baird AN editors: *Sheep & goat medicine*, ed 2, St. Louis, MO, 2012, Elsevier.
2. Craigmill AL, Rangel-Lugo M, Riviere JE: Extralabel use of tranquilizers and general anesthetics, *J Am Vet Med Assoc* 211:302, 1997.
3. Fajt VR: Label and extra label drug use in small ruminants, *Vet Clin North Am Food Anim Pract* 2:553, 1986.
4. Riebold TW: Ruminants. In Grimm, KA, Lamont LA, Tranquilli, WJ, et al, editors: *Veterinary anesthesia and analgesia: the fifth edition of Lumb and Jones*, Ames, IA, 2015, John Wiley & Sons.
5. Tranquilli WJ: Techniques of inhalation anesthesia in ruminants and swine, *Vet Clin North Am Food Anim Pract* 2:593–619, 1986.
6. Stewart SL, Secrest JA, Norwood BR, et al: A comparison of endotracheal tube cuff pressures using estimation techniques and direct intracuff measurement, *AANA J* 71:443–447, 2003.
7. Morrison, JD: Drugs used in neuroleptanalgesia, *Int Anesthesiol Clin* 7:141–158, 1969.
8. Taylor PM: Anaesthesia in sheep and goats, *In Pract* 13:31–36, 1991.
9. Rankin DC: Sedatives and tranquilizers. In Grimm, KA, Lamont LA, Tranquilli, WJ, et al, editors: *Veterinary anesthesia and analgesia: the fifth edition of Lumb and Jones*, Ames, IA, 2015, John Wiley & Sons.
10. Caulkett N, Haigh JC: Deer (Cervids). In West G, Heard D, Caulkett N editors: *Zoo animal & wildlife immobilization and anesthesia*, Ames Iowa, 2007, Blackwell.
11. Read M, Caulkett NA, McCallister M: Evaluation of zooclopenthixol acetate to decrease handling stress in wapiti, *J Wildl Dis* 36:450–459, 2000.
12. Stegmann GF, Bester L: Sedative-hypnotic effects of midazolam in goats after intravenous and intramuscular administration, *Vet Anes Analg* 28:49–55, 2001.
13. Grandy JL, McDonell WN: Evaluation of concentrated solutions of guaifenesin for equine anesthesia, *J Am Vet Med Assoc* 176:619–622, 1980.
14. Thurmon JC: Injectable anesthetic agents and techniques in ruminants and swine, *Vet Clin North Am Food Anim Pract* 2:567–592, 1986.
15. KuKanich B, Wiese AJ: Opioids. In Grimm, KA, Lamont LA, Tranquilli, WJ, et al, editors: *Veterinary anesthesia and analgesia: the fifth edition of Lumb and Jones*, Ames, IA, 2015, John Wiley & Sons.
16. Valverde A, Doherty TJ. Anesthesia and analgesia in ruminants. In: Fish R, Danneman PJ, Brown M, et al, editors: *Anesthesia and analgesia in laboratory animals*, ed 2, London, 2008, Academic Press.
17. Katzung BG, editor: *Basic and clinical pharmacology*, ed 9, New York, 2004, McGraw Hill.
18. Greene SA, Thurmon JC: Xylazine—a review of its pharmacology and use in veterinary medicine, *J Vet Pharmacol Ther* 11:295, 1988.
19. Celly CS, McDonell WN, Young SS et al: The comparative hypoxaemic effect of four alpha2 adrenoceptor agonists (xylazine, romifidine, detomidine and medetomidine) in sheep, *J Vet Pharmacol Ther* 20: 464–471, 1997.

20. Celly CS, McDonell WN, Black WD: Comparative cardiopulmonary effects for four α-2 adrenoceptor agonists in sheep, *Vet Surg* 22:545, 1993.
21. Celly CS, McDonell WN, Black WD: Histopathologic alterations induced in the lungs of sheep by use of alpha2-adrenergic receptor agonists, *Am J Vet Res* 60:154–161, 1999.
22. Kastner SBR: α2-agonists in sheep: a review, *Vet Anaesth Analg* 33:79, 2006.
23. Kastner SBR, Keller K, Rechenberg BV, et al: Comparison of medetomidine and dexmedetomidine as premedication in isoflurane anaesthesia for total hip replacement in domestic sheep, *J Vet Med Assoc* 48:231–241, 2001.
24. Hsu WH, Schaffer DD, Hanson CE: Effects of tolazoline and yohimbine on xylaine-induced central nervous system depression, bradycardia, and tachypnea in sheep, *J Am Vet Med Assoc* 190:423–426, 1987.
25. Eisenach JG: Intravenous clonidine produces hypoxemia by a peripheral alpha 2 adrenergic mechanism, *J Pharmacol Exp Ther* 244: 247–252, 1988.
26. Nolan A, Livingston A, Waterman A: The effects of alpha2 adrenoceptor agonists on airway pressure in anaesthetized sheep, *J Vet Pharmacol Ther* 9:157–163, 1986.
27. Read MR, Duke T, Toews AR: Suspected tolazoline toxicosis in a llama, *J Am Vet Med Assoc* 216:227, 2000.
28. Lin HC, Riddell MG: Tolazoline: dose responses and side effects in non-sedated Holstein calves, *Bov Practitioner* 42:86, 2008.
29. Galatos AD: Anesthesia and analgesia in sheep and goats, *Vet Clin Food Anim* 27:47–59, 2011.
30. Carroll GL, Hartsfield SM: General anaesthetic techniques in ruminants, *Vet Clin North Am Food Anim Pract* 12:627–661, 1996.
31. Hall LW, Clarke KW, Trim CM: Anaesthesia of sheep, goats and other herbivores. In: *Veterinary anaesthesia,* ed 10, London, 2001, W. B. Saunders.
32. Gray PR, McDonell WN: Anaesthesia in goats and sheep. Part II. General anesthesia, *Compend Contin Educ Pract Vet* 8(Suppl): S127–S135, 1986.
33. Ghurashi, MAH, Seri HI, Bakheit, AH, et al: Evaluation of ketamine/diazepam anaesthesia for performing surgery in desert goats under field conditions, *Aust J Basic and Appl Sci* 3:455–459, 2009.
34. Berry, S: Injectable Anesthetics. In Grimm, KA, Lamont LA, Tranquilli, WJ, editors: *Veterinary anesthesia and analgesia: the fifth edition of Lumb and Jones*, Ames, IA, 2015, John Wiley & Sons.
35. White PR, Way WI, Trevor AJ: Ketamine—its pharmacology and therapeutic uses, *Anesthesiology* 56:119–136, 1982.
36. Zhuo, M: Plasticity of NMDA receptor NR2B subunit in memory and chronic pain, *Mol Brain* 2(1):4–15, 2009.
37. Dzikiti TB, Stegmann, GF, Dzikiti LN, Hellebrekers LJ: Total intravenous anaesthesia (TIVA) with propofol-fentanyl and propofol-midazolam combinations in spontaneously breathing goats, *Vet Anaesth Analg* 37:519–525, 2010.
38. Goodchild CS, Serrao JM: Cardiovascular effects of propofol in the anaesthetized dog, *Br J Anaesth* 63(1):87–92, 1989.
39. Brussel T, Theissen JL, Vigfusson G, et al: Hemodynamic and cardiodynamic effects of propofol and etomidate: negative inotropic properties of propofol, *Anesth Analg* 69(1):35–40, 1989.
40. Muir WW, Gadawski JE: Respiratory depression and apnea induced by propofol in dogs, *Am J Vet Res* 59(2):157–161, 1998.
41. Prassinos NN, Galatos AD, Raptopoulos D: A comparison of propofol, thiopental or ketamine as induction agents in goats, *Vet Anaesth Analg* 32:289–296, 2005.
42. Ferre, PJ, Pasloske K, Whittem T, et al: Plasma pharmacokinetics of alfaxalone in dogs after an intravenous bolus of Alfaxan-CD RTU, *Vet Anesth Analg* 33:229–236, 2006.
43. Suarez MA, Dzikiti BT, Stegman FG, et al: Comparison of alfaxalone and propofol administered as total intravenous anaesthesia for ovariohysterectomy in dogs, *Vet Anesth Analg* 28:49–55, 2012.
44. Andaluz A, Felez-Ocana N, Santos L, et al: The effects on cardiorespiratory and acid-base variables of the anaesthetic alfaxalone in a 2-hydroxypropyl-β-cyclodextrin (HPCD) formulation in sheep, *Vet J* 191:389–392, 2012.
45. Child KJ, Currie JP, Dis B, et al: The pharmacological properties in animals of CT1341-A new steroid anaesthetic agent, *Brit J of Anaesthesia* 43:2–13, 1971.
46. Sear JW, Phillips KC, Andrews CJH, et al: Dose-response relationships for infusions of Althesin or methohexitone *Anesthesia* 38:931-936, 1983.
47. Abrahamsen EJ: Ruminant field anesthesia, *Vet Clin Food Anim Pract* 24:429–441, 2008.
48. Dzikiti TB: Intravenous anaesthesia in goats: a review, *J S Afr Vet Assoc* 84(1):E1–E8, 2013. doi:10.4102/jsava.v84i1.499.
49. Beths T: *Total intravenous anaesthesia in dogs: development of a target-controlled infusion (TCI) scheme for propofol.* PhD thesis, Department of Companion Animal Sciences, University of Glasgow, 2008.
50. Waelbers T, Vermoere P, Polis I: Total intravenous anaesthesia in dogs. A review, *Vlaams Diergeneeskundie Tijdschrift* 78:160–169, 2009.
51. Steffey EP, Mama KR, Brosnan RJ: Inhalation Anesthetics. In Grimm, KA, Lamont LA, Tranquilli, WJ, et al, editors: *Veterinary anesthesia and analgesia: the fifth edition of Lumb and Jones*, Ames, IA, 2015, John Wiley & Sons.
52. Palahniuk RJ, Shnider SM, Eger EI II: Pregnancy decreases the requirement for inhaled anesthetic agents, *Anesthesiology* 41:82–83, 1974.
53. Doherty TJ, Rohrbach BW, Geiser DR: Effect of acepromazine and butorphanol on isoflurane mi in goats, *J Vet Pharmacol Ther* 25:65–67, 2002.
54. Doherty TJ, Will WA, Rohrbach BW, Geiser DR: Effect of morphine and flunixin meglumine on isoflurane minimum alveolar concentration in goats, *Vet Anaesth Analg* 31(2):97–101, 2004.
55. Hikasa Y, Okuyama K, Kakuta T, et al: Anesthetic potency and cardiopulmonary effects of sevoflurane in goats: comparison with isoflurane and halothane, *Can J Vet Res* 62:299–306, 1998.
56. Haskins SC: Monitoring anesthetized patients. In Grimm, KA, Lamont LA, Tranquilli, WJ, et al, editors: *Veterinary anesthesia and analgesia: the fifth edition of Lumb and Jones*, Ames, IA, 2015, John Wiley & Sons.
57. Aarnes T, Hubbell JAE, Lerche P, Bednarski R: Comparison of invasive and oscillometric blood pressure measurement techniques in sheep, goats, and cattle anesthetized for surgery [Abstract]. In: Proceedings of the American College of Veterinary Anesthesiologists Meeting, San Antonio, TX, 2012.
58. McDonell WN, Kerr CL: Physiology, pathophysiology, and anesthetic management of patients with respiratory disease. In Grimm, KA, Lamont LA, Tranquilli, WJ, et al, editors: *Veterinary anesthesia and analgesia: the fifth edition of Lumb and Jones*, Ames, IA, 2015, John Wiley & Sons.
59. Gallivan GJ, McDonell WN, Forrest JB: Comparative ventilation and gas exchange in the horse and cow, *Res Vet Sci* 46:331–336, 1989.
60. Hubbell AE, Muir WW: Monitoring anesthesia, In Muir WW, Hubbell JAE, editors: *Equine anesthesia monitoring and emergency therapy*, ed 2, St. Louis, 2009, Elsevier.
61. Heesch CM: Reflexes that control cardiovascular function, *A J Physiol* 277:S234–S243, 1999.
62. Wagner AE, Bednarski RM, Muir WW: Hemodynamic effects of carbon dioxide during intermittent positive pressure ventilation in horses, *Am J Vet Res* 51:1922–1929, 1990.
63. Guyton GC, Hall JE, editors: *Guyton and hall textbook of medical physiology*, Philadelphia, PA, 2016, Elsevier.
64. Mitchell B, Williams JT: Respiratory function changes in sheep associated with lying in lateral recumbency and with sedation by xylazine, *Proc Assoc Vet Anaesth Great Br Ire* 6:30, 1976–1977.
65. Stafford KJ: Recognition and assessment of pain in ruminants. In Egger CM, Love L, Doherty T, editors: *Pain management in veterinary practice,* Ames, 2014, John Wiley & Sons.
66. Molony V, Kent JW, McKendrick, IJ: Validation of a method for assessment of an acute pain in lambs, *Appl Anim Behav Sci* 76:215–238, 2002.
67. National Research Council (US) Committee on Recognition and Alleviation of Pain in Laboratory Animals: *Recognition and alleviation of pain in laboratory animals*, Washington, DC, 2009, National Academies Press. Available at: https://www.ncbi.nlm.nih.gov/books/NBK32658/. doi:10.17226/12526.

68. Staffieri F, Driessen B, Lacitignola L, et al: A comparison of subarachnoid buprenorphine or xylazine as an adjunct to lidocaine for analgesia in goats, *Vet Anaesth Analg* 36:502–511, 2009.
69. Valverde A: Treatment of acute and chronic pain in ruminants. In Egger CM, Love L, Doherty T, editors: *Pain management in veterinary practice,* Ames, 2014, John Wiley & Sons.
70. Nolan A, Livingston A, Waterman AE: Investigation of the antinociceptive activity of buprenorphine in sheep, *Br J Pharmacol* 92: 527–533, 1987.
71. Nolan A, Livingston A, Waterman AE: The correlation of the thermal and mechanical antinociceptive activity of pethidine hydrochloride with plasma concentrations of the drug in sheep, *J Vet Pharm Ther* 11:94–102, 1988.
72. Waterman AE, Livingston A, Amin A: The antinociceptive activity and respiratory effects of fentanyl in sheep, *J Assoc Vet Anaesth* 17:20–23, 1990.
73. Waterman AE, Livingston A, Amin A: Analgesic activity and respiratory effects of butorphanol in sheep, *Res Vet Sci* 51:19–23, 1991.
74. Waterman AE, Livingston A, Amin A: Further studies on the antinociceptive activity and respiratory effects of buprenorphine in sheep, *J Vet Pharm Ther* 14:230–234, 1991.
75. Ahern BJ, Soma LR, Rudy JA, et al: Pharmacokinetics of fentanyl administered transdermally and intravenously in sheep, *Am J Vet Res* 71:1127–1132, 2010.
76. Christou C, Oliver RA, Rawlinson, J, et al: Transdermal fentanyl and its use in ovine surgery, *Res Vet Sci,* 100:252–256, 2015.
77. Ahern BJ, Soma LR, Boston RC, et al: Comparison of the analgesic properties of transdermally administered fentanyl and intramuscularly administered buprenorphine during and following experimental orthopedic surgery in sheep, *Am J Vet Res* 70:418–422, 2009.
78. Carroll GL, Hooper RN, Boothe DM, et al: Pharmacokinetics of fentanyl after intravenous and transdermal administration in goats, *Am J Vet Res* 60:986–981, 1999.
79. Jen KY, Dyson MC, Lester PA: Pharmacokinetics of a transdermal fentanyl solution in Suffolk sheep (Ovis aries), *J Amer Assoc Lab Anim Sci* 56:550–557, 2017.
80. Papich MG, Messenger K: Non-Steroidal anti-inflammatory drugs. In Grimm, KA, Lamont LA, Tranquilli, WJ, et al, editors: *Veterinary anesthesia and analgesia: the fifth edition of Lumb and Jones,* Ames, IA, 2015, John Wiley & Sons.
81. Plummer PJ, Schleining JA: Assessment and management of pain in small ruminants and camelids, *Vet Clin Food Anim* 29:185–208, 2013.
82. Shukla M, Singh G, Sindhura BG, et al: Comparative plasma pharmacokinetics of meloxicam in sheep and goats following intravenous administration, *Comp Bio-Chem Physiol C Toxicol Pharmacol* 45(4): 528–532, 2007.
83. Ingvast-Larsson C, Hogberg M, Mengistu U, et al: Pharmacokinetics of meloxi-cam in adult goats and its analgesic effect in disbudded kids, *J Vet Pharmacol Ther* 34(1):64–69, 2011.
84. Stock ML, Coetzee JF, KuKanich B, et al: Pharmacokinetics of intravenously and orally administered meloxicam in sheep, *Am J Vet Res* 74:779–783, 2013.
85. Garcia ER: Local anesthetics. In Grimm, KA, Lamont LA, Tranquilli, WJ, et al, editors: *Veterinary anesthesia and analgesia: the fifth edition of Lumb and Jones,* Ames, IA, 2015, John Wiley & Sons.
86. Liu SS, Joseph RS: Local anesthetics. In: Barash PG, Cullen BF, Stoelting RK, editors: *Clinical anesthesia,* ed 5, Philadelphia, PA: Lippincott Williams & Wilkins, 2006.
87. Komai H, McDowell TS: Local anesthetic inhibition of voltage-activated potassium currents in rat dorsal root ganglion neurons, *Anesthesiology* 94:1089–1095, 2001.
88. Olschewski A, Hempelmann G, Vogel W, et al: Blockade of Na+ and K + currents by local anesthetics in the dorsal horn neurons of the spinal cord, *Anesthesiology* 88:172–179, 1998.
89. Xiong ZL, Strichartz GR: Inhibition by local anesthetics of Ca2+ channels in rat anterior pituitary cells, *Eur J Pharmacol* 363:81–90, 1998.
90. Sugiyama K, Muteki T. Local anesthetics depress the calcium current of rat sensory neurons in culture. *Anesthesiology* 80:1369–1378, 1994.
91. Scholz A: Mechanisms of (local) anaesthetics on voltage-gated sodium and other ion channels, *Br J Anaesth* 89:52–61, 2002.
92. Butterworth JF: Clinical pharmacology of local anesthetics. In: Cousins MJ, Carr DB, Horlocker TT, editors: *Cousins & bridenbaugh's neural blockade in clinical anesthesia and pain medicine,* ed 4, Philadelphia, 2009, Lippincott Williams & Wilkins.
93. Feldman HS, Arthur GR, Covino BG: Comparative systemic toxicity of convulsant and supraconvulsant doses of intravenous ropivacaine, bupivicaine, and lidocaine in the conscious dog, *Anesth Analg* 69:794–801, 1989.
94. Copeland SE, Ladd LA, Gu SQ, et al: The effects of general anesthesia on the central nervous and cardiovascular system toxicity of local anesthetics, *Anesth Analg* 106:1429–1439, 2008.
95. Gomoll AH, Kang RW, Williams JM, et al: Chondrolysis after continuous intra-articular bupivacaine infusion: an experimental model investigating chondrotox-city in the rabbit shoulder, *Arthroscopy* 22:813–819, 2006.
96. Karpie JC, Chu CR: Lidocaine exhibits dose- and time-dependent cytotoxic effects on bovine articular chondrocytes in vitro, *Am J Sports Med* 35:1621–1627, 2007.
97. Park J, Sutradhar BC, Hong G, et al: Comparison of the cytotoxic effects of bupivacaine, lidocaine, and mepivacaine in equine articular chondrocytes, *Vet Anaesth Analg* 38:127–133, 2011.
98. Dragoo JL, Braun HJ, Kim HJ, et al: The in vitro chondrotoxicity of single-dose local anesthetics, *Am J Sports Med* 40:794–799, 2012.
99. Hansen BP, Beck CL, Beck EP, et al: Postarthroscopic glenohumeral chondrolysis, *Am J Sports Med* 35:1628–1634, 2007.
100. Shafford HL, Hellyer PW, Turner AS: Intra-articular lidocaine plus bupivacaine in sheep undergoing stifle arthrotomy, *Vet Anaesth Analg* 31:20–26, 2004.
101. Krohm P, Levionnois O, Ganster M, et al: Antinociceptive activity of pre- versus post-operative intra-articular bupivacaine in goats undergoing stifle arthrotomy, *Vet Anaesth Analg* 38:363–373, 2011.
102. Valverde A, Sinclair M. ruminant and swine local anesthetic and analgesic techniques. In Grimm, KA, Lamont LA, Tranquilli, WJ, et al, editors: *Veterinary anesthesia and analgesia: the fifth edition of Lumb and Jones,* Ames, IA, 2015, John Wiley & Sons.
103. Caulkett N, Arnemo JM: Cervids (deer). In West G, Heard D, Caulkett N editors: *Zoo animal & wildlife immobilization and anesthesia,* ed 2, Ames, IA, 2014, John Wiley & Sons.
104. Kreeger TJ, Arnemo JM: *Handbook of wildlife chemical immobilization,* ed 4, Wheatland, TJ, 2012, Kreeger.
105. Cattet MRL, Caulkett NA, Wilson C, et al: Intranasal administration of xylazine to reduce stress in elk captured by net gun, *J Wildl Dis* 40:562–565, 2004.
106. Caulkett N: Anesthesia for North American cervids, *Can Vet J* 38:389–390, 1997.
107. Murray S, Monfort SL, Ware L, et al: Anesthesia in female white-tailed deer using telazol and xylazine, *J Wildl Dis* 36(4):670–675, 2000.
108. Monteith KL, Monteith KB, Delger JA, et al: Immobilization of white-tailed deer with Telazol, ketamine, and xylazine, and evaluation of antagonists, *J Wildl Manag* 76(7):1412–1419, 2012.
109. Moresco AM, Larson JM, Sleeman MA, et al: Use of naloxone to reverse carfentanil citrate-induced hypoxemia and cardiopulmonary depression in rocky mountain wapiti, *J Zoo Wildl Med* 32:81–89, 2001.
110. Read MR, Caulkett NA, Symington A, et al: Treatment of Hypoxemia during xylazine-tiletamine-zolazepam immobilization of wapiti, *Can Vet J* 42:661–664, 2001.
111. Wilson PR, Stafford KJ, Thomas DJ, et al: Evaluation of techniques for lignocaine hydrochloride analgesia of the velvet antler of adult stags. *N Z Vet J* 48:182–187, 2000.

19

Herd and Flock Health

LIONEL J. DAWSON, CLIFFORD F. SHIPLEY, ROGER MERKEL, AND DAVID G. PUGH

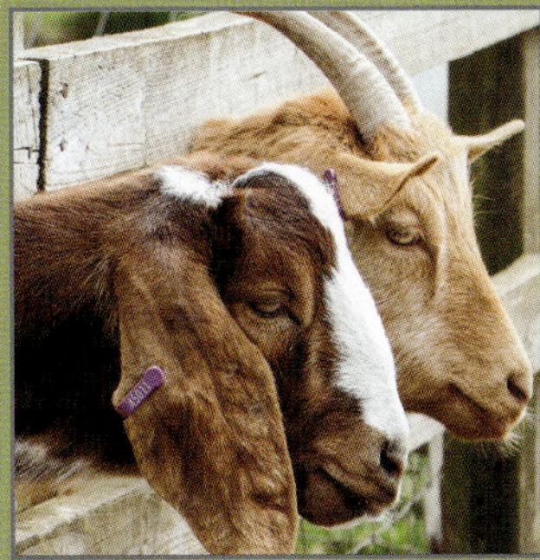

Introduction

Flock/herd health considers the health and wellbeing of the herd/flock, not individual animals. The main goal of a herd health program is to improve overall health and welfare, thereby decreasing production losses from diseases, increasing productivity, and maximizing profitability. Flock/herd health improved through general husbandry, nutrition, parasite control, vaccination, and environmental management. A veterinarian should understand the various management practices and common diseases seen on the farm to accomplish this goal.

The majority of small ruminant herds in the United States are managed as groups of 5 to 100 animals. While there are large sheep flocks in the southern and western regions of the United States such as Texas, California, Colorado, Wyoming, and Utah, there are few large commercial goat herds with numbers above 500 head. Large small ruminant herds usually have health problems associated with high animal density and continuous animal turnover. Small herds tend to have higher ratios of nonproductive to productive animals due to owners often keeping favorite animals that are less productive. Often, the net result for small herd owners is maintaining animals with chronic illnesses that may serve as reservoirs of various diseases. A veterinarian should be cognizant of these issues when working with clients to develop herd health programs.

The production of deer and other cervids for products, tourism, and hunting ranches is a growing industry in North America. Both native and imported species of cervids are farmed in different parts of North America. Due to the wild nature of deer and other cervids, many locales place restrictions on production, facilities, and management not seen with other farm animals. Further, their wild behavior requires changes in the basic handling techniques and treatment options normally used with small ruminants. The availability of drugs approved for deer and other cervid species makes designing and conducting a herd health program more difficult.

Since each flock/herd is different, a veterinarian should work with each client to develop an individual herd health plan, the exact makeup of which depends on the herd/flock size, purpose, and the farm's production goals. The clinician should have sound knowledge of small ruminant diseases, management, husbandry, nutrition, show animals, and the industry to advise their clients on ways to enhance production.

Producer education should be a component of any health program. Although many small ruminant producers have extensive livestock experience with sheep and goats or large ruminants, some producers new to small ruminants have little knowledge of animal management, nutrition, or health issues. These producers must learn safely and properly conduct basic management practices from hoof trimming to giving vaccinations. In today's environment, all producers have access to web-based information, blogs, chat rooms, newsletters, etc., some of which may present incorrect or misleading information. Providing producers with online resources of reliable, scientific-based production and health information will help both producer and veterinarian. Web-based training programs can be important avenues for producers to increase their knowledge of small ruminant production.

Clients should keep good records for each animal regarding medications, vaccinations, anthelmintic used, diseases diagnosed, breeding history, culling, etc., and use this information with their veterinarian to plan their health program as well as to analyze farm success. Many diseases have similar symptoms, and a veterinarian should work with clients to recognize and treat common conditions and diseases seen at their farm while working to prevent future occurrences. Preventive medicine is less expensive than treating the disease, as the highest economic returns are realized when disease problems are at a minimum. Many clients are not full-time farmers and work off-farm. These farmers are only able to spend time with their animals on weekends or in the evenings. This can present challenges in terms of timely disease recognition and treatment.

Establishing and maintaining a good relationship with clients cannot be overstressed. This is particularly important since most pharmaceuticals used in small ruminants are extra-label, being prescribed within the context of a valid veterinarian-client-patient relationship. Periodic visits to the farm help establish and nurture this relationship (Table 19.1). Farm visits during critical times in the production cycle (prebreeding, mid to late lactation, and postlambing) allow time to examine and provide recommendations to prevent problems. Other times to potentially visit are the breeding period when involved with artificial insemination, late first trimester or early second trimester for pregnancy diagnosis and separation of females having more than two fetuses, and the postweaning period to evaluate the dams and offspring. Table 19.1 lists some of the activities that a veterinarian may conduct during these visits in addition to basic evaluation for small ruminants. Assessment can be done with the owner/caretaker and can focus on behavior, body condition, pasture management, grazing rotation, health issues, nutrition, and feeding management. Animals showing poor body condition score (BCS), poor appetite, diarrhea, respiratory issues, lameness, etc., should be examined and isolated. A written report detailing the visit, which

TABLE 19.1 Generic Veterinary Farm Visits for Small Ruminants.

Production Cycle	Activities Performed During Farm Visits	Husbandry Activities Performed During This Period
1. Prebreeding period	• BCS • BSE—rams and bucks • Ewe and doe selection for breeding	• FAMACHA (impractical for cervids in most cases)/FEC • Deworm > 3 • Trim feet • Vaccination • Flushing • Cull—nonproductive ewes, does, bucks, and rams
2. Breeding period	• Natural service—ram/buck-to-ewe/doe ratio • AI—LAI in ewe/does TCAI—does	• Observe marking • Synchronization • Prepare animals for AI
3. Postbreeding period	• U/S = 45–70 days • BCS • Health of the flock	• Separate—non-pregnant ewes/does • Separate—ewes/does > fetuses
4. Prelambing/kidding period	• BCS • FAMACHA • U/S ewes/does not showing signs of pregnancy	• Shearing—ewes • Vaccination • Deworming > 3 • Nutrition • Look for pregnancy toxemia signs in ewes/does
5. Weaning period	• BCS • FAMACHA (sheep and goats) • Kids/lambs/fawns—observe for health	• Feet • Nutrition • Vaccination • FAMACHA/FEC • Deworming
6. Post weaning	• Cull—ewes/does poor mothering ability, udder conformation, age, lameness, poor BCS, etc.	• Shearing • FAMACHA/FEC • Deworming • BCS—flushing

This health care outline maybe modified for species, animal use, location, etc.

AI, Artificial Insemination; *BCS*, body condition score; *BSE*, Breeding Soundness Evaluation; *FAMACHA*, FAffa MAlan CHArt; *FEC*, Fecal Egg Count; *LAI*, Laparoscopic Artificial Insemination; *TCAI*, Trans-Cervical Artificial Insemination; *U/S*, Ultrasound evaluation.

comprises of observations of the facility and animals, examination results, and any laboratory reports on samples submitted, is sent to the client.

General Herd Health Considerations

An obvious key to a successful small ruminant operation is having a healthy, productive herd. The health of small ruminants is affected by a number of factors, including genetics, disease prevalence, environment, nutrition, and management, among others. The greatest disease threat is an animal introduced from another farm. Clients must be educated on how to select healthy animals and how to integrate these animals into their herds. This begins at the time of purchase. Producers should buy only from reputable sources to minimize the chance of buying diseased animals or animals carrying unapparent disease. If animals are purchased at an auction where comingling occurs, one can usually expect problems. Prior to purchase, the client should ask the animal owner about his/her disease history, current disease status, and vaccination protocols. Animals can undergo disease testing prior to final purchase. The exact diseases tested will vary depending on the operation. If purchasing milking sheep or goats, milk samples from the bulk tank or individual animals are tested both for the presence of bacteria and for white blood cell count/numbers. Test results may be negative and desired animals are purchased, or the results may find diseases that a client does not wish to import onto the farm. Anthelmintic used and likelihood of resistance should be considered.

If the desired animals pass all serological testing prior to purchase, the importance of an adequate quarantine and isolation period for the purchased animals is stressed to the client. Too often, producers may quarantine newly purchased animals for only 2 weeks prior to introducing them to the herd. An ideal quarantine period should be a minimum of 30 days and can be up to 60 days. This period allows any diseases to express themselves; provides adaptation time for new animals before being exposed to a new herd; and gives the owner time to deworm, administer vaccinations, and perform other preventive health measures according to his/her established health protocol. During this time, disease testing or retesting can also occur.

If purchased animals are moved across state lines, a certificate of veterinary inspection (health paper) is usually required. This is a common procedure and should not be difficult to obtain. State requirements vary. To view your state's requirements, log on to http://www.aphis.usda.gov/import_export/animals/animal_import/animal_imports_states.shtml.

Once animals are on the farm, providing a healthy environment, proper nutrition, and preventive health care is essential in maintaining herd health. However, animals are affected by a variety of conditions and diseases under different management conditions, and no matter how well animals are cared for, diseases will occur. Early detection of sick animals or animals undergoing nutritional or other stress falls on the owner or caretaker and is accomplished by daily observation. Small ruminants show mild to moderate behavioral changes before showing obvious signs of a condition or disease. Cervids are especially adept at hiding clinical signs of disease. The producer should be educated to observe unrestrained animals in order to learn how they look and behave in a normal manner. This includes general appearance and movement, normal behavior patterns, fecal consistency, eating behavior, teeth, body parts, etc. Any deviation from that "normal" appearance and behavior should be cause for concern and a veterinarian should be contacted for further investigation.

When changes in behavior do occur, consider that it may be a herd/flock health problem rather than an individual animal problem. This is because small ruminants tend to stay close to one another, which can promote the spread of any infectious conditions.

The following steps should be undertaken when dealing with a potential disease outbreak.

1. Isolate any affected animals.
2. Determine if the condition is a single occurrence or the start of a bigger problem.
3. Check all animals carefully to identify sick ones.
4. Submit any mortality for a postmortem examination as soon as possible or take appropriate tissues from the animal for diagnosis at a state or other diagnostic laboratory facility.

Of special note on purchasing new stock, pay close attention for any disease regulated by the state or federal government, e.g., brucellosis, tuberculosis (TB), scrapie, and chronic wasting disease (CWD). Programs associated with these diseases may determine whether animals should be moved farm to farm or if a farm's disease status will change should animals be imported. These rules may be complicated (e.g., in CWD) and vary greatly from state to state and day by day. Efforts should be made to follow all current regulations with respect to reporting, disease control, animal disposal methods, etc.

Biosecurity

Each producer, in conjunction with their veterinarian, should create a biosecurity plan to keep diseases off the farm and prevent disease transmission from animal to animal or animal to humans. The process begins with a risk assessment listing already present diseases and then diseases that the producer does not wish to have. Procedures and protocols to prevent disease entry through management, disease testing, quarantine procedures, etc., need to be established. In addition to keeping diseases off the farm, producers must also have a plan to deal with animals that contract a disease to prevent further spread within the farm (biocontainment). Producers may not know all of the routes that diseases can be introduced to the farm or passed to animals or farm workers. Even protective measures, such as gloves, boots, and clothing, do not work if used improperly. As an example, workers on a dairy goat farm wore examination gloves when cleaning pens of kids having cryptosporidiosis. However, while wearing gloves, the workers checked messages on their cell phones, contaminating the screen. Use of the phone later without cleaning the screen led to employees contracting the disease. This stresses the need for producer education on zoonotic diseases, modes of disease transmission, prevention, and sanitation procedures.

Realistically, few producers will ever have a totally closed herd, as purchase of breeding animals is commonly practiced. For producers who wish to maintain a closed herd, new genetics can be introduced using advanced reproductive technology such as artificial insemination or embryo transfer. Biosecurity measures begin with the selection and purchase of only healthy animals through getting health history and disease and parasite testing. Once on the farm, strict quarantine protocols are followed. Much has been written on biosecurity plans and their components. The basics of a small ruminant herd biosecurity plan are listed in the following.

1. **Establish a biosecurity plan for the farm.** Reduce the risk of diseases entering and spreading within the farm and prevent diseases or conditions in your animals from leaving the farm. Evaluate the farm operation, feed deliveries, visitors, animal replacements, show animals returning to the farm, stray animals, rodents, birds, and others and plan accordingly.
2. **Minimize or avoid contact with animals outside the farm.** Avoid contact with animals outside the farm at a show or fence line. Consider pasture and grazing area location in relation to neighboring farms. If new facilities are planned for the farm, consider drainage and proper fencing. Clean and disinfect animal trailers between use when taken or brought to the farm and do not haul animals other than those on the farm.
3. **Establish a quarantine protocol for animals entering the farm**. Prevent diseases from entering the farm by proper purchasing strategies. Obtain health records and prior disease history of farm of origin. A minimum quarantine period for new arrivals of at least 30 days is ideal, with 60 days even better. Design a protocol for vaccinations, diagnostic tests, and deworming. Equipment and feed from the quarantine area are not moved to the main farm. Having footbaths, equipment, footwear, and clothing used only in the quarantine area and not used on the main farm is essential.
4. **Establish a protocol for farm visitors.** Control traffic and have designated parking areas so that feed trucks, livestock trailers, etc., will not contaminate the farm with dirt or manure. Visitors should have a designated entrance with a footbath. Provide a method of hand sanitation so that visitors can wash their hands upon entry and exit.
5. **Do not allow persons on your farm who have traveled to foreign countries and have had contact with livestock or stepped on a farm for a period of 10 days after their arrival in the United States.** There are countries that have diseases that are not present in the United States, such as foot and mouth disease, which are important to keep out of the United States.

Quarantine

All farms need a place to quarantine newly acquired animals and animals returning from shows. Animals are quarantined for at least 30 days, during which time a complete physical examination should be done along with other testing and giving vaccinations. The quarantine area should be a dry lot without grass or a concrete area where animals can be confined and separated from other animals by at least 100 feet. Tests to consider during quarantine include serological tests for caprine arthritis encephalitis (CAE), ovine progressive pneumonia (OPP), caseous lymphadenitis (CL), Johne's disease, TB, and brucellosis, among other diseases encountered endemically. Quarantined dairy animals are tested for mastitis-causing organisms. Considerations are given for deworming and fecal egg counts. To test for resistant parasites, take a fecal sample prior to deworming for fecal egg count. After 14 days, perform a second fecal egg count to see the effectiveness of the anthelmintic. Animals with low to zero fecal egg counts may be added to the grazing pasture. Animals that still have high fecal egg counts are not to be added, to avoid introducing anthelmintic resistant worms to the farm.

Zoonotic Diseases

Animals can transmit a number of zoonotic diseases, many of which producers may not be aware that can have serious health effects on humans. The elderly, the young, and those with compromised immune systems are most at risk for contracting these diseases. With the rise in agro-tourism, buying local meat and dairy products, visiting days to the farm as part of marketing strategies, and other farm visit activities, livestock owners need to know how to recognize and prevent disease transmission from animals to humans. Hand-washing stations, disposable boots or boot covers, and visitor education are essential tools in fighting zoonotic disease spread. Veterinary practitioners should be familiar with the One Health initiative as they work with producers to safeguard animals, people, and the environment.

Euthanasia and Carcass Disposal

Livestock producers realize that there will be times when euthanasia is needed. Clinicians should be prepared to discuss strategies with their clients as to acceptable and unacceptable methods of euthanasia following American Veterinary Medical Association (AVMA) guidelines. Acceptable means for on-farm use include injection of barbiturates by a veterinarian or penetrating or non-penetrating captive bolt or firearm with an adjunctive method such as exsanguination or anesthetic injection. In addition to the physical aspects of euthanasia, clinicians should be aware of emotional reactions and ethical concerns of livestock owners or caretakers.

Producers also need to have a plan to handle farm mortality. The five legal means of carcass disposal are: burial following state guidelines; landfills where permitted; incineration in an appropriate facility; rendering; and composting. Individual state guidelines and requirements vary, and the state veterinarian should be contacted to see which methods could be used, particularly in the case of wild or exotic cervid species.

Strategies to Control Internal Parasites

Gastrointestinal parasite management, especially for *Haemonchus contortus*, is a primary concern for all small ruminant producers. Gastrointestinal parasites cause significant economic losses worldwide and are one of the top three important conditions causing high mortality in sheep and goats. The development of dewormer resistance to nearly all three classes of anthelmintics available in the United States has made control difficult and has promoted alternative management strategies. Dewormer resistance indicates when there is less than 95% reduction in fecal egg count 14 days after administration. Resistance has arisen due to overuse of anthelmintics, too frequent anthelmintic drug rotation, and underdosing (see Chapter 6).

H. contortus thrives in warm and humid conditions and has the ability to undergo hypobiosis, or become metabolically inactive, within the host during unfavorable weather conditions, emerging when conditions improve. The survival time of infective larvae (L3) is short during hot summer months (30–60 days) but prolonged during cooler, wet months (> 4 months). Periparturient egg rise seen in early spring promotes shedding of a large number of eggs in the feces. A good working knowledge of parasite life cycles is necessary to create control programs.

Sheep, goats, and cervids are adaptable in their feeding behavior. Sheep are more inclined to be grazers, whereas goats and cervids prefer browsing. This has implications for parasite control, as when animals graze, they are in close contact with parasite larvae. When animals graze close to the ground and nutritional input is marginal, gastrointestinal parasite infestation may escalate and animals will show clinical signs of parasitism, especially during periods of stress due to production (e.g., pregnancy, lactation, etc.) or environment (e.g., weather extremes, sparse vegetation, etc.). Internal parasite control is tailored to a particular region of the country, whether the farm is confined, pastured, or rotationally grazed. Although susceptible to many of the same gastrointestinal parasites, a bunk-fed deer population with good BCSs (3–4 on a 1–5 scale; e.g., https://www.purinamills.com/deer-feed/education/detail/body-condition-score-for-deer) will usually be relatively free of most gastrointestinal nematode parasites. If cervids are maintained in a densely populated area with sheep and/or goats, then exposure to nematode parasites may be increased, and parasitism becomes more of a problem. To adequately control and manage internal parasites, veterinarians must work with producers to develop integrated approaches by looking at the specifics of the host, parasite, and environmental interactions (Table 19.2). Control strategies must rely on the smart use of dewormers. This means treating only those animals that need to be dewormed and keeping a pool of susceptible worms, called refugia, in the group. These susceptible worms will mate with resistant ones to help prolong the use of anthelmintics. Smart deworming strategies for blood-sucking worms *(Haemonchus)* use the FAMACHA system to score the color of mucous membranes of the eye, evaluating anemia or blood loss. Another strategy useful for other worms is a five-point check (bottle jaw, hair coat, diarrhea, body condition, and nasal secretion for nasal bots). Aspects of successful control programs include regular monitoring of the efficacy of anthelmintics by performing fecal egg count and fecal egg reduction test after deworming, monthly FAMACHA scoring, maintaining refugia on the farm, rotational grazing, smart drenching, grazing cattle and horses on unoccupied pastures before small ruminants are turned out to graze, and selecting nematode resistant animals.

Periparturient deworming has been a mainstay of many internal parasite control programs. Deworming all the periparturient animals in early spring leaves minimal refugia in the pasture and can speed resistance. It is better not to deworm 15 to 25% of animals not showing clinical signs to provide enough refugia.

Due to the increased dewormer resistance seen in goats compared to sheep, combining two or three classes of wormers at their appropriate dosages at the same time has been used with a fair amount of success. Selective deworming using a combination of different classes at the appropriate dosages at the same time is beneficial to promote refugia, but it can also promote resistance to all wormers available (see Chapter 6 and Appendix 1).

The three classes of anthelmintics currently available are: (1) benzimidazoles (oxfendazole, febantel, fenbendazole, and albendazole); (2) macrocyclic lactones—(a) avermectins (ivermectin, doramectin, and eprinomectin) and (b) milbemycins; and (3) cholinergic agonists—(a) imidazothiazoles [levamisole] and

TABLE 19.2 Alternative Internal Parasite Control Methods for Sheep and Goats.

Pasture Management	Selective Deworming	Selecting Resistant Animals	Quarantine

• Maintain forage height greater than 2 inches
• Provide areas of browse (brush, shrubs, small trees, etc.)
• Maintain low stocking rate
• Graze sheep and goats with cattle or in a rotation with cattle or horses
• Provide tannin-rich forages
• Harvest hay off pastures
• Avoid wet patches in a pasture, such as from a leaky water trough
• Fence-off naturally wet areas
• Low stocking rate
• Pasture rotation suited for the farm's environment
• Leave the pasture unoccupied 30 to 60 days in summer; 120 days in cooler weather
• After deworming, move the animals, preferably to a clean pasture in 24 to 48 hours
	• Use FAMACHA (*Haemonchus contortus*)/fecal egg count
	• Treat only animals with symptoms of anemia
	• Maintain a large pool of refugia
	• Reduce the use of dewormers and slow development of resistance
	• Control periparturient egg rise: 15–30 days before kidding
	  • Deworm > 3 on FAMACHA
	  • 5 point check
		• Several breeds show resistance to internal parasites
		• Individual animals can demonstrate resistance to parasites
		  • Resistant animals have a lower host parasite burden and are not negatively affected by the parasites (do not show signs of parasitism, remain productive)
		  • FAMACHA scores can be helpful for selection
			• Quarantine new animals
			• Use a dry lot
			• On arrival, deworm with all three classes of wormer
			• FEC in 14 days
			• Make sure they are clean before they are exposed to the pasture

Some of these programs may be applicable to farmed deer.
FAMACHA, FAffa MAlan CHArt; *FEC*, Fecal Egg Count.

(b) tetrahydropyrimidines [pyrantel and morantel]. Fenbendazole is used under a zoo label for cervidae, but other than that, nothing has been approved for cervids. Veterinarians should consult with the Food Animal Residue Avoidance Databank (FARAD) (http://www.farad.org) periodically to see if there are any changes regarding the use of these pharmaceuticals (see Chapter 6 and Appendix 1).

Copper oxide wire particles have been shown to be significantly effective (70–90% fecal egg count reduction) against *Haemonchus*. Although doses are low, caution is needed with sheep as they accumulate copper in the liver and are susceptible to copper poisoning. There is a very narrow safety range for dietary copper in sheep, with maintenance requirements being 10 ppm, while a level of 25 ppm can be toxic (see Chapter 6).

Producers need to be advised that good nutrition is important in reducing the severity of internal parasitism. Literature reports the positive effect of supplemental protein, and in particular bypass or rumen undegradable protein, on enhancing the resistance to internal parasites. Protein aids in tissue repair and provides essential amino acids to stimulate an immune response.

Cervids raised in confined situations with abnormally high animal densities will be as susceptible to internal parasites as are goats. However, many cervid farms provide supplemental bunks feeding to the most susceptible animals (i.e., fawns, weanlings, late gestational animals, etc.), thus reducing possible parasite exposure. Periodic parasite egg counts of cervids need to be monitored.

External Parasites

Arthropod pests limit production in small ruminants. External parasites like lice, nose bots, keds, mites, fleas, and ticks can cause skin irritations, wounds, and discomfort to the animals. Biting and sucking lice, keds, and nose bots are prevalent external parasites of sheep. Biting and sucking lice and mites, especially chorioptic mites, are seen in goats. Depending upon the number of animals involved, the animal and the premises need to be treated. Cervids are susceptible to external parasites, but there is much variation between regions of the country. Familiarity with the parasites, especially ticks, is very important for treatment and control (see Chapter 10).

Shearing

Wool sheep, Angora goats, and cashmere goats undergo shearing one to two times annually. Shearing is a stressful experience for animals. The location of the area used for shearing, weather, stage of the production cycle, and competence of the shearer all affect the amount of stress undergone by the animals. Stress can be minimized by an efficient shearing area or shed design to facilitate easy handling of animals. To avoid abortions due to stress, shear at least 4 weeks away from parturition. Preparturition shearing may decrease the incidence of pregnancy toxemia, encourage pregnant females to take shelter on cold or hot days, decrease the maintenance requirements for ewes/does with heavy fiber coats, and enhance the visibility of teats for nursing newborns. Angora goats, in particular, appear to be susceptible to stress such as shearing, ice or snow storms, cold weather, transportation, etc., during pregnancy, and producers need to know what signs to look for and what to do should problems arise.

Antler Collection

Antler removal is a procedure performed occasionally on cervids and is described in Chapter 10.

Herd and Flock Health

Herd/Flock Health at Different Production Stages

Small ruminants have different health needs according to their stage of production. Providing for these health needs will increase your chances of having a healthy, productive farm. General recommendations apply for all small ruminants.

Prebreeding. To achieve a healthy gestation and parturition, a producer must attend to breeding animal condition prior to mating. An easy and practical way to assess the nutritional, and indirectly the health, status of the herd is through the BCS. It is the best simple indicator of available fat reserves that can be used by the animal in periods of high energy demand, stress, or suboptimal nutrition (see Table 19.3, Chapter 1, Table 1.1 and Chapter 2, Figure 2.1). Scoring is performed in small ruminants using a BCS ranging from 1.0 to 5.0, with 0.5 increments. A BCS of 1.0 is an extremely thin animal with no fat reserves, and a BCS of 5.0 is a very overconditioned (obese) animal. In most cases, healthy small ruminants should have a BCS of 2.5 to 4.0. A BCS of 2.0 or lower indicates a management or health problem. Severe obesity is most commonly seen in animals that are considered pets or in show animals.

To assign a BCS, palpate the lumbar area behind the ribs containing the loin and score this area based on the amount of fat over and around the vertebrae. Lumbar vertebrae have a vertical protrusion (spinous process) and two horizontal protrusions (transverse process). Both processes are used in determining BCS. The second body area to feel is the fat covering on the sternum (breastbone). Score this area based upon the amount of fat that can be palpated. A third area is the rib cage and fat cover on the ribs and intercostal (between ribs) spaces. With practice, evaluating the BCS of an animal will take only

TABLE 19.3 Body Condition Scoring in Goats.

Body Condition Scoring of Goats

Body condition scoring (BCS) is a quick, easy method of describing how thin or fat goats are, using a numerical score from 1 to 5. A goat may be given a half score, such as 2.5, if it is between BCS 2 and BCS 3. Assigning a BCS cannot be done by looking at the goat; one must feel for muscle and fat cover. An appropriate BCS range for goats is from BCS 2 to BCS 4, as seen on the reverse side. Goats that are too thin (BCS 1) may have nutritional or health problems, reducing productivity. Overly fat goats (BCS 5) have reduced fertility, increased birthing problems, and health problems.

BCS is commonly assessed in the loin area. Feel the amount of tissue covering the ends of the spinous and transverse processes of the vertebrae. Feel any loin muscle and fat filling the space between the backbone and horizontal bones. In very thin goats the bones can feel "sharp." As the animal gains condition, the thicker tissue covering makes the bone ends feel more rounded and smooth.

Recommendations

Does

- BCS between 2.5 to 3.5 at breeding
- BCS of 3 to 3.5 prior to wintering and prior to kidding (does may drop 0.5 or more in BCS during lactation, regaining condition after weaning with sufficient nutrition.)

Bucks

- BCS 3 to 3.5 prior to the breeding season

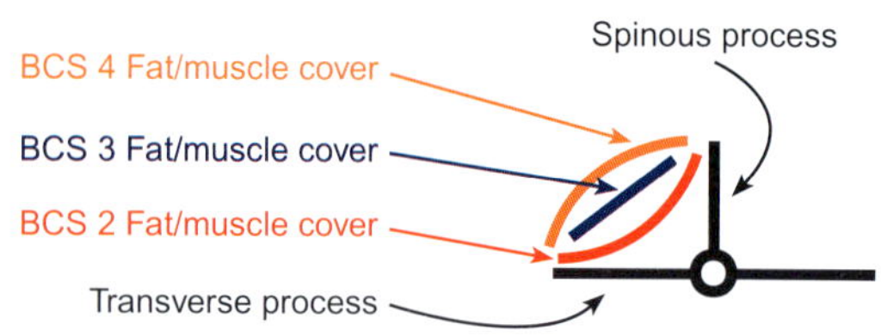

http://www.luresext.edu/?q=content/body-condition-score

The Cooperative Extension Program at Langston University provides educational programs to individuals regardless of race, color, national origin, religion, sex, age disability or status as a veteran. Issued in furtherance of Agricultural Extension Work Act of September 29, 1977, in cooperation with the U.S. Department of Agriculture.

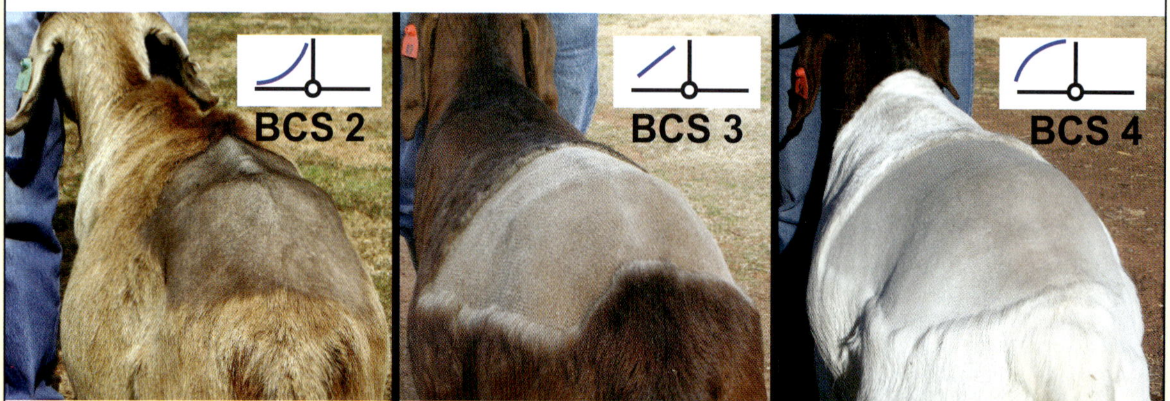

BCS 2	BCS 3	BCS 4
BCS 2 - Spinous process is felt as a ridge. A depression is felt between the spinous and transverse processes. Little muscle and fat can be felt. If bone ends are sharp and individual vertebrae felt, the BCS is 1.	BCS 3 - Spinous process does not feel like a ridge, but smooth with small ripples indicating the bones. Area between spinous and transverse processes is filled with muscle and fat cover and felt as a straight or slightly bowed out slope.	BCS 4 - Spinous process feels smooth but not buried in tissue. Individual bones are difficult to feel. Area between the spinous and transverse processes feels full and rounded. If bones are buried in tissue and not felt, the BCS is 5.

(Permission from Langston University. April 2018)

about 10 to 15 seconds. When overall herd body condition starts to decrease, managerial intervention such as supplemental feeding, deworming, pasture rotation, etc., needs to be taken. Conversely, when overall body condition starts to increase in the herd to above recommended levels, the producer should reduce supplemental feeding. Ignoring an animal's body condition and waiting to intervene until they become either too thin or too fat may result in production and animal losses or decreased profits from overfeeding.

Ideally, does and ewes at prebreeding should have a BCS of 2.5 to 3.5. Females having a BCS less than 2.0 should be supplemented (flushed) with grain 2 to 4 weeks before breeding, which may improve their pregnancy rates. Abrupt fence line exposure to males in the late fall transition period can help bring about cycling (see Chapter 8).

Breeding Does and Ewes. Thirty to 60 days before the breeding season, examine animals for udder and teat conformation, dentition (teeth), musculoskeletal problems, feet, and body condition. Cull does and ewes that have severe problems or do not meet herd conformation goals. Some common conditions seen in breeding females include lameness, chronic mastitis, bad teats, and poor body condition due to chronic diseases, parasitism, old age, or other causes. Doelings/ewe lambs should be at least 65 to 70% of their estimated mature weight before their first breeding. Does/ewes should have fair to good body condition at the time of breeding (BCS 3–3.5). They need to be vaccinated for common diseases and conditions seen at the farm, FAMACHA scored and dewormed if necessary, and have their feet trimmed.

Breeding Bucks and Rams. Bucks and rams are often neglected or not examined during routine herd health procedures. Some common conditions seen are urinary calculi (stones), lameness, urine scalding around the prepuce, damage to horns/antlers due to fighting, and injury due to a dominant buck/ram in the pen. In the case of urinary scald, wash the affected area and apply petroleum jelly to help protect that area. To prevent urinary calculi, maintain a 2:1 to 2.5:1 ratio of dietary calcium to phosphorous and provide a high level of salt (up to 4%) to encourage water consumption. Adding 1 to 2% ammonium chloride in the diet to acidify urine can also help prevent urinary calculi.

At least 4 weeks before the breeding season, evaluate bucks'/rams' body condition and adjust feeding program as needed. Conduct a breeding soundness examination, assess the buck's/ram's overall condition and capacity to serve does/ewes by evaluating the health history, checking physical soundness of feet and legs, and inspecting the external genitalia for abnormalities. Palpate the scrotum to ensure that it is firm, testes are similar in size and freely movable in the scrotum, and the epididymis is normal. Rams should have minimum scrotal measurements for their age (see Chapter 8). There are no standards for buck scrotal circumference, but a scrotal circumference of 23 to 25 cm minimum measurement is desirable. Bucks/rams should be vaccinated at the same time as the females and for the same diseases. As breeding season approaches, extremely aggressive and dominant bucks/rams may need to be penned separately to prevent injury. Monitor fecal egg counts or FAMACHA score and deworm as needed.

Breeding Season. Watch does/ewes and bucks/rams carefully during the breeding season. This is a particularly strenuous and active time for bucks/rams, and lame or sick sires will not be able to breed adequate numbers of does/ewes. Fertility drastically decreases in hot weather. Do everything you can to cool the buck/ram. This may include shade and fans during the day in very hot climates. To prevent overexertion, maintain a proper male-to-female ratio. In pasture conditions, a mature goat buck or ram can be expected to breed 30 to 50 does/ewes during the breeding season. Definitive numbers for a cervid/buck-to-doe ratio range from 10 to 25 depending on pen size and the age of the buck. Have some means of monitoring breeding activity, such as a marking harness for goats and sheep. A breeding season of 45 to 55 days is common. If artificial insemination is practiced on the farm, heat detection and timing of insemination are very important. Teaser animals, teasing aprons, or fence line exposure can be used to identify does/ewes in heat. Producers should have training in estrus detection and timing of insemination, as well as the insemination technique itself and semen handling.

Gestation

Preparturition. Fulfilling the health and nutritional needs of the doe/ewe during gestation promotes a normal parturition, healthy kid/lamb/fawn, and sufficient colostrum and milk production after parturition. Provide an adequate diet and have clean, cool water and free-choice trace-mineralized salt available. Pregnant does/ewes should be body condition scored in early pregnancy and again 6 weeks prior to kidding/lambing and should have a BCS of 3.0 to 3.5 just prior to parturition. Monitor feed quantity and quality in the last one-third of gestation, as most fetal growth occurs during this time. Very thin or fat older sheep/goats carrying triplets or quadruplets may experience a decline in feed intake during this time, making them highly at risk for developing pregnancy toxemia. Booster vaccinations for *Clostridium perfringens* type C and D and tetanus toxoid be administered no later than 3 to 4 weeks prior to kidding/lambing and should be considered on some fenced deer production units (Table 19.6). Vitamin E/selenium injections are given to does/ewes during the dry period to prevent white muscle disease in kids/lambs/fawns, especially in areas where soils are selenium deficient and supplementation is inadequate. However, a nutrition program designed to provide adequate dietary selenium is preferable to providing injections. Provide other vaccinations or boosters for diseases causing abortion. Monitor fecal egg counts or FAMACHA score and deworm as needed.

The majority of does/ewes experience no severe problems during gestation. However, vaginal prolapses, hernia, ruptured prepubic tendon, acute mastitis, and pseudo-pregnancy can occur. Vaginal prolapses are not very common in goats but may be seen occasionally in prepartum pygmy does. Vaginal prolapses in ewes are more common. Factors that contribute to vaginal prolapses in ewes are genetics, body condition of the ewe, quality of roughage fed, location of tail docking, etc. Abdominal hernia is seen usually in late gestation or due to trauma or postsurgical complications. Postsurgical complications may arise from a caesarian section or from an embryo transfer performed on a donor doe. Ruptured prepubic tendon is seen in older does/ewes in late gestation.

Vaccinations for chlamydia, campylobacter, and leptospirosis are included, if they are diagnosed as a problem of reproductive failure and abortions on the farm. Prebreeding booster vaccinations are usually done at least 3 to 4 weeks prior to breeding (Table 19.6). There is a *Chlamydophila* vaccine approved for sheep available as a single antigen or in combination with campylobacter. A number of goat operations have started using the *Chlamydophila* vaccine to control abortions and to avoid feeding tetracycline. Abortions can occur anytime during gestation for a variety of reasons. Early-term abortions may go unnoticed and the doe/ewe is categorized as having failed to conceive rather than aborted. Late-term abortion storms are mainly infectious in nature as summarized in Table 19.4. Sporadic abortions in does may be due to stress-related causes like weather changes, transportation, shearing etc.

Text continued on page 490

TABLE 19.4 Summary of Infectious Abortions in Sheep and Goats (With Some Cervid Notes).

Disease	Transmission	Clinical Features	Diagnosis	Diagnostic Aids	Control
1. **Enzootic abortion** (EAE, *Chlamydia* or *Chlamydophila abortion*): *caused by Chlamydophila abortus* cause late-term abortions.	Transmission is mainly by ingesting contaminated feed, water, and the environment with vaginal secretions, placenta, and aborted fetuses. Spread is more rapid when females are confined. Many carriers seen in endemic herds. Infection at birth in kids kept as replacement does may be carriers through to their first pregnancy.	Late-term abortions, stillbirths, and birth of weak infected progeny are the most common clinical signs encountered. Fetal mummification occasionally seen. Female fetuses exposed in utero may abort during their first pregnancy; does infected in the last month of pregnancy may not abort until the next gestation period.	A chorionitis with chorionic epithelial cells packed with elementary bodies appears to be the essential lesion. Cotyledons are pale, grayish white, and necrotic with a dark brown exudate. Intercotyledonary areas are necrotic, thickened, opaque, and leathery.	Impression smears of the cotyledon, placenta, and vaginal discharge (but not fetal stomach) stained by the modified Ziehl-Nielsen or Gimenez stain. Organisms can be cultured in yolk sac of embryonating chicken eggs. PCR techniques on placental trophoblasts, spleen, and liver are useful. Serology on the dam is unrewarding. Detecting antibodies in the fetal fluids is also useful.	Vaccines are given to males and females 4–6 weeks prior to breeding or use 150 mg of tetracyclines per head per day in the feed for 2–3 weeks prior to breeding: may continue this in their feed through the first half of gestation. Controlling abortion outbreak with tetracyclines (limited success): 400 mg/head/day in feed or water for the last 60 days of gestation. Use slow-release tetracycline (LA 200) 20 mg/kg injectable every 10 days to start during the last 60 days of gestation. Treat weak newborns with tetracycline. Isolate aborting females and those with weak born kids. **Prevention:** LA oxytetracycline, 90 days and 120 days of gestation is very effective in preventing abortions. Onset of therapy after the start of abortions will only reduce abortion rate. OTC or aureomycin orally (400 mg/head/day).
2. **Toxoplasmosis:** *Toxoplasma gondii* affects a wide range of animals. Cats and other Felidae considered the primary host and excrete oocysts.	Oocysts excreted in the feces of young or immune-compromised cats provide the major source of infection. Congenital transmission from does to kids has been established. Further epidemiologic knowledge is required to establish how the disease spreads during an epidemic.	Early embryonic loss, fetal mummification (often only one of a twin pair), twin or triplet abortions with variation in fetal ages, and/or perinatal losses. Congenitally affected neonates may survive. Adult are generally asymptomatic. Occasionally, adults show developing CNS signs. In endemic areas only younger females usually are affected and may show the above clinical signs.	Placental changes may be the only gross lesions observed. Gross lesions of the cotyledons (numerous gray-white foci 1–3 mm in diameter) are indicative of the disease. Not all cotyledons are equally affected, and such lesions be differentiated from non-specific calcification. Focal neurologic lesion in the CNS of stillborns, or neonates dying shortly after birth is a common finding.	**Histology** of the cotyledon to demonstrate local areas of necrosis, mineralization, and the organisms. Histology of fetal brain to demonstrate foci of glial cells. Microscopy of the brain and cotyledonary villi sections to see tachyzoites, and immunohistochemistry for antibodies is necessary to confirm your diagnosis. Precolostral serology of the kids is useful. Maternal serology is usually unrewarding.	**Prevent exposure to cats, particularly kittens or immunosuppressed adult cats.** Do not allow cats to consume aborted fetuses in a toxoplasma abortion. Treatment: Decoquinate 2 mg/kg/day or Monensin 15–30 mg/kg/head/day throughout gestation

3. ***Campylobacter fetus, Campylobacter jejuni* and *Campylobacter lari:*** Can infect and cause abortions in both sheep and goats and have been reported in some species of cervids. Sheep appear to be more susceptible to *Campylobacter* infection and abortions.	Transmission is mainly oral, through aborted material and feces contaminating feed and water from carrier animals. The organism colonizes the intestinal tract of the adult animal usually without clinical signs of diarrhea. Bacteremia may occur in susceptible pregnant animals with extension to the uterus and placenta.	Abortion storms occur when susceptible does or ewes brought into a herd with *Campylobacter*-infected herd mates. This organism is highly contagious, resulting in most of the flock infected at the time the abortion storm begins. Ewes that abort are often immune to reinfection. Usually will not abort again when re-exposed to these organisms. Abortion followed by septic metritis and maternal death may occur.	Cotyledons are enlarged, yellowish, and covered with a brownish/red suppurative exudate. Intercotyledonary areas are often edematous and hyperemic. Aborted fetuses may be fresh or autolyzed. Meconium staining of the fetus and placental tissues may occur. Serosanguinous fluid and fibrin is present in the thorax and abdomen. Multifocal white to yellowish brown areas of necrosis observed on liver surface.	**Histologically** chorionic villi are necrotic with variable numbers of neutrophils, lymphocytes, and macrophages. Numerous colonies of small gram negative, rod-shaped bacteria present in the trophoblasts and placental stroma. The liver has multifocal coagulative necrosis, with mononuclear and neutrophilic infiltrates. Bacterial culture—placenta, lungs, liver, and abomasum. IHC and FA testing—rapid diagnosis. Abomasal contents and cotyledon—dark field and phase contrast microscopy.	Prevent exposure to aborted material and contaminated feed. Vaccine available and is given prebreeding and, if necessary, midgestation. Aborted animal—long-acting oxytetracycline 20 mg/kg every 72 hours—Two treatments Treat the other ewes 20 mg/kg every 7 days, until all of them have lambed or kidded. Or 300–400 mg/kg/day in the feed to the rest of the pregnant does or ewe, until all of them have lambed or kidded. Vaccine used prebreeding and midgestation may aid in control of abortions in endemic herds.
4. **Salmonellosis** (Paratyphoid Abortion): *Salmonella abortus ovis, Salmonella typhimurium, and Salmonella dublin* have been associated with abortion in goats, but other species may potentially be susceptible.	Ingestion of contaminated food and water usually shed from carrier animals. Does and ewes in late pregnancy appear more susceptible. Overcrowding and other forms of stress favor an outbreak. Infection seldom causes clinical disease in the absence of some other predisposing factors resulting in stress.	Abortions, stillbirths, births of weak infected progeny that usually die within 7 days of birth. Does and ewes may show high fever before aborting; most recover, but some may succumb to metritis and/or septicemia. Some does and newborn kids show diarrhea; in the kids/lambs, this is usually fatal. Kids/lambs up to 2 weeks of age may show bronchopneumonia. When infection is endemic, abortions are confined to the younger ewes and does.	No specific placental lesions seen. Swollen, pale hemorrhagic cotyledons with necrosis. Aborted fetuses show usual signs of intrauterine death. Septicemic lesions seen in kids/lambs dying during or shortly after birth.	Culture of organisms from fetus, placenta, and uterine discharge.	Antibiotic treatment on flock basis is seldom effective and is very expensive. Avoid overcrowding or stressing of does. Do not feed on the ground unless a new area used each day. For valuable individuals, supportive therapy (fluids) and antibiotics recommended.
5. **Brucellosis:** *Brucellosis melitensis* affects goats, sheep, and other species including man. Brucella abortus occasionally affects does and ewes. *Brucella ovis* affects rams—epididymitis, can cause infertility, early and late-term abortions, stillbirths, and weak kids.	Ingestion is the main method of transmission, especially during the kidding period. Droplet inhalation and entry both through the conjunctival membrane and broken skin occasionally occurs. Venereal transmission following natural mating is rare.	Abortions in late pregnancy, stillbirths, and birth of weak infected kids/lambs may occur. Congenital infections may persist throughout life (especially *B. melitensis*). Systemic effects may be seen in the dam with fever, lameness (associated with joint swellings), and central nervous system (CNS) signs.	The main lesion is placentitis, with edema and necrosis of cotyledons. The intercotyledons' membrane may be thickened, yellow-brown necrotic areas, often with adjacent hemorrhage. Mucopurulent material may be adherent to the allantochorion. Fetus shows usual signs of intrauterine death.	Culture and direct microscopy used to identify organisms that are plentiful in the placenta, fetal stomach, and vaginal discharge of the doe. Modified Ziehl-Nielsen technique is satisfactory for staining for direct microscopy. Complement fixation ELISA, CF, and PCR are available on sera of aborting does and ewes.	Test and slaughter policy is necessary when the disease is prevalent. Testing of replacement animals. General hygiene at kidding.

Continued

TABLE 19.4 Summary of Infectious Abortions in Sheep and Goats (With Some Cervid Notes).—cont'd

Disease	Transmission	Clinical Features	Diagnosis	Diagnostic Aids	Control
6. **Listeriosis:** *(Listeria monocytogenes or Listeria ivanovii)*	Mainly ingestion.	Abortion, stillbirths, weak kids/lambs, and/or autolyzed fetuses may occur. Abortion occurs from day > 50 of gestation. Some born alive but die. Metritis and septicemia common in females. Placentitis, around the cotyledon and intercotyledon areas. (Note: Kids/lambs grafted to the aborting females can contract Listeriosis through the milk, develop septicemia and die.)	Necrotic, greyish white foci (1 or 2 mm diameter) seen in in the liver, spleen, kidneys, lungs, heart, and adrenals. Leathery placenta.	Culture from fetal stomach, liver, and placenta. Fluorescent antibody test on the placenta.	**Isolation** of aborting females. Do not feed spoiled silage or poorly fermented silage. During outbreak administration of long acting tetracycline at 20 mg/kg every 72 hours. Chlortetracycline in the feed 300 mg/head/day.
7. **Leptospirosis:** *Leptospira icterohaemorrhagiae, Leptospira grippotyphosa, Leptospira pomona, Leptospira hardjo, Leptospira canicola, Leptospira castellonis,* and *Leptospira bratislava* been reported as primary causes of abortions in goats and ewes.	Secreted in the urine. Transmission is through skin or mucosal abrasions.	Clinical signs seen primarily in primiparous does. They include metritis after abortions, anorexia, anemia, jaundice, hemoglobinuria, and death.	Fetal organs will be hemosiderin stained due to autolysis. Some edema of the intercotyledonary regions.	Dark field microscopy, immunofluorescence testing and silver stains on placenta, fetal tissue, and fluids. FA on the kidney. PCR on the urine. Paired serum samples from aborting does.	Vaccination, rodent control, clean water supply **Isolation** of aborting females. During outbreak, administration of long-acting tetracycline at 20 mg/kg every 72 hours. Chlortetracycline in the feed 300–500 mg/herd/day during the outbreak.
8. **Q-Fever** *(Coxiella burnetii):* It affects sheep, goats, cattle, and other wildlife. This organism shed heavily in placentas, birth fluid, colostrum, and milk.	Inhaling dust, grazing contaminated pastures, and tick bites. Infected does can shed in the feces after parturition.	Abortion primarily in the naïve animals. Late-term abortions. Fresh fetuses. Some kids born alive. Aborting does usually retain their placenta.	Late-term abortion and stillbirth. Placentitis with intercolyedonary areas thickened and leathery. Cotyledons diffusely thickened with multiple areas of necrosis, covered with grayish/white to brownish/red exudate.	Serological testing is of little use. Paired serum samples may give a retrospective study of the flock. IFA is commonly used. ELISA along with IFA would strongly suggest *Coxiella* infection.	Producers should burn or bury the placenta. Oral chlortetracycline 300 mg/head/day for 3 weeks. Long-acting tetracycline 20 mg/kg given SC or IM every 3 days for 5 treatments.
9. **Caprine herpes virus**	Direct—nasal and genital routes. Latent infection in adults and spread during stress.	**Kids**—viremia and enteritis. Ulcerative and necrotic lesions the entire GI tract. **Adults**—vulvovaginitis, balanoposthitis, respiratory disease, and abortions.	Multifocal white necrosis in liver, spleen, kidney and lungs, mesenteric lymph nodes, thymus and liver.	BoHV-1 positive virus isolation on nasal and vaginal swab. PCR—blood and swabs. Intranuclear inclusion bodies in the placenta and internal organs of the aborted fetus.	Avoid stress. Buy animals from a clean herd. Avoid commingling with calves and sheep. BoHV-1 Infect sheep and goats but they are subclinical. CpHv-1 can infect sheep and calves and become latent. Reactivation has not been successful in sheep and calves.

10. **Border disease (hairy shaker disease):** The cause is infection of the pregnant ewe and doe with a pestivirus closely related to, if not identical with bovine viral diarrhea (BVD) virus. Several strains appear to be involved.	Vertical transmission from ewe to lamb during gestation is well established, and venereal spread of the disease seems likely. Surviving lambs can transmit the virus both vertically and laterally for years. Most of the more obvious clinical signs result from infection of pregnant ewes in the first half of gestation. Severe loss is likely if susceptible pregnant ewes introduced to infected flocks or if infected ewes mixed with resident ewes having no immunity to the disease.	A loss of potential progeny at any stage during pregnancy and in the postnatal period occurs. Infertility with a marked increase in barren ewes, fetal mummification and/or maceration, abortions, stillbirths, and losses of lambs born alive are all features of the disease. When the fleece has developed, it tends to be hairy and pigmented. If born alive, lambs may show muscular tremors causing incoordination and difficulty in nursing.	Cotyledons tend to be small for fetal age; they occasionally show areas of focal necrosis (1–3 mm). Abortions and mummification; hairy/pigmented coats if the wool has developed; fetus small for gestational age; muscular tremors and incoordination if lambs are born alive. When late gestation fetuses or young lambs encounter the disease, nodular periarteritis, which is slow to resolve, may occur.	CNS signs seen in live lambs with hypomyelinogenesis and the skin shows characteristic lesions on histologic studies. BVD-neutralizing antibodies in the serum of dam or lamb to virus isolation PCR.	Prevent commingling of pregnant ewes with cattle.
11. **Bovine viral diarrhea:** A pestivirus has been implicated in pigs, alpacas, sheep, goats, and deer. Causes abortion in sheep and goats.	Commingling with cattle. Persistent infection of lambs, kids, and calves born when mothers infected during pregnancy.	Stillbirths. Weak kids do not survive. Shaker kids with no changes in hair coat. Abortions at any stage. Skeletal defects on aborted fetus—arthrogryposis, anasarca, and mummified fetuses. PI kids possible when a pregnant doe exposed to PI calf—Swiss symposium.	Necrotizing placenta	Virus isolation PCR Serology—ELISA or SN	Prevent commingling of pregnant does with cattle.
12. **Cache Valley virus and Akabane virus:** Cache Valley Virus is common in the United States	Arthropod borne disease—mainly by mosquitoes and flies (Culicoides)	Infection in early pregnancy can result in wide range of deformities in the fetus, microencephaly, hydrocephalus, arthrogryposis, and muscle atrophy. Joint malformation may cause dystocia. Late gestation can cause premature and stillborn kid.	Clinical signs Serology—precolostral serum or fetal serum for antibodies.	Serology on the doe. Virus isolation on the aborted kids may be difficult.	Control. Fly and mosquito control.
13. **Bluetongue virus:**	Culicoides	Goats are subclinical, infected ewes are febrile, swollen discolored tongue, mucosal ulceration, pulmonary edema, lameness and abortions. Early in gestation leads to fetal resorption. Affected late term may cause abortions, stillbirths, weak kids, and kids with neural and ocular defects.	Clinical signs. Abortion and placenta is normal. Fetuses—lesions in the brain.	Serology—Sera from aborted fetuses and precolostral serum tested for antibodies to BTV. Virus isolation and PCR.	Fly control and vaccination.

Diagnosis of abortion and fetal loss should be confirmed via an accredited diagnostic lab.

Note: Drugs, route of administration, and/or dosages listed may not be approved in your location, for the listed, condition or for species listed—see Appendix 1 and Chapter 8.

BTV, Bluetongue virus; *CF*, Complement Fixation; *CNS*, Central Nervous System; *EAE*, Enzootic Abortion in Ewes; *ELISA*, enzyme-linked immunosorbent assay; *FA*, Florescent Antibody test; *GI*, gastrointestinal; *IFA*, Immunofluorescent assay; *IHC*, ImmunoHistoChemistry; *IM*, intramuscularly; *OTC*, Over The Counter; *PCR*, polymerase chain reaction; *PI*, Persistently Infected; *SC*, subcutaneously; *SN*, Serum Neutralization test.

Parturition (Kidding/Lambing). The doe/ewe should kid/lamb in a clean environment, either a well-drained clean pasture or a stall bedded with straw or other absorbent material. Prior to birth, the kid/lamb/fawn has existed in a germ-free environment, and parturition exposes them to common disease organisms to which a mature animal has developed resistance. The kidding/fawning/lambing stall or pasture should be located near a well-traveled area so that the does/ewes are observed at frequent intervals for dystocia. Few adult sheep, goats, or cervids require assistance at the time of parturition, although problems are always a possibility. First-freshening does or ewe lambs should be closely watched, especially if bred to bucks/rams known to sire large kids/lambs/fawns.

Signs of impending parturition include udder engorgement, swelling of the vulva, restlessness, and vulva mucus discharge. The ligaments in the pelvic area will relax and the udder secretions will change from clear honey-like to thick white/yellow milk (colostrum). The doe/ewe may also lose appetite. Stage one of parturition consists of uterine contraction and cervical dilation, may last from 3 to 6 hours or more, and ends with the rupture of the amnion. Stage two is the active stage of labor exhibited by abdominal contractions and birth, lasting 30 minutes to 1 hour. If the doe/ewe is straining or birth is delayed for more than 30 minutes in an adult doe/ewe, or greater than 1 hour in first time kidding does or ewe lambs, assistance maybe needed. Stage three consists of expulsion of the placenta and usually occurs within a few hours after the last fetus is born.

Problems in Parturition. Most does/ewes will kid/lamb/fawn with little to no assistance required; however, problems can occur. The most common problems encountered are an oversized single fetus; abnormal presentation, position, and posture; or two fetuses entering the birth canal at the same time. In a normal birth presentation, the fetus will be in an anterior presentation, dorsosacral position with their front feet extended into the birth canal. Posterior presentation, dorsosacral position, with their hindlimbs extended, is seen where the rear legs enter the birth canal first. See Chapter 8 for specifics on parturition and dystocia management.

Kid/Lamb Management at Birth. After birth, two management practices are critical to the future health and survival of the newborn. The navel cord should be dipped in a solution of iodine (1 or 2% is now preferred to 7% tincture of iodine due to tissue damage) or 2% chlorhexidine solution to prevent entry of disease-causing organisms, especially for neonates born in confinement or small lots with high populations. Make sure the entire cord is immersed in the iodine or chlorhexidine solution.

The other critical practice is the feeding of colostrum ideally within 2 to 4 hours of birth. If a newborn neonate does not or cannot nurse, the colostrum should be bottle-fed or tube fed to insure adequate consumption. Neonates should receive 15% of their body weight during the first 24 hours of life. For example, a 6-lb (2.7 kg) kid/lamb should receive 15 oz (400 mL) of colostrum within 24 hours of birth, and the colostrum should be divided into at least three to four feedings, due to the size of the abomasum. As a general rule of thumb, feed a minimum of 2 oz/lb (2.7 kg – 360 mL or 1 kg – 150 mL or 2.7 kg – 375 mL) of body weight within 24 hours. Excess colostrum may be collected and frozen for use to supplement orphaned/abandoned kids/lambs/fawns (see Chapter 8).

CAE virus and OPP are transmitted from the doe/ewe to the kid/lamb mainly through colostrum and milk. Methods to prevent transmission include feeding colostrum frozen from does and ewes tested and shown to be CAE/OPP-free, feeding heat-treated colostrum and pasteurized milk, feeding bovine colostrum and milk, or feeding commercially available artificial colostrum replacer. Colostrum can be heat treated by raising the temperature to 133° F (56° C) for 60 minutes or 165° F (74° C) for 15 seconds. Milk should be pasteurized by treating at 145° F (63° C) for 30 minutes or 161° F (72° C) for 15 seconds. The temperature is critical for colostrum because a higher temperature will denature colostral proteins that provide disease immunity and a lower temperature will not kill the virus. Heat treat colostrum or pasteurize milk by using a water bath with an accurate thermometer or by equipment purchased for the task. If a herd is infected with CAE, producers should not feed kids unpasteurized milk even from test-negative does.

Under certain conditions, newborn kids/lambs may benefit from injections of vitamins A and D within 4 days of birth. A vitamin E/selenium injection given within 72 hours may be beneficial in areas of selenium-deficient soils. If supplementation is necessary, feeding dietary supplements in the ration in appropriate levels will usually prevent deficiencies. Fat-soluble vitamins and minerals are toxic if given in excess.

Examine neonates carefully at birth for any physical deformities or congenital abnormalities. The most common congenital defects include cleft palate (Figure 19.1), umbilical hernia, cyclops, parrot mouth (under shot jaw), and atresia ani (no anal sphincter). Diarrhea and pneumonia can cause high mortality rates in neonates. A clean, dry, draft-free environment is an excellent preventive measure.

Artificial Rearing of Neonates. Milk is the principal dietary component for neonates. The majority of meat goat kids, fawns, and lambs will nurse their dam until weaning. However, commercial milk replacer is used in orphans, kids/lambs/fawns from young does and ewes that have lactation problems, does/ewes with more than two offspring, and does/ewes who have abandoned their young. Dairy kids are taken away from their dam as soon as they are born. Typically, milk replacers contain 22 to 30% protein and 28 to 30% fat (on a dry matter basis). A species-specific milk replacer needs to be used if possible. If no other milk replacer is available, calf milk replacers may be used as

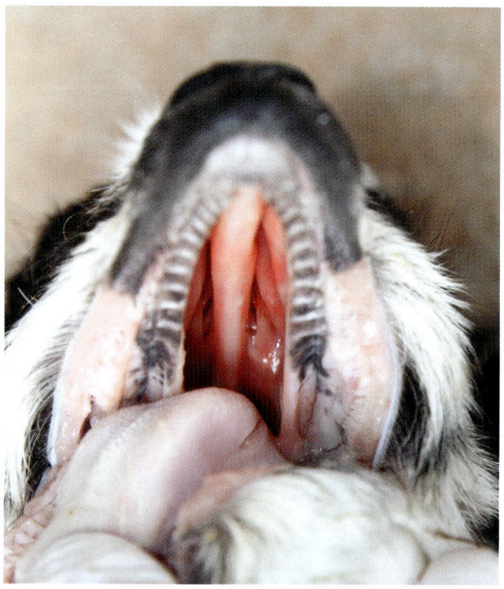

• **Fig. 19.1** A cleft palate is shown in an Alpine kid 3 hours old.

a last resort. Maintaining milk replacer quality after mixing is very important when neonates are fed ad libitum.

Milk is fed using bottles, pails, or self-feeder units depending upon size of the farm, available labor, and personal preference (Figures 19.2 and 19.3). With any system of feeding, the health of the neonate, sanitation, and available labor are the major factors to consider.

Under natural suckling, neonates consume small amounts of milk at very frequent intervals. Ideally, artificial rearing should mimic natural suckling, but labor constraints often preclude frequent feeding. Nevertheless, neonates are ideally fed three to five times daily for the first 1 to 2 weeks and two to three times daily thereafter. Bottle-feeding is labor intensive, but neonates receive more individual attention and are easier to handle post-weaning than kids, lambs, and fawns suckling does.

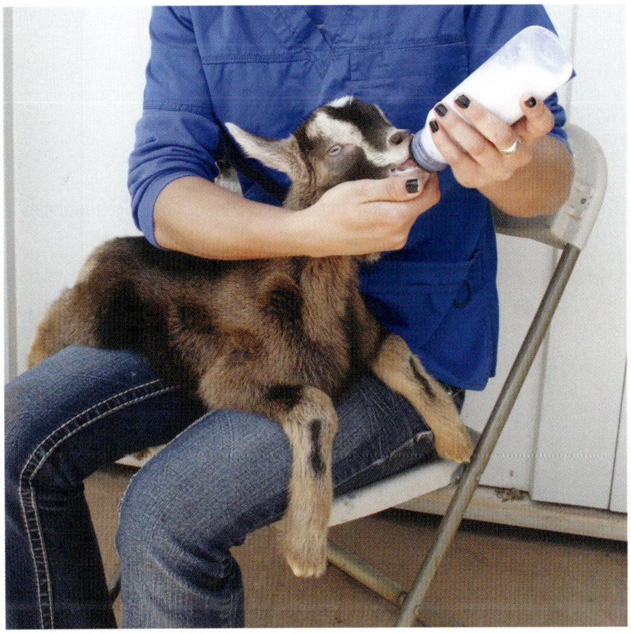

• **Fig. 19.2** A 1-week-old Alpine kid being bottle fed.

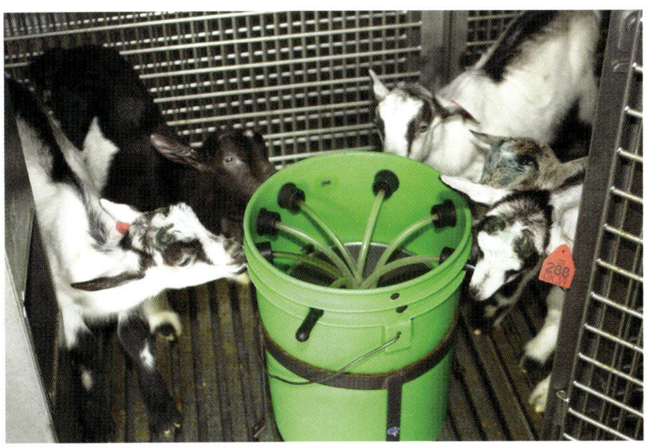

• **Fig. 19.3** Two-week-old Alpine kids nursing a "lamb bar."

For larger herds, self-feeder units may successfully reduce labor. The key factor in this system is maintaining a low milk temperature (40° F, < 5° C) to limit excessive intake by a kid/lamb/fawn at any one time. Small, frequent feedings increase digestibility and decrease digestive disturbances. Rapid consumption of large quantities of milk may lead to fatal bloat due to milk entering the reticulo-rumen space. Rapid passage of milk through the abomasum and small intestines can result in diarrhea or nutritional scours.

A strict feeding schedule should be followed when using a milk replacer to bottle feed kids, lambs, or fawns (Table 19.5). Frequently, neonates become "pets," and there is a tendency to feed them as much milk as they will consume each feeding. By leaving them on a milk replacer too long, these neonates extend the time they take to start eating solid feeds and may result in bloat and sudden death due to enterotoxaemia or diarrhea. It is a common practice with fawns to keep them on a milk replacer to increase growth rate and keep them as tame as possible. Longer nursing periods generally occur with fawns rather than with lambs or kids. Early vaccination for *C. perfringens* is necessary for bottle-fed or artificially reared neonates (Table 19.6).

Dam-Raised Neonates. Most neonates are raised with their dams on pasture. While this removes the need for feeding milk replacer, these kids/lambs/fawns should not be neglected in terms of nutritional and health needs. Producers must remember that since these animals are raised in the same environment as their dams, they are also exposed to the same health, disease, management, and grazing conditions. If internal parasites are a problem in the dams, expect the same in the neonates and take management steps to reduce exposure to internal parasites through pasture rotation or other means. If housed at any time, avoid crowding and have clean bedding and adequate ventilation. Neonates are naturally curious and will begin to explore and nibble on various items in their pens and surroundings early in their life. If there are toxic substances or plants, plastic, or other harmful materials lying around, chances are some neonates will eat them. If pasture is of very poor quality, neonates that are beginning to nibble on grass or hay will not receive much nutritional benefit. This can slow down early growth (see Chapter 8).

Early access to a creep feed or pasture containing lush, nutritious forage will benefit neonates and get them accustomed

TABLE 19.5 Feeding Schedule for Bottle-Fed Small Ruminants.

Age	Amount of Feeding	Feeding Schedule
1 to 3 days	4–6 oz	Three times a day
3 days to 2 weeks	8 oz 12 oz	Three times a day Twice a day
Kids separated depending on their weights. Gradually increase the milk with lamb bar (12 oz/kid or lamb) twice a day (Figure 19.3)		
2 weeks to 3 months	16–20 oz Lamb bar	Twice a day Offer creep feed and hay
3 months to 4 months	20 oz/kid Lamb bar	Twice a day Increase creep feed and hay

TABLE 19.6 **Vaccination Schedule for Small Ruminants.**

Vaccination Schedule for Small Ruminants

Dam—*3–4 weeks prior to parturition*

- CD&T vaccine to help increase antibodies against enterotoxaemia and tetanus in the colostrum. In areas or regions deficient in selenium and supplementation is inadequate, BoSe to raise selenium levels and prevent white muscle disease in kids and retained placenta in the does and ewes. Providing a proper mineral nutrition program to ensure adequate consumption of all minerals is preferable.

Lamb/kid/fawns—*birth to first week*

- BoSe + vitamins A and D—use depends on soil in the region and the diet of the dam. Kids raised indoors in a barn, recommended vitamin A and D injection.

Lamb/Kid—3 *weeks—begin coccidiosis prevention*

- Coccidiostat in the creep feed.
- Once a month for 5 days amprolium and sulfadimethoxine in the water or milk.
- 4 and 8 weeks—BoSe—repeat if in selenium-deficient area.
- 6 to 8 weeks—begin monitoring for parasites and deworm as needed, especially if kid has access to outdoors.

Period	Time to Vaccinate	Disease	Booster
Meat and fiber kids, preweaning lambs Dairy/orphan kids Fawns	4 and 8 weeks of age 2, 4, and 8 weeks of age (bottle fed) As practical, birth, 2, 4 and 8 weeks	*Clostridium perfringens* C and D *C. tetanus*—toxoid *C. perfringens* C and D *C. tetanus*—toxoid	Yearly prebreeding and prekidding booster (replacements) Yearly prebreeding and prekidding booster (replacements) Yearly when handling
Show animals	4, 8, and 16 weeks of age	*C. perfringens* C and D *C. tetanus*—toxoid	60 days before the first show
Show animals	6 to 8 weeks before the show	Contagious ecthyma	Show animals Adult animals vaccinated if there is a problem in the herd
Dairy and meat kids	8 and 12 weeks of age	Caseous lymphadenitis	If there is a problem in the herd Yearly prebreeding booster
Companion sheep and goats	16 weeks of age	Rabies	If rabies is a concern Yearly booster
Prebreeding Young females and males	60 and 30 days prior to breeding	Chlamydia Campylobacter Leptospirosis	If a problem in the herd
Older females and males	30 days prior to breeding (booster)	Chlamydia Campylobacter Leptospirosis	If a problem in the herd Yearly prebreeding booster
		C. perfringens C and D *C. tetanus*—toxoid	Prebreeding
Gestation Ewes/does	30 days prior to parturition	*C. perfringens* C and D *C. tetanus*—toxoid	Booster prebreeding and prekidding yearly
Dairy animals	**Females** 30 days prior to breeding or prebreeding	Chlamydia Campylobacter Leptospirosis	If a problem in the herd Yearly prebreeding booster
	Females	*C. perfringens* C and D *C. tetanus*—toxoid	Prebreeding, midlactation, and prekidding
	Males	Chlamydia Campylobacter Leptospirosis	If a problem in the herd Yearly prebreeding booster
	Males	*C. perfringens* C and D *C. tetanus*—toxoid	Yearly prebreeding booster
Flock/herd	Prebreeding	Rabies	Endemic areas—yearly booster

CD&T, Clostridium perfringens C & D and C. tetanus vaccine.

to eating solid food and enhance the development of their gastrointestinal tract, promoting early growth. Entry into the area containing creep feed or pasture should be restricted to neonates by fencing or gates that prevent access by adult animals. Coccidiostats can be mixed in the creep feed and in grower rations for lambs and kids. There are no coccidiostats approved for use in cervids at this time. Treatment and prevention should be discussed with the attending veterinarian for alternatives in fawns that may include individual treatment with standard ruminant coccidia medicaments or feed or water treatments prescribed within a valid veterinarian/client/patient relationship.

Weaning. In raising kids and lambs, increases in size and weight are not the only measure of success. A well-formed skeleton and proper development of internal organs are often neglected or overlooked. Dry-feed consumption is important in developing body capacity that leads to increased feed intake and digestion.

In bottle-fed young over 2 weeks of age, limiting daily milk consumption to about 48 oz will encourage daily consumption of dry feed. Begin offering a creep feed no later than 3 to 4 weeks of age. As creep feed consumption increases, gradually reduce the amount of milk fed. Research has shown that at 2 months of age, a weaned kid has a reticulo-ruminal capacity five times as large as suckling kids/lambs of the same age do.

Kids/lambs on pasture should be consuming forages such as pasture or hay by 2 weeks of age and grain within 4 weeks. Give careful attention to the formulation of a concentrate supplement for preweaning animals. Palatability is of primary concern. Molasses at the rate of 10% of total dry matter, corn (preferably ground or rolled), and whole or rolled oats make up the energy "core" of a good preweaning diet. Balance the crude protein needs by adding cottonseed or soybean meal or another high quality protein source. Crude protein in the preweaning ration should range from 14 to 18%. Ground alfalfa may be added up to 5% or less to provide additional stimulation for reticulo-ruminal development (see Chapter 2).

Several factors should be considered when deciding to wean. The most important consideration is whether the average daily consumption of concentrate and forage is adequate for growth and development to continue in the absence of milk. Fixed weaning ages are less desirable than weight goals such as 2.0 to 2.5 times birth weight. When a kid/lamb is eating 0.25 lb of grain per day, plus some hay, and is drinking water from a bucket, it is time to wean. Adding coccidiostats in the creep feed and in the grower ration will help control coccidiosis in lambs and kids, but there are no products approved for fawns at this time. Most fawns are weaned in the late summer, when they are approximately 3 to 4 months old. Fawns should be consuming feed by this time. As lactation needs decrease, cervid does have adequate time to rebuild body condition prior to the breeding season beginning in the very late fall to early winter depending on the region of the United States in which they live.

Postweaning. The postweaning period is a critical time due to the stress of removing offspring from their dams. Hand-reared neonates seem to be less stressed when weaned from a milk source as compared to neonates that have been nursing their dams. Neonates that have started consuming creep feed and hay prior to weaning tolerate weaning stress better than those that do not consume appreciable amounts of solid feed. Common diseases encountered during the weaning period include pneumonia, coccidiosis, gastrointestinal parasitism, polioencephalomalacia, and enterotoxaemia. To reduce the incidence of respiratory diseases at weaning, avoid overcrowding, maintain proper barn ventilation, and observe animals daily to ensure adequate feed and water intake as well as early detection of disease signs. To control coccidiosis, reduce the number of oocytes in the environment by reducing stocking densities and removing soiled bedding. Keep hay and feed racks above the ground and incorporate a coccidiostat in the feed (sheep/goats). Regular pen and pasture rotation can decrease exposure to coccidia.

On initial exposure to fresh pasture in late spring or summer, weanlings may incur heavy internal parasite exposure. To avoid exposing them to an infested pasture, place weanlings in a clean pasture that has had no small ruminant presence for at least 2 months. Give booster injections of CD&T and FAMACHA score weaned lambs and kids monthly until the first freeze in fall. Depending on the history of anthelmintic used, kids and lambs with a FAMACHA score greater than 3 should be dewormed with an appropriate dewormer or a combination of different classes of wormer.

In meat goat/lamb finishing programs or feedlots, be aware of the potential for bloat, enterotoxemia, and urinary calculi. Prevent bloat by gradually increasing grain over a 10- to 14-day period. Follow proper vaccination program to prevent enterotoxemia. Polioencephalomalacia incidences can be reduced by gradually increasing grain in the diet, decreasing sulfur/sulfate content in the ration, providing clean water, early detection and treatment with amprolium and sulfa drugs, and monitoring animals after deworming. Castrated and intact males are prone to urinary calculi as young as 3 months of age. Prevent by providing a continuous supply of clean fresh water, including 4% salt in the diet, or giving a salt block. Continuous or pulse dose feeding of urinary acidifiers like ammonium chloride helps to acidify the urine and prevent stone formation.

Basic Vaccination Recommendations for Goats and Sheep

A vaccination program in a herd health plan depends on the conditions or diseases likely be encountered on a particular farm. A minimum basic vaccination schedule should include *Clostridium* C and D and *Clostridium tetani*. Multivalent Clostridial vaccines containing antigens that cause black leg, malignant edema, bacillary hemoglobinuria, big head, and black disease are commonly used in many parts of the United States on a routine basis where those diseases are prevalent. Vaccines should be given subcutaneously in the axillary region or in the neck to minimize lameness and swelling and to prevent excess trimming of meat at slaughter (Table 19.6).

Vaccinate against contagious ecthyma (sore mouth, Orf, contagious pustular dermatitis) if the disease has been diagnosed in a herd or if animals are participating in livestock shows where they may contract it. Contagious ecthyma vaccine is a live-virus vaccine, and it serves as a means of introducing the virus to the herd. Once introduced, through an outbreak or vaccination, the contagious ecthyma virus will persist for a long time. Once the herd has been exposed to the virus by natural infection or vaccination and is subsequently immune, the producer or owner may consider implementing a vaccination protocol for lambs and kids only. This is a zoonotic disease and may cause painful lesions to people who contract it.

The majority of U.S. goats have been exposed to *Corynebacterium pseudotuberculosis*, the agent causing CL or abscesses. The external form of CL involving the lymph nodes is commonly seen in goats, whereas the internal form of CL is more frequently seen in sheep. The bacteria in the purulent material may contaminate the environment, where it persists for months. Commercial vaccines are available for sheep and goats. Autogenous vaccine is manufactured from the bacteria isolated during the culturing process. These vaccines promote humoral response and are not effective in animals already exposed to this bacterium. Vaccinating kids and lambs at a young age may help in reducing the severity of the disease. Cervids do not commonly get CL.

Vaccines used in sheep for abortion-causing *Campylobacter* and *Chlamydia* are not approved for goats or cervids. If these organisms are found to have caused abortions in goats, sheep vaccines have been used off-label with limited success because of variations in biotypes. For *Leptospira* abortions, cattle vaccines have been used with mixed results, anecdotally. Foot rot in sheep and goats is caused by the synergistic actions of *Fusobacterium necrophorum* and *Dichelobacter nodosus* or by either organism alone. Using a cattle vaccine containing *Fusobacterium* has met with mixed results in sheep and goats.

Vaccination programs for cervids are controversial at best. They commonly contract *Clostridium* type C and D, so this vaccine is the most common vaccine given. *Clostridium* type A is also frequently diagnosed, and a commercial cattle vaccine is used or an autogenous vaccine given. Fusobacteria cause a number of conditions in cervids, and autogenous vaccines or cattle vaccines have been used with some success. Hemorrhagic disease causes large losses on many farms, but there has been limited success with autogenous vaccines due to multiple serotypes and lack of cross-protection, as well as the difficulty of implementing a vaccination program to animals prior to the vector season. Other bacteria for which autogenous vaccines are used include *Trueperella pyogenes*, *Bibersteinia trehalosi*, *Pasteurella multocida* type A, and *Mycoplasma bovis*. Management and environment can exacerbate many of these diseases, and as such, a holistic approach to herd health should be used.

Herd/flock health programs are normally developed to prevent common diseases and develop management strategies to minimize the risk factors. A good vaccination program needs to be included to prevent some of the common diseases affecting the animals in that farm. Table 19.6 gives a basic vaccination program that can be used in a sheep and goats.

Basic Vaccination Recommendations for Cervids

Vaccination programs for farmed cervids should be designed for specific farms, endemic diseases, feeding programs, etc. Does late in gestation are prone to injury and stress when moved through handling facilities, thus reducing the use of prefawning vaccinations. As with many cervids, white-tailed deer bucks in velvet are very susceptible to antler injury, thus reducing handling from April through September, for example. Handling these bucks past mid-October in North America may prove problematic, as they are prone to fight and injure nearing or during "rut." Small fawns are very difficult to catch and, if moved through handling facilities with adults, can be injured. Darting vaccines and medications can be effective but may increase injury, costs, etc.

The most commonly used vaccinations in North American cervid farms are as follows:

1. *C. perfringens* type C, D, and A yearly (e.g., commercially available multivalent clostridial vaccines). Does and bucks are traditionally vaccinated in late winter early spring, prior to late gestation and after antler drop, respectively. Alternatively, bucks may be handled on some facilities after antlers have hardened, but prior to rut, where possible. Bottle-fed fawns can effectively be vaccinated like lambs or kids (see Table 19.6). Fawns raised by the doe are usually vaccinated at 3 to 4 months of age.
2. *F. necrophorum* and *Fusobacterium varium*, *Escherichia coli*, and leptospirosis when needed for specific farms should be considered at 6 to 8 weeks of age and a booster in 2 to 4 weeks. As with Clostridiums, fawns raised by the doe are usually vaccinated at 3 to 4 months of age.
3. Epizootic hemorrhagic disease virus (EHDV)—At the time of this writing, the most commonly used vaccines used for epizootic hemorrhagic disease control used in North America are killed viral products containing EHDV type 1 or 2 antigens or bluetongue virus 10 or 17 or other serotypes. These vaccines need two initial doses prior to the vector season, which is late spring early fall until a frost. An annual booster prior to the vector season is recommended. Anecdotal information suggests that the commonly used vaccine to control EHDV may have limited efficacy to poor efficacy in many areas, depending on the viral biotype.

Presently, no commercial vaccines are approved for use for cervids in North America.

Reproductive Management

Goats, sheep, and cervids are generally classified as seasonally polyestrous or short day breeders in the United States. The degree of seasonality varies among breeds and their location (latitude). The annual reproductive cycle of goats in a temperate region can be divided into a breeding season or period, a nonbreeding season or physiologic anestrous period, and a transitional period (see Chapter 8).

Estrus synchronization is increasingly being used as an effective tool in reproductive management for meat and dairy goats, particularly with the demand for year-round milk supply. Synchronizing estrus early in the breeding season allows an increased proportion of does to become pregnant early. Kids born to these does are older and are of more uniform size at weaning to take advantage of niche markets during religious events and rising price trends in the market. Out-of-season breeding will enable the producer to take their kid crop to market when prices are higher and have year-round milk production in dairy animals and increases the number of kids born to the doe during her lifetime. Estrus synchronization techniques include altering light patterns, manipulating social interaction with buck exposure early in the breeding season, and manipulating the estrous cycle by extending or shortening the luteal phase of the cycle (see Chapter 8).

Annual Health Management Practices

Creating and using a management calendar are good methods to ensure the maintenance of flock health. The calendar should be designed on the herds' needs and production cycle. Table 19.7 outlines a basic herd/flock management program. Although much of the information is aimed at sheep and goat flocks/herds, it has some applications for cervid production.

CWD, TB, and brucellosis are of special concern for cervid producers in North America. The veterinarian and producer consider both individual state and federal supervision guidelines prior to implementing a monitoring/reporting program. Most such programs involve animal identification and sampling of obex, lymph nodes, and tonsils on animals over a specific age at death. TB accreditation and brucellosis certification programs are important for state-to-state movement. With cervids, testing in rut or late pregnancy should be avoided. Johne's disease is a quarantinable disease in some states and could result in a producer being unable to move or market animals. Ovine for of malignant catarrhal fever is of concern for some cervids. White-tailed deer appear extremely sensitive to the virus, with mortalities reaching 100% in herds. Sheep are inapparent carriers, with up to 60% of lambs (from 4–12 months of age) shedding the virus in some parts of North America. Minimizing sheep/cervid contact will minimize the incidence of this disease on a cervid farm. A well-planned and well-operated handling facility, with a long-term

TABLE 19.7 **Small Ruminant Herd Health Calendar.**

Small Ruminant Herd Health Calendar

A custom-designed calendar is an excellent way to ensure the health of a herd is maintained. A calendar can be designed based upon your specific herd's production cycle. Veterinarians with their client can formulate a herd health program for individual herd needs. Cervids present a special challenge due to their temperament, physiology (antler growth cycle), and handling needs sometimes outweighing the health benefits or timing of a procedure.

Planning Calendar for Goat Herd Health

Stage	Suggested Health Practices	Additional Practices
Prebreeding (30–60 days)	**Males** • Be aware of heat stress. • Breeding soundness evaluation done. • Vaccinate for *Clostridium perfringens* type C and D, plus tetanus toxoid. • Vaccinate for chlamydia, campylobacter and leptospirosis, if necessary. • Trim feet. • Body condition score, flushing the bucks and adjust management accordingly. • Deworm based upon fecal egg counts or FAMACHA score. **Females** • Vaccinate for *C. perfringens* type C and D, plus tetanus toxoid. • Vaccinate for chlamydia, campylobacter, and leptospira if necessary. • Trim feet. • Body condition score, flushing the females, and adjust management accordingly. • Deworm based upon fecal egg count or FAMACHA score at least 2 weeks before breeding. • Dry the dairy does if they are producing less than 1 lb of milk a day. • Final cull of does based on production records, udders, feet, and type.	• Vitamin E and selenium given to does 30–45 days before breeding in selenium-deficient areas. • See vaccination schedule. • Put males next to female pens. The "buck and ram effect" will bring transitional does and ewes into heat.
Breeding	**Males** • Provide additional feed. • Be aware of heat stress and provide shade and fresh water • Proper buck-to-doe ratio. • Provide marking harnesses and change colors every 14 days (not practical for cervids). **Females** • Observe for heat or use marking harness on males. • Record the markings.	• Make sure cats are not defecating in feed to prevent toxoplasmosis. • Perform fecal egg count or check FAMACHA score and deworm if necessary. • Treat for flukes if a problem in the herd.
Gestation	• Blood test for PSP $>$ 30 days after breeding if necessary. • Check for pregnancy at 45–60 days with ultrasound. • Separate the ones with more than two fetuses and feed accordingly if practical • Breeding $\rightarrow$ midgestation. Does with BCS $>$ 3.0 are fed good-quality hay and trace minerals. If BCS $<$ 3.0, supplement with grain 0.5–1 lb/day. • Last trimester: supplement with grain accordingly. BCS 3 or greater 1 lb/day. BCS $< 3 = 2$ lb a day.	
Preparturition (15–30 days)	• Booster C. perfringens type C and D, plus tetanus toxoid. • Deworm based upon fecal egg counts or FAMACHA score. • Body condition scoring, adjust management and feeding. • Watch for pregnancy toxemia. Urine ketone testing done if needed. • Does need proper exercise. • Dairy doe udders clipped. • Dairy doe teats tapped for accidental nursing of kids.	• Perform fecal egg count or check FAMACHA score and deworm if necessary. • Begin to collect supplies for birthing.

Parturition	**Dams**
	• Observe three to five times per day.
	• Assist if needed.
	• Kidding pens similar to lambing pens used for doelings.
	Neonates
	• Clip, dip, and strip:
	  ◦ Clip navel cord to 2–4 inches.
	  ◦ Dip navel in appropriate iodine/chlorhexidine solution.
	  ◦ Strip small amount of milk to make sure the teat ends are open. (Not cervids.)
	  ◦ Make sure neonates are nursing.
	  ◦ If the dam has more than 2 or 3 offspring, cross fostering within 24 hours after birth is necessary.
	  ◦ Vitamin E/selenium given within 72 hours in deficient areas.	

Continued

TABLE 19.7 Small Ruminant Herd Health Calendar.—cont'd

Stage	Suggested Health Practices	Additional Practices
Nursing/lactation	**Dams** • Feed extra feed to dams with multiple kids. • Monitor somatic cell counts—bulk and individual. • FAMACHA scoring every month. Not practical in cervids. Deworm if necessary. **Neonates** • Observe daily for signs of diarrhea or respiratory disease. • Vaccinate—*C. perfringens* type C and D and tetanus, revaccinate at 4 weeks and booster 4 weeks later. • Castrate males before 3 months of age. Do not castrate cervids unless there is a specific reason. • Dairy kids dehorned and castrated within 10 days. • Start creep feeding by 2 weeks of age.	See Vaccination Schedule for Small Ruminants.
Weaning	• Weaning at 3–4 months, marketed or kept as replacements. • Weaning is determined if the kids/lambs consuming ¼ lb of grain/day and grazing. • Check for internal parasites and deworm if needed.	• Coccidiostat in creep feed and postweaning feed.
Postweaning/drying	• FAMACHA score every 4 weeks; check for internal parasites and deworm as needed. Not practical for cervids. • Reduce feed to does just before weaning. • May want to reduce water availability for a day or two after weaning. • Flushing if necessary. • Dry treat the mammary glands in dairy does when the milk production drops below a pound a day or before the start of the breeding season or 2 months before kidding.	Select appropriate antibiotic for dry treatment, also give the mammary gland time to recuperate from the previous lactation.
Dairy females and males	• Yearly TB testing. • Yearly brucellosis testing.	Performed by an accredited veterinarian Any suspects on TB testing on the caudal fold at 72 hours are notified to the APHIS office in the state immediately.
Dairy females and males	**Does** • Prekidding vaccination—*C. perfringens* type C and D, plus tetanus toxoid. • Midlactation—*C. perfringens* type C and D, plus tetanus toxoid. • Prebreeding vaccination—*C. perfringens* type C and D, plus tetanus toxoid. • Prebreeding vaccination—vaccinate for chlamydia, campylobacter, and leptospira if necessary. **Bucks** • Prebreeding vaccination—C. perfringens type C and D, plus Tetanus toxoid. • Prebreeding vaccination—vaccinate for chlamydia, campylobacter, and leptospira if necessary.	 Yearly booster—prekidding Yearly booster—midlactation Yearly booster—prebreeding Yearly booster—prebreeding Yearly booster—prebreeding Yearly booster—prebreeding

APHIS, Animal and Plant Health Inspection Service; *BCS*, Body Condition Score; *FAMACHA*, FAffa MAlan CHArt; *PSP*, Pregnancy Specific Protein; *TB*, tuberculosis.

view of potential animal movement, is critical to disease prevention and testing. These factors are magnified when working with nondomesticated animals.

Table 19.8 lists some of the production goals ideal for a sheep flock.

Milk Quality Assessment in Dairy Goats and Sheep

The goal for dairy animals is to produce quality milk as efficiently as possible. This is an area of utmost importance in a herd health evaluation. Management changes can affect milk production and quality very quickly. Milk quality assessment begins with the bulk tank reports and tests that the creamery sends to the producer. Most often, the processor will offer premiums above base price for milk components such as butterfat, protein, and solids, as well as for quality reflected in bacteria and somatic cell counts. Individual records will show which does are earning their spot in the milking string.

Bacteria count in the bulk tank sample is primarily a measure of sanitation. It is rare that individual mastitis infections will seriously raise bacteria counts. If counts are elevated, the rate that the milk is been cooled needs to be checked, along with the cleaning system and procedures for cleaning the milking units. The temperature of the water heater needs to be checked regularly to make

TABLE 19.8 Production Goals in Sheep.

Pregnancy	
Ewes	More than 95%
Ewe lambs	More than 75%
Visible abortion	Less than 5%
Lambing	
Ewes	More than 90%
Ewe lambs	More than 70%
Stillbirths	Less than 2%
Weaning	More than 95%

sure it is hot enough when used for cleaning. A visual inspection of hoses, pipelines, milking units, and bulk tank after cleaning is necessary. Correct any deficiencies, and if a high bacteria count persists, the milking equipment maintenance technician should be notified. Somatic cell counts are used to monitor milk quality for all dairy animals. There are state, national, and international standards that need to be met. Regulatory officials link somatic cell count levels to the incidence of clinical and subclinical mastitis in the herd. It is felt that high levels of bacteria in the milk will result in shorter shelf life and increase the chance of milk spoilage, causing human health issues. Goats normally have higher somatic cell counts than cows do as measured by the machines used to screen milk. Small ruminants secrete milk using an apocrine system, resulting in the presence of cytoplasmic particles that can register as somatic cells. Also during the time of year when goats are cycling and declining in milk production, their cell counts are greatly elevated. CAE and CL will cause elevated counts not linked to mastitis. For these reasons, a dairyman will want to monitor cell counts (see Chapter 15).

Dairy Herd Improvement (DHI) tests are probably best at monitoring the whole herd. Individual does and ewes should be tested with the California mastitis test (CMT). This test involves placing an equal amount of milk and CMT solution in a test well, mixing and reading the degree of gel formation after 30 to 45 seconds. This test is not very sensitive. Milk needs to have more than 750,000 cells to react, but it will identify problem mammary glands and may aid in determining if treatment is necessary. The PortaSCC goat milk test is an owner-run test that is more accurate than the CMT in that it only measures white blood cells and seldom other particles. The test is interpreted by comparing the test strip to a color chart (see Chapter 15). Another monitoring tool for mastitis control is to have routine bulk tank cultures taken. This test will give colony counts for both contagious and environmental forms of mastitis. The number of colonies can be correlated to the number of goats or ewes infected with a particular type of organism. The test is never negative as there are always some environmental bacteria, but it designates acceptable, moderate, and high levels for each class of bacteria. This allows the producer and/or consulting veterinarian to establish goals to improve udder health. Individual mastitis cultures with a sensitivity test should be run periodically to allow for a rational selection of the appropriate antibiotic used as a treatment in the herd. This also allows the correct dry treatment to be used if necessary. Many types of bacteria can be cultured from milk.

Bacteria causing mastitis are divided into contagious and environmental groups. Contagious mastitis in goats is mainly limited to *Staphylococcus aureus* and *Mycoplasma* spp. During milking, contagious organisms easily spread from animal to animal via hands or milking equipment. Environmental mastitis encompasses all bacteria that can invade the udder from where lactating animals are housed or kept, or that occur naturally on their skin. When contagious mastitis shows up, prompt action is required to prevent a small problem from quickly growing into an immense problem putting your dairy at risk of failure. *Mycoplasma* comes in a variety of species. It is untreatable at present time by any approved products. Identification of infected individual goats through culture is important. A culture of pooled samples of 10 animals can lower the cost but will prolong the time needed to identify infected animals. When a ewe or doe is identified with *Mycoplasma* mastitis, she needs to be removed from the milking group, either culled or kept in isolation, if she is a valuable animal. *S. aureus*–infected dairy animals must be identified and either culled or segregated. Identification can be made by culture, *S. aureus* polymerase chain reaction test, or by a technology called matrix-assisted laser desorption ionization–time of flight. This enables a faster identification of bacteria based upon detecting unique protein profiles of individual bacteria. If there are too many infected animals, it will be difficult to cull them all; they should be identified with leg bands, either be milked as a final group or have a designated milking machine that is used only on *S. aureus* goats. Remember the hands of the person milking can be the vector for spreading *S. aureus*. Gloves should be used so they can be sanitized or disposed of after handling infected goats or ewes.

Most environmental mastitis organisms are treatable. About 85% of mastitis cases are caused by a skin bacterium, *Staphylococcus epidermidis*. Rarely does it cause inflammation but will cause one-half of the udder to atrophy and gradually cease to lactate. This organism is responsible for most of the elevation of bulk tank cell counts. It is often identified as a "coagulase negative staph" on culture reports and must be differentiated from *S. aureus*, a "coagulase positive staph." It is treatable if identified early. If not, it will cause fibrosis of the gland and that half of the udder will not milk during future lactations.

Milking ewes and does can be treated by intramammary infusion like a cow. An alcohol wipe is used to sanitize the end of the teat, after which the tip of the infusion tube is partially inserted. Opening the teat canal with your thumb and forefinger may help start the tube into the canal. Infuse the entire tube as it is contaminated and a partial tube will transmit the organism to the next goat. Milking goats or sheep with a history of mastitis or chronic somatic cell count should be dry treated with an appropriate product as identified by culture and sensitivity tests. Animals without mastitis should not be dry treated as the infuser tip will cause damage to the keratin plaques lining the teat orifice and canal. These structures form a natural barrier to bacterial invasion, and removing them with the cannula may invite infection. Mastitis is further divided into groups, by degree of severity, into peracute, acute, clinical, and subclinical. Subclinical mastitis is detectable but does not make the goat systemically ill. Treatment of mastitis is often frustrating, so the priority should be prevention. Use appropriate milking protocols. Udder cleanliness prior to and after milking is important and pre- and post-dips can be effective. In particular, a post-dip should remain on the teat end until the orifice closes to prevent bacterial invasion. If environmental mastitis is a problem, a pre-dip is recommended. If contagious mastitis is a problem, then a post-milking dip is recommended. It is preferable if the person milking wears disposable gloves, as the hands are a good source of bacteria (see Chapter 15).

Recommended Reading

Johnson J: Goat herd health. In Pugh DG, Baird AN, editors: *Sheep and goat medicine*, ed 2, Maryland Heights, Missouri, USA, 2012, Elsevier, pp 545–566.

Sharko P: Flock and herd health. In Pugh DG, Baird AN, editors: *Sheep and goat medicine*, ed 2, Maryland Heights, Missouri, USA 2012, Elsevier, pp 539–545.

Dawson LJ, Boileau M: Meat goat herd health: procedures and prevention. *Meat goat production handbook*, ed 2, American Institute for Goat Research. Langston University, 2015, pp 81–114.

Boileau M, Dawson LJ: Meat goat herd health: common diseases. *Meat goat production handbook*, ed 2, American Institute for Goat Research. Langston University, 2015, pp 115–139.

Boileau M, Dawson LJ: Dairy goat herd health, common diseases. *Dairy Goat Production Handbook*, American Institute for Goat Research. Langston University, 2016, pp 73–108.

Duemler C: Dairy goat herd health: procedures and prevention. *Dairy Goat Production Handbook*, American Institute for Goat Research. Langston University, 2016, pp 39–56.

Haigh J, Hudson R: *Farming wapiti and red deer*, St. Louis, Mo, 1993, Mosby.

Alexander T, Buxton D: *Management and diseases of deer*, ed 2, Loanhead, Midlothian, 1994, The Veterinary Deer Society, J.A. Spence.

AWMDA—body condition scoring for whitetail and mule deer, Available at: http://www.albertadeer.com/uploads/1/2/5/9/125989078/awmda-body-condition-scoring.pdf.

PennState Extension: *White-tailed Deer Production*, 2015. Available at: https://extension.psu.edu/white-tailed-deer-production.

PennState Extension: *Red deer production*, 2005. Available at: https://extension.psu.edu/red-deer-production.

20

Field Necropsy and Diagnostic Tests

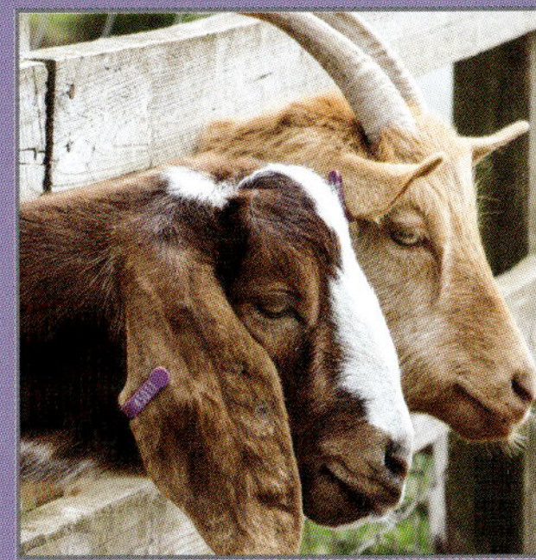

HEATHER WALZ, JENNY POPE, AND DAVID G. PUGH

Indications for postmortem examination vary with each individual owner or producer. Finding a cause of death can assist with future treatment and culling decisions, help with dietary and nutritional modifications for the herd, and initiate a search for toxins like toxic plants in the area. Additionally, for some sheep and goat clients, there is an emotional attachment, and finding the cause of death provides a sense of closure for the owner.

Postmortem examination can be equally rewarding and frustrating for veterinary practitioners and pathologists. Practitioners and pathologists both have the common goal of identifying the cause of morbidity and mortality. However, the diagnostic process can be slower than owners and producers expect, and additional deaths may occur before initial test results can be completed. To prevent frustration, it is important for deaths in a herd to be investigated early on, as owners and producers occasionally wait until multiple animals have died before submitting the first animal for necropsy. To improve the diagnostic process, a clear line of communication should exist between owners, veterinarians, and the diagnostic laboratory. If a practitioner does not know what tissues to submit, or what tests to request, calling or emailing a pathologist at the laboratory for recommendations ahead of time can help ensure a better chance of a diagnosis. Additionally, this communication can be helpful so that pathologists know the clinical signs, herd morbidity or mortality rate, and time period in which problems have arisen. Pathologists also appreciate clinical pathology data, physical examination findings, and digital photographs to help guide the diagnostic process. A brief description of the lesions observed at necropsy (simple descriptors are often better than interpretations) or a statement of no gross lesions observed is also helpful. Pathologists and practitioners have the same goal, which is to find meaningful and timely answers to explain sickness and death losses. Appropriate samples and pertinent information can make the difference in getting a diagnosis. Although there are diseases like tetanus for which a definitive diagnosis cannot be made at necropsy, necropsy can still be helpful for ruling out other causes of disease or finding supportive lesions. The clinician may find complimentary information with respect to necropsy procedures in Chapter 20, Necropsy, by Dr. JF Roberts in the second edition of this text.[24]

A field necropsy can be performed similar to a laboratory necropsy, but the main objective is to leave the skin attached, and viscera within the body cavity for easier cleanup and disposal. Elements needed for a successful gross necropsy examination include a thorough history, all necessary equipment, and a location conducive for performing a necropsy. Procedures for a field necropsy are much more challenging than performing a necropsy at a laboratory as laboratory necropsies have readily accessible utensils, necropsy tables, and easier methods of carcass disposal. The location of the field necropsy should be away from other animals, high-traffic areas, and areas where there can be human exposure. Performing the necropsy on a cement pad allows for easy cleanup if a water source is available. A tarp can also help contain bodily fluids. The capability of removing contaminated soil may be indicated if certain pathogens are later identified from necropsy samples. Veterinarians performing the necropsy should have maintain adequate rabies prophylaxis. The necropsy clinician should take all precautions and be cognizant of other potential zoonotic diseases (e.g., goat/sheep placentas and fetuses after abortions caused by *Chlamydia* sp. and *Coxiella* sp.).

Personal Protective Equipment and Equipment for the Necropsy Procedure

In most instances, coveralls, boots, and gloves are sufficient for the necropsy examination. However, enhanced personal protective equipment (PPE) should be worn if handling fetal membranes or performing a necropsy on an aborted fetus. A face mask, protective eye goggles, and double gloving are recommended in these situations.

Recommended equipment:

- Rubber or synthetic gloves: wrist or mid-arm length
- Tarp
- Permanent marker
- Ruler
- Digital camera or phone for photographic documentation
- Bacterial culture swabs, portable culture tubes, synthetic or cotton swabs without bacterial growth media
- Leak-proof jars containing 10% neutral buffered formalin: maintain a formalin to tissue ratio of $> 10\times$
- Boning knife, knife sharpener, polished steel, forceps, scissors, loppers/rib cutter, hand saw, small hatchet

- Disinfectant
- Scissors, forceps
- Leak-proof bags

Materials for Polymerase Chain Reaction, Bacterial Culture

- Submission of tissues is preferred over swabs.
- Swabs with wooden shafts are contraindicated for polymerase chain reaction (PCR), as wood splinters can break off. Each laboratory prefers particular swab types (work with a local laboratory), and generally, synthetic swab materials are preferred for PCR. Viral transport media may be requested by some laboratories.
- Swabs should not be submitted dry, and a bacteriology transport media such as Stuarts or Amies media should be used to cultivate potential bacteria in the sample and to prevent desiccation.
- Twine—Tying off a segment of bowel with twine prevents gastrointestinal (GI) content spilling onto other tissues, and luminal content will be preserved.
- Whirl-Paks (Manufacturer: Nasco) are ideal to avoid sample leakage, but plastic baggies can be used by double bagging samples.

General Recommendations for Sample Collection

The authors' recommendations for sample collection are listed here, with more detail available in each section throughout the necropsy procedure and in Table 20.1. Collection of all main tissues, placement in formalin, and submission for histopathology, regardless of presence or absence of gross lesions, are recommended to ensure the best chance of a diagnosis. Collection of any additional tissues that are considered abnormal and submission for histopathology should also be done. Tissues submitted for histopathology should be less than 1 cm (0.5 cm is recommended) sections to permit full tissue fixation. Fixation of tissues is recommended prior to submission to prevent autolysis, which may prevent detailed assessment. Aside from tissues submitted for histopathology, which can be submitted in a single jar containing 10% formalin, other tissues should be submitted in separate bags or containers. Collection of ocular fluid (both aqueous and vitreous), large pieces of liver and kidney, and rumen contents is necessary for toxicology/mineral testing. Aqueous and vitreous humor are often used as approximation for blood levels. Collection of spleen, lung, liver, kidney, small intestine, half of the brain, and

TABLE 20.1 Routine Sample Submissions for Necropsies[a].

Test Section	Samples	Potential tests
Histopathology	**Fixed tissue**	Microscopic examination
	Any abnormal tissue, lung, liver, kidney, heart, brain, spleen, gastrointestinal segments (rumen, abomasum, small intestine [multiple including ileum], colon), ileocecal lymph node	
Bacteriology	**Fresh tissue**	
	Lung, liver, kidney ± other tissues with concern for infection: intestine/colon, spleen, brain, lymph node, joint fluid, mammary gland, skin, base of antler/horn	Aerobic culture Anaerobic culture
	Fresh Tissue Submission for Cultures Requiring Special Media/Preparation	
	Liver, mediastinal lymph node, intestine	Salmonella
	Ileum, ileocecal lymph node	Johne's
	Brainstem	Listeria
	Rumen, lung, other	Fungal
Molecular/Virology	**Fresh tissue**	
	Spleen, lung, liver, kidney, brain, small intestine	PCR for viral testing, PCR for mycoplasma, Johne's disease
	Ear notch	BVD ELISA
	Oral/muzzle/teat lesions consistent with contagious ecthyma	FA/PCR for parapoxvirus
Serology	Serum (red top tube)	CAE, OPP
Toxicology	**Fresh tissue/feed**	
	Liver	Selenium, copper
	Kidney	Arsenic, lead
	Rumen contents	Insecticides, cyanide, pH
	Aqueous humor	Nitrate, ammonia
	Vitreous humor	Magnesium, calcium
	Feed	Mycotoxins, ionophores, botulism

BVD, Bovine Viral Diarrhea virus; *CAE*, Caprine Arthritis and Encephalitis; *ELISA*, enzyme-linked immunosorbent assay; *FA*, Fluorescent Antibody; *OPP*, ovine progressive pneumonia; *PCR*, polymerase chain reaction.

[a]Can vary between diagnostic laboratories, so calling ahead will ensure appropriate sample submission.

ear notch are necessary for PCR/virology testing. Collection of lung, liver, kidney ± spleen, intestine, brain, or other potentially infected organs are recommended for culture. Collection of feces is recommended for a McMaster's egg count. Collection of serum is recommended for serologic tests and can be collected from blood present when cutting the jugular veins in the neck or from the heart.

Necropsy Procedure

Positioning of the animal can vary based on preference of the examiner; however, it is best to position each species of animal the same way every time a necropsy is performed. Generally, there is a preference for ruminants to be in left lateral recumbency to prevent the rumen from obstructing the view of tissues and organs.

External Examination

External examination encompasses evaluation of the eyes, ears, oral cavity, dorsal and ventral aspects of the tongue, perineum for evidence of diarrhea, mammary gland, external genitalia, joints, and feet. Body condition of the animal and state of preservation should be recorded for each necropsy. Documentation of animal identification numbers, including state (chronic wasting disease [CWD], depending on each state) and federal ID numbers (scrapie), is essential. Any lesions found externally on the animal should be documented and photographed. A careful external examination may be the only chance for a diagnosis of conditions like lightning strike (singed hair) or documentation of supportive lesions for a diagnosis of tetanus (wounds). If erosions or vesicular lesions are found in the oral cavity, on the lips or muzzle, around the eyes or feet, and coronary bands, photographs and a full history should be shared with the local diagnostic laboratory and/or the state veterinarian or state animal health representative. If regulatory officials believe it is warranted, collection of vesicular fluid in a tube, swabbing a vesicular lesion, or collecting tissue-containing vesicles may be performed by the state veterinary authorities or a veterinary medical officer with the U.S. Department of Agriculture (USDA).

Skin

Collection of ear notch samples from sheep and goats for bovine viral diarrhea virus (BVDV) is recommended. Antigen capture enzyme-linked immunosorbent assay (ELISA) testing on deer ear notch samples has been not been validated for use in white-tailed deer.[1]

Ocular Fluids

Collect aqueous and vitreous samples at this time and place them in labeled red-top tubes. Aqueous samples can be submitted for nitrate testing, or testing can be done on site with the water-quality test strips used for pools, which are readily available. Calcium, potassium, sodium, and magnesium levels can be evaluated in vitreous samples. Other tests that can be performed on ocular fluids, dependent on the specific laboratory, include evaluation of electrolytes, urea nitrogen, and ammonia nitrogen.[2]

Mammary Tissue

Assess the mammary glands for color, symmetry, and presence of milk. Cut into the mammary tissue and assess again for color, texture, presence of fibrosis, as well any changes to the milk and submit for culture as needed (see Chapter 15).

Antlers and Horns

Assess antlers and horns for fractures and any changes to the surrounding tissue. If dehorning is recent, carefully assess these areas for extension through the skull.

Musculoskeletal System

Assess joints for swelling, particularly in neonates. Remove synovial fluid with a needle for culture if bacterial infection is suspected and cut into multiple joints (particularly the carpus and tarsus) to assess for the presence of fibrin, pus, and excess fluid, as well as the color and viscosity of fluid. There may also be swelling in goats or sheep with chronic lentiviral arthritis.[3] Collection of synovium for histopathology, culture, and PCR for mycoplasma is recommended if there is pus or fibrin in the joint. Cut into muscles to assess for necrosis or mineralization associated with diseases like capture myopathy in deer,[4] vitamin E/selenium deficiency, or plant toxicities like *Senna* spp. Assessment of musculature over the spine can help determine the potential for trauma in ataxic animals particularly if the spinal cord cannot be removed (see Chapter 11).

Reflection of the Limbs and Removal of Skin and Subcutis

For animals in left lateral recumbency, begin by incising the axillary region, pulling the leg upward, while simultaneously cutting and reflecting the right forelimb dorsally until the limb lies on the ground above the animal. Similarly, incise the right inguinal region, cut through the right coxofemoral joint, incise the round ligament of the femur, and transect musculature while pulling the leg upward then dorsally until the limb has been reflected above the animal. Figure 20.1 shows the right front limb of a deer reflected and a focally extensive region of hemorrhage in the subcutis of the neck associated with epizootic hemorrhagic disease (EHD). Dissect skin and subcutis and associated musculature from the right axilla moving caudally to remove skin over the thoracic wall, continue to dissect skin and subcutis of the right body wall to connect to the incised area of the right femur. Reflect skin of the thorax and right body wall upward and continue to the level of the vertebrae to extend the dissected skin dorsally to lie above the

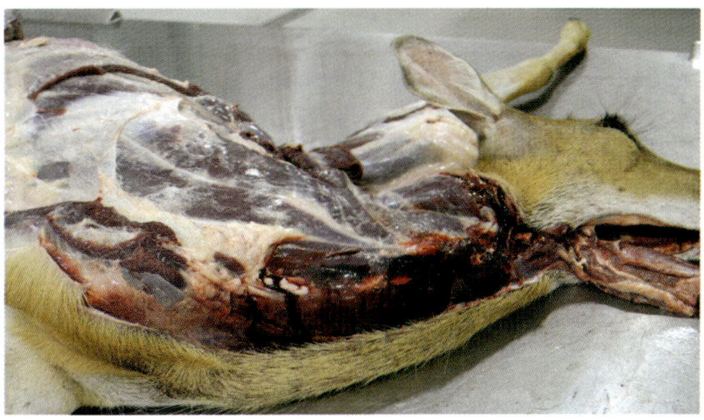

• **Fig. 20.1** Deer with the right leg reflected dorsally. Skin and subcutis have been dissected and removed. Ventral cervical hemorrhage is also present, and this corresponds with polymerase chain reaction detection of epizootic hemorrhagic disease virus for this case. (Courtesy Kelley Steury, Auburn, AL.)

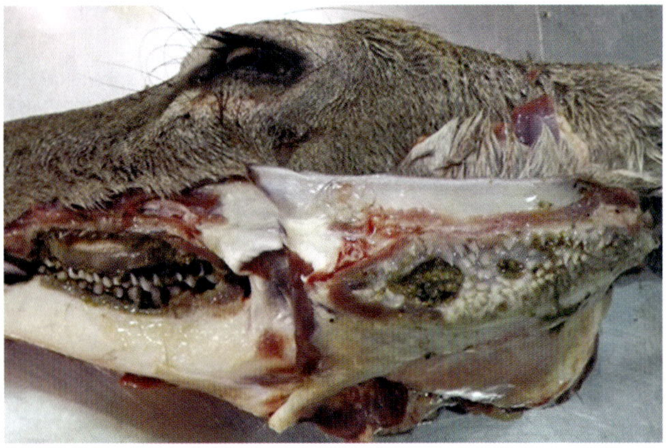

• **Fig. 20.2** Deer with buccal abscess.

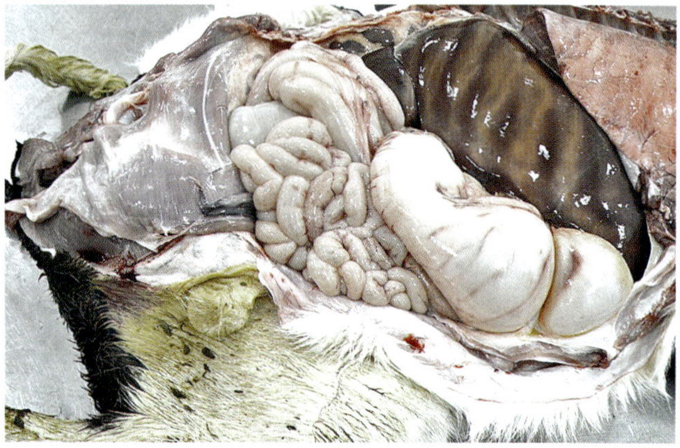

• **Fig. 20.3** Goat with pale musculature and viscera. The striped appearance of the liver capsule is secondary to compression by the overlying ribcage. (Courtesy Kelley Steury, Auburn, AL.)

animal. This is also a good time to assess the subcutis for color changes such as yellowing (icterus) associated with hemolytic disease and to assess the blood for thinning (anemia) or color changes such as those associated with nitrate toxicity (chocolate blood).

Oral Cavity

Evaluate the teeth for wear and breakage, pull the tongue laterally and expose the dorsal and ventral surfaces to evaluate for vesicles, erosions, and ulcers. Cut at the lateral commissures of the mouth and extend the skin caudally and dorsally to evaluate the buccal region for abscesses or foreign bodies entrapped within the mucosa. Figure 20.2 shows a buccal abscess in a white-tailed deer. Continue cutting the skin and underlying musculature so the base of the tongue can be evaluated (see Chapter 4).

Exposing the Larynx, Esophagus, and Trachea

Bilaterally remove the skin and subcutis behind the jaw to the thorax, extending caudally to the level of the thoracic inlet. Bilaterally, dissect lateral and dorsal to the larynx and cut the larynx, trachea, and esophagus. For a field necropsy, the pluck does not have to be removed, and incising the larynx, trachea, and esophagus in situ to the level of the thoracic inlet is acceptable. If the veterinarian prefers to have the entire pluck removed during the procedure, cut the hyoid bones, forming a V-shape on both sides, then connect this cut with the incisions being made caudally along the lateral aspects of the pharynx. Continue simultaneously cutting and pulling the tongue, trachea, esophagus, and associated musculature caudally until the soft tissue has been cut to the thoracic inlet, and free the lateral and dorsal aspects of the esophagus and trachea. Leave the trachea, esophagus, larynx, pharynx, and tongue and place aside until the thoracic cavity is ready to be opened. Evaluation of cervical lymph nodes for lesions of caseous lymphadenitis (crumbly or pasty white material in lymph nodes) caused by *Corynebacterium pseudotuberculosis* and collection for culture are best completed at this step as well. Assessment for lymph node enlargement and cutting into the lymph node will give the most information. Lymph nodes should have a smooth homogenous texture and slight color variation between the cortex and medulla. Evaluation of the thyroid glands, particularly size, is recommended at this step, especially in fetuses or neonates, which are susceptible to goiter (see Chapter 4 and 9).

Opening the Abdominal Cavity

Gently incise the musculature along the caudal aspect of the last rib by making a superficial dorsal-to-ventral incision, being careful not to cut into the abdominal viscera. Extend the incision from the dorsal thoracic vertebral region to the midventral abdominal cavity, then course caudally then dorsally again to free the musculature and fascia overlying the abdominal wall and reflect this layer of musculature dorsally. Evaluate the abdominal contents and look for displacements, obstructions, areas of discoloration, fibrin or feed covering abdominal viscera, the volume and character of abdominal fluid, and the overall color of the visceral organs and incised musculature. Abomasal rupture due to *Clostridium septicum* (braxy) or *Sarcina*-like bacteria[5] can occur, and anaerobic culture and microscopic examination, respectively, are required for identifying the exact cause. Reddening, coating with fibrin, and thickening of the abomasal wall with edema is consistent with premortem rupture. Figure 20.3 depicts a goat with pale viscera and musculature. Check the fat reserves around the kidneys and intestine and evaluate the size of the liver for atrophy. Weighing the liver is a nonsubjective method to assess liver size, but this is primarily feasible when a necropsy facility is available. A prominent looking gallbladder is a good indicator of hepatic atrophy.

Opening the Thoracic Cavity

Evaluate the abdominal side of the diaphragm to ensure that there is no evidence of a diaphragmatic hernia, gastric displacement or rupture, or nodular thickening of the diaphragm as can be found with parasitic diseases. Figure 20.4 shows larval cestodes present in the diaphragm of a wild white-tailed deer. Incise the diaphragm and listen carefully for negative pressure. Cut the ribs with rib cutters moving caudally to cranially along the dorsal and ventral aspects of the ribs, then connect the two cuts at the thoracic inlet while avoiding cutting into the trachea. Pull the ribs off and set them on the ground. Evaluate the parietal pleura covering the rib cage, taking note of any adhesions, how difficult the adhesions are to remove, areas of hemorrhage, or presence of exudate. Evaluate the amount and character of thoracic fluid, amount and character of thymic tissue located cranially within the thoracic inlet (or also extending to the ventral cervical neck region), lungs, tracheobronchial

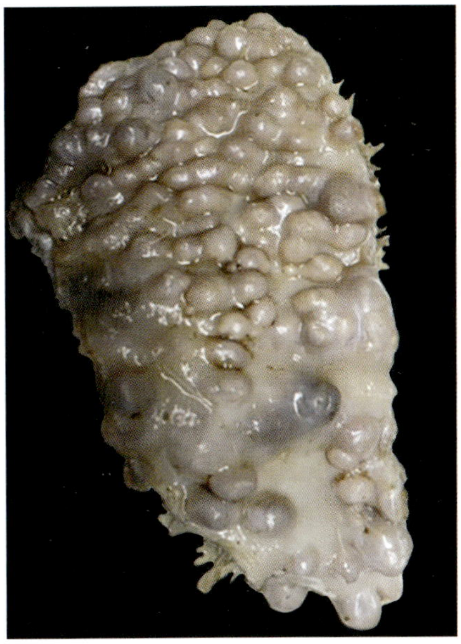

• **Fig. 20.4** Wild, white tailed deer, diaphragm. Multifocal to coalescing, smooth nodules expand the diaphragm. Histologic findings were consistent with larval cestodiasis. (Specimen submitted by Terry Slaten, Hanceville, AL.)

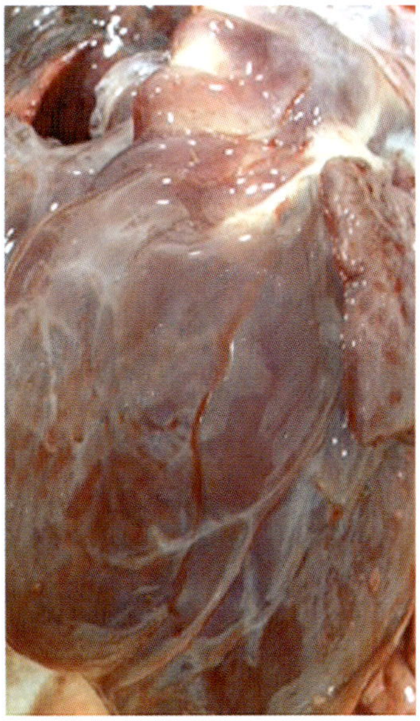

• **Fig. 20.6** Pericardial fat has been replaced by clear gelatinous material (serous atrophy of fat).

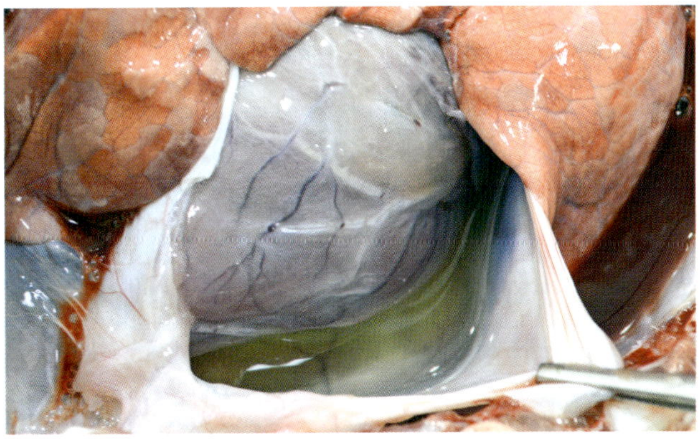

• **Fig. 20.5** Goat; pericardium is distended by clear, pale yellow fluid (hydropericardium) and there is serous atrophy of epicardial fat. (Courtesy Travis Heskett, Auburn, AL.)

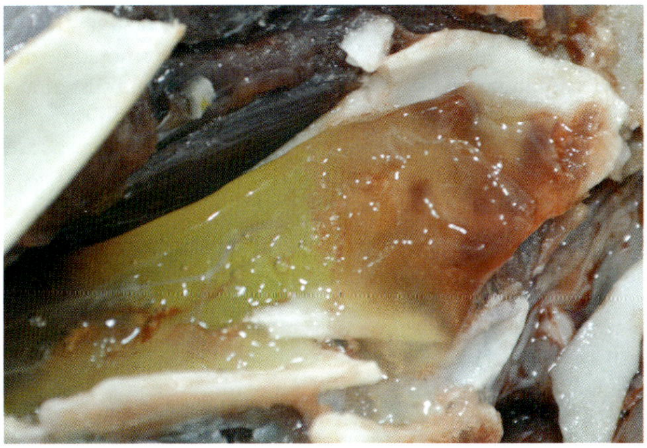

• **Fig. 20.7** Goat; bone marrow is replaced by yellow gelatinous material (serous atrophy). (Courtesy Travis Heskett, Auburn, AL.)

lymph nodes, heart, and pericardium, including any evidence of pericardial distention. Figure 20.5 shows hydropericardium in a deer with abundant abomasal *Haemonchus* spp. Evaluate the serosal aspects of the esophagus and trachea, thoracic aorta, and thoracic side of the diaphragm. Evaluate the amount of epicardial fat and whether the fat is gelatinous (serous atrophy). Epicardial fat is replaced by gelatinous material in Figure 20.6. If there is serous atrophy of epicardial fat and reduction in visceral fat, bone marrow fat should be evaluated for serous atrophy, which is important for establishing the chronicity of negative energy balance. Figure 20.7 shows no fat within the marrow cavity of this adult goat, only gelatinous material. The general color of the carcass is also important, as pale viscera, pale musculature, and pale gums are often indicative of anemia associated with endoparasitism or yellowing of the carcass can be associated with hemolytic disease like that from copper toxicity.

If loppers/rib cutters are not available, assessment of the thoracic cavity can still be completed. Incise the diaphragm as described earlier and reach into the thoracic cavity as far as possible to cut the trachea and esophagus. Once this is completed, peel the lungs and heart out through the diaphragm, cutting as necessary.

Thoracic Cavity

After performing a full evaluation for lesions within the thoracic and abdominal cavities, some pathologists and practitioners prefer to collect tissues for bacteriology and virology prior to removing viscera to decrease the number of surface bacteria on samples submitted for testing. First, remove and collect thoracic specimens, and then collect fresh tissues from abdominal visceral organs, leaving evaluation of the GI tract for last. If concerned about airway-associated bacterial disease, collecting the right cranial ventral lung for bacterial culture is indicated, especially if there is evidence of pulmonary discoloration, a firm to meaty consistency,

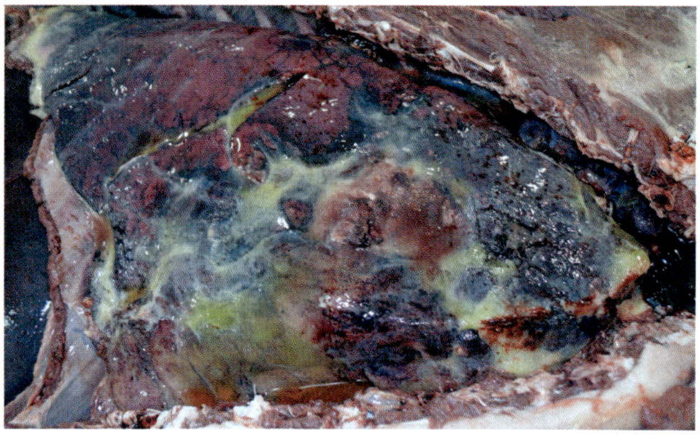

• **Fig. 20.8** Deer with pleuropneumonia. Lungs are consolidated with multifocal hemorrhages. There is abundant yellow fibrin on the visceral pleura of the lung. Reddened, translucent thoracic fluid is also present. (Courtesy Kelley Steury, Auburn, AL.)

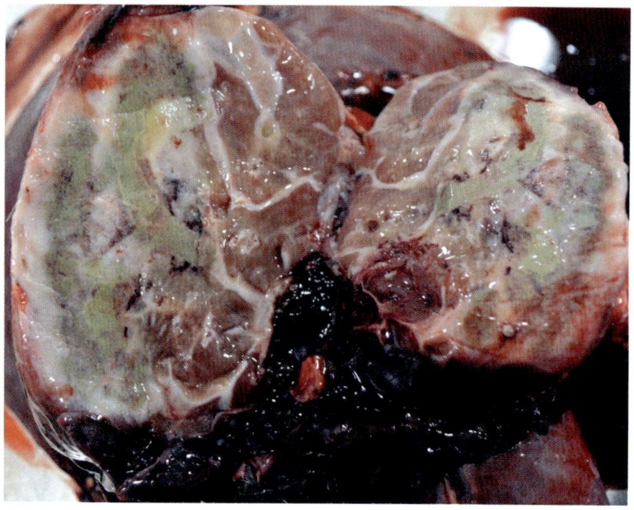

• **Fig. 20.10** Deer; cut section of lung with yellow to green areas and abundant fibrosis due to a fungal granuloma. (Courtesy of Kelley Steury, Auburn, AL.)

fibrin along the visceral pleura of the lungs, as in Figure 20.8, or if pleural adhesions were evident on the rib cage. If the history warrants concern about sepsis or embolic pneumonia, collecting lung from the caudal lung lobes may be indicated. Lungworms can also form small nodules in the caudal lung lobes, so this may be a good area to collect if these are a concern. Collection of lung samples should not be from the peripheral aspects of the lung, and every attempt should be made to collect pulmonary tissue with major airway, as ample respiratory epithelium will be present in these samples. In addition, infectious agents causing pneumonia (*Mycoplasma* spp., respiratory viruses, and bacterial agents such as *Pasteurella multocida, Trueperella pyogenes, Bibersteinia trehalosi*, and *Mannheimia haemolytica*) will have major airway involvement. Sampling at the junction of normal and abnormal tissue will give the most active part of the lesion. Also note whether the pieces of lung sink in formalin as this can help document the extent of the pneumonia. If abscesses are noted, especially in deer, lung should be submitted for mycoplasma PCR (Figure 20.9). Some laboratories may accept swabs or respiratory mucus for mycoplasma PCR, but lung tissue is recommended, as multiple tests can be performed on tissue while the sample volume for swabs can be limiting. If pulmonary nodules suggestive of tuberculosis are found, the level of PPE being worn during the procedure should be increased, and the bacteriology laboratory should know in advance both for biosafety concerns and to select appropriate media. Tissues collected for bacteriology preferably should be collected with cold disinfected or autoclaved instruments, and organ and tissue sections approximately 3 cm diameter should be submitted to enable the laboratory to sear the tissue and sample the central aspect of the lesion. Fungal culture is indicated in some captive white-tailed deer necropsies but may be encountered in other small ruminants. These cases often have green to yellow exudate that has been walled off in a thick layer of fibrous connective tissue affecting one lung lobe, as in Figure 20.10. Refrigeration can kill fungi, but prolonged time at room temperature or above can allow for overgrowth of bacteria, which can compete for and outgrow fungi on media. If abscesses or dark gray to brown fluid are found, as in Figure 20.11, anaerobic culture may be warranted. Some of the pulmonary isolates from cases of deer pneumonia have identified anaerobes. Reports of pneumonia in captive deer have identified *Fusobacterium varum* and *Fusobacterium necrophorum* with different antimicrobial sensitivity patterns.[6]

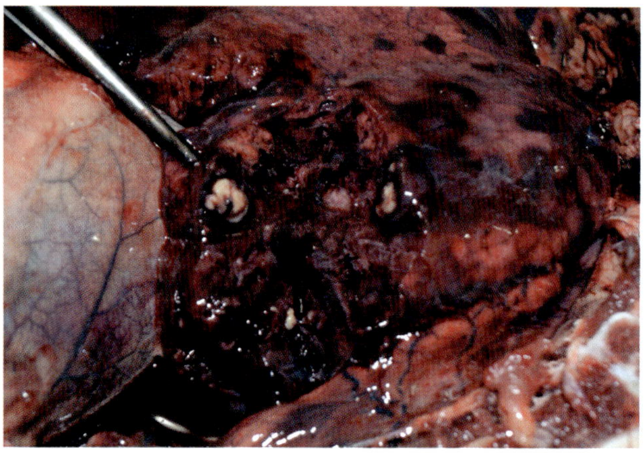

• **Fig. 20.9** Deer with multifocal, discrete yellow to tan abscesses randomly distributed throughout the pulmonary parenchyma.

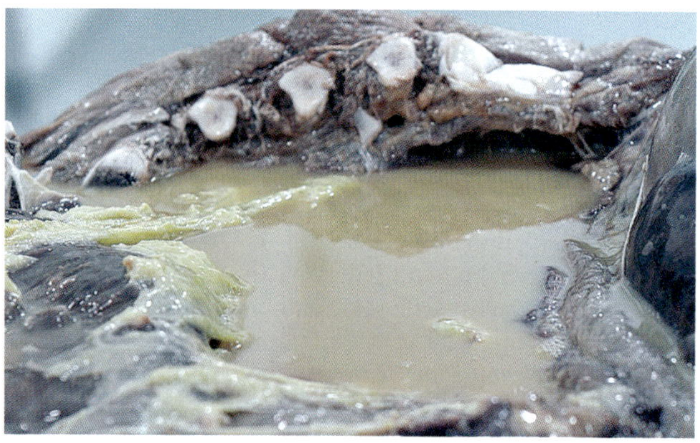

• **Fig. 20.11** Deer; incising a large fluctuant pulmonary abscess revealed copious amounts of thin brown fluid with multiple large aggregates of fibrin. (Courtesy Kelley Steury, Auburn, AL.)

Cranial mediastinum and heart

Evaluation of the thymus should be performed before there is further dissection, followed by collection of thymus for virology or PCR and histopathology. Any enlarged lymph nodes in the thoracic cavity should also be noted and collected for virology, PCR, and histopathology. Evaluate the pericardium and carefully incise and evaluate the amount and consistency of pericardial fluid before the content escapes from the pericardial sac. Evaluate the epicardium for evidence of hemorrhage, pale regions, fibrin, or exudate. Epicardial hemorrhage in deer is often associated with EHD virus (EHDV), but PCR testing is necessary for a confirmatory diagnosis. Prominent epicardial hemorrhage is found at the base of the heart in Figure 20.12. If removing the pluck, the tongue, trachea, and esophagus can be removed by cutting and pulling caudally simultaneously while extending cuts to the dorsal aspect of the thoracic wall to include the aorta and thoracic portions of the trachea and esophagus to the level of the diaphragm. The same approach should be taken to cut ventral lung attachments, free the heart, and cut the lungs ventrally to the diaphragmatic surface. Finally, cut the caudal lung attachments from the thoracic wall and diaphragm and transect the trachea and esophagus on the cranial side of the diaphragm. Pull the pluck out of the thoracic cavity and place on a nearby surface to evaluate. Collect additional tissue from the left lung lobes that were previously unexposed if indicated. If there is evidence of bronchopneumonia, estimate the percent consolidation and make a note in the report. This will help determine if pneumonia was the cause of death or if an early case of pneumonia was detected. After evaluating the pharynx and larynx, incise the esophagus to the terminal aspect. Evaluate the mucosa for vesicles or ulcers and a bloat line. As frothy bloat dissipates over time, this may be the best chance for a diagnosis of bloat in some cases. Now incise the trachea to the terminal aspect and evaluate for reddening, froth, or exudate in tracheal lumen. Figure 20.13 shows the opened distal trachea of a deer with fungal tracheitis. Follow the trachea along its length to the tracheal bifurcation, mainstream, and bronchi and continue to incise along major airways until the terminal aspects of the airway are reached. This is especially important due to the potential for lungworms. Foam in the trachea and wet, heavy lungs indicate pulmonary edema, which can occur with many different diseases (see Chapter 7).

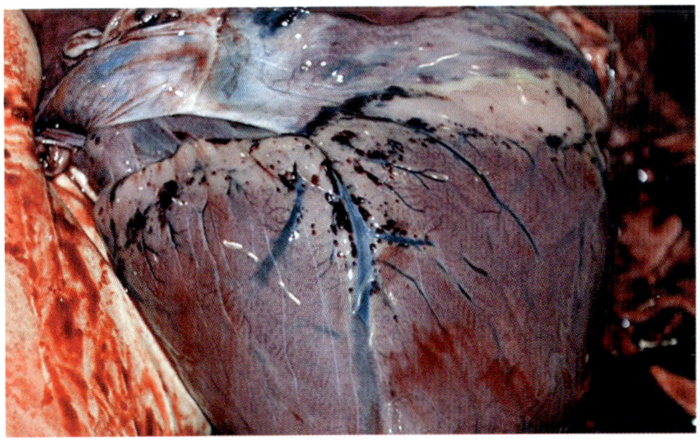

• **Fig. 20.12** Deer; multifocal petechial hemorrhages present at the base of the heart. This deer tested positive for epizootic hemorrhagic disease, but Clostridial enterotoxemia and sepsis can be differentials for these lesions. (Courtesy Kelley Steury, Auburn, AL.)

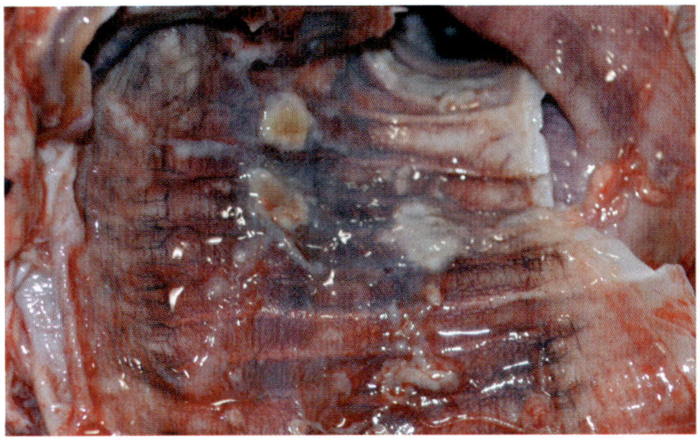

• **Fig. 20.13** Distal trachea of a captive white-tailed deer is reddened, and the tracheal mucosa is covered by nodular aggregates of tan exudate. (Courtesy Kelley Steury, Auburn, AL.)

Now evaluate the heart, following the flow of blood originating from the caudal vena cava to the right atrium, right ventricle, right atrioventricular (AV) valve, and chordae tendineae.[7] Transect the moderator band (trabecula septomarginalis), then cut the rostral wall of the right ventricle, and follow the pulmonic outflow tract and associated pulmonary valve, and pulmonary artery.[7] Evaluate the ductus arteriosus in neonates; follow the intrapulmonary branches of the pulmonary artery and pulmonary vein going back to the heart.[7] Open the left atrium; examine the interatrial septum, foramen ovale, and left AV valve; and cut the left ventricle from the base to apex of the free wall.[7] Evaluate the left AV valve, cut chordae tendineae and follow the left ventricular outflow tract to the aortic valve and aorta.[7] It is critical to evaluate the interventricular septum for ventricular septal defects and to evaluate for a patent foramen ovale in neonates. Several sections from the right and left ventricular free walls, which include papillary muscle, and interventricular septum should be submitted for microscopic examination. Sections for histopathology should include the epicardium, myocardium, and endocardium. Heart is not typically submitted for routine culture and virology/PCR, but this varies for each individual case and is dependent on the clinical history and gross necropsy lesions. For cases with grossly evident heart lesions such as endocarditis, bacterial culture of the lesion and adjacent endocardium and myocardium at the edge of the lesion can identify the specific etiology. Identifying the same type of bacteria from lesions found in several locations can be helpful to help determine the underlying source of entry in some cases. This deer with vegetative valvular endocarditis (Figure 20.14) also had a fractured antler with thick yellow purulent exudate in multiple areas of the subcutis under the antler, behind the eye, and within the musculature behind the optic nerve. As the same bacteria were isolated in both locations, fighting with other bucks was considered the likely initiating cause of the antler fracture leading to antler infection, bacteremia, and endocarditis (see Chapter 17).

Liver

Evaluate the liver for symmetry, rounded edges or borders, overall color, and areas of discoloration or nodules. Generalized color changes can indicate anemia (pallor), acute right sided congestive heart failure (dark red), or lipidosis (yellow). Repetitive patterns

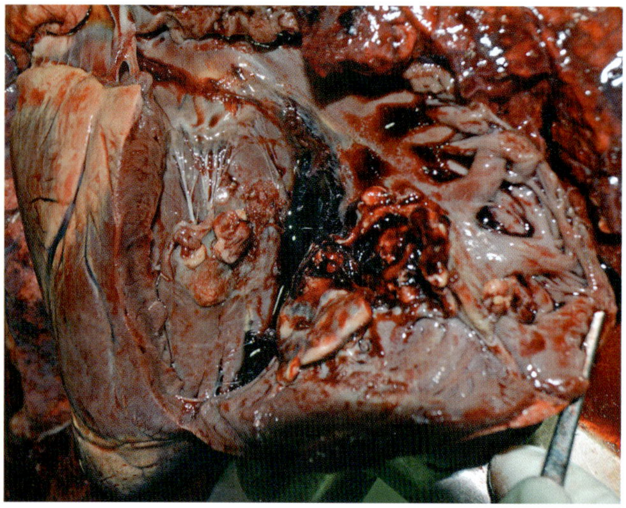

• **Fig. 20.14** Deer buck with vegetative valvular endocarditis on the right atrioventricular valve leaflets.

of light and dark often referred to as nutmeg liver can also indicate chronic right-sided congestive heart failure or targeted necrosis. If lesions are found, sampling the junction of the lesion and normal parenchyma for culture and histopathology are indicated. Sampling multiple lobes is recommended for microscopic examination. Nodular lesions that appear to be an abscess or area of necrosis should be submitted for both aerobic and anaerobic culture (evaluating for *T. pyogenes* and *F. necrophorum*), especially in captive deer, which are inclined to have ruminal hyperkeratosis, ruminal dysbiosis, and rumen acidosis when fed grain-based diets. Additionally, irregular nodular enlarged livers with areas of black pigment should be submitted for anaerobic culture as death could be due to *Clostridium novyi* associated with migrating flukes. Nodular lesions found in the livers of goats and sheep can have a variety of etiologies, but Figure 20.15 shows *Rhodococcus equi* infection in a goat with discrete nodules in the lung and liver.

Liver and mediastinal lymph nodes (also intestine) are good samples for *Salmonella* culture, and this is recommended for all species, but particularly deer. The major vessels of the liver should be incised, and the entire liver should be serially sectioned. Assess the texture of the liver on the cut section (not through the capsule). Moderate pressure of the fingertips should go through a normal liver. If similar results occur with light pressure, this could indicate autolysis, necrosis, or lipidosis. If increased pressure is required, this can indicate fibrosis. Autolysis can result in gas bubbles in the liver, and these should not be mistaken for a significant lesion. If the cause of death is not apparent, or there is a concern about toxicity, a large Whirl-Pak bag should be filled with liver until approximately two thirds full and held for toxicology testing. In cases of acute hepatic necrosis, there may be no easily discernable gross lesions. Copper, zinc, and selenium require liver for analysis. Smaller section(s) of liver (1.0–1.5 cm or less to facilitate tissue homogenization) should be held for virology/PCR. Proceed to evaluate perihepatic lymph nodes and the gall bladder. Liver can also be an excellent sample to evaluate for viral-associated lesions. This was particularly noteworthy in several cases of malignant catarrhal fever (MCF) found in captive deer. Of the numerous positive MCF cases evaluated, portal hepatitis was consistently found. Other tissues with lesions included kidney, lung, and brain.

Spleen and Lymph Nodes

Pull the rumen and forestomachs dorsally and locate the spleen attached to the ventral portion of the rumen. Spleen is the ideal tissue sample for viral diseases, including BVDV, bluetongue (BT) virus, and EHDV. Capsular splenic hemorrhages can be suggestive of EHDV, BT, and clostridial enterotoxemia but most often corresponds with EHDV in areas of the United States with a high incidence (Figure 20.16). For sheep and goats, spleen, thymus, and lymph nodes are needed to test for most viral diseases and

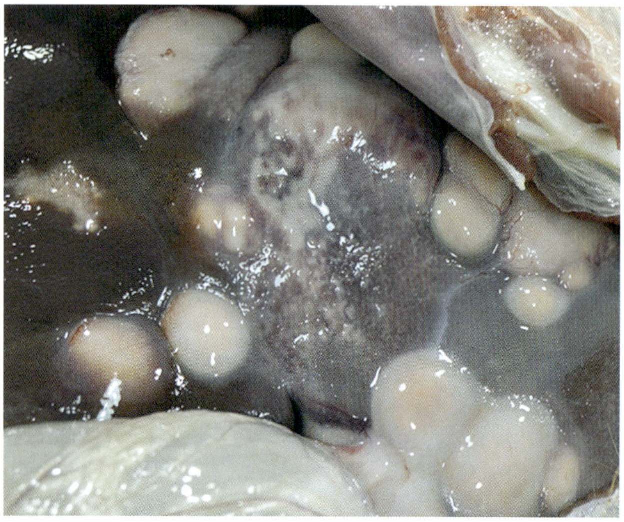

• **Fig. 20.15** Goat liver. *Rhodococcus equi* was isolated from the liver of this goat, and histopathology identified multiple pyogranulomas with intracellular, pleomorphic gram positive rods. (Courtesy of Travis Heskett, Auburn, AL.)

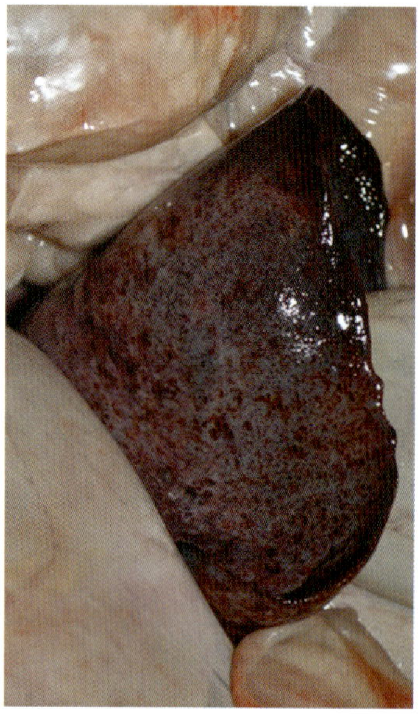

• **Fig. 20.16** Fawn spleen with multifocal capsular hemorrhages. This fawn was positive for epizootic hemorrhagic disease virus (EHDV), and both young and adult deer are susceptible to EHDV. (Courtesy Kelley Steury, Auburn, AL.)

some bacterial diseases. Splenic enlargement can be found with a variety of causes, including barbiturate euthanasia, salmonellosis, hemolytic disease, and babesiosis.[8] Mesenteric lymph nodes often appear enlarged in young animals due to antigenic stimulation rather than disease but should still be submitted. Enlarged mesenteric lymph nodes in an animal with poor body condition may be indicative of Johne's disease caused by *Mycobacterium avium* subspecies *paratuberculosis* and can provide a diagnosis particularly if the intestinal tract is poorly preserved. Collect lymph nodes for bacterial culture, PCR, and histopathology, particularly if abnormal (see Chapter 16).

Urogenital System

Prior to removal of the kidneys, evaluate the ureter for dilation, trace caudally, then incise and evaluate the mucosal surface. The right kidney is accessible when the animal is in left lateral recumbency, and the kidney will be visible following dissection through the dorsal perirenal fat behind the liver. The GI tract should be pulled dorsally and reflected over the spine to allow for removal and evaluation of the left kidney. Note the color of the kidney. A "gun metal" gray kidney may point to copper toxicity. Kidneys are susceptible to autolysis, particularly in overweight or obese animals, which can affect color and texture. Assess for perirenal edema, which may indicate acute renal necrosis due to toxins like oak. Serous atrophy of fat can have a gelatinous appearance and should not be confused with perirenal edema. Remove the renal capsule, noting if it is difficult to remove in the necropsy report. Incise the kidney along the long axis and then evaluate cortex to pelvis. Submit a section of kidney (1 cm or less) for virology/PCR, a 2- to 3-cm section for bacteriology, and provide a capsular to pelvic section of kidney for histopathology ideally 0.5 cm, but less than 1 cm thick. The pelvis is often overlooked and is important to evaluate for ascending infections, tubular mineralization, and toxicities. The cortex is important to evaluate for toxicities including copper and oxalates as well as for glomerular disease. Figure 20.17 shows white to tan nodular foci in the renal cortex of a deer kidney. Histologic evaluation of kidneys with culture is often rewarding in deer because does with no clinical signs can have severe ascending pyelonephritis. MCF may demonstrate systemic lesions in white-tailed deer, but the kidneys, liver, lungs, and brain seem to be targets for perivascular lymphoproliferation and vasculitis with occasional intranuclear viral inclusion bodies (based on histologic examination of a captive deer farm with an approximately 40–50% mortality rate). The remaining renal tissue not submitted for other tests should be submitted for toxicology as kidney is required for heavy metal analysis like lead and arsenic. Evaluate the urinary tract by examining the serosal surface of the urinary bladder and following the ureters to the kidneys. Urinary bladder is a dynamic organ, and the thickness of the wall can vary depending on distention with urine. A full distended urinary bladder with serosal or mucosal color changes (red to black) can indicate urinary blockage.

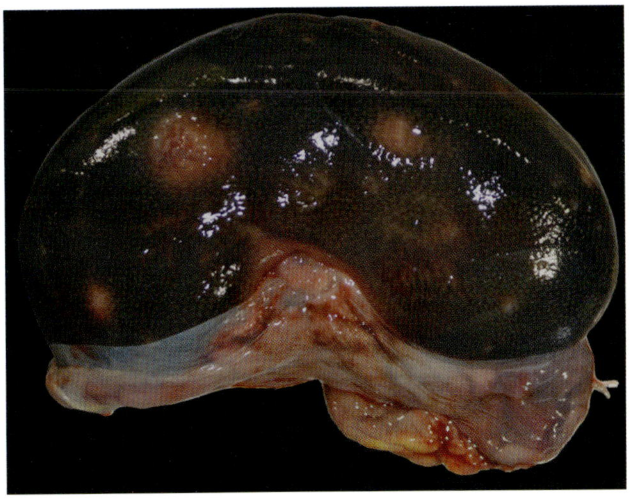

• **Fig. 20.17** Deer kidney. Multifocal, variably sized tan nodular foci are visible on the capsular surface of the kidney. Evenly distributed small white circular regions represent glomeruli. (Courtesy Kelley Steury, Auburn, AL.)

Evaluate the urinary bladder and collect urine if indicated for culture or toxicology testing. The color of the urine (red brown to brown) can help determine the potential for capture myopathy, copper toxicity, or other hemolytic diseases. Quantifying compounds to determine if a deer died from excess anesthetic administered by dart or if there was an adverse reaction to anesthetic may be requested despite our inability to provide a clear answer in these cases. A few laboratories perform illicit drug testing on tissues and urine, and it is always beneficial to call in advance to make sure you have the correct samples saved. Finally, evaluate the urinary bladder for uroliths. If uroliths are present in the urinary bladder or there are other changes as described previously, evaluate the urethra, particularly the penile urethra at the sigmoid flexure and vermiform process for presence of uroliths. Submit uroliths from any location in the urogenital tract for analysis to determine if they are diet related, as is typical, or if they could be due to excess minerals, particularly calcium from a water source.

Causes of death associated with genital tract lesions are typically related to urinary blockage in bucks, rams, or wethers or endometritis, pregnancy toxemia, or dystocia in does and ewes. However, evaluation of testicles in bucks and rams may be warranted for farms having problems with infertility or screening for agents like *Brucella ovis*. Death due to hemorrhage following castration can occasionally happen, and hemorrhage can occur in the scrotum or abdomen depending on retraction of the vessel. In pregnant does or ewes, measurement of the fetus or fetuses and determination of sex is recommended even if not determined to be the cause of death as this may be of interest to the owner. Additionally, gestational age and number of fetuses may make pregnancy toxemia a more or less likely diagnosis. Assessing the non-pregnant uterus, particularly if enlarged, can be helpful for determining time since parturition as well as for potential infections (see Chapter 8).

Abortions

Abortions are some of the most frustrating cases for pathologists, veterinarians, and owners alike. Many times (often over 50%), abortion cases have no diagnosis. Reasons for no diagnosis can vary and may include submission of inappropriate samples, including lack of placenta, abortions due to toxic plants, or abortions due to maternal factors such as stress or disease. A definitive diagnosis is also less likely with a single abortion versus multiple abortions on a farm. However, even with no definitive diagnosis, information can be gained from submission of an abortion, and various infectious agents or other factors can be ruled out. As stated previously, necropsy of an aborted goat or sheep fetus should include additional PPE. Most fetuses have some fluid in the abdomen and thoracic cavity and are often a dark red color. Additional steps to take when necropsying a fetus include measuring from crown to rump, weighing if possible, estimation of gestational age, noting presence or absence of meconium staining, and noting whether lungs sink in formalin (determines if a breath was taken). Collection of blood or thoracic fluid for serologic tests is particularly helpful in a fetus. Collection of maternal blood and testing are also recommended. Additional samples in a fetus to take for microscopic examination include tongue, muscle, diaphragm, umbilicus along with umbilical arteries and vein, skin and/or eyelid, and placenta if available. Evaluation of thyroids for enlargement (goiter) is recommended. Submission of tissues for bacteriology includes typical samples of liver, lung, kidney, ± spleen as well as placenta and abomasal fluid. Abomasal fluid in a fetus best mimics the fetal environment with the least amount of contamination and is particularly helpful if no placenta is available. Collection of abomasal fluid using a needle and syringe prior to opening will prevent any iatrogenic contamination. Special cultures should be requested for *Brucella*, *Listeria*, *Campylobacter*, and *Salmonella*, as these require special media. Capability of testing for *Leptospira* spp., *Chlamydia*, and *Toxoplasma gondii* varies by laboratory, and contacting the laboratory to determine appropriate samples to submit is recommended. Some laboratories rely on serology, while others have the capability for PCR on tissues. Submission of spleen, lung, liver, and placenta for virology/molecular is recommended. Submission of liver, kidney, aqueous, and vitreous humor for toxicology is also recommended, particularly to test for nitrate toxicity or selenium deficiency. Nitrate levels are slightly higher in fetuses and neonates than adults, and this must be taken into consideration during interpretation of results.[9,10] See Table 20.2 for additional information regarding collection of samples at necropsy for an abortion (see Chapter 8).

Evaluation of the GI Tract

Evaluation of the esophagus is done along with the pluck, as described earlier.

Note if there are any abnormalities along the GI tract serosa by examining each segment from the duodenum to the terminal colon. If there is diarrhea or a history of GI disease, a more detailed tissue collection protocol of the GI tract should be followed. Dependent on the personal preference of the individual performing the necropsy, the small intestine is pulled ventrally toward the pathologist while cutting the mesenteric attachments along the entire length. Incise the cranial duodenum, compress the gallbladder, and look for bile duct patency at the major duodenal papillae along the serosal aspect of the duodenum. Transect at the cranial (orad) duodenum (in ruminants). Push terminal colonic content cranially to avoid spillage into the abdomen, then transect the terminal colon. Remove the small intestine to terminal colon and set aside until last. Incise the intestine and look for intraluminal hemorrhage, pseudomembranes, obstructions, and parasites. Isolate the ileum by identifying entry into the cecum and collect ileocecal lymph node for histopathology and culture if enlarged. A segment of ileum should be collected for histopathology and Johne's culture if clinical history fits. Sheep and goats may not show gross evidence of mucosal thickening like cattle but may still be positive for *M. avium* subspecies *paratuberculosis*. Some laboratories may not perform Johne's cultures for sheep and goats, so calling ahead before sending the sample is advised. Samples can also be requested to be sent to the National Veterinary Services Laboratory (NVSL) for PCR and semiquantitative results regarding shedding. Ileum is a valuable area for tissue collection due to Peyer's patches and the affinity of some organisms, such as *Salmonella* spp., to invade the ileal mucosa. Coccidiosis can cause thickening and irregular nodular lesions in

TABLE 20.2 Additional Samples and Specific Testing in Aborted Fetuses.[16] *(see Chapter 19)*

Test Section	Samples	Test	Comments
Histopathology	As in Table 20.1 Also collect: diaphragm, tongue, skeletal muscle, placenta, conjunctiva	Microscopic examination	Adequate sections of brain and skeletal muscle can aid in diagnosis of *Toxoplasma* abortions Microscopic lesions may only be present in the placenta with abortions (include both cotyledonary and intercotyledonary areas)
Bacteriology	Abomasal fluid Placenta Lung, liver, kidney, spleen	Cultures: Aerobic Salmonella Listeria Brucella Campylobacter Fungal	Abomasal fluid most closely mimics the fetal environment with the least contamination and should be collected with a sterile needle and syringe
Molecular/virology	As in Table 20.1 Also collect placenta	PCR for viruses, *Leptospira* spp., chlamydia	Spleen is particularly important
Serology	Serum or thoracic fluid from fetus Maternal serum	Viral titers Brucella and Leptospira titers	All titers should be interpreted in light of vaccination status
Toxicology	Liver Aqueous humor	Selenium Nitrate	Nitrate levels are normally higher in fetus/neonates than adults[9]

PCR, Polymerase chain reaction.

the small intestine and colon and *Oesophagostomum* spp. can cause nodular lesions along the serosa. In young animals, Peyer's patches may be prominent and visible through the intestinal serosa, which is a normal finding. Distal colon fecal content should be collected and placed in a fecal cup for parasitology for sheep, goats, and captive white-tailed deer. Parasitology samples should be taken from the most distal portion of GI with contents if no feces are present in the colon. Even young captive-raised fawns can have an unexpected level of parasitism (Cryptosporidium, *Strongyloides* spp.), and adult captive deer with *Haemonchus* spp.–associated mortality can be a surprise to some owners (see Chapter 6).

Forestomachs and Abomasum

Evaluation of the forestomachs and abomasum is often performed toward the end of the necropsy procedure due to the potential for spillage of ruminal or abomasal content into the necropsy field. The serosa of all four tissues should be evaluated for areas of hemorrhage, edema, congestion, or serosal abscesses. Evaluate rumen size and content. Postmortem bloat is common, but a full rumen with liquid contents is suggestive of rumen acidosis. A screening test for rumen acidosis can be done in the field with pH paper. Rumen pH will rise slightly and then fall back to the initial pH during the 24 hours following death, documented in cattle.[11] Therefore, rumen acidosis may still be present in an animal with borderline pH. Submission of rumen for histopathology along with pH is critical for determining whether acute rumen acidosis resulting in death is present or if subacute rumen acidosis is present. A high rumen pH can also increase the suspicion for ammonia/urea toxicity, leading to further testing. Luminal inspection of all mucosal surfaces should be performed after feed content has been removed. Ruminal content is required for insecticide testing, and this is also a recommended specimen for botulism testing (other recommended samples for botulism include fecal, GI, and feed samples). Areas of reddening involving the rumen, and possibly other forestomachs, may be suggestive of EHD in deer. Sloughing of rumen mucosa is common with autolysis and should not be confused as a lesion. In neonates, evaluation for milk curd is critical, particularly as some laboratories may not be able to perform immunoglobulin G testing on serum from species other than cattle. Close inspection of the abomasal mucosa for nematode worms should be performed in all sheep, goats, and deer. If nematodes are not readily visible, abomasal content should be placed in a small foam tray or disposable dish and mixed with water, and this often helps remove feed material to see the worms as in Figure 20.18. If the animal is particularly anemic, the worms may be mostly white, lacking the characteristic barber pole appearance, and difficult to see.[10] Additionally, owners may deworm animals near death, so worms may not be present even in an animal with characteristic lesions (emaciation, tricavitary effusion, edema, serous atrophy of fat, and thin blood) for *Haemonchus* spp. infection. We often see a prominent vascular pattern with central red foci surrounded by circumscribed pale zones (nutmeg liver) with long-standing parasitism due to centrilobular hepatic congestion and necrosis, which is interpreted as centrilobular hypoxic damage due to anemia (see Chapter 5).

Evaluation of the Central Nervous System

The right limb has already been reflected dorsally. If not, reflecting a limb will facilitate removal of the head. Remove skin on the back of the neck. Cut behind the caudal aspect of both ears and

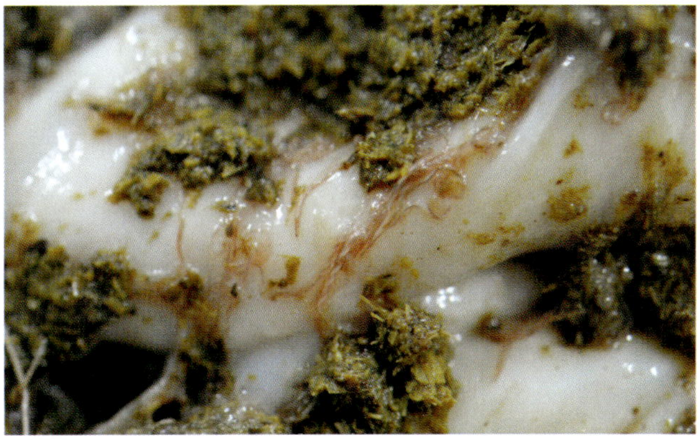

• **Fig. 20.18** Goat abomasum. Feed is intermixed with *Haemonchus* adults. (Courtesy of Dr John Roberts, University of Florida, College of Veterinary Medicine)

leave ears intact and attached to the head. Continue deeper cuts through the cervical musculature behind the vertical ramus of the mandible. Continue cutting musculature behind the base of each ear until you reach the ventral atlanto-occipital membrane between the occipital condyles rostrally and the facets of the atlas caudally. Then, cut through the dura, transect the spinal cord, and disarticulate at the atlanto-occipital joint.

To remove the brain whole, the skin overlying the cranium to the rostral nasal cavity will have to be removed, but leave the ears and associated skin. Using a hand saw or ax, follow the natural landmarks around the cranial vault to cut a semicircle around the edges of the skull bilaterally and coursing cranially to connect the two lateral cut sides with a cut in the occipital bone at the rostral brain behind the eye (distance behind the eye depends on the species). After the calvarium is pried upward from the underlying brain, evaluate, and then remove the dura mater. There will be tight attachments of dura mater that can be cut from the inner aspect of the cranium, between the cerebral hemispheres (falx cerebri), and between the cerebrum and caudal cerebral hemispheres (tentorium cerebelli).[12] The head can be tilted in a ventral to dorsal orientation, and gravity should help the prosector transect cranial nerves and any attachments to the skull. The sulci of the cerebrum should be evaluated for cloudiness or a hint of exudate. In some cases, close examination is not required, as in Figure 20.19, which shows a brain abscess in a captive white-tailed deer buck. Most brain abscesses in bucks are associated with fighting, and there may also be abscessation of the base of the antler. Many diseases causing neurologic signs like polioencephalomalacia, meningeal worm, listeria, viral encephalitis, or even septic meningitis may have no or extremely subtle gross lesions.[10]

If examination of the brain is warranted based on clinical signs, but an ax or handsaw is not available, the head can be removed as described earlier and submitted to a diagnostic laboratory for evaluation. Alternatively, a brain spoon used primarily for collection for CWD or scrapie samples can be used to collect at least a portion of the brain. With this method, cerebral cortex would not be available for evaluation for polioencephalomalacia, but evaluation for *Listeria monocytogenes* infection and, possibly, meningitis may still be accomplished. Removal of the spinal cord is difficult and time-consuming but can be completely by removing muscle overlying the spinous processes of the vertebrae and cutting on either side of the dorsal spinous process with the saw. Some diseases, such as enzootic ataxia (caused by copper deficiency) or meningeal worm, may primarily affect the spinal cord.

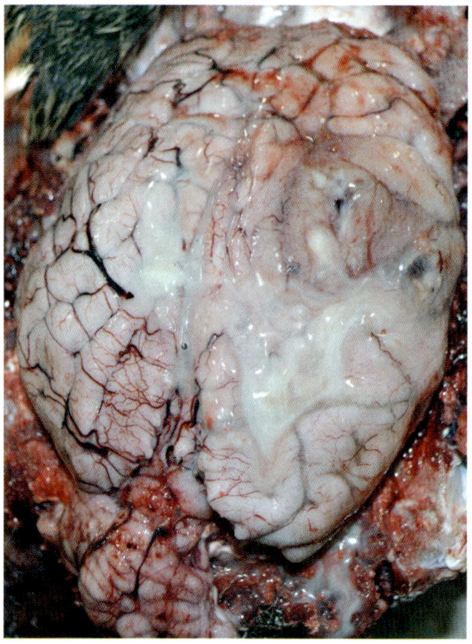

• **Fig. 20.19** Captive deer buck. Thick purulent exudate covers the leptomeninges and escapes from a few discrete gray to tan abscesses. (Courtesy Kelley Steury, Auburn, AL.)

Alternatively, at least a small piece of cervical spinal cord can be removed where the head was removed by cutting the dura and cutting with a scalpel or brain spoon (see Chapter 13).

Rabies Tissue Collection

Since some rabies cases may not have widespread viral antigen and spread may be unilateral, a complete cross-section of the brainstem is required.[13] A full cross-section of fresh brainstem can be collected at the level of the pons, medulla, or midbrain. Other brain sections necessary for rabies testing include cerebellum and hippocampus. Cerebellum and brainstem provide the greatest amount of diagnostic value, but the hippocampus can be evaluated if the cerebellum is not present in the submission. Freezing is not recommended for rabies samples, and transport to the laboratory within 48 hours is preferred.

CWD Tissue Collection

The Animal Plant Health Inspection Service (APHIS) CWD Herd Certification Program[14] requires brainstem with obex and both medial retropharyngeal lymph nodes, and samples must be submitted within 7 days of collection. Testing for CWD should be done in any deer over 1 year of age.

The APHIS Sampling Procedure for obex is as follows[14]:

1. Incise the head at the atlanto-occipital joint. Cut behind the back of the ears and extend the incision around and through the front of the larynx. During this process, cut the brainstem caudally as much as possible.
2. Position the head ventrally and the brainstem will be visible caudally within the foramen magnum and bordered laterally by the occipital condyles. Trim the dura mater circumferentially around the brainstem and cut attached cranial nerve trunks.
3. Carefully lift the brainstem with forceps and insert the spoon into the dorsal aspect of the foramen magnum between the brainstem and dorsal calvarium.
4. Advance the spoon 2 to 3 inches rostrally until it contacts bone and the cerebellum is severed.

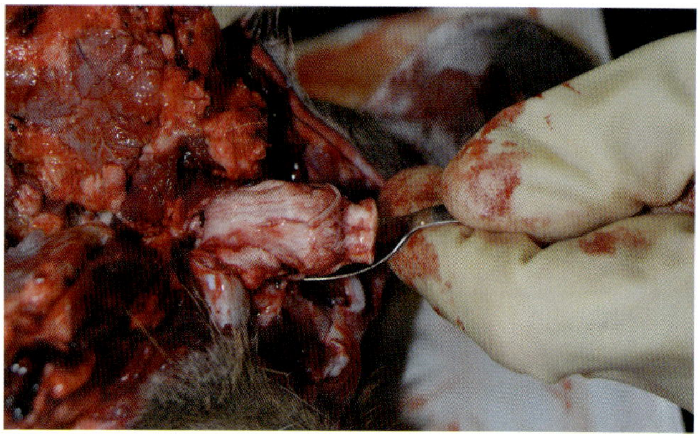

• **Fig. 20.20** Brainstem is being removed with a brain spoon. The brain spoon is inserted dorsally within the foramen magnum, and the spoon is pushed rostrally between the brainstem and the dorsal calvarium.

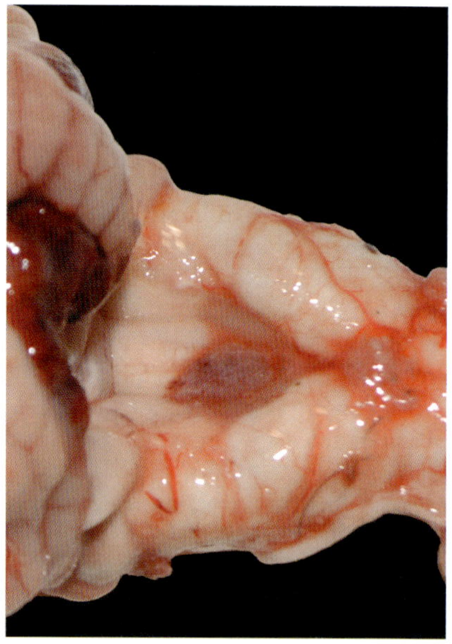

• **Fig. 20.21** High magnification of brainstem with obex. Obex is a delicate layer of connective tissue found at the V-shaped bifurcation of the brainstem, located between the medulla oblongata and the spinal cord. Paired dorsal motor nuclei of the vagus nerve are found in the obex.

5. Reposition the spoon in the ventral aspect of the foramen magnum between the brainstem and ventral calvarium. Advance the spoon until it contacts bone and severs the brainstem transversely.
6. Using the spoon and forceps, remove the brainstem with the brain spoon (Figure 20.20) and examine for the presence of the Y-shaped bifurcation with connective tissue (obex) (Figure 20.21).
7. For adequate fixation, trim the brainstem by cutting transversely 3/4 inch in front of the bifurcation, and also an equal distance behind the bifurcation.
8. While the head is positioned with the ventral side up, a portion of trachea and larynx (approximately 1 inch, depending on the initial cut) may need to be removed, as well as some fascia and fat, to see the medial retropharyngeal lymph nodes and permit for removal of both lymph nodes (Figure 20.22).

Testing options are dependent on the laboratory that will be used for the submission, and only APHIS/National Animal Health Laboratory Network–approved laboratories at state or federal

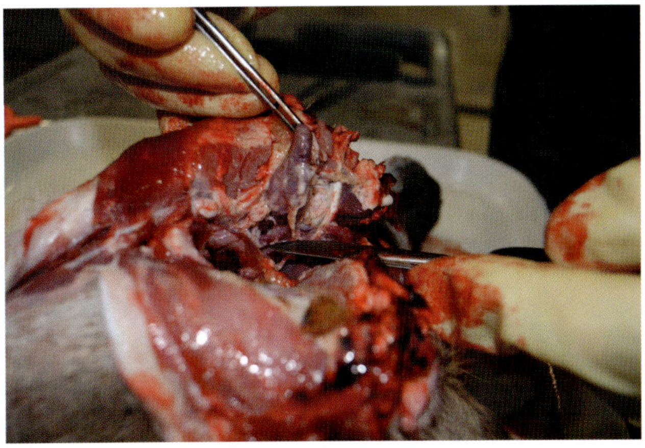

• **Fig. 20.22** One medial retropharyngeal lymph node is being removed in the photo.

TABLE 20.3 CWD Testing Sample Requirements (Including Updated CWD Herd Certification Information, Fall 2018).[14]

POSTMORTEM TISSUES TO BE SUBMITTED	
Fresh Samples	**Formalin-Fixed Samples**
For ELISA, DNA analysis, Western blot	For histopathology, IHC
Single container/each animal	Single container/each animal
Chilled or frozen	Do not freeze
Skin (ear or hide attached to ear tag; quarter-size, approx. 1 × 1 inch)	None
One-half of each medial retropharyngeal lymph node	One-half of each medial retropharyngeal lymph node
One-half obex with 1–2 cm brainstem	One-half obex with 1–2 cm brainstem
Tonsils are optional	Tonsils are optional

CWD, Chronic wasting disease; *ELISA*, enzyme-linked immunosorbent assay; *IHC*, immunohistochemistry.

veterinary diagnostic laboratories or universities can perform testing. Accredited veterinarians should check with state and federal regulatory authorities for sample requirements and sample submission if samples will be collected from farmed deer or elk. Sample collection from hunter harvested deer can also be performed by accredited veterinarians, but coordination with the state wildlife agency or the state department of agriculture is recommended. Some laboratories perform ELISA, immunohistochemistry, or both. ELISA samples can be chilled or frozen. All CWD samples must be submitted with ear tags that have been removed from the animal, and a fresh section of skin (ear) is also required for the current CWD Herd Certification Program (Table 20.3).

Scrapie Tissue Collection in Sheep and Goats[15,10]

Testing should be done on any sheep or goat over 14 months of age. The sample collection procedure is dependent upon the presence or absence of clinical signs and if there is a history of exposure (Table 20.4). All submissions require the animal identification tags with a quarter-sized section of skin (ear, tail web tattoo) in formalin (USDA protocol).

TABLE 20.4 Scrapie Testing Sample Requirements (Based on Clinical Signs).[15,10]

Postmortem Tissues to Be Submitted for Routine Submissions: Animals With No Clinical Signs or History of Exposure
Formalin-fixed samples
For histopathology, IHC
Single container/each animal
Do not freeze
Entire brainstem with obex
One retropharyngeal lymph node
Cerebellum (2 g)
Skin (ear or hide attached to ear tag; quarter-size, approx. 1 × 1 inch)

Postmortem Tissues to Be Submitted: Animals With Known Exposure or Less Specific Clinical Signs	
Formalin-fixed samples	**Fresh samples**
For histopathology, IHC	For ELISA, DNA analysis, Western blot
Single container/each animal	Single container/each animal
Do not freeze	Chilled or frozen
Obex with 1–2 cm brainstem	Remainder of brainstem
One retropharyngeal lymph node	One retropharyngeal lymph node
Cerebellum (2 g)	Cerebellum, separate bag or container
Skin (ear or hide attached to ear tag; quarter-size, approx. 1 × 1 inch)	None
Tonsils (optional)	Tonsils

ELISA, Enzyme-linked immunosorbent assay; *IHC*, immunohistochemistry.

Routine submission for animals without clinical signs and no history of exposure requires formalin fixed tissues, to include 1 retropharyngeal lymph node, entire brainstem including obex, and cerebellum (approximately 2 g).

Animals that are exposed or have less specific clinical signs, such as being nonambulatory, being unthrifty, wool/hair loss suggestive of rubbing, biting at the legs or side, lip smacking, or intense rubbing without bare areas, requires submission of formalin fixed tissue and fresh tissue. The remainder of the brainstem, one retropharyngeal lymph node, one tonsil, and the cerebellum are submitted fresh.

If the sheep or goat is also a rabies suspect, please contact the diagnostic laboratory or state animal health animal official for recommendations since rabies testing protocols vary by state.

Diseases and Necropsy Findings

See Table 20.5 for select diseases and findings at necropsy in captive white-tailed deer in the southeastern United States, Table 20.6 for select diseases in sheep and goats and findings at necropsy, and Table 20.7 for diseases that may have no gross findings at necropsy.

TABLE 20.5 Select Diseases in Captive White-Tailed Deer in the Southeastern United States. *Clinical Presentation or Disease, Findings at Necropsy, Potential Etiologies*

DISEASES IN CAPTIVE WHITE-TAILED DEER IN THE SOUTHEASTERN UNITED STATES		
Clinical presentation or Disease	**Findings at Necropsy**	**Etiology(ies) and Comments**
Sudden death (especially late summer and fall)[a]	Hemorrhages on serosa of rumen and intestines and epicardium, pulmonary edema, large, pulpy spleen with capsular hemorrhages, intestinal hemorrhage	Epizootic hemorrhagic disease virus (EHDV) or bluetongue virus
Pneumonia[a]	Fibrin coating the lungs, dark red meaty cranioventral lung lobes ± abscesses or thoracic fluid	*Pasteurella multocida, Trueperella pyogenes, Bibersteinia trehalosi, Mannheimia haemolytica, Mycoplasma* spp., *Fusobacterium necrophorum*, or *Fusobacterium varum*[6]
	Marked enlargement of a single lung lobe, extensive fibrosis and green to yellow on cut section	Fungal, NOS, may have generalized thickening of metatarsals (hypertrophic osteopathy)
Haemonchus infection (emaciation, anemia)[a]	Subcutaneous edema, tricavitary effusion (yellow, serous), serous atrophy of fat, nematode worms in abomasum, nutmeg liver (centrilobular necrosis)	*Haemonchus* spp. Pneumonia, other chronic diseases, and poor dentition or husbandry can also result in emaciation
Brain abscess	Broken antler, subcutaneous edema, pus, fibrin in area of antler, pus in the brain	Fighting
Trauma	Subcutaneous hemorrhages/edema, puncture wounds, broken neck, fractures	Fighting Running into fences
Capture myopathy[4]	Skeletal muscle or myocardial hemorrhage, muscle pallor (necrosis) or mineralization, brown urine May only be microscopic lesions (multiorgan necrosis) in peracute cases	Darting/handling Being chased
Rumen acidosis[a]	Distended fluid-filled rumen, possible areas or red or black on the mucosa, pH < 5.5, ± abscesses in liver	Excess grain or carbohydrates
Diarrhea in fawns[a]	Fecal staining of perineum, no formation of fecal pellets, watery contents in small intestine	Parasites: *Strongyloides*, *Cryptosporidium*, Coccidia Rotavirus *Escherichia coli* or other bacteria
	Pseudomembranes, luminal casts	*Salmonella* spp.
Malignant catarrhal fever	High mortality in herd (50%) May have no gross lesions Microscopic lesions of lymphoproliferation and vasculitis (brain, liver, lung, kidney)	Ovine herpes virus 2 Caprine herpes virus 2 Alcelaphaline herpes virus 1 and 2 Malignant catarrhal fever virus of white-tailed deer
Neonatal death[a]	Reddening or pus around the umbilicus/umbilical arteries/veins Redding or possible exudate meninges, swollen joints with thin fluid, fibrin, or pus, cloudy eyes, possible pinpoint white foci: lung, liver, kidney	Failure of passive transfer *E. coli* and other bacteria

NOS, Not otherwise specified.
[a]Diseases that commonly occur in goats and sheep as well.

TABLE 20.6 Select Diseases in Sheep and Goats, not Otherwise Described in Table 20.5. *Clinical Signs and/or Disease, Findings at Necropsy, and Etiology(ies)/Comments*

DISEASES IN SHEEP AND GOATS		
Clinical presentation and/or Disease	**Findings at Necropsy**	**Etiology(ies)/Comments**
Diarrhea in an adult, weight loss (Johne's disease)	Thickening of small intestine, particularly ileum, Enlarged ileocecal lymph node ± Tan nodules in liver Findings associated with emaciation as in Table 20.5	*Mycobacterium avium* spp. *paratuberculosis*
Diarrhea, may be bloody (coccidiosis)	Thickened small intestine/colon with irregular raised nodules in the mucosa	*Eimeria* spp.

TABLE 20.6 Select Diseases in Sheep and Goats, not Otherwise Described in Table 20.5. *Clinical Signs and/or Disease, Findings at Necropsy, and Etiology(ies)/Comments—cont'd*

DISEASES IN SHEEP AND GOATS		
Clinical presentation and/or Disease	**Findings at Necropsy**	**Etiology(ies)/Comments**
Copper toxicity	Generalized icterus, thin anemic blood, yellow-orange liver, "gun metal grey kidneys," brown urine	Sheep especially susceptible (decreased ability to excrete copper in bile)[17]
Pregnancy toxemia	Yellow fatty liver, may float in formalin, pregnant with twins or triplets, excess body fat	Twins or triplets with excess body fat
Hemorrhagic enteritis	Bloody intestinal contents, dark red intestinal serosa and mucosa	*Clostridium perfringens* type C or A (also causes yellow lamb disease, can be normal gastrointestinal inhabitant), associated with diet changes and excess carbohydrates[18]
Urinary blockage	Distended urinary bladder with hemorrhages mucosa/serosa, thickening of wall with edema, urolith in penile urethra	Submit uroliths for analysis
Caseous lymphadenitis	Enlarged lymph nodes, particularly in cervical region with white pasty or crumbly material	*Corynebacterium pseudotuberculosis*
Contagious ecthyma	Vesicles, ulcers, proliferative lesions muzzle, oral cavity, teats, possible rumen lesions[19]	Parapoxvirus Zoonotic
Lentiviral pneumonia	Wet heavy white to gray lungs, rubbery, do not collapse, rib impressions	Small ruminant lentivirus[3]
Thymoma	Mass mediastinum or ventral cervical region (can be cystic), yellow or red tinged thoracic fluid	Common tumor in some goat breeds[20]
Lymphoma	Enlarged lymph nodes, soft, white masses multiple organs (liver, kidney, lung, etc.)	Most common tumor in goats in one study Can be associated with bovine leukemia virus[8]
Nutritional myopathy	Skeletal muscle or myocardial pallor with pinpoint white gritty foci (mineralization)	Vitamin E/selenium deficiency

TABLE 20.7 Diseases That May Have No Gross Necropsy Lesions.

Disease (organism)	Notes
Tetanus *(Clostridium tetani)*	Diagnosis based on clinical signs and supporting lesions such as wounds (may or may not be present), recent castration, etc.
Listeriosis *(Listeria monocytogenes)*	Diagnosis requires brainstem, may see red pinpoint foci at necropsy, special culture requirements, characteristic microscopic lesions
Meningeal worm *(Parelaphostrongylus tenuis)*[22]	Microscopic lesions may only be present in spinal cord
Meningitis (various bacteria causing sepsis)	May or may not see exudate in meninges; culturing multiple organs and umbilicus may help identify entry point
Encephalitis (lentiviruses, West Nile virus,[23] eastern equine encephalitis virus[24])	Differentiation may require additional testing like PCR and/or serology
Rabies	Zoonotic, use additional PPE, may submit whole head to diagnostic laboratory or department of public health
Polioencephalomalacia	Requires cerebral cortex for microscopic diagnosis; causes include sulfur toxicity (can test levels in food or water), lead toxicity (test kidney), thiamine deficiency, ingestion of thiaminase-containing plants, overgrowth of thiaminase-producing bacteria (concurrent rumen acidosis), salt toxicity/water intoxication
Focal symmetric encephalomalacia (*Clostridium perfringens* type D)	Often no signs of enteritis; "pulpy kidneys" likely represent rapid postmortem autolysis, toxin detection in intestinal contents[18]

Continued

TABLE 20.7 **Diseases That May Have No Gross Necropsy Lesions.—cont'd**

Disease (organism)	Notes
Toxins (insecticides, ammonia/urea, nitrate, cyanide, etc.)	Submit rumen contents, liver, kidney, aqueous humor, and vitreous humor in cases of suspected toxicity, high rumen pH > 7.5 (ammonia toxicity), chocolate brown blood (nitrate)
Botulism *(Clostridium botulinum)*	Can test gastrointestinal contents or feed
Anthrax *(Bacillus anthracis)*	Zoonotic, blood for diagnosis, "bloody" fluid from nostrils not due to anthrax infection common in autolyzed animals during the summer
Lightning strike	Diagnosis may be more circumstantial based on sudden death in relation to reported storms and excluding other causes, may see singed hair
Mineral imbalances (calcium, magnesium, selenium, etc.)	Submit liver, kidney, aqueous humor, and vitreous humor for testing
CWD/scrapie	See Tables 20.3 and 20.4

CWD, Chronic wasting disease; *PCR*, polymerase chain reaction; *PPE*, personal protective equipment.

Carcass Disposal

The Food and Drug Administration now regulates rendering plants for barbiturates in the raw materials stream. Due to the risk for scrapie in sheep and goats and the potential for CWD in deer, these species cannot be rendered (regulation details may depend on the individual rendering company and state). The ideal method of disposal is chemical digestion, but incineration is an alternative. If the animal is identified as positive for scrapie or CWD, retrieval of the carcass for chemical digestion is indicated. Deep burial with ear tags is recommended in case CWD is detected. Retrieval of carcasses from the landfill is problematic, and prior to disposal all carcasses should be held until scrapie and CWD results have been received.

Packaging Samples for Shipment

Formalin fixed tissues should be submitted in a wide necked container approved for use with formalin. Sealing the lid with paraffin wrap or masking tape can also reduce the likelihood of spills. All fresh tissues should be placed in leak-proof bags such as a Whirl-Pak and double bagged. If submitting breakable items such as serum tubes, wrapping the tubes in paper towels or other padded/absorbent material and enclosing within a Whirl-Pak or Ziplock bag is recommended. Overnight transport of fresh samples is vital for adequate tissue preservation, and overnight shipping also helps reduce issues with samples decaying on the mail carrier's truck or at the postal facility over a weekend. Even with overnight transport, multiple ice packs are required to cool the specimen in an insulated container, especially during warm months. External packaging should be sufficient that contents should not leak outside the container. Filling most of the available space in the insulated container with ice packs is recommended during summer months, as we have seen that one to two small ice packs do not sufficiently cool specimens during summer months. Virology and PCR samples can be frozen prior to transport, but it is important that samples requiring bacterial culture remain at a temperature close to refrigeration prior and during transport. Some fungal agents can be difficult to isolate if refrigerated (Pythium and some Zygomycetes). It is also beneficial to place submission forms in a separate leak-proof plastic bag (Ziplock bag).

References

1. Passler T, Ditchkoff SS, Walz PH: Bovine viral diarrhea virus in white-tailed deer (*Odocoileus virginianus*), *Front Microbiol* 7:945, 2016.
2. Osweiler GD: *Toxicology: the national veterinary medical series for independent study*, Ch. 4, Philadelphia, PA, 1996, Williams & Wilkins, pp 37–40, 1996.
3. Centers for Disease Control, Protocol for Postmortem Diagnosis of Rabies in Animals by Direct Fluorescent Antibody Testing. A Minimum Standard for Rabies Diagnosis in the United States. Electronic Material. Available at: https://www.cdc.gov/rabies/pdf/rabiesdfapv2/pdf.
4. Wolfe, BA: Bovidae (except sheep and goats) and Antilocapridae. In Miller RE, Fowler ME, editors: *Fowler's zoo and wild animal medicine*, ed 8, vol 8, Ch. 63, St. Louis, Missouri, USA, 2019, Elsevier Inc., pp 626–644.
5. Hill, JA, Fubini, SL, Hackett, RP: Clinical features, treatment, and outcome in goats with thymomas: 13 cases (1990–2014), *J Am Vet Med Assoc* 251(7):829–834, 2017.
6. Brooks JW, Kumar A, Narayanan S, et al: Characterization of Fusobacterium isolates from the respiratory tract of white-tailed deer (*Odocoileus virginianus*), *J Vet Diagn Invest* 26(2):213–220, 2014.
7. Robinson WF, Robinson NA: Cardiovascular system. In Maxie MG, editor: *Jubb, Kennedy and Palmer's pathology of domestic animals*, ed 6, vol 3, Ch. 1, London, UK, 2016, Saunders, An Imprint of Elsevier, pp 12–13.
8. Valli, VEO, Kiupel, M, Bienzle, D: Hematopoietic system. In Maxie MG, editor: *Jubb, Kennedy, and Palmer's pathology of domestic animals*, ed 6, vol 3, Ch. 2, London, UK, 2016, Saunders, An Imprint of Elsevier, pp 12–13.
9. Yang, D, Lang U, Greenberg SG, et al: Elevation of nitrate levels in pregnant ewes and their fetuses, *Am J Obstet Gynecol* 174(2): 573–577, 1996.
10. Roberts, JF: Chapter 20, in In Pugh DG, Baird AN, editors: *Sheep and goat medicine*, ed 2, Kansas City, Maryland Heights, MO, 2012, Elsevier.
11. Löhr, CV: One hundred two tumors in 100 goats (1987–2011), *Vet Pathol* 50(4):668–685, 2013.
12. Caswell JL, Williams KJ: Respiratory system. In Maxie MG, editor: *Jubb, Kennedy, Palmer's pathology of domestic animals*, ed 6, vol 2, Philadelphia, PA: 2016, Elsevier, pp 558–559.
13. Cullen, JM and Stalker, MJ: Liver and biliary system. In Maxie MG, editor: *Jubb, Kennedy, and Palmer's pathology of domestic animals*, ed 6, vol 2, ch. 1, 2016, pp. 258–352.

14. Animal Plant Health Inspection Service (APHIS): *CWD Herd Certification Program, CFR-2016*, vol 1, 2016, title 9, part 55.
15. USDA, Animal and Plant Health Inspection Service: *Scrapie*, Jul 11, 2017. Available at: https://www.aphis.usda.gov/aphis/ourfocus/animalhealth/nvap/NVAP-Reference-Guide/Control-and-Eradication/Scrapie.
16. Moeller RB Jr: Disorders of sheep and goats. In Njaa BL, editor: Ch. 3 *Kirkbride's diagnosis of abortion and neonatal loss in animals*, ed 4, Hoboken, New Jersey, USA, 2012, John Wiley & Sons, Ltd.
17. Dobey, CL, Grunenwald C, Newman SJ, et al: Retrospective study of central nervous system lesions and association with *Parelaphostrongylus* species by histology and specific nested polymerase chain reaction in domestic camelids and wild ungulates, *J Vet Diagn Invest* 26(6):748–754, 2014.
18. Uzal, FA, Songer JG: Diagnosis of *Clostridium perfringens* intestinal infections in sheep and goats, *J Vet Diagn Invest* 20(3):253–265, 2008.
19. Uzal, FA, Plattner, BL, Hostetter, JM: Alimentary system. In Maxie MG, editor: *Jubb, Kennedy, and Palmer's pathology of domestic animals*, ed 6, vol 2, Ch. 1, London, UK, 2016, Saunders, An Imprint of Elsevier, pp 1–257.
20. Lee TL, Thomson DU, Wileman BW: Stability of rumen pH measurements obtained postmortem, *Bov Pract* 45(1):52–56, 2011.
21. Mason GL, Madden DJ: Performing the field necropsy examination, In Callan, RJ, editor: *Veterinary clinics of North America, food animal practice, ruminant diagnostic medicine*, vol 23, no. 3, Philadelphia, PA, Nov. 2007, Elsevier Inc.
22. Edwards, GT, Woodger NG, Barlow AM, et al: Sarcina-like bacteria associated with bloat in young lambs and calves, *Vet Rec* 163(13): 391–393, 2008.
23. Rimoldi, G, Mete A, Adaska JM, et al: West Nile virus infection in sheep, *Vet Pathol* 54(1):155–158, 2017.
24. Schmitt SM, Cooley TM, Fitzgerald SD, et al: An outbreak of Eastern equine encephalitis virus in free-ranging white-tailed deer in Michigan, *J Wildl Dis* 43(4):635–644, 2007.

Appendix 1

Commonly Used Drugs and Veterinary Feed Directive in Sheep, Goats, and Cervids

Virginia R. Fajt, Kenneth R. Brown, and David G. Pugh

Drug and Dosages

Some of the drugs and uses listed in this appendix may be illegal, unavailable, or extra-label in the United States or other countries. It is the responsibility of attending veterinarians to be familiar with the laws governing drugs in their practice areas. The clinician should therefore be cognizant of, and take steps to reduce, drug residues in food animals.

If a dose is provided only for sheep and not for goats or cervids, unless the drug appears to be contraindicated or toxic to goats or cervids, the sheep dose usually can be extrapolated for use in goats or cervids, or vice versa. Some of the dosages listed here are the same as seen in other chapters and are referenced as such. After reviewing Chapter 18, where dosages for anesthetics appear different, the clinician can then compare the two, and decide the best dosage for the situation based on referenced materials (Table 1).

In an effort to provide an evidence-based approach and confidence level for the dosages presented in this Appendix, superscripted alphabets[a–d] have been included to indicate the level of support for each dosage recommendation. Based on the GRADE approach to assessing the strength of a recommendation, type of study and quality of the study are assimilated to provide an overall assessment.[1,2] The type of study leads to an initial assessment, because, for example, randomized controlled studies provide stronger evidence than case series due to likelihood of bias. Quality of study then modifies the strength of the study based on risk of bias, precision of effect estimates, and other internal and external validity factors.[3] All evidence assessments derive from an unpublished analysis of the data (by V.R.F) and have not been subjected to peer review. For some dosages, the cited references do not constitute the only evidence but rather are provided as examples of relevant published data. The presented levels of evidence are based only on the studies cited and should not be construed as clinical recommendations, because clinical recommendations also require balancing of adverse effects, costs, and client factors with the strength of evidence for efficacy.

Veterinary Feed Directive for Sheep, Goats, and Cervids

In the United States, the Food and Drug Administration (FDA) has undertaken steps to reduce the use of drugs in food and water fed to food-producing animals. Medically important antibiotics, as determined by the FDA, are now restricted in the use of feed and water and the effort is to eliminate the use of all such drugs when used in a production environment to improve growth or feed efficiency. The veterinarian is now primarily responsible for the judicious use of such drugs and for using them therapeutically and according to label limitations. The Veterinary Feed Directive (VFD) has become a major part of the FDA's effort to restrict antibiotic use in feed. The initial phase of investigation and education to enforce the rule, effective in 2015, has not moved into enforcement with the states being an active partner with the FDA in the enforcement effort; scrutiny at the distributor level will be expanded to include the veterinarian and the producer (end user of the VFD). Further information can be obtained at the FDA website, with specific attention given to GFI #120, GFI #231, GFI #233, and the Final VFD Rule.

The VFD Rule authorizes the use of VFD drugs as well as creates a framework to authorize veterinarians to use medically important antimicrobials in feed when needed for a specific, identified animal-health purpose. The framework includes the requirement that any VFD only be issued in the context of a valid veterinarian-client-patient-relationship (VCPR) and that this relationship includes the following elements with the client (producer) at a minimum: (1) assume responsibility to make decisions regarding animal health; (2) have sufficient knowledge of the patient by physical visits to the facility and examination of the patient; (3) provide for follow-up care if necessary. State VCPR requirements must also be followed and the FDA will defer to those requirements so long as they contain the minimum FDA requirements.

Currently, the following drugs when used alone or combined with other drugs and added to feed are VFD drugs (Table 2) and require a valid VFD order (the most current list can be found on the FDA website). VFD drugs cannot be used extra-label (actual or intended use of a drug in an animal in a manner that is not in accordance with the approved labeling).

The following drugs are not considered medically important and are not within the VFD limitations: ionophores such as monensin or lasalocid, bacitracin, bambermycins, and carbadox. In addition, drugs that are not antimicrobials are not limited by the VFD and include antithelmintics, beta agonists, and coccidiostats (including decoquinate).

The VFD itself is a written statement (not verbal) issued by a licensed veterinarian in the course of the veterinarian's professional

TABLE 1 **Some Drug Dosages.**

Drug	Sheep	Goats	Cervids
Abamectin			0.2 mg/kg[d4]
Acepromazine maleate	0.05–0.10 mg/kg IM[a5–7]	0.05–0.10 mg/kg IM[a5–8] 0.2 mg/kg IM tetany[d9]	0.05–0.10 mg/kg IM[b5]
Acetic acid (5% solution)	0.5–1.0 L/head PO for ammonia toxicosis[b10–12]	0.5–1.0 L/head PO for ammonia toxicosis[b10–12]	
Albendazole	7.5 mg/kg PO for flukes and nematodes[a13–15] 10 mg/kg PO for cestodes[b19]	7.5 mg/kg PO for nematodes[16–18] 10 mg/kg PO for flukes[a13] 10 mg/kg PO for cestodes[b19,20]	10 mg/kg PO for nematodes[c]
Alfaxalone	1.2–2.6 mg/kg IV for induction[c21,22]	1.75–3.0 mg/kg IV for induction[c23]	
Amikacin			7.5 mg/kg IM every 4–6 h[d24]
Ammonium chloride	0.5–1.0% of diet for prevention of urinary calculi[a25–32]	0.5–1.0% of diet for prevention of urinary calculi[a25–33]	
Ammonium molybdate	100 mg/head/day PO in combination with sodium sulfate to increase elimination of copper[a34–36]	300 mg/head/day PO in combination with sodium thiosulfate to increase elimination of copper[b37,38]	
Ammonium tetrathiomolybdate	3.4 mg/kg IV once daily for 4 days[b39,40]		
Amoxicillin-clavulanic acid	20 mg/kg (amoxicillin component) IV BID to TID[c41,42] 7 mg/kg IM for prevention of pneumonia[c43] 200 mg amoxicillin and 50 mg clavulanate per quarter IMM[c44]	20 mg/kg (amoxicillin component) IV BID to TID[c41,42] 200 mg amoxicillin and 50 mg clavulanate per quarter[c]IMM[45]	
Amoxicillin trihydrate	10 mg/kg IM BID to TID[c46,47]	10 mg/kg IM BID to TID[c46,47]	
Ampicillin sodium	10 mg/kg IV TID to QID[c46,48]	10 mg/kg IV TID to QID[c46,48]	
Ampicillin-sulbactam	13.3 mg/kg (ampicillin component) IM once a day or BID[c49]	13.3 mg/kg (ampicillin component) IM once a day or BID[c49]	
Ampicillin trihydrate	10 mg/kg IM[c50]	10 mg/kg IM[c50]	
Amprolium	50 mg/kg PO for 5 days for treatment[b51] 55 mg/kg PO BID for 21 days for treatment[b53] 15 mg/kg in feed for prevention[c58]	100 mg/kg PO for 5 days for treatment[b51,52] 50 mg/kg PO for 5 days[54,55] or 21 days for treatment[b56,57]	
Aspirin	100 mg/kg PO BID[c59–61]	100 mg/kg PO BID[c59–61]	
Atipamezole	0.1–0.2 mg/kg IV slowly[b62,63] 0.005 μg/kg IV slowly following intrathecal or subarachnoid alpha$_2$-agonists[b64,65]	0.1–0.2 mg/kg IV slowly[b62,63] 0.005 μg/kg IV slowly following intrathecal or subarachnoid alpha$_2$-agonists[b64,65]	
Atropine	0.05–0.2 mg/kg IV to prevent bradycardia during anesthesia[b66] 0.15–0.5 mg/kg IV for organophosphate toxicity[b67–69] (some recommendations are to give one-half to one-third of the dose IV and the rest IM or SC but there are no published data on the efficacy of this approach)	0.05–0.2 mg/kg IV to prevent bradycardia during anesthesia[b66] 0.15–0.5 mg/kg IV for organophosphate toxicity[b67–69] (some recommendations are to give one-half to one-third of the dose IV and the rest IM or SC but there are no published data on the efficacy of this approach)	
Azithromycin	20 mg/kg IV or IM[c70–73]	20 mg/kg IV or IM[c70–73]	
Buprenorphine	0.01–0.03 mg/kg IM every 6–8 h[b74–76] 0.5 mg/kg SC[c77] 6 μg/kg IV[c78]		

TABLE 1 Some Drug Dosages—cont'd.

Drug	Sheep	Goats	Cervids
Butorphanol	0.2–0.5 mg/kg IM or SC for sedation and analgesia[b7,77,79,80]	0.2–0.5 mg/kg IM for sedation and analgesia[b7,23,79,80] 0.1 mg/kg IV for reducing stress response[b81]	
Calcium borogluconate	50–100 mL of 20% solution IV or SC for hypocalcemia[b83–85]	50 to 100 mL of 20% solution IV or SC for hypocalcemia[b83–85]	
Calcium gluconate	11 mg/kg IV (approximately 1 g/200 lb) for hypocalcemia[b82]	11 mg/kg IV (approximately 1 g/200 lb) for hypocalcemia[b82]	
Carprofen	4 mg/kg SC or IM[a75,86–88] 8 mg/kg PO[c89]	4 mg/kg SC or IM[b75,86–88]	
Cefquinome	1–2 mg/kg IM once a day[c90–94]	1–2 mg/kg IM or IV once a day[c90–92,95–97]	
Ceftiofur crystalline-free acid	6.6 mg/kg SC in neck[b105]	6.6 mg/kg SC behind elbow or in neck[b106,107]	1–2.2 mg/kg IM every 24 h[d108]
Ceftiofur hydrochloride			3.6 mg/kg IM every 12 h[d98]
Ceftiofur sodium	1.0–2.2 mg/kg IM every 24 h [[a]for respiratory disease;[b] for all other indications][99–102]	1.0–2.2 mg/kg IM every 24 h [[a]for respiratory disease;[b] for all other indications][99–103]	2.5 mg/kg IM every 12 h[d104]
Cefuroxime	250 mg IMM every 12 h for 3 doses[c109]	250 mg IMM every 12 h for 3 doses[c110]	
Cephapirin benzathine	300 mg dry cow syringe intramammary in dry ewes[b111,112]	300 mg dry cow syringe intramammary in dry does[b113]	
Charcoal (activated)	500 g in 4 L of fluid[c114]	500 g in 4 L of fluid[c114]	
Chloral hydrate	100–150 mg/kg IV reported in calves[c115,116]		
Chlortetracycline	80 mg/head/day to reduce the incidence of abortion caused by susceptible *Campylobacter fetus*[c117,118]		
Clopidogrel	6 mg/kg PO loading dose first day, 3 mg/kg daily after loading[c119,120]	7 mg/kg PO loading dose first day, 3 mg/kg daily after loading[c119,120]	
Cloprostenol	100–125 µg IM at 7–11 day interval for estrus synchronization and for early pregnancy termination[a121–126]	100–125 µg IM at 7–11 day interval for estrus synchronization and for pregnancy termination[a121–124,127–129] 100 µg IM followed by 50 µg IM 10 h later for induction of parturition[b130]	100–500 µg IM[c131]
Clorsulon	7–21 mg/kg PO for flukes[b132–134]	7–15 mg/kg PO for flukes[b135,136]	
Clostantel	7.5–10 mg/kg PO for nematodes[b137–139] 10 mg/kg PO for flukes and *Oestrus ovis*[b140–143]	15 mg/kg PO for flukes[b144]	
Danofloxacin	6 mg/kg SC or IV q24h[b145,146]	6 mg/kg SC or IV q24h[b146,147]	
Decoquinate	0.5 mg/kg in feed for at least 28 days for prevention of coccidiosis[a148,149] 2 mg/kg in feed during pregnancy to prevent abortion and decrease lamb mortality caused by *Toxoplasma gondii*[b149,150]	0.5 mg/kg in feed for at least 28 days for prevention of coccidiosis[a148]	
Detomidine	0.01 mg/kg intrathecal[b64] 0.01–0.02 mg/kg IM[a152,154,155] 0.02 mg/kg IV followed by 0.60 mg/kg/hr CRI[b156]	0.01–0.04 mg/kg IM[a151–153]	

Continued

TABLE 1 Some Drug Dosages—cont'd.

Drug	Sheep	Goats	Cervids
Dexamethasone	15 mg IM for pregnancy termination[b157,158] 0.05–0.44 mg/kg IM as an anti-inflammatory[b160–162]	10 mg IM for induction of parturition[a159] 0.44 mg/kg IV once as an antiinflammatory[b163] (higher doses or more than one dose may result in immunosuppression[164])	
Dexamethasone sodium phosphate	5–6 mg/kg IV for shock[c165,166]	5–6 mg/kg IV for shock[c165,166]	
Dextrose (glucose)	4–10 g IV for pregnancy toxemia[c167,168] 10 mL/kg of 20% solution IP for weak lambs[c169]	4–10 g IV for pregnancy toxemia[c167,168]	
Diazepam	0.3–0.4 mg/kg IV[b74,170–172] 1 mg/kg IV for tetany[c173]	0.3–0.4 mg/kg IV[b74,170–172] 1 mg/kg IV for tetany[c173] 0.06 mg/kg IV to stimulate appetite[c174]	
Diclazuril	1 mg/kg PO[a175–177]	1 mg/kg PO[b178]	
Dinoprost (prostaglandin $F_{2}\alpha$)	15 mg IM twice at 10 day interval for estrus synchronization[a179,180] 10 mg to terminate early pregnancy[b185]	5–10 mg IM for induction of parturition, treatment of hydrometra, and luteolysis and estrus synchronization[a181–184]	
Dopamine	5–20 µg/kg/min IV to increase blood pressure[b186–189]	5–20 µg/kg/min IV to increase blood pressure[b186–189]	
Doramectin	200 µg/kg IM for gastrointestinal nematodes and *Oestrus ovis*[b190] 300 µg/kg IM or SC for *Psoroptes* and gastrointestinal nematodes[b191,192]	400 µg/kg PO[c193]	200 µg/kg PO[d194]
Doxapram	5.5 mg/kg IV[c195]	1 mg/kg IV[c196]	
EDTA (calcium EDTA)	100–110 mg/kg IV for lead poisoning for 4 days[c197–199]		
Enrofloxacin	5 mg/kg IV, IM, or SC every 24 h[b200–202]	5–7.5 mg/kg IM or SC[c201,203]	
Epinephrine	0.01 mg/kg IV, IM, or SC[c204]	0.01 mg/kg IV, IM, or SC[c204]	
Eprinomectin	0.5–1 mg/kg topically for gastrointestinal and lung nematodes and *Oestrus ovis*[b205–207]	0.5–1 mg/kg topically for gastrointestinal nematodes and *Sarcoptes*[b208–211]	
Erythromycin	10 mg/kg IM once a day or BID[b212–215]	10 mg/kg IM once a day or BID[b212–215]	
Estradiol cypionate		0.2 mg/kg IM after GnRH for induction of estrus[c216]	
Etomidate	1 mg/kg IV[c217]		
Febantel	5–12 mg/kg PO[b218–220]	5 mg/kg PO[c221]	
Fenbendazole	5 mg/kg PO[b222] (Anecdotal reports suggest that this dosage may not be clinically effective and 10–20 mg/kg PO may be required to control nematode parasites in sheep and goats[223])	5 mg/kg PO[b222] (Anecdotal reports suggest that this dosage may not be clinically effective and 10–20 mg/kg PO may be required to control nematode parasites in sheep and goats[223])	
Fenprostalene		0.5 mg SC for pregnancy termination[c224]	
Fentanyl transdermal patch on clean shaved skin	2 µg/kg/h[b74,225,226]	2.5 µg/kg/h[b227]	

TABLE 1 Some Drug Dosages—cont'd.

Drug	Sheep	Goats	Cervids
Florfenicol	20–30 mg/kg IM[b228,229] 40 mg/kg SC[b229,230]	20 mg/kg IM[b231–233]	20 mg/kg IM[d108] 40 mg/kg SC[d108,234]
Flumazenil	20 μg/kg IV to reverse benzodiazepines[c235]		
Flunixin meglumine	1 mg/kg IV[c236] 2.0 mg/kg IM[b102] 2.5 mg/kg SC[c88,109]	2.5 mg/kg IM[b110]	
Follicle-stimulating hormone	See Chapter 8	See Chapter 8	
Furosemide	0.5–1.0 mg/kg IV or PO for heart failure or diuresis[b237–239]	0.5–1 mg/kg IV or PO for heart failure or diuresis[b237–239]	
Gamithromycin			6 mg/kg SC[d108]
Glycopyrrolate	0.01 mg/kg IV[b66]	0.01 mg/kg IV[b66]	
Griseofulvin	7.5 mg/kg PO for 7 days[c240]		
Guaifenesin	50 mg/kg IV[c241]		
Heparin	200 IU/kg bolus for anticoagulation[c119]	350 to 400 IU/kg bolus for anticoagulation[c119]	
Hyaluronate sodium	20 mg intra-articularly weekly for 5 weeks[c242,243]		
Hypertonic saline (7%)	4 mL/kg IV over 5–10 minutes[b244–246]	4 mL/kg IV over 5–10 minutes[b244–246]	
Ibuprofen	12.5–15 mg/kg IV[c247,248]	14–25 mg/kg IV or 50 mg/kg PO[c247–249]	
Imidocarb	1.2 mg/kg IM twice separated by 10–14 days[c250]		
Insulin	0.4 IU/kg SC of intermediate acting insulin for pregnancy toxemia[c168]		
Ivermectin	200 μg/kg PO[b251] (anecdotal reports suggest that this dosage may be clinically ineffective in sheep and goats, and more than 300 μg/kg may be needed for nematode parasite control)	200 μg/kg PO[b251] (anecdotal reports suggest that this dosage may be clinically ineffective in sheep and goats, and more than 300 μg/kg may be needed for nematode parasite control)	200 μg/kg PO or SC[d252,253]
Ketamine	See Chapter 18	See Chapter 18	
Ketoprofen	3 mg/kg IV[a154,254–256]	3 mg/kg IV[a154,254,255]	
Lasalocid	15–70 mg/head/day (20–30 g/ton in feed) for prevention of coccidiosis[a257,258]		
Levamisole	8 mg/kg PO[b259,260] (anecdotal reports suggest that this dosage may be clinically ineffective for nematode parasite control in sheep and goats, and 12 mg/kg PO may be needed)	8 mg/kg PO[b259,260]	
Lidocaine	3–4 mg/kg epidural[b170,261] 0.5–0.6 mg/kg caudal epidural[c262] 3 mg/kg IV as anti-arrhythmic[b265]	3 mg/kg epidural[b263,264]	
Lincomycin hydrochloride	10 mg/kg IM every 24 h[d266]	10 mg/kg IM every 24 h[d266]	
Lincomycin/spectinomycin	5 mg/kg lincomycin/10 mg/kg spectinomycin[c267,268 269]		
Lipid emulsion		1.5 mL/kg of 20% solution IV slowly[c270]	

Continued

TABLE 1 Some Drug Dosages—cont'd.

Drug	Sheep	Goats	Cervids
Magnesium	200–400 mg/kg IV or SC for treatment of hypomagnesemic tetany[c271,272]		
Mannitol	0.3–2 mg/kg IV over 5 to 10 minutes[b273–275]	0.3–2 mg/kg IV over 5–10 minutes[b273–275]	
Mebendazole	15 mg/kg PO[a276–281]	15 mg/kg PO[a276–281]	
Medetomidine	0.005–0.020 mg/kg IV[b62,282]	0.005–0.020 mg/kg IV[b62,282,283]	
Melengestrol acetate	0.125 BID or 0.25–0.3 mg per day in feed for 7–10 days for estrus synchronization[a284–287]		1–2 mg per day in feed[d288]
Meloxicam	0.5 mg/kg IV[c289] 1 mg/kg buccal formulation[c290] 1 mg/kg PO[d291]	0.5 mg/kg IM, PO, or SC[c292,293]	
Methocarbamol	22 mg/kg IV for tetany[d9]	22 mg/kg IV for tetany[d9]	
Methohexitone (methohexital)	3–5 mg/kg IV[c294,295]		
Methylene blue	2–15 mg/kg IV (depending on severity) for treatment of nitrate toxicity[b296–301]	2–4 mg/kg IV (depending on severity) for treatment of nitrate toxicity[b296–301]	
Metoclopramide	0.5 mg/kg IM or IV[c302,303]	0.5 mg/kg IM or IV[c302,303]	
Midazolam	0.3–0.4 mg/kg IV[b] 0.5 mg/kg IM[c304]	0.3–0.6 mg/kg IV[b7,235,305–310]	
Mineral oil	0.5–1.0 L PO for treatment of bloat, effective in cattle[c311,312]		
Monensin sodium	15 mg/head/day throughout gestation to prevent abortion and improved lamb birth weight caused by *Toxoplasma gondii*[b313,314] 11–22 ppm for coccidiosis control[b258,315]		
Morantel tartrate	1.0 lb of medicated ration (0.44 g of morantel)/45 kg body weight[a316] 10 mg/kg PO[a317]	1.0 lb of medicated ration (0.44 g of morantel)/45 kg body weight[a316] 10 mg/kg PO[a317]	
Moxidectin	200–500 μg/kg PO or SC[a318,319]	200–400 μg/kg SC[b193,320–322]	200 μg/kg SC[c323]
Naltrexone			100 mg/mg carfentanil for reversal[c324]
Nandrolone	1–1.5 mg/kg/week for adjunctive therapy of anemia[d325,326]	1–1.5 mg/kg/week for adjunctive therapy of anemia[d325,326]	
Neomycin soluble powder	22 mg/kg BID PO in water or milk replacer for a maximum of 14 days for treatment and control of colibacillosis caused by *Escherichia coli* susceptible to neomycin[a327,328]	22 mg/kg BID PO in water or milk replacer for a maximum of 14 days for treatment and control of colibacillosis caused by *E. coli* susceptible to neomycin[a327,328]	
Neostigmine methylsulfate	0.02–0.03 mg/kg SC[b329]	0.02–0.03 mg/kg SC[b329]	
Netobimin	7.5 mg/kg PO for adult nematodes[b330,331] 15–20 mg/kg PO for L4 larvae or flukes[b330,332–334]	10 mg/kg PO for 2 days or 7.5 mg/kg PO for 3 days for gastrointestinal and lung nematodes[c335]	
Niclosamide	75 mg/kg for cestodes[b336,337]	75 mg/kg for cestodes[c20,336]	
Nitrooxinil	10 mg/kg SC for flukes[b140,338,339]		
Norgestomet without or with estradiol valerate or benzoate and other hormones	See Chapter 8		

TABLE 1 Some Drug Dosages—cont'd.

Drug	Sheep	Goats	Cervids
Oxfendazole	5–10 mg/kg PO for nonresistant nematodes and cestodes[b278,340] 30–60 mg/kg PO once a week for several weeks for cystic echinococcosis or flukes[b341–345]	5–10 mg/kg PO for nonresistant nematodes and cestodes[b278,346]	
Oxyclozanide	15 mg/kg PO for flukes[b140,338] 20 mg/kg PO twice 72 h apart for *Paraphistomum*[c347]		
Oxytetracycline injectable	10 mg/kg IV or IM q24h for 7–10 days for listeriosis[c348]		
Oxytetracycline (long-acting)	20 mg/kg IM (once, every 72 h, or weekly depending on therapeutic need)[a349–357]	20 mg/kg IM[b355,356,358,359]	30 mg/kg SC[d108,360]
Oxytetracycline (in water)	22 mg/kg q24h PO for up to 14 days[b361]	22 mg/kg q24h PO for up to 14 days[b361]	
Oxytetracycline (in feed)	22 mg/kg q24h PO for 7–14 days[b362] 100–150 mg/head/day prebreeding to prevent Chlamydial abortion[c363] 400–500 mg/head/day for an outbreak of chlamydial abortion[c363]	22 mg/kg q24h PO for 7–14 days[b362] 100–150 mg/head/day prebreeding to prevent chlamydial abortion[c363] 400–500 mg/head/day for an outbreak of chlamydial abortion[c363]	
Oxytocin	20–50 IU IV, IM, or SC for obstetric use and retained placenta[a364,365]	20–50 IU IV, IM, or SC for obstetric use and retained placenta[a364,366]	
Penicillamine	50 mg/kg/day PO to increase elimination of copper[b34,367,368]	50 mg/kg/day PO to increase elimination of copper[c37]	
Penicillin G sodium or potassium	20,000–40,000 IU/kg IV every 4 to 6 h[c369,370]	20,000–40,000 IU/kg IV every 4 to 6 h[c369,370]	
Penicillin G procaine	10,000 IU/kg IM every 24 h[b371–373] 50,000 IU/kg SC q24h for 7–14 days for listeriosis[c374] 15,000 IU/kg IM q8h for 7–10 days for listeriosis or Clostridium haemolyticum[c348,375]	10,000 IU/kg IM every 24 h[b371–373] 50,000 IU/kg SC q24h for 7–14 days for listeriosis[c374] 15,000 IU/kg IM q8h for 7–10 days for listeriosis[c348]	
Penicillin-novobiocin dry cow therapy	½ syringe of 200,000 IU penicillin/200 mg novobiocin[c376]		
Pentobarbital (pentobarbitone)	10–30 mg/kg IV[b295,377] 6–75 mg/kg IV to control tetany or seizures[b378,379]		
Phenylbutazone	4 mg/kg IV or PO[b380–382]	4–10 mg/kg IV or PO[b382,383]	
Poloxalene	3 g/50 kg in feed to prevent bloat[c384]		
Ponazuril		10 mg/kg PO[b54]	
Praziquantel	3.75 mg/kg PO[c385]	60 mg/kg PO for *Schistosoma bovis*[c386]	
PMSG or eCG	See Chapter 8		
Prednisolone		1 mg/kg IM every 12 h for immunosuppression until remission, then 1 mg/kg IM every 48 h[c387,388]	
Propofol	2.0–6.0 mg/kg IV for induction[b7,282,389] 0.1–0.3 mg/kg/min IV for constant rate infusion[b389,390]	2.0 to 6.0 mg/kg IV for induction[b7,282,389] 0.1–0.3 mg/kg/min IV for constant rate infusion[b389,390]	

Continued

TABLE 1 Some Drug Dosages—cont'd.

Drug	Sheep	Goats	Cervids
Propylene glycol	30–100 mL PO[b391–393,394]	30–100 mL PO[b391,392,394]	
Pyrantel	25 mg/kg PO[a278,395–398]	20–40 mg/kg PO[b399]	
Salinomycin	0.5–2.0 mg/kg PO in cattle[c400] 10-30 ppm in feed[c401]		
Sodium bicarbonate	2 to 3 L of isotonic (1.3%, 156 mmol/L) solution IV for pregnancy toxemia (60–70 kg/ewe)[c402] 0.5–1.0 L of 5% solution for acidosis[c403] 50 mL of 8.4% solution for Drunken Lamb syndrome[c404]	23–63 mL of 5% solution IV for Floppy Kid Syndrome[c405]	
Sodium iodide	3 g IV or 70 mg/kg at weekly intervals[c406,407]		
Sodium nitrite	20 mg/kg IV for cyanide poisoning in combination with sodium thiosulfate[c408–410]		
Sodium propionate	12.5 g PO for pregnancy toxemia[c168]		
Sodium sulfate	1 g/head/day PO in combination with ammonium molybdate to increase elimination of copper[b34–36]		
Sodium thiosulfate	500 mg/kg IV for cyanide poisoning in combination with sodium nitrite[c408–410]	300 mg/head/day in combination with ammonium molybdate to increase elimination of copper[c37]	
Stanozolol	25–50 mg IM weekly for adjunctive therapy of anemia[d325,326]	25–50 mg IM weekly for adjunctive therapy of anemia[d325,326]	
Sulfadiazine	100 mg/kg IV[c411]		
Sulfadimethoxine	50 mg/kg PO for 5 days to reduce coccidial oocyst shedding[c412]		
Sulfamethazine	200 mg/kg PO for several days to reduce coccidial oocyst shedding[c413]	200 mg/kg PO for several days to reduce coccidial oocyst shedding[c413]	
Sulfaquinoxaline	1 tsp of 24% powder/125 lb bodyweight in drinking water for 3 to 5 days (approximately 125 mg/kg) approved in cattle[b414,415]	1 tsp of 24% powder/125 lb bodyweight in drinking water for 3 to 5 days (approximately 125 mg/kg) approved in cattle[b414,415]	
Testosterone propionate	25 mg IM three times/week for adjunctive therapy of anemia[d325]	25 mg IM three times/week for adjunctive therapy of anemia[d325]	
Thiabendazole	44 mg/kg PO[c416] (anecdotal reports suggest that this drug may only rarely be clinically effective for sheep and goats)	44 mg/kg PO[c416] (anecdotal reports suggest that this drug may only rarely be clinically effective for sheep and goats)	
Thiamine	10 mg/kg IV or 25 mg/kg BID or 75 mg/kg SC daily as an adjunct for lead poisoning[b197,417–419] 10 mg/kg IV or SC for polioencephalomalacia[b420,421]	10 mg/kg IV or 25 mg/kg BID or 75 mg/kg SC daily as an adjunct for lead poisoning[b197,417–419] 10 mg/kg IV or SC for polioencephalomalacia[b420,421]	
Thiopental (thiopentone) sodium	13–20 mg/kg IV[b422,423]	6–8 mg/kg IV[b241,424]	
Tiletamine-zolazepam (Telazol)	1.1–5.5 mg/kg IV[b80,425,426]	1.1–5.5 mg/kg IV[b80,425,426]	
Tilmicosin	10 mg/kg SC for bacterial pneumonia[a427,428] 10 mg/kg SC for mastitis[b429]	(anecdotal reports suggest that the use of this drug may result in death in some goats)	
Tolazoline	2 mg/kg IV[b377,430]	2.2 mg/kg IV[b431]	4 mg/kg IV[c432]
Toltrazuril	20 mg/kg PO once[a433–436]	20 mg/kg PO once[b437–439]	

TABLE 1 **Some Drug Dosages—cont'd.**

Drug	Sheep	Goats	Cervids
Triclabendazole	10–20 mg/kg PO for flukes[b440–444]	5–12 mg/kg PO for flukes[b440,445]	
Trimethoprim-sulfadiazine	30 mg/kg IM in pre-ruminant lambs[c446]	20 mg/kg IM in pre-ruminant goats[c447]	
Tulathromycin	2.5 mg/kg SC[b448–451]	2.5 mg/kg SC[b448–450,452,453]	2.5 mg/kg SC[c454]
Tylosin	20 mg/kg IM every 12–24 h[c455,456]	20 mg/kg IM[c457]	
Vitamin B_{12} (cyanocobalamin)	0.05–0.2 mg IM or 2 mg SC for deficiency[b458–462]		
Vitamin K_1 (phylloquinone)	1.1 mg/kg IM or 2.2 mg/kg IV reported in cattle[c463–465]	1.1 mg/kg IM or 2.2 mg/kg IV reported in cattle[c463–465]	
Xylazine	0.05–0.22 mg/kg IV or IM[b155,170,466–468]	0.05–0.22 mg/kg IV or IM[b306,469,470]	
Yohimbine	0.2–0.25 mg/kg IV[b65,430,471,472]	0.2–0.25 mg/kg IV[b65,471,472]	

The Authors Wish to Acknowledge Stephanie Morel for Help With This Table.
[a]High quality: further research is unlikely to change our confidence in the dosage.
[b]Moderate quality: further research is likely to have an important impact in our confidence in the dosage and may change it.
[c]Low quality: further research is very likely to have an important impact in our confidence in the dosage and is likely to change it.
[d]Very low quality: dosage estimate is very uncertain.
CRI, constant rate infusion; *eCG*, equine chorionic gonadotropin; *EDTA*, Ethylenediaminetetraacetic acid; *GnRH*, gonadotropin-releasing hormone; *IM*, intramuscular; *IP*, intra-peritoneal; *IV*, intravenous; *PMSG*, pregnant mare serum gonadotropin; *PO*, per os; *q24h*, every 24 hrs; *QID*, 4 times per day; *SC*, subcutaneous; *TID*, 3 times per day.

TABLE 2 **Drugs Affected by VFD or Guidance 213**

AFFECTED FEED-USE ANTIMICROBIALS	
Antimicrobial Class	**Specific Drugs Approved for use in Feed**
Aminoglycosides	Apramycin, hygromycin B, neomycin, streptomycin
Diaminopyrimidines	Ormetoprim
Lincosamides	Lincomycin
Macrolides	Erythromycin, oleandomycin, tylosin
Penicillins	Penicillin
Streptogramins	Virginiamycin
Sulfas	Sulfadimethoxine, sulfamerazine, sulfamethazine, sulfaquinoxaline
Tetracycline	Chlortetracycline, oxytetracycline
AFFECTED WATER-USE ANTIMICROBIALS	
Antimicrobial Class	**Specific Drugs Approved for use in Water**
Aminoglycosides	Apramycin, gentamicin, neomycin, spectinomycin, streptomycin
Lincosamides	Lincomycin
Macrolides	Carbomycin, erythromycin, tylosin
Penicillins	Penicillin
Streptogramins	Virginiamycin
Sulfas	Sulfachloropyrazine, sulfachlorpyridazine, sulfadimethoxine, sulfamerazine, sulfamethazine, sulfaquinoxaline
Tetracycline	Chlortetracycline, oxytetracycline, tetracycline

VFD, Veterinary feed directive.

practice that orders the use of a VFD drug or combination VFD drug in or on an animal feed or in water (Box 1). The written statement authorizes the client or other caretaker to obtain and use animal feed containing a VFD drug or combination VFD drug to treat the client's animals only in accordance with the conditions for use in compliance with FDA limitations. A copy of the written order must be kept for a period of 2 years by the veterinarian, client, and mill or distributor.

- Veterinarian's name, address, and telephone number.
- Client's name, business or home address, and telephone number.
- Premises at which the animals specified in the VFD are located (may also use GPS coordinates or specify pen, barn, stall, tank, or other description).

• BOX 1 General Label Information for VFD

Labels for VFD drugs will include a cautionary statement stating "Federal law restricts medicated feed containing this VFD drug to use by or on the order of a licensed veterinarian." Information that is required on a VFD order is:

- Veterinarian and client information
- Premise information: where the animals specified in the VFD are located
- Date of VFD issuance
- Expiration date of the VFD
- Name of the VFD drug(s)
- Species and production class of animals to be fed the VFD feed
- Approximate number of animals to be fed the VFD feed by the expiration date of the VFD
- Indication for which the VFD is issued
- Level of VFD drug in the feed and duration of use
- Withdrawal time, special instructions and cautionary statements
- Number of reorders authorized
- Statement: "Use of feed containing this VFD drug in a manner other than as directed on the labeling is not permitted"
- An affirmation of intent for combination VFD drugs as described in 21 CFR 558.6(b)(6)

VFD, *Veterinary feed directive.*

Contains Nonbinding Recommendations

Veterinary Feed Directive

Veterinarian: ____________________ **Client:** ____________________
Address: ____________________ **Address:** ____________________
____________________ (business or home) ____________________
Phone: ____________________ **Phone:** ____________________
Fax or email (optional): ____________________ **Fax or email** (optional): ____________________

Drug(s) Name: __________ **Drug(s) Level:** __________ **g/ton Duration of use:** __________
Species and Production class: __________ **Number of reorders (refills) authorized** (if permitted by the drug approval): _____
Indications for use (as approved): ____________________
Caution (related to this medicated feed, if any): ____________________

USE OF FEED CONTAINING THIS VETERINARY FEED DIRECTIVE (VFD) DRUG IN A MANNER OTHER THAN AS DIRECTED ON THE LABELING (EXTRA-LABEL USE) IS NOT PERMITTED

Approximate Number of Animals: ____________________
Premises: ____________________
Other Identification (e.g., age, weight) (optional): ____________________
Special Instructions (if any): ____________________

Affirmation of intent (for combination VFD Drugs) (check one box)*:
('For VFD drugs for which there are no approved VFD combinations, only the first affirmation statement should be included on the VFD)

☐ This VFD only authorizes the use of the VFD drug(s) cited in this order and is not intended to authorize the use of such drug(s) in combination with any other animal drugs.

☐ This VFD authorizes the use of the VFD drug(s) cited in this order in the following FDA-approved, conditionally approved, or indexed combination(s) in medicated feed that contains the VFD drug(s) as a component:

Drug(s)	Drug Level(s) and any Special Instructions

☐ This VFD authorizes the use of the VFD drug(s) cited in this order in any FDA-approved, conditionally approved, or indexed combination(s) in medicated feed that contains the VFD drug(s) as a component.

Withdrawal Time (if any): This VFD Feed must be withdrawn ________ days prior to slaughter

VFD Date of Issuance: _____ **(Month/Day/Year)** **VFD Expiration Date:** ______ **(Month/Day/Year)** (As specified in the approval; cannot exceed 6 months after issuance)

Veterinarian's Signature: ____________________

All parties must retain a copy of this VFD for 2 years after the date of issuance. 21 CFR 558.6(a)(4)

• **Fig. 1** A sample VFD from FDA GFI #233. (*FDA*, U.S. Food and Drug Administration; *VFD*, veterinary feed class.)

- Date of VFD issuance.
- Expiration date of the VFD.
- Name of the VFD drug(s).
- Species and production class of animals to be fed the VFD feed (age and weight range optional).
- Approximate number of animals to be fed the VFD feed by the expiration date of the VFD.
- Indication for which the VFD is issued.
- Level of VFD drug in the feed and duration of use.
- Withdrawal time, special instructions, and cautionary statements necessary for use of the drug in conformance with the approval.
- Number of reorders (refills) authorized, if permitted by drug approval, conditional approval, or index listing.
- The statement: "Use of feed containing this Veterinary Feed Directive (VFD) drug in a manner other than as directed on the labeling (extra-label use), is not permitted".
- An affirmation of intent for combination VFD drugs as described in 21 CFR 558.6(b)(6).

Either

(i) "This VFD only authorizes the use of the VFD drug(s) cited in this order and is not intended to authorize the use of such drug(s) in combination with any other animal drugs." OR

(ii) "This VFD authorizes the use of the VFD drug(s) cited in this order in the following FDA-approved, conditionally approved, or indexed combination(s) in medicated feed that contains the VFD drug(s) as a component." [List specific approved, conditionally approved, or indexed combination medicated feeds following this statement.] OR

(iii) "This VFD authorizes the use of the VFD drug(s) cited in this order in any FDA-approved, conditionally approved, or indexed combination(s) in medicated feed that contains the VFD drug(s) as a component."

- Veterinarian's electronic or written signature.

Practice pointers to bear in mind when working with a VFD are:

- The expiration date is the last date the feed may be fed.
- Dates are calculated by calendar date, not days, July 10 to January 10, or for an end of month, August 31 to February 28 (or 29) for example, even though there are fewer days in the ending month.
- An expiration date is 6 months, but the veterinarian may reduce this time period.
- Duration of use is separate from expiration date; the expiration date is the time frame to obtain and use the VFD feed and the actual time used is determined by the labeled use period for the VFD drug.
- Approximate number of animals means the potential number of animals to be fed the feed identified at the premises and over the time period stated on the VFD.
- A copy of the VFD to the distributor in hardcopy may be sent directly or via the client and may also be sent by facsimile (fax), or by electronic means.
- There is no provision to allow a VFD for an over-the-counter (OTC) drug; only VFD drugs pursuant to a VFD order may be used on feed or in water.

In order for a VFD to be lawfully issued, the veterinarian issuing the VFD must comply with the following:

- Must be licensed to practice veterinary medicine (21 CFR 558.6(b)(1)(i)).
- Must be operating in the course of the veterinarian's professional practice and in compliance with all applicable veterinary licensing and practice requirements (21 CFR 558.6(b)(1)(ii)).
- Must write VFD orders in the context of a veterinarian-client-patient relationship (VCPR) (21 CFR 558.6(b)(1)(ii)).
- Must only issue a VFD that is in compliance with the conditions for use approved, conditionally approved, or indexed for the VFD drug or combination VFD drug (21 CFR 558.6(b)(2)).
- Must prepare a written (nonverbal) VFD (21 CFR 558.6(b)(7)) that includes the veterinarian's electronic or written signature (21 CFR 558.6(b)(3)(xv)).
- Must ensure the VFD includes all required information specified in the VFD regulation (21 CFR 558.6(b)(3)).
- May enter additional discretionary information to more specifically identify the animals to be treated/fed the VFD feed (21 CFR 558.6(b)(4)).
- Must include certain drug-specific information for each VFD drug when the veterinarian is authorizing the use of a drug combination that includes more than one VFD drug (21 CFR 558.6(b)(5)).
- For VFD drugs approved for use alone or in combination with one or more OTC drugs, must include on the VFD order an affirmation of intent either to restrict authorized use only to the VFD drug cited on the VFD or to allow the use of the cited VFD drug in an approved combination with one or more OTC drug(s) (21 CFR 558.6(b)(6)).
- Must provide the distributor with a copy of the VFD order (21 CFR 558.6(b)(8)).
- Must provide the client with a copy of the VFD order (21 CFR 558.6(b)(9)).
- Must retain the original VFD for 2 years (21 CFR 558.6(a)(4)).
- Must provide VFD orders for inspection and copying by FDA upon request (21 CFR 558.6(a)(5)).

Many distributors and drug suppliers will have available online a VFD from for veterinarians' use (Figure 1).

References

1. Guyatt GH, Oxman AD, Kunz R, et al: What is "quality of evidence" and why is it important to clinicians? *BMJ*. 2008:336(7651);995–998.
2. Guyatt GH, Oxman AD, Vist GE, et al: GRADE: an emerging consensus on rating quality of evidence and strength of recommendations. *BMJ*. 2008:336(7650);924–926.
3. O'Connor A, Fajt V: Evaluating treatment options for common bovine diseases using published data and clinical experience. *Vet Clin North Am Food Anim Pract*. 2015:31(1);1–15, v.
4. Žele D, Tavcar Kalcher G, Kobal S, Vengust G, Vengust A, Grabnar I: Plasma pharmacokinetics of abamectin in fallow deer (Cervus dama dama) following subcutaneous administration. *J Vet Pharmacol Ther*. 2011:34(5);455–459.
5. Acepromazine maleate, Atravet 10 mg injectable. Accessed December 1, 2009. https://dailymed.nlm.nih.gov/dailymed/drugInfo.cfm?setid=e1039978-b318-4611-9fdc-fe7ab10e3246, accessed Sept. 1, 2019. The product is just Acepromazine Maleate, so take out Atravet.
6. Doherty TJ, Rohrbach BW, Geiser DR: Effect of acepromazine and butorphanol on isoflurane minimum alveolar concentration in goats. *J Vet Pharmacol Ther*. 2002:25(1);65–67.
7. Dzikiti TB, Stegmann GF, Hellebrekers LJ, Auer RE, Dzikiti LN: Sedative and cardiopulmonary effects of acepromazine, midazolam, butorphanol, acepromazine-butorphanol and midazolam-butorphanol on propofol anaesthesia in goats. *J South African Vet Assn*. 2009:80(1);10–16.
8. Casas-Díaz E, Marco I, López-Olvera J, Mentaberre G, Lavín S: Use of acepromazine for stress control in Spanish ibex (Capra pyrenaica) captured by drive-net. *Vet J (London, England 1997)*. 2010:183(3);332–336.

9. Smith MC, Sherman DM: Nervous system in *Goat Medicine*. 2nd ed., Smith MC, Sherman DM, Eds.; Ames, Iowa: Wiley-Blackwell, 2009.
10. Halliburton JC. Nonprotein nitrogen-induced ammonia toxicosis in ruminants, in *Current Veterinary Therapy 4*: Food Animal Practice. Howard JL, Smith RA, Eds., Philadelphia: W.B. Saunders Company, 242–243, 1999.
11. Word JD, Martin LC, Williams DL, et al: Urea toxicity studies in the bovine. *J Anim Sci.* 1969:29(5);786–791.
12. Ortolani EL, Mori CS, Rodrigues Filho JA: Ammonia toxicity from urea in a Brazilian dairy goat flock. *Vet Human Toxicol.* 2000:42(2);87–89.
13. United States Food and Drug Administration Center for Veterinary Medicine: Code of Federal Regulation; Part 520 Oral Dosage Form New Animal Drugs; Section 520.45a; Albendazole Suspension. Accessed November 2, 2009.
14. Moreno L, Echevarria F, Munoz F, Alvarez L, Sanchez Bruni S, Lanusse C: Dose-dependent activity of albendazole against benzimidazole-resistant nematodes in sheep: relationship between pharmacokinetics and efficacy. *Exp Parasitol.* 2004:106(3–4);150–157.
15. Darabus GH, Indre D, Morariu S, Mederle N, Imre M: The efficacy of an albendazole based product in lambs gastrointestinal nematode parasitism. *Lucrari Stiintifice Medicina Veterinara.* 2013:46(3);41–45.
16. M. F, Gammaz H, Abdel-Daim M, Muzamil Y, Mohammed SK: Efficacy and safety of Albendazole against Haemonchus contortus infestation in goats. Paper presented at: 5th Animal Wealth Research Conference 2012; Middle East & North Africa.
17. Kumbhakar NK, Sanyal PK, Rawte D, Kumar D, Kerketta AE, Pal S: Efficacy of pharmacokinetic interactions between piperonyl butoxide and albendazole against gastrointestinal nematodiasis in goats. *J Helminthol.* 2016:90(05);624–629.
18. Kerketta AE, Sanyal PK, Pal S, Baghel KR: Dose-dependent plasma disposition kinetics of albendazole in goats. *Indian J Small Ruminants.* 2017:23(2);213–218.
19. Morris DL, Richards KS, Clarkson MJ, Taylor DH: Comparison of Albendazole and Praziquantel therapy of Echinococcus granulosus in naturally infected sheep. *Vet Parasitol.* 1990:36(1–2);83–90.
20. Smith MC, Sherman DM: Digestive system, in *Goat Medicine*. 2nd ed., Smith MC, Sherman DM, Eds., Ames, IA: Wiley-Blackwell; 2009.
21. del Mar Granados M, Domínguez JM, Fernández Sarmiento A, et al. Anaesthetic and cardiorespiratory effects of a constant-rate infusion of alfaxalone in desflurane-anaesthetised sheep. *Veterinary record.* 2012:171(5):125-125.
22. Torres. Effects of an intravenous bolus of alfaxalone versus propofol on intraocular pressure in sheep. *Veterinary record.* 2012:170(9):226.
23. Dzikiti TB, Zeiler GE, Dzikiti LN, Garcia ER: The effects of midazolam and butorphanol, administered alone or combined, on the dose and quality of anaesthetic induction with alfaxalone in goats. *JSouth African VetAssn.* 2014:85(1);1–8.
24. Heatley JJ, Boothe DM, Jensen JM: Disposition of amikacin in fallow deer (Dama dama) following a single intramuscular dose. *J Zoo Wildl Med.* 1996:27(2);227–233.
25. Romanowski RD: Biochemistry of urolith formation. *J Am Vet Med Assoc.* 1965:147(12);1324–1326.
26. Manning RA, Blaney BJ: Epidemiological aspects of urolithiasis in domestic animals in Queensland. *AustrVet J.* 1986:63(12);423–424.
27. Stewart SR, Emerick RJ, Pritchard RH: Effects of dietary ammonium chloride and variations in calcium to phosphorus ratio on silica urolithiasis in sheep. *J Anim Sci.* 1991:69(5);2225–2229.
28. Stewart SR, Emerick RJ, Pritchard RH: High dietary calcium to phosphorus ratio and alkali-forming potential as factors promoting silica urolithiasis in sheep. *J Anim Sci.* 1990:68(2);498–503.
29. Bushman DH, Emerick RJ, Embry LB: Effect of various chlorides and calcium carbonate on calcium, phosphorus, sodium, potassium and chloride balance and their relationship to urinary calculi in lambs. *J Anim Sci.* 1968:27(2);490–496.
30. Jones ML, Streeter RN, Goad CL: Use of dietary cation anion difference for control of urolithiasis risk factors in goats. *Am J Vet Res.* 2009:70(1);149–155.
31. Crookshank HR, Keating FE, Burnett E, Jones JH, Davis RE: Effect of chemical and enzymatic agents on the formation of urinary calculi in fattening steers. *J Anim Sci.* 1960:19;595–600.
32. Stratton-Phelps M, House JK: Effect of a commercial anion dietary supplement on acid-base balance, urine volume, and urinary ion excretion in male goats fed oat or grass hay diets. *Am J Vet Res.* 2004:65(10);1391–1397.
33. Mavangira V, Cornish JM, Angelos JA: Effect of ammonium chloride supplementation on urine pH and urinary fractional excretion of electrolytes in goats. *J Am Vety Med Assn.* 2010:237(11);1299–1304.
34. Hidiroglou M, Heaney DP, Hartin KE: Copper poisoning in a flock of sheep. Copper excretion patterns after treatment with molybdenum and sulfur or penicillamine. *Can Vet J.* 1984:25(10);377–382.
35. Kupper J, Bidaut A, Waldvogel A, Emmenegger B, Naegeli H: Treatment of chronic copper poisoning in dairy sheep with oral ammonium molybdate and sodium sulphate. *Schweizer Archiv fur Tierheilkunde.* 2005:147(5);219–224.
36. Ross DB: The effect of oral ammonium molybdate and sodium sulphate given to lambs with high liver copper concentrations. *Res Vet Sci.* 1970:11;295–297.
37. Cornish J, Angelos J, Puschner B, Miller G, George L: Copper toxicosis in a dairy goat herd. *J Am Vet Med Assn.* 2007:231(4);586–589.
38. Zhou S, Zhang C, Xiao Q, et al: Effects of different levels of molybdenum on rumen microbiota and trace elements changes in tissues from goats. *Biol Trace Element Res.* 2016:174(1);85–92.
39. Ortolani EL, Antonelli AC, de Souza Sarkis JE: Acute sheep poisoning from a copper sulfate footbath. *Vet Human Toxicol.* 2004: 46(6);315–318.
40. Suttle NF: Responsiveness of prehaemolytic copper poisoning in sheep from a specific pathogen-free environment to a relatively high dose of tetrathiomolybdate. *Vet Rec.* 2012:171(10);246–246.
41. Escudero E, Carceles CM, Vicente S: Pharmacokinetics of amoxicillin/clavulanic acid combination and of both drugs alone after intravenous administration to goats. *Brit VetJ.* 1996:152(5);551–559.
42. Carceles CM, Escudero E, Vicente MS, Serrano JM, Carli S: Pharmacokinetics of amoxicillin/clavulanic acid combination after intravenous and oral administration in goats. *Vet Q.* 1995:17(4);134–138.
43. Gilmour NJ, Gilmour JS, Quirie M, Donachie W: Treatment of experimental pasteurellosis in lambs with clavulanic acid and amoxycillin. *Vet Rec.* 1990:126(13);311.
44. Buswell JF, Barber DM: Antibiotic persistence and tolerance in the lactating sheep following a course of intramammary therapy. *Brit Vet J.* 1989:145(6);552–557.
45. Buswell JF, Knight CH, Barber DM: Antibiotic persistence and tolerance in the lactating goat following intramammary therapy. *Vet Re.* 1989:125(11);301–303.
46. Fernandez C, Modamio P, Mestorino N, Errecalde JO, Marino EL: Pharmacokinetics of sodium and trihydrate amoxicillin in sheep after intravenous and intramuscular administration. *J Vet Pharmacol Ther.* 2007:30(3);263–266.
47. Elsheikh HA, Taha AA, Khalafalla AE, Osman IA, Wasfi IA: Pharmacokinetics of amoxicillin trihydrate in Desert sheep and Nubian goats. *Vet ResCommun.* 1999:23(8);507–514.
48. Craigmill AL, Pass MA, Wetzlich S: Comparative pharmacokinetics of amoxicillin administered intravenously to sheep and goats. *J Vet PharmacolTher.* 1992:15(1);72–77.
49. Escudero E, Espuny A, Vicente S, Carceles CM: Pharmacokinetics of an ampicillin-sulbactam combination after intravenous and intramuscular administration to sheep. *Can JVet Res.* = Revue Canadienne de Recherche Veterinaire. 1999:63(1);25–30.
50. Elsheikh HA, Osman IA, Ali BH: Comparative pharmacokinetics of ampicillin trihydrate, gentamicin sulphate and oxytetracycline hydrochloride in Nubian goats and desert sheep. *J Vet Pharmacol The.* 1997:20(4);262–266.
51. Horak IG, Raymond SM, Louw JP: The use of amprolium in the treatment of coccidiosis in domestic ruminants. *J South African Vet Med Assn.* 1969:40;293–299.

52. Sharma D, Agnihotri RK, Moudgil AD, Mandial RK, Katoch A: Comparative efficacy of sulphadimidine and amprolium against natural coccidiosis in Chegu goats. *J Vet Parasitol.* 2011:25(2); 175–176.
53. Hammond DM: Amprolium for control of experimental coccidiosis in lambs. *Cornell Vet.* 1967:57;611–623.
54. Gibbons P, Love D, Craig T, Budke C: Efficacy of treatment of elevated coccidial oocyst counts in goats using amprolium versus ponazuril. *Vet Parasitol.* 2016:218;1–4.
55. Iqbal A, Tariq KA, Wazir VS, Singh R: Antiparasitic efficacy of Artemisia absinthium, toltrazuril and amprolium against intestinal coccidiosis in goats. *J Parasit Dis.* 2013:37(1);83–93.
56. Fitzsimmons WM: Amprolium as a coccidiostat for goats. *Vet Rec.* 1967:80(1);24–26.
57. Avais M, Rashid G, Ijaz M, et al: Evaluation of furazolidone, sulfadimidine and amprolium to treat coccidiosis in beetal goats under field conditions. *Pakistan J Pharmaceut Sci.* 2016:29(2);485–487.
58. Talmon P, Jager LP, de Leeuw WA, Timmer WJ: [Coccidiosis in lambs: observations in the preventive use of an amprolium-containing medicated feed]. *Tijdschrift voor Diergeneeskunde.* 1989:114(11);611–617.
59. Ali BH: Comparative pharmacokinetics of salicylate in camels, sheep and goats. *Eur J Drug Metab Pharmacokinet.* 2003:28(2);125–128.
60. Coetzee JF, Gehring R, Bettenhausen AC, et al: Attenuation of acute plasma cortisol response in calves following intravenous sodium salicylate administration prior to castration. *J Vet Pharmacol Ther.* 2007:30(4);305–313.
61. Gingerich DA, Baggot JD, Yeary RA: Pharmacokinetics and dosage of aspirin in cattle. *J Am Vet Med Assoc.* 1975:167(10);945–948.
62. Carroll GL, Hartsfield SM, Champney TH, Geller SC, Martinez EA, Haley EL: Effect of medetomidine and its antagonism with atipamezole on stress-related hormones, metabolites, physiologic responses, sedation, and mechanical threshold in goats. *Vet Anaesthes Analges.* 2005:32(3);147–157.
63. Ranheim B, Arnemo JM, Stuen S, Horsberg TE: Medetomidine and atipamezole in sheep: disposition and clinical effects. *J Vet Pharmacol Thers.* 2000:23(6);401–404.
64. Christina Haerdi-Landerer M, Schlegel U, Neiger-Aeschbacher G: The analgesic effects of intrathecal xylazine and detomidine in sheep and their antagonism with systemic atipamezole. *Vet Anaesthes Analges.* 2005:32(5);297–307.
65. Kinjavdekar P, Amarpal GR, Pawde AM, Aithal HP, Gupta OP: Influence of yohimbine and atipamezole on haemodynamics and ECG after lumbosacral subarachnoid administration of medetomidine in goats. *JVet Med.* 2003:50(8);424–431.
66. Pablo LS, Webb AI, McNicholas WT, Jr: The effects of atropine and glycopyrrolate on heart rates in conscious mature goats. *Vet Surg.* 1995:24(6);531–534.
67. Bakima M, Baudet HM, Lekeux P, Lomba F: Respiratory and pulmonary haemodynamic changes during experimental organophosphate poisoning in goats. *Vet Res Commun.* 1989:13(2);127–133.
68. Boermans HJ, Black WD, Chesney J, Robb R, Shewfelt W: Terbufos poisoning in a dairy herd. *Can Vet J.* 1984:25(9);335–338.
69. Younger RL, Wright FC: Acute coumaphos toxicosis in cattle: antidotal therapy with pralidoxime chloride and atropine, and related alterations of blood and serum enzymatic activities. *Am J Vet Res.* 1971:32(7);1053–1063.
70. Carceles CM, Font A, Escudero E, Espuny A, Marin P, Fernandez-Varon E: Pharmacokinetics of azithromycin after i.v. and i.m. administration to sheep. *J Vet Pharmacol Ther.* 2005:28(5);475–479.
71. Carceles CM, Font A, Espuny A, Fernandez-Varon E, Serrano JM, Escudero E: Pharmacokinetics of azithromycin after intravenous and intramuscular administration to goats. *J VetPharmacol Ther.* 2005:28(1);51–55.
72. Kemp MW, Miura Y, Payne MS, et al: Maternal intravenous administration of azithromycin results in significant fetal uptake in a sheep model of second trimester pregnancy. *Antimicrob Agents Chemother.* 2014:58(11);6581–6591.
73. Miura Y, Payne MS, Keelan JA, et al: Maternal intravenous treatment with either azithromycin or solithromycin clears ureaplasma parvum from the amniotic fluid in an ovine model of intrauterine infection. *Antimicrob Agents Chemother.* 2014:58(9);5413–5420.
74. Ahern BJ, Soma LR, Boston RC, Schaer TP: Comparison of the analgesic properties of transdermally administered fentanyl and intramuscularly administered buprenorphine during and following experimental orthopedic surgery in sheep. *Am JVety Res.* 2009: 70(3);418–422.
75. Schauvliege S, Narine K, Bouchez S, et al: Refined anaesthesia for implantation of engineered experimental aortic valves in the pulmonary artery using a right heart bypass in sheep. *Lab Animals.* 2006:40(4);341–352.
76. Walkowiak KJ, Graham ML: Pharmacokinetics and antinociceptive activity of sustained-release buprenorphine in sheep. *J Am Assn Lab Animal Sci*2015:54(6);763–768.
77. O'Hair KC, Dodd KT, Phillips YY, Beattie RJ: Cardiopulmonary effects of nalbuphine hydrochloride and butorphanol tartrate in sheep. *Lab Animal Sci.* 1988:38(1):58-61.
78. Nolan A, Livingston A, Waterman AE: Investigation of the antinociceptive activity of buprenorphine in sheep. *Brit J Pharmacol.* 1987:92(3);527–533.
79. Waterman AE, Livingston A, Amin A: Analgesic activity and respiratory effects of butorphanol in sheep. *Res Vet Sci.* 1991:51(1);19–23.
80. Howard BW, Lagutchik MS, Januszkiewicz AJ, Martin DG: The cardiovascular response of sheep to tiletamine-zolazepam and butorphanol tartrate anesthesia. *Vet Surg.* 1990:19(6);461–467.
81. Carroll GL, Hartsfield SM, Champney TH, Slater MR, Newman JA: Stress-related hormonal and metabolic responses to restraint, with and without butorphanol administration, in pre-conditioned goats. *Lab Animal Sci.* 1998:48(4);387–390.
82. Doze JG, Donders R, van der Kolk JH: Effects of intravenous administration of two volumes of calcium solution on plasma ionized calcium concentration and recovery from naturally occurring hypocalcemia in lactating dairy cows. *Am JVet Res.* 2008:69(10); 1346–1350.
83. Farningham DA: Formation of calcium complexes by borogluconate in vitro and during calcium borogluconate infusion in sheep. *Res Vet Sci.* 1985:39(1);70–74.
84. Melendez P, Donovan A, Risco CA, Hall MB, Littell R, Goff J: Metabolic responses of transition Holstein cows fed anionic salts and supplemented at calving with calcium and energy. *J D Sci.* 2002:85(5);1085–1092.
85. Elias E, Shainkin-Kestenbaum R: Hypocalcaemia and serum levels of inorganic phosphorus, magnesium parathyroid and calcitonin hormones in the last month of pregnancy in Awassi fat-tail ewes. *Reprod NutrDev.* 1990:30(6);693–699.
86. Paull DR, Lee C, Colditz IG, Fisher AD: Effects of a topical anaesthetic formulation and systemic carprofen, given singly or in combination, on the cortisol and behavioural responses of Merino lambs to castration. *Austr Vet J.* 2009:87(6);230–237.
87. Colditz IG, Lloyd JB, Paull DR, et al: Effect of the non-steroidal anti-inflammatory drug, carprofen, on weaned sheep following non-surgical mulesing by intradermal injection of cetrimide. *Australian Vet J.* 2009:87(1);19–26.
88. Paull DR, Lee C, Colditz IG, Atkinson SJ, Fisher AD: The effect of a topical anaesthetic formulation, systemic flunixin and carprofen, singly or in combination, on cortisol and behavioural responses of Merino lambs to mulesing. *Austr Vet J.* 2007:85(3);98–106.
89. Marini D, Pippia J, Colditz IG, Hinch G, Petherick JC, Lee C: Randomised trial of the bioavailability and efficacy of orally administered flunixin, carprofen and ketoprofen in a pain model in sheep. *Austr Vet J.* 2015:93(8);265–270.
90. Shpigel NY, Levin D, Winkler M, Saran A, Ziv G, Bottner A. Efficacy of cefquinome for treatment of cows with mastitis experimentally induced using Escherichia coli. *Journal of dairy science.* 1997:80(2): 318-323.

91. Errecalde C, Prieto G, Puelles I, Luders C, Garcia Ovando H. Plasma disposition of cefquinome in goats after intramuscular application. *Investigacion Veterinaria.* 2001:3(1/2):89-94.
92. El-Hewaity M, El Latif AA, Soliman A, Aboubakr M. Comparative Pharmacodynamics of Cefquinome (Cobactan 2.5%) following Repeated Intramuscular Administrations in Sheep and Goats. *Journal of Veterinary Medicine.* 2014:2014.
93. Rana MP, Sadariya KA, Thaker AM. Effect of tolfenamic acid co-administration on pharmacokinetics of cefquinome following intramuscular administration in sheep. *Veterinarski Arhiv.* 2015:85(3):283-292.
94. Tohamy MA. Age-related intramuscular pharmacokinetics of cefquinome in sheep. *Small Ruminant Research.* 2011:99(1):72-76.
95. Dumka VK, Dinakaran V, Ranjan B, Rampal S. Comparative pharmacokinetics of cefquinome following intravenous and intramuscular administration in goats. *Small Ruminant Research.* 2013: 113(1):273-277.
96. El-Badawy SA, Amer AM, Kamel GM, Eldeib KM, Constable PD. Comparative pharmacokinetics using a microbiological assay and high performance liquid chromatography following intravenous administration of cefquinome in lactating goats with and without experimentally induced Staphylococcus aureus mastitis. *Small Ruminant Research.* 2015:133:67-76.
97. Rashmi S, Mudasir S, Dumka VK, Mir AH, Prashant, Sahrish C: Pharmacokinetics and dosage regimen of cefquinome in healthy female goats following intravenous administration. *J Vet Pharmacol Toxicol.* 2015:14(2);74–78.
98. Kottwitz J, Blue McLendon A, Monarski C, Jensen J, Boothe D: Disposition of ceftiofur and its active metabolites in fallow deer (Dama dama) following single-dose intravenous and intramuscular administration. *J Zoo Wildlife Med.* 2015:46(2);255–261.
99. United States Food and Drug Administration Center for Veterinary Medicine: Code of Federal Regulation; Part 522 Implantation or Injectable Dosage Form New Animal Drugs; Section 522.313c; Ceftiofur Sodium. Accessed November 2, 2009.
100. Courtin F, Craigmill AL, Wetzlich SE, Gustafson CR, Arndt TS: Pharmacokinetics of ceftiofur and metabolites after single intravenous and intramuscular administration and multiple intramuscular administrations of ceftiofur sodium to dairy goats. *J Vet Pharmacol Ther.* 1997:20(5);368–373.
101. Craigmill AL, Brown SA, Wetzlich SE, Gustafson CR, Arndt TS: Pharmacokinetics of ceftiofur and metabolites after single intravenous and intramuscular administration and multiple intramuscular administrations of ceftiofur sodium to sheep. *J Vet Pharmacol Ther.*1997:20(2);139–144.
102. Upjohn P: Freedom of Information Summary, Naxcel Sterile Powder (ceftiofur sodium), Supplement to NADA 140-338. 2001:1-9.
103. Fernandez-Varon E, Carceles-Garcia C, Serrano-Rodríguez JM, Carceles-Rodriguez CM: Pharmacokinetics (PK), pharmacodynamics (PD), and PK-PD integration of ceftiofur after a single intravenous, subcutaneous and subcutaneous-LA administration in lactating goats. *BMC Vet Res.* 2016:12;232.
104. Drew M, Waldrup K, Kreeger T, Craigmill A, Wetzlich S, Mackintosh C: Pharmacokinetics of ceftiofur in red deer (Cervus elaphus). *J Vet Pharmacol Theraps.* 2004:27(1);7–11.
105. Rivera-Garcia S, Angelos JA, Rowe JD, et al: Pharmacokinetics of ceftiofur crystalline-free acid following subcutaneous administration of a single dose to sheep. *Am J Vet Res.* 2014:75(3);290–295.
106. Dore E, Angelos JA, Rowe JD, et al: Pharmacokinetics of ceftiofur crystalline free acid after single subcutaneous administration in lactating and nonlactating domestic goats (Capra aegagrus hircus). *J Vet Pharmacol Ther.* 2011:34(1);25–30.
107. Waraich GS, Sidhu PK, Daundkar PS, Kaur G, Sharma SK: Pharmacokinetic and pharmacodynamic characterization of ceftiofur crystalline-free acid following subcutaneous administration in domestic goats. *J Vet Pharmacol Thers.* 2017:40(5);429–438.
108. Wagner D: Cervid Field Medicine & Surgery. Paper presented at American Veterinary Medical Association 2011 Conference2011; St. Louis.
109. Fthenakis GC: Field evaluation of flunixin meglumine in the supportive treatment of ovine mastitis. *J Vet Pharmacol Therap.* 2000: 23(6);405–407.
110. Mavrogianni VS, Alexopoulos C, Fthenakis GC: Field evaluation of flunixin meglumine in the supportive treatment of caprine mastitis. *J Vet Pharmacol Ther.* 2004:27(5);373-375.
111. Hernandez F, Elvira L, Fernández B, et al: Effects of intramammary antibiotic therapy during the dry period on the performance of Lacaune dairy sheep under intensive management. *J Dairy Res.* 2014:82(1);95–101.
112. Spanu C, Berger YM, Thomas DL, Ruegg PL: Impact of intramammary antimicrobial dry treatment and teat sanitation on somatic cell count and intramammary infection in dairy ewes. *Small Ruminant Res.* 2011:97(1–3);139–145.
113. Fox LK, Hancock DD, Horner SD: Selective intramammary antibiotic therapy during the nonlactating period in goats. *Small Ruminant Res.* 1992:9(3);313–318.
114. Pass MA, Stewart C: Administration of activated charcoal for the treatment of lantana poisoning of sheep and cattle. *J Appl Toxicol.* 1984:4(5);267–269.
115. Berger JA: comparison of some anaesthetic techniques in young calves. *Brit Vet J.* 1966:122(2);65–73.
116. Singh J, Prasad B, Mirakhur KK, Kohli RN: Oxygen environment and acid–base status of the jugular, portal and renal veins and brain sinus of bovines in the conscious and sedated states. *Zentralblatt fur Veterinarmedizin.* 1981:28(7);559–568.
117. United States Food and Drug Administration Center for Veterinary Medicine: Code of Federal Regulations; 21 CFR 558.128; New Animal Drugs for Use in Animal Feeds; Chlortetracycline. Vol July 1, 20182018:421-425.
118. Washburn K, Fajt VR, Plummer P, Coetzee JF, Wulf LW, Washburn S: Pharmacokinetics of oral chlortetracycline in nonpregnant adult ewes. *J Vet Pharmacol Ther.* 2014:37(6);607–610.
119. Connell JM, Khalapyan T, Al–Mondhiry HA, Wilson RP, Rosenberg G, Weiss WJ: Anticoagulation of juvenile sheep and goats with heparin, warfarin, and clopidogrel. *Asaio J.* 2007: 53(2);229–237.
120. Weigand A, Boos AM, Ringwald J, et al: New aspects on efficient anticoagulation and antiplatelet strategies in sheep. *BMC Vet Res.* 2013:9(192):(3October2013).
121. Challis JR, Forster CS, Furr BJ, Robinson JS, Thorburn GD: Production of prostaglandin Falpha in ewes following luteal regression induced with a prostaglandin analogue, Estrumate (cloprostenol; I.C.I. 80996). *Prostaglandins.* 1976:11(3);537–543.
122. Fernandez-Moro D, Veiga-Lopez A, Ariznavarreta C, Tresguerres JA, Encinas T, Gonzalez-Bulnes A: Preovulatory follicle development in goats following oestrous synchronization with progestagens or prostaglandins. *Reprod Domestic Animals* = Zuchthygiene. 2008:43(1);9–14.
123. Nuti LC, Bretzlaff KN, Elmore RG, et al: Synchronization of estrus in dairy goats treated with prostaglandin F at various stages of the estrous cycle. *Am J et Res.* 1992:53(6);935–937.
124. Reid RN, Crothers I: Prostaglandin F2 alpha for oestrus synchronisation or abortion in Polwarth ewes. *AustrVet J.* 1980:56(1);22–24.
125. Nancarrow CD, Evison BM, Connell PJ: Effect of embryos on luteolysis and termination of early pregnancy in sheep with cloprostenol. *Biol Reprod.* 1982:26(2);263–269.
126. de Carvalho Menezes de Almeida SF, Souza-Fabjan JMG, Balaro MFA, et al: Use of two doses of cloprostenol in different intervals for estrus synchronization in hair sheep under tropical conditions. *Trop Animal Health Prod.* 2018:50(2);427–432.
127. Day AM, Southwell SR: Termination of pregnancy in goats using cloprostenol. *N ZVet J.* 1979:27(10);207–208.
128. Tyrrell RN, Lane JG, Nancarrow CD, Connell PJ: Termination of early pregnancy in ewes by use of a prostaglandin analogue and subsequent fertility. *Austr Vety J.* 1981:57(2);76–78.
129. Maia ALRS, Brandao FZ, Souza-Fabjan JMG, et al: Reproductive parameters of dairy goats after receiving two doses of d-cloprostenol at different intervals. *Animal Reprod Sci.* 2017:181;16–23.

130. Maule Walker FM: Lactation and fertility in goats after the induction of parturition with an analogue of prostaglandin F2 alpha, cloprostenol. *Res Vet Sci.* 1983:34(3);280–286.
131. Fisher MW, Asher GW, Meikle LM, Newman RE: Cloprostenol-induced luteolysis in the red deer hind: the effects of age, dose, number of corpora lutea and the later stages of the oestrous cycle. *Animal Reprod Sci.* 1994:35(1–2);99–109.
132. Conboy GA, Stromberg BE, Schlotthauer JC: Efficacy of clorsulon against Fascioloides magna infection in sheep. *J Am Vet Med Assoc.* 1988:192(7);910–912.
133. Zimmerman GL, Wallace DH, Schons DJ, Hoberg EP: Efficacy of clorsulon against mature, naturally acquired Fasciola hepatica infections in cattle and sheep. *Am J Vet Res.* 1986:47(8);1665–1667.
134. Foreyt WJ: Evaluation of clorsulon against immature Fascioloides magna in cattle and sheep. *Am J VetRes.* 1988:49(7);1004–1006.
135. Sundlof SF, Bliss EL, Greiner EC, Tran TQ, Wertenberger MA: Efficacy of clorsulon for the treatment of experimentally induced infections of Fasciola hepatica in goats. *Am J VetRes.* 1991:52(1);111–114.
136. Rehbein S, Visser M: Efficacy of an injectable ivermectin/clorsulon combination against Fasciola hepatica in sheep. *Vet Rec.* 1999: 145(16);468.
137. Tramboo SR, Shahardar RA, Allaie IM, Wani ZA, Abbas M: Efficacy of ivermectin, closantel and fenbendazole against gastrointestinal nematodes of sheep in Kashmir valley. *J Parasitic Dis: Offic Organ Indian Soc Parasitol.* 2017:41(2);380–382.
138. Westers T, Jones-Bitton A, Menzies P, Van Leeuwen J, Poljak Z, Peregrine AS: Efficacy of closantel against ivermectin- and fenbendazole-resistant Haemonchus sp. in sheep in Ontario, Canada. *Vet Parasitol.* 2016:228;30–41.
139. Costa CT, Bevilaqua CM, Maciel MV, et al: Anthelmintic activity of Azadirachta indica A. Juss against sheep gastrointestinal nematodes. *Vet Parasitol.* 2006:137(3–4);306–310.
140. Mooney L, Good B, Hanrahan JP, Mulcahy G, de Waal T: The comparative efficacy of four anthelmintics against a natural acquired Fasciola hepatica infection in hill sheep flock in the west of Ireland. *Vet Parasitol.* 2009:164(2–4);201–205.
141. Coles GC, Rhodes AC, Stafford KA: Activity of closantel against adult triclabendazole-resistant Fasciola hepatica. *Vet Record.* 2000:146(17);504.
142. Dorchies P, Alzieu JP, Cadiergues MC: Comparative curative and preventive efficacies of ivermectin and closantel on Oestrus ovis (Linne 1758) in naturally infected sheep. *Vet Parasitol.* 1997: 72(2);179–184.
143. Suarez VH, Busetii MR, Miranda AO, Prevot F, Jacquiet P: Epidemiology of Oestrus ovis infection of sheep in Argentina's Western Pampas. *Parasite (Paris, France).* 2004:11(4);405–410.
144. Shrimali RG, Patel MD, Patel RM: Comparative efficacy of anthelmintics and their effects on hemato-biochemical changes in fasciolosis of goats of South Gujarat. *Vet World.* 2016:9(5);524–529.
145. Godinho K, Benchaoui HA, Tilt N, et al: Efficacy of danofloxacin in the treatment of pneumonic pasteurellosis in specific pathogen-free lambs. *Vet Rec.* 2007:160(22);770–771.
146. Escudero E, Carceles CM, Fernandez-varon E, Marin P, Benchaoui H: Pharmacokinetics of danofloxacin 18% in lactating sheep and goats. *J Vet Pharmacol Ther.* 2007:30(6);572–577.
147. Ozdemir U, Loria GR, Godinho KS, et al: Effect of danofloxacin (Advocin A180) on goats affected with contagious caprine pleuropneumonia. *Trop Animal Health Product.* 2006:38(7–8);533–540.
148. United States Food and Drug Administration Center for Veterinary Medicine: Code of Federal Regulation; Part 558 New Animal Drugs for Use in Animal Feeds; Section 558.195; Decoquinate. Accessed November 2, 2009.
149. Anonymous: Deccox 6% Premix for Medicated Feeding Stuff for Sheep and Cattle, http://www.noahcompendium.co.uk/Alpharma_Belgium_bvba/documents/S3341.html. Accessed November 28, 2009.
150. Buxton D, Brebner J, Wright S, Maley SW, Thomson KM, Millard K: Decoquinate and the control of experimental ovine toxoplasmosis. *Vet Rec.* 1996:138(18);434–436.
151. Clark TP, Purohit RC, Wilson RC: Evaluation of sedative and analgesic properties of detomidine in goats. *Agri-Practice.* 1993: 14(4);29–33.
152. Carroll GL, Hooper RN, Slater MR, Hartsfield SM, Matthews NS: Detomidine-butorphanol-propofol for carotid artery translocation and castration or ovariectomy in goats. *Vet Surg.* 1998:27(1);75–82.
153. Singh AP, Peshin PK, Singh J, Sharifi D, Patil DB: Evaluation of detomidine as a sedative in goats. *Acta Vet Hungarica.* 1991:39 (3–4);109–114.
154. Stafford KJ, Chambers JP, Sylvester SP, et al: The stress caused by laparoscopy in sheep and its alleviation. *N Z Vet J.* 2006: 54(3);109–113.
155. Waterman AE, Nolan A, Livingston A: Influence of idazoxan on the respiratory blood gas changes induced by alpha 2-adrenoceptor agonist drugs in conscious sheep. *Vet Rec.* 1987:121(5);105–107.
156. de Moura RS, Bittar IP, da Silva LH, et al: Sedative and cardiorespiratory effects of detomidine constant rate infusion in sheep. *Lab Animals.* 2018:52(1);51–58.
157. Bosc MJ: The induction and synchronization of lambing with the aid of dexamethasone. *J Reprod Fertil.* 1972:28(3);347–357.
158. Edey TN, Thwaites CJ, Baillie ND, Bremner GJ: Dose rate, time of injection and litter size effects on dexamethasone-induced parturition in Border Leicester x Merino ewes. *Austr Vet J.* 1985: 62(3);104–105.
159. Thakur MS, Verma SK: Use of dexamethasone for induction of parturition in goats. *Archiv Experimentelle Veterinarmedizin.* 1990:44(3);459–463.
160. Lohuis JA, Van Leeuwen W, Verheijden JH, Van Miert AS, Brand A: Effect of dexamethasone on experimental Escherichia coli mastitis in the cow. *J Dairy Sci.* 1988:71(10);2782–2789.
161. Lohuis JA, Van Leeuwen W, Verheijden JH, Brand A, Van Miert AS: Effect of steroidal anti-inflammatory drugs on Escherichia coli endotoxin-induced mastitis in the cow. *J Dairy Sci.* 1989:72(1);241–249.
162. Anderson KL, Hunt E. Anti-inflammatory therapy in acute endotoxin-induced bovine mastitis. *Vet Res Commun.* 1989:13(1);17–26.
163. Anderson KL, Hunt E, Davis BJ: The influence of anti–inflammatory therapy on bacterial clearance following intramammary Escherichia coli challenge in goats. *Vet Res Commun.* 1991: 15(2):147-161.
164. Zamri-Saad M, Effendy AW, Israf DA, Azmi ML. Cellular and humoral responses in the respiratory tract of goats following intranasal stimulation using formalin-killed Pasteurella haemolytica A2. *Vet Microbiol.* 1999:65(3);233–240.
165. Schuler JJ, Erve PR, Schumer W: Glucocorticoid effect on hepatic carbohydrate metabolism in the endotoxin-shocked monkey. *Ann Surg.* 1976:183(4);345–354.
166. Shatney CH, Lillehei RC: Serum complement levels in canine endotoxin shock: relation to survival and to corticosteroid therapy. *Adv Shock Res.* 1983:9;265–274.
167. Van Saun RJ: Pregnancy toxemia in a flock of sheep. *J Am Vet Med Assoc.* 2000:217(10);1536–1539.
168. Henze P, Bickhardt K, Fuhrmann H, Sallmann HP: Spontaneous pregnancy toxaemia (ketosis) in sheep and the role of insulin. *Zentralblatt fur Veterinarmedizin.* 1998:45(5);255–266.
169. Eales FA, Small J, Gilmour JS: Resuscitation of hypothermic lambs. *Vet Rec.* 1982:110(6);121–123.
170. Vesal N, Oloumi MM: A preliminary comparison of epidural lidocaine and xylazine during total intravenous anaesthesia in Iranian fat-tailed sheep. *Zentralblatt fur Veterinarmedizin.* 1998:45(6–7);353–360.
171. Celly CS, McDonell WN, Black WD, Young SS: Cardiopulmonary effects of clonidine, diazepam and the peripheral alpha 2 adrenoceptor agonist ST-91 in conscious sheep. *J Vet Pharmacol Ther.* 1997:20(6);472–478.
172. Coulson NM, Januszkiewicz AJ, Dodd KT, Ripple GR: The cardiorespiratory effects of diazepam-ketamine and xylazine-ketamine anesthetic combinations in sheep. *LabAnimal Sci.* 1989:39(6);591–597.

173. McKeough VL, Collett MG, Parton KH: Suspected Vestia foetida poisoning in young goats. *N Z Vet Jl.* 2005:53(5);352–355.
174. Van Miert AS, Koot M, Van Duin CT: Appetite-modulating drugs in dwarf goats, with special emphasis on benzodiazepine-induced hyperphagia and its antagonism by flumazenil and RO 15-3505. *J Vety Pharmacol Ther.* 1989:12(2);147–156.
175. Mundt HC, Dittmar K, Daugschies A, Grzonka E, Bangoura B: Study of the comparative efficacy of toltrazuril and diclazuril against ovine coccidiosis in housed lambs. *Parasitol Res.* 2009: 105(Suppl 1):S141–150.
176. Diaferia M, Veronesi F, Morganti G, Nisoli L, Fioretti DP: Efficacy of Toltrazuril 5% suspension (Baycox®, Bayer) and diclazuril (Vecoxan®, Janssen-Cilag) in the control of Eimeria spp. in lambs. *Parasitol Res.* 2013:112(S1);163–168.
177. Saratsis A, Karagiannis I, Brozos C, et al: Lamb eimeriosis: Applied treatment protocols in dairy sheep production systems. *Vet Parasitol.* 2013:196(1–2);56–63.
178. Ruiz A, Guedes A, Muñoz M, et al: Control strategies using diclazuril against coccidiosis in goat kids. *Parasitol Res.* 2012:110(6); 2131–2136.
179. Godfrey RW, Collins JR, Hensley EL, Wheaton JE: Estrus synchronization and artificial insemination of hair sheep ewes in the tropics. *Theriogenology.* 1999:51(5);985–997.
180. Godfrey RW, Gray ML, Collins JR: A comparison of two methods of oestrous synchronisation of hair sheep in the tropics. *Animal Reprod Sci.* 1997:47(1–2);99–106.
181. Alan M, Tasal I: Efficacy of prostaglandin F2alpha and misoprostol in the induction of parturition in goats. *Vet Rec.* 2002:150(25);788–789.
182. Bretzlaff KN, Hill A, Ott RS: Induction of luteolysis in goats with prostaglandin F2 alpha. *Am J Vet Res.* 1983:44(6);1162–1164.
183. Hesselink JW: Hydrometra in dairy goats: reproductive performance after treatment with prostaglandins. *Vet Rec.* 1993: 133(8);186–187.
184. Souza JMG, Maia ALRS, Brandão FZ, et al: Hormonal treatment of dairy goats affected by hydrometra associated or not with ovarian follicular cyst. *Small ruminant research.* 2013:111(1–3):104-109.
185. Audicana L, Harvey MJ: Termination of early pregnancy in sheep with dinoprost or cloprostenol: comparison of two commercial preparations. *Vet Rec.* 1993:133(23);574–576.
186. Rolbin SH, Levinson G, Shnider SM, Biehl DR, Wright RG: Dopamine treatment of spinal hypotension decreases uterine blood flow in the pregnant ewe. *Anesthesiology.* 1979:51(1);37–40.
187. Bernstein D, Crane C: Comparative circulatory effects of isoproterenol and dopamine in lambs with experimental cyanotic heart disease. *Pediatr Res.* 1991:29(4 Pt 1);323–328.
188. Sun Q, Tu Z, Lobo S, et al: Optimal adrenergic support in septic shock due to peritonitis. *Anesthesiology.* 2003:98(4):888-896.
189. Brew N, Azhan A, den Heijer I, et al: Dopamine treatment during acute hypoxia is neuroprotective in the developing sheep brain. *Neuroscience.* 2016:316:82-93.
190. Dorchies P, Jacquiet P, Bergeaud JP, et al: Efficacy of doramectin injectable against Oestrus ovis and gastrointestinal nematodes in sheep in the southwestern region of France. *Vet Parasitol.* 2001: 96(2);147–154.
191. Hertzberg H, Meyer A, Kohler L, Falconi F, Ochs H: [Effect of a single injection of doramectin on gastrointestinal nematode infections of sheep grazing on alpine pastures.]. *Schweizer Archiv fur Tierheilkunde.* 2001:143(6);305–311.
192. Zaman MA, Rehman TU, Abbas RZ, et al: Theraputic potential of Ivermectin, doramectin and trichlorophan against Psoroptes ovis in sheep and cattle of Cholistan. *Pakistan Vet J.* 2017:37(2);233–235.
193. Terrill TH, Kaplan RM, Larsen M, Samples OM, Miller JE, Gelaye S: Anthelmintic resistance on goat farms in Georgia: efficacy of anthelmintics against gastrointestinal nematodes in two selected goat herds. *Vet Parasitol.* 2001:97(4);261–268.
194. Pound JM, Miller JA, Oehler DD: Depletion rate of Doramectin from blood serum of penned female white-tailed deer. *J Med Entomol.* 2004:41(5);942–945.
195. Bairam A, Blanchard PW, Bureau MA, Laudignon N, Cote A, Aranda JV: Interactive ventilatory effects of two respiratory stimulants, caffeine and doxapram, in newborn lambs. *Biol Neonate.* 1992:61(3);201–208.
196. Haw A, Meyer L, Greer J, Fuller A: Ampakine CX1942 attenuates opioid-induced respiratory depression and corrects the hypoxaemic effects of etorphine in immobilized goats (Capra hircus). *Vet AnaesthesAnalges.* 2016:43(5);528–538.
197. Olkowski AA, Gooneratne SR, Christensen DA: The effects of thiamine and EDTA on biliary and urinary lead excretion in sheep. *Toxicol Lett.* 1991:59(1–3);153–159.
198. Meldrum JB, Ko KW: Effects of calcium disodium EDTA and meso-2,3-dimercaptosuccinic acid on tissue concentrations of lead for use in treatment of calves with experimentally induced lead toxicosis. *Am J Vet Res.* 2003:64(6);672–676.
199. Aronson AL, Hammond PB, Strafuss AC: Studies with calcium ethylenediaminetetraacetate in calves; toxicity and use in bovine lead poisoning. *Toxicol. Appl Pharmacol.* 1968:12(3);337–349.
200. Rahal A, Kumar A, Ahmad AH, Malik JK, Ahuja V: Pharmacokinetics of enrofloxacin in sheep following intravenous and subcutaneous administration. *J Vet Pharmacol Ther.* 2006:29(4);321–324.
201. Elsheikh HA, Taha AA, Khalafallah AI, Osman IA: Disposition kinetics of enrofloxacin (Baytril 5%) in sheep and goats following intravenous and intramuscular injection using a microbiological assay. *Res Vet Sci.* 2002:73(2);125–129.
202. Attili AR, Preziuso S, Ngu Ngwa V, Cantalamessa A, Moriconi M, Cuteri V: Clinical evaluation of the use of enrofloxacin against Staphylococcus aureus clinical mastitis in sheep. *Small Ruminant Res.* 2016:136;2–77.
203. Ramesh S, Rao GS, Malik JK: Pharmacokinetic disposition of subcutaneously administered enrofloxacin in goats. *Vet Res Commun.* 2002:26(7);563–569.
204. Burchfield DJ, Preziosi MP, Lucas VW, Fan J: Effects of graded doses of epinephrine during asphxia-induced bradycardia in newborn lambs. *Resuscitation.* 1993:25(3);235–244.
205. Cringoli G, Rinaldi L, Veneziano V, Capelli G: Efficacy of eprinomectin pour-on against gastrointestinal nematode infections in sheep. *Vet Parasitol.* 2003:112(3);203–209.
206. Habela M, Moreno A, Gragera-Slikker A, et al: Efficacy of eprinomectin pour-on in naturally Oestrus ovis infested merino sheep in Extremadura, South-West Spain. *Parasitol Res.* 2006:99(3);275–280.
207. Hamel D, Bosco A, Rinaldi L, et al: Eprinomectin pour-on (EPRINEX Pour-on, Merial): efficacy against gastrointestinal and pulmonary nematodes and pharmacokinetics in sheep. *BMC Vet Res.* 2017:(13);148.
208. Chartier C, Etter E, Pors I, Alvinerie M: Activity of eprinomectin in goats against experimental infections with Haemonchus contortus, Teladorsagia circumcincta and Trichostrongylus colubriformis. *Vet Rec.* 1999:144(4);99–100.
209. Hamel D, Visser M, Kellermann M, Kvaternick V, Rehbein S: Anthelmintic efficacy and pharmacokinetics of pour-on eprinomectin (1mg/kg bodyweight) against gastrointestinal and pulmonary nematode infections in goats. *Small Ruminant Res.* 2015: 127;74–79.
210. Katoch R, Yadav A, Sharma RK, Kour R, Tazeen. Efficacy of eprinomectin pour on against natural infestation of sarcoptic mange in goats. *Vet Practitioner.* 2010:11(2);99–100.
211. Rehbein S, Kellermann M, Wehner T: Pharmacokinetics and anthelmintic efficacy of topical eprinomectin in goats prevented from grooming. *Parasitol Res.* 2014:113(11);4039–4044.
212. Rendell DK, Callinan AP: Comparison of erythromycin and oxytetracycline for the treatment of virulent footrot in grazing sheep. *Austr Vet J.* 1997:75(5);354.
213. Ambros L, Montoya L, Kreil V, et al: Pharmacokinetics of erythromycin in nonlactating and lactating goats after intravenous and intramuscular administration. *J Vet Pharmacol Ther.* 2007:30(1);80–85.
214. Goudah A, Sher Shah S, Shin HC, Shim JH, Abd El-Aty AM: Pharmacokinetics and mammary residual depletion of erythromycin in healthy lactating ewes. *J Vet M.* 2007:54(10);607–611.

215. Piriz S, Pobel T, Jimenez R, et al: Comparison of erythromycin and oxytetracycline for the treatment of ovine footrot. *Acta Veterinaria Hungarica.* 2001:49(2);131–139.
216. Mizinga KM, Verma OP. LHRH-Induced ovulation and fertility of anestrous goats. *Theriogenology.* 1984:21(3);435–446.
217. Fresno L, Andaluz A, Moll X, Cristofol C, Arboix M, García F: Placental transfer of etomidate in pregnant ewes after an intravenous bolus dose and continuous infusion. *Vet J.* 2008:175(3);395–402.
218. Burger HJ. Efficacy of febantel in sheep experimentally infected with five species of gastrointestinal nematodes. *Vet Rec.* 1978: 103(26–27);572–574.
219. Thomas H: The efficacy of febantel on gastrointestinal nematodes in sheep. *Res Vet Sci.* 1978:25(3);290–293.
220. Lyons ET, Drudge JH, Tolliver SC: Activity of febantel on natural infections of gastrointestinal helminths in lambs in a controlled test. *Am J Vet Res.* 1988:49(6);901–902.
221. Chartier C, Kulo A, Cabaret J, Pors I, Benoit C: Individual fluctuations in efficacy of febantel against Muellerius capillaris in goats. *Vet Res.* 1995:26(2);116–123.
222. United States Food and Drug Administration Center for Veterinary Medicine: Code of Federal Regulation; Part 520 Oral Dosage Form New Animal Drugs; Section 520.905a; Fenbendazole Suspension. Accessed November 2, 2009.
223. Peña Espinoza M, Thamsborg S, Demeler J, Enemark H: Field efficacy of four anthelmintics and confirmation of drug-resistant nematodes by controlled efficacy test and pyrosequencing on a sheep and goat farm in Denmark. *Vet Parasitol.* 2014:206(3–4);208–215.
224. Haibel GK, Hull BL: Induction of parturition in goats with fenprostalene. *Theriogenology.* 1988:30(5);901–903.
225. Christou C, Oliver RA, Rawlinson J, Walsh WR: Transdermal fentanyl and its use in ovine surgery. *Res Vet Sci.* 2015:100;252–256.
226. Ahern B, Soma L, Rudy J, Uboh C, Schaer T: Pharmacokinetics of fentanyl administered transdermally and intravenously in sheep. *Am J Vet Res.* 2010:71(10);1127–1132.
227. Burke MJ, Soma LR, Boston RC, Rudy JA, Schaer TP: Evaluation of the analgesic and pharmacokinetic properties of transdermally administered fentanyl in goats. *J VetEmer Critl Care.* 2017: 27(5);539–547.
228. Shen J, Li X, Jiang H, Hsu WH: Bioavailability and pharmacokinetics of florfenicol in healthy sheep. *J Vet Pharmacol Ther.* 2004:27(3);163–168.
229. Balcomb C, Angelos J, Chigerwe M, et al: Comparative pharmacokinetics of two florfenicol formulations following intramuscular and subcutaneous administration to sheep. *Am J Vet Res.* 2018: 79(1);107–114.
230. Lane VM, Villarroel A, Wetzlich SE, Clifford A, Taylor I, Craigmill AL: Intravenous and subcutaneous pharmacokinetics of florfenicol in sheep. *J Vet Pharmacol Ther.* 2004:27(4);191–196.
231. Ali BH, Al-Qarawi AA, Hashaad M: Comparative plasma pharmacokinetics and tolerance of florfenicol following intramuscular and intravenous administration to camels, sheep and goats. *Vet Res Commun.* 2003:27(6);475–483.
232. Atef M, el-Gendi AY, Amer AM, Abd El-Aty AM: Disposition kinetics of florfenicol in goats by using two analytical methods. *J Ve Med.* 2001:48(3);129–136.
233. Elitok OM, Elitok B, Konak S, Demirel HH: Clinical efficacy of florfenicol on caprine pasteurellosis. *Small Ruminant Res.* 2015:125;142–145.
234. Alcorn J, Dowling P, Woodbury M, Killeen R: Pharmacokinetics of florfenicol in North American elk (Cervus elaphus). *J Vet Pharmacol Ther.* 2004:27(5);289–292.
235. Kyles AE, Waterman AE, Livingston A: Antinociceptive activity of midazolam in sheep. *J Vet Pharmacol Ther.* 1995:18(1);54–60.
236. Stubsjoen SM, Flo AS, Moe RO, et al: Exploring non-invasive methods to assess pain in sheep. *PhysiolBehav.* 2009:98(5);640–648.
237. Larvor P, Rayssiguier Y: Hypomagnesaemia following theophylline or furosemide injection in ewes: renal versus extrarenal effect. *J Physiol.* 1972:227(2);365–375.
238. Rademaker MT, Fitzpatrick MA, Charles CJ, et al: Comparison of chronic neutral endopeptidase inhibition and furosemide in an ovine model of heart failure. *J CardiovascPharmacol.* 1996: 27(3);439–446.
239. English PB, Becvar WE: Effects of furosemide on the external balances of water, sodium, potassium, and chloride in sheep. *Am J Vet Res.* 1971:32(9);1371–1379.
240. Power SB, Malone A: An outbreak of ringworm in sheep in Ireland caused by Trichophyton verrucosum. *Vet Rec.* 1987:121(10); 218–220.
241. Guedes AG, Pluhar GE, Daubs BM, Rude EP: Effects of preoperative epidural administration of racemic ketamine for analgesia in sheep undergoing surgery. *Am JVet Res.* 2006:67(2);222–229.
242. Cake MA, Smith MM, Young AA, Smith SM, Ghosh P, Read RA: Synovial pathology in an ovine model of osteoarthritis: effect of intraarticular hyaluronan (Hyalgan). *Clin Exp Rheumatol.* 2008: 26(4);561–567.
243. Tytherleigh-Strong G, Hurtig M, Miniaci A: Intra-articular hyaluronan following autogenous osteochondral grafting of the knee. *Arthroscopy.* 2005:21(8):999-1005.
244. do Nascimento P, Jr., Vaid SU, Hoskins SL, Espana JM, Kinsky MP, Kramer GC: Hypertonic 15% sodium pyruvate offers no initial resuscitation advantage compared with 8% hypertonic NACl in sheep with multiple hemorrhages. *Shock (Augusta, Ga.)* 2007: 27(5);565–571.
245. Svensen CH, Waldrop KS, Edsberg L, Hahn RG: Natriuresis and the extracellular volume expansion by hypertonic saline. *J Surg Res.* 2003:113(1);6–12.
246. Ogino R: Effects of hypertonic saline and dextran 70 on cardiac diastolic function after hemorrhagic shock. *J Surg Res.* 2002: 107(1);27–36.
247. Demling RH, LaLonde C, Goad ME: Effect of ibuprofen on the pulmonary and systemic response to repeated doses of endotoxin. *Surgery.* 1989:105(3);421–429.
248. Emau P, Giri SN, Bruss ML, Zia S: Ibuprofen prevents Pasteurella hemolytica endotoxin-induced changes in plasma prostanoids and serotonin, and fever in sheep. *J Vet Pharmacol Ther.* 1985:8(4);352–361.
249. DeGraves FJ, Anderson KL, Aucoin DP: Pharmacokinetics of ibuprofen in lactating dairy goats. *Am J Vet Res.* 1993:54(3);434–437.
250. McHardy N, Woollon RM, Clampitt RB, James JA, Crawley RJ: Efficacy, toxicity and metabolism of imidocarb dipropionate in the treatment of Babesia ovis infection in sheep. *Res Vet Science.* 1986:41(1);14–20.
251. United States Food and Drug Administration Center for Veterinary Medicine: Code of Federal Regulations; 21 CFR 520.1195; Oral Dosage Form New Animal Drugs; Ivermectin Liquid. Vol July 1, 20182018:171-172.
252. Oksanen A, Asbakk K, Raekallio M, Niemenen M: The relative plasma availabilities of Ivermectin in reindeer following subcutaneous and two different oral formulation applications. *Acta Vet Scand.* 2014:56;76.
253. Oksanen A, Norberg H, Nieminen M, Bernstad S: Influence of route of administration on the plasma concentrations of ivermectin in reindeer. *Res Vet Sci.* 1995:58(3);286–287.
254. Lizarraga I, Chambers JP: Involvement of opioidergic and alpha2-adrenergic mechanisms in the central analgesic effects of non-steroidal anti-inflammatory drugs in sheep. *Res VetSci.* 2006:80(2);194–200.
255. Arifah AK, Landoni MF, Lees P: Pharmacodynamics, chiral pharmacokinetics and PK-PD modelling of ketoprofen in the goat. *J Vet Pharmacol Ther.* 2003:26(2);139–150.
256. Rahmani Shahraki A, Pourjafar M, Chalmeh A, et al: Attenuating the endotoxin induced acute phase response by pentoxifylline in comparison with dexamethasone and ketoprofen in sheep. *Small Ruminant Res.* 2016:136;156–160.
257. United States Food and Drug Administration Center for Veterinary Medicine: Code of Federal Regulations; 21 CFR 558.311; New Animal Drugs for Use in Animal Feeds; Lasalocid. Vol July 1, 20182018:449-457.

258. Horton GM, Stockdale PH: Lasalocid and monensin in finishing diets for early weaned lambs with naturally occurring coccidiosis. *Am J Vet Res.* 1981:42(3);433–436.
259. United States Food and Drug Administration Center for Veterinary Medicine: Code of Federal Regulations; 21 CFR 520.1242a; Oral Dosage Form New Animal Drugs; Levamisole Powder for Oral Solution. Vol July 1, 20182018:175-176.
260. United States Food and Drug Administration Center for Veterinary Medicine: Code of Federal Regulations; 21 CFR 520.1242b; Oral Dosage Form New Animal Drugs; Levamisole Hydrochloride Tablet or Oblet (Bolus). Vol July 1, 20182018:176.
261. Habibian S, Bigham AS, Aali E: Comparison of lidocaine, tramadol, and lidocaine–tramadol for epidural analgesia in lambs. *Res Vet Sci.* 2011:91(3);434–438.
262. Scott PR, Gessert ME: Evaluation of caudal epidural lignocaine injection during dystocia correction in ewes. *Vet Rec.* 1996: 138(1);19–20.
263. Dehkordi S, Bigham Sadegh A, Gerami R: Evaluation of anti-nociceptive effect of epidural tramadol, tramadol-lidocaine and lidocaine in goats. *Vet Anaesth Analges.* 2012:39(1);106–110.
264. Mpanduji DG, Ndossi DG: Comparison of analgesia and cardio-pulmonary effects of epidural injection of pethidine and lidocaine in small East African goats. *Res Opinions AnimalVet Sci.* 2013:3(2);30–34.
265. Edjtehadi M, Mehrabani D: Prevention of epinephrine-induced arrhythmias with lidocaine during thiopental and methoxyflurane anesthesia in sheep. *J Appl Anim Res.* 2005:27;55–59.
266. Plenderleith RW: Treatment of cattle, sheep and horses with lincomycin: case studies. *Vet Rec.* 1988:122(5);112–113.
267. Marcus S, Ziv G, Glickman A, Ozbonfil D, Bartoov B, Klein A: Lincomycin and spectinomycin in the treatment of breeding rams with semen contaminated with ureaplasmas. *Res Vet Sci.* 1994: 57(3);393–394.
268. Venning CM, Curtis MA, Egerton JR: Treatment of virulent footrot with lincomycin and spectinomycin. *Austr Vet J.* 1990: 67(7);258–260.
269. Jordan D, Venning CM. Treatment of ovine dermatophilosis with long-acting oxytetracycline or a lincomycin-spectinomycin combination. *Austr VetJ.* 1995:72(6);234–236.
270. Bischoff K, Smith MC, Stump S: Treatment of pieris ingestion in goats with intravenous lipid emulsion. *J Med Toxicol.* 2014:10(4);411–414.
271. Richards IS: The effect of magnesium sulphate on convulsions induced by annual ryegrass toxicity. *Austr Vet J.* 1982:58(3);115–117.
272. West DM, Bruere AN: Hypomagnesaemic tetany in sheep. *N Z Vet J.* 1981:29(6);85–87.
273. Towstoless MK, Congiu M, Coghlan JP, Wintour EM: Placental and renal control of plasma osmolality in chronically cannulated ovine fetus. *Am J Physiol.* 1987:253(3 Pt 2);R389–395.
274. Herin P, Kim JK, Schrier RW, Meschia G, Battaglia FC: Ovine fetal response to water deprivation: aspects on the role of vasopressin. *Q JExp Physiol (Cambridge, England).* 1988:73(6);931–940.
275. Rabinowitz L, Gunther RA: Renal concentrating ability in sheep during urea, mannitol, and methylurea diuresis. *Am J Physiol.* 1972:222(4);801–806.
276. Bauer C, Conraths FJ: Comparative efficacy of moxidectin and mebendazole against gastrointestinal nematodes in experimentally infected lambs. *Vet Rec.* 1994:135(6);136–138.
277. Kelly JD, Chevis RA, Whitlock HV: The anthelmintic efficacy of mebendazole against adult Fasciola hepatica and a concurrent mixed nematode infection in sheep. *N Z Vet J.* 1975:23(5);81–84.
278. Lyons ET, Drudge JH, Tolliver SC, Stamper S: Controlled tests of activity of several antiparasitic compounds against natural infections of Haemonchus contortus and other helminths in lambs from a flock established in 1962. *Am VetRes.* 1993:54(3);406–410.
279. Taylor MA, Hunt KR, Wilson CA, Quick JM: Effectiveness of strategic anthelmintic dosing in controlling Haemonchus contortus infections in sheep in the United Kingdom. *Vet Rec.* 1991:129(9);189–192.
280. Uhlinger C, Fetrow J, Johnstone C: A field evaluation of benzimidazole and nonbenzimidazole drugs in a herd of dairy goats. *J Vet Internal Medicine/Am Coll Vet Internal M.* 1988:2(3);113–116.
281. Van der Westhuizen B, Newcomb K, Guerrero J: Anthelmintic efficacy of mebendazole suspension against induced helminth infections in South African sheep and cattle. *Am J Vet Res.* 1984:45(4);779–782.
282. Kastner SB, Kutter AP, von Rechenberg B, Bettschart-Wolfensberger R: Comparison of two pre-anaesthetic medetomidine doses in isoflurane anaesthetized sheep. *VetAnaesthes Analges.* 2006:33(1);8–16.
283. Kalhoro AB, Memon AQ: Sedative/analgesic efficacy of medetomidine in goats. *Pakistan Vet J.* 2011:31(3);257–259.
284. Windorski EJ, Schauer CS, Wurst AK, Inskeep EK, Luther JS: Effects of melengestrol acetate and P.G. 600 on fertility in Rambouillet ewes outside the natural breeding season. *Theriogenology.* 2008:70(2);227–232.
285. Safranski TJ, Lamberson WR, Keisler DH: Use of melengestrol acetate and gonadotropins to induce fertile estrus in seasonally anestrous ewes. *J Animal Sci.* 1992:70(10);2935–2941.
286. Jabbar G, Umberger SH, Lewis GS: Melengestrol acetate and norgestomet for the induction of synchronized estrus in seasonally anovular ewes. *J Anim Sci.* 1994:72(12);3049–3054.
287. Powell MR, Kaps M, Lamberson WR, Keisler DH: Use of melengestrol acetate-based treatments to induce and synchronize estrus in seasonally anestrous ewes. *J Animal Sc.* 1996:74(10);2292–2302.
288. Raphael B, Kalk P, Thomas P, Calle P, Doherty J, Cook R: Use of melengestrol acetate in feed for contraception in herds of captive ungulates. *Zoo Biol.* 2003:22(5);455–463.
289. Shukla M, Singh G, Sindhura BG, Telang AG, Rao GS, Malik JK: Comparative plasma pharmacokinetics of meloxicam in sheep and goats following intravenous administration. *Compar Biochem Physiol Toxicol Pharmacol: CBP.* 2007:145(4);528–532.
290. Small AH, Marini D, le Floch M, Paull D, Lee C: A pen study evaluation of buccal meloxicam and topical anaesthetic at improving welfare of lambs undergoing surgical mulesing and hot knife tail docking. *Res Vet Sci.* 2018:118;270–277.
291. Stock ML, Coetzee JF, KuKanich B, Smith BI: Pharmacokinetics of intravenously and orally administered meloxicam in sheep. *Am J Vet Res.* 2013:74(5);779–783.
292. Karademir U, Erdogan H, Boyacioglu M, Kum C, Sekkin S, Bilgen M: Pharmacokinetics of meloxicam in adult goats: a comparative study of subcutaneous, oral and intravenous administration. *N Z Vet J.* 2016:64(3);165–168.
293. Ingvast-Larsson C, Hogberg M, Mengistu U, Olsen L, Bondesson U, Olsson K. Pharmacokinetics of meloxicam in adult goats and its analgesic effect in disbudded kids. *J Vet Pharmacol Ther.* 2011:34(1);64–69.
294. Voss LJ, Ludbrook G, Grant C, Upton R, Sleigh JW: A comparison of pharmacokinetic/pharmacodynamic versus mass-balance measurement of brain concentrations of intravenous anesthetics in sheep. *Anesthes Analges.* 2007:104(6):1440–1446, table of contents.
295. Collan R: Anesthetic and paraoperative management of sheep for total heart replacement. *Anesthes Analges.* 1970:49(2);336–343.
296. Wendel WB: The control of methemoglobinemia with methylene blue. *JClin Invest.* 1939:18(2);179–185.
297. Neilson FJ: Nitrite and nitrate poisoning with special reference to 'grasslands tama' ryegrass. *N Z Vet J.* 1974:22(1–2);12–13.
298. Burrows GE, Horn GW, McNew RW, Croy LI, Keeton RD, Kyle J: The prophylactic effect of corn supplementation on experimental nitrate intoxication in cattle. *J Anim Sc.* 1987:64(6);1682–1689.
299. Mondal DB, Pandey NN. Dosing regimen of methylene blue and its comparative efficacy with tolonium chloride and ascorbic acid in induced acute nitrate toxicity in goats. *Indian J Anim Sci.* 2000: 70(6);572–575.
300. Burrows GE: Nitrate intoxication. *J Am Vet Med Assoc.* 1980:177(1);82–83.
301. Burrows GE: Methylene blue: effects and disposition in sheep. *J Vet Pharmacol Ther.* 1984:7(3);225–231.

302. Huhn JC, Nelson DR: The quantitative effect of metoclopramide on abomasal and duodenal myoelectric activity of goats. *Zentralblatt fur Veterinarmedizin.* 1997:44(6);361–371.
303. Stafford KJ, Leek BF: Dopamine-sensitive receptors that evoke rumination and modify reticulo-ruminal activity in sheep. *J Vet Pharmacol Ther.* 1988:11(2);171–176.
304. Simon B, Scallan E, O O, et al: Pharmacokinetics and pharmacodynamics of midazolam following intravenous and intramuscular administration to sheep. *Am JVet Res.* 2017:78(5);539–549.
305. Upton RN, Martinez AM, Grant C: Comparison of the sedative properties of CNS 7056, midazolam, and propofol in sheep. *Brit J Anaesthes.* 2009:103(6);848–857.
306. Stegmann GF: Observations on some cardiopulmonary effects of midazolam, xylazine and a midazolam/ketamine combination in the goat. *JSouth Afr Vet Assn.* 1999:70(3);122–126.
307. Stegmann GF: Observations on the use of midazolam for sedation, and induction of anaesthesia with midazolam in combination with ketamine in the goat. *J South Afr Vet Assn.* 1998:69(3);89–92.
308. Dzikiti TB, Stegmann GF, Hellebrekers LJ, Auer REJ, Dzikiti LN: Sedative and cardiopulmonary effects of acepromazine, midazolam, butorphanol, acepromazine-butorphanol and midazolam-butorphanol on propofol anesthesia in goats. *J South Afr VetAssn.* 2009:80(1);10–16.
309. Dzikiti TB, Zeiler GE, Dzikiti LN, Garcia ER: The effects of midazolam and butorphanol, administered alone or combined, on the dose and quality of anaesthetic induction with alfaxalone in goats. *J South Afr Vet Assn.* 2014:85(1).
310. Vishnugurubaran D, Kathirvel S, Kumar SS, Balasundaram K, Dharmaceelan S: Isoflurane sparing effect of diazepam and midazolam to xylazine-ketamine induction and isoflurane maintenance in goats. *Indian J Anim Res.* 2017:51(4);762–763.
311. Min BR, Pinchak WE, Mathews D, Fulford JD: In vitro rumen fermentation and in vivo bloat dynamics of steers grazing winter wheat to corn oil supplementation. *Animal Feed Sci Technol.* 2007:133;192–205.
312. Miltimore JE, Pidgen WJ, Mcarthur TM, Anstey TH: Bloat investigations. I. Reduction of bloat incidence in dairy cattle with penicillin and antifoaming agents. *Can J Animal Sci.* 1964:44;96–101.
313. Buxton D, Blewett DA, Trees AJ, McColgan C, Finlayson J: Further studies in the use of monensin in the control of experimental ovine toxoplasmosis. *J Compar Pathol.* 1988:98(2);225–236.
314. Buxton D, Donald KM, Finlayson J: Monensin and the control of experimental ovine toxoplasmosis: a systemic effect. *Vet Rec.* 1987: 120(26);618–619.
315. Horton GM, Stockdale PH. Oocyst discharge, rumen metabolism and performance of early weaned lambs with naturally occurring coccidiosis fed monensin. *Can Vet J.* 1981:22(6);175–178.
316. United States Food and Drug Administration Center for Veterinary Medicine: Code of Federal Regulation; Part 558 New Animal Drugs for Use in Animal Feeds; Section 558.360; Morantel Tartrate. Accessed November 2.
317. Reinemeyer CR, Pringle JK: Evaluation of the efficacy and safety of morantel tartrate in domestic goats. *Vet Human Toxicol.* 1993:35 Suppl 2;57–61.
318. United States Food and Drug Administration Center for Veterinary Medicine: Code of Federal Regulations; 21 CFR 520.1454; Oral Dosage Form New Animal Drugs; Moxidectin Solution. Vol July 1, 20182018:190.
319. O'Brien DJ, Brown D, Parker LD, McAuliffe A, Pike K, Murphy TM: Evaluation of the persistent activity of injectable endectocides against Psoroptes ovis. *Vet Rec.* 2001:149(17);522–523.
320. Pomroy WE, Whelan N, Alexander AM, et al: Multiple resistance in goat-derived Ostertagia and the efficacy of moxidectin and combinations of other anthelmintics. *N Z Vet J.* 1992:40(2);76–78.
321. Varady M, Praslicka J, Corba J: Efficacy of moxidectin against multiple resistant Ostertagia spp. in lambs. *N Z Vet J.* 1995:43(3);89–90.
322. Giadinis ND, Farmaki R, Papaioannou N, Papadopoulos E, Karatzias H, Koutinas AF: Moxidectin efficacy in a goat herd with chronic and generalized sarcoptic mange. *Vet Med Int.* 2011:2011;476348.
323. Mackintosh CG, Cowie C, Fraser K, Johnstone P, Mason PC: Reduced efficacy of moxidectin and abamectin in young red deer (Cervus elaphus) after 20 years of moxidectin pour-on use on a New Zealand deer farm. *Vet Parasitol.* 2014:199(1);81–92.
324. Miller MW, Wild MA, Lance WR: Efficacy and safety of naltrexone hydrochloride for antagonizing carfentanil citrate immobilization in captive Rocky Mountain elk (Cervus elaphus nelsoni). *J Wildl Dis.* 1996:32(2);234–239.
325. Constable PD: Therapeutic management of cardiovascular diseases, in *Current Veterinary Therapy 4: Food Animal Practice*. Howard JL, Smith RA, Eds. Philadelphia: W.B. Saunders, 1999.
326. Navarro JF, Mora C. In-depth review effect of androgens on anemia and malnutrition in renal failure: implications for patients on peritoneal dialysis. *Perit Dial Int.* 2001:21(1):14–24.
327. United States Food and Drug Administration Center for Veterinary Medicine: Code of Federal Regulation; Part 558 New Animal Drugs for Use in Animal Feeds; Section 558.364; Neomycin Sulfate. Accessed November 2, 2009.
328. United States Food and Drug Administration Center for Veterinary Medicine: Code of Federal Regulation; Part 520 Oral Dosage Form New Animal Drugs; Section 520.1484; Neomycin Sulfate. Accessed November 2, 2009.
329. United States Food and Drug Administration Center for Veterinary Medicine: Code of Federal Regulation; Part 522 Implantation or Injectable Dosage Form New Animal Drugs; Section 522.1503; Neostigmine Methylsulfate Injection. Accessed November 2, 2009.
330. Richards LS, Zimmerman GL, Hoberg EP, Schons DJ, Dawley SW: The anthelmintic efficacy of netobimin against naturally acquired gastrointestinal nematodes in sheep. *Vet Parasitol.* 1987:26 (1–2):87–94.
331. Rinaldi L, Morgan ER, Bosco A, Coles GC, Cringoli G: The maintenance of anthelmintic efficacy in sheep in a Mediterranean climate. *Vet Parasitol.* 2014:203(1);139–143.
332. Richards LS, Zimmerman GL, Nelson MJ, Schons DJ, Dawley SW: The anthelmintic efficacy of netobimin against experimental infections of Fasciola hepatica in sheep. *Vet Parasitol.* 1987:26 (1–2);71–77.
333. Bauer C, Hafner M: Efficacy of two formulations of netobimin against gastrointestinal helminths in sheep. *Vet Rec.* 1990:127 (25–26);621–622.
334. Arias MS, Suárez JL, Hillyer GV, et al: A recombinant-based ELISA evaluating the efficacy of netobimin and albendazole in ruminants with naturally acquired fascioliasis. *Vet Jl.* 2009:182(1);73–78.
335. Cabaret J: Efficacy of netobimin against Muellerius capillaris and resistant strain of digestive tract strongyles in dairy goats. *Am J Vet Res.* 1991:52(8);1313–1315.
336. Elliott DC: Tapeworm (Moniezia expansa) in sheep: anthelmintic treatment studies to assess possible pathogenic effects and production loss in young infected animals in the field. *N Z V J.* 1984:32(11);185–188.
337. Pavan Kumar C, Syaama Sundar N, Devi Prasad V: Outbreak of immature paramphistomosis in Nellore Jodipi sheep. *J Parasitic Dis: Offic Organ Indian Soc Parasitol.* 2016:40(2);533–535.
338. Coles GC, Stafford KA: Activity of oxyclozanide, nitroxynil, clorsulon and albendazole against adult triclabendazole-resistant Fasciola hepatica. *Vet Rec.* 2001:148(23);723–724.
339. Martínez-Valladares M, del Rosario Famularo M, Fernández-Pato N, Castañón-Ordóñez L, Cordero-Pérez C, Rojo-Vázquez FA: Efficacy of nitroxynil against Fasciola hepatica resistant to triclabendazole in a naturally infected sheep flock. *Parasitol Res.* 2010: 107(5);1205–1211.
340. Kistner TP, Wyse D: Efficacy of oxfendazole against an ovine isolate of benzimidazole resistant Haemonchus contortus. *Austr V J.* 1978:54(10);469–470.
341. Gavidia CM, Gonzalez AE, Lopera L, et al: Evaluation of nitazoxanide and oxfendazole efficacy against cystic echinococcosis in naturally infected sheep. *Am J Trop Med Hyg.* 2009:80(3); 367–372.

342. Dueger EL, Moro PL, Gilman RH: Oxfendazole treatment of sheep with naturally acquired hydatid disease. *Antimicrob Agents Chemother.* 1999:43(9);2263–2267.
343. Gavidia CM, Gonzalez AE, Barron EA, et al: Evaluation of oxfendazole, praziquantel and albendazole against cystic echinococcosis: a randomized clinical trial in naturally infected sheep. *PLoS Neglected Trop Dis.* 2010:4(2);e616.
344. Gomez-Puerta LA, Gavidia C, Lopez-Urbina MT, Garcia HH, Gonzalez AE: Short report: efficacy of a single oral dose of oxfendazole against Fasciola hepatica in naturally infected sheep. *Am J Trop Med Hyg.* 2012:86(3);486–488.
345. Khan MN, Sajid MS, Rizwan HM, Qudoos A, Abbas RZ, Riaz M, and Khan MK: Comparative efficacy of six anthelmintic treatments against natural infection of Fasciola species in sheep. *Pakistan Vet J.* 2016:37(1)65–68.
346. Elliott DC: Removal of Haemonchus contortus, Ostertagia circumcincta and Trichostrongylus spp. from goats, by morantel citrate, levamisole hydrochloride, fenbendazole, and oxfendazole. *N Z Vet J.* 1987:35(12);208–210.
347. Sanabria R, Moreno L, Alvarez L, Lanusse C, Romero J: Efficacy of oxyclozanide against adult Paramphistomum leydeni in naturally infected sheep. *VetParasitol.* 2014:206(3);277–281.
348. Schweizer G, Ehrensperger F, Torgerson PR, Braun U: Clinical findings and treatment of 94 cattle presumptively diagnosed with listeriosis. *Vet Rec.* 2006:158(17);588–592.
349. Joussellin W, Valentin-Smith A: La Terramycine Longue Action – Son emploi dans les pneumopathies bovines, ovines et porcines et la prevention de la chlamydiose ovine. *Bull Soc Vet Prat de France.* 1983:67(7);459–480.
350. Rodolakis A, Souriau A, Raynaud JP, Brunault G: Efficacy of a long-acting oxytetracycline against chlamydial ovine abortion. *Annales de Recherches Veterinaires.* 1980:11(4);437–444.
351. Wilsmore AJ, Dawson M, Arthur MJ, Davies DC: The use of a delayed hypersensitivity test and long-acting oxytetracycline in a flock affected with ovine enzootic abortion. *Brit Vet J.* 1986:142(6);557–561.
352. Gilmour NJ, Sharp JM, Gilmour JS: Effect of oxytetracycline therapy on experimentally induced pneumonic pasteurellosis in lambs. *Vet Rec.* 1983:111(5);97–99.
353. Kaler J, Daniels SLS, Wright JL, Green LE: Randomized clinical trial of long-acting oxytetracycline, foot trimming, and flunixine meglumine on time to recovery in sheep with footrot. *J Vet Intern Med.* 2010:24;420–425.
354. Thornsberry RM: Goat foot rot infection clinical trial. *N Engl J Large Animal Health.* 2002:Winter;26–27.
355. Escudero E, Carceles CM, Ponferrada C, Baggot JD: The pharmacokinetics of a long-acting formulation of oxytetracycline in sheep and goats. *J Vet Pharmacol Ther.* 1996:19(1);75–77.
356. Escudero E, Carceles CM, Serrano JM: Pharmacokinetics of oxytetracycline in goats: modifications induced by a long-acting formulation. *Vet Rec.* 1994:135(23)548–552.
357. Strobel H, Lauseker M, Forbes AB. Targeted antibiotic treatment of lame sheep with footrot using either oxytetracycline or gamithromycin. *Vet Rec.* 2014 Jan 11;174(2):46.
358. Giadinis ND, Petridou EJ, Sofianidis G, et al: Mortality in adult goats attributed to Mycoplasma capricolum subspecies capricolum. *Vet Re.* 2008:163(9);278–279.
359. Aktas İ, Yarsan E: Pharmacokinetics of conventional and long-acting oxytetracycline preparations in Kilis goat. *Frontiers Vet Scie.* 2017:4;229.
360. Haigh JC, Dowling PM, Smits JG: Pharmacokinetics of long-acting oxytetracycline in fallow deer (Dama dama). *J Vet Pharmacol Ther.* 1997:20(3);243–245.
361. United States Food and Drug Administration Center for Veterinary Medicine: Code of Federal Regulations; 21 CFR 520.1660d; Oral Dosage Form New Animal Drugs; Oxytetracycline Powder. Vol July 1, 20182018:196–198.
362. United States Food and Drug Administration Center for Veterinary Medicine: Code of Federal Regulations; 21 CFR 558.450; New Animal Drugs for Use in Animal Feeds; Oxytetracycline. Vol July 1, 20182018:488–490.
363. Hall RF, Waldham DG, DeLong WJ. The prevention of chlamydial abortion in sheep and goats. Paper presented at Third International Conference on Goat Production and Disease 1982, Tucson, AZ.
364. United States Food and Drug Administration Center for Veterinary Medicine; Code of Federal Regulations; 21 CFR 522.1680; Implantation or Injectable Dosage Form New Animal Drugs; Oxytocin Injection. Vol July 1, 20182018:300.
365. Majeed AF, Taha MB. Obstetrical disorders and their treatment in Iraqi Awassi ewes. *Small Rumin Res.* 1995:17(1);65–69.
366. Majeed AF: Obstetrical problems and their management in Iragi goats. *Small Rumin Res.* 1994:14(1):73–78.
367. Humann-Ziehank E, Bickhardt K: Effects of D-penicillamine on urinary copper excretion in high-copper supplemented sheep. *J Vet Med.* 2001:48(9);537–544.
368. Botha CJ, Naude TW, Swan GE, Dauth J, Dreyer MJ, Williams MC: The cupruretic effect of two chelators following copper loading in sheep. *Vet Human Toxicology.* 1993:35(5);409–413.
369. Ziv G, Shani J, Sulman FG: Pharmacokinetic evaluation of penicillin and cephalosporin derivatives in serum and milk of lactating cows and ewes. *Am J Vet Res.* 1973:34(12);1561–1565.
370. Cooke IM, Bevill RP, Nelson DR, Koritz GD: Pharmacokinetics of penicillin G in plasma and interstitial fluid collected with dialysis fiber bundles in sheep. *Vet Res.* 1996:27(2);147–159.
371. McCarthy FD, Lindsey JB, Gore MT, Notter DR: Incidence and control of subclinical mastitis in intensively managed ewes. *J Animal Sci.* 1988:66(11);2715–2721.
372. Oukessou M, Benlamlih S, Toutain PL: Benzylpenicillin kinetics in the ewe: influence of pregnancy and lactation. *Res Vet Sci.* 1990: 49(2);190–193.
373. Phukan A, Dutta GN, Kalita D, Das BC: Experimental production of enterotoxaemia in goats and its treatment. *Int J Animal Sci.* 2000:15(2);233–236.
374. Kumper H: [Therapy of central nervous system listeriosis in sheep]. *Tierarztliche Praxis.* 1991:19(4);369–372.
375. Randhawa SS, Sharma DK, Randhawa CS, Gill BS, Brar RS, Singh J: An outbreak of bacillary haemoglobinuria in sheep in India. *Trop Animal Health Prod.* 1995:27(1);31–36.
376. Gonzalo C, Tardaguila JA, De La Fuente LF, San Primitivo F: Effects of selective and complete dry therapy on prevalence of intramammary infection and on milk yield in the subsequent lactation in dairy ewes. *J Dairy Res.* 2004:71(1);33–38.
377. Hsu WH, Hanson CE, Hembrough FB, Schaffer DD: Effects of idazoxan, tolazoline, and yohimbine on xylazine-induced respiratory changes and central nervous system depression in ewes. *Am J Vet Res.* 1989:50(9);1570–1573.
378. Panter KE, Baker DC, Kechele PO: Water hemlock (Cicuta douglasii) toxicoses in sheep: pathologic description and prevention of lesions and death. *J Vet Diagn Invest.* 1996:8(4);474–480.
379. Peterson DW, Penny RH, Day JB, Mantle PG: A comparative study of sheep and pigs given the tremorgenic mycotoxins verruculogen and penitrem A. *Res Vet Sci.* 1982:33(2);183–187.
380. Cheng Z, McKeller Q, Nolan A: Pharmacokinetic studies of flunixin meglumine and phenylbutazone in plasma, exudate and transudate in sheep. *J VetPharmacol Ther.* 1998:21(4);315–321.
381. Cheng Z, Nolan AM, McKellar QA: Measurement of cyclooxygenase inhibition in vivo: a study of two non-steroidal anti-inflammatory drugs in sheep. *Inflammation.* 1998:22(4):353–366.
382. Cheng Z, Welsh E, Nolan A, McKellar QA: Pharmacokinetic and pharmacodynamic studies on phenylbutazone and oxyphenbutazone in goats. *Vet Rec.* 1997:140(2);40–43.
383. Eltom SE, Guard CL, Schwark WS: The effect of age on phenylbutazone pharmacokinetics, metabolism and plasma protein binding in goats. *JVet Pharmacol Ther.* 1993:16(2);141–151.
384. Lippke H, Vetter RL, Jacobson NL: Poloxalene for bloat prevention in lambs. *J Animal Sci.* 1969:28(6);819–821.
385. Strobel H, de Ponte M, Knoppe TN, Bhushan C: Comparison of three different treatment schedules for praziquantel (Cestocur®, Bayer) in the treatment of tapeworm infections (Moniezia spp.)

and their impact on body weight gains in a German sheep flock. *Parasitol Res.* 2013:112(1);139–147.
386. Monrad J, Soren K, Johansen MV, Lindberg R, Ornbjerg N: Treatment efficacy and regulatory host responses in chronic experimental Schistosoma bovis infections in goats. *Parasitology.* 2006:133(2);151–158.
387. Valdez RA, Gelberg HB, Morin DE, Zuckermann FA: Use of corticosteroids and aurothioglucose in a pygmy goat with pemphigus foliaceus. *J Am Vet Med Assoc.* 1995:207(6);761–765.
388. Janzen AM, Wiles D, Myers S, Marqués FJ: Pemphigus foliaceus in a juvenile Cashmere goat, and outcome after prednisolone and methylprednisolone therapy. *Can Vet J.* 2011:52(12);1345–1349.
389. Larenza MP, Bergadano A, Iff I, Doherr MG, Schatzmann U: Comparison of the cardiopulmonary effects of anesthesia maintained by continuous infusion of ketamine and propofol with anesthesia maintained by inhalation of sevoflurane in goats undergoing magnetic resonance imaging. *Am JVet Res.* 2005:66(12);2135–2141.
390. Dzikiti B, Stegmann F, Cromarty D, Dzikiti L, Hellebrekers L: Effects of propofol on isoflurane minimum alveolar concentration and cardiovascular function in mechanically ventilated goats. *Vet Anaesthes Analges.* 2011:38(1);44–53.
391. Wierda A, Verhoeff J, van Dijk S, Dorresteijn J, Wensing T: Effects of trenbolone acetate and propylene glycol on pregnancy toxaemia in ewes. *Vet Rec.* 1985:116(11);284–287.
392. Andrews AH: Effects of glucose and propylene glycol on pregnancy toxaemia in ewes. *Vet Rec.* 1982:110(4);84–85.
393. Silva SDA, Cal-Pereyra LG, Benech A, et al: Evaluation of a fibrate, specific stimulant of PPAR alpha, as a therapeutic alternative to the treatment of clinical ovine pregnancy toxaemia. *J Vet Pharmacol Ther.* 2016:39(5);497–503.
394. Edmondson MA, Pugh DG: Pregnancy toxemia in sheep and goats. In *Current Veterinary Therapy: Food Animal Practice.* 5th ed., Anderson DE, Rings DM, Eds., St. Louis, MO: Saunders Elsevier,144–145, 2009.
395. Hordegen P, Hertzberg H, Heilmann J, Langhans W, Maurer V: The anthelmintic efficacy of five plant products against gastrointestinal trichostrongylids in artificially infected lambs. *Vet Parasitol.* 2003:117(1–2);51–60.
396. Cornwell RL: Field trials in sheep with the anthelmintic pyrantel tartrate. Comparative trials in the prevention of Nematodirus infection in lambs. *Vet Rec.* 1966:79(22);626–629.
397. Cornwell RL, Jones RM, Berry J, et al: Field trials in sheep with the anthelmintic pyrantel tartrate. IV. Comparison of pyrantel tartrate and tetramisole in the prevention of parasitic gastro-enteritis. *Vet Rec.* 1967:80(23);676–679.
398. Cornwell RL, Jones RM, Berry J, et al: Field trials in sheep with the anthelmintic pyrantel tartrate. 3. Comparison of pyrantel and tetramisole in the prevention of Nematodirus infection in lambs. *Vety Rec.* 1967:80(14);434–436.
399. Chartier C, Pors I, Benoit C: Efficacy of pyrantel tartrate against experimental infections with Haemonchus contortus, Teladorsagia circumcincta and Trichostrongylus colubriformis in goats. *Vet Parasitol.* 1995:59(1);69–73.
400. Benz GW, Ernst JV: Efficacy of salinomycin in treatment of experimental Eimeria bovis infections in calves. *Am J Vety Res.* 1979:40(8);1180–1186.
401. McAllister TA, Annett CB, Olson ME, Morck DW, Cheng KJ: Effect of salinomycin on giardiasis and coccidiosis in growing lambs. *J Animal Sci.* 1996:74(12);2896–2903.
402. Kronfeld DS: Ketosis in pregnant sheep and lactating cows. A review. *Austr Veterinary J.* 1972:48(12);680–687.
403. Braun U, Rihs T, Schefer U: Ruminal lactic acidosis in sheep and goats. *Vet Rec.* 1992:130(16);343–349.
404. Angell JW, Jones GL, Voigt K, Grove-White DH: Successful correction of D-lactic acid neurotoxicity (drunken lamb syndrome) by bolus administration of oral sodium bicarbonate. *Vety Re.* 2013:173(8);193–193.
405. Bleul U, Schwantag S, Stocker H, et al: Floppy kid syndrome caused by D-lactic acidosis in goat kids. *J Vet Intern Medicine/Amn Coll Vety Int Med.* 2006:20(4);1003–1008.
406. Taylor AW: Actinobacillosis in sheep. *J Compar Pathol.* 1944: 54;228–237.
407. Smith BP. Actinomycosis (lumpy jaw), in *Large Animal Internal Medicine.* 3rd ed., Smith BP, Ed., St. Louis: Mosby, 699–700, 2002.
408. Soto-Blanco B, Stegelmeier BL, Gorniak SL: Clinical and pathological effects of short-term cyanide repeated dosing to goats. *J Appl Toxicol.* 2005:25(6);445–450.
409. Burrows GE: Cyanide intoxication in sheep; therapeutics. *Vet Human Toxicol.* 1981:23(1);22–28.
410. Burrows GE, Way JL: Cyanide intoxication in sheep: enhancement of efficacy of sodium nitrite, sodium thiosulfate, and cobaltous chloride. *Am J VetRes.* 1979:40(5);613–617.
411. Youssef SA, El-Gendi AY, El-Sayed MG, Atef M, Salam SA; Some pharmacokinetic and biochemical aspects of sulphadiazine and sulphadimidine in ewes. *J Vet Pharmacol Ther.* 1981:4(3);173–182.
412. Alzieu JP, Mage C, Maes L, de Muelenaere C: Economic benefits of prophylaxis with diclazuril against subclinical coccidiosis in lambs reared indoors. *Vet Rec.* 1999:144(16);442–444.
413. Gjerde B, Helle O: Effects of leucocyte extract, levamisole and sulphadimidine on natural coccidial infections (Eimeria spp.) in young lambs. *Acta Vet Scand.* 1987:28(1);33–45.
414. United States Food and Drug Administration Center for Veterinary Medicine: Code of Federal Regulations; 21 CFR 520.2325a; Oral Dosage Form New Animal Drugs; Sulfaquinoxaline Drinking Water. Vol July 1, 20182018:227–228.
415. Whitten LK. Further field experiments on the use of coccidiostatic drugs in unweaned lambs. *N Z Vet J.* 1956:4;25–26.
416. United States Food and Drug Administration Center for Veterinary Medicine: Code of Federal Regulation; Part 520 Oral Dosage Form New Animal Drugs; Section 520.2380b; Thiabendazole Drench or Oral Paste. Accessed November 2, 2009.
417. Bratton GR, Zmudzki J, Kincaid N, Joyce J: Thiamin as treatment of lead poisoning in ruminants. *Mod Vet Pract.* 1981:62(6):441–446.
418. Dey S, Swarup D, Kalicharan, Singh B: Treatment of lead toxicity in calves. *Vet Human Toxicol.* 1995:37(3);230–232.
419. Najarnezhad V, Aslani MR, Balali-Mood M: The therapeutic potential of thiamine for treatment of experimentally induced subacute lead poisoning in sheep. *Compar Clin Pathol.* 2010:19(1);69–73.
420. Ramos JJ, Ferrer LM, Garcia L, Fernandez A, Loste A: Polioencephalomalacia in adult sheep grazing pastures with prostrate pigweed. *Can Vet J.* 2005:46(1);59–61.
421. Low JC, Scott PR, Howie F, Lewis M, FitzSimons J, Spence JA: Sulphur-induced polioencephalomalacia in lambs. *Vet Rec.* 1996:138(14);327–329.
422. Hikasa Y, Saito K, Takase K, Ogasawara S; Clinical, cardiopulmonary, hematological and serum biochemical effects of sevoflurane and isoflurane anesthesia in oxygen under spontaneous breathing in sheep. *Small Rumin Res.* 2000:36(3);241–249.
423. Edjtehadi M: Effects of thiopentone sodium, methoxyflurane and halothane on haematological parameters in sheep during prolonged anaesthesia. *Clin Expl PharmacolPhysiol.* 1978:5(1);31–40.
424. Prassinos NN, Galatos AD, Raptopoulos D: A comparison of propofol, thiopental or ketamine as induction agents in goats. *Vet Anaesthes Analges.* 2005:32(5);289–296.
425. Carroll GL, Hartsfield SM, Hambleton R: Anesthetic effects of tiletamine-zolazepam, alone or in combination with butorphanol, in goats. *J Am Vet Med Assoc.* 1997:211(5);593–597.
426. Doherty TJ, Rohrbach BW, Ross L, Schultz H: The effect of tiletamine and zolazepam on isoflurane minimum alveolar concentration in goats. *J Vet Pharmacol Ther.* 2002:25(3);233–235.
427. United States Food and Drug Administration Center for Veterinary Medicine: Code of Federal Regulations; 21 CFR 522.2471; Implantation or Injectable Dosage Form New Animal Drugs; Tilmicosin. Vol July 1, 20182018:317.
428. Naccari F, Giofre F, Pellegrino M, Calo M, Licata P, Carli S: Effectiveness and kinetic behaviour of tilmicosin in the treatment of respiratory infections in sheep. *VetRec.* 2001:148(25);773–776.

429. Croft A, Duffield T, Menzies P, Leslie K, Bagg R, Dick P: The effect of tilmicosin administered to ewes prior to lambing on incidence of clinical mastitis and subsequent lamb performance. *Can Vet J.* 2000:41(4);306–311.
430. Hsu WH, Schaffer DD, Hanson CE: Effects of tolazoline and yohimbine on xylazine-induced central nervous system depression, bradycardia, and tachypnea in sheep. *J Am Vet Med Assoc.* 1987:190(4);423–426.
431. Mpanduji DG, Bittegeko SB, Batamuzi EK, Mgasa MN, Shami CL: Comparison of the effects of atipamezole and tolazoline on analgesia, cardiopulmonary and rectal temperature changes induced by lumbosacral epidural injection of medetomidine in goats. *Small Rumin Res.* 2001:40(2);117–122.
432. Mortenson J, Robison J: Tolazoline-induced apnea in mule deer (Odocoileus hemionus). *J Zoo Wildl Med.* 2011:42(1);105–107.
433. Gjerde B, Helle O: Chemoprophylaxis of coccidiosis in lambs with a single oral dose of toltrazuril. *Vet Parasitol.* 1991:38(2–3); 97–107.
434. Scala A, Varcasia A, Dore F, et al: Evaluation of efficacy of toltrazuril and diclazuril in the control of subclinical eimeriosis in weaned lambs. *Small Ruminant Res.* 2014:120(2–3);242–246.
435. Scala A, Varcasia A, Dore F, et al: Evaluation of efficacy of toltrazuril and diclazuril in the control of subclinical eimeriosis in weaned lambs. *Small Ruminant Res.* 2014:120(2);242–246.
436. de Souza Rodrigues F, Cezar AS, de Menezes FR, Sangioni LA, Vogel FSF, de Avila Botton S: Efficacy and economic analysis of two treatment regimens using toltrazuril in lambs naturally infected with Eimeria spp. on pasture. *Parasitol Res.* 2017:116(11);2911–2919.
437. Iqbal A, Wazir VS, Singh R: Comparative studies on the efficacy of toltrazuril and amprolium in the treatment of caprine coccidiosis. *Intas Polivet.* 2013:14(1);102–104.
438. Iqbal A, Tariq KA, Wazir VS, Singh R: Antiparasitic efficacy of Artemisia absinthium, toltrazuril and amprolium against intestinal coccidiosis in goats. *J Parasit Dis: OfficOrgan Indian Soc Parasitol.* 2013:37(1);88–93.
439. Arunvipas P, Ratanapob N, Phimprapahai W: Comparative study on the efficacy of toltrazuril for coccidiosis control in meat goats raised in Chainat province. *Kasetsart Veterinarians.* 2013:23(3); 132–137.
440. Wolff K, Eckert J, Schneiter G, Lutz H: Efficacy of triclabendazole against Fasciola hepatica in sheep and goats. *Vet Parasitol.* 1983:13(2);145–150.
441. Boray JC, Crowfoot PD, Strong MB, et al: Treatment of immature and mature Fasciola hepatica infections in sheep with triclabendazole. *Vet Rec.* 1983:113(14);315–317.
442. Smeal MG, Hall CA: The activity of triclabendazole against immature and adult Fasciola hepatica infections in sheep. *Austr Vet J.* 1983:60(11);329–331.
443. Foreyt WJ: Efficacy of triclabendazole against experimentally induced Fascioloides magna infections in sheep. *Am J Vet Res.* 1989:50(3);431–432.
444. Stansfield DG, Lonsdale B, Lowndes PA, Reeves EW, Schofield DM: Field trials of triclabendazole against mixed age infections of Fasciola hepatica in sheep and cattle. *Vet Rec.* 1987:120(19);459–460.
445. S. K, Islam MS, Aktaruzzaman M, et al: Effects of triclabendazole and nitroxynil on EPG, hematological parameters and body weight against fascioliasis in goats at government goat development farm, Sylhet, Bangladesh. *Int J Nat Sci.* 2015:5(2);46-51.
446. Batzias GC, Delis GA, Koutsoviti-Papadopoulou M: Bioavailability and pharmacokinetics of sulphadiazine, N4-acetylsulphadiazine and trimethoprim following intravenous and intramuscular administration of a sulphadiazine/trimethoprim combination in sheep. *Vety Res Communs.* 2005:29(8);699–712.
447. Tras B, Elmas M, Yazar E, Bas AL, Keskin E, Dasci Z: Concentrations of sulfadoxine and trimethoprim in plasma, lymph fluids and some tissues 24 h after intramuscular administration to Angora goats. *Vet Q.* 1998:20(2);62–64.
448. Robb EJ, Tucker CM, Corley L, et al: Efficacy of tulathromycin or enrofloxacin for initial treatment of naturally occurring bovine respiratory disease in feeder calves. *Vet Ther.* 2007:8(2);127–135.
449. Washburn KE, Bissett W, Fajt V, et al: The safety of tulathromycin administration in goats. *J Vet Pharmacol The.* 2007:30(3);267–270.
450. United States Food and Drug Administration Center for Veterinary Medicine: Code of Federal Regulations; 21 CFR 522.2630; Implantation or Injectable Dosage Form New Animal Drugs; Tulathromycin. Vol July 1, 20182018:322–323.
451. Washburn K, Fajt VR, Coetzee JF, Rice S, Wulf LW, Washburn S: Pharmacokinetics of tulathromycin in nonpregnant adult ewes. *JVet Pharmacol Thers.* 2015:38(4);414–416.
452. Amer AMM, Constable PD, A.Goudah, El Badawy SA: Pharmacokinetics of tulathromycin in lactating goats. *Small Ruminant Res.* 2012:108(1);137–143.
453. Clothier KA, Leavens T, Griffith RW, et al: Pharmacokinetics of tulathromycinafter single and multiple subcutaneous injections in domestic goats (Capra aegagrus hircus). *J Vet Pharmacol Ther.* 2010:34;448–454.
454. Bachtold KA, Alcorn JM, Boison JO, Matus JL, Woodbury MR: Pharmacokinetics and lung and muscle concentrations of tulathromycin following subcutaneous administration in white-tailed deer (Odocoileus virginianus). *J Vet Pharmacol Ther.* 2016:39(3);292–298.
455. Ball HJ, Logan EF, Campbell JN: Mycoplasma californicum mastitis in ewes as an experimental model for antibiotic treatment. *Epidemiol Infect.* 1987:98(3);369–378.
456. Ball HJ, McCaughey WJ: Experimental intramuscular inoculation of tylosin in the elimination of ureaplasmas from ewes. *Vet Rec.* 1987:120(23);557–558.
457. El Hassan SM, Harbi MS, Abu Bakr MI: Treatment of contagious caprine pleuropneumonia. *Vet Re Commun.* 1984:8(1);65–67.
458. Smith SE, Koch BA, Turk KL: The response of cobalt-deficient lambs to liver extract and vitamin B12. *J Nutr.* 1951:44(3);455–464.
459. Marston HR, Smith RM: Control of cobalt-deficiency in sheep by injection of vitamin B12. *Nature.* 1952:170(4332):792–793.
460. Anderson JP, Andrews ED: Response of vitamin B12 of grazing cobalt-deficient lambs. *Nature.* 1952:170(4332);807.
461. Shallow M, Ellis NJ, Judson GJ: Sex-related responses to vitamin B12 and trace element supplementation in prime lambs. *Austr Vet J.* 1989:66(8);250–251.
462. Grace ND, West DM, Sargison ND: The efficacy of a subcutaneous injection of soluble Vitamin B12 in lambs. *N Z Vet J.* 1998: 46(5);194–196.
463. Dwyer CJ, Downing GM, Gabor LJ: Dicoumarol toxicity in neonatal calves associated with the feeding of sweet vernal (Anthoxanthum odoratum) hay. *Austr Vet J.* 2003:81(6);332–335.
464. Goplen BP, Bell JM: Dicoumarol studies: IV. Antidotal and antagonistic properties of Vitamin K1 and K3 in cattle. *Can J Animal Sci.* 1967:47(2);91–100.
465. Alstad AD, Casper HH, Johnson LJ: Vitamin K treatment of sweet clover poisoning in calves. *J Am Vet Med Assoc.* 1985:187(7);729–731.
466. Nolan A, Livingston A, Waterman A: Antinociceptive actions of intravenous alpha 2-adrenoceptor agonists in sheep. *J Vet Pharmacol Ther.* 1987:10(3);202–209.
467. Lin HC, Wallace SS, Tyler JW, Robbins RL, Thurmon JC, Wolfe DF: Comparison of tiletamine-zolazepam-ketamine and tiletamine-zolazepam-ketamine-xylazine anaesthesia in sheep. *Austr Vet J.* 1994:71(8);239–242.
468. Ludbrook G, Grant C, Upton R, Penhall C: A method for frequent measurement of sedation and analgesia in sheep using the response to a ramped electrical stimulus. *J Pharmacol Toxicol Meth.* 1995:33(1);17–22.
469. Kumar A, Thurmon JC: Cardiopulmonary, hemocytologic and biochemical effects of xylazine in goats. *Lab Animal Sci.* 1979:29(4);486–491.
470. Liu DM, Zhou ZY, Ding Y, et al: Physiologic effects of electroacupuncture combined with intramuscular administration of xylazine to provide analgesia in goats. *Am J Vet Res.* 2009:70(11);1326–1332.
471. Mohammad FK, Zangana IK, Abdul-Latif AR: Reversal of medetomidine sedation in sheep by atipamezole and yohimbine. *Vet Human Toxicol.* 1995:37(2);97–99.
472. Ndeereh DR, Mbithi PM, Kihurani DO: The reversal of xylazine hydrochloride by yohimbine and 4-aminopyridine in goats. *J South Afr Vet Assn.* 2001:72(2);64–67.

Appendix 2

Reference Intervals and Conversions

Eric J. Fish and David G. Pugh

Reference intervals (RIs) are often erroneously referred to as the "normal range," but it must be stressed that RIs are merely a statistical calculation that includes approximately 95% of normal patient values.[1] It is both possible for a healthy patient to have an "abnormal" value for no pathologic reason, as well as a value within the RI that is inappropriate and indicative of disease. Whenever possible, reference intervals should be generated de novo for a sufficiently large and representative patient population.[1]

However, this is not always possible for financial and/or logistical reasons. In place of de novo RIs, published RIs can provide guidance when more appropriate RIs are unavailable. If published RIs are to be used, it is recommended that the (1) reference population used for the intervals, (2) sample collection and handling procedures, and (3) instruments and assay methodologies (including reagents) are well defined and similar to the patient testing circumstances.

Some selected population variables that may affect reference intervals and interpretation of a patient's data include animal age, sex, species, breed, function, diet, and pregnancy and lactation status.[1] Although the values in this appendix come from respected sources, the essential background information on reference population and test method is usually lacking. If the RIs contained in this appendix are the best source available for interpreting patient data, clinicians should be aware of these significant caveats, and consultation with the testing laboratory may be helpful. Results presented in different units can be corrected using the included conversion tables. The "deer" RI data in this appendix are drawn from multiple studies that include a combination of many different deer breeds, including white-tailed, red, Rusa, fallow, and chital.

• BOX 1 Celsius to Fahrenheit and Fahrenheit to Celsius

To change Celsius to Fahrenheit, multiply the degrees in Celsius by 1.8, then add 32 to the number.
Example: 40°C
(1.8) (40) + 32 = 104°F

To change Fahrenheit to Celsius, subtract 32 from the degrees in Fahrenheit, then multiply that number by 0.556.
Example: 104°F
(104 – 32) (0.556) = 40°C

TABLE 1 Erythrocyte Parameters.

	SHEEP		GOATS		DEER	
Parameter	**Range**	**Mean**	**Range**	**Mean**	**Range**	**Mean**
Hematocrit (packed cell volume [PCV]) %	27–45	35	22–38	28	27.6–54.4[4]	40.8
Hemoglobin (Hb) g/dL	9–15[2,3]	11.5	8–12[2,3]	10	7.9–18.7[4]	14
Erythrocytes (red blood cells [RBCs]) $10^6/\mu L$	9–15[2,3]	12	8–18[2,3]	13	6.2–14.27[4]	10.9
Mean corpuscular volume (MCV) fl	28–40[2,3]	34	16–25[2,3]	19.5	27.7–58.1[4]	38.6
Mean corpuscular hemoglobin (MCH) pg	8–12[2,3]	10	5.2–8[2,3]	6.5	9.8–21.9[4]	13.4
Mean corpuscular hemoglobin concentration (MCHC) g/dL	31–34[2,3]	32.5	30–36[2,3]	33	27.7–37.6[4]	
Platelet count, N × $10^3/\mu L$	205–705[3] 800–1100[2]	500	300–600[2,3]	450	233–482[4]	
Red blood cell (RBC) diameter (μm)	3.2–6.0[2]	4.5	2.5–3.9	3.2		
RBC life (days)	125	140–150			125–149	
Myeloid:erythroid ratio (M/E)	0.71	0.77–1.7[2]				
	0.8–1.7[3]	0.7–1[3]				
Notes					Deer erythrocytes may assume sickle shape in vitro after phlebotomy	

fL, means femtoliter(s) and it is a unit of volume measurement; *pg,* is picogram(s), a measure of mass.

TABLE 2 Leukocyte Parameters, Plasma Protein, and Fibrinogen.

	SHEEP			GOATS			DEER	
Parameter	Percentage	Range	Mean	Percentage	Range	Mean	Range	Mean
White blood cell count (WBC) n/μL		4000–12,000[3]			4000–13,000[3]		2600–8400[4]	4800
Segmented neutrophils (seg) (%) n/μL	10–50[3]	700–6000[2,3]	2400	30–48[2]	1200–7200[2,3]	3,250	540–581[4]	2199
Banded neutrophils (band) (%) n/μL		0			0		0	
Lymphocytes (lymph) (%) n/μL	40–75[3]	2000–9000[2,3]	5000	50–70[2]	2000–9000[2,3]	5000	1040–2741[4]	2164
Monocytes (mono) (%) n/μL	6–6[3]	0–750[1,2]	200	0–4[2]	0–550[2,3]	250	20–230[4]	126
Eosinophils (eos) (%) n/μL	0–10[3]	0–1000[3]	400	1–8[2]	50–650[2,3]	450	50–181[4]	130
Basophils (baso) (%) n/μL	0–3[3]	0–300[2,3]	50	0–1[2]	0–120[2,3]	50	0–20[4]	5
Plasma protein (PP) g/dL	6–7.5[2,3]		6.0–7.5[2,3]					
Fibrinogen (mg/dL)	100–500[2,3]				100–400[2,3]			

n = number, used to express a cell concentration

TABLE 3 Coagulation Parameters (Goats).[5]

		GOATS		
Parameter	Units	Mean	SD	RI
Prothrombin time (PT)	Seconds	12.8	0.99	15.7–19.8
Activated partial thromboplastin time (APTT)	Seconds	20.3	2	16.2–24.3
D-dimer	mg/mL	0.27	0.25	0–0.68
Antithrombin (AT III)	%	133.2	11.8	108.6–156.5
Fibrinogen	mg/dL	203.7	52.8	89.5–303.2

TABLE 4 Serum Biochemical Values.

Value	Sheep	Goats	Deer
Acetone mmol/L	0–1.72[6]		
Acetylcholinesterase U/L	640[6]	270[6]	
Albumin, g/dL	2.4–3.0[3,6]	2.7–3.9[3,6]	3.47–4.25[7]
Alkaline phosphatase (ALP) U/L	68–387[3,6]	93–387[3,6]	
Arginase (ARG) U/L	0–14[6]		
Aspartate aminotransferase (AST, SGOT) U/L	60–280[3,6]	167–513[3,6]	22.00–60.00[7]
β-Hydroxybutyrate (β-OHB) mmol/L	Normal: < 0–7 Moderate: 0.8–1.6 Severe underfeeding: 1.7–3.0 Pregnancy toxemia: > 6.5		
Bicarbonate (HCO_3^-) mmol/L	20–25[6]		
Bilirubin, total mg/dL	0.1–0.5[3,6]	0.10–1.71[6]	0.03–0.76[7]
Bilirubin, unconjugated (UCB) mg/dL	0–0.12[6]		

TABLE 4 **Serum Biochemical Values.—cont'd**

Value	Sheep	Goats	Deer
Bilirubin, conjugated (direct) mg/dL	0–0.27[3,6]		
Cholesterol mg/dL	52–76[2]	80–130[2]	91.11–122.95[7]
Carbon dioxide, total (TCO_2) mmol/L	21–28[6]	25.6–29.6[6]	
Creatinine phosphokinase (CPK) U/L	8–13[6]	0.8–9[3,6]	
Creatinine mg/dL	1.2–1.9[6]	1–1.82[3,6]	1.44–2.54[7]
Gamma-glutamyl transferase (GGT) U/L	44 ± 11[3] 20–52[6]	20–56[6]	
Globulin g/L, g/dL	3.5–5.7[6]	2.7–4.1[6]	2.15–3.55[7]
Glucose mg/dL	50–80[3,6]	50–75[3,6]	78.87–107.61[7]
Glutamate dehydrogenase (GD) U/L	20[6]		
Hemoglobin mg/dL	90–140[6]	80–120[6]	
Icterus index	2–5[6]	2–5[6]	
Isocitrate dehydrogenase (ICD) U/L	0.4–8.0[6]		
Lactate dehydrogenase (LDH) U/L	238–440[3] 88–487	123–392[3,6]	
Lactate mmol/L	1–1.33[6]		
Protein, total serum g/dL	6–7.9[6]	6.4–7[3,6]	5.90–7.73[7]
Sorbitol dehydrogenase U/L	5.8–27.9[6]	14–23.6[6]	
Blood urea nitrogen (BUN) mg/dL	8–20[3,6]	10–20[3,6]	15.33–33.33[7]

TABLE 5 **Serum Electrolyte and Mineral Concentrations.**

Parameter	Sheep	Goats	Deer
Calcium mg/dL	11.5–12.8[3]	8.9–11.7[3]	8.9–11.76[7]
Phosphate mg/dL	5.0–7.3[3]	4.2–9.1[3]	6.57–11.74[7]
Magnesium mg/dL	2.2–2.8[3]	2.8–3.6[3]	
Sodium mEq/L	139–152[3]	142–155[3]	
Chloride mEq/L	95–103[3]	99–110.3[3]	97.35–109.66[7]
Potassium mEq/L	3.9–5.4[3]	3.5–6.7[3]	
Bicarbonate (HCO_3^-) mEq/L	20–25[3]		
Iron μmol/L	29.7–39.7[6]		
μg/dL	162–222[6]		
Copper μmol/L	9.13–25.2[6]		
Lead μmol/L	0.24–1.21[6]	0.24–1.21[6]	
μg/dL	5–25[6]	5–25[6]	

TABLE 6 **Vitamins and Minerals in Serum and Liver (Sheep).**

Measured Element	Deficient	Adequate	Toxic
Vitamin A (serum) ng/m[9]	Newborn < 20 Yearling < 150 Adult < 150	30–100 225–00 225–500	
Vitamin A (liver) µg/g dry weight[9]	Newborn < 20 Yearling < 40 Adult< 40	50,100 100–500 3,0011,00	
Vitamin E (liver) µg/dL dry weight[9]	Newborn < 3 Yearling < 10 Adult< 10	7–35 20–40 20–40	
Selenium (serum) ng/mL[9]	Newborn < 20 Yearling < 50 Adult < 50	50–90 80–120 110–160	
Zinc (serum) ppm	0.22–0.45[10]	0.8–2[9,10]	30–50
Zinc (liver) mg/kg (dry weight)		10–250	400
Copper (serum) mg/kg	< 0.6	0.7–2.0[9,10]	3.3–20
Copper (liver) mg/kg (dry weight)	0.5–4.0	88–350[9]	250–400
Iron (serum) mg/kg (as soluble element)		1.6–2.2[9]	
Iron (liver) mg/kg (dry weight)		105–1050	
Manganese		7–15	
Molybdenum		1.5–6	

TABLE 7 **Cerebrospinal Fluid.[6]**

Parameter	Sheep	Goats
White blood cells (WBC) number/µL	0–5	0–4
Erythrocytes number/µL		
Calcium mg/dL	5.1–5.5	4.6
Magnesium mg/dL	2.2–2.8	2.3
Chloride mg/dL	128–148	116–130
Phosphorus mg/dL	1.2–2	
Potassium mg/dL	3.0–3.3	3.0
Sodium mg/dL	145–157	131
Hydrogen ion (pH)	7.3–7.4	
Glucose mg/dL	52–85	70
Total protein mg/dL	29–42	12

TABLE 8 **Urinalysis.[15]**

Test	Normal Results
Color	Pale yellow
Glucose	Negative
Ketones	Negative
Protein	Negative to trace
Specific gravity	1.015–1.045
Bilirubin	Negative
Turbidity	Clear
Crystals	Rare
Casts	Occasional hyaline
Epithelial cells	Occasional
Gamma-glutamyl transferase (GGT)	< 40 U/L
Red blood cells (RBC)	< 5
White blood cells (WBC)	< 5

TABLE 9 Paracentesis.[8,11]

Characteristic	Normal Value
Odor	None
Color	Colorless to yellow
Turbidity	Clear to slightly turbid
Total nucleated cell count (cells/μL) Total protein (g/dL)	200–3,600[12] 0.5–3.2 g/dL
Neutrophils	< 10,000
Specific gravity	< 1.018
Glucose (mg/dL)	45–66[12]

TABLE 10 Synovial Fluid.[13]

Characteristic	Normal	Inflammation Or Low-Grade Infection	Septic	Degenerative Joint Disease
Color	Clear	Yellow to red	Yellow to red	Yellow
Clarity	Transparent	Translucent	Cloudy	Transparent
Leukocytes/μL	< 200	2000–10,000	30,000–100,000	200–2000
Neutrophils %	< 25	> 75	> 75	25
Viscosity	Very viscous	Poor	Poor	Variable

TABLE 11 Conversions.[14]

Prefix	Value
Milli-	1/1000
Centi-	1/100
Deci-	1/10
Deca-	10
Necto-	100
Kilo-	1000

TABLE 12 Miscellaneous Conversions.[14]

Conversion	Multiply By
Grain to milligrams	64.799
Ounces to grams	28.35
Pounds to grams	453.6
Pounds to kilograms	0.4536
Tons to metric tons	0.9
Grams to ounces	0.035
Kilograms to pounds	2.205
Metric tons to tons	1.102
mg/lb to g/ton	2
g/lb to g/ton	2000
lb/ton to g/ton	453.6
mg/g to mg/lb	453.6
mg/kg to mg/lb	0.4536
μg/kg to g/lb	0.4536
ppm to mg/lb	0.4536
mg/lb to ppm	2.2046
ppm to g/ton	0.907
g/ton to g/lb	0.0005
g/ton to lb/ton	0.0022
g/ton to %	0.00011
% to g/ton	9072.2
g/ton to ppm	1.1
% to ppm	Divide by 10,000
ppm to %	10,000

TABLE 13 Imperial to Metric and Metric to Imperial Conversion.

Value	Converted Equivalent
1 oz	28.5 g
1 lb	16 oz
1 kg	1000 g
1 ton	2000 lb 1.07 kg
1 metric ton	1000 kg 2205 lb 1.102 ton
1 mg/kg	1 ppm

TABLE 14 Equivalent Values for Capacity or Volume.[14]

Value	Equivalent
1 cubic cm 1 U.S. pint	1 mL 28.875 cubic inches 0.5 quarts 0.47316 L
1 U.S. quart	57.75 cubic inches 2 U.S. pints 0.9463L
1 U.S gallon	231 cubic inches 8 U.S. pints 4 U.S. quarts 3.7853 L
1 L	2.1134 U.S. pints 1.057 U.S. quarts 0.2642 U.S. gallon
1 bushel	2150.42 cubic inches 1.244 cubic feet 9.309 U.S. gallons

References

1. Friedrichs KR, Harr KE, Freeman KP, et al: ASVCP reference interval guidelines: determination of de novo reference intervals in veterinary species and other related topics, *Vet Clin Pathol* 41(4):441–453, 2012.
2. Byers SR, Kramer JW: Normal hematology of sheep and goats. In Weiss DJ, Wardrop KJ, editors: *Schalm's veterinary hematology,* ed 6, Ames, IA, 2010, Blackwell Publishing Ltd. [chapter 108].
3. Duncan JR, Prasse KW: *Veterinary laboratory medicine – clinical pathology*, ed 2, Ames, IA, 1986, Iowa State University Press.
4. Boes KM: Hematology of cervids. In Weiss DJ, Wardrop KJ, editors: *Schalm's veterinary hematology*, ed 6, Ames, IA, 2010, Blackwell Publishing Ltd. [chapter 116].
5. Zersen KM, Moore AR, Olver CS, Mathis JC: Reference intervals for coagulation variables in healthy adult domestic goats *(Capra aegagrus hircus)*, *Vet Clin Pathol* 47(3):396–399, 2018. https://doi.org/10.1111/vcp.12621.
6. Kaneko JJ, Harvey JW, Bruss ML: *Clinical biochemistry of domestic animals*, ed 6, San Diego, CA, 2008, Academic Press.
7. Gupta AR, Patra RC, Saini M, Swarup D: Haematology and serum biochemistry of chital *(Axis axis)* and barking deer *(Muntiacus muntjak)* reared in semi-captivity, *Vet Res Commun* 31;801–808, 2007.
8. Belknap EB, Navarre CB: Differentiation of gastrointestinal diseases in adult cattle, *Vet Clin North Am Food Anim Pract* 16(1):63, 2000.
9. Braselton WE: *Personal communication, Animal Health Diagnostic Laboratory*, East Lansing, Michigan State University, 2010.
10. D'Andrea G, Robert S: *Personal communication*, Veterinary *Diagnostic Laboratory,* Auburn, AL, Auburn University, 2009.
11. Kopcha M, Schultze AE: Peritoneal fluid. Part II. Abdominocentesis in cattle and interpretation of non neoplastic samples, *Comp Cont Ed Pract Vet* 13(4):703, 1999.
12. Al-Rukibat RK, Bani Ismail ZA, Al-Majali AM, Al-Zghoul MB: Peritoneal fluid analysis in adult, nonpregnant Awassi sheep, *Vet Clin Pathol* 35(2):215–218, 2006.
13. Orsini JA: Septic arthritis (infectious arthritis). In Smith BP, editor: *Large animal internal medicine,* ed 2, St Louis, 1996, Mosby.
14. Ensminger ME, Oldfield JE, Heinemann WW: *Feeds and nutrition*, ed 2, Clovis, CA, 1990, Ensminger Publishing.
15. Christian J, Pugh DG: Appendix II — Reference intervals and conversions. In Pugh DG, Baird NN, editors: *Sheep and goat medicine*, ed 2, St. Louis, 2012, Elsevier.

Index

O

P